The 5-Minute Sports Medicine Consult

4th EDITION

The 5-Minute Sports Medicine Consult

4th EDITION

EDITORS-IN-CHIEF

Kenneth S. Taylor, MD, FAAFP, CAQSM
Clinical Professor of Family Medicine/Sports Medicine
University of California, San Diego, School of Medicine
Chief, Primary Care Sports Medicine
Director, UCSD Primary Care Sports Medicine Fellowship
Head Primary Care Sports Physician, San Diego Padres
Team Physician, UCSD Tritons
Team Physician, US Olympic Training Center
San Diego, California

Suraj A. Achar, MD, FAAFP, CAQSM
Clinical Professor of Family Medicine
University of California, San Diego, School of Medicine
Director of UCSD School of Medicine Sports Medicine Selective
Associate Director UCSD Primary Care Sports Medicine Fellowship
Team Physician, US Olympic Training Center, UCSD Tritons
Lead Physician, Rady Children's Hospital 360 Sports Medicine
Department of Pediatric Orthopedics
San Diego, California

ASSISTANT EDITORS

Alec Gabriel Contag, MD
Sports Medicine Fellow
Department of Family and Sports Medicine
University of California, San Diego
San Diego, California

Arthur Davis Daniel, MD, CAQSM
Primary Care Sports Medicine
Department of Orthopedics
United States Navy
Agana Heights, Guam

Priya Sharma, DO
Physician
Department of Family and Sports Medicine
Family Health Centers of San Diego, UC San Diego Health
San Diego, California

Wolters Kluwer

Philadelphia • Baltimore • New York • London
Buenos Aires • Hong Kong • Sydney • Tokyo

5MinuteConsult™

Director, Medical Practice: Brian Brown
Associate Director of Medicine Content Development: Anne Malcolm
Acquisitions Editor: Joe Cho
Development Editor: Cindy Yoo
Editorial Assistant: Kristen Kardoley
Marketing Manager: Kirsten Watrud
Senior Production Specialist: Bridgett Dougherty
Manager, Graphic Arts & Design: Stephen Druding
Manufacturing Coordinator: Lisa Bowling
Prepress Vendor: Absolute Service, Inc.

4th edition

9 8 7 6 5 4 3 2 1

Printed in the United States of America

Library of Congress Cataloging-in-Publication Data available from the Publisher upon request.

ISBN-13: 978-1-9752-3794-3

shop.lww.com

MPP1125

This book is dedicated to the entire team of health care professionals who work with athletes of all ages and abilities, often in time-sensitive environments where accurate diagnoses and treatment plans are critical. *The 5-Minute Sports Medicine Consult* in both printed and web-based format is ideal for this setting.

It is our hope that the information contained in this body of work will help guide you and your patients along the path to recovery and peak performance.

PREFACE

Since the publication of the 3rd and 4th edition of *The 5-Minute Sports Medicine Consult*, technology has changed our lives. As computer and mobile devices permeate our professional and personal lives, health care professionals have increasingly turned to web-based formats as a source of medical information in our busy practices. Building on our success with the first two editions of *The 5-Minute Sports Medicine Consult*, progress with the 3rd and 4th edition was streamlined by using the expertise of sports medicine authors and editors from around the country and now world. Users of the first three editions will be pleased to note that the format has remained by and large the same with new focused chapters and updated evidence-based information. In addition, the book is now available in the LWW Health Library in Family Medicine, a new web-based, mobile-friendly platform for institutions that makes searches and cross-referencing information easier.

The basic concept for this book parallels teaching techniques from our collaborative sports medicine fellowship at the University of California, San Diego (UCSD). As part of our regular weekly Sports Medicine didactics program, fellows and faculty from four separate Accreditation Council for Graduate Medical Education (ACGME)-approved sports fellowships are asked to present lectures on topics in sports medicine clinical practice covering the essential elements in the diagnosis and management of problems as seen through the eyes of a primary care sports physician. The audience consists of experienced clinicians, including orthopedic surgeons, radiologists, physical therapists, athletic trainers, and other members of the "Sports Medicine Team." The organization and presentation of these didactics follow those found in this book with an emphasis on evidence-based medicine and clinical relevance.

We would like to express our sincerest gratitude to the late Mark Bracker, MD, who founded the UCSD sports medicine fellowship and who led the effort to create the first edition in 2001. We also want to thank our section editors and authors who used their expertise to provide organized and useful reviews on each topic in the book. Additional gratitude and recognition go toward our assistant editors: Arthur Davis Daniel, MD; Alec Gabriel Contag, MD; and Priya Sharma, DO. Drs. Contag, Daniel, and Sharma worked diligently reviewing chapters, communicating with the team of section editors, finding new authors, as well as working closely with the publisher and authors to keep this project moving forward and completed on time. We hope you enjoy this updated edition, and it further streamlines your ability to provide the best and most up-to-date information while caring for your patients.

KENNETH S. TAYLOR, MD, FAAFP, CAQSM
SURAJ A. ACHAR, MD, FAAFP, CAQSM

CONTRIBUTORS

Jivan Achar, BA
Case Western Reserve School of Medicine
Cleveland, Ohio

Suraj A. Achar, MD, FAAFP, CAQSM
Clinical Professor of Family Medicine
University of California, San Diego, School of Medicine
Director of UCSD School of Medicine Sports Medicine Selective
Associate Director UCSD Primary Care Sports Medicine Fellowship
Team Physician, US Olympic Training Center, UCSD Tritons
Lead Physician, Rady Children's Hospital 360 Sports Medicine
Department of Pediatric Orthopedics
San Diego, California

Ayo Adu, MD, DC, CAQSM
Sports Medicine and Pain Management
Victoria, Texas

Arturo J. Aguilar, MD, FAAFP, CAQSM
Head Team Physician
Medical Director of Student Health Services
Student Health Services/Athletic Training
Boston University
Boston, Massachusetts

Muath Alammar, MBBS, SBFM, ABFM, JBFM
Associate Professor
Department of Family Medicine
McGill University
Montreal, Canada

Kathryn M. Alfonso, DO
Clinical Assistant Professor
Physical Medicine and Rehabilitation
University of Florida
Gainesville, Florida

Claudia Alvarez, DO
Doctor of Osteopathic Medicine
Family Medicine Specialist
Harbor-UCLA Medical Center
Los Angeles, California

Soroosh Amanat, MD
Family Medicine and Sports Medicine Physician
Department of Family Medicine
Scripps Coastal
San Diego, California

Edwin Amirianfar, DO
Physician
Department of Anesthesiology
University of Louisville
Louisville, Kentucky

Laura Anderson, MD
Assistant Professor
Department of Emergency Medicine
Lahey Hospital and Medical Center
Burlington, Massachusetts

Mitchell P. Anderson, MD
Physical Medicine and Rehabilitation Sports Medicine Physician
VA Northern California
Stockton, California

William Andrew, DO, CAQSM
Assistant Clinical Professor
Department of Family Medicine, Division of Sports Medicine
University of California, San Diego
San Diego, California

Victoria Andros, DO, CAQSM
Staff Physician
Department of Student Wellness
University of Chicago
Chicago, Illinois

Marcus Anthony, MD
Primary Care Sports Medicine Fellow
Department of Orthopedic Surgery
NYU Grossman School of Medicine
New York, New York

Brandon Arehart, DO
Physician
Department of Emergency Medicine
OhioHealth
Columbus, Ohio

Cesar S. Arguelles, MD, CAQSM
Program Director
Primary Care Sports Medicine Fellowship—Quincy
Family and Community Medicine
Southern Illinois University
Quincy, Illinois

Brian Atkinson, MD, CAQSM, DipABLM
Assistant Program, Director
Sports Medicine Fellowship
Mountain Area Health Education Center
Asheville, North Carolina

Alvin Au-Yeung, DO, MPH†
Primary Care Sports Medicine Fellow
Family Medicine/Sports Medicine
The University of Chicago/Northshore University
Chicago, Illinois

Jackson Bagby, DO, MS
Primary Care Sports Medicine Fellow
Department of Family Medicine
University of Nebraska Medical Center
Omaha, Nebraska

David Bakal, MD
Assistant Clinical Professor
Department of Orthopedic Surgery
University of California
San Diego School of Medicine
La Jolla, California

Larry Balle II, MD, MPH, CAQSM
Assistant Professor
Department of Orthopedics
University of Arkansas for Medical Sciences
Fayetteville, Arkansas

Ilona Barash, MD, PhD, CAQSM
Department of Emergency Medicine
Scripps Torrey Pines Urgent Care
University of California, San Diego
San Diego, California

Erin S. Barnes, MD
Assistant Professor
Department of Physical Medicine and Rehabilitation
MetroHealth/Case Western Reserve University
Cleveland, Ohio

Kenneth P. Barnes, MD, MSc, CAQSM, FACP, FACSM, FAMSSM
Non-operative Musculoskeletal Sports Medicine Physician
Department of Sports Medicine
The Orthopedic Institute
Gainesville, Florida

Brandon W. Barsky, MD, FAAP, CAQSM
Sports Medicine Physician
Rady Children's Hospital
San Diego, California

Briana Beach, DO
Associate Program Director
Department of Family and Community Medicine
Virginia Tech Carilion Clinic
Roanoke, Virginia

Holly Beach, MD, CAQSM
Sports Medicine Fellowship Director
Department of Family and Community Medicine
University of Arizona
Tucson, Arizona

Samuel Bell, MD
Resident Physician
University of California, Irvine
Orange, California

Thomas P. Bell, MD
Family Medicine Resident
Department of Family Medicine
University of Tennessee Health Science Center College of Medicine
University of Tennessee Graduate School of Medicine
Knoxville, Tennessee

Holly J. Benjamin, MD, FAMSSM, FACSM
Professor of Orthopedic Surgery, Rehabilitation
Department of Medicine and Pediatrics
Director of Primary Care Sports Medicine
University of Chicago
Chicago, Illinois

Annemarie Beran, DO
Family Medicine Resident
Blacksburg, Virginia

Kenneth M. Bielak, MD, MBA, FAAFP, FACSM
Professor *(Retired)*
Department of Family Medicine
University of Tennessee Medical Center
University of Tennessee Graduate School of Medicine
Knoxville, Tennessee

W. Scott Black, MD, MS
Clinical Director
University Health Service
University of Kentucky
Lexington, Kentucky

Katherine Boehm, DO
San Diego Sports Medicine
San Diego, California

Delmas J. Bolin, MD, PhD, FACSM
Professor
Department of Sports and Family Medicine
Via College of Osteopathic Medicine—Virginia Campus
Blacksburg, Virginia

Lyndsey N. Booker, MD, CAQSM
Clinical Assistant Professor
Department of Rehabilitation Medicine
Division of Sports and Spine
University of Washington
Seattle, Washington

James R. Borchers, MD, MPH
Professor
Department of Family Medicine/Sports Medicine
The Ohio State University
Columbus, Ohio

Christopher S. Bossart, MD
Assistant Professor
Department of Emergency Medicine
University of New Mexico
Albuquerque, New Mexico

Benjamin L. Boswell, DO
Assistant Professor and Attending Physician
Drusinsky Sports Medicine Institute
University Hospitals
Cleveland, Ohio

Anne S. Boyd, MD, FAAFP, FACSM
Clinical Assistant Professor
Department of Family Medicine
Thomas Jefferson University
Sidney Kimmel Medical College
Philadelphia, Pennsylvania

Dana W. Brooks, DO, CAQSM
Primary Care Sports Medicine Physician
Cone Health OrthoCare
Cone Health Sports Medicine Fellowship
Greensboro, North Carolina

Elizabeth E. Brown, MD
Sports Medicine Fellow
Department of Musculoskeletal Medicine
Northwestern Feinberg School of Medicine
Chicago, Illinois

Chau Bui, DO
USA Rugby Team Physician
Department of Family Medicine
Northridge Hospital Medical Center
Northridge, California

Kimberly Burbank, MD
Resident Physician
Department of Family Medicine
Wake Forest University School of Medicine
Winston-Salem, North Carolina

Kevin J. Burnham, MD, CAQSM
Health Sciences Clinical Professor
Department of Internal Medicine, Physical Medicine and Rehabilitation
University of California Davis Health
Sacramento, California

Kevin E. Burroughs, MD, CAQSM, FAMSSM
Professor, Wake Forest University School of Medicine
Department of Family and Community Medicine
Co-Chief, Primary Care Sports Medicine Atrium Health Musculoskeletal Institute
Director, Cabarrus Sports Medicine Fellowship
Concord, North Carolina
Head Team Physician, Catawba College
Kannapolis Cannon Ballers, AL
Kannapolis, North Carolina
Brown High School
Team Physician, Charlotte FC
Charlotte, North Carolina

Jeffrey R. Bytomski, DO, FAOASM, FAMSSM
Head Medical Training Physician
Department of Family Medicine and Community Health
Duke University
Durham, North Carolina

Elizabeth A. Callahan, DO
Fellow, Physical Medicine and Rehabilitation
Northwestern McGaw Medical Center/Shirley Ryan AbilityLab
Chicago, Illinois

Greg Canty, MD
Medical Director, Sports Medicine
UMKC Department of Orthopedic Surgery
Children's Mercy Kansas City
Kansas City, Missouri

Nathan Cardoos, MD, CAQSM
Sports Medicine Physician
Boston Medical Center
Boston University
Boston, Massachusetts

David Carfagno, DO, CAQSM
Scottsdale Sports Medicine
Scottsdale, Arizona

Rebecca L. Carl, MD, MSCI
Associate Professor of Pediatrics
Department of Pediatrics
Ann and Robert H. Lurie Children's Hospital of Chicago
Chicago, Illinois

Catherine Carragee, MD
Resident Physician
Department of Family Medicine and Sports Medicine
University of California, San Diego
San Diego, California

Rachel E. Chamberlain, MD, CAQSM
Program Director, Sports Medicine Fellowship
Assistant Professor
Department of Family and Community Medicine
University of New Mexico
Albuquerque, New Mexico

Anthony Chang, MD†
Resident Physician
Department of Family Medicine
UC Irvine School of Medicine
Irvine, California

Lawrence Chang, DO, MPH
Non-operative Sports Medicine
Department of Orthopaedics
Rothman Orthopaedics Institute
New York University
New York, New York

John Cheng, MD
Clinical Director
Department of Family Medicine
Harbor-UCLA Medical Center
Torrance, California

Karen Yik Ting Cheng, MD
Assistant Professor of Clinical Radiology
Department of Radiology
University of California, San Diego
San Diego, California

Joseph Chin, MD, CAQSM
Physical Medicine and Rehabilitation/Sports Medicine
Kaiser Clovis
Clovis, California

Weng Leong Choy, MD
Family Medicine Physician
Department of Family Medicine
University of Tennessee Medical Center
Knoxville, Tennessee

Adam T. Chrusch, MD, CAQSM
Assistant Clinical Professor
Department of Community and Family Medicine
Rothman Orthopaedics
Philadelphia, Pennsylvania

Julie Chuan, MD, FAAFP, CAQSM
Department of Family and Sports Medicine
Overlake Medical Center
Bellevue, Washington

Peter Clements, MD
Physician
Family Medicine and Primary Care Sports Medicine
San Diego Sports Medicine and Family Health Center
San Diego, California

Amity Clow, MD
Family Medicine and Sports Medicine
Sharp Rees-Stealy Medical Group
San Diego, California

Rachel A. Coel, MD, PhD, FAAP, CAQSM
Pediatric and Adolescent Sports Medicine
Department of Pediatrics
University of Hawaii
Kapiolani Medical Center for Women and Children
Honolulu, Hawaii

Douglas Comeau, DO, FAAFP, FAMSSM
Director
University Health Services and Primary Care Sports Medicine
Boston College
Chestnut Hill, Massachusetts

Rosalynn R. Z. Conic, MD, PhD, MPH
Pain Fellow
Mayo Clinic
Jacksonville, Florida

Alec Gabriel Contag, MD
Sports Medicine Fellow
Department of Family and Sports Medicine
University of California, San Diego
San Diego, California

David J. Cormier, DO, DPT, CAQSM, FAAPMR
Associate Director
University Health Services and Sports Medicine
Coston College
Chestnut Hill, Massachusetts

Allison Cotter, MD
Resident Physician
UC San Diego Health
San Diego, California

Steven Cuff, MD, FAAP, CAQSM
Associate Professor of Pediatrics
Department of Sports Medicine
Nationwide Children's Hospital
The Ohio State University
Columbus, Ohio

Adam Culver, MD, CAQSM
Primary Care Sports Medicine Physician
Novant Health
Waxhaw, North Carolina

Claudia Dal Molin, DO, RMSK, FAMSSM
Director of MSK US Education
Department of Orthopedics
University of Maryland Medical School
Baltimore, Maryland

Arthur Davis Daniel, MD, CAQSM†
Primary Care Sports Medicine
Department of Orthopedics
United States Navy
Agana Heights, Guam

Kayla Daniel, MD
Assistant Professor
Department of Orthopedic Surgery
Washington University in St. Louis
St. Louis, Missouri

James M. Daniels, MD, MPH, PhD, RMSK, FAAFP, FACOEM, FACPM, FAMSSM
Professor
Department of Family and Community Medicine and Orthopedic Surgery
Southern Illinois University School of Medicine
Quincy, Illinois

Rachel Danzig, MD, FAAP
Fellow
Department of Pediatric Emergency Medicine
Comer Children's Hospital
University of Chicago
Chicago, Illinois

C. Trent Davis, MD†
Resident Physician
Department of Family Medicine
Mayo Clinic, Florida
Jacksonville, Florida

Nardos Dawit, MD
Family Medicine Physician
University of Minnesota
Minneapolis, Minnesota

Dayken Dawson, MD
Physician
Department of Physical Medicine and Rehabilitation
UC Davis Health
Sacramento, California

Sandra de Mel, MD
Physician
Department of Physical Medicine and Rehabilitation
University of Miami/Jackson Health System
Miami, Florida

Alexei DeCastro, MD, FAAFP, CAQSM
Director, Sports Medicine Fellowship Program
Department of Family Medicine/Orthopedics and Physical Medicine
Medical University of South Carolina
Charleston, South Carolina

Marjorie Delo, MD, CAQSM, RMSK
President/Owner
Delo Sports Medicine and Interventional Orthopedics
Green Bay, Wisconsin

Brendan Dempsey, MD
Primary Care Sports Medicine Fellow
University of Maryland
Baltimore, Maryland

Kevin deWeber, MD, FAMSSM, FAAFP, FACSM, RMSK
COL, USA, MC
Department of Family Medicine and Sports Medicine
PeaceHealth Family Medicine of Southwest Washington
Vancouver, Washington

Michelle Doscas, MD, CAQSM
Primary Care Sports Medicine Physician
Silicon Valley Sports Medicine
Campbell, California

Bridget Doyle, DO, MPH
Primary Care Sports Medicine Physician
The Georgia Institute of Technology
Atlanta, Georgia

Drew Duerson, MD, RMSK
Assistant Professor
Department of Pediatrics
Nationwide Children's Hospital
Columbus, Ohio

Rachel T. Duong, MD
Resident Physician
Department of Family Medicine
UC Irvine Health
Orange, California

Angelina R. Edwards, MD, FASN
Fellowship Program Director
Division of Nephrology
Department of Internal Medicine
Houston Methodist Hospital
Houston, Texas

David S. Edwards, MD, CAQSM
Associate Professor
Assistant Team Physician and Medical Director
Department of Family and Community Medicine
Texas Tech University Health Sciences Center
Lubbock, Texas

Tanner Craig Eiben, DO, CAQSM
Assistant Professor
Associate Program Director, Quincy Sport
Department of Family and Community Medicine
Southern Illinois University Medicine
Quincy, Illinois

Griffin Elbert, DO, CAQSM
Department of Family and Sports Medicine
Community Memorial Healthcare
Ventura, California

Angelene M. Elliott, DO
Primary Care Sports Medicine Physician
Boston, Massachusetts

Mackenzie Erdmann, MD
Assistant Professor
Department of Sports Medicine
Cincinnati Children's Hospital Medical Center
Cincinnati, Ohio

Hans A. Erickson, MD
Resident Physician
Department of Internal Medicine/Pediatrics
University of Massachusetts
Worcester, Massachusetts

Lisa Falotico, DO, CAQSM
Family Medicine
Parkview Physician Group
Fort Wayne, Indiana

Marcus Farrand, DO
Physician
St. Joseph Health System
Mishawaka, Indiana

Connor Farrell, DO
Clinical Instructor
Family Medicine/Sports Medicine
Oregon Health & Science University
Portland, Oregon

Melissa Faubert, DO, CAQSM
Physician
Department of Family Medicine
Sauk Prairie Healthcare
Lodi, Wisconsin

Marcia Faustin, MD, CAQSM, FAAFP
Assistant Clinical Professor
Department of Family and Community Medicine
UC Davis Health
Sacramento, California

Jeffrey P. Feden, MD, FACEP, CAQSM
Professor and Clinical Educator
Department of Emergency Medicine
Alpert Medical School of Brown University
Providence, Rhode Island

Karl B. Fields, MD, CAQSM, FAMSSM
Professor of Family Medicine and Sports Medicine
University of North Carolina
Faculty Sports Medicine Fellowship
Cone Health
Greensboro, North Carolina

Rebekah Fiers, MD
Resident Physician
Department of Family Medicine
University of Minnesota
Minneapolis, Minnesota

Diana Filtz, MD, FAAP, CAQSM
Urgent Care Physician
Cook Children's Medical Center
Fort Worth, Texas

Anastasia Fischer, MD, FAAFP, FACSM
Clinical Professor of Pediatrics
Department of Sports Medicine
Nationwide Children's Hospital
The Ohio State University
Columbus, Ohio

Ryan C. Fowler, MD, CAQSM
Sports Medicine Physician
Fowler Medical Group
Temple, Texas

Alexandra M. Frank, MD
M4
University of Wisconsin School of Medicine and Public Health
Madison, Wisconsin

Caroline M. Fryar, MD
Sports Medicine Physician
Department of Physical Medicine and Rehabilitation
University of Florida
Gainesville, Florida

Samuel J. Galloway, MD, CAQSM
Assistant Clinical Professor
Department of Family and Sports Medicine
UC San Diego Health
San Diego, California

Shaun P. Garff, DO
Sports Medicine Physician Director
Department of Sports Medicine
Methodist Health System
Dallas, Texas

Anne M. Garrison, DO, CAQSM
Occupational Medicine Physician
Occupational Medicine Specialty Centers
HCA CareNow Urgent Care
Houston, Texas

Corey T. Gatewood, MD
Physician
Department of Physical Medicine and Rehabilitation
UC Davis Health
Sacramento, California

Kevin B. Gebke, MD
President, Indiana University Health Community Medicine
Department of Family Medicine
Indiana University
Indianapolis, Indiana

Christopher A. Gee, MD, MPH, FACEP, CAQSM
Associate Professor
Department of Orthopedics
University of Utah
Salt Lake City, Utah

Shane Geffe, MD
Chief Sports Medicine Fellow
Department of Orthopedics
Emory University
Atlanta, George

Alecia Gende, DO, CAQSM, FACEP, FAAEM
Assistant Professor of Orthopedics
Department of Sports Medicine, Emergency Medicine
Mayo Clinic Health System
La Crosse, Wisconsin

Margaret E. Gibson, MD, FAMSSM
Professor
Department of Community and Family Medicine
University of Missouri Kansas City
Kansas City, Missouri

Joshua Goldman, MD, MBA
Associate Clinical Professor
Department of Family Medicine and Orthopedic Surgery
University of California, Los Angeles
Los Angeles, California

Hernan Goldsztein, MD
Section Chief
Department of Otolaryngology Head and Neck Surgery
Pacific ENT Medical Group/Scripps Memorial Hospital La Jolla
San Diego, California

Scott Goodsell, DO
Sports Medicine Fellow
Department of Primary Care Sports Medicine
University of Nebraska Medical Center
Omaha, Nebraska

Aaron D. Gray, MD
Physician
Department of Orthopaedics
University of Missouri
Columbia, Missouri

Steven A. Greer, MD, CAQ, FAAFP
Medical Director
St. Joseph's/Candler Sports Medicine
St. Joseph's/Candler Bone Joint and Muscle Care
Savannah, Georgia

Andrew J.M. Gregory, MD, FAAP, FACSM
Associate Professor, Clinical Educator Track
Department of Orthopedics, Pediatrics and Neurosurgery
Vanderbilt University Medical Center
Nashville, Tennessee

Claire Gross, MD, CAQSM
Sports Medicine Physician
Intermountain Health
Salt Lake City, Utah

Alexander T. Grover, DO
Primary Care Sports Medicine Fellow
Jameson Crane Sports Medicine Institute
The Ohio State University Wexner Medical Center
Columbus, Ohio

Sunny Gupta, DO
Clinical Assistant Professor
Department of Family and Community Medicine, Sports Medicine
Sidney Kimmel Medical College
Thomas Jefferson University
Philadelphia, Pennsylvania

Mario Gutierrez, MD, CAQSM
Vice President
Pride Sports Medicine
Fresno, California

Jack Haberl, MD, MBA
Resident Physician
Rehabilitation and Regenerative Medicine
Columbia University College of Physicians and Surgeons
New York, New York

Mark E. Halstead, MD
Professor
Department of Orthopedics and Pediatrics
Washington University School of Medicine
St. Louis, Missouri

Argin Haritounian, DO
Primary Sports Medicine Physician
Harbor-UCLA Medical Center
Harbor City, California

Kimberly G. Harmon, MD
Professor
Department of Family Medicine and Orthopedics
University of Washington
Seattle, Washington

Brandon Hassid, MD
Assistant Clinical Professor
Department of Physical Medicine and Rehabilitation
UC Davis Health
Sacramento, California

Daniel C. Herman, MD, PhD, FAAPMR, FACSM, FISBS, CAQSM
Associate Professor
Department of Physical Medicine and Rehabilitation
UC Davis Health
Sacramento, California

Vihangi Hindagolla, DO
Physician
Department of Family Medicine/Sports Medicine
Providence Health
Portland, Oregon

Peter Hoang, MD
Physician
Department of Family Medicine
University of California, Irvine
Orange, California

Quynh Hoang, MD, FAAP, CAQSM
Pediatric Sports Medicine
Adolescent and Children's Orthopedic Surgeons, Inc.
Encino, California

Dana Hong, DO, CAQSM
Family Medicine Physician and Primary Care Sports Medicine Fellow Physician
Department of Family Medicine and Sports Medicine
University of California, San Diego
San Diego, California

Michal Kalli Hose, MD
Clinical Professor of Medicine
University of California, San Diego
San Diego, California

Antonio Howard, MBBS, MSc, FAAPMR, CAQSM
Clinical Assistant Professor
Orthopedic Surgery and Rehabilitation
Wake Forest School of Medicine
Charlotte, North Carolina

Connie Hsu, MD
Sports Medicine Fellow
Department of Orthopedics and Sports Medicine
University of Chicago
Chicago, Illinois

Shane Hudnall, MD, CAQSM
Associate Program Director
Cone Health Sports Medicine Fellowship
Greensboro, North Carolina

Tudor Hesketh Hughes, MD
Professor of Radiology
Department of Radiology
University of California, San Diego
San Diego, California

Andrew Hurvitz, MD, FAAOS
Associate Professor of Orthopedic Surgery
Department of Orthopedic Surgery
University of California, San Diego
San Diego, California

Julia Louisa Iafrate, DO
Assistant Professor
Director of Musculoskeletal Ultrasound Education
Department of Orthopedic Surgery, Rehabilitation Medicine
NYU Langone Health
New York, New York

Tyler D. Ingersoll, DO, CAQSM, ABOFP
Department of Primary Care Sports Medicine
Texas Health Resources
Fort Worth, Texas

Haruki Ishii, MD, CAQSM
Clinical Assistant Professor
Department of Rehabilitation Medicine
New York University
New York, New York

Tyson A. Jackson, MD
Emergency/Sports Medicine Physician
University of New Mexico
Albuquerque, New Mexico

Jeswin Jacob, DO
Sports Medicine Fellow
Department of Sports Medicine
UPMC
Harrisburg, Pennsylvania

Shaheen Jadidi, DO
Attending Physician
Department of Orthopedics
Edward-Elmhurst/NorthShore University Health System
Chicago, Illinois

Maria Janakos, MD, FAAPMR, CAQSM
Clinical Assistant Professor
Department of Rehabilitation Medicine
NYU Grossman School of Medicine
New York, New York

Patrick Jenkins III, MD
Physician
Atrium Health Barnett Family Medicine
Indian Land, South Carolina

Matthew J. Jepson, MD, MS, CAQSM
The Centers for Advanced Orthopaedics —MMI Division
Frederick, Maryland

Kevin C. Jillson, MD, CAQSM
Medical Director, Primary Care Sports Medicine
Department of Orthopedics, Internal Medicine-Pediatrics
University of Massachusetts, Memorial Health-Milford Regional Medical Center
Milford, Massachusetts

Amy B. Jones, MD
Primary Care Sports Medicine Fellow
Houston Methodist
Houston, Texas

Christopher Jordan, MD, ATC, CAQSM
Director of Sports Medicine
St. Joseph Health System
Mishawaka, Indiana

Vijay Jotwani, MD
Assistant Professor of Clinical Family Medicine
Department of Orthopedic Surgery
Houston Methodist Hospital
Houston, Texas

Kimberly Kaiser, MD, CAQSM
Associate Professor
Department of Orthopedic Surgery and Sports Medicine
University of Kentucky
Lexington, Kentucky

Sravya Kamarajugadda, BS[†]
University of Florida College of Medicine
Gainesville, Florida

Donald Kasitinon, MD, CAQSM, RMSK
Assistant Professor
Physical Medicine and Rehabilitation
University of Texas Southwestern Medical Center
Dallas, Texas

Jack Keeley, MD
Physician
Department of Family Medicine
Wake Forest Baptist
Winston-Salem, North Carolina

Sarah Kennedy, DO, CAQSM
Primary Care Sports Medicine Physician
Sideline Orthopedics and Sports Medicine
Arlington, Texas

Julie M. Kerr, MD, CAQSM
Associate Professor of Clinical, Pediatrics
Department of Orthopedics and Sports Medicine
Akron Children's Hospital
Akron, Ohio

Razib Khaund, MD
Director of Sports Medicine
Care New England
Providence, Rhode Island

Daniel Kiehl, DO
Resident Physician
Department of Physical Medicine and Rehabilitation
University of Florida
Gainesville, Florida

John M. Kiel, DO, MPH
Associate Professor of Emergency Medicine
Department of Emergency Medicine
USF Morsani College of Medicine/TGH
Tampa, Florida

Amie Kim, MD, CAQSM
Associate Professor
Department of Emergency Medicine, Physical Rehabilitation Medicine
Icahn School of Medicine Mount Sinai
New York, New York

Brian Young Kim, MD, MS, CAQSM
Associate Clinical Professor
Program Director
Primary Care Sports Medicine
Department of Family Medicine
University of California, Irvine
School of Medicine
Irvine, California

Christina Kim, MD, CAQSM, FAAFP
Sports Medicine Physician
Boston College
Chestnut Hill, Massachusetts

Yuka Kobayashi, DO
Assistant Professor
Department of Orthopedic Surgery
Medical College of Wisconsin
Milwaukee, Wisconsin

Sujith Kochat, MD
Sports Medicine Fellow
Department of Sports Medicine
Advocate Lutheran General Hospital
Chicago, Illinois

Clarence Kong, MD
Resident Physician
Department of Emergency Medicine
Zucker School of Medicine at Hofstra/Northwell—North Shore University Hospital
Long Island Jewish Medical Center
New Hyde Park, New York

Neel Kotrappa, MD
Sports Medicine Physician
Eisenhower Sports Medicine Clinic
Eisenhower Health
Rancho Mirage, California

Chris Koutures, MD, FAAP
Pediatric and Sports Medicine Specialist
ActiveKidMD
Orange, California

Christopher A. Kroner, MD, MPH
Associate Clinical Professor
Department of Family Medicine
University of California, Irvine
Irvine, California

Jason A. Krystofiak, MD, CAQSM
Medical Director of Sports Medicine
Medical Director of the Matthew J. Morahan III Center
RWJ Barnabas Health
Department of Orthopedic and Sports Medicine
Livingston, New Jersey
Team Physician, Rutgers Athletics
Clinical Assistant Professor
Department of Family Medicine and Community Health
Rutgers Robert Wood Johnson Medical School
Newark, New Jersey

Anthony Kwon, MD
Physician
Department of Family Medicine
University of Hawaii
Honolulu, Hawaii

Michael Ladewski, DO, FAAFP, CAQSM
Medical Director
Ascension Resurrection Family Medicine Residency Center
Ascension Resurrection Medical Center
Chicago, Illinois

Lindsay A. Lafferty, MD
Assistant Professor
Department of Family and Community Medicine and Orthopedics and Rehabilitation
Pennsylvania State University College of Medicine
Hershey, Pennsylvania

Mark E. Lavallee, MD, CSCS, FACSM, FAMSSM
Faculty
UPMC Central PA Sports Medicine Fellowship
UPMC Central PA
Harrisburg, Pennsylvania

Kurtis Lawton, DO
Primary Care Sports Medicine Fellow
Department of Sports Medicine
Medical College of Wisconsin
Milwaukee, Wisconsin

Justin Leasure, MD
Fellow
Department of Sports Medicine
Nationwide Children's Hospital
Columbus, Ohio

Ryley Lee, MD
Resident
Department of Family Medicine
Kaiser
Orange County, California

Bryan Leek, MD
Associate Clinical Professor
Department of Orthopedic Surgery
University of California, San Diego
San Diego, California

Jeffrey C. Leggit, MD, CAQSM[†]
Vice Chair
Department of Family Medicine
Uniformed Services University
Bethesda, Maryland

Terrance L. Leighton III, BS, DO[†]
Dive Medical Officer
United States Navy
San Diego, California

Nicole L. Leonard, MD[†]
Physician
UC Davis Health
Sacramento, California

Amy Leu, DO, FAAFP, CAQSM
HS Clinical Professor
Division of Sports Medicine
Department of Family Medicine
UC San Diego School of Medicine
San Diego, California

Jina Libby, DO, FAAPMR
Physical Medicine and Rehabilitation and Sports Medicine Physician
Department of Sports Medicine and Physical Medicine and Rehabilitation
NYU Langone Health
New York, New York

Whitney Liehr, DO
Physician
Department of Physical Medicine and Rehabilitation
UC Davis Health
Sacramento, California

Ryan J. Lingor, MD, AT-C, RD, CSCS
Primary Sports Physician
Department of Primary Sports Medicine
Hospital for Special Surgery
New York, New York

Laura J. Lintner, DO, CAQSM
Assistant Professor
Department of Family and Community Medicine
Wake Forest University School of Medicine
Winston Salem, North Carolina

Justin Lockrem, MD, CAQSM
Assistant Director
Department of Sports Medicine
Boston College
Boston, Massachusetts

Jayson Loeffert, DO
Physician
Associate Professor
Department of Family and Community Medicine and Orthopedics and Rehabilitation
Penn State Milton S. Hershey Medical Center
Hershey, Pennsylvania

Joshua F. Loiseau, MD
Sports Medicine Fellow
South Bend-Notre Dame Sports Medicine Fellowship
Mishawaka, Indiana

Brian Lowell, MD, CAQSM
Teacher Clinician
Department of Family Medicine of Southwest Washington
PeaceHealth
Vancouver, Washington

Jordan W. Lyons, MD, MBA, FAAFP
Fellow
Department of Sports Medicine
NMRTC Camp Pendleton
Oceanside, California

Kevin Machino, DO
Physical Medicine and Rehabilitation and Sports Medicine Physician
Department of Physical Medicine and Rehabilitation and Sports Medicine
Intermountain Health
Las Vegas, Nevada

Nicole Madrilejo, MD
Primary Care Sports Medicine Fellow
Department of Family and Sports Medicine
University of California, San Diego
San Diego, California

Aimee Madsen, MD
Physical Medicine and Rehabilitation Resident
Physical Medicine and Rehabilitation
University of Florida
Gainesville, Florida

Navid Mahooti, MD, MPH, CAQSM
Clinical Instructor, Sports Medicine
Mass General Brigham—Salem Hospital
Boston, Massachusetts

Stefany J. K. Malanka, MD
Fellow, Primary Care Sports Medicine
University of Chicago/NorthShore University Health System
Chicago, Illinois

Britt Marcussen, MD, FAAFP, CAQSM
Clinical Professor
Program Director Primary Care Sports Medicine Fellowship
Department of Family Medicine
University of Iowa Hospitals and Clinics
Iowa City, Iowa

Christopher Mariano, DO
Resident
Family and Community Medicine
Virginia Tech Carilion Clinic
Roanoke, Virginia

Janelle Marra, DO, FAAFP, CAQSM†
Assistant Professor
Department of Family Medicine
Uniformed Services University of the Health Sciences
Bethesda, Maryland

Vincent Marshall, DO
Clinical Fellow
Department of Emergency Sports Medicine
Mass General Brigham
Boston, Massachusetts

Anthony Martin, MD, CAQSM
Associate Program Director, Sports Medicine Fellowship
Department of Family Medicine
Atrium Health
Charlotte, North Carolina

Robert D. Martin, MD
Orthopedic Surgeon
Associate Professor of Orthopedic Surgery
University of Arkansas for Medical Sciences
Little Rock, Arkansas

Brianna Martinez, MD
Primary Care Sports Medicine Fellow
University of California, San Diego
San Diego, California

Julio A. Martinez-Silvestrini, MD, FAAPMR, CAQSM
Medical Director
Baystate Rehabilitation Care
Baystate Health
Springfield, Massachusetts

Jonathan Mason, DO, CAQSM, RMSK
Clinical Professor, Sports Medicine
Musculoskeletal Institute
The University of Texas at Austin—Dell Medial School
Austin, Texas

Brandan Mayer-Blackwell, MD
Department of Sports Medicine
Kaiser Permanente
San Diego, California

David McClaskey, MD, ATC
Primary Care Sports Medicine Physician
Department of Family Medicine
Kaiser Permanente
San Diego, California

Christopher McGrew, MD, FACSM, CAQSM
Professor
Department of Family and Community Medicine and
Department of Orthopedics and Rehabilitation
University of New Mexico Health Sciences Center
Albuquerque, New Mexico

Ian D. McKeag, MD, MS, CAQSM
Assistant Professor
Program Director UAB Sports and Exercise Medicine Fellowship
Department of Family and Community Medicine
University of Alabama at Birmingham (UAB)
Birmingham, Alabama

Sean McKeown, MS, PT, Cred MDT
Director of Quality Care
Physical Rehabilitation Network
Carson City, Nevada

Bailey J. Meccariello, DO, CAQSM
Primary Care Sports Medicine Physician
Cone Health Sports Medicine Fellowship Faculty
Murphy Wainer Orthopedics and Cone Health
Greensboro, North Carolina

Jaison Medayil, DO
Sports Medicine Fellow
Department of Emergency Medicine and Sports Medicine
University of New Mexico
Albuquerque, New Mexico

Joseph Medellin, MD, MPH, MBA
Medical Director
Department of Sports Medicine
Henry Ford Health Jackson
Jackson, Michigan

Paul Meirick, MD
Sports Medicine Physician
St. Cloud Orthopedics
Sartell, Minnesota

Sarah Merrill, MD, CAQSM
Sports Medicine Physician
Department of Family and Sports Medicine
University of California, San Diego
San Diego, California

Brent H. Messick, MD, MS, FAAFP, FASCM, CAQSM
Associate Professor
Department of Family and Community Medicine Wake Forest University School of Medicine
Atrium Health Musculoskeletal Institute
Concord, North Carolina

Christopher Miles, MD, CAQSM
Associate Professor
Family and Community Medicine
Wake Forest University School of Medicine
Winston-Salem, North Carolina

Jennifer J. Mitchell, MD, FAAFP, CAQSM, FAMSSM
Professor, Sports Medicine Fellowship Director
Department of Family and Community Medicine
Texas Tech University Health Sciences Center School of Medicine
Lubbock, Texas

Kelly T. Mitchell, MD
Professor and Ophthalmology Residency Director
Department of Ophthalmology and Visual Sciences
Texas Tech University Health Sciences Center School of Medicine
Lubbock, Texas

Mary Mitchell, DO
Team Physician and Assistant Professor
Department of Family and Sports Medicine
Edward Via College of Osteopathic Medicine
Virginia Tech
Blacksburg, Virginia

Jeffrey M. Mjaanes, MD, CAQSM, FAAP, FACSM
Assistant Professor
Director of Sports Medicine
Department of Orthopedic Surgery
Northwestern University, Feinberg School of Medicine
Evanston, Illinois

Caitlyn C. Mooney, MD, FAAP, CAQSM
Assistant Professor, Orthopedics
Vanderbilt University Medical Center
Nashville, Tennessee

Carly Morgan, DO, ATC
Primary Care Sports Medicine Fellow
TriHealth
Cincinnati, Ohio

Kinshasa Morton, MD, CAQSM
Assistant Professor
Department of Family Medicine and Community Health
Rutgers University
Piscataway, New Jersey

Ryan Muehling, MD, CAQSM
Sports Medicine Physician
University of Nevada, Reno
Reno, Nevada

Thomas Munro, MD
Pediatric Sports Medicine Specialist and General Pediatrician
Priority Care Pediatrics
Kansas City, MO

John Munyak, MD
Emergency Medicine/Sports Medicine Physician
Walk-in Orthopedics and Sports Medicine
New York Bone and Joint Specialists
New York, New York

Laura Murphy, DO, CAQSM
Core Faculty
Ventura County Medicine Center, Family Medicine Residency
Ventura, California

Tenley Murphy, MD, FAAFP, CAQSM
Assistant Director of Sports Medicine
Clemson University
Clemson, South Carolina

Chadwick C. Nabors, DO, CAQSM
Sports Medicine Fellow
Atrium Health
Concord, North Carolina

William C. Nace, DO
Primary Care Sports Medicine Fellow
Department of Sports Medicine
The Ohio State University
Columbus, Ohio

Dhiren J. Naidu, MD, FRCPC, Dip. Sport Med.
Professor
Division of Physical Medicine and Rehabilitation
University of Alberts
Edmonton, AB, Canada

Hirotaka Nakagawa, MD
Fellow
Department of Sports Medicine
UC Davis Medical Center
Sacramento, California

Greg Nakamoto, MD, FACP
Department of Orthopedics and Sports Medicine
Clinical Assistant Professor of Medicine
Department of Medicine
University of Washington School of Medicine
Seattle, Washington

Jonathan Napolitano, MD, FAAPMR
Attending Physician, Assistant Professor
Department of Physical Medicine and Rehabilitation, Pediatrics
Division of Sports Medicine
Nationwide Children's Hospital and The Ohio State University
Columbus, Ohio

Kevin Nasre-Esfahani, DO, MS
Physician
Department of Physical Medicine and Rehabilitation
UC Davis Health
Sacramento, California

Melissa Nayak, MD, CAQSM
Senior Staff Physician
Department of Orthopedics
Henry Ford Health
Detroit, Michigan

Sara L. Neal, MD, MA, CAQSM
Program Director
Family Medicine Residency
Cone Health
Greensboro, North Carolina

Giorgio A. Negron, MD
Sports Medicine Physician

Chris Nelson, MD, CAQSM
Assistant Professor
Department of Family and Community Medicine
Wake Forest University School of Medicine
Winston Salem, North Carolina

Tammy Ng, MD
Physician
UC Davis Health
Sacramento, California

Tu Dan Nguyen, MD, CAQSM
Director of Sports Medicine
Clinical Assistant Professor
Department of Family Medicine
Memorial Family Medicine Residency Program, UTHealth Houston McGovern Medical School
Houston, Texas

Mark W. Niedfeldt, MD
Clinical Associate Professor
Department of Family and Community Medicine
Medical College of Wisconsin
Milwaukee, Wisconsin

Srikanth Nithyanandam, MBBS, MS, CAQSM
Assistant Professor
Orthopedics and Sports Medicine
University of Kentucky
Lexington, Kentucky

Andrew Nobe, MD, CAQSM
Assistant Clinical Professor
Department of Family Medicine and Orthopedic Surgery
University of California, Irvine
Irvine, California

Laika M. Nur, MD
Clinical Assistant Professor
Department of Orthopedic Surgery, Division of Sports Medicine
Scripps Clinic Medical Group
San Diego, California

Rathna R. Nuti, MD, CAQSM, FAAFP
Sports Medicine Physician
DFW Sports Medicine
McKinney, Texas

Jennifer Oberstar, MD, CAQSM
Physician
Department of Family Medicine
University of Minnesota
Minneapolis, Minnesota

Richard A. Okragly, MD, FAMSSM
Director of Sports Medicine
TriHealth Sports Medicine Fellowship Program
Cincinnati, Ohio

Tony Olmert, MD, MPhil
Physician
Department of Family Medicine
University of California, San Diego
La Jolla, California

David E. Olson, MD, CAQSM, FACSM
Assistant Professor
Department of Family Medicine
University of Minnesota
Minneapolis, Minnesota

Irie Paul Padua, MD
Sports Medicine Fellow
Department of Family Medicine
University of California, Irvine
Irvine, California

Scott L. Paradise, MD, CAQSM, FAAFP[†]
Assistant Professor
Department of Family Medicine
Uniformed Services University of the Health Sciences
Bethesda, Maryland

Jun Hwan Park, MD
PGY-3 Family Medicine Resident
University of Illinois College of Medicine at Peoria
Peoria, Illinois

Sona Patel, MD, FAAP
Independent Consultant
Miami, Florida

Austin Patterson, DO
Sports Medicine Fellow
Department of Sports Medicine
Texas Tech University
Lubbock, Texas

Bernadette Pendergraph, MD
Sports Medicine Fellowship Director
Department of Family Medicine
Harbor-UCLA Medical Center
Harbor City, California

Andrew Pennock, MD
Rady Children's Health
San Diego, California

Evan D. Perez, MD, CAQSM
Assistant Professor
Surgical Specialty and MSK Integrated Service Unit
University of Texas Rio Grande Valley School of Medicine
Edinburg, Texas

Michael Jake Peterson, MD
Pediatric Resident
Department of Pediatrics
UC Davis Health
Sacramento, California

Shawn Phillips, MD, MSPT
Associate Professor
Department of Family and Community Medicine and Orthopedics
Penn State College of Medicine
Hershey, Pennsylvania

Brent Pickett, DO
Team Physician, Utah State University Athletics
Intermountain Healthcare, Logan Regional Orthopedics
Logan, Utah

Craig Pille, MD
Primary Care Sports Medicine Fellow
Department of Primary Care Sports Medicine
Maryland School of Medicine
Baltimore, Maryland

Wikien Hung Pinto, MD
Clinical Fellow/Instructor
Division of Pediatric Sports Medicine
Department of Orthopedic Surgery
Vanderbilt University Medical Center
Nashville, Tennessee

Katherine M. Pohlgeers, MD, MS, CAQSM[†]
Associate Program, Director
University of Louisville
Louisville, Kentucky

Thomas L. Pommering, DO, FAAFP, FAMSSM
Division Chief
Department of Sports Medicine
Nationwide Children's Hospital
The Ohio State University College of Medicine
Columbus, Ohio

Nandakumar Ponnusamy, MBBS, MD, FASA
Medical Director
Pain Management Clinic
Department of Anesthesiology
Baystate Medical Center
Springfield, Massachusetts

Steven K. Poon, MD, CAQSM
Primary Care Sports Medicine Physician
Department of Orthopedic Surgery
Mayo Clinic Arizona
Tempe, Arizona

Salvador Portugal, DO, MBA, FAAPMR, CAQSM
Assistant Professor
Department of Rehabilitation Medicine
NYU Grossman School of Medicine
NYU Langone Health
New York, New York

Morgan Potter, MD
Emergency Medicine Physician
Sports Medicine Fellow
Department of Emergency Medicine
The Mount Sinai Hospital
New York, New York

Abdullah Hasan Pratt, MD
Assistant Professor
Emergency Medicine Physician
University of Chicago
Chicago, Illinois

Denice Praxidio, DO
Primary Care Sports Medicine Fellow
Family Medicine/Sports Medicine
Oregon Health & Science University
Portland, Oregon

Patrick J. Prazak, DO, CAQSM
Primary Care Sports Medicine Physician
Orthopedics and Sports Medicine
Houston Methodist Sugar Land
Sugar Land, Texas

Michael Prestgard-Duke, MD
Sports Medicine Fellow
Department of Family Medicine
PeaceHealth Family Medicine of Southwest Washington
Vancouver, Washington

David E. Price, MD, FAMSSM
Professor
Department of Family Medicine
Department of Orthopedics
Atrium Health
Charlotte, North Carolina

Tricia Prince, DO, MS, AOCPMR
Assistant Professor
Department of Primary Care medicine and Rehabilitation
University of Miami, Miller School of Medicine
Miami, Florida

Erika Pruss, MD
Assistant Clinical Professor
Department of Orthopedics
University of California, San Diego
San Diego, California

George G. A. Pujalte, MD, FACSM, FAMSSM, FAAFP
Consultant
Department of Family Medicine, and Orthopedics and Sports Medicine
Mayo Clinic
Jacksonville, Florida

Anna P. Quan, MD
Clinical Professor of Medicine
Department of Internal Medicine, Primary Care
University of California, San Diego
San Diego, California

Kristina Quirolgico, MD, FAAPMR
Assistant Attending Physiatrist
Clinical Assistant Professor
Department of Physiatry, Rehabilitation Medicine
Hospital for Special Surgery
New York Presbyterian/Weill Cornell Medical Center
New York, New York

Matthew Rachwalski, DO
Sports Medicine Physician
Department of Orthopedics and Sports Medicine
Franciscan Physician Network
Michigan City, Indiana

Hunter Rafoth, MD
Physician
Department of Sports Medicine
Cone Health
Greensboro, North Carolina

Navdeep Rai, MD, MS
Physician
Department of Family and Sports Medicine
Palo Alto Medical Foundation
San Jose, California

Sara N. Raiser, MD, FAAPMR, CAQSM
Assistant Professor
Department of Physical Medicine and Rehabilitation
University of Virginia
Charlottesville, Virginia

Reno Ravindran, MD, FAAFP, CAQSM
Sports Medicine Physician
Charlottesville, Virginia
Sports Medicine
Nationwide Children's Hospital
Columbus, Ohio

Ziad Fahad Rayes, MBBS, MBA, Ccfp(Sem), Dip Sport Med(Casem)
King Faisal Specialist Hospital and Research Center
Riyadh, Saudi Arabia

Steven Reece, MD, CAQSM
Physician
Department of Sports Medicine
OrthoVirginia
Richmond, Virginia

Kari J. Rezac, DO
Sports Medicine Fellow
Physical Medicine and Rehabilitation
University of California, Davis
Sacramento, California

Brittney M. Richardson, MD, CAQSM
Physician
Department of Family and Geriatric Medicine
University of Louisville School of Medicine
Louisville, Kentucky

Shelby Rider, MD, MS
General Surgery Resident
Department of General Surgery
LSUHS-Shreveport
Shreveport, Louisiana

Diego Riveros, MD
Assistant Professor
Emergency Medicine and Sports Medicine
University of South Florida Morsani College of Medicine
Tampa, Florida

Tara Robbins, MD
Physician
Department of Family Medicine
Scripps Clinic Medical Group
San Diego, California

Richard E. Rodenberg Jr., MD, FAAP, CAQSM
Program Director
Division of Sports Medicine
Nationwide Children's Hospital
Columbus, Ohio

Natalie Ronshaugen, MD, CAQSM
Sports Medicine Physician
Associate Professor
University of Nebraska Medical Center
Omaha, Nebraska

Daryl Rosenbaum, MD
Associate Professor
Department of Family Medicine
Wake Forest University School of Medicine
Winston-Salem, North Carolina

Eric A. Rosson, DO, MBA†
Senior Medicine Officer
USS Tripoli
United States Navy
San Diego, California

Justin Rouintan, DO
Physician
Kingman Regional Medical Center
Kingman, Arizona

Gregory Rubin, DO, CAQSM
Department of Sport Medicine
Hospital for Special Surgery
Naples Community Hospital
Naples, Florida

Chelsea Rubis, DO†
Sports Medicine Physician
Edwar Via College of Osteopathic Medicine
Blacksburg, Virginia

Alana Ryan, DO, CAQSM
Sports Medicine Physician
Samaritan Medical Group
Corvallis, Oregon

Rhiannon Ryan, DO†
Primary Care Sports Medicine Fellow
Department of Sports Medicine
University of California, San Diego
San Diego, California

Anthony J. Saglimbeni, MD, CAQSM
Team Physician
West Coast Sports Institute
Santa Clara University
San Jose, California

Glenn H. Sapp II, MD
Physician
Medstar National Rehabilitation Network
Washington DC

Uziel Sauceda, MD, CAQSM
Program Director, RUHS/UCR Sports Medicine Fellowship
Department of Family Medicine
Riverside University Health System/UC Riverside
Riverside, California

Fouad Sayde, MD, ABIM, ABEM, FACP
Sports Medicine Physician
Toronto, Canada

Brandon Schabacker, MD
University of California, San Diego
San Diego, California

Daniel Schlegel, MD, MHA
Associate Professor
Department of Family and Community Medicine
Penn State Milton S. Hershey Medical Center
Hershey, Pennsylvania

Joshua Schulte, MD
Resident Physician
UT Southwestern
Dallas, Texas

Rohan M. Sebastian, MD, MBA
Physician
Department of Sports Medicine
Dallas Methodist Health Systems
Dallas, Texas

LaRae L. Seemann, MD
Assistant Professor
Department of Family Medicine
Mayo Clinic
Jacksonville, Florida

Nilesh Shah, MD, FAAFP, CAQSM
Medical Director and Fellowship Director
Department of Sports Medicine
Summa Health
Akron, Ohio

Stephen Shaheen, MD, CAQSM, FACEP
Assistant Professor
Department of Orthopedics and Emergency Medicine
Duke University Medical Center
Durham, North Carolina

Alan Shahtaji, DO, CAQSM
Clinical Professor
Department of Family Medicine
University of California at San Diego Health
San Diego, California

Priya Sharma, DO
Physician
Department of Family and Sports Medicine
Family Health Centers of San Diego, UC San Diego Health
San Diego, California

Zainab Shirazi, MD
Chief Resident
Department of Physical Medicine and Rehabilitation
NYPH Columbia and Cornell
New York, New York

Anant Shukla, MD
Emergency Medicine Physician and Sports Medicine Fellow
Division of Sports Medicine
Vanderbilt University Medical Center
Nashville, Tennessee

Matthew L. Silvis, MD, FAMSSM
Professor, Sports Medicine Division Chief
Department of Family and Community Medicine and Orthopedics and Rehabilitation
Penn State Health
Hershey, Pennsylvania

Zachary Sitton, MD
Resident Physician
Department of Family and Community Medicine
Atrium Health Wake Forest Baptist
Winston-Salem, North Carolina

Kristy Smith, MD
Associate Clinical Professor
Department of Community Health and Family Medicine
University of Florida
Gainesville, Florida

Neil L. Sparks, DO, MS, FAAFP
Assistant Professor
Department of Family and Community Medicine
Wake Forest University School of Medicine
Winston-Salem, North Carolina

Jason J. Stacy, MD
Director of Sports Medicine and Physical Therapy
Department of Student Health Services
University of South Carolina
Columbia, South Carolina

Mark Stovak, MD
Professor and Acting Chair
Department of Family and Community Medicine
University of Nevada, Reno School of Medicine
Reno, Nevada

Keith A. Stuessi, MD, CAQSM
Physician Subject Matter Expert in Traumatic Brain Injury
General Dynamics Information Technology
Bremerton, Washington

James Suchy, MD, CAQSM
Department of Primary Care and Sports Medicine
Hoag
Irvine, California

Theodora L. Swenson, MD
Sports Medicine Fellow
Department of Orthopedics and Pediatrics
Vanderbilt University Medical Center
Nashville, Tennessee

Jeremy Swisher, MD
Department of Family Medicine
Wake Forest University School of Medicine
Winston-Salem, North Carolina

Adrian Tabares, MD, CAQSM, RMSK
Physician
Department of Family Medicine and Orthopedics
Sutter Medical Group
Sacramento, California

Kenneth S. Taylor, MD, FAAFP, CAQSM
Clinical Professor of Family Medicine/ Sports Medicine
University of California, San Diego, School of Medicine
Chief, Primary Care Sports Medicine
Director, UCSD Primary Care Sports Medicine Fellowship
Head Primary Care Sports Physician, San Diego Padres
Team Physician, UCSD Tritons
Team Physician, US Olympic Training Center
San Diego, California

Michelle A. Tedrowe, DO
Sports Medicine Fellow
Department of Sports Medicine
Cone Health
Greensboro, North Carolina

Alexandra Tee, MD, CAQSM
Primary Care and Sports Medicine Physician
Department of Sports Medicine and Orthopedic Surgery
Kaiser Permanente
South San Francisco, California

Surein Theivakumar, DO, CAQSM, RMSK
Physician
Department of Rehabilitation
NYU School of Medicine
New York University
New York, New York

Timothy Tiu, MD, FAAPMR, CAQSM
Assistant Professor
Department of Physical Medicine and Rehabilitation
University of Miami
Miami, Florida

Jessica C. Tomazic, MD, CAQSM
Staff Physician
Department of Sports Medicine
Cleveland Clinic Foundation
Cleveland, Ohio

Alex Tomesch, MD, BCEM, CAQSM
Assistant Professor of Emergency Medicine
Department of Emergency Medicine
University of Nebraska Medical Center
Omaha, Nebraska

Christopher C. Trigger, MD, FACEP, CAQSM
Attending Physician, EM Residency Core Faculty
Department of Emergency Medicine
Corewell Health Lakeland
St. Joseph, Michigan

Michael Troy, DO
Sports Medicine Fellow
University of California, San Diego
San Diego, California

Priscilla Tu, DO, FAOASM, FAAP, FAAMA, FACOFP
Associate Program Director and Director of Osteopathic Education
Department of Family and Community Medicine
Virgina Tech, Carilion Clinic
Roanoke, Virginia

Philipp J. Underwood, MD, FAAEM, FACEP, FAAFP, CAQSM, RDMS
Program Director, Sports Medicine Fellowship
Department of Emergency Medicine
North Shore University Hospital
Manhasset, New York

Saif Usman, MD, FAMSSM, FAAFP
Sports Medicine Physician
Facey Medical Group
Valencia, California

Haris Vakil, MD
Primary Care Sports Medicine Fellow
Department of Orthopedics and Sports Medicine
Houston Methodist Hospital
Houston, Texas

Edgar M. VanHorne, MD
Sports Medicine Fellow/Undersea Medical Officer (UMO)
Naval Hospital Camp Pendleton
Oceanside, California

Ricardo Villanueva Alvarez, MD
Family Medicine PGY-3
Department of Family Medicine
LSU Health Shreveport
Shreveport, Louisiana

Kenneth Vitale, MD, FACSM, FAAPMR
Professor
Department of Orthopedic Surgery
University of California, San Diego
La Jolla, California

Matthew Waldrop, MD
Department of Family Medicine
Wake Forest University School of Medicine
Winston-Salem, North Carolina

Elizabeth Walker, DO
Sports Medicine Fellow
Assistant Professor of Family Medicine
Edward Via College of Osteopathic Medicine, Virginia Tech Sports Medicine
Blacksburg, Virginia

Jacob Walker, MD
Physician
St. Joseph Health System
Mishawaka, Indiana

Bryant Walrod, MD, CAQSM
Professor
Department of Family and Community Medicine
The Ohio State University
Columbus, Ohio

Keifer P. Walsh, DO, MS
Sports Medicine Physician
Naval Hospital Camp Pendleton
Oceanside, California

John C. Walton, MD, MSL
Sports Medicine Physician
Department of Orthopedics
University of Chicago
Chicago, Illinois

Austin Jinwei Wang, DO
Physician
Department of Physical Medicine and Rehabilitation
UC Davis Medical Center
Sacramento, California

David A. Wang, MD
Assistant Attending Physician
Department of Primary Sports Medicine Service
Hospital for Special Surgery
New York, New York

Kevin Waninger, MD, MS, FAAFP, FACEP, FACSM, FAMSSM, CAQSM
Physician
Lehigh Valley Hospital and Health Network
Allentown, Pennsylvania

Alexandra E. Warrick, MD, CAQSM
Assistant Professor
Department of Physical Medicine and Rehabilitation, Sports Medicine
University of California Davis School of Medicine
Sacramento, California

Charles W. Webb, DO, FAMSSM, FAAFP, CAQSM
Director, Division of Sports Medicine
Department of Family Medicine
LSU Health Science Center Shreveport
Shreveport, Louisiana

Kathleen Weber, MD, MS
Director
Primary Care Sports Medicine
Department of Orthopedics
Rush University Medical Center
Midwest Orthopedics in at Rush University
Chicago, Illinois

Matthew Wessinger, MD, MPH[†]
Resident Physician
Department of Emergency Medicine
UPMC Harrisburg
Harrisburg, Pennsylvania

William H. West, MD, CAQSM
Department of Primary Care Sports Medicine
Kadlec Northwest Orthopedic and Sports Medicine
Richland, Washington

Keenan Wheeler, DO
Department of Internal Medicine and Sports Medicine
Carlsbad, California

Alec Wilhelmi, MD, CAQSM
Primary Care Sports Medicine Physician
Aurora Health Care
Adjunct Clinical Professor
Department of Family Medicine
University of Wisconsin—Madison
De Pere, Wisconsin

Elizabeth A. Williams, DO
Physician
San Diego Sports Medicine and Family Health Center
San Diego, California

Kristina Wilson, MD, MPH, FAAP, CAQSM
Medical Director
Department of Primary Care Sports Medicine
Children's Hospital of Colorado
University of Colorado
Aurora, Colorado

Amanda T. Wise, DO, CAQSM
Assistant Professor
Department of Physical Medicine and Rehabilitation
UT Southwestern Medical Center
Dallas, Texas

Matthew W. Wise, DO, CAQSM
Assistant Professor
Department of Family and Community Medicine and Orthopaedic Surgery
UT Southwestern Medical Center
Dallas, Texas

Jason P. Womack, MD
Associate Professor
Department of Family Medicine and Community Health
Rutgers—Robert Wood Johnson Medical School
New Brunswick, New Jersey

Gillian G. Wooldridge, DO, CCD, FAOASM
Physician
Department of Orthopedics and Sports Medicine
Houston Methodist Hospital
Houston, Texas

Rukmini Yakkanti, DO
Primary Care Sports Medicine Physician
Department of Orthopedics
University of Louisville
Louisville, Kentucky

Jarrod Yamanaka, MD, CAQSM
Sports Medicine Physician
Fairview
Blaine, Minnesota

Ramon Ylanan, MD, CAQSM
Fellowship Program Director
University of Arkansas for Medical Sciences NW Primary Care Sports Medicine Fellowship
Assistant Professor for Family and Community Medicine
Assistant Professor Department of Orthopedics
University of Arkansas for Medical Sciences
Fayetteville, Alaska

Craig C. Young, MD
Professor
Department of Orthopedic Surgery and Community and Family Medicine
Medical College of Wisconsin
Milwaukee, Wisconsin

Rachel Young, DO, ATC
Sports Medicine Fellow
TriHealth Bethesda Sports Medicine Fellowship
Cincinnati, Ohio

Warren Young, MD, FAAP
Assistant Attending Physician
Department of Primary Sports Medicine
Hospital for Special Surgery
New York, New York

Eric Yuan, MD, FAAFP, CAQSM[†]
Physician
Department of Primary Care and Sports Medicine
University of California, San Diego
San Diego, California

Jason L. Zaremski, MD, CAQSM, FAAPMR, FACSM, FAMSSM
Clinical Associate Professor of Sports Medicine and Physical Medicine and Rehabilitation
Department of Physical Medicine and Rehabilitation
University of Florida
Gainesville, Florida

Carrie B. Zaslow, MD
Clinical Assistant Professor of Ophthalmology
Northwell Health Physicians Partners—Hofstra University
Bayside, New York

Tracy L. Zaslow, MD, FAAP, CAQSM
Primary Care Sports Medicine Physician
Cedars Sinai
Los Angeles, California

Roman Zolotoy, DO
Physician
West Michigan Pain
Big Rapids, Michigan

[†] *The views expressed are those of the authors and do not reflect the official policy of the Department of the Army, Department of the Navy, Department of the Air Force, the Department of Defense, or the United States Government.*

THIRD EDITION AUTHOR ACKNOWLEDGMENTS

The editors and authors of the third edition gratefully acknowledge the past contributions of the following previous edition authors:

Jessalyn Adam
Giselle Aerni
Sonya Ahmed
Ibraheem Algarni
Joseph E. Allen
Kamel Azhar
Amanda Babcock
Rebecca Bacharach
Aaron Baggish
Marwan A. Bakarman
Robert J. Baker
Aleem Bakhtiar
Evan Bass
David Bazzo
Brandon Bockewitz
William W. Briner Jr.
David L. Brown
Steven Brown
Sean Bryan
Randall Burgett
Nick Cardinale
Stephen Carek
Corey Carson
Scott Chandler
Amanda Chaney
Andrew Cheung
Alicia Chitanand
Jin Choi
Joseph N. Chorley
Dwaipayan Choudhury
Matthew H. Chung
Philip H. Cohen
Ryan P. Cole
William M. Collins
Michael Connolly
Timothy Dekker
Rania L. Dempsey
William W. Dexter
Mark Diamond
Joshua Dilley
Douglas J. DiOrio
Laura M. Distel
William Dixon
Ryan Draper
Timothy R. Draper
Brandon Eck
Dina Elnaggar
Johnnie Faircloth
Cody Franzen
Jordan F. Geroski
Chad Giles
Kory Gill
Rodney S. Gonzalez
Miranda Gordon-Zigel
Tarek Hadla
John Hariadi
Mark D. Harris
Fernando E. Hernandez
Marc P. Hilgers
David M. Hirschi III
Brandon Hockenberry
Matthew Horn
Robert G. Hosey
Robert Howard
Yaffa Ilyaguyeva
Krishna Israni
Dominic Jacobelli
Bjorn A. Jacobson
Carrie A. Jaworski
David Johnson
Robert L. Jones
Amy Kakimoto
Rahul Kapur
Misha Khalighi
Spencer S. Kirk
Jennifer Scott Koontz
David W. Kruse
Geoffrey Kuhlman
Daniel T. Kuo
Bittu Kuruvilla
Andrea Kussman
Mike LaGrange
Christopher P. Lake
Se Won Lee
Emily Levy
Michael M. Linder
Fernando Liquido
Kelsey Logan
Frank E. Lorch
James H. Lynch
Adam Lyons
Gary E. Means
Kyle Meyer
Daniel Murphy
Laura Murphy
Priya Nagarajan

Dusty Marie Narducci
Mark Nelson
Vicki Nelson
Rochelle M. Nolte
David Olson
Ross Osborn
Stephen Paul
Timothy Perdue
David J. Pohl
Steve Poon
Emily Porter
Shannon Powers
Aaron J. Provance
James C. Puffer
Margaret E. Pusateri
Tracy Ray
Ryan Reese
Brent S. E. Rich
James C. Ritchey
Stephen J. Rohrer
Yaqoob Sayed
Andrew Schleihauf
W. Franklin Sease Jr.
Michael K. Seifert
Nicholas R. Sgrignoli
David C. Shin
Stephen Simons
Shawn Skarpnes
Andrew Smith
Drew Smith
Michael Seth Smith
M. Kyle Smoot
Ryan Sorell
Isaac Syrop
Johnny C. Tenegra
Thomas Trojian
JP Valette
Gerardo Vazquez
Andrew M. Warner
Anna Waterbrook
William West
Nancy White
Justin M. Wright
Michael Yang
Ramon Ylanan

CONTENTS

ABDOMINAL MUSCLE STRAINS

Brittney M. Richardson, MD, CAQSM

BASICS

DESCRIPTION

Injury to the abdominal wall musculature, including the rectus abdominis, internal/external obliques, and transverse abdominis muscles:

- Typically a noncontact injury but may be caused by trauma
- Acute injury typically is the result of an abrupt movement of the trunk.
- Subacute injury caused by repetitive activity
- A specific variant known as a side strain most commonly involves the internal oblique at or near the inferior rib attachments.

EPIDEMIOLOGY

Somewhat uncommon injuries, but specific sports have a higher prevalence:

- Account for <2% of athletic injuries (1)
- Sports with repetitive trunk rotation have higher rates:
  - Soccer, tennis, baseball, ice hockey, gymnastics, pole vault, cricket, bowling (2)
- Seen in runners because the abdominal muscles are used for pelvic stabilization
- Attributed to weight training and abdominal workouts as well

ETIOLOGY AND PATHOPHYSIOLOGY

Acute or chronic muscle-tendon injury of the abdominal wall musculature from a sudden intrinsic eccentric contraction of the abdominal musculature (3)

RISK FACTORS

- Poorly conditioned abdominal musculature or deficits in core strength
- Previous abdominal wall muscle strain/tear
- Poor weight training or conditioning techniques
- Participation in activities that require abrupt and/or repetitive movements of the torso early in the sport season

GENERAL PREVENTION

Appropriate weight training and conditioning techniques with attention to core strength

DIAGNOSIS

HISTORY

- Abdominal wall pain associated with stretching or twisting mechanism
- Direct trauma associated with a minority of these injuries
- Pain usually focal and exacerbated by specific movements or positions
- Pain with active contraction of affected muscle during sneezing or coughing
- Symptoms generally subside in the absence of activity.
- In throwing or overhead athletes typically on the side contralateral to the throwing arm, in baseball batters contralateral to the dominant batting side (4)

PHYSICAL EXAM

- Appearance is typically normal with swelling, and evidence of contusion rare in the absence of preceding trauma.
- Splinting may be noted if pain is severe.
- Tenderness of the abdominal wall is usually focal and discrete but may be more diffuse in overuse injuries.
- Muscle defect may be notable if an associated tear or herniation is present.
- Peritoneal signs are absent.
- Symptoms are reproduced by contraction of the affected muscle.

DIFFERENTIAL DIAGNOSIS

- Abdominal wall contusion
- Abdominal wall hematoma:
  - Swelling, periumbilical contusion, and a mass with rigidity and/or guarding are signs of a rectus sheath hematoma.
- Abdominal wall hernia (umbilical, spigelian)
- Intra-abdominal injury (contusion, laceration, perforation)
- Intra-abdominal process (e.g., infection, mass)
- Iliac apophysitis
- Nerve entrapment
- Osteitis pubis

DIAGNOSTIC TESTS & INTERPRETATION

- Typically not indicated (5)[C]
- Plain films, computed tomographic (CT) scan indicated if there is concern for rib fracture or intra-abdominal process
- Magnetic resonance imaging (MRI) can be used to assess for muscle tear or to assess the extent of injury (6):
  - Reserved for more severe injuries
- Musculoskeletal ultrasound (US) can help confirm the diagnosis of muscle tear or hematoma and aid in clinical follow-up (3),(6)[C].

TREATMENT

Acute treatment:

- Remove the athlete from the offending activity.
- Ice
- Compressive wrap
- Nonsteroidal anti-inflammatory drugs (NSAIDs) or acetaminophen PRN only
- Once pain subsides, a rehabilitation program may be initiated (1)[C].

MEDICATION

First Line

NSAIDs or acetaminophen:

- Avoid NSAIDs if there is concern for bleeding or hematoma.

Second Line

Low-dose opioids or muscle relaxants may be used for more severe injuries but are rarely needed (5). Use should be limited to 3 days.

ADDITIONAL THERAPIES

- Rehabilitation:
  - Assess abdominal muscle strength and core strength/stability.
  - Initiate a rehab program once pain has subsided:
    - Start with passive stretching.
    - Advance to strengthening activities as tolerated with isometrics starting 5 to 7 days; concentrics at day 12; and advancement to eccentrics, core strength, and plyometrics (4)[C].
    - Progress to sport-specific activities (1),(6)[C].
- Thoracic spine mobilization may help restore unrestricted motion.
- Platelet-rich plasma injection at the site of injury may help improve pain relief and introduce growth factors to the injured muscle group (3)[C].
- Corticosteroid injection at the site of muscle tear/strain may be considered for acute pain relief or refractory cases.
- Trigger point injections with or without US guidance can help provide symptoms relief for abdominal wall pain caused by nerve entrapment or myofascial pain (5),(6).
- Local anesthetic
- Corticosteroid
- Botox
- Phenol

SURGERY/OTHER PROCEDURES

Surgery may be necessary in cases of rectus sheath hematoma, hernia, or intra-abdominal process.

- Transversus abdominis release (TAR) is a surgical procedure that repairs complex abdominal wall defects, including tears of the transversus abdominis muscle.

ONGOING CARE

FOLLOW-UP RECOMMENDATIONS

- The athlete may return to activity once pain subsides and they can engage in sport specific activity.
- Side strain–type injury has been reported to take up to 30 days in some athletes.

PROGNOSIS

Overall prognosis for recovery is excellent:

- Duration of symptoms is variable and may persist for months.
- Recurrence rates are high (>20%).

REFERENCES

1. Johnson R. Abdominal wall injuries: rectus abdominis strains, oblique strains, rectus sheath hematoma. *Curr Sports Med Rep*. 2006;5(2):99–103.
2. Nealon AR, Cook JL. Trunk side strain has a high incidence in first-class cricket fast bowlers in Australia and England. *Clin J Sport Med*. 2018;28(3):284–288.
3. Dauty M, Menu P, Dubois C. Uncommon external abdominal oblique muscle strain in a professional soccer player: a case report. *BMC Res Notes*. 2017;7:684.
4. Nealon AR, Kountouris A, Cook JL. Side strain in sport: a narrative review of pathomechanics, diagnosis, imaging and management for the clinician. *J Sci Med Sport*. 2017;20(3):261–266.
5. Shian B, Larson ST. Abdominal wall pain: clinical evaluation, differential diagnosis, and treatment. *Am Fam Physician*. 2018;98(7):429–436.
6. Gundersen A, Borgstrom H, McInnis KC. Trunk injuries in athletes. *Curr Sports Med Rep*. 2021;20(3):150–156.

CLINICAL PEARLS

- Athletes can return to play when there is minimal to no tenderness, normal muscle strength and stamina, and can perform sport-specific tasks.
- Usual duration of symptoms varies from weeks to months.

ACHILLES TENDINOPATHY

Craig C. Young, MD ▪ Mark W. Niedfeldt, MD

BASICS

DESCRIPTION

- Achilles tendinopathy is an overuse injury of the Achilles tendon that causes pain in the posterior calf and heel.
- Synonym(s): Achilles tendinosis; Achilles tendinitis

EPIDEMIOLOGY

- Accounts for 6.5–18% of injuries in runners
- Accounts for up to 4% of patients in sports medicine clinics
- Found in ~4% of youth basketball players
- Most common site is midportion (80–90%); pure insertional is rare (5%).
- Although most patients will improve, a significant number (up to 20%) will have some continuing symptoms.

Incidence

- Lifetime incidence in competitive athletes is estimated to be 24%.
- Athletes in running and jumping sports are especially at risk:
  - Lifetime incidence in competitive runners may be as high as 50%.

ETIOLOGY AND PATHOPHYSIOLOGY

- Higher risk areas:
  - Musculotendinous junction
  - The region of distal Achilles tendon that is 2 to 6 cm proximal to insertion. This is a region with a relative lack of mesotenon and intratendinous vessels.
- Tendinosis: Chronic degenerative condition is more common than tendinitis, which is an inflammatory condition.
- Disruption of normal tendon architecture:
  - Chronic intratendinous degeneration, collagen disorientation, and increases in mucoid ground substance
  - Neovascularization and increase in sympathetic nerve ingrowth around the ventral surface of the Achilles tendon

RISK FACTORS

- Training errors: recent increase in distance, intensity, or length of activity
- Worn and/or old shoes
- Inflexibility, especially tight heel cords
- Higher body mass index (BMI)
- Hypertension
- Diabetes
- Hypothyroidism
- Older patients: decreased tensile strength and increased stiffness of tendon
- Malalignment of the leg (excessive genu valgum, external tibial torsion) or ankle/foot (pes planus)
- Medications:
  - Fluoroquinolones: Recent use of these antibiotics has been associated with increased risk for Achilles tendinopathy and rupture.
  - Glucocorticoids
  - Aromatase inhibitors
  - Statins have been theorized to cause tendinopathy and have been shown in some animal models.

COMMONLY ASSOCIATED CONDITIONS

- Retrocalcaneal bursitis
- Posterior ankle impingement syndrome
- Superficial Achilles bursitis ("pump bump" or Haglund deformity)
- Achilles tendon rupture: Chronic changes in tendon may predispose to rupture.

DIAGNOSIS

HISTORY

- Pain that initially subsides with use but returns with continued use or after use suggests an overuse injury.
- Morning stiffness is a hallmark of Achilles tendinitis.
- Training errors are a factor in a large percentage of cases.
- Worn or old shoes: Shoes need to be changed every 250 to 500 miles because of shoe padding breakdown:
  - Older shoes, even new, unused shoes, may have decreased shock absorption from age-related breakdown of the shock-absorbing materials.
- Patients may report weakness and intermittent swelling.

PHYSICAL EXAM

- Pain and stiffness 2 to 6 cm above Achilles tendon insertion
- Pain with running, especially sprinting
- Tenderness over the distal Achilles tendon (2 to 6 cm above the insertion):
  - Tenderness near insertion suggests insertional Achilles tendinopathy (enthesopathy) or bursitis.
- Thickening of distal Achilles tendon in chronic cases
- Tenderness with resisted plantar flexion
- Weakness with repetitive single leg heel raises
- Crepitus with ankle motion
- Negative Simmonds-Thompson test: Compression of the calf will cause normal passive plantar flexion of the foot:
  - A positive test (absence of plantar flexion with calf compression) suggests complete Achilles tendon rupture.
- Decreased ankle dorsiflexion (from tight heel cord)

DIFFERENTIAL DIAGNOSIS

- Retrocalcaneal bursitis
- Superficial Achilles bursitis
- Calcaneal apophysitis (Sever condition) in adolescents
- Haglund deformity: prominent superior tuberosity of calcaneus
- Achilles tendon rupture
- Gastrocsoleus tear
- Plantaris tendinopathy
- Overuse myositis
- Chronic exertional compartment syndrome
- Os trigonum irritation or posterior ankle impingement syndrome
- Vascular/neurogenic claudication
- Deep venous thrombosis
- Hematoma
- Infection

DIAGNOSTIC TESTS & INTERPRETATION

- Not usually needed for initial evaluation. X-rays should be obtained if other potential injuries are suspected (e.g., fracture or tumor) or if injury is not responding to appropriate treatment.
- Standard ankle series (anteroposterior, lateral, and mortise) may show calcification of tendon; however, presence of calcification does not affect initial treatment.
- Ultrasound:
  - Hypoechoic regions, intratendinous calcifications, disorganization of fibers, fusiform expansion, intrasubstance/partial-thickness tears, and neovascularization may be seen with Achilles tendinopathy:
    - Degenerative changes may be seen in ~60% of healthy uninjured persons.
      - Higher activity individuals are more likely to have changes.
      - Studies have shown that these abnormalities are related to an increased risk of future tendinopathy (1)[A], but that resolution of these changes is not necessarily related to resolution of symptoms (2)[B].
    - Neovascularization at baseline does not predict clinical outcome of nonoperative treatment.
- MRI shows thickening of the tendon with intratendinous changes.

TREATMENT

GENERAL MEASURES

- Relative rest: Especially eliminate sprinting, speed work, and running hills or stairs. Overall decrease in running intensity, duration, and/or frequency.
- Ice after activity; proper warm-up prior to activity
- Use properly fitted, activity-appropriate shoes.
- Stretching: Ensure athlete is on appropriate conditioning program, preactivity warm-up, and postactivity cool-down programs.
- Strengthening: Include a gastrocnemius and soleus strengthening program with emphasis on eccentric exercises (1)[A],(2)[A],(3)[A].

MEDICATION

- Nonsteroidal anti-inflammatory drugs (NSAIDs): may be useful as an adjunct for pain control particularly in cases of acute injury but do not change long-term outcome
- Consider topical nitroglycerin for chronic, noninsertional Achilles tendinopathy—studies show conflicting evidence on effectiveness.
- Injections:
  - Autologous blood or platelet-rich plasma: theoretically makes the environment of fibroblasts more conducive to healing; however, results of studies are equivocal (2)[A],(4)[A],(5)[A]
  - Injection of sclerosing agents to destroy the sensory nerves that travel with the blood vessels of neovascularization
  - Avoid injection of cortisone into the Achilles tendon because of risk of rupture.

ISSUES FOR REFERRAL

Consider referral for surgical débridement for individuals whose symptoms have not responded to 3 to 6 or more months of nonoperative treatment.

- Minimally invasive techniques result in clinical outcomes equivalent to traditional open techniques but with lower complications (3)[A].

ADDITIONAL THERAPIES

- Short-term immobilization (7 to 10 days) with walking boot for severe acute symptoms or recalcitrant symptoms
  - Alternatively, a heel lift (or high-heeled shoes):
    - Use of heel lifts or high heels often can acutely decrease symptoms. However, chronic use of these devices may increase risk of developing symptoms in the future.
- Night splints may also be useful in patients with recalcitrant symptoms; physical therapy with emphasis on lower extremity flexibility and gastrocsoleus strengthening:
  - Progression to eccentric exercise programs has been shown to shorten time to return to full activity.
  - Aggressive or instrument-assisted soft tissue mobilization: techniques thought to break up scar tissue and stimulate healing
- Gait retraining: Consider converting forefoot strikers to rearfoot strikers.
- Modalities: Although some studies have shown that these modalities are useful in returning an athlete to activity sooner, they also show no long-term benefit:
  - Ultrasound
  - Low-level laser therapy: thought to modulate inflammation and regeneration of collagen
- Orthotics or arch supports may be useful in patients with pes planus and those who overpronate.
- Extracorporeal shock wave therapy: thought to induce neovascularization and new inflammatory process that leads to tissue healing. Studies have shown this treatment may be a useful adjunct to eccentric exercises (2)[A],(3)[A],(6)[A].

ONGOING CARE

- Gradual return to activity: gradual increase in running intensity, duration, and/or frequency. General rule of thumb is no >10% increase per week.
- New shoes: Avoid shoes with high heel counters or other structures that place pressure over irritated area. Running shoes should be changed every 250 to 500 miles.

REFERENCES

1. Arora NK, Sharma S, Sharma S, et al. Physical modalities with eccentric exercise are no better than eccentric exercise alone in the treatment of chronic Achilles tendinopathy: a systematic review and meta-analysis. *Foot*. 2022;53:101927.
2. Jarin I, Backer HC, Vosseller JT. Meta-analysis of noninsertional Achilles tendinopathy. *Foot Ankle Int*. 2020;41(6):744–754.
3. Zhi X, Liu X, Han J, et al. Nonoperative treatment of insertional Achilles tendinopathy: a systematic review. *J Orthop Surg*. 2021;16(1):233.
4. Masiello F, Pati I, Veropalumbo E, et al. Ultrasound-guided injection of platelet-rich plasma for tendinopathies: a systematic review and meta- analysis. *Blood Transfus*. 2023;21(2):119–136.
5. Nauwelaers AK, Van Oost L, Peers K. Evidence for the use of PRP in chronic midsubstance Achilles tendinopathy: a systematic review with meta-analysis. *J Foot Ankle Surg*. 2021;27(5):486–495.
6. Yusof TNBT, Seow D, Vig KS. Extracorporeal shockwave therapy for foot and ankle disorders: a systematic review and meta-analysis. *J Am Podiatr Med Assoc*. 2022;112(3):18–191.

ADDITIONAL READING

- Challoumas D, Kirwan PD, Borysov D, et al. Topical glyceryl trinitrate for the treatment of tendinopathies: a systematic review. *Br J Sports Med*. 2019;53(4):251–262.
- Chen J, Wan Y, Jiang H. The effect of platelet-rich plasma injection on chronic Achilles tendinopathy and acute Achilles tendon rupture. *Platelets*. 2022;33(3):339–349.
- Cushman DM, Petrin Z, Eby S, et al. Ultrasound evaluation of the patellar tendon and Achilles tendon and its association with future pain in distance runners. *Phys Sportsmed*. 2021;49(4):410–419.
- Desai N, Baker JF, Bucci J, et al. Ultrasound evaluation of the Achilles enthesis in inflammatory and non-inflammatory processes: a systematic review and meta-analysis. *Clin Exp Rheumatol*. 2023;41(1):24–31.
- Eliasson P, Dietrich-Zagonel F, Lundin AC, et al. Statin treatment increases the clinical risk of tendinopathy through matrix metalloproteinase release—a cohort study design combined with an experimental study. *Sci Rep*. 2019;9(1):17958.
- Horterer H, Oppelt S, Bocker W, et al. Patient-reported outcomes of surgically treated insertional Achilles tendinopathy. *Foot Ankle Int*. 2021;42(12):1565–1569.
- Jarin IJ, Backer HC, Vosseller JT. Functional outcomes of insertional Achilles tendinopathy treatment: a systematic review. *JBJS Rev*. 2021;9(6).
- Kearney RS, Ji C, Warwick J, et al. Effect of platelet-rich plasma injection vs sham injection on tendon dysfunction in patients with chronic midportion Achilles tendinopathy: a randomized clinical trial. *JAMA*. 2021;326(2):137–144.
- Kirschner JS, Cheng J, Hurwitz N, et al. Ultrasound-guided percutaneous needle tenotomy (PNT) alone versus PNT plus platelet-rich plasma injection for the treatment of chronic tendinosis: a randomized controlled trial. *PM&R*. 2021;13(12):1340–1349.
- Knapik JJ, Pope R. Achilles tendinopathy: pathophysiology, epidemiology, diagnosis, treatment, prevention, and screening. *J Spec Oper Med*. 2020;20(1):125–140.
- Ko VM, Cao M, Qiu J, et al. Comparative short-term effectiveness of non-surgical treatments for insertional Achilles tendinopathy: a systematic review and network meta-analysis. *BMC Musculoskelet Dis*. 2023;24(1):102.
- Lagas IF, Tol JL, Weir A, et al. One fifth of patients with Achilles tendinopathy have symptoms after 10 years: a prospective cohort study. *J Sports Sci*. 2022;40(22):2475–2483.
- Malmgaard-Clausen NM, Jorgensen OH, Hoffner R, et al. No additive clinical or physiologic effects of short-term anti-inflammatory treatment to physical rehabilitation in the early phase of human Achilles tendinopathy: a randomized controlled trial. *Am J Sports Med*. 2021;49(7):1711–1720.
- Mansur NSB, Matsunaga FT, Carrazzone OL, et al. Shockwave therapy plus eccentric exercises versus isolated eccentric exercises for Achilles insertional tendinopathy: a double-blinded randomized clinical trial. *J Bone Joint Surg Am*. 2021;103(14):1295–1302.
- Nuhmani S, Khan MH, Ahsan M, et al. Dry needling in the management of tendinopathy: a systematic review of randomized control trials. *J Bodyw Mov Ther*. 2023;33:128–135.
- Owoeye OBA, Palacios-Derflingher L, Pasanen K, et al. The burden and risk factors of patellar and Achilles tendinopathy in youth basketball: a cohort study. *Int J Environ Res Public Health*. 2021;18(18):9840.
- Rabusin CL, Menz HB, McClelland JA, et al. Efficacy of heel lifts versus calf muscle eccentric exercise for mid-portion Achilles tendinopathy (HEALTHY): a randomised trial. *Br J Sports Med*. 2021;55(9):486–492.
- Saltychev M, Johansson J, Kemppi V, et al. Effectiveness of topical glyceryl trinitrate in treatment of tendinopathy—systematic review and meta-analysis. *Disabil Rehabil*. 2022;44(20):5804–5810.
- Steere HK, DeLuca S, Borg-Stein J, et al. A narrative review evaluating extracorporeal shockwave therapy as a potential regenerative treatment for musculoskeletal conditions in military personnel. *Mil Med*. 2021;186(7–8):682–706.
- van der Vlist AC, Winters M, Weir A, et al. Which treatment is most effective for patients with Achilles tendinopathy? A living systematic review with network meta-analysis of 29 randomised controlled trials. *Br J Sports Med*. 2021;55(5):249–256.
- von Rickenbach KJ, Borgstrom H, Tenforde A, et al. Achilles tendinopathy: evaluation, rehabilitation, and prevention. *Curr Sports Med Rep*. 2021;20(6):327–334.
- Van Schaik KD, Lee KS. Orthobiologics: diagnosis and treatment of common tendinopathies. *Semin Musculoskel Radiol*. 2021;25(6):735–744.

CLINICAL PEARLS

- Because of the high stresses placed on the Achilles tendon with weight-bearing activities and the risk of rupture, corticosteroid injection into the Achilles tendon should be avoided.
- Categorization of the problem into paratendinopathy, insertional tendinopathy, or midportion tendinopathy may be helpful in guiding treatment decisions.
- A walking boot, night splint, or heel lift may be useful for pain relief especially in cases of acute injury.

ACHILLES TENDON RUPTURE

Katherine Boehm, DO

BASICS

- Achilles tendon ruptures are caused by laceration or by indirect forces applied to the tendon.
- Three types of indirect forces have been described:
  - Pushing off with the weight-bearing forefoot while extending the knee, such as with sprint starts and the push off in basketball
  - Sudden, unexpected dorsiflexion of the ankle, as when the foot slips in a hole
  - Forceful dorsiflexion of a plantarflexed foot, as with a fall from a height

DESCRIPTION

- Achilles tendon rupture is a complete disruption of the Achilles tendon, usually occurring 2 to 6 cm proximal to its calcaneal insertion, where blood supply is the poorest.
- It can be associated with preexisting tendon degeneration and microtrauma.
- It most commonly occurs in 30- to 40-year-old men.
- Synonym(s): heel-cord rupture; Achilles tear

EPIDEMIOLOGY

- >75% of Achilles tendon ruptures occur in patients 30 to 40 years old while they partake in sports activities.
- Males > females: Ratio ranges from 2:1 to 19:1.
- Left Achilles > right Achilles: thought to be due to higher prevalence of right-side dominant individuals using left lower limb to push off during activity
- Yearly incidence is around 40 patients per 100,000 patient population annually and increasing.
- Common in gymnastics, football, soccer, basketball, tennis, jumping, and running—however, a third of patients do not engage in intensive physical activity.

ETIOLOGY AND PATHOPHYSIOLOGY

- Is the largest tendon in the human body and is designed to endure stresses up to 10 times the body's weight
- Is formed by the confluence of the tendons of the gastrocnemius and soleus muscles. The gastrocnemius medial and lateral heads originate from the medial and lateral femoral condyles, respectively. The soleus originates from a large attachment on the posterior tibia and fibula. Together, these tendons insert onto the calcaneus and form the Achilles tendon.
- Receives its blood supply intrinsically from both the musculotendinous junction and the osteotendinous insertion site
- Additional vascular supply comes from an external source known as the paratenon. The paratenon is a thin layer of areolar tissue that encases the Achilles tendon. The further the tendon is from its musculotendinous origin and calcaneal insertion, the more it relies on the paratenon for vascular support.
- The area with the poorest vascular supply is ~2 to 6 cm proximal to the calcaneal insertion site.
- Prior to inserting into the calcaneus, the Achilles tendon internally rotates approximately 90 degrees, which imparts a structural torque stress in the tendon. This is thought to contribute to decreased vascularity in the tendon and ensuing tendon failure.

RISK FACTORS

- Disease processes: connective tissue disorders, seronegative spondylopathies, rheumatoid arthritis, collagen vascular disease, diabetes mellitus, gout, hyperparathyroidism, hypothyroidism, renal insufficiency, lupus, and infections
- Disuse atrophy and sedentary lifestyle
- Prolonged immobilization
- Advanced age
- History of Achilles tendonitis/tendinosis, regardless of history of injection therapy
- Mechanical imbalances (i.e., decreased flexibility of gastrocnemius-soleus complex, cavus foot, tibia vara)
- Body weight/obesity
- Possibility of genetic predisposition (possibility of association with human leukocyte antigen [HLA]-B27, blood group 0)

ALERT

Medications: Anabolic steroids or prolonged oral corticosteroid as well as fluoroquinolone antimicrobial usage leads to degradation of collagen fibrils and decreased Achilles tendon strength. Corticosteroid injections weaken tendon structure.

DIAGNOSIS

HISTORY

- Sudden, sharp pain behind the ankle
- Patients commonly report feeling as if they have been kicked or struck in the back of the heel, only to find no one is nearby.
- May feel or hear a "pop" or snap, or notice giving way sensation in heel after pushing off
- Pain with weight-bearing
- Weakness or stiffness of posterior ankle
- May give history of chronic Achilles tendinitis with or without history of injection therapy

PHYSICAL EXAM

- Swelling and/or ecchymosis
- "Hatchet strike" defect: painful, palpable defect, usually 2 to 6 cm from the tendon insertion site
- Positive Thompson test is diagnostic. Have patient lie prone or kneel with ankles clear of the table. Perform on uninvolved side first for comparison. Squeeze bulk of calf muscle and observe for plantarflexion. Absence of plantarflexion is consistent with complete tendon rupture (sensitivity 0.96, specificity 0.93) (1).

ALERT

Note that for the Achilles to function normally, only 25% of the fibers are needed; therefore, partial tears may be missed on manual examination. Overall, Achilles tendon ruptures may be missed in >20% of patients on initial evaluation (2),(3).

- Plantarflexion strength and ability to toe rise may be decreased compared to unaffected side.
- Passive dorsiflexion may be increased compared to unaffected side.
- These signs may be absent because of recruitment of other intact muscles, such as tibialis posterior, plantaris, peroneus longus and brevis, and flexor digitorum and hallucis longus.

DIFFERENTIAL DIAGNOSIS

- Achilles tendinitis
- Ankle or calcaneal fracture
- Ankle impingement syndrome
- Ankle sprain
- Calcaneal avulsion
- Gastrocnemius or soleus muscle strain or rupture
- Peritendinitis
- Retrocalcaneal bursitis
- Superficial Achilles bursitis
- Periostitis
- Plantaris tendon rupture

DIAGNOSTIC TESTS & INTERPRETATION

- Routine plain films should be obtained to avoid missing a calcaneal avulsion rupture, which would require surgical treatment. This finding usually can be appreciated on the lateral ankle radiograph.
- Ultrasound (US) and magnetic resonance imaging (MRI) should be reserved for when the diagnosis of a complete rupture is questionable.
- US should be first line to diagnose as it is a dynamic evaluation and more effective at identifying location of tear, the gap in the tendon, as well as partial versus complete tear (3).

TREATMENT

- Analgesia should be based on the patient's degree of pain.
- Rest, elevation, pain control, and functional bracing should be used in the initial treatment of complete and partial tears.
- Controversy in the literature exists as to the best treatment approach for Achilles tendon rupture.
- Careful patient selection is based on the patient's activity level and goals.
- Nonoperative treatment:
  - Fewer complications than surgery (infection, risk of deep vein thrombosis [DVT], sural nerve injury) (4)[A],(5)[A]

- Nonoperative treatment is targeted to ruptures with <1 cm of gapping on US examination.
- Partial tears, or a tear in continuity diagnosed by MRI, also treated conservatively
- Traditionally, nonoperative treatment was almost exclusively used by older, more sedentary patients, or those with medical contraindications to surgery. Now more young, active people are undergoing nonoperative treatment with comparable results.
- Older studies show risk of rerupture greater than with surgical repair: 12.6% for nonsurgical versus 3.5% for surgical repair (3).

ALERT
Early weight-bearing and functional rehabilitation have improved outcomes and decreased risk of rerupture in randomized control trials, equivalent to that of operative repair (2)[A],(3)[A],(4)[A].

ALERT
When early functional rehabilitation was not used, surgical repair reduced the absolute rerupture rate by 8.8% (number needed to treat [NNT] = 12) (4)[A].

- The option exists to use a functional dorsal block splint that restricts dorsiflexion and gradually increases the amount of plantarflexion. Functional splints have been shown to help prevent gastrocnemius atrophy, quicker return to full dorsiflexion, and better tolerance by patients.

ADDITIONAL THERAPIES

ALERT
Both treatment approaches should be followed by a well-outlined rehabilitation program.

- Advances in therapy should be supervised by the treating physician.
- Cardiovascular fitness during treatment can be sustained through arm ergometer use and then recumbent cycling once no longer using crutches.
- Once the cast or boot is removed (nonoperative treatment), active movement is initiated with the knee bent to 90 degrees; wound care and edema reduction is administered if patient underwent surgical treatment.
- Progress to passive movement, but focus on limiting maximum stretch on the tendon as to not let ankle progress past neutral for at least 12 to 16 weeks (1)[A].
- Slowly start strength exercises with isometrics and then progress to resisted range-of-motion exercises.
- To restore functional activity, progress to closed kinetic chain exercises focusing on eccentric gastrocnemius strength.

SURGERY/OTHER PROCEDURES

Open repair or closed, percutaneous technique:

- Associated with a lower incidence of rerupture compared to nonoperative with no early functional training
- Increased restoration of calf strength/less loss of push-off power (6)
- Surgical complications can include infection, DVT, pulmonary embolism, and death (4),(5).
- Other postoperative risks include delayed healing, scar adhesions, infection, persistent equinus, overlengthening, and fistulas and sural nerve injury in percutaneous techniques.
- Usually recommended for high-level athletes, those returning to high-risk activities (basketball, tennis, soccer, and sprinting), and for treatment of rerupture
- Injectable therapies do not currently have high level of evidence supporting their use.
- Corticosteroid injections are contraindicated as they weaken tendon structure.
- Platelet-rich plasma (PRP) has not been proven to improve plantarflexion strength of the ankle or pain after Achilles tendon rupture. In studies, PRP has positive effects on a few factors including dorsiflexion angle, dorsal extension strength of the ankle, and calf circumference; however, more research is required in this area.

ONGOING CARE

FOLLOW-UP RECOMMENDATIONS

Return-to-activity guidelines in nonoperative treatment with functional rehabilitation available (1)[A]:

- 0 to 2 weeks: equinus cast in 15 to 20 degrees plantarflexion and non–weight-bearing with crutches
- 2 to 6 weeks: removable controlled ankle motion (CAM) boot with 1- to 2-inch heel lift. Partial weight-bearing with crutches progressing to full weight-bearing as tolerated (WBAT) by week 4. Boot should be removed for active unrestricted plantar flexion and dorsiflexion to neutral.
- 6 to 8 weeks: full weight-bearing in the boot. Decrease heel lift by 25% each week. Start resisted plantarflexion exercises with resistance bands, gentle dorsiflexion stretching with belt.
- 8 to 12 weeks: Discontinue boot 1 week after ambulation with no heel lift; physical therapist to guide patient through strengthening, range of motion, and proprioception
- 16 weeks: Start low-impact activities and progression to run-walk program and continue strengthening.
- 6 months: Return to full activity. Continue aggressive rehab focused on calf muscle recovery as this usually does not progress after 1 year post injury (3).

REFERENCES

1. Cooper MT. Acute Achilles tendon ruptures: does surgery offer superior results (and other confusing issues)? *Clin Sports Med.* 2015;34(4):595–606.
2. Tarantino D, Palermi S, Sirico F, et al. Achilles tendon rupture: mechanisms of injury, principles of rehabilitation and return to play. *J Funct Morphol Kinesiol.* 2020;5(4):95.
3. Park SH, Lee HS, Young KW, et al. Treatment of acute Achilles tendon rupture. *Clin Orthop Surg.* 2020;12(1):1–8.
4. Soroceanu A, Sidhwa F, Aarabi S, et al. Surgical versus nonsurgical treatment of acute Achilles tendon rupture: a meta-analysis of randomized trials. *J Bone Joint Surg Am.* 2012;94(23):2136–2143.
5. Myhrvold SB, Brouwer EF, Andresen TKM, et al. Nonoperative or surgical treatment of acute Achilles' tendon rupture. *N Engl J Med.* 2022;386(15):1409–1420.
6. Mansfield K, Dopke K, Koroneos Z, et al. Achilles tendon ruptures and repair in athletes—a review of sports-related Achilles injuries and return to play. *Curr Rev Musculoskelet Med.* 2022;15(5):353–361.

ADDITIONAL READING

- Glazebrook M, Rubinger D. Functional rehabilitation for nonsurgical treatment of acute Achilles tendon rupture. *Foot Ankle Clin.* 2019;24(3):387–398.
- Ochen Y, Beks RB, van Heijl M, et al. Operative treatment versus nonoperative treatment of Achilles tendon ruptures: systematic review and meta-analysis. *BMJ.* 2019;364:k5120.
- Wang C, Fan H, Li Y, et al. Effectiveness of platelet-rich plasma injections for the treatment of acute Achilles tendon rupture: a systematic review and meta-analysis. *Medicine (Baltimore).* 2021;100(41):e27526.

CLINICAL PEARLS

- New literature is emerging suggesting nonoperative treatment with early functional rehabilitation has similar rerupture rates to surgical treatment; however, overall power is reduced by about 10% with nonoperative treatment.
- Nonoperative treatment has less complication overall compared to surgery.
- Early weight-bearing and range of motion are preferred for ruptures <1 cm, but it is best to discuss surgical treatment approaches with your local sports medicine or orthopedic group to determine their philosophy.

ACL INJURIES

Suraj A. Achar, MD, FAAFP, CAQSM • Kenneth S. Taylor, MD, FAAFP, CAQSM

BASICS

DESCRIPTION

- The anterior cruciate ligament (ACL) is a critical stabilizer of the knee.
- The ACL provides stability against anterior translation of the knee and is a secondary stabilizer of tibial rotation.
- The ACL has two important bundles: The posterolateral bundle is tight in extension, whereas the anteromedial bundle is tight in flexion.
- ACL tears can occur with trauma but occur more often with noncontact hyperextension or twisting injuries (1)[B],(2),(3).

EPIDEMIOLOGY

- The ACL is the most commonly injured knee ligament accounting for almost half of knee injuries in sport (4).
- An estimated 200,000 ACL injuries occur annually in the United States with ~100,000 ACL reconstructions.
- The incidence of ACL injury is greater in active adults and children participating in cutting sports such as basketball, football, skiing, soccer, and gymnastics.
- Female gender confers the higher risk. A meta-analysis in 2007 noted a roughly 3 to 4 times greater incidence of ACL tears in female gymnastics, soccer, and basketball players versus male athletes. Year-round female athletes who play soccer and basketball have an ACL tear rate approaching 5% (2)[A].
- In a retrospective review of children <12 years old, boys sustained a higher rate of ACL injury than girls (5).

RISK FACTORS

- High-risk sports and female gender are the primary risk factors for ACL injuries (1)[B]:
  - ~70% of ACL injuries occur in the high-risk sports, such as football (i.e., soccer), American football, basketball, volleyball, gymnastics, and downhill skiing.
  - Female risk factors being evaluated include differences in quadriceps-dominant deceleration, increased valgus angle of the knee (knock-kneed position) when pivoting, decelerating, or landing, different strength-to-weight ratios, joint laxity, and muscle recruitment patterns. No convincing evidence exists to support an association between the Q angle and ACL injury. The impact of hormones remains controversial.
  - Kinematics and electromyography studies suggest that females prepare for landing with decreased hip and knee flexion, increased quadriceps activation, and decreased hamstring activation, which may result in increased ACL loading and injury.
- Factors that increase traction have been associated with a higher incidence of ACL tears:
  - Early studies of artificial turf ("AstroTurf") in the National Football League noted an increased risk.
  - Cleats that have a predominant grip on the periphery may also increase the risk, especially when used with artificial turf.
  - Research in American football players found a significantly lower rate of ACL injuries when playing on wet surfaces.

GENERAL PREVENTION

- Neuromuscular training programs:
  - Neuromuscular training significantly reduces ACL incidence in athletes ($p < .0001$). High-intensity plyometrics, sessions 3 times a week for 15 to 20+ minutes, and a minimum 6-week duration are key. Comprehensive protocols should include plyometrics, landing feedback, balance, stretching, and strengthening exercises (3)[B].
- Bracing:
  - Bracing has been used to reduce knee injuries in American football for many years.
  - Randomized and observational studies suggest that prophylactic bracing does not prevent ACL tears or reduce retears in ACL reconstructed knees.

COMMONLY ASSOCIATED CONDITIONS

- Injuries to the medial and lateral meniscus are commonly associated with an ACL tear.
- ~50% of ACL injuries are associated with meniscal tears (most often lateral initially and medial when the ACL injury is chronic).
- Chondral and subchondral injuries are often noted.

DIAGNOSIS

HISTORY

- Many patients with an ACL tear feel a "pop" in their knee, followed by an acute swelling of the knee within hours.
- In the absence of bony trauma, an immediate effusion is believed to have a strong correlation with an ACL injury of some degree.
- Symptoms of an ACL-deficient knee include feeling of "giving out" and instability aggravated by squatting, pivoting, and stepping laterally or bearing the entire body weight when walking down stairs.

PHYSICAL EXAM

- If evaluated within 12 hours of an acute injury, the athlete will have difficulty bearing weight and will have an effusion.
- Loss of full knee extension can occur when an ACL stump gets caught in the intercondylar notch, an associated bucket meniscal tear is present, or a loose body fragment gets stuck.
- Examination should begin with inspection to look for an effusion and examination of the uninjured knee.
- Palpation of bony structures is important to evaluate for associated tibial plateau fractures or growth plate injuries in the case of growing adolescents.
- Palpation of the joint line is critical to evaluate for meniscal tears or medial collateral ligament (MCL) injuries.
- Valgus stress testing can be of further help in evaluating the MCL.
- Specific tests to determine an ACL tear include the Lachman test, the pivot shift test, the anterior drawer test, and the flexion-rotation drawer examination:

ALERT

The anterior drawer test was found to be only 50% positive, especially if the posterior horn of the medial meniscus is intact. It is important to first examine for posterior translation, which can occur with a posterior cruciate ligament (PCL) injury.

  - The flexion-rotation drawer/pivot shift examination is performed by cradling the calf and flexing the knee. A posteriorly directed force on the tibia will cause reduction of the tibia as the femur rotates from an externally rotated position.
  - The pivot shift test, although useful, is often painful and leads to guarding so if done it needs to be the last test performed.
  - The Lachman test is an accurate predictor of anterior cruciate injury. The sensitivity of this test decreases with hemarthrosis, guarding, and experience of the performer but is still reported to have a pooled sensitivity of 85%. One key to using the Lachman test is to first examine the uninjured side for comparison. Patients may have increased laxity that is not pathologic (6)[A].
  - The Lachman test, involves:
    - Patient position: hip externally rotated, knee slightly flexed for relaxation
    - Hand placement: One hand grasps the femur, and the other below the joint grasps the tibia.
    - Knee flexion: around 20 to 30 degrees
    - Action: quick, firm anterior pull on the tibia while stabilizing the femur
    - Interpretation: Assess translation and endpoint quality. A soft endpoint or >3 mm side-to-side laxity asymmetry suggests an ACL tear. Focus on positive/negative interpretation, not just laxity quantification.

DIAGNOSTIC TESTS & INTERPRETATION

Initial Tests (lab, imaging)

- Standard radiography:
  - Plain radiography should be performed on all patients suspected of acute ACL tears because of the risk of fractures.
  - X-ray studies have a pivotal role in the evaluation of adolescents and children because of the risk of growth plate fractures and tibial spine fractures.
  - In children, plain x-rays should be performed before aggressive maneuvers are performed, especially in the case of decreased active range of motion (ROM) or tenderness at the distal femoral physis.
  - X-rays should include anteroposterior (AP); lateral; and sometimes, oblique views to better visualize fractures. In some cases, 1–2%, an avulsion fracture of the anterolateral tibial plateau at the attachment of the lateral capsular ligament (Segond fracture) is noted.
  - The lateral femoral notch sign (LFNS) has been described as a sign of chronically ACL-deficient knees. Researchers have defined the LFNS as a depression >1.0 mm deep in the lateral femoral condyle (7).
- Advanced imaging:
  - Magnetic resonance imaging (MRI) should be used to evaluate for other concomitant injuries and, in some cases, either to confirm the diagnosis or help to plan surgery.
  - The surgical consent and plan will depend on associated injuries, such as meniscal or MCL injuries.
  - MRI, if used for evaluation of a presumed ACL tear, should be non–contrast-enhanced.
  - The accuracy and sensitivity of MRI are excellent when compared with arthroscopic findings.
  - Sonography is another modality that can be used to assess the ACL; has limited use in the United States owing to the widespread use of MRI

TREATMENT

- Most patients with an ACL injury are active in sports, and surgical reconstruction is an elective procedure, with many maintaining active lifestyles without it. However, high-level athletes and young individuals often experience instability without surgery or cross bracing with healing of the ACL. Adolescent patients with open growth plates present a challenge due to potential growth plate damage from tunnels, although this risk is very low.
- A novel approach, the Cross Bracing Protocol (CBP), has shown promising results for nonsurgical ACL healing. A study demonstrated an 89.5% success rate of regaining normal ACL anatomy and function without surgery using this protocol (8). This method offers a potential alternative for select patients seeking to avoid reconstructive surgery. This study found that 90% of patients managed with the CBP showed evidence of ACL healing on 3-month MRI. For those with a higher degree of healing (anterior cruciate ligament osteoarthritis score [ACLOAS] grade 1), 92% returned to preinjury sport.
- To date, there is a lack of evidence to support a protective role of reconstructive surgery of the ACL against osteoarthritis development. At 10 to 20 years, 50% of those diagnosed with an ACL tear have osteoarthritis and functional impairment—"the young patient with an old knee"(9).
- No studies have shown that bracing an ACL-deficient knee will prevent episodes of instability when an athlete returns to cutting and pivoting sports. The data on bracing do show a decrease in anterior tibial translation at low levels of force. Activity modification provides the best method outside of surgery to prevent "giving way" episodes. If an athlete attains and maintains full ROM and at least 90% strength of the contralateral lower extremity, low-risk sports such as running, bicycling, and swimming can be performed.

- An athlete's inability to return to sports determines whether that athlete elects surgery or successfully participates in cross bracing program leading to healing of the ACL. Dynamic functional testing (a series of hopping tests) may be a useful adjunct to predict who may be a "coper" and can continue nonoperative treatment.
- In most cases, incomplete or partial tears of the ACL can be managed nonoperatively. A hinged knee brace can be worn during the early stages of rehab.

SURGERY/OTHER PROCEDURES

- ACL reconstruction aims to restore normal stability and full ROM. Although primary ACL suturing has largely been abandoned due to its inability to restore stability, an exception exists for bony avulsions, common in adolescents. A newer, innovative approach is the bridge-enhanced ACL repair (BEAR) procedure, which helps the torn ACL heal itself instead of replacing it with a graft.
- Graft selection:
  - Autogenous tissue:
    - Patellar tendon (with bone attached both proximally and distally)
    - Hamstring tendons
    - Quadriceps tendon
  - Allograft tissue: Most allografts are taken from the patellar tendon, or Achilles from cadaver donors. However, hamstring and quadriceps tendons can also be used. The use of synthetic materials such as Dacron and Gore-Tex have been abandoned because of long-term failure.
- Patellar tendon autograft: The patellar tendon autograft is an example of bone-to-bone ACL reconstruction and has been used more for high-demand athletes. Of all the procedures, it appears to have the least laxity on KT-1000 testing on follow-up. The potential bone-to-bone fixation promotes earlier graft fixation. Long-term follow-up shows no difference in return to full participation for either autograft procedure.
- Hamstring tendon autograft: The hamstring graft has several advantages. Use of the hamstring tendon avoids patellar tendon morbidity. Studies have shown a decrease in anterior knee pain among those who undergo a hamstring autograft compared with those undergoing bone-to-bone fixation (relative risk 0.49, 95% confidence interval 0.32–0.76, $p = .001$, $I^2 = 0\%$). Hamstring donor-site pain heals within 3 months while hamstring strength returns within 12 months (10)[A].
- Allografts, often secondary options for ACL reconstruction, carry extremely low infection risks (<1% bacterial, no HIV/hepatitis reported post-2002 due to testing/irradiation). Although offering decreased surgical morbidity and easier rehab, new data suggests higher failure rates compared to hamstring or patellar tendon autografts.
- Timing of surgery:
  - The timing of surgery is controversial because some surgeons perform surgery at the site where patients are injured (i.e., the ski area).
  - Negative outcomes, especially arthrofibrosis, are not directly associated with surgical timing but rather with signs of inflammation marked by periarticular swelling, effusion, and hyperthermia.
  - Other factors that predict arthrofibrosis include decreased ROM and perioperative pain.
  - Surgery should be delayed until these factors are improved (often >3 weeks).
  - Early surgery is absolutely indicated only in bony avulsions.

ONGOING CARE

- Patients are now returning to activity sooner after reconstruction. Return to sport depends more on strength and proprioception than on time from surgery. Usual return to sport may fall between 6 and 12 months or longer after surgery. Early return prior to full proprioception and strength may lead to prolonged instability and possible reinjury (11)[A],(12).
- Therapy protocols may be divided into four categories:
  - Phase 1: preoperative; maintain ROM
  - Phase 2 (0 to 2 weeks): Achieve full extension; maintain quadriceps strength, reduce swelling, and achieve flexion to 90 degrees
  - Phase 3 (3 to 5 weeks): Maintain full extension and increase flexion up to full ROM; stair climbers and stationary cycle may be used.
  - Phase 4 (6 weeks to 9 months): Increase strength and agility; progressive return to sports
- Prior to return to sport, athletes should meet discharge criteria including isokinetic strength, running T-test, single hop, triple hop, and crossover tests.
- The use of custom ACL bracing has also been controversial. A systemic review of several randomized, controlled trials (level I evidence, 12 trials) found no evidence that pain, ROM, graft stability, or protection from subsequent injury was affected by postoperative bracing (13)[A].
- Patients who have ACL healing with CBP returned to sport at 9 to 12 months but further research is needed to monitor long term outcomes.

FOLLOW-UP RECOMMENDATIONS

- If arthrofibrosis is evident after surgery, early surgical intervention (<1 year) improves the outcome.
- Full ROM should be achieved to prevent degenerative joint disease.

PROGNOSIS

- Most patients with ACL injuries do well with activities of daily living even after follow-up in the range of 5 to 15 years. Most can participate in some sports activity if they are inclined to do so, but most will have some limitations in vigorous sports, and only a few will be entirely asymptomatic.
- The presence of clinically significant chondral and meniscal injuries that occur at the time of injury or after injury determines long-term prognosis more than the ACL injury itself. Over time, the prevalence of meniscal injuries increases, leading to increasing disability, surgery, and arthrosis in high-risk patients.
- Ligament reconstruction has not been shown to prevent arthrosis, but in prospective studies, it appears to reduce the risk of subsequent meniscal injury and to facilitate return to high-level sporting activities (11).

REFERENCES

1. Chappell JD, Creighton RA, Giuliani C, et al. Kinematics and electromyography of landing preparation in vertical stop-jump: risks for noncontact anterior cruciate ligament injury. *Am J Sports Med.* 2007;35(2):235–241.
2. Prodromos CC, Han Y, Rogowski J, et al. A meta-analysis of the incidence of anterior cruciate ligament tears as a function of gender, sport, and a knee injury-reduction regimen. *Arthroscopy.* 2007;23(12):1320.e6–1325.e6.
3. Sugimoto D, Myer GD, McKeon JM, et al. Evaluation of the effectiveness of neuromuscular training to reduce anterior cruciate ligament injury in female athletes: a critical review of relative risk reduction and numbers-needed-to-treat analyses. *Br J Sports Med.* 2012;46(14):979–988.
4. Musahl V, Karlsson J. Anterior cruciate ligament tear. *N Engl J Med.* 2019;380(24):2341–2348.
5. Bloom DA, Wolfert AJ, Michalowitz A, et al. ACL injuries aren't just for girls: the role of age in predicting pediatric ACL injury. *Sports Health.* 2020;12(6):559–563.
6. Benjaminse A, Gokeler A, van der Schans CP. Clinical diagnosis of an anterior cruciate ligament rupture: a meta-analysis. *J Orthop Sports Phys Ther.* 2006;36(5):267–288.
7. Lodewijks PCAM, Delawi D, Bollen TL, et al. The lateral femoral notch sign: a reliable diagnostic measurement in acute anterior cruciate ligament injury. *Knee Surg Sports Traumatol Arthrosc.* 2019;27(2):659–664.
8. Filbay SR, Dowsett M, Chaker Jomaa M, et al. Healing of acute anterior cruciate ligament rupture on MRI and outcomes following non-surgical management with the Cross Bracing Protocol. *Brit J Sports Med.* 2023;57(23):1490–1497.
9. van Meer BL, Meuffels DE, van Eijsden WA, et al. Which determinants predict tibiofemoral and patellofemoral osteoarthritis after anterior cruciate ligament injury? A systematic review. *Br J Sports Med.* 2015;49(15):975–983.
10. Poolman RW, Farrokhyar F, Bhandari M. Hamstring tendon autograft better than bone patellar-tendon bone autograft in ACL reconstruction: a cumulative meta-analysis and clinically relevant sensitivity analysis applied to a previously published analysis. *Acta Orthop.* 2007;78(3):350–354.
11. Czuppon S, Racette BA, Klein SE, et al. Variables associated with return to sport following anterior cruciate ligament reconstruction: a systematic review. *Br J Sports Med.* 2014;48(5):356–364.
12. Kyritsis P, Bahr R, Landreau P, et al. Likelihood of ACL graft rupture: not meeting six clinical discharge criteria before return to sport is associated with a four times greater risk of rupture. *Br J Sports Med.* 2016;50(15):946–951.
13. Wright RW, Fetzer GB. Bracing after ACL reconstruction: a systematic review. *Clin Orthop Relat Res.* 2007;455:162–168.

CLINICAL PEARLS

- Nearly all patients with an acute ACL tear have an effusion.
- Noncontact injuries account for the majority of ACL tears.
- ACL reconstruction does not protect against the development of osteoarthritis.
- A novel Cross Bracing Protocol can lead to healing of complete ACL tears without surgery with excellent outcomes and return to play. Long-term results are pending.

ACL TEAR: MANAGEMENT IN SKELETALLY IMMATURE ATHLETES

Holly J. Benjamin, MD, FAMSSM, FACSM • Victoria Andros, DO, CAQSM • Michael Ladewski, DO, FAAFP, CAQSM

BASICS

DESCRIPTION

- Acute injury sustained by known mechanism that leads to knee instability with significant effect on the athlete's ability to perform at the highest levels of sport
- Considerable variation exists regarding specific treatment in the skeletally immature population with early operative treatment becoming more favorable when compared to nonoperative or delayed operative treatment (1).
- New research now suggests the possibility of healing the anterior cruciate ligament (ACL) with a cross bracing protocol.

EPIDEMIOLOGY

- 1.4 times higher risk in female athletes than in male athletes per athlete exposure (2)
- The higher incidence in females is thought to be due to differences in biomechanics, joint laxity, hormonal influences, intercondylar notch size, smaller, ligament diameter, and neuromuscular factors.
- Sporting activity associated with ACL injury involves cutting, pivoting, and sudden deceleration.

Incidence

- Risk of ACL injury by sex highest in girls' soccer and boys' football (2)
- ACL injury >9 and 7 times more likely to occur in match versus practice setting for female and male athletes, respectively (2)
- 0.084/1,000 athlete exposure (one game or practice) in females (2)
- 0.060/1,000 athlete exposure in males (2)

ETIOLOGY AND PATHOPHYSIOLOGY

- Midsubstance tear most common
- Tibial spine avulsion fracture more frequent in the skeletally immature athletes
- Femoral ACL avulsion fractures are rare causes of ACL injury.
- Mechanisms of injury:
  - Hyperextension, sudden deceleration, or a valgus and rotator force with a planted foot
  - External rotation of the femur on a fixed tibia combined with a valgus load often the result of a noncontact pivoting injury

GENERAL PREVENTION

- Neuromuscular balance training and core strengthening have been shown to decrease the incidence in athletes of various ages.
- Lower body strength exercises (i.e., Nordic hamstrings, lunges, and heel-calf raises) as part of ACL neuromuscular training program with specific focus on landing stabilization (jump/hop and hold) (3)
- Jump training to land in less knee valgus and more knee flexion
- Increasing hamstring strength to decrease quadriceps dominance ratio

COMMONLY ASSOCIATED CONDITIONS

- Bone contusion: lateral compartment more common than medial compartment
- Meniscus tears: lateral more commonly in acute knee injury; medial more common in athlete with chronic ACL deficiency
- Associated medial meniscus tears and medial collateral ligament (MCL) injury in patient with valgus stress mechanism

DIAGNOSIS

HISTORY

- May be a "pop" sensation at the time of injury
- Describe turn with fixed foot
- Effusion usually develops acutely.
- Athlete unable to continue play
- Sensation of instability less frequent in skeletally immature
- Variable pain; may increase days after injury

PHYSICAL EXAM

- It can be difficult to perform an accurate physical exam after significant hemarthrosis develops.
- Loss of normal knee contour secondary to effusion is often present.
- Limited range of motion (ROM)
- Quadricep avoidance gait: Avoid active knee extension.
- The Lachman test is the most sensitive physical examination test and is the "gold standard" for diagnosis.
- Anterior drawer and pivot-shift tests are positive but are less sensitive tests.
- Evaluation of the uninjured knee can help establish a baseline when compared to the injured knee.
- Testing for other ligamentous, tendon, and meniscal injury is indicated.
- Palpate the distal femur and proximal tibia physis for tenderness that might indicate the presence of a physeal fracture.
- Tenderness at the ends of long bones is a fracture until proven otherwise in skeletally immature patients.
- Perform a complete neurologic and vascular exam of the lower extremity.

DIFFERENTIAL DIAGNOSIS

- Tibial spine avulsion fractures
- Physeal fractures of the distal femur or proximal tibia
- Meniscal injury
- Articular cartilage injury
- Patellar subluxation
- Other ligamentous injury of the knee

DIAGNOSTIC TESTS & INTERPRETATION

Initial Tests (lab, imaging)

- Knee radiographs (anteroposterior [AP], lateral, sunrise/merchant/skyline view) to rule out tibial spine avulsion fracture, physeal fractures, Segond fracture, and osteochondral fractures
- Magnetic resonance imaging (MRI) to evaluate ACL and concomitant meniscal, posterior cruciate ligament, collateral ligament, and chondral injuries:
  - Tear imaging shows increased signal intensity with a disrupted pattern.
  - The prevalence of bone bruise in pediatric patients with ACL tears is high; about 70% of cases

Diagnostic Procedures/Other

- Diagnostic arthroscopy is sometimes required when physical exam and imaging studies are equivocal.
- KT-1000 device may be helpful in quantifying relative ACL laxity.

TREATMENT

GENERAL MEASURES

- Compression
- Ice
- Pain management
- Weight-bearing as tolerated unless physeal fracture is suspected

- Arthrocentesis can be performed for both therapeutic and diagnostic purposes in the case of traumatic effusion.
- If fat is noted in the hemarthrosis, then a fracture is present.

ISSUES FOR REFERRAL

- Patients with suspected ACL injuries should be referred to an orthopedic or sports medicine specialist.
- Preference for specialist with experience in surgical techniques in the skeletally immature athlete

ADDITIONAL THERAPIES

Nonoperative therapy may be considered depending on physical demands and age of athlete:

- Restoration of ROM
- Strengthening quadriceps and hamstrings
- Activity modification
- May be recommended if ACL reconstruction delayed owing to skeletal immaturity, low demand, or for partial ACL tears
- Specific physical therapies and bracing can significantly improve functional status of injured knee.
- High rates of residual knee instability, increased risk of meniscal and articular cartilage damage, and comparatively low rates of return to sports with nonoperative treatment (4)[A]
- Bracing with derotational ACL-stabilizing brace does not restore stability when athlete returns to high-demand sport.
- ACL cross bracing protocol done within 1 month of injury has high rates of healing the ACL without surgery (5).

SURGERY/OTHER PROCEDURES

Variation related to approach and risk for early physeal closure:

- Degree of knee instability is primary driving force to pursue early surgical treatment (1)[B].
- Options include physeal sparing, partial transphyseal, and complete transphyseal ACL reconstruction (1)[A],(6)[A].
- Degree of skeletal maturity is a factor in decision making for treatment (1)[C],(6)[C].
- Undertaken only after restoration of ROM and resolution of joint effusion
- Delaying ACL reconstruction for >12 weeks significantly increased the risk of meniscal injury and irreparable meniscal tears (4)[A].
- Both early and delayed operative treatment achieved satisfactory knee stability (4)[A].

ONGOING CARE

FOLLOW-UP RECOMMENDATIONS

- Patients will require substantial physical therapy to regain ROM and strength as well as to address functional and sports-specific mechanics to address prevention of recurrence.
- Use of postsurgical ACL bracing may be more effective in pediatric compared to adult patients possibly due to compliance with activity restriction guidelines and therapy protocols (1)[C],(6)[C].
- Consistent clinical follow-up post-ACL reconstruction until skeletal maturity for complication surveillance

PROGNOSIS

- Typical postoperative recovery and rehabilitation period is usually 9 to 12 months, prolonged period of rehab of possible benefit for skeletally immature.
- Return to preinjury level of competition rate can be as high as 90% after operative treatment (1)[C],(6)[C].
- Natural history of the ACL-deficient knee is chronic instability, chondral injury, subsequent meniscal pathology, pain, and joint arthrosis.

COMPLICATIONS

- Associated MCL and meniscal injuries
- Surgical complications:
  - Graft failure
  - Premature physeal closure
  - Leg length discrepancy
  - Limb malalignment
  - Angular deformity
  - Slow recovery in ROM
  - Usual risks of infection and anesthesia

REFERENCES

1. Popkin CA, Wright ML, Pennock AT, et al. Trends in management and complications of anterior cruciate ligament injuries in pediatric patients: a survey of the PRiSM society. *J Pediatr Orthop*. 2018;38(2):e61–e65.
2. Bram JT, Magee LC, Mehta NN, et al. Anterior cruciate ligament injury incidence in adolescent athletes: a systematic review and meta-analysis. *Am J Sport Med*. 2021;49(7):1962–1972.
3. Petushek EJ, Sugimoto D, Stoolmiller M, et al. Evidence-based best-practice guidelines for preventing anterior cruciate ligament injuries in young female athletes: a systematic review and meta-analysis. *Am J Sports Med*. 2019;47(7):1744–1753.
4. James EW, Dawkins BJ, Schachne JM, et al. Early operative versus delayed operative versus non-operative treatment of pediatric and adolescent anterior cruciate ligament injuries: a systematic review and meta-analysis. *Am J Sports Med*. 2021;49(14):4008–4017.
5. Filbay SR, Dowsett M, Chaker Jomaa M, et al. Healing of acute anterior cruciate ligament rupture on MRI and outcomes following non-surgical management with the cross bracing protocol. *Br J Sports Med*. 2023;57(23):1490–1497.
6. Anderson CN, Anderson AF. Management of the anterior cruciate ligament-injured knee in the skeletally immature athlete. *Clin Sports Med*. 2017;36(1):35–52.

ADDITIONAL READING

- Dekker TJ, Rush JK, Schmitz MR. What's new in pediatric and adolescent anterior cruciate ligament injuries? *J Pediatr Orthop*. 2018;38(3):185–192.
- Kay J, Memon M, Marx RG, et al. Over 90% of children and adolescents return to sport after anterior cruciate ligament reconstruction: a systematic review and meta-analysis. *Knee Surg Sports Traumatol Arthrosc*. 2018;26(4):1019–1036.

CLINICAL PEARLS

- Injury that is increasing in incidence in the skeletally immature population
- ACL cross bracing protocol has significant promise for healing ACL tears non surgically and needs further study.
- Type of ACL reconstruction and timing of surgery in the skeletally immature athlete vary widely, and cases should be decided on an individual basis.
- Primary and secondary prevention programs have been shown to be effective.

ACROMIOCLAVICULAR SEPARATIONS (TYPES 1–6)

Anne S. Boyd, MD, FAAFP, FACSM

BASICS

- Disruption of the joint formed by the clavicle and acromion due to injury of the acromioclavicular (AC) and coracoclavicular (CC) ligaments
- Classified based on radiographic findings, indicating severity of injury to the capsular and extracapsular ligaments and supporting structures (types I to VI) (1)
- The capsule and AC and CC ligaments provide static stability to the joint and are responsible for maintaining the joint in physiologic position (2).
- AC ligament joins the acromion to the distal clavicle and is the main static stabilizing force for the AC joint in the anteroposterior (AP) direction (2),(3):
  - This ligament blends with the trapezius and deltoid fascia to form the AC capsule.
  - The AC ligament complex usually fails first, whereas the CC ligament resists larger forces (2).
- CC ligament connects the clavicle to the coracoid process of the scapula and is a vertical and rotational stabilizing force at the AC joint (2):
  - The CC ligament involves two components: the trapezoid and conoid ligaments.
- Synonym(s): shoulder separation; shoulder sprain; AC sprain; AC dislocation
- Note: The term *shoulder dislocation* primarily refers to glenohumeral dislocation, not disruption of the AC joint.

DESCRIPTION

The 1984 Rockwood classification system is the most widely used classification method:

- Type I:
  - Sprain or partial tear of the AC ligament, some fiber disruption
  - Intact CC ligament and AC joint capsule
  - No displacement appreciated on radiograph
- Type II:
  - Complete tear of the AC ligament
  - Sprained or partially torn CC ligaments
  - Minimally, widened AC joint on radiograph
- Type III:
  - Complete tear of both AC and CC ligaments
  - Dislocated AC joint
  - Superior displacement of distal clavicle (CC distance increased ≤100%)
- Type IV:
  - Complete tear of both the AC and CC ligaments
  - Dislocation of AC joint
  - Posterior displacement of distal clavicle through the trapezius muscle
  - High probability of detachment of deltoid and trapezius muscle from distal clavicle

ALERT

Axillary view is the gold standard. Radiographs demonstrate posterior displacement of distal clavicle in relation to the acromion. Type IV injury may be missed without this view (3),(4).

- Type V:
  - Complete tear of both the AC and CC ligaments
  - Dislocated AC joint
  - >100% superior displacement of distal clavicle
  - Considered an exaggerated type III with 100–300% widening of CC interval
  - High probability of detachment of deltoid and trapezius muscle from distal clavicle
- Type VI: rare
  - Complete tear of AC and CC ligaments
  - Dislocated AC joint
  - Inferior displacement of the distal clavicle relative to the acromion or coracoid (subacromial or subcoracoid)
  - Often damage to the fascia of the trapezium or the deltoid muscle (2)
  - Position of clavicle: 100% inferior AC joint displacement, usually with distal clavicle wedged underneath coracoid process. There is potential damage to the underlying brachial plexus and subclavian vessels.

EPIDEMIOLOGY

- Commonly occurs during sports involving direct contact (2),(3),(4)
- Commonly occurs during sports participation, especially contact sports such as football, hockey, wrestling, and rugby
- Mechanism of injury is primarily by direct impact over the superolateral shoulder (e.g., tackling or direct blow to "point" of shoulder), forcing the AC joint inferiorly (2),(4), causing depression of the scapular complex (not elevation of the clavicle) and disruption of the AC and CC ligaments (3).
- Secondary mechanism of injury is indirect trauma such as a fall on ipsilateral adducted or outstretched extremity, causing the humeral head to be driven upward into the inferior aspect of the AC joint (2).

Incidence

- Common, representing 9% of all shoulder injuries (1),(2)
- Majority of injuries occur between ages 20 and 40 years, with men suffering the injury 8.5 times more than women (2).
- Nearly 50% of all AC dislocations occur to individuals in their 20s (1),(3).
- Males are up to 8.5 times more likely to suffer injuries than females (1),(2).
- Types I and II injuries account for most AC separations.

COMMONLY ASSOCIATED CONDITIONS

- Fracture injuries are associated with types III to V AC separations in 5% of patients.
- Intra-articular injuries are associated with types III to V AC dislocations in 18% of patients (3).
  - Shoulder labrum/superior labrum anterior and posterior (SLAP) tears reported in 5–14%
  - Rotator cuff tears reported in ~4%

DIAGNOSIS

HISTORY

- Present following a fall on the shoulder or collision and pain at the AC joint
- Exact mechanism of injury is helpful to identify severity of the injury and potential for associated injuries.
- Always assess for neurologic or vascular symptoms (which indicate a more severe injury and may require immediate surgical intervention).

PHYSICAL EXAM

- Inspection should be done bilaterally for comparison to the uninjured side.
- Inspection may show asymmetry of the shoulders or swelling at the AC joint.
- Deformity (step-off) of AC joint with type III injuries and higher (2); swelling may obscure the degree of injury.
- Palpation reproduces localized point tenderness of the affected AC joint.
- Type III injuries often have additional tenderness of the CC ligaments.
- Types III and V may show instability of the lateral clavicle when depressed manually ("piano key" phenomenon) (3).
- Range of motion is typically decreased in the acute postinjury period due to pain.
- Adduction of the shoulder is often painful, as is shoulder abduction and flexion.
- Cross body adduction test (77% sensitivity) involving forward flexion of shoulder to 90 degrees, and then assisted adduction across chest, reproduces pain over the AC joint (3).
- Careful neurovascular examination should always be performed with any significant musculoskeletal injury.

DIFFERENTIAL DIAGNOSIS

- Fractures of the coracoid, acromion, or clavicle
- AC joint or shoulder arthritis
- Rotator cuff injuries
- SLAP/shoulder labrum lesion
- Glenohumeral dislocation
- Distal clavicle osteolysis
- Biceps tendinopathy
- Adhesive capsulitis
- Burner/stinger (neurogenic)
- Cervical spine injuries
- Pneumothorax (rare)
- Gorham disease or massive osteolysis
- Gout
- Neoplasm (multiple myeloma)

DIAGNOSTIC TESTS & INTERPRETATION

Initial Tests (lab, imaging)

- Radiographs: True AP, scapular Y lateral, and an axillary view are the initial images of choice for this injury (1)[B],(3)[C],(4)[C].
- In most cases, plain radiographs are sufficient for AC injury grading, although computed tomography (CT) or magnetic resonance imaging (MRI) may be useful if suspected injury surpasses visible injury on radiographs.

- The AC joint is visible on standard AP shoulder radiographs, but the joint is angulated and superficial, so typically over penetrated on standard films. An AP angulated (Zanca) view is preferred for more accurate assessment of the AC joint and clavicle.
  - Zanca view: The beam is centered over the AC joint and tilted cephalad 10 to 15 degrees with a reduced beam. This optimizes penetration, improves joint detail, and decreases overlap of the clavicle and scapula (3),(4). Zanca views of both shoulders provide superior AC joint evaluation while avoiding the superimposition of the acromion on the distal clavicle.
  - Helps to identify fractures of the clavicle, acromion, or coracoid and to preliminarily evaluate AC joint separation and CC ligament disruption
- Vertical displacement of the distal clavicle may be seen on the AP view, whereas AP displacement may be evident on the axillary view.
- If suspecting posterior dislocation, consider adding a lateral view of the acromion.
- Axillary lateral is essential to distinguish a type III from a type IV injury. A type IV injury will show the scapula anterior to the clavicle.
  - Axillary view may be uncomfortable and take some time to obtain.
- A wide plate should be used with AP and Zanca views to incorporate bilateral shoulders for direct comparison views on a single cassette (4).
- Stress views (weighted views) can be used to differentiate types I to III, but are not recommended, because the results do not affect treatment, and disruption of the CC ligament (larger space between coracoid and clavicle on the affected side) can be seen on the standard AP (4).
- The average distance between the inferior aspect of the clavicle and the coracoid is 1.1 to 1.3 cm. This value can vary, so it is important to compare to the unaffected side.
- Stryker notch views to assess for coracoid fracture when indicated

Diagnostic Procedures/Other

- CT scan has not been shown to improve diagnostic reliability (1)[B].
- MRI in coronal oblique plane parallel to the CC ligament may be used to identify higher grade or additional injuries if surgical intervention is being considered (1)[B].

TREATMENT

GENERAL MEASURES

The Rockwood classification assists with guiding treatment:

- Types I and II:
  - Types I and II injuries involve minimal disruption of the joint and are stable. Treatment is conservative (nonoperative) (2)[A].
  - Conservative treatment includes a sling and activity modification for comfort, ice, and analgesics until symptoms subside and range of motion is comfortable.
  - Shoulder sling for 1 to 2 weeks with early range of motion and weaning the sling as pain permits
  - Ice and analgesics for pain and swelling:
    - Due to the superficial nature of the joint, ice should be applied for 15 minutes every 4 to 6 hours as needed.
    - Generally, <1 to 2 weeks of analgesia is needed.
  - Range of motion exercises are recommended as soon as they can be tolerated.
  - Early range of motion exercises (e.g., pendulum exercises) help to maintain joint mobility and flexibility and avoid adhesive capsulitis.
  - Type II injuries receive similar treatment as those with type I injuries but generally require addition of an early rehabilitation program with passive and active shoulder range of motion exercises.
  - Rotator cuff, scapular stabilization, and trunk strengthening exercises are introduced as pain resolves.
  - Return to activity varies from days to weeks, depending on the extent of injury. Complete healing may take up to 4 to 6 weeks.
  - Heavy lifting and contact activities to resume only once the extremity is pain free and symmetric range of motion and strength are achieved.
- Type III:
  - Some controversy regarding management
  - Most can be managed nonsurgically with ice, temporary sling immobilization, and analgesic medication.
  - Studies demonstrate 80% of type III injuries have excellent outcomes so initial conservative management is often encouraged, resorting to surgery if the nonoperative management fails (2).
  - Some type III injuries are unstable, unresponsive to conservative treatment, or will not withstand a high-demand lifestyle (athletes, laborers, some military personnel) and may benefit from surgical intervention (2),(3),(4),(5).
  - Most studies show comparably high satisfaction and long-term functional outcomes with operative and nonoperative treatment yet higher incidence of complications in those treated surgically (2)[A],(6)[B].
  - Activity progression and rehabilitation may be prolonged.
  - Return to full activities when full range of motion and strength have resumed which may take 6 to 12 weeks.
- Types IV to VI (2)[A],(3)[A],(4)[A]:
  - Surgical referral for reduction and stabilization
  - Some studies have demonstrated good return to activity results with conservative management of type V injuries. Further studies are needed.
  - Any indication of vascular or neurologic compromise requires urgent surgical referral.

ADDITIONAL THERAPIES

- Types I and II: Shoulder range of motion exercises should be started as pain eases, followed by a strengthening program for the rotator cuff and scapular stabilizers. Return to contact when full, painless range of motion and normal strength resumes.
- Type III: Shoulder strengthening exercises are introduced when range of motion and pain are improved. Return to contact sports usually is anticipated in 6 weeks to 6 months, depending on resumption of full painless range of motion and normal strength.

SURGERY/OTHER PROCEDURES

Types IV to VI usually require operative treatment.

ONGOING CARE

- If types IV to VI, refer to orthopedics.
- Refer type III AC separations for discussion of surgical options for high-level athletes, patients refusing conservative therapy, heavy manual laborers, patients unable to tolerate the deformity, and patients who have failed nonoperative treatment after 6 months (2),(3).

PROGNOSIS

- In most cases, pain resolves, and an athlete may return to sports within several weeks. Recovery generally takes 6 weeks for type II and 12 weeks for type III injuries.
- Reports suggest that up to 40% of individuals with type I or II injuries will go on to develop osteoarthritis at the AC joint.

COMPLICATIONS

- Persistent instability or residual pain with activity
- Cosmetic deformity and AC joint arthritis are common complications.
- Some patients note intermittent pain and/or clicking, often referred to as nuisance symptoms. These symptoms may require an injection or further physical therapy.
- Although uncommon, severe, persistent symptoms may require surgical intervention (2),(5),(6).
- Rarely, distal clavicle osteolysis may occur.

REFERENCES

1. Gorbaty JD, Hsu JE, Gee AO. Classifications in brief: Rockwood classification of acromioclavicular joint separations. *Clin Orthop Relat Res*. 2017;475(1):283–287.
2. Nolte PC, Lacheta L, Decker TJ, et al. Optimal management of acromioclavicular dislocation: current perspectives. *Orthop Res Rev*. 2020;12:27–44.
3. Van Bergen CJA, Van Bemmel AF, Alta TDW, et al. New insights in the treatment of acromioclavicular separation. *World J Orthop*. 2017;8(12):861–873.
4. Lee S, Bedi A. Shoulder acromioclavicular joint reconstruction options and outcomes. *Curr Rev Musculoskelet Med*. 2016;9(4):368–377.
5. Tamaoki MJ, Lenza M, Matsunaga FT, et al. Surgical versus conservative interventions for treating acromioclavicular dislocation of the shoulder in adults. *Cochrane Database of Syst Rev*. 2019;10(10):CD007429.
6. Joukainen A, Kröger H, Niemitukia L, et al. Results of operative and nonoperative treatment of Rockwood types III and V acromioclavicular joint dislocation: a prospective, randomized trial with an 18- to 20-year follow-up. *Orthop J Sports Med*. 2014;2(12):2325967114560130.

CLINICAL PEARLS

- Types I and II AC separations generally do well with conservative treatment.
- Management of type III injuries should be made on a case-by-case basis.
- In general, full return to contact sports is possible when painless range of motion and normal, symmetrical strength are achieved.
- Cosmetic deformity and AC joint arthritis are common complications.

ADDUCTOR TENDON INJURY

Sara N. Raiser, MD, FAAPMR, CAQSM • Daniel C. Herman, MD, PhD, FAAPMR, FACSM, FISBS, CAQSM

BASICS

DESCRIPTION

- Medial thigh/groin pain and weakness resulting from injury to muscle-tendon unit
- The hip adductors include adductor longus, magnus, and brevis; gracilis; obturator externus; and pectineus.
- Adductor longus is the most commonly injured adductor muscle; other muscles involved in groin injuries may include gracilis, iliopsoas, rectus femoris, sartorius, and/or abdominal muscles.
- Three-tier grading system: (i) mild partial tear with pain but minimal loss of strength or range of motion; (ii) moderate partial tear with pain, +/− swelling, and noticeable decrease in strength and range of motion without complete loss of function; (iii) complete tear with severe limitation or complete loss of function, +/− retraction
- Synonym(s): groin strain; pulled groin

EPIDEMIOLOGY

Most common cause of groin pain in athletes, but symptoms overlap with a wide differential.

ETIOLOGY AND PATHOPHYSIOLOGY

- Eccentric loading of adductor muscle (muscle is passively being stretched while it is contracting) is usual mechanism of injury.
- Sudden acceleration/deceleration, change of direction, kicking, jumping, and/or overstretching are commonly involved mechanisms.

RISK FACTORS

- Increasing age
- Previous adductor injury
- Weak, inactive, or fatigued adductor muscles have less ability to absorb energy and are more likely to undergo acute strain.
- Reduced hip rotational range of motion
- Core muscle weakness

DIAGNOSIS

HISTORY

- Acutely, often a stretch injury with an abrupt cutting motion as in soccer, basketball, or a straddling injury as in gymnastics, cheerleading, or horseback riding
- Usually an acute episode is reported, but symptoms may become chronic after initial injury if undertreated and repeatedly strained.
- Chronic injury may also result from overuse through repetitive activity such as skating, kicking, or rollerblading.
- Typically unilateral but may become bilateral
- May have only minor discomfort with walking, but pain and weakness are noticeable with cutting or running.
- An unusual presentation, nocturnal pain, or lack of response to appropriate treatment may be concerning for a nonmusculoskeletal etiology.

PHYSICAL EXAM

- Classic triad of tenderness to palpation of the muscle and its bony attachments (proximal third of medial thigh and tendinous origin in pubic region), pain with passive stretching (hip abduction), and pain with resisted contraction (hip adduction), tested both with straight legs and with knees bent (1)[C]
- Swelling, ecchymosis, and significant weakness increase suspicion for tear.
- With complete rupture, palpable depression and retraction of torn muscle may be present.

DIFFERENTIAL DIAGNOSIS

- Osteitis pubis
- Bone stress injury of femoral neck, femoral shaft, or pubic ramus
- Iliopsoas or rectus femoris tendonitis, iliopsoas bursitis
- Avascular necrosis of femoral head
- Core muscle injury (sports hernia, Gilmore groin, athletic pubalgia)
- Femoroacetabular impingement, labral tear, osteochondral lesion, and/or osteoarthritis
- Myositis ossificans
- Pubic apophysitis and/or avulsion fracture in skeletally immature athlete
- Slipped capital femoral epiphysis (usually seen in early teens)
- Inguinal hernia
- Nerve entrapment (e.g., obturator nerve)
- Referred pain from spine
- Conjoined tendon lesions
- Nonmusculoskeletal considerations include urologic, gynecologic, and gastrointestinal disorders as well as malignancies (1)[C].

DIAGNOSTIC TESTS & INTERPRETATION

ALERT

- Straightforward cases may not require imaging.
- Hip and pelvis films should be obtained for the following concerns: pubic ramus tenderness; persistent pain despite conservative treatment; or suspicion of hip joint involvement, myositis ossificans following direct trauma, or avulsion fracture in an adolescent.
- Bone scan or magnetic resonance imaging (MRI) if bone stress injury is suspected
- MRI may also be used (2)[C].
- Musculoskeletal ultrasound (US) may be used to evaluate for tendon fiber discontinuity (1)[C] or hematoma if there is a palpable mass or retraction (2)[C], and to periodically monitor during the recovery phase.

TREATMENT

GENERAL MEASURES

- Protection, rest, ice, compression, and elevation (PRICE) is beneficial.
- Gentle compression with compression shorts, neoprene sleeve, or elastic wrap
- Strict immobilization generally is not recommended, and rehabilitation should be initiated early within the first few days.
- Limited activity as tolerated for 1 to 2 weeks, longer for more protracted cases

- If pain with ambulation, use crutches for weight-bearing as tolerated while symptomatic.
- Pain is usually controlled with over-the-counter (OTC) analgesics and/or restricted weight-bearing.

ISSUES FOR REFERRAL
- Skeletally mature pelvic avulsion fractures should be referred to an orthopedic surgeon.
- If suspicion for nonmusculoskeletal etiology exists, refer to the appropriate specialist for further workup and treatment.

ADDITIONAL THERAPIES
- A pain-limited independent progression of basic exercises including isometric strengthening should be instituted as symptoms allow (3)[B],(4)[A].
- Avoid excessive passive stretching.
- Progress as tolerated to dynamic, eccentric strengthening, balance training, and proprioceptive exercises of hip and groin musculature (3)[B],(4)[A],(5)[C],(6)[A].
- When active range of motion reaches at least 50% of the noninjured side with good muscle activation and pain free with exercises, may increase to full loading for conditioning (4)[A]
- Strength and range of motion should be nearly 100% and pain free prior to return to sport (4)[A],(6)[A].
- Conservative care has shown successful return to play in complete adductor longus avulsions (3)[B].

SURGERY/OTHER PROCEDURES
- Peritendinous adductor corticosteroid injections are not recommended given no evidence of long-term benefit.
- Regenerative therapies may potentially play a role in adductor injury treatment, although there is currently no evidence specifically regarding use with adductor injuries.
- Surgical repair may be indicated for complete avulsion from the femur/pubis or complete muscle/tendon tears (6)[A].
- Early repair is generally recommended if surgery is deemed appropriate.
- Adductor tenotomy for chronic adductor tendonitis is considered when conservative treatments have failed. This means things like rest, physical therapy, pain medications, and injections have not provided sufficient relief.

ONGOING CARE

PATIENT EDUCATION
- Correction of predisposing factors, such as hip muscle tightness, weakness, or imbalance, should be addressed (5)[C],(6)[A].
- Adequate stretching and warm-up may help prevent reinjury.
- Decision on return to play is dependent on extent of injury and underlying predisposing factors. Pain is usually a fair measure, so unrestricted play is generally permitted if pain free.

PROGNOSIS
- Prognosis is generally favorable.
- Early identification and treatment is essential for preventing a protracted course or chronic injury (1)[C].
- Healing of an adductor strain may take from 1 to 3 weeks for a grade 1 injury, up to 4 to 8 weeks for grade 3 injuries, and longer for chronic injuries.
- Average return to play following an acute grade 1 or 2 tendon tear treated with physical therapy is 1 to 7 weeks, depending on severity.
- Nonsurgical treatment of complete avulsion may take 2 to 3 months (3)[B] and up to a 14-week average return to play following surgical treatment of a grade 3 injury (6)[A].
- With appropriate treatment, average recurrence rate is 5% (6)[A].

REFERENCES

1. Thorborg K, Reiman MP, Weir A, et al. Clinical examination, diagnostic imaging, and testing of athletes with groin pain: an evidence-based approach to effective management. *J Orthop Sports Phys Ther*. 2018;48(4):239–249.
2. Lee SC, Endo Y, Potter HG. Imaging of groin pain: magnetic resonance and ultrasound imaging features. *Sports Health*. 2017;9(5):428–435.
3. Serner A, Hölmich P, Arnaiz J, et al. One-year clinical and imaging follow-up after exercise-based treatment for acute complete adductor longus tendon avulsions in athletes: a prospective case series. *Am J Sports Med*. 2021;49(11):3004–3013.
4. Hölmich P, Uhrskou P, Ulnits L, et al. Effectiveness of active physical training as treatment for long-standing adductor-related groin pain in athletes: randomised trial. *Lancet*. 1999;353(9151):439–443.
5. Thorborg K. Current clinical concepts: exercise and load management of adductor strains, adductor ruptures and longstanding adductor-related groin pain. *J Athl Train*. 2022;58(7–8):589–601.
6. Farrell SG, Hatem M, Bharam S. Acute adductor muscle injury: a systematic review on diagnostic imaging, treatment, and prevention. *Am J Sports Med*. 2023;51(13):3591–3603.

ADDITIONAL READING

- Branci S, Thorborg K, Nielsen MB, et al. Radiological findings in symphyseal and adductor-related groin pain in athletes: a critical review of the literature. *Br J Sports Med*. 2013;47(10):611–619.
- Chaudhari AMW, Jamison ST, McNally MP, et al. Hip adductor activations during run-to-cut maneuvers in compression shorts: implications for return to sport after groin injury. *J Sports Sci*. 2014;32(14):1333–1340.
- Gilmore J. Groin pain in the soccer athlete: fact, fiction, and treatment. *Clin Sports Med*. 1998;17(4):787–793, vii.
- Tyler TF, Silvers HJ, Gerhardt MB, et al. Groin injuries in sports medicine. *Sports Health*. 2010;2(3):231–236.
- Weir A, Homlich P, Thorborg K. Groin pain. In: Hutchinson M, Brukner P, Khan K, et al, eds. *Brukner & Khan's Clinical Sports Medicine*. Vol 1. 5th ed. McGraw-Hill; 2017:629–658.

CLINICAL PEARLS

- Although initial symptoms may not be debilitating enough to impair performance, pain is a marker for injury.
- Inadequately treated adductor strains can become chronic and ultimately take longer to rehabilitate or fail to fully recover.
- A history of prior groin injury is the greatest risk factor for subsequent injury.
- The clinical examination is neither sensitive nor specific for identifying the exact etiology of athletic groin pain in the majority of cases.
- Return to full competitive play should not occur until the athlete is pain free due to the high risk of chronic pain or complications.

ANAPHYLAXIS

Kristina Wilson, MD, MPH, FAAP, CAQSM

BASICS

- The causative agent in anaphylaxis remains unknown in up to 1/3 of cases.
- Food is the most common causative agent (about 1/3 of known cases) in children.
- Pharmacotherapeutic agents are the most common cause in adults.
- Other common causes include Hymenoptera stings and latex.
- Key to management and treatment is early recognition and immediate initiation of appropriate medical therapy.
- Only 55% of health care professionals recognized anaphylaxis without cutaneous involvement.
- Gastrointestinal (GI) symptoms more common in children
- Epinephrine is the undisputed initial therapy for anaphylaxis; administration should never be delayed.
- Failure to inject epinephrine promptly has been identified as the most important factor contributing to death.
- Only one-half of patients presenting to the emergency department (ED) who meet the National Institute of Allergy and Infectious Diseases/Food Allergy and Anaphylaxis Network diagnostic criteria for anaphylaxis receive treatment with epinephrine.

DESCRIPTION

- Serious, life-threatening generalized or systemic hypersensitivity reaction:
  - Rapid in onset
  - Involves airway, breathing, or circulatory problems
  - Usually associated with skin and mucosal changes
- Allergic type mediated by immunoglobulin E (IgE):
  - Involves the respiratory and/or cardiovascular systems
  - Patients may have a history of less severe reaction previously on exposure to relevant allergen.
- Exercise-induced anaphylaxis (EIAn):
  - Occurs in response to physical exertion
  - Subset of patients must have associated food trigger—food-dependent exercise-induced anaphylaxis (FDEIAn).
- Cold urticaria:
  - Reproducible, rapid onset of erythema, pruritus, and edema after exposure to cold
  - Most idiopathic
  - Occasionally involves abnormal circulating proteins (i.e., cryoglobulins or cryofibrinogens); agglutinates or precipitates at lower temperatures

EPIDEMIOLOGY

Death rates from the most common causes of anaphylaxis have varied:

- Food induced has increased 0.03 to 0.32 per million per year.
- Insect sting has declined 0.09 to 0.13 per million per year.
- Drug induced has increased 0.05 to 0.51 per million per year.
- Recurrence 26.5–54% in follow-up time 1.5 to 25 years

Incidence

- 50 to 112 episodes per 100,000 person-years (1)
- 1 to 761 per 100,000 person-years in children (1)
- Wide variation due to differences in sample populations, data-collection methods, and varying definitions of anaphylaxis

Prevalence

Lifetime prevalence of 0.3–5.1% globally (1)

ETIOLOGY AND PATHOPHYSIOLOGY

- Allergic: IgE-mediated: drugs, venom, latex, vaccines, food
- Nonallergic: direct basophil/mast cell–mediated: radiocontrast dye, opioid drugs

RISK FACTORS

- Prior anaphylaxis event can predict subsequent anaphylaxis:
  - Particularly with food, latex, aeroallergens, Elan, Hymenoptera, or idiopathic
  - 14% of anaphylaxis admissions for peanut sensitivity have a prior history of anaphylaxis.
  - Often occurs following a previous mild allergic reaction to the same allergen
- Most proposed risk factors have limited value owing to a low specificity:
  - Coexisting atopic disease; especially poorly controlled asthma
  - Older age at first reaction to food allergy
- Clinical risk factors for fatality in anaphylactic reactions (2): severe or uncontrolled asthma, cardiovascular disease, mastocytosis

GENERAL PREVENTION

- Avoidance of known allergen
- No available tests exist to predict the likelihood of a person developing anaphylaxis.
- Neither size of skin prick test wheal nor the level of serum-specific IgE correlate with reaction severity.
- Immunotherapy:
  - Hymenoptera venom and penicillin: currently available
  - Oral immunotherapy (OIT) milligram doses or sublingual immunotherapy (SLIT) microgram doses over months
  - Milk, egg, and peanut
  - 20% drop out due to serious side effects such as anaphylaxis.
  - Temporary tolerance maintained with regular ingestion
  - Permanent immunologic tolerance difficult to demonstrate
  - Only available in controlled trials
- Cold-induced anaphylaxis:
  - Avoidance of cold water and air; cold food and beverages

- Promising outlooks: characterization of β-cell epitope responses:
  - Specific allergenic epitopes may correlate with severity of reaction.
  - Individuals have a unique fingerprint of IgE-specific allergenic epitopes, and characterization of profile may help determine risk of anaphylaxis.

DIAGNOSIS

- Diagnosis is made based on clinical symptoms:
  - Do not underestimate the potential severity of an allergic reaction in its early stages.
  - Symptoms may progress rapidly.
- Suspicion of anaphylaxis requires immediate medical intervention—do not delay for diagnostic tests.
- Biphasic reactions occur in up to 20% of reactions.
- Clinical criteria for diagnosing anaphylaxis (1)[C]:
  - Acute onset of an illness (minutes to several hours) with involvement of the skin, mucosal tissue, or both (e.g., generalized hives; pruritus or flushing; swollen lips, tongue, and/or uvula) and *at least one* of the following:
    - Respiratory compromise (e.g., dyspnea, wheeze/bronchospasm, stridor, reduced peak expiratory flow [PEF], hypoxemia)
    - Reduced blood pressure (BP) or associated symptoms of end organ dysfunction (e.g., hypotonia/collapse, syncope, incontinence)
    - Severe GI symptoms (e.g., severe crampy abdominal pain, repetitive vomiting) especially after exposure to nonfood allergens
  - Acute onset of hypotension or bronchospasm or laryngeal involvement after exposure to a known or highly probably allergen for that patient, even in the absence of typical skin involvement
    - Infants and children: low systolic BP (age specific) or >30% decrease in systolic BP
    - Adults: systolic BP of <90 mm Hg or >30% decrease from that person's baseline

HISTORY

- Previous history of anaphylaxis—treatments/effects
- Symptoms: fatigue, pruritus, urticaria, angioedema, wheezing, rhinitis, GI distress, cardiovascular collapse
- Time from exposure/suspected exposure to event
- Recent changes in baseline health
- Contributing environmental factors: extremes of temperature, elevated humidity, increased pollen count
- Contributing personal factors: physical exertion, ethanol consumption, insect sting, food consumption, stress, menses, fever
- Medications: nonsteroidal anti-inflammatory drugs (NSAIDs), aspirin, antibiotics, angiotensin-converting enzyme (ACE) inhibitors
- Comorbid medical conditions: asthma, chronic obstructive pulmonary disease (COPD), cardiovascular disease, mastocytosis

PHYSICAL EXAM

- Respiratory: bronchospasm, laryngeal edema
- Cardiovascular: hypotension, dysrhythmias, myocardial ischemia
- GI: nausea, vomiting, diarrhea
- Cutaneous: urticaria, angioedema
- Hematologic: activation of intrinsic coagulation pathway → disseminated intravascular coagulation (DIC), thrombocytopenia
- Neurologic: seizures
- Death can occur from airway obstruction or circulatory collapse.

DIFFERENTIAL DIAGNOSIS

- Pulmonary embolism
- Acute myocardial infarction
- Airway obstruction
- Asthma
- Syncope
- Anxiety/panic attack
- Shock—hypovolemic/cardiogenic/distributive/septic
- Hereditary angioedema
- Vocal cord dysfunction
- Systemic mastocytosis
- Pheochromocytoma
- Carcinoid syndrome

DIAGNOSTIC TESTS & INTERPRETATION

Initial Tests (lab, imaging)

- There are no specific tests to make the diagnosis of anaphylaxis, and evaluation should not delay diagnosis and treatment.
- For respiratory distress after administration of epinephrine, an arterial blood gas analysis may be helpful in evaluating ventilatory status.
- These changes can be noted during anaphylaxis:
  - Elevation of plasma histamine level
  - Increase in hematocrit due to fluid extravasation
- Tryptase levels helpful in making official diagnosis (2):
  - Draw 30 minutes to 2 hours of symptom onset.
  - Must be placed on ice
  - Rarely elevated in food-induced anaphylaxis

Diagnostic Procedures/Other

Electrocardiogram (ECG): abnormalities including dysrhythmias, ischemic changes, infarction

TREATMENT

- Prehospital:
  - Airway, breathing, and circulation (ABCs)
  - Remove trigger (i.e., stinger from insect).
  - Early administration of epinephrine intramuscular (IM) in the anterolateral thigh positively affects outcome (3)[B]:
    - If preloaded epinephrine is available, administer prior to emergency personnel arriving if anaphylaxis is suspected.
    - May be administered every 5 to 15 minutes as needed based on patient's condition
    - Call 911 for emergent transfer to hospital.

– Recumbent position with legs elevated (3)[B]
– Albuterol: metered-dose inhaler (MDI) or nebulized solution if bronchospasm not relieved by administration of epinephrine: every 20 minutes or continuously
– Diphenhydramine: Cochrane Review 2007 of H_1 antihistamines in anaphylaxis:
  ○ No evidence to support use (4)[B]
  ○ Long onset of action—1 to 2 hours
  ○ Relieves pruritus, urticaria, and angioedema
  ○ Works synergistically with epinephrine
  ○ Does not relieve upper or lower respiratory tract obstruction or circulatory collapse
  ○ Does not prevent fatality
- ED treatment:
  – Continuous cardiac/vitals monitoring until stable
  – Persistent bronchospasm can be treated with β-agonist bronchodilators.
  – Hypotension should be treated with isotonic volume. Vasopressors and Trendelenburg positioning are useful adjuncts.
  – Antihistamines (both H_1 and H_2 blockers) helpful in preventing histamine interactions with target tissues:
    ○ *Now* a third-line treatment
    ○ Does not treat life-threatening symptoms of anaphylaxis (4)[B]
    ○ Most helpful treating cutaneous symptoms
  – Corticosteroids have never been shown in placebo-controlled trials to affect the course of anaphylaxis but are used to treat associated conditions (e.g., asthma, allergic rhinitis):
    ○ Long onset 4 to 6 hours
    ○ May decrease the chance of having a biphasic reaction:
      ▪ Second episode of anaphylaxis after treatment for first episode
      ▪ Occurs 2 to 72 hours after onset of first episode
      ▪ 80% occur within the first 4 hours of initial episode.
  – Glucagon is useful in epinephrine-resistant anaphylaxis from β-adrenergic blocking agents.

MEDICATION

First Line

Epinephrine (EpiPen):

- Adult: 0.3 to 0.5 mg (Use 1:1,000 dilution for subcutaneous [SC] route.)
- Children: 0.01 mg/kg SC (maximum dose 0.3 mg)
- Preloaded syringe: 0.15 mg per injector (EpiPen Jr) and 0.30 mg per injector (EpiPen)
- Refractory hypotension:
  – Epinephrine drip 0.1 to 1.0 μg/kg/min (maximum 10 μg/min)
  – Titrated based on clinical effect; must be on cardiac monitor owing to risk of lethal cardiac arrhythmias

Second Line

- β-Agonist: albuterol: MDI, continuous nebulizer treatment
- Oxygen: respiratory distress/hypoxia
- H_2 antagonist:
  – Ranitidine: adult: 50 mg IV *or*
  – Cimetidine: 300 mg IV; children: 1 to 2 mg/kg (maximum dose 75 to 150 mg)
- Glucagon: for refractory hypotension, especially if patient is on a β-blocker:
  – Adult: 1 mg IV
  – Children: 20 to 30 μg/kg (maximum dose 1 mg) given over 5 minutes; followed by an infusion of 5 to 15 μg/min titrated to effect
- Corticosteroids (controversial):
  – Methylprednisolone: severe reactions:
    ○ Adult: 125 mg IV
    ○ Children: 1 to 2 mg/kg IV (maximum single dose 60 to 80 mg)
  – Prednisone: mild reactions:
    ○ Adult: 60 mg PO
    ○ Children: 1 to 2 mg/kg PO (maximum single dose 60 to 80 mg)
  – Hydrocortisone:
    ○ Adults: 500 mg IV
    ○ Children: 4 to 8 mg/kg per dose IV

Third Line

H_1 antagonist: diphenhydramine:

- Adult: 50 mg IV
- Children: 1 to 2 mg/kg slow IV pump (IVP)

ADMISSION, INPATIENT, AND NURSING CONSIDERATIONS

- Initial stabilization:
  – ABCs:
    ○ Ensure adequate ventilation.
    ○ Endotracheal intubation may be required but is difficult because of laryngeal edema or spasm.
    ○ Transtracheal jet insufflation or cricothyrotomy may be necessary to control the airway.
  – Epinephrine IM

- Aggressive volume resuscitation with crystalloids to maintain BP; transfer of as much as 50% of the intravascular fluid into the extravascular space may occur within 10 minutes.
- In volume-refractory hypotension, may need continuous IV epinephrine or other vasopressors (e.g., vasopressin or dopamine)
- Monitor for biphasic reaction.

- Admission criteria:
  - Intubated patients, patients in respiratory distress, and patients with refractory hypotension should be admitted to an intensive care unit (ICU) setting.
  - Monitored bed may be necessary if there has not been a substantial response to initial therapy.
  - Patients with significant generalized reactions and persistent symptoms should be admitted for observation for 24 hours.
- Discharge criteria:
  - Individualized based on the following criteria (5)[C]:
    - Initial presentation
    - Response to therapy
    - Availability of close observation at home
    - Accessibility of a medical facility from home
  - Patients with complete resolution of symptoms, okay to discharge after 4 to 6 hours of ED observation:
    - Epinephrine duration—1 hour
    - Majority of biphasic reactions occur within the first 4 hours of initial episode.
  - Continue H_1 antagonist, H_2 antagonist, and corticosteroids for minimum 48 hours after discharge.
  - Follow up within 48 hours of discharge to evaluate effectiveness of outpatient therapy.
  - Severity of the reaction should be emphasized to each patient and family.
  - Anaphylaxis action plans (5)[C]:
    - Education about prevention and prehospital management
    - Prescription for self-administered epinephrine and instruction on its use
    - Patients with a known trigger counseled on strict avoidance of that trigger
    - Limited evidence on impact on recurrence of anaphylaxis or reduction in fatal events (5)[B]
  - Follow-up visit with an allergist is also recommended for consideration of allergy testing exercise ± food provocation test.

REFERENCES

1. Cardona V, Ansotegui IJ, Ebisawa M, et al. World allergy organization anaphylaxis guidance 2020. *World Allergy Organ J*. 2020;13(10):100472.
2. Pflipsen MC, Vega Colon KM. Anaphylaxis: recognition and management. *Am Fam Physician*. 2020;102(6):355–362.
3. Muraro A, Worm M, Alviani C, et al. EAACI guidelines: anaphylaxis (2021 update). *Allergy*. 2022;77(2):357–377.
4. Sheikh A, ten Broek VM, Brown SGA, et al. H1-antihistamines for the treatment of anaphylaxis with and without shock. *Cochrane Database Syst Rev*. 2007;(1):CD006160.
5. Nurmatov U, Worth A, Sheikh A. Anaphylaxis management plans for the acute and long-term management of anaphylaxis: a systematic review. *J Allergy Clin Immunol*. 2008;122(2):353–361, 361.e1–361.e3.

ADDITIONAL READING

- Clark E, Tanno LK, Vo T, et al. Anaphylaxis management in a French pediatric emergency department: lessons from the ANA-PED study. *Clin Transl Allergy*. 2023;13(8):e12289.
- Eller E, Muraro A, Dahl R, et al. Assessing severity of anaphylaxis: a data-driven comparison of 23 instruments. *Clin Trans Allergy*. 2018;8:29.
- Muraro A, Ferandez-Rivas M, Beyer K, et al. The urgent need for a harmonized severity scoring system for acute allergic reactions. *Allergy*. 2018;73(9):1792–1800.
- Pumphrey RSH. When should self-injectible epinephrine be prescribed for food allergy and when should it be used? *Curr Opin Allergy Clin Immunol*. 2008;8(3):254–260.
- Sheikh A, Shehata YA, Brown SGA, et al. Adrenaline for the treatment of anaphylaxis: Cochrane systematic review. *Allergy*. 2009;64(2):204–212.

CLINICAL PEARLS

- Epinephrine is the undisputed initial therapy for anaphylaxis, and its administration should never be delayed.
- There are no specific tests to make the diagnosis of anaphylaxis, and evaluation should not delay diagnosis and treatment.
- Failure to inject epinephrine promptly has been identified as the most important factor contributing to death in patients experiencing anaphylaxis.

ANKLE IMPINGEMENT

Marcia Faustin, MD, CAQSM, FAAFP • Kari J. Rezac, DO • Michael Jake Peterson, MD

BASICS

DESCRIPTION

- Impingement is a clinical syndrome of end-range joint pain or restricted motion caused by direct abutment and/or compression of bone or soft tissues.
- Ankle impingement syndromes are heterogenous group of conditions, divided broadly into intra-articular and extra-articular types as well as location around the ankle (1).
- Classifications: based on type of impingement:
  - Posttraumatic synovitis
  - Bony spur
  - Intra-articular fibrous band/scar
  - Capsular scarring
- Classifications: based on location:
  - Anterior
  - Anterolateral
  - Anteromedial (less common)
  - Posterior
  - Posteromedial (less common)

EPIDEMIOLOGY

- 1–2% of ankle inversion injuries lead to symptomatic impingement syndrome (1),(2).
- Common in athletes who play on grass or turf (3)
- 14–25% of the population have os trigonum (1).
- Os trigonum appears to be symptomatic only with coinciding trauma (2),(4).

ETIOLOGY AND PATHOPHYSIOLOGY

- Arises from either traumatic or repetitive hyperdorsiflexion (anterior impingement) or hyperplantarflexion (posterior impingement)
- Microtrauma from repetitive movements such as kicking soccer ball can lead to spur formation.
- Initial ankle injuries in the subacute or chronic phase can lead to the development of abnormal osseous or soft tissue thickening.
- Pain generators are typically the soft tissue caught between bony spurs; however, this differs for purely anterior impingement syndromes, as direct bony spur contact is a common pain generator (1),(5)[C].
- Anterior impingement is typically easier to diagnose than posterior impingement due to superficial location:
  - Anterior impingement:
    - Anterior lateral gutter—damage to lateral collateral ligament complex and joint capsule, resulting in synovitis, irregular thickening, and/or scarring of ligaments after inversion ankle sprain
    - Anterior:
      - Repeated capsuloligamentous traction or microtrauma in plantar flexion may induce spur formation (kicking a ball).
      - Tibial or talar bony spurs impinge soft tissue.
  - Anteromedial—rare; secondary to inversion injury with rotational component that leads to stretching of the capsule and anterior tibial ligament (1)[C]
  - Posterior impingement: spectrum of disorders characterized by posterior ankle pain after acute fracture or recurrent plantar flexion or hyperplantarflexion. Symptoms can arise due to impingement and mechanical irritation of the soft tissues between these posterior structures:
    - Os trigonum (accessory ossicle connected by a fibrous band to the posterolateral tubercle of the talus) (4)[C]
    - Talar compression syndrome
    - Prominent posterolateral process of talus (Stieda process)
    - Prominent medial malleoli process
    - Prominent posterior process of calcaneus

RISK FACTORS

- Anterior impingement:
  - Risk factors include sports requiring recurrent forceful dorsiflexion of the ankle, recurrent ankle sprains (supination and plantar flexion) and/or chronic ankle instability, and acute ankle sprains/fractures (1),(3),(4),(5)[C].
  - Athletes: soccer players, gymnasts, basketball players, football players, high jumpers, running uphill (1)[C]
- Posterior impingement (1),(2),(3),(5)[C]:
  - Risk factors include acute or recurrent hyperplantarflexion (ballet on pointe), recurrent ankle sprains, or ankle instability.
  - Athletes: ballet dancers ("en pointe" and "demi pointe"), cheerleaders, cricketers, javelin throwers, long jumpers, running downhill (forced plantar flexion)
  - Poor shoe wear without appropriate support
  - Overuse injury is more common than traumatic injury (2)[C].

GENERAL PREVENTION

- Preventing recurrent ankle sprains
- Early exercise protocol for acute ankle sprain (1),(2),(3),(4),(6)[C]
- Proper rehabilitation, including ankle strengthening, range of motion, and proprioception (1),(2),(3),(4),(6)[C]
- Proper footwear/orthotics (3),(4)[C]
- Recognizing the condition early to allow early rest and rehabilitation (6)[C]

DIAGNOSIS

HISTORY

- Typically, a clinical diagnosis of exclusion
- Prior history of single or multiple episodes of traumatic ankle injuries (typically inversion injuries)
- Mild swelling or effusion after activity (2),(4),(5)[C]
- Anterior impingement (2),(3),(4),(6)[C]:
  - Pain with activities requiring ankle in dorsiflexion (uphill running/walking)
  - Pain with kicking a soccer ball, especially a dead ball
  - Popping or snapping sensation of isolated soft tissue lesions
  - Subjective feeling of limited range of motion or blocking on dorsiflexion
- Exacerbating factors: climbing stairs, ascending ladders, and deep squat (2),(3),(4),(6)[C]
- Posterior impingement:
  - Pain is difficult to localize, typically at the posterior joint line anterior to the Achilles tendon (6)[B].
  - Pain described as consistent, sharp, dull, and/or radiating
  - Prior history of inversion (supination) and plantar flexion injury
  - Posterior ankle pain exacerbated by either plantar flexion (compression of soft tissues or bony prominence) or dorsiflexion (stretching of the posterior capsule and ligaments)
- History of repetitive push off or plantar flexion maneuvers (i.e., downhill running/walking, descending stairs, and high-heeled shoe wear) (2),(3),(4),(5),(6)[C]

PHYSICAL EXAM

- Complete neurovascular exam, strength, and range of motion
- Possible soft tissue swelling or effusion
- Anterior impingement (2),(3),(4),(5)[C]:
  - Tenderness to palpation over the anterior, anterolateral, or anteromedial ankle (most important clinical finding)
  - Pain in the anterior aspect of the ankle with either forced plantar flexion or dorsiflexion
  - Possible palpable mass with tenderness to palpation
- Posterior impingement (2),(3),(4),(5)[C]:
  - Tenderness to palpation in the posterior aspect of ankle, typically anterior to and not involving the Achilles tendon
  - Possible palpable soft tissue thickening with tenderness to palpation
  - Positive plantar flexion test: pain in posterior ankle with plantar flexion (pathognomonic)
  - Reproducible pain with pressure over posteromedial aspect of the ankle during passive inversion and plantar flexion
- Pain with dorsiflexion (stretching of the capsule and ligament) (2),(3),(4)[C].

DIFFERENTIAL DIAGNOSIS

- Anterior impingement (2),(3),(4),(5)[A]:
  - Lateral ankle ligament sprain
  - Synovial thickening/synovitis
  - Loose/intra-articular bodies, avulsion fragments
  - Chondral or osteochondral lesions of anterior tibial plafond or talar dome
  - Osteoid osteoma of the talus
  - Ganglion cyst
  - Osteoarthritis
- Posterior impingement (2),(3),(4),(5),(6)[C]:
  - Deltoid ligament sprain
  - Posterior tibial tendonitis/tenosynovitis

- Flexor hallucis tendonitis/tenosynovitis
- Achilles tendonitis/tenosynovitis
- Peroneal tendonitis/tenosynovitis
- Retrocalcaneal bursitis
- Haglund deformity
- Tarsal coalition
- Thickening of posteromedial ankle capsule
- Tarsal tunnel syndrome
- Osteochondral lesions of talar dome (medial)
- Shepherd fracture (acute fracture of the posterolateral process of the talus)
- Ganglion cyst
- Chronic regional pain syndrome
- Sural neuralgia
- Osteoarthritis

DIAGNOSTIC TESTS & INTERPRETATION

Initial Tests (lab, imaging)

- Weight-bearing ankle x-rays:
  - Anteroposterior (AP), lateral, oblique (4)[C]
- Anterior impingement:
  - Oblique anterior impingement view: beam tilted in 45-degree craniocaudal direction with leg in 30-degree external rotation and foot in plantar flexion (1),(4),(5)[C]
- Posterior impingement:
  - Posterior impingement view: lateral, 25-degree external rotation, oblique view (os trigonum) (1),(4),(5)[C]

Follow-Up Tests & Special Considerations

- Magnetic resonance imaging (MRI) (evaluates osseous and soft tissue) (1),(3),(4),(5)[C]
- Ultrasound (evaluates osseous structures, soft tissue, and tendons statically and dynamically) (1)[C]
- Computed tomography (CT) (evaluates osseous pathologies and for surgical planning) (1),(3),(4)[C]
- MRI versus magnetic resonance (MR) arthrogram (3)[C]

Diagnostic Procedures/Others

Ultrasound-guided injection of local anesthetic and/or corticosteroid or ketorolac into (1),(3),(4),(6)[C]:

- Anterolateral gutter
- Area of synovitis or focal capsular thickening (anterior or posterior impingement)
- Os trigonum synchondrosis

Test Interpretation

- X-ray (1),(5),(6)[C]:
  - Most useful to diagnose osseous lesions, degeneration, alignment
  - Negative radiographs do not rule out impingement syndrome.
- MRI (1),(2),(3)[C]:
  - Most useful to diagnose soft tissue pathology and excluding other pathology (such as an osteochondral lesion)
  - Bone marrow edema, fracture line, fluid in synchondrosis (in case of os trigonum fracture), posterior capsular or ligament thickening with intermediate to low intensity on T2-weighted images

TREATMENT

GENERAL MEASURES

- Rest, avoid provocative activities, ice (2),(3),(4),(6)[C]
- Cast immobilization (severe cases) (2),(3),(4),(6)[C]
- Shoe modifications, heel lifts, orthotics (3),(4)[C]
- Physical therapy with emphasis on (1),(2),(3),(4),(6)[C]:
  - Range-of-motion exercises, proprioceptive (balance) training, and strengthening exercises to improve ankle stability
  - Address core/gluteal weakness.
  - Modalities: electrotherapy, transcutaneous electrical nerve stimulation (TENS) unit, deloading taping, soft tissue massage

MEDICATION

First Line

- Acetaminophen
- Nonsteroidal anti-inflammatory drugs (NSAIDs)

Second Line

Ultrasound-guided local anesthetic and/or corticosteroid or ketorolac injection (diagnostic and therapeutic) (1),(3),(4),(6)[C]

ISSUES FOR REFERRAL

- 3 to 6 months of failed conservative treatment affected normal daily activities or athletic performance and correlated physical exam and imaging findings (2),(3),(4),(6)[C]
- Posteromedial impingement typically fails conservative treatment, which leads to surgical débridement (2)[C].

SURGERY/OTHER PROCEDURES

- Surgical goals are to improve function and pain by removing offending pathologic bony and/or soft tissue lesions.
- Arthroscopic (more common) or open procedures (2),(5),(6)[B]
- Prognosis decreases with higher degree of tibiotalar osteoarthritis (4),(5)[A].

COMPLEMENTARY & ALTERNATIVE MEDICINE

Limited data suggests the use of dry needling targeted at abnormal synovial or scar tissue, and biologic injections such as with platelet-rich plasma (PRP) (5)[C].

ONGOING CARE

FOLLOW-UP RECOMMENDATIONS

Postsurgical treatment (3),(4),(5),(6)[A]:

- Weight-bearing as tolerated immediately postoperative with early range of motion
- Physical therapy focuses on increasing available joint space for more mobility and less pain during activity.
- Ankle immobilization is recommended if there is intraoperative evidence of extensive osseous injury (2)[A].
- Return to play 6 to 16 weeks depending on type and level of sport.

PROGNOSIS

- The majority of patients have resolution of symptoms with conservative/nonoperative care (2),(5)[C].
- Posterior impingement secondary to overuse has a better prognosis than traumatic injury (2),(4)[C].

Pediatric Considerations

Pediatric patients will present with similar symptoms and exam findings as adults. In patients with open physis, posterior impingent may be misdiagnosed, as os trigonum may be small or cartilaginous with normal radiographs. Impingement syndromes in children are typically treated conservatively; if they fail nonoperative management, surgical treatment may be indicated (6)[C].

REFERENCES

1. Armstrong TM, Rowbotham E, Robinson P. Update on ankle and foot impingement. *Semin Musculoskelet Radiol*. 2023;27(3):256–268.
2. Russo A, Zappia M, Reginelli A, et al. Ankle impingement: a review of multimodality imaging approach. *Musculoskelet Surg*. 2013;97(Suppl 2):S161–S168.
3. Lavery KP, McHale KJ, Rossy WH, et al. Ankle impingement. *J Orthop Surg Res*. 2016;11(1):97.
4. van Dijk CN. Anterior and posterior ankle impingement. *Foot Ankle Clin*. 2006;11(3):663–683.
5. Carreira DS, Ueland TE. Ankle impingement: a critical review analysis. *JBJS Reviews*. 2020;8(5):pe0215.
6. Kushare I, Kastan K, Allahabadi S. Posterior ankle impingement: an underdiagnosed cause of ankle pain in pediatric patients. *World J Orthop*. 2019;10(10):364–370.

ADDITIONAL READING

- John S, Mendicino R, Catanzariti A. Mastering ankle impingement syndromes. *Podiatry Today*. 2007;(20) 8:52–60.
- McMurray TP. Footballer's ankle. *J Bone Joint Surg Br*. 1950;32(1):68–69.
- Witjes S, Gresnigt F, van den Bekerom MP, et al. The ankle trial (ankle treatment after injuries of the ankle ligaments): what is the benefit of external support devices in the functional treatment of acute ankle sprain? A randomized controlled trial. *BMC Musculoskelet Disord*. 2012;13:21.
- Zbojniewicz AM. Impingement syndrome of the ankle and hindfoot. *Pediatr Radiol*. 2019;49(12):1691–1701.

CLINICAL PEARLS

- An ankle impingement is classified according to type of impingement and location of impingement.
- Largely a clinical diagnosis of exclusion
- Arises from either traumatic or repetitive hyperdorsiflexion (anterior impingement) or hyperplantarflexion (posterior impingement)
- Typically, conservative treatment will resolve most cases.

ANKLE SPRAINS, LATERAL

Christopher A. Gee, MD, MPH, FACEP, CAQSM

BASICS

DESCRIPTION

- Lateral ankle sprains are the most common injury sustained by athletes (1) and comprise approximately 14% of all sports-related injuries (2).
- >80% of ankle sprains are due to an inversion type of injury that damages the lateral ankle ligaments.
- Whereas the medial side of the ankle has the broad, strong deltoid ligament as a restraint, the lateral side of the ankle has three smaller ligaments that act as the static restraint system.
- Bony support of the distal fibula assists the deltoid ligament in restricting eversion stress to the ankle.
- Primary static restraints to ankle inversion:
  - Anterior talofibular ligament (ATFL): passes from the tip of the fibula to the lateral talar neck; taut in plantar flexion; most commonly injured
  - Calcaneofibular ligament (CFL): passes inferior and posterior from the tip of the fibula to the lateral calcaneus; usually injured along with the ATFL
  - Posterior talofibular ligament (PTFL): passes posteriorly from the fibula to the talus; injured less often
- These ligaments are injured in a sequential pattern as extreme inversion and plantarflexion forces are placed on the ankle. The ATFL is injured first (isolated ATFL injuries occur in approximately 2/3 of injuries). After the small ATFL is injured, the CFL then is stressed and injured, followed by the PTFL. The ankle joint capsule is also sprained during an inversion injury. Given this pattern, isolated CFL injuries are uncommon.
- Increasing inversion force leads to more damage to lateral ligaments and capsule.
- The smaller medial malleolus provides less protection and allows inversion stress to injure the lateral ankle ligaments more easily.
- Ankle sprain grading:
  - Grade 1: stretch or partial tearing of ligaments but no gross laxity
  - Grade 2: partial tear of ligaments with increased laxity of ankle but still firm end point
  - Grade 3: complete rupture of ligaments; gross laxity of ankle with no end point

EPIDEMIOLOGY

Incidence

Very common injury in athletes and the general population, with around 2 million cases each year in the United States (3)

ETIOLOGY AND PATHOPHYSIOLOGY

Lateral ankle sprains occur when the ankle is stressed with extreme inversion and plantarflexion forces that overcome the static restraints (ligaments, capsule). Spraining and tearing of the ligaments leads to pain, swelling, and varying degrees of disability.

RISK FACTORS

- Athletes (especially those involved in sports with jumping near other players and quick "cutting" motions, e.g., basketball, soccer, football) (4)
- Dancers
- Congenital tarsal coalition (allows less "give" in the foot and results in more stress to ankle)
- Prior ankle injury (Previously injured or stretched ligaments provide less overall stability.) (5)
- Hypermobility syndromes may predispose to sprains.

DIAGNOSIS

HISTORY

Patients report history of inversion-type injury often with an audible pop. This is followed by rapid swelling, pain, and an inability to walk.

PHYSICAL EXAM

- Physical examination reveals ecchymosis and diffuse swelling but not effusion about the ankle joint.
- Tenderness to palpation is noted along the course of injured ligaments and can be diagnostic of which ligaments are injured.
- Palpation of the anterior ankle joint and the talar dome with the foot in full plantarflexion can help to diagnose other forms of pathology (e.g., osteochondral defects, cartilage injuries).
- It is important to palpate both the medial and lateral malleoli, proximal fibula, talus, and the base of the 5th metatarsal to examine for possible fracture (e.g., Ottawa Ankle Rules) (6).
- Occasionally, the ankle ligaments can be disrupted, and the stress passed up the tibiofibular syndesmosis. This leads to syndesmotic injuries or the so-called high ankle sprain. In extreme cases, the force can fracture out the proximal fibula causing a Maisonneuve fracture.
- Assess neurovascular status by feeling distal pulses (dorsalis pedis, posterior tibialis) and manually testing appropriate muscle groups.
- Grading of ankle injury can be accomplished by testing the integrity of various ligaments. Examiner also should take into account the fact that prior ankle sprains may have left residual laxity on either side; can use other ankle as comparison for general laxity
- Inversion tilt: tests stability of CFL; performed by holding the distal tibia and moving the foot from a neutral position to an inversion position. Increased laxity compared with opposite side indicates a tear of the CFL.
- Posterior drawer: tests stability of the PTFL; performed by holding the distal tibia and pushing the ankle backward in the joint. Increased laxity without an endpoint can indicate a tear.
- Anterior drawer:
  - Tests stability of ATFL; performed by holding the distal tibia and pulling the heel forward. Increased laxity relative to the opposite side indicates a tear of the ATFL. The anterior drawer test in the ankle has poor sensitivity and specificity.

DIFFERENTIAL DIAGNOSIS

- Tibia fracture (shaft, malleolus, etc.)
- Pilon fracture
- Fibula fracture (malleolus, Maisonneuve)
- Avulsion fracture (malleolus, 5th metatarsal)
- Osteochondral defect in talar dome/tibial plafond
- Anterior ankle impingement
- Os trigonum syndrome
- Talus fracture including lateral process of talus fractures
- Calcaneal fracture
- Peroneal subluxation, tear
- Bimalleolar/trimalleolar fracture

DIAGNOSTIC TESTS & INTERPRETATION

- Plain radiographs of affected ankle (including anteroposterior, lateral, and mortise views) to evaluate for fracture (weight-bearing if able)
- May not need to perform x-rays if patient does not have tenderness along posterior 6-cm edge of lateral and medial malleoli and can bear weight initially after injury (Ottawa Ankle Rules) (6)
- Computed tomography (CT) scans may be performed to evaluate for occult fracture.
- Magnetic resonance imaging (MRI) is rarely useful in ankle sprains but may be useful in assessing integrity of various ligaments in patients with chronic ankle instability or in evaluation of osteochondral defects that are not apparent on radiographs.
- Musculoskeletal ultrasound is a helpful modality to identify disruption of ligaments; very operator dependent

TREATMENT

GENERAL MEASURES

- Initial therapy focuses on PRICE (protection [bracing], rest, ice, compression, elevation) protocol to decrease pain and swelling.
- Crutches can be used until patient is able to bear weight as tolerated.
- Various kinds of braces, compression devices, stirrup splints, and walking boots can be used to provide protection and support and to encourage walking.
- Should advise patients to begin gentle range of motion as soon as pain allows and to keep limb elevated to decrease swelling
- Severe sprains may be best treated with more motion restriction in devices such as casts or walking boots. Continued bracing may help to reduce risk of sprains in high-risk athletic population (7).
- Progressive therapy through a three-phase approach may best promote rapid recovery:
  - Phase 1 consists of PRICE protocols to improve pain and swelling (often weeks 1 to 2).
  - Phase 2 consists of progressive range of motion exercises to improve motion and decrease swelling. Patients should continue to use a protective brace when walking to prevent further injury. Patients should be working toward full weight-bearing during this stage (weeks 2 to 4).
  - Phase 3 begins more aggressive strengthening and rehabilitation exercises. Specifically, patients should work on proprioception and endurance. This can be a formalized physical therapy program as needed (weeks 4 to 6).

MEDICATION

Acetaminophen or nonsteroidal anti-inflammatory drugs (NSAIDs) can be used after initial injury for pain but limited to no more than 10 days. NSAIDs should be avoided in patients at risk for gastrointestinal (GI) bleeding.

ADDITIONAL THERAPIES

- Physical therapy can be used to assist patients in strengthening and generally rehabilitating the injured ankle.
- Balance exercises have been shown to improve speed to return to play and reduce reinjury rates by as much as 50%.
- Electrical stimulation and iontophoresis may have a role in pain and swelling control.

SURGERY/OTHER PROCEDURES

- In general, most patients recover spontaneously and are able to go back to activities as pain allows. More unstable joints, recurrent injuries, and higher level athletes may need formal physical therapy.
- Often, general rehabilitation principles and conservative therapy are adequate to return athletes to their sport without more aggressive interventions. Patients rarely need primary repair of ligaments after an acute lateral ankle sprain.
- Occasionally, severe or ongoing chronic laxity of lateral ankle restraints may lead to recurrent ankle injuries and chronic ankle instability. These patients may benefit from ligament repair or ankle reconstruction to improve stability.

ONGOING CARE

FOLLOW-UP RECOMMENDATIONS

Patient Monitoring

- Patients may return to play once they have achieved a full range of motion and strength as well as being able to perform their sport-specific activities without limitations. Some may be able to return to play with a supportive device to protect from further injury depending on the sport and the patient's position.
- Depending on the sport, certain patients may need to go through a progression of sport-specific activities to return to play.

PROGNOSIS

- Prognosis depends on the extent of injury and any concurrent injuries, but for most patients, prognosis is excellent. More severe injuries may require more extensive rehabilitation for a patient to return to full function and prevent recurrence.
- Patients with recurrent instability and those in high-risk sports (e.g., volleyball, basketball) may benefit from functional bracing or taping.
- Patients who fail to undergo proper rehabilitation are often left with chronic instability and recurrent ankle injuries.

COMPLICATIONS

- Stiffness from prolonged immobilization
- Recurrent instability
- Osteochondral defects
- Fractures
- Chronic regional pain syndromes

REFERENCES

1. Roos KG, Kerr ZY, Mauntel TC, et al. The epidemiology of lateral ligament complex ankle sprains in National Collegiate Athletic Association sports. *Am J Sports Med.* 2017;45(1):201–209.
2. Fong DT, Chan YY, Mok KM, et al. Understanding acute ankle ligamentous sprain injury in sports. *Sports Med Arthrosc Rehabil Ther Technol.* 2009;1:14.
3. Herzog MM, Kerr ZY, Marshall SW, et al. Epidemiology of ankle sprains and chronic ankle instability. *J Athl Train.* 2019;54(6):603–610.
4. Nelson AJ, Collins CL, Yard EE, et al. Ankle injuries among United States high school sports athletes, 2005–2006. *J Athl Train.* 2007;42(3):381–387.
5. Chen ET, Borg-Stein J, McInnis KC. Ankle sprains: evaluation, rehabilitation, and prevention. *Curr Sports Med Rep.* 2019;18(6):217–223.
6. Stiell IG, Greenberg GH, McKnight RD, et al. A study to develop clinical decision rules for the use of radiography in acute ankle injuries. *Ann Emerg Med.* 1992;21(4):384–390.
7. Bellows R, Wong CK. The effect of bracing and balance training on ankle sprain incidence among athletes: a systematic review with meta-analysis. *Int J Sports Phys Ther.* 2018;13(3):379–388.

CLINICAL PEARLS

- Extremely common injury that can present with swelling, ecchymosis, and inability to walk.
- Thorough exam and proper imaging (when indicated) can help to avoid missing associated fractures.
- Musculoskeletal ultrasound can be diagnostic of level of ligament injury.
- Treatment involves progression from PRICE protocol to progressive weight-bearing and range of motion and finally to strengthening and proprioceptive exercises.

ANKLE SPRAINS, MEDIAL

Kari J. Rezac, DO ▪ Giorgio A. Negron, MD ▪ Daniel C. Herman, MD, PhD, FAAPMR, FACSM, FISBS, CAQSM

BASICS

DESCRIPTION

- Injury to the deltoid ligament complex of the medial ankle occurs when the foot is forced into eversion and external rotation.
- Medial ankle sprains are less common than their lateral counterpart due to the vast strength of the deltoid ligament (1),(2):
  - Deltoid ligament complex is composed of four superficial and two deep components (1),(3).
- Grade I sprain results from mild stretching of the deltoid ligament with microscopic tears (1). Patients have mild swelling and tenderness. There is no joint instability on exam, and the patient is able to bear weight and ambulate with minimal pain. Owing to their benign nature, these injuries are not seen frequently in the office.
- Grade II sprain is a more severe injury involving an incomplete tear of the deltoid ligament. Patients have moderate pain, swelling, tenderness, and ecchymosis (1). There is mild to moderate joint instability on exam with some restriction in the range of motion and loss of function. Weight-bearing and ambulation are painful.
- Grade III sprain involves a complete tear of the deltoid ligament (1). Patients have severe pain, swelling, tenderness, and ecchymosis. There is significant mechanical instability on exam and significant loss of function and motion. Patients are unable to bear weight or ambulate.
- May progress to chronic ankle instability (constant sensation of ankle "giving away") if lingering symptoms persist a year after initial ankle sprain (1),(3)
- Synonym(s): medial ankle sprain; deltoid ligament sprain

EPIDEMIOLOGY

- The majority (85%) of ankle sprains are of lateral etiology (2).
- Deltoid ligament sprains are often accompanied by a lateral malleolar fracture and/or syndesmotic injury (4).

RISK FACTORS

- Previous ankle sprain
- High-risk sports, including football, basketball, and long jumping
- Valgus-flat foot deformity (2)
- Low arch of the foot (i.e., pes planus) (2)
- Dysfunction of the spring ligament
- Dysfunction of the posterior tibialis tendon
- Extreme fatigue of peroneus (fibularis) longus muscle
- High body mass index (BMI) (2)

GENERAL PREVENTION

- Exercise therapy and taping/bracing are effective in the management of primary and recurrent ankle sprains (4),(5).
- Proprioceptive training appears to be effective in secondary prevention of ankle injuries (4),(5).

COMMONLY ASSOCIATED CONDITIONS

- Syndesmosis disruption
- Fracture of the fibula and/or tibia
- Avulsion fracture of the medial malleolus
- Bimalleolar and trimalleolar fractures
- Severe lateral ligament injury
- Spring ligament injury
- Posterior tibial tendon injury
- Flexor hallucis longus injury
- Posterior tibial and/or saphenous nerve traction injury

DIAGNOSIS

HISTORY

- Mechanism of injury: Athletes typically report an off-balanced, pronated foot landing, which leads to forced valgus stress in external rotation, abduction, and eversion (1),(3),(6).
- One should inquire about previous ankle injury and history of "giving way." This would suggest that there is an acute injury superimposed on chronic ankle instability (3),(6).

PHYSICAL EXAM

- Signs and symptoms include (1),(6):
  - Medial ankle pain
  - Swelling on the medial aspect of the ankle
  - Ecchymosis around the medial aspect of the ankle
  - Sensation of a "pop"
  - Inability to bear weight
- Physical examination (1),(4):
  - Evaluation of the ability to bear weight
  - Careful palpation to identify tender structures
  - Determination of tenderness over the deltoid ligament
  - A check for tenderness over the anterior syndesmosis ligament, the anterior process of the calcaneus, Achilles tendon, lateral ankle, and fibula (distal and proximal)
  - Check posterior tibial tendon function with resisted inversion strength testing.
  - Check extensor hallucis longus tendon function with resisted extension of the great toe.
  - Assess range of motion of the ankle joint.
  - Check flexor hallucis longus tendon function with resisted flexion of the great toe.
  - An eversion stress test determines the stability of the deltoid ligament; this is done with passive eversion of the ankle.
  - A squeeze test and external rotation test are highly specific tests to rule out syndesmotic injury.
  - An anterior drawer test may evaluate anterior and medial subluxation with deltoid ligament injury.
  - Examine the patient's gait and while standing for valgus-flat foot deformity.

DIFFERENTIAL DIAGNOSIS

- Syndesmosis tear or sprain
- Posterior tibial tendon tear or subluxation
- Flexor hallucis longus tendon tear or sprain
- Distal tibia fracture
- Osteochondral fracture of the talar dome
- Fracture of the calcaneus
- Fracture of the lateral process of the talus
- Medial ankle sprain with associated proximal fibular fracture (Maisonneuve fracture)

DIAGNOSTIC TESTS & INTERPRETATION

- In the setting of acute injury, follow the Ottawa Ankle Rules to determine if radiographs are indicated (inability to bear weight, tenderness over posterior edge or tip of lateral/medial malleolus, the base of the 5th metatarsal, or navicular bone) (1),(4)[A].
- Anteroposterior, lateral, and mortise weight-bearing views of the injured ankle are essential to rule out fracture when indicated (3),(4)[B].
- $>$3 mm of medial clear space between the lateral border of the medial malleolus and the medial border of the talus at the level of the talar dome is abnormal and suggestive of a deltoid ligament disruption (6)[C].
- Consider a valgus talar tilt stress radiograph to assess for significant instability and possible surgical treatment: $>$10 degrees difference in abduction tilt of the talus compared with the opposite ankle is abnormal (perform this test *only* if there are no associated fractures) (3),(6)[C].
- Magnetic resonance imaging (MRI) has high sensitivity and high specificity for injury to superficial/deep deltoid ligaments. Consider MRI if deltoid ligament rupture is unclear (partial vs. complete) and surgical treatment is being considered (1),(3),(4)[C].
- Ultrasonography may be an alternative when MRI is not readily available (high sensitivity and high specificity) (1),(4)[C].

TREATMENT

GENERAL MEASURES

Prehospital:

- PRICE protocol: protection from further injury, rest, ice, compression, and elevation for up to 1 to 3 weeks depending on symptom severity (1),(2),(3)[C]
- Protection can be achieved through an Aircast or a boot with a bladder to restrict inversion/eversion stress while also maintaining sagittal plane motion.
- Rest is achieved by limiting weight-bearing by having patients use crutches or other assistive devices until they are able to walk with a normal gait.
- Ice or cold-water immersion is recommended for 15 to 20 minutes q2–3h for the first 48 hours or until swelling improves, whichever comes first.
- Compression to control and decrease swelling should be applied early, usually with a compressive wrap or stirrup brace. Compression should be supportive but not constrictive.
- The injured ankle should be kept elevated above the level of the heart to further alleviate swelling.

ISSUES FOR REFERRAL

- >4 mm of medial clear space on the mortise view (weight-bearing)
- Significant instability on reverse talar tilt stress radiograph or weight-bearing views (4)[C]
- Grade III injury may need operative repair to prevent long-term complications (1),(4)[C].
- Medial malleolus fracture
- Displaced lateral malleolus fracture (may be functionally a bimalleolar fracture)
- Wound penetrating into the joint
- Nonsurgical treatment has failed for >12 months and the injury has progressed to chronic ankle instability (1),(2),(3)[C].
- Patients with neurovascular compromise
- Uncertain diagnosis

ADDITIONAL THERAPIES

- Grade I sprain: functional rehabilitation and possibly a splint or a brace, with the recognition that return to sports generally is more delayed (3 to 6 weeks) than with a lateral sprain (1 to 3 weeks) (1),(6)[C]
- Grade II sprain: same as grade 1, but in addition, may need a short period prior of immobilization in posterior splint or walking boot (3 to 4 weeks) (1)[C]
- Grade III sprain: Treatment is controversial; requires immobilization (6 to 8 weeks) or may need operative repair (see "Issues for Referral") (1),(5)[C]
- Nonsteroidal anti-inflammatory drugs (NSAIDs) are the first-line medication for pain control (4),(5)[A].
- After pain and swelling subside, patient can be transitioned to lace up ankle stabilization brace and begin course of stabilization, proprioception, and strength training to prevent chronic instability (3)[C].
- The exercises should begin as soon as the initial pain and swelling have subsided sufficiently to allow the patient to perform simple exercises and should continue until the patient has returned to pain-free activity (4),(5)[A].
- Exercises can include:
  - Achilles tendon stretch
  - Foot circles
  - Alphabet exercises: Although leg is stable, patient should use the great toe and foot to "write" the letters of the alphabet in the air.
  - Isometric and isotonic plantar flexion, dorsiflexion, inversion, eversion, and toe curls
  - Marble pickups (using toes)
  - Heel walks
  - Toe walks
  - Circular wobble board
  - Walking on different surfaces
  - Walk–jog, jog–run
- Splinting, bracing, and taping help to reduce instability and protect the ankle from further injury (4),(5)[A].
- Return to sport may be aided by further foot and ankle support with orthotics (3)[C].

COMPLEMENTARY & ALTERNATIVE MEDICINE

- Neither ultrasound therapy, low-level laser therapy, nor hyperbaric therapy appears to be effective in the treatment of medial ankle sprains (5)[B].
- Platelet-rich plasma (PRP) injection for ankle sprains may decrease pain scores and allow for quicker return to play, but more research is needed (4)[C].

ONGOING CARE

PROGNOSIS

- Pain decreases rapidly during the first 2 weeks following injury:
  - Up to 70% of patients report residual symptoms or recurrence (2).
- Ongoing, refractory medial ankle symptoms and instability after significant conservative management may require surgical management. However, further research needs to be performed on surgical outcomes of medial ankle instability operative management (3),(6)[B].

COMPLICATIONS

Deltoid ligament injury generally is a more serious injury than lateral ankle sprain and frequently is associated with concomitant injury to the lateral ligaments or fibula (3),(4)[C].

Geriatric Considerations

Higher age and low baseline activity level are associated with poor recovery in ankle sprains (2)[B]. Due to this, aggressive nonsurgical measurements should be started including low threshold for imaging, delayed weight-bearing, and consideration of immobilization/bracing.

REFERENCES

1. Czajka CM, Tran E, Cai AN, et al. Ankle sprains and instability. *Med Clin North Am.* 2014;98(2):313–329.
2. Ferreira JN, Vide J, Mendes D, et al. Prognostic factors in ankle sprains: a review. *EFORT Open Rev.* 2020;5(6):334–338.
3. Pflüger P, Valderrabano V. Sprain of the medial ankle ligament complex. *Foot Ankle Clin.* 2023;28(2):355–367.
4. Chen ET, Borg-Stein J, McInnis KC. Ankle sprains: evaluation, rehabilitation, and prevention. *Curr Sports Med Rep.* 2019;18(6):217–223.
5. Doherty C, Bleakley C, Delahunt E, et al. Treatment and prevention of acute and recurrent ankle sprain: an overview of systematic reviews with meta-analysis. *Br J Sports Med.* 2017;51(2):113–125.
6. Gopinath R, Pigott M, Lindsey B, et al. Medial ankle instability: review of anatomy, evaluation, and treatment. *Foot Ankle Spec.* 2022;15(6):573–578.

ADDITIONAL READING

- Birrer RB, Fani-Salek MH, Totten VY, et al. Managing ankle injuries in the emergency department. *J Emerg Med.* 1999;17(4):651–660.
- Mei-Dan O, Kahn G, Zeev A, et al. The medial longitudinal arch as a possible risk factor for ankle sprains: a prospective study in 83 female infantry recruits. *Foot Ankle Int.* 2005;26(2):180–183.

CLINICAL PEARLS

- An athlete may return to full activity once he or she is able to do a progressive rehabilitation program without pain and instability. Return to sports may be prolonged over several months depending on the degree of injury.
- To prevent future injuries, athlete should wear an ankle brace for sporting activities and complete rehabilitation.
- Untreated, severe sprain may result in chronic pain, instability, and the possibility of ankle arthritis.
- Effect of external ankle support on performance:
  - Dependent on the specific brace or method (such as taping) used
  - Decrease in performance ≤5%

ANKYLOSING SPONDYLITIS

Kevin deWeber, MD, FAMSSM, FAAFP, FACSM, RMSK

BASICS

DESCRIPTION

- Ankylosing spondylitis (AS) is a chronic inflammatory, autoimmune arthritis characterized by inflammatory back pain (IBP).
- Most common and potentially severe subtype of spondyloarthritis (SpA)
- Causes inflammation of the sacroiliac (SI) joints, peripheral joints, and entheses (sites where ligaments or tendons attach to bone)
- Common sites for enthesitis include:
  - Calcaneus (Achilles and plantar fascia insertions)
  - Patella
  - Tibial tubercle
  - Vertebral bodies
- Vertebral body enthesitis leads to the characteristic findings of syndesmophytes (vertical bony growths) and eventual fusion, which are responsible for the classic radiographic "bamboo" appearance of the spine in advanced disease.

EPIDEMIOLOGY

Incidence

- Overall incidence: 0.5 to 8.2/100,000 per year
- Incidence rate varies directly with prevalence of human leukocyte antigen (HLA)-B27 in given population.
- Commonly presents in young adulthood
- Predominant age:
  - 80% with AS develop symptoms before age 30 years.
  - <5% of patients with AS present after age 45 years.
- Predominant gender: male > female (~3:1)

Prevalence

- Prevalence of AS is 9 to 30/10,000 depending on HLA-B27 prevalence in the population (1).
- Higher in Alaskan Eskimos and some Native American populations owing to higher than average HLA-B27 rate
- Lower in African Americans secondary to a lower HLA-B27 rate
- Up to 5% of patients evaluated for chronic low back pain are ultimately diagnosed with AS.

ETIOLOGY AND PATHOPHYSIOLOGY

- A clear etiologic pathway has not been established.
- Speculated that an environmental/infectious trigger in a genetically susceptible individual leads to an inflammatory (T cell and macrophage) immune response that specifically targets SI, peripheral joint, and enthesis inflammation, eventually causing bony proliferation, erosions, sclerosis, and joint destruction

Genetics

- Expression of HLA-B27 antigen is clearly linked to the development of AS, but the exact mechanism is unknown.
- 90% of persons with AS are HLA-B27 positive, but HLA-B27–positive persons have 5% chance of having AS.
- Prevalence of HLA-B27 in Caucasians is 8%, and African Americans 2–4%.

RISK FACTORS

- Positive family history of SpA or HLA-B27
- Reactive arthritis triggered by *Chlamydia trachomatis* and certain enteric infections (e.g., *Shigella*, *Salmonella*, *Yersinia*, and *Campylobacter* spp.) predisposes to development of AS.

GENERAL PREVENTION

- Currently no preventive therapies or screening tests
- Early recognition and initiation of treatment can prevent disease progression and complications; unfortunately, it is common for there to be 5 to 6 years delay in diagnosis.

COMMONLY ASSOCIATED CONDITIONS

- Enthesitis—29% (e.g., calcaneus, patella, tibia) (2)
- Uveitis/iritis—23%
- Psoriasis—10%
- Dactylitis—6%
- Inflammatory bowel disease (IBD)—4%
- Rarely, cardiac valve/aortic root involvement

DIAGNOSIS

- Diagnosis is primarily based on history of IBP (see "History") and exam findings with imaging used to confirm diagnosis.
  - Clinical criteria:
    - Low back pain with onset <45 years for at least 3 months duration, with stiffness that improves with exercise but is not relieved by rest
  - Radiologic criteria (anteroposterior [AP] pelvis):
    - Bilateral sacroiliitis grades 2 to 4 *or*
    - Unilateral sacroiliitis grade 3 or 4
- If both clinical and radiologic criteria are positive, the patient has AS.
- If radiographs are negative, the Assessment for SpondyloArthritis International Society (ASAS) criteria are helpful (3)[A]:
  - Age of onset <45 years and >3 months of back pain
  - Sacroiliitis on imaging + one SpA feature *or* positive HLA-B27 + two SpA features:
    - SpA features: IBP, arthritis, enthesitis, uveitis, dactylitis, psoriasis, IBD, responds to nonsteroidal anti-inflammatory drugs (NSAIDs), family history of SpA, HLA-B27 positive, elevated C-reactive protein (CRP)
  - 82.9% sensitive, 84.4% specific for SpA
- AS without confirmed radiographic findings is classified as nonradiographic axial spondyloarthropathy (nr-axSpA) and has similar outcomes and response to treatment.

HISTORY

- 3 months of back pain with insidious onset
- IBP: morning stiffness >30 minutes, improves with exercise but not with rest, alternating buttock pain, back pain at night

PHYSICAL EXAM

Physical exam should include assessment of:

- Entire spine: range of motion, tenderness (although clinical spinal mobility measurements do not correlate with degree of inflammation or radiographic measure of spinal mobility):
  - Decreased lumbar motion is often severe. Quantify with Schober test: Mark area on patient's midline of back at L5 and 10 cm above that point. Have patient bend forward and then remeasure that distance. Normal is >15 cm in flexion.
  - Decreased cervical motion may be present.
- Peripheral joints, especially in the lower extremity: limited range of motion, inflammatory signs such as effusion, warmth, tenderness
- Major entheses: calcaneus for Achilles and plantar fascia attachments, patella, tibial tubercle
- Eyes: inflammatory changes (may require slit-lamp exam; consider ophthalmology referral)
- Skin: rash characteristic of psoriasis

DIFFERENTIAL DIAGNOSIS

- Mechanical low back pain
- Myofascial low back pain
- SI joint dysfunction
- Herniated nucleus pulposus
- Degenerative spinal disease
- Spondylolysis/spondylolisthesis
- Discitis
- Other causes of SpA
  - Reactive (Reiter) arthritis
  - IBD associated spondylitis
  - Psoriatic spondylitis

DIAGNOSTIC TESTS & INTERPRETATION

Initial Tests (lab, imaging)

- If the history suggests chronic IBP, initial testing should include blood tests for HLA-B27, CRP, and erythrocyte sedimentation rate (ESR); and plain radiographs of the lumbar spine and SI joints.
- HLA-B27: See "Genetics."
- CRP and ESR can be elevated in 50–70% of patients with AS, but normal values do not negate presence of disease. Levels in patients with established disease do not correlate with disease activity.
- Sacroiliitis on radiographs is a hallmark of disease, but its absence does not rule out inflammation or AS.
  - Severity is graded 1 (suspicious), 2 (minimal), 3 (moderate), or 4 (ankylosis).
  - Structural changes may take several years to show on radiographs.
  - In established AS, 95% of patients have detectable structural changes.

Follow-Up Tests & Special Considerations

- Magnetic resonance imaging (MRI) (T2 and short-tau inversion recovery [STIR]):
  - Useful to identify early inflammatory changes before structural changes are apparent on plain radiographs
  - Less sensitive than plain radiographs to assess degree of structural changes
- Computed tomography (CT) scan:
  - Can detect chronic changes in SI joints, although role is limited due to high radiation exposure and the high sensitivity of the other imaging modalities

TREATMENT

GENERAL MEASURES

- A multidisciplinary approach of drug therapy along with exercise/physiotherapy helps decrease disease activity and progression while improving function.
- Treatment is generally lifelong and divided into active versus stable disease.

- Recent literature reviews performed by American College of Rheumatology, Spondylitis Association of America, and Spondyloarthritis Research and Treatment Network have provided the latest guidelines for treatment and are reviewed here.
- Treatment same for AS and nr-axSpA

MEDICATION

Depending on location and severity of disease, the following treatment modalities may be indicated:

- NSAIDs
- Disease-modifying antirheumatic drugs (DMARDs):
  - Tumor necrosis factor inhibitors (TNFi)
  - Interleukin-17A inhibitors
  - Janus kinase (JAK) inhibitors (classified as targeted synthetic DMARDs)
  - Conventional synthetic (cs) DMARDs
- Corticosteroid injections into inflamed joints:
  - No role for systemic glucocorticoids

First Line

NSAIDs (4)[A]:

- No one NSAID recommended over another
- Use full dose and regular scheduling to maximize symptom relief for active disease; use as needed for stable disease.
- Beneficial for both axial (spine) and peripheral (joint, enthesis) involvement
- Data suggest that long-term therapy may have disease-controlling properties evidenced by suppression of radiographic progression.
- Trial of two NSAID classes for 1 to 2 months each prior to moving onto second-line therapy
- Monitor for gastrointestinal (GI), cardiovascular, renal, and hepatic side effects.

Second Line

- TNFi (4)[A]:
  - Infliximab, adalimumab, etanercept and others
  - No clear recommendation for one TNFi versus another; infliximab and adalimumab considered for recurrent iritis or concomitant IBD
  - With extended therapy, up to 1/3 of patients may develop remission.
  - TNFi increases risk for infection; screen for tuberculosis, HIV, and hepatitis before initiating. Ensure vaccinations are up to date; do not give live vaccines while on therapy.
- Interleukin-17A inhibitor (5)[A]
  - Recommended if no response to NSAIDs and one TNFi
  - Secukinumab has shown significant reduction in signs/symptoms of disease.
  - Ixekizumab has shown to improve signs/symptoms in patients not previously treated with csDMARDs.
- JAK inhibitor (6)[C]:
  - U.S. Food and Drug Administration (FDA)-approved for treatment with upadacitinib and tofacitinib in patients without benefit or intolerance of ≥1 TNFi
- csDMARDs (e.g., sulfasalazine) (4)[A]:
  - Consider use prior to TNFi after failure to NSAID in patients with predominant peripheral joint disease.
  - No role for methotrexate

ISSUES FOR REFERRAL

- Early rheumatology referral for patients with IBP may help prevent a delay in diagnosis and can help with initiating biologics.
- Refer to ophthalmology if signs/symptoms of iritis, which may consider prescription of topical steroids to use PRN for flares.

ADDITIONAL THERAPIES

- Physical therapy helps improve spinal mobility and overall function (7)[A].
- Supervised training and home exercises improve long-term functional outcomes when compared to no intervention or educational/behavioral intervention.

SURGERY/OTHER PROCEDURES

- Local corticosteroid injections: for isolated sacroiliitis or peripheral joint disease if more than three joints involved
- Hip arthroplasty as indicated for progressive arthropathy
- Thoracolumbar osteotomy can be considered for severe kyphotic disease, or cervicothoracic osteotomy for chin to chest deformity to restore horizontal gaze, but should be performed at specialized spine centers.

ONGOING CARE

FOLLOW-UP RECOMMENDATIONS

Patient Monitoring

- Monitor response to treatment using CRP and validated AS disease activity measures (Bath Ankylosing Spondylitis Disease Activity Index [BASDAI], Bath Ankylosing Spondylitis Functional Index [BASFI], or Ankylosing Spondylitis Disease Activity Score [ASDAS]) (8)[A].
- The BASDAI is a valid and appropriate composite to quantify disease activity during treatment:
  - Five major symptoms (fatigue, spinal pain, joint pain/swelling, areas of tenderness, and duration/severity of morning stiffness) are individually rated on 0 to 10 scale.

PROGNOSIS

- The key to good outcomes and prevention of disease progression and severe complications is early recognition and initiation of treatment.
- AS has an unpredictable clinical course independent of age of onset or sex.
- Most patients have a fluctuating course with flares and periods of relative remission.

COMPLICATIONS

- Fusion of vertebrae leading to loss of function or restrictive lung disease
- Aortitis or aortic insufficiency (rare)
- Hip arthritis with refractory pain or disability requiring arthroplasty

REFERENCES

1. Wang R, Ward MM. Epidemiology of axial spondyloarthritis: an update. *Curr Opin Rheumatol.* 2018;30(2):137–143.
2. de Winter JJ, van Mens LJ, van der Heijde D, et al. Prevalence of peripheral and extra-articular disease in ankylosing spondylitis versus non-radiographic axial spondyloarthritis: a meta-analysis. *Arthritis Res Ther.* 2016;18(1):196.
3. Sieper J, van der Heijde D, Landewé R, et al. New criteria for inflammatory back pain in patients with chronic back pain: a real patient exercise of the Assessment in SpondyloArthritis International Society (ASAS). *Ann Rheum Dis.* 2009;68(6):784–788.
4. Ward MM, Deodhar A, Akl EA, et al. American College of Rheumatology/Spondylitis Association of America/Spondyloarthritis Research and Treatment Network 2015 recommendations for the treatment of ankylosing spondylitis and nonradiographic axial spondyloarthritis. *Arthritis Rheumatol.* 2016;68(2):282–298.
5. Ward, MM, Deodhar A, Gensler LS, et al. 2019 Update of the American College of Rheumatology/Spondylitis Association of America/Spondyloarthritis Research and Treatment Network recommendations for the treatment of ankylosing spondylitis and nonradiographic axial spondyloarthritis. *Arthritis Rheumatol.* 2019;71(10):1599–1613.
6. van der Heijde D, Baraliakos X, Sieper J, et al. Efficacy and safety of upadacitinib for active ankylosing spondylitis refractory to biological therapy: a double-blind, randomised, placebo-controlled phase 3 trial. *Ann Rheum Dis.* 2022;81(11):1515–1523.
7. Braun J, Baraliakos X, Deodhar A, et al. Effect of secukinumab on clinical and radiographic outcomes in ankylosing spondylitis: 2-year results from the randomised phase III MEASURE 1 study. *Ann Rheumatic Dis.* 2017;76(6):1070–1077.
8. Dagfinrud H, Kvien TK, Hagen KB. Physiotherapy interventions for ankylosing spondylitis. *Cochrane Database Syst Rev.* 2008;(1):CD002822.

ADDITIONAL READING

- Braun J, Sieper J. Ankylosing spondylitis. *Lancet.* 2007;369(9570):1379–1390.
- Sieper J, Rudwaleit M, Khan MA, et al. Concepts and epidemiology of spondyloarthritis. *Best Pract Res Clin Rheumatol.* 2006;20(3):401–417.

CLINICAL PEARLS

- Diagnosing AS requires a history of chronic IBP (significant stiffness after immobilization, improvement after exercise, responsive to NSAIDs) with supporting findings of positive HLA-B27, positive inflammatory blood markers, and imaging showing sacroiliitis.
- Not all AS fits this paradigm, and some AS takes years to develop all criteria.
- If SI radiographs are normal, MRI can show early inflammation.
- Early diagnosis may be critical to control symptoms, slow disease progression, and prevent irreversible changes.
- Treatment is multimodal and typically includes NSAIDs ± DMARDs, physical therapy, and home exercises.

ANTERIOR INTEROSSEOUS SYNDROME

Jennifer Oberstar, MD, CAQSM ▪ Jarrod Yamanaka, MD, CAQSM

BASICS

- The anterior interosseous nerve (AIN) is a motor branch of the median nerve that innervates the pronator quadratus (PQ), flexor pollicis longus (FPL), and flexor digitorum profundus serving the index finger.
- Forearm pain that progresses to palsy of deep forearm muscles and weakness of thumb and/or index finger flexion
- *Anterior interosseous syndrome* (AIS) is a "catch-all" term for neuropathies that result in paralysis of these muscles secondary to several causes.
- Rare, comprising <1% of all upper limb nerve syndromes (1)
- Associated with diabetes, HIV, nutritional deficiencies
- Form of neuralgic amyotrophy, immune-mediated process (2)
- Acute fascicular axonopathy presenting with a prodrome of severe shoulder, arm, or elbow pain followed by clinical and electrodiagnostic palsy of ≥1 AIN-innervated muscle (2)
- Overall, AIS is a rare condition with a paucity of research (3).

ETIOLOGY AND PATHOPHYSIOLOGY

The most frequent causes of AIS occurrence are direct traumatic nerve damage and external compression. Insidious onset of the condition thought to be a transient neuritis, although pathophysiology remains unclear (1).

- Traumatic causes:
  - Penetrating trauma
  - Blunt injury
  - Traction injury
  - Chronic vibration (cyclists)
  - Fracture (supracondylar fracture in children)
  - Surgery
  - Venipuncture
  - Injection
  - Cast pressure
- External compression:
  - Bulky, tendinous origin of the deep head of the pronator teres
  - Soft tissue mass such as lipoma, ganglion, hematoma, or tumor
  - Accessory muscle
  - Fibrous band originating from the superficial flexor
  - Vascular abnormality
  - Pregnancy

DIAGNOSIS

HISTORY

- Pain in the forearm
- Sensory loss not present
- Weakness noted as difficulty with writing or with fine-pinch activities

PHYSICAL EXAM

- The signature finding is weakness of the FPL, flexor digitorum profundus (index finger and partial innervation of the 3rd digit), as well as PQ.
- Weakness of the FPL and flexor digitorum profundus to the index finger is indicated by an inability to make the "OK sign." Rather, the distal interphalangeal (DIP) joint of the index finger and interphalangeal (IP) joint of the thumb are hyperextended during attempted tip-to-tip pinch.
- The PQ is difficult to isolate clinically. Weakness may be detected by asking the patient to forcibly pronate the forearm against resistance with the elbow flexed at 90 degrees (3)[C].
- Negative Phalen and Tinel tests at the wrist
- The AIN provides no sensory fibers to the skin; therefore, abnormal sensation testing suggests another etiology (3)[C].

DIFFERENTIAL DIAGNOSIS

- Tendon rupture
- Brachial plexus neuritis (Parsonage-Turner syndrome)
- Congenital absence of the flexor digitorum longus and FPL
- Partial lesion of the median nerve

DIAGNOSTIC TESTS & INTERPRETATION

- Electrodiagnostic testing (2)[C]:
  - Electromyography (EMG) demonstrates abnormal activity in FPL and PQ.
  - No motor fascicles of the median nerve, which exceeds the territory of the AIN, were observed to be affected.
  - Should include EMG of the FPL, PQ, and flexor digitorum profundus (index and long finger)
  - The latency and amplitude of compound muscle action potential are compared with those of the unaffected side.
  - Sensory nerve action potentials are normal.
- Imaging modalities:
  - Both magnetic resonance imaging (MRI) and ultrasound (US) may be helpful in confirming the clinical diagnosis of AIS.
  - MRI findings of edema in the muscles innervated by the AIN on T2-weighted fat-suppressed images

– MRI 45% revealed increased signal intensity in the non-AIN innervated muscles.
  ○ High-resolution MRI—mononeuropathy of AIN motor fascicles that exists within the median nerve at the upper arm level
– The AIN may appear swollen on US when compared with the normal contralateral nerve.
– US of the AIN-innervated muscles may show a loss of bulk, increased reflectivity, reduced perfusion on Doppler sonography, and lack of active contraction of the affected muscles.

TREATMENT

- Once an accurate diagnosis of AIS is made, treatment must be guided by the underlying etiology (1)[C].
- Penetrating trauma suggests nerve disruption or compression and is best treated with surgical exploration and nerve decompression or repair.
- With blunt trauma, an EMG suggestive of a complete lesion may mandate early surgical exploration. Partial injuries may be given an opportunity to recover spontaneously. If no improvement is noted after 6 to 12 weeks of nonsurgical management, surgical exploration is necessary (4)[C].
- The typical nonsurgical treatment regimen includes rest, splinting, and observation.
- Spontaneous paralysis of the AIN may be treated nonsurgically for 12 weeks with surgical exploration if no clinical or EMG improvement is evident (4)[C].
- Spontaneous recovery is not ensured.
- Some advocate nonsurgical management for at least 6 months before proceeding with surgical exploration in cases of transient neuritis.
- Consider alternative causes of neuritis if lack of resolution after 6 months.
- Tendon transfers allow functional reconstruction of the thumb and index finger should the AIN fail to recover, fail tendon reconstruction, or irreversible muscle atrophy is present after prolonged muscle denervation.

REFERENCES

1. Li N, Russo K, Rando L, et al. Anterior interosseous nerve syndrome. *Ortho Rev*. 2022;14(4):38678.
2. Krishnan KR, Sneag DB, Feinberg JH, et al. Anterior interosseous nerve syndrome reconsidered: a critical analysis review. *JBJS Rev*. 2020;8(9):e2000011.
3. Rodner CM, Tinsley BA, O'Malley MP. Pronator syndrome and anterior interosseous nerve syndrome. *J Am Acad Orthop Surg*. 2013;21(5):268–275.
4. Pham M, Bäumer P, Meinck H, et al. Anterior interosseous nerve syndrome: fascicular motor lesions of median nerve trunk. *Neurology*. 2014;82(7):598–606.

ADDITIONAL READING

- Dang AC, Rodner CM. Unusual compression neuropathies of the forearm, part II: median nerve. *J Hand Surg Am*. 2009;34(10):1915–1920.
- Dunn AJ, Salonen DC, Anastakis DJ. MR imaging findings of anterior interosseous nerve lesions. *Skeletal Radiol*. 2007;36(12):1155–1162.
- Na K, Jang D, Lee Y, et al. Anterior interosseous nerve syndrome: is it a compressive neuropathy? *Indian J Orthop*. 2020;54(Suppl 1):193–198.
- Singh V, Ericson WB. Median nerve entrapments. In: Trescot AM, ed. *Peripheral Nerve Entrapments: Clinical Diagnosis and Management*. Springer; 2016:369–382.
- Sneag DB, Arányi Z, Zusstone EM, et al. Fascicular constrictions above elbow typify anterior interosseous nerve syndrome. *Muscle Nerve*. 2020;61(3):301–310.

CLINICAL PEARLS

- Dysfunction of the AIN is characterized by weakness of the PQ, FPL, and flexor digitorum profundus of the index finger.
- On examination, the patient cannot make the "OK sign" with the thumb and index finger.
- The AIN does not provide sensory nerves to the skin; therefore, abnormal sensation suggests an alternative diagnosis.
- Penetrating trauma or blunt trauma with an EMG suggestive of a complete AIN lesion mandates surgical exploration.
- Insidious onset of condition can signify transient neuritis; usually resolves in 6 months
- Intense rehabilitation is first-line treatment.

ANTERIOR METATARSALGIA

Thomas P. Bell, MD ▪ Kenneth M. Bielak, MD, MBA, FAAFP, FACSM

BASICS

DESCRIPTION

- Pain in the plantar aspect of the metatarsal (MT) heads
- Metatarsalgia can be thought of as a symptom rather than a specific disease.
- Primary metatarsalgia develops from intrinsic factors, such as a long first ray, hallux valgus, or other congenital deformities.
- Secondary metatarsalgia may result from trauma, infectious process, inflammatory process, overuse, or poor footwear.

EPIDEMIOLOGY

Athletes in high-impact sports involving the lower extremities (dancing, running, jumping)

ETIOLOGY AND PATHOPHYSIOLOGY

- Repetitive/excessive stress combined with intrinsic and extrinsic factors
- The 1st MT head usually carries 30% of the load in weight-bearing. A normal MT arch ensures this balance by providing adequate padding around the 1st MT head. A pronated or splayfoot can disturb this balance, resulting in an abnormally high pressure over the 2nd through 5th MT heads. Over time, reactive tissue can form a callus around the MT heads, which further compounds pain.
- Abnormal biomechanics in the gait cycle can result in MT pain and are identified in the different stages of the gait cycle (1)[C].
- Biomechanical factors explain 90% of all cases of metatarsalgia (2)[C].

RISK FACTORS

- Foot deformities: overpronation, pes planus, pes cavus, hallux valgus, prominent MT heads, hammertoe deformity, Morton foot (short 1st MT and a relatively long 2nd MT)
- Muscle imbalance or soft tissue dysfunction: tight Achilles tendon or toe extensors, weak toe flexors, laxity in the Lisfranc ligament
- Extrinsic factors: obesity, high heels, poorly fitted or worn-down shoes
- Dermatologic issues: calluses and warts
- Fat pad atrophy or displacement
- Iatrogenic changes from surgeries resulting in unequal force distribution

GENERAL PREVENTION

- Wear properly fitted shoes with adequate padding.
- Gradual progression of weight-bearing exercise programs

COMMONLY ASSOCIATED CONDITIONS

- Intrinsic foot muscle weakness
- Calluses and warts
- Hallux valgus or rigidus
- Hammertoe or claw toe
- Morton syndrome (long 2nd MT)
- Freiberg infraction (aseptic necrosis of an MT head, most commonly the 2nd, as seen in adolescent sprinters)

DIAGNOSIS

HISTORY

- Pain over the plantar surface of the MT heads, typically described as walking with a "pebble in the shoe"
- Pain is typically gradual and chronic in onset rather than acute.
- Pain is worse in midstance and propulsion phases of walking and running.

PHYSICAL EXAM

- Inspect for the presence of callus, edema, erythema, deformity, and skin breaks.
- Palpate for tenderness, which is typically located over the distal half of the MT shaft and head.
- Pain in the interdigital space or positive MT squeeze test suggests interdigital neuroma.
- Range of motion of the phalanges, metatarsophalangeal (MTP) joint, and ankle, especially to dorsiflexion, to evaluate tight gastrocsoleus complex
- Gait analysis should be performed.

DIFFERENTIAL DIAGNOSIS

- Neuroma (plantar or Morton neuroma)
- Idiopathic MTP joint synovitis
- Freiberg disease: ischemic epiphyseal necrosis of the 2nd MT
- Inflammatory arthritis of MT joint (rheumatoid arthritis, seronegative spondyloarthropathy, crystalline-induced arthritis, osteoarthritis, septic arthritis)
- Stress fracture
- Salter I fracture (pediatric population)
- Sesamoiditis or sesamoid fracture
- Lisfranc injury
- Traumatic arthritis
- Foreign body
- Cellulitis or infection (diabetic foot, Lyme disease)
- Ganglion cyst
- Vasculitis (diabetes)
- Tumor (rare)

DIAGNOSTIC TESTS & INTERPRETATION

Initial Tests (lab, imaging)

- Lab usually not required but may be considered based on differential diagnosis
- White blood cell (WBC) count and erythrocyte sedimentation rate (ESR) may be elevated in infection or inflammatory arthritis.
- Consider testing for:
  - Gout—uric acid level
  - Pseudogout—synovial fluid
  - Systemic disease—rheumatoid factor
- Imaging usually not required but may be considered based on differential diagnosis
- Weight-bearing anteroposterior (AP), lateral, and oblique films often normal but may demonstrate foot deformities that may predispose to metatarsalgia
- Bone scan or magnetic resonance imaging (MRI) may be considered based on suspicion for stress fracture.
- Ultrasonography can be used to evaluate for neuromas, bursitis, and joint effusions.

Diagnostic Procedures/Other

- Diagnostic injection (MTP joint) with local anesthetic can help differentiate intra-articular pathology (synovitis/capsulitis) from extra-articular pathology (neuroma).
- Plantar pressure distribution analysis may help to distinguish patterns of pressure distribution due to malalignment.

TREATMENT

- Acute:
  - Ice and rest with activity modification
  - Well-cushioned, correctly fitted athletic shoes
  - Analgesics such as acetaminophen or nonsteroidal anti-inflammatory drugs (NSAIDs)

- Calluses should be pared down, preferably after soaking the foot in warm water and using a stone or emery board.
- An MT pad may be placed just proximal to the MT heads to relieve pressure (avoid the pad directly beneath MT heads).
- Stretching a tight Achilles tendon
- Long-term treatment:
  - Prescriptive orthotics are beneficial:
    - Pes cavus
    - Hallux valgus
    - Intermetatarsal bursitis (3)[B]
  - Arch support and a well-fitted, low-heel shoe for daily wear
  - Weight loss decreases the load on the MT pads.
  - Energy-absorbing running shoes, which are replaced every 350 miles or when showing early wear
  - Maintenance of gastrocsoleus flexibility
  - Physical therapy for the correction of postural or gait imbalance
  - Avoid hard surfaces and prolonged standing.

MEDICATION

Analgesics, NSAIDs, or acetaminophen for symptom control

ISSUES FOR REFERRAL

- Athletes may warrant early podiatric or orthopedic evaluation.
- If no improvement with conservative therapy for 3 to 6 months, consider referral to foot/ankle orthopedist or surgical podiatrist.
- Multiple types of osteotomies with varying success rates have been described as surgical interventions for metatarsalgia.
- The Weil osteotomy, which is a shortening osteotomy performed to decrease pressure on a prominent MT head and performed by shifting the MT head back toward the heel, appears to be a safe and effective surgical procedure for the treatment for metatarsalgia of the 2nd and 3rd MT (4)[B].
- More recently, percutaneous surgical techniques have been developed, which in retrospective analysis, show significantly better long-term outcomes and lower rates of late metatarsalgia compared to open procedures (5)[B].
- Proximal medial gastrocnemius release (PMGR) helps to relieve tension in the Achilles-calcaneus-plantar system, useful in second rocker metatarsalgia (6)[C].

ADDITIONAL THERAPIES

Corticosteroid injection should be avoided because it may cause fat pad atrophy.

ONGOING CARE

PATIENT EDUCATION

- Instruct patient about wearing proper shoes and gradual return to activity.
- Cross training until symptoms subside

COMPLICATIONS

- Back, knee, and hip pain owing to compensatory gait change
- Transfer metatarsalgia following surgical intervention as stress transfers to other areas.

REFERENCES

1. Lopez V, Slullitel G. Metatarsalgia: assessment algorithm and decision making. *Foot Ankle Clin*. 2019;24(4):561–569.
2. Besse JL. Metatarsalgia. *Orthop Traumatol Surg Res*. 2017;103(1S):S29–S39.
3. Albano D, Bonifacini C, Zannoni S, et al. Plantar forefoot pain: ultrasound findings before and after treatment with custom-made foot orthoses. *Radiol Med*. 2021;126(7):963–970.
4. Pérez-Muñoz I, Escobar-Antón D, Sanz-Gómez TA. The role of Weil and triple Weil osteotomies in the treatment of propulsive metatarsalgia. *Foot Ankle Int*. 2012;33(6):501–506.
5. Bauer T, Gaumetou E, Klouche S, et al. Metatarsalgia and Morton's disease: comparison of outcomes between open procedure and neurectomy versus percutaneous metatarsal osteotomies and ligament release with a minimum of 2 years of follow-up. *J Foot Ankle Surg*. 2015;54(3):373–377.
6. Gamba C, Álvarez Gomez C, Martínez Zaragoza J, et al. Proximal medial gastrocnemius release: surgical technique. *JBJS Essent Surg Tech*. 2022;12(1):e20.00039.

ADDITIONAL READING

- Baker CL, Flandry F, Henderson JM, eds. Reactive synovitis of the foot—metatarsalgia. In: *The Hughston Clinic Sports Medicine Field Manual*. Williams & Wilkins; 1996:270.
- Besse JL. Metatarsalgia. *Orthop Traumatol Surg Res*. 2017;103(1S):S29–S39.
- DiPreta JA. Metatarsalgia, lesser toe deformities, and associated disorders of the forefoot. *Med Clin North Am*. 2014;98(2):233–251.
- Espinosa N, Maceira E, Myerson MS. Current concept review: metatarsalgia. *Foot Ankle Int*. 2008;29(8):871–879.
- Federer AE, Tainter DM, Adams SB, et al. Conservative management of metatarsalgia and lesser toe deformities. *Foot Ankle Clin*. 2018;23(1):9–20.
- Gregg J, Marks P. Metatarsalgia: an ultrasound perspective. *Australas Radiol*. 2007;51(6):493–499.
- Gregg JM, Schneider T, Marks P. MR imaging and ultrasound of metatarsalgia—the lesser metatarsals. *Radiol Clin North Am*. 2008;46(6):1061–1078.
- Johansen JK, Jordan M, Thomas M. Clinical and radiologic outcomes after Weil osteotomy compared to distal metatarsal metaphyseal osteotomy in the treatment of metatarsalgia—a prospective study. *Foot Ankle Surg*. 2019;25(4):488–494.
- Labidi M, Seyani M. Sporting foot and ankle injuries in older athletes. *Orthop Trauma*. 2024;38(1):51–55.
- Maceira E, Monteagudo M. Transfer metatarsalgia post hallux valgus surgery. *Foot Ankle Clin*. 2014;19(2):285–307.
- Tóth K, Huszanyik I, Kellermann P, et al. The effect of first ray shortening in the development of metatarsalgia in the second through fourth rays after metatarsal osteotomy. *Foot Ankle Int*. 2007;28(1):61–63.
- Weber PC. Resolution of metatarsalgia following oblique osteotomy. *Clin Orthop Relat Res*. 2007;458:248.

CLINICAL PEARLS

- Pain of the plantar surface of the forefoot, usually over the MT heads
- May be caused by abnormal pressure distribution over the plantar surface of the MT heads
- Common in athletes involved in high-impact sports (running, jumping, dancing)
- Athletes may warrant early referral to podiatry or orthopedic surgery.

ATHLETIC HEART SYNDROME

Evan D. Perez, MD, CAQSM ▪ Tu Dan Nguyen, MD, CAQSM ▪ Gillian G. Wooldridge, DO, CCD, FAOASM

BASICS

DESCRIPTION

- A benign reversible physiologic condition caused by adaptations to increased cardiac workload
- Associated with normal systolic and diastolic function
- Characteristics may overlap with pathologic conditions.
- Synonym(s): athlete's heart; physiologic cardiac hypertrophy; exercise-induced cardiac remodeling; exercise-related cardiac remodeling

EPIDEMIOLOGY

- Physiologic cardiac adaptations are common in highly trained athletes.
- Electrocardiography (ECG) changes have been observed in individuals who engage in intense or vigorous exercise for at least 4 h/wk.
- Can be mistaken for pathologic conditions

ETIOLOGY AND PATHOPHYSIOLOGY

- Physiologic hypertrophic hearts have preserved or increased contractile function along with the following characteristics (1)[C]:
  - Fully reversible and adaptive
  - Increased cardiomyocyte size
  - Increased/sufficient capillary network for nourishment
  - Unchanged myofibroblast activation
  - Unchanged type 1 collagen levels
  - Unchanged or decreased fetal genes
  - No maladaptive remodeling
  - No progression to heart failure
  - No interstitial fibrosis
  - No replacement fibrosis
- Cardiac dimensions rarely exceed upper limits of normal.
- Changes in cardiac structure vary based on type of exercise (2)[C],(3)[C].
- Dynamic or isotonic exercise (e.g., distance running, swimming) (2)[C],(3)[C]:
  - Increased cardiac output with normal or decreased peripheral vascular resistance creates volume overload
  - Increased left ventricular (LV) end-diastolic diameter with proportional increases in septal and free-wall thickness leading to largely eccentric remodeling
- Static exercise (e.g., weight lifting, bodybuilding) (2)[C]:
  - Increased peripheral resistance with smaller increases in heart rate and cardiac output
  - Increased septal and free-wall thickness without an increase in LV end-diastolic diameter
- Combined exercise (e.g., cycling, rowing) (2)[C]:
  - Extreme volume and pressure load
  - Largest increase in LV end-diastolic diameter, septal wall, and free-wall thickness without an increase in LV end-diastolic diameter leading to concentric remodeling

RISK FACTORS

- Regular participation in at least 4 h/wk of intense exercise (3)[C]
- Genetic predisposition

DIAGNOSIS

HISTORY

- Differentiate benign physiologic change from pathologic conditions.
- History of chest pain, dizziness, impaired exercise capacity, palpitations, presyncope, or syncope with exercise may be suggestive of pathology.
- Inquire about heart disease risk factors, including hypertension (HTN), hyperlipidemia, tobacco use, family history of sudden cardiac death (SCD), or other family history of cardiac conditions (hereditary, electrical, or structural abnormalities).
- History of cardiac murmur should be investigated along with history of cardiac surgeries.

PHYSICAL EXAM

- Decreased body fat and increased muscle mass
- Bradycardia (sinus bradycardia or bradycardia with 1st- and 2nd-degree blocks).
- Grade 1 or 2 midsystolic murmurs (benign functional ejection murmur, which resolves with Valsalva maneuver)
- Third and fourth heart sounds are common (benign filling).
- Blood pressure (BP) remains normal.
- Point of maximal ventricular impulse displaced lateral to the midclavicular line.

DIFFERENTIAL DIAGNOSIS

- Hypertensive cardiac hypertrophy
- Hypertrophic cardiomyopathy (HCM)
- Dilated cardiomyopathy (DCM)
- Arrhythmogenic right ventricular cardiomyopathy (ARVC)
- Myocarditis
- Left ventricular noncompaction (LVNC)
- Mitral valve prolapse (MVP)
- Bicuspid aortic valve (BAV)
- Coronary artery anomalies
- Aortic stenosis (AS)

DIAGNOSTIC TESTS & INTERPRETATION

Initial Tests (lab, imaging)

- ECG normal findings (4)[C]:
  - Increased vagal tone:
    - Sinus bradycardia:
      - 40 to 60 beats/min at rest is common; 30 to 40 beats/min in highly trained athletes
      - Sinus pauses <3 seconds
    - Early repolarization:
      - J-point elevation, ST elevation, J waves, or terminal QRS slurring in the inferior and/or lateral leads
      - Normal when present in isolation
    - "Black athlete heart" (African/Afro-Caribbean descent):
      - J-point elevation, convex ST segment elevation followed by T-wave inversion in leads V_1 to V_4
    - Juvenile T-wave pattern (<16 years old):
      - T-wave inversion in leads V_1 to V_3
    - Sinus arrhythmia:
      - Physiologic heart rate variation associated with respirations (increased with inspiration; decreased with expiration)
      - Resolves with onset of exercise
    - Junctional escape rhythm:
      - QRS rate faster than resting P wave
      - Regular R-R interval
      - Sinus rhythm should resume with activity.
    - Ectopic atrial rhythm:
      - Morphologically different ectopic P waves from the sinus P wave
      - Sinus rhythm should resume with exercise.
    - Atrioventricular (AV) blocks:
      - 1st-degree AV block present only at rest; P-R interval normalizes with exercise.
      - Mobitz type I (Wenckebach) 2nd-degree AV block: present only at rest; common in marathon runners.
  - Increased chamber size:
    - Voltage criteria for the following:
      - LV hypertrophy
      - Right ventricular hypertrophy, common in dynamic athletes
      - Incomplete right bundle branch block (RBBB)
- ECG borderline findings (4)[C]:
  - Isolated borderline ECG findings do not warrant further investigation (if asymptomatic and negative cardiac family history).
  - Two or more of the following borderline ECG findings need further investigation:
    - Left axis deviation:
      - −30° to −90°

- Left atrial enlargement:
  - Prolonged P wave duration of >120 milliseconds in leads I or II with negative portion of the P wave ≥1 mm in depth and ≥40 milliseconds in duration in lead V_1
- Right axis deviation:
  - 120°
- Right atrial enlargement:
  - P wave ≥2.5 mm in II, III, or aVF
- Complete RBBB:
  - rSR′ pattern in lead V_1 and an S wave wider than R wave in lead V_6 with QRS duration ≥120 milliseconds

- Echocardiography (2)[C],(5)[C]:
  - Biventricular hypertrophy
  - LV wall hypertrophy with LV wall thickness 11 to 13 mm is common in athletes.
  - LV wall thickness measuring 13 to 16 mm considered a "gray zone"
  - LV wall thickness ≥15 mm suggestive of HCM; requires a multimodality evaluation
  - Diastolic dysfunction is suspicious for pathology.
  - High-dynamic athletes:
    - Eccentric hypertrophy with increased left and right ventricular wall thickness
    - Left and right ventricular chamber dilation
    - Normal to mildly enlarged left and right atria
    - Supranormal LV diastolic indices
    - Normal to low normal systolic function
  - High-static athletes:
    - Mild symmetric LV concentric hypertrophy with normal to subnormal chamber size
    - Normal right ventricle dimensions
    - Normal to mildly enlarged left atrium
    - May be more pronounced in high-static athletes with HTN
  - Exercise echocardiogram has good sensitivity and specificity to determine athletic heart versus DCM in gray zone athletes (6)[C]:
    - In endurance athletes with reduced ejection fraction at rest, an increase of 5% with exercise suggests physiologic remodeling as a cause of LV and/or right ventricular dilation (5)[C].
  - Speckle tracking echocardiography (5)[C]:
    - Can detect decreased contractile reserve measured by limited increase in LV global longitudinal strain with exercise, indicating cardiomyopathy
  - Combined static/dynamic athletes (2)[C]:
    - Eccentric LV hypertrophy with a balanced increase in wall thickness and chamber size
- Cardiac magnetic resonance imaging (MRI) (2)[C],(5)[C]:
  - Considered the gold standard for precise assessment of chamber size, myocardial mass, and systolic function
  - Presence of pathologic fibrosis suggesting HCM can be identified by late gadolinium enhancement, native T1 and extracellular volume mapping.
  - Not influenced by body habitus
  - Useful in differentiating athlete's heart versus pathologic morphology
- Cardiac computed tomography (CCT) (5)[C]:
  - Can be used when MRI is contraindicated
  - Can assess for anomalous coronary arteries, aortic root dilation, and estimate LV parameters (volume, ejection etc.)

Diagnostic Procedures/Other

Prescribed detraining (2)[C],(3)[C],(5)[C]:

- Leads to a decrease in wall thickness and a reversal of ECG and echocardiographic abnormalities
- Atrophy rate of ~1%/wk can be seen in complete bed rest.
- Reversible after temporary (3 months) detraining
- Can be used to differentiate from HCM or ARVC if other methods are unrevealing

TREATMENT

GENERAL MEASURES

- Unwarranted discontinuation of exercise may have unintended psychological ramifications to the athlete.
- Reassure the athlete that the observed changes are normal physiologic adaptations to exercise and encourage the athlete to continue exercising.

ISSUES FOR REFERRAL

Patients with overlapping features of athletic heart and pathologic features (i.e., exertional symptoms, family history, LV wall thickness "gray zone") should be evaluated by a cardiologist prior to returning to physical activity.

ONGOING CARE

FOLLOW-UP RECOMMENDATIONS

- Many of the physiologic adaptations observed in athletic heart syndrome resolve when exercise is stopped.
- The adaptations that occur in resistant or static athletes are similar to those caused by chronic HTN.
- Routine follow-up is recommended especially in gray zone athletes as pathologic changes can potentially develop over time.

REFERENCES

1. Nakamura M, Sadoshima J. Mechanisms of physiological and pathological cardiac hypertrophy. *Nat Rev Cardiol*. 2018;15(7):387–407.
2. Baggish AL, Battle RW, Beckerman JG, et al. Sports cardiology: core curriculum for providing cardiovascular care to competitive athletes and highly active people. *J Am Coll Cardiol*. 2017;70(15):1902–1918.
3. Danielian A, Shah AB. Differentiating physiology from pathology: the gray zones of the athlete's heart. *Clin Sports Med*. 2022;41(3):425–440.
4. Sharma S, Drezner JA, Baggish A, et al. International recommendations for electrocardiographic interpretation in athletes. *Eur Heart J*. 2018;39(16):1466–1480.
5. D'Andrea A, Sperlongano S, Russo V, et al. The role of multimodality imaging in athlete's heart diagnosis: current status and future directions. *J Clin Med*. 2021;10(21):5126.
6. Millar LM, Fanton Z, Finocchiaro G, et al. Differentiation between athlete's heart and dilated cardiomyopathy in athletic individuals. *Heart*. 2020;106(14):1059–1065.

ADDITIONAL READING

- Baggish AL. Exercise-induced cardiac remodeling: competitive athletes are just the tip of the iceberg. *Circ Cardiovasc Imaging*. 2016;9(8):e005321.
- Drezner JA, O'Connor FG, Harmon KG, et al. AMSSM position statement on cardiovascular preparticipation screening in athletes: current evidence, knowledge gaps, recommendations, and future directions. *Clin J Sport Med*. 2016;26(5):347–361.
- Hill B, Grubic N, Williamson M, et al. Does cardiovascular preparticipation screening cause psychological distress in athletes? A systematic review. *Br J Sports Med*. 2023;57(3):172–178.
- Martinez MW, Kim JH, Shah AB, et al. Exercise-induced cardiovascular adaptations and approach to exercise and cardiovascular disease: JACC state-of-the-art review. *J Am Coll Cardiol*. 2021;78(14):1453–1470.

CLINICAL PEARLS

- Physiologic response to exercise; no increased risk with participation
- Given that SCD is the leading cause of sport/exercise related mortality, it is crucial to be able to differentiate athletic heart syndrome from pathologic conditions.
- ECG and other cardiac imaging modalities may help distinguish physiologic from pathologic changes.
- Detraining can aid in differentiation.

ATLANTOAXIAL INSTABILITY

Rebecca L. Carl, MD, MSCI

BASICS

DESCRIPTION

- Atlantoaxial instability (AAI) is the term for increased motion at the joint between the 1st and 2nd cervical vertebrae (the atlas and the axis).
- Congenital, inflammatory, traumatic, or infectious conditions may weaken the structures supporting the C1–C2 joint leading to AAI.
- Many patients who meet the radiographic definition of AAI are asymptomatic and at low risk for neurologic sequelae.
- Synonym(s): atlantoaxial subluxation

EPIDEMIOLOGY

- The incidence of radiographic/asymptomatic AAI in individuals with Down syndrome is estimated between 10% and 20%.
- The incidence of symptomatic AAI is much lower at ~2.6%.
- Incidence of AAI increases with age, and progression may occur during growth spurts.
- For individuals with Down syndrome, males aged >10 years are most likely to have progression of AAI.

RISK FACTORS

- Down syndrome
- Rheumatoid arthritis
- Juvenile idiopathic arthritis
- Many forms of dwarfism/skeletal dysplasia
- Marfan syndrome: increased incidence of C1–C2 hypermobility, but symptoms are rare

DIAGNOSIS

Lateral cervical radiographs with flexion and extension views are used for screening. AAI is defined radiographically as an increased distance between the odontoid process and the anterior arch of the axis.

- Obtaining screening x-rays for AAI in asymptomatic patients with Down syndrome is controversial:
  - Because of poor radiographic reproducibility and because many radiographic signs of AAI often resolve over time in asymptomatic patients, the American Academy of Pediatrics does not endorse routine radiographic screening (1)[A],(2)[C].
  - The Special Olympics requires a history and physical evaluation that includes screening for AAI. Individuals with symptoms that could represent AAI must have a comprehensive workup (3)[C].

HISTORY

- Most individuals with AAI are asymptomatic.
- AAI can be acute or chronic. However, acute AAI without a history of preceding symptoms is rare:
  - Patients with acute AAI often present after injury. Injury can be due to direct or indirect trauma. Mechanisms of injury include hyperextension, hyperflexion, and direct loading.
  - In patients who have an acute worsening of AAI, participation in organized sports is an uncommon triggering event.
  - Patients with chronic AAI often present with gait changes, progressive weakness, and fatigue. Neck pain, bowel and bladder incontinence, ataxia, spasticity, and quadriplegia can be present with long-standing, severe chronic AAI (4)[B].

PHYSICAL EXAM

- Hyperreflexia
- Sensory changes
- Weakness
- Gait changes
- Cervical spine range of motion is often normal.

DIAGNOSTIC TESTS & INTERPRETATION

- Lateral neck radiographs with flexion/extension views:
  - AAI is defined as a space of 5 mm or more between the odontoid process of the axis and the anterior arch of the atlas.
- Further evaluation with computed tomography (CT) or magnetic resonance imaging (MRI) in cervical flexion and extension is often needed to assess for spinal cord compression in patients with AAI on plain radiographs.

DIFFERENTIAL DIAGNOSIS

- Neck sprain/strain
- Cervical disc herniation
- Torticollis
- Vertebral fracture
- Ligamentous laxity
- Spinal contusion
- Epidural hemorrhage

TREATMENT

GENERAL MEASURES

- Management of athletes with acute worsening of AAI symptoms
- If worsening occurs with trauma, assume a potentially unstable injury is present until proven otherwise.
- The cervical spine must be stabilized in the field.
- Protect the airway if respiratory difficulties arise.

ADDITIONAL THERAPIES

Anesthesia administration:

- Blind endotracheal intubation of a patient with AAI should be avoided.
- Tracheal intubation with a flexible bronchoscope under topical anesthesia avoids neck flexion and maintains cervical spine stability.
- For elective procedures, consider regional anesthesia with minimal sedation (5)[C].

SURGERY/OTHER PROCEDURES

- Atlantoaxial fusion should be considered for patients with progressive, symptomatic AAI and/or cervical myelopathy (4)[B].
- Because atlantoaxial fusion is a very high-risk procedure, nonoperative management is recommended for patients without neurologic symptoms.

ONGOING CARE

Long-term management:

- Individuals who exhibit signs and symptoms should be restricted from contact sports and other activities that place stress on the neck (4)[B].
- Restriction of asymptomatic patients with only radiographic evidence of AAI is somewhat controversial, particularly for noncontact activities.
- Special Olympics restricts individuals with AAI from participating in the following:
  - Gymnastics
  - Butterfly stroke
  - Diving (including diving starts in swimming)
  - Pentathlon
  - High jump
  - Squat lifts
  - Equestrian sports
  - Artistic gymnastics
  - Soccer
  - Alpine skiing
  - Judo
  - Snowboarding

FOLLOW-UP RECOMMENDATIONS

- Primary care physicians should counsel families of patients with Down syndrome, rheumatoid arthritis, juvenile inflammatory arthritis, and skeletal dysplasia about possible signs and symptoms of AAI (2)[C],(6)[C].
- Physicians should counsel parents of children with Down syndrome about the increased risk of AAI and potential spinal cord injury with contact sports and activities with a high risk of collision or fall (e.g., trampoline) (2)[C].

REFERENCES

1. Cremers MJ, Bol E, de Roos F, et al. Risk of sports activities in children with Down's syndrome and atlantoaxial instability. *Lancet*. 1993;342(8870):511–514.
2. Bull MJ, Trotter T, Santoro SL, et al. Health supervision for children and adolescents with Down syndrome. *Pediatrics*. 2022;149(5):e2022057010.
3. Special Olympics Medical Form. Updated April 2021. Accessed August 11, 2025. https://media.specialolympics.org/resources/leading-a-program/registration-forms/SOI-Medical-Form-US-Programs-April-2021-English.pdf?_ga=2.146079604.1172780706.1628011465-23375062.1628011465
4. Atlantoaxial instability in Down syndrome: subject review. American Academy of Pediatrics Committee on Sports Medicine and Fitness. *Pediatrics*. 1995;96(1 Pt 1):151–154.
5. Lewanda AF, Matisoff A, Revenis M, et al. Preoperative evaluation and comprehensive risk assessment for children with Down syndrome. *Paediatr Anaesth*. 2016;26(4):356–362.
6. Sudoł-Szopińska I, Herregods N, Doria AS, et al. Advances in musculoskeletal imaging in juvenile idiopathic arthritis. *Biomedicines*. 2022;10(10):2417.

ADDITIONAL READING

- Torg JS, Ramsey-Emrhein JA. Suggested management guidelines for participation in collision activities with congenital, developmental, or postinjury lesions involving the cervical spine. *Med Sci Sports Exerc*. 1997;29(Suppl 7):S256–S272.
- Wills BP, Dormans JP. Nontraumatic upper cervical spine instability in children. *J Am Acad Orthop Surg*. 2006;14(4):233–245.
- Winell J, Burke SW. Sports participation of children with Down syndrome. *Orthop Clin North Am*. 2003;34(3):439–443.

CLINICAL PEARLS

- Athletes with radiographic evidence of AAI who are asymptomatic appear to be at low risk for experiencing acute worsening during participation in organized sports (particularly noncontact activities) (1)[B].
- Each individual athlete should discuss sports participation guidelines with his or her physician(s) (2)[C].

AURICULAR HEMATOMAS

Steven K. Poon, MD, CAQSM ▪ Kimberly G. Harmon, MD

BASICS

ALERT

Failure to diagnose and promptly treat this condition with evacuation of the hematoma may lead to permanent deformation of the ear.

DESCRIPTION

- Auricular hematoma is an injury caused by trauma or friction of the ear that often occurs in contact sports such as wrestling, rugby, boxing, and judo.
- Trauma or continuous friction to the auricle leads to bleeding into the soft tissues of the ear.
- Bleeding often occurs anteriorly at the junction of the perichondrium and elastic cartilage of the ear.
- Recognition of this condition led to the development of treatments during the latter half of the 20th century.

EPIDEMIOLOGY

Incidence

Most injuries occur while engaged in combat sports such as wrestling while not wearing protective headgear.

Prevalence

Studies estimate ear injuries account for up to 23.4% of all reported wrestling related injuries.

ETIOLOGY AND PATHOPHYSIOLOGY

- The condition is caused by trauma owing to a direct blow or frictional forces to the auricle.
- Bleeding into the auricle, specifically between the skin and auricular cartilage, results in a hematoma in this space.
- Untreated, the hematoma can cause pressure, necrosis, and scarring of the auricular cartilage leading to a "cauliflower ear," which is the name given to the characteristic deformity to the ear:
  - Neocartilage formation at the site of the clot also plays a role in the associated deformity.
  - This deformity is disfiguring and permanent.

RISK FACTORS

Failure to wear headgear while participating in sports such as wresting, rugby, or martial arts disciplines such as judo may increase the risk of ear trauma.

GENERAL PREVENTION

- General prevention is based on proper use of headgear during participation.
- Ill-fitting headgear may provide inadequate protection to the auricle.
- Awareness of the importance and use of proper fitting headgear by athletes, coaches, and athletic training staff may prevent this injury.

COMMONLY ASSOCIATED CONDITIONS

- Auricle laceration
- Rupture of tympanic membrane owing to associated trauma
- Concussions related to head trauma
- Cellulitis and perichondritis may mimic or be associated with this disorder.

DIAGNOSIS

- Diagnosis is made based on clinical exam and history of trauma/excessive friction to the ear (1)[C].
- The absence of associated factors which may lead to cellulitis of the ear may aid in the correct diagnosis.

HISTORY

- History of direct and recent trauma to the auricle with resulting hematoma
- Lack of protective headgear while participating in high-risk sports for this injury should raise level of suspicion.
- The athlete complains of a painful ear and may have associated hearing loss.

PHYSICAL EXAM

- Examination of the auricle reveals a soft hematoma with tenderness of the auricle presenting within a few hours after the inciting injury.
- Loss of the normal architecture of the auricle compared with the contralateral side
- Exam should include an assessment of the athlete's hearing.
- Associated ear drainage should prompt consideration for rupture of the tympanic membrane.
- Assessment to rule out signs and symptoms of concussion should be performed.

DIFFERENTIAL DIAGNOSIS

- Ear laceration
- Cellulitis of ear
- Perichondritis

DIAGNOSTIC TESTS & INTERPRETATION

Diagnosis of this condition is based on history and clinical exam:

- No specific lab tests confirm diagnosis.
- Complete blood count (CBC) or erythrocyte sedimentation rate (ESR) may aid in the diagnosis of associated infection.

TREATMENT

GENERAL MEASURES

- Once frictional and/or direct pressures have resulted in a hematoma between the skin and auricular cartilage, the initial goal in treatment is to aspirate this area to prevent further complications.
- Following anesthesia with lidocaine without epinephrine, aspiration can be attempted with an 18- to 22-gauge needle and syringe (2)[C]:
  - This aspiration must be done in the acute phase when the hematoma is palpable.
- If left untreated, the hematoma can lead to neocartilage formation, scarring, and necrosis, all of which can lead to permanent deformity.
- Antibiotics are sometimes given as a preventive measure because infection of the auricle will result in further poor outcomes. See below.

MEDICATION

- Consider antibiotics for prophylactic coverage (e.g., cephalexin × 7 days). If suturing or incision and drainage are done, antibiotics definitely should be used (3)[B].
- Nonsteroidal anti-inflammatory drugs (NSAIDs) and aspirin should be avoided to minimize hematoma recurrence risk.

ADDITIONAL THERAPIES

- The importance of acute aspiration of hematoma has been described as well as the possible need for attempted hematoma evacuation with a larger bore needle.
- On occasion, a pressure dressing may not be needed if the hematoma does not recur within 1 hour of successful aspiration.
- To prevent reaccumulation of the hematoma and the need for additional aspirations, a compression dressing commonly is placed over the area:
  - Compression must stay over the ear until it is fully healed.
  - Compression dressing may be needed for 3 days or more.
- Multiple reports have described using through-and-through mattress sutures for better cosmetic outcomes and lower risk of hematoma reaccumulation (3),(4)[B]:
  - Anesthesia is achieved by using an auricular block and lidocaine 1% without epinephrine.
  - Incision and drainage is performed with a number 15 blade scalpel over the area of fluid accumulation and allowing for full evacuation of hematoma. Hemostats may be needed to break up loculations.
  - After copious irrigation, horizontal mattress sutures are placed through and through the ear cartilage with 4-0 or 5-0 absorbable sutures.
  - Cover the suture and incision site with topical antimicrobial ointment and start oral antibiotics as described above.
  - Sutures remain in place for 7 to 10 days.
  - This can be done in a training room setting but may require referral to ear, nose, and throat (ENT) if provider is not comfortable with this procedure.
- Thermoplastic splints can be used to provide additional compression to reduce reaccumulation of hematoma (3)[B].

SURGERY/OTHER PROCEDURES

The possibility of surgery may be entertained, as mentioned earlier, in consultation with ENT or plastic surgery.

ONGOING CARE

FOLLOW-UP RECOMMENDATIONS

Daily follow-up is needed to observe for signs of hematoma redevelopment, pressure necrosis, allergic reaction to materials, and infection.

Patient Monitoring

Follow-up with ENT or plastic surgery after acute treatment is recommended because of the risk of poor cosmetic result even with proper treatment of the condition.

PATIENT EDUCATION

- Return to play too early, prior to fully healing of the injury, will increase the risk of a poor outcome:
  - No definitive return-to-play protocol exists.
  - Some authors recommend no competition while wearing ear compression dressing, whereas others allow full activity with ear protection being worn.
  - Bolsterless mattress suture repair often allows for immediate return to activity.
  - The decision should be made in consultation with the athlete, recognizing the potential for poor cosmesis with recurrence of the injury.
- Ear protectors and headgear always should be worn in high-risk sports.
- Ice and pressure applied at the end of practices and matches may help to prevent recurrence of injury.

PROGNOSIS

- Best prognosis is achieved by prompt aspiration and compression.
- Poorer outcomes are associated with repeated need for aspiration and earlier return to contact sports/reinjury.
- Recurrence rates remain high but can be reduced with the use of bolster dressings instead of aspiration alone (5)[B].

COMPLICATIONS

- Permanent scarring and cosmetic deformity referred to as "cauliflower ear"
- Chondritis and perichondritis
- Prompt treatment, including aseptic technique, may prevent these consequences.

REFERENCES

1. Cassaday K, Vazquez G, Wright JM. Ear problems and injuries in athletes. *Curr Sports Med Rep.* 2014;13(1):22–26.
2. Kiningham R, Monseau A. Caring for wrestlers. *Curr Sports Med Rep.* 2015;14(5):404–412.
3. Yerlikaya HS, Akyildiz I, Ugurlu BN, et al. Use of thermoplastic splint for the treatment of auricular hematoma. *J Craniofac Surg.* 2020;31(8):2310–2312.
4. Giles WC, Iverson KC, King JD, et al. Incision and drainage followed by mattress suture repair of auricular hematoma. *Laryngoscope.* 2007;117(12):2097–2099.
5. Dalal PJ, Purkey MR, Price CPE, et al. Risk factors for auricular hematoma and recurrence after drainage. *Laryngoscope.* 2020;130(3):628–631.

ADDITIONAL READING

- Hewett TE, Pasque C, Heyl R, et al. Wrestling injuries. *Med Sport Sci.* 2005;48:152–178.
- Skidmore K, Gossman WG. *Ear, Cauliflower Ear.* StatPearls Publishing; 2018.

CLINICAL PEARLS

- Diagnosis of this condition is based on history and clinical exam.
- Early recognition and treatment of this condition with hematoma aspiration may prevent long-term sequelae and disfigurement.
- Return to contact sports without sufficient time for injury to fully heal/allow adequate retreatment increases the risk for a poor cosmetic result.
- Compression treatment options include bolsters and horizontal mattress suture repair.
- ENT/plastic surgery consultation may be required.
- Use of ear protection/headgear is effective in prevention of this condition.

AXILLARY NERVE INJURY

Alexander T. Grover, DO • James R. Borchers, MD, MPH

BASICS

DESCRIPTION

- Originates from the C5–C6 rami (and occasionally C4) and is a branch of the posterior cord of the brachial plexus (1)
- Courses from the brachial plexus and below the coracoid process along the anterior surface of the subscapularis and then travels posteriorly and through the quadrilateral space (1)
- The quadrilateral space is an anatomic entity created by the teres minor muscle inferiorly, the long head of the triceps medially, the neck of the humerus laterally, and the subscapularis and teres major muscles superiorly. The axillary nerve and posterior humeral circumflex artery travel within this space (1).
- Once through the space, the nerve travels further posteriorly and branches into an anterior and posterior trunk.
- The anterior trunk courses around the posterolateral (surgical) neck of the humerus to innervate the anterior and middle deltoid.
- The posterior trunk bifurcates into a motor branch, the teres minor and posterior deltoid muscles, and a sensory branch innervating the superolateral brachial cutaneous nerve, which innervates the lateral upper extremity.

EPIDEMIOLOGY

An axillary nerve mononeuropathy is a rare event, occurring in about 0.3–6% of all brachial plexus injuries (2).

Incidence

True incidence rates are unknown owing to under recognition of the diagnosis.

ETIOLOGY AND PATHOPHYSIOLOGY

- Traction injury to the nerve during an anterior dislocation or fracture (2)
- Presumed compression injury of the nerve as a result of a direct blow to the anterolateral deltoid (2)
- Quadrilateral space syndrome: Proposed mechanisms include compression of the nerve by fibrous bands, hypertrophied muscles that border the space, any space-occupying lesion (e.g., aneurysm or cyst), or shear between the teres minor and major (2).
- Iatrogenic damage to the nerve during shoulder surgery (2)

RISK FACTORS

- Anterior shoulder (glenohumeral) dislocation
- Humeral neck fracture
- Direct blunt trauma to the anterior lateral deltoid, which is common in contact sports such as hockey, football, or rugby
- Repetitive overhead sports (e.g., volleyball, tennis, or baseball): This can lead to quadrilateral space syndrome.
- Iatrogenic damage (e.g., shoulder instability surgery, rotator cuff surgery, and rarely, shoulder arthroscopy)

COMMONLY ASSOCIATED CONDITIONS

- Anterior glenohumeral dislocation
- Humeral neck fracture

DIAGNOSIS

Nerve injury should be suspected in any athlete with anterior shoulder dislocation or humeral neck fracture.

HISTORY

- Easy fatigability weakness with overhead activities or heavy lifting (2)
- Decreased strength with shoulder abduction (2)
- Paresthesias or loss of sensation in the lateral upper arm (Sensation is spared after anterior shoulder dislocation.)
- Quadrilateral space syndrome: vague, nonspecific aching or burning of the posterolateral shoulder and/or generalized weakness with overhead activities (1)

PHYSICAL EXAM

- Assess for deltoid or teres minor atrophy compared with the unaffected side (more common in chronic cases).
- Active and passive range of motion (ROM) about the shoulder, including abduction, forward elevation, and external rotation
- Strength testing of abduction and forward elevation (deltoid function) and external rotation (teres minor function)
- Neurovascular exam, especially assessing for sensation over the lateral deltoid area known as the "sergeant's patch"
- Perform the Spurling maneuver (rotate the patient's head to the affected side and hyperextend the neck) to assess for cervical radiculopathy.
- Tenderness to palpation of the posterior shoulder at the quadrilateral space (often the only positive finding in quadrilateral space syndrome)

DIFFERENTIAL DIAGNOSIS

- Brachial plexus syndromes:
  - Thoracic outlet syndrome
  - Neuralgic amyotrophy (Parsonage-Turner syndrome)
- Quadrilateral space syndrome
- Cervical spine lesions
- Aneurysm, neoplasm, or cystic mass along the distribution of the axillary nerve

DIAGNOSTIC TESTS & INTERPRETATION

Initial Tests (lab, imaging)

- Plain x-rays of the shoulder to evaluate glenohumeral dislocation or evidence of fracture (2)
- Consider cervical spine x-rays to rule out cervical spine causes of deltoid paresthesias, weakness, or atrophy (1).
- Magnetic resonance imaging (MRI) can be helpful in chronic cases to identify a combined nerve injury, to determine prognosis of functional recovery by evaluating fatty replacement of the muscle, or to evaluate other soft tissue causes of shoulder weakness but is often not needed (2).

Diagnostic Procedures/Other

- Electromyography (EMG) and nerve conduction velocity (NCV) should be obtained no sooner than 4 weeks after injury to establish baseline dysfunction (2),(3)[A].
- Repeat EMG and NCV after 12 weeks to assess for nerve recovery if no clinical improvement in deltoid function (2),(3)[A].
- Arteriogram of the posterior circumflex humeral artery to evaluate for quadrilateral space syndrome but there are conflicting recommendations regarding the use of this test (1)[B]

TREATMENT

GENERAL MEASURES

- Nonoperative treatment is preferred initially (2),(3)[A].
- Emphasize active and passive ROM of the shoulder.
- Relative rest
- Strengthening exercises of the shoulder
- Avoidance of exacerbating triggers or activities
- Emergency department (ED) treatment:
  - Reduction of glenohumeral dislocation or treatment of fracture

ADDITIONAL THERAPIES

Electrical stimulation of the deltoid is an option to prevent atrophy while the nerve is recovering (2)[C].

SURGERY/OTHER PROCEDURES

- Appropriate interval for surgical intervention is unclear, but there is some evidence to suggest that surgery within 6 months of injury yields superior return of function and strength (2)[B].
- Generally indicated if no improvement using nonoperative treatments or if EMG/NCV shows no interval nerve recovery in 3 to 12 months postinjury (2)[A]
- Operative procedures include (2),(4),(5)[A]:
  - Neurolysis
  - Sural nerve grafting
  - Neurorrhaphy
  - Nerve transfer
  - Neurotization
- Surgical decompression can be performed for quadrilateral space syndrome to release fibrous bands (2)[B].

ONGOING CARE

FOLLOW-UP RECOMMENDATIONS

- Routine clinical follow-up every 4 to 8 weeks while patient is undergoing therapy to assess for return of strength and sensation
- Repeat EMG/NCV if no improvement in 3 months.
- Return to contact sports once full ROM and adequate strength of the shoulder are achieved.

PROGNOSIS

- Depends on mechanism and severity of nerve damage
- Functional shoulder recovery is usually excellent (2).
- 85–100% of axillary nerve injury owing to fracture or dislocation will recover fully by 6 to 12 months with nonoperative treatment (1).
- Poorer prognosis for functional recovery in symptomatic patients who undergo surgical intervention >12 months after date of injury (2)

REFERENCES

1. Safran MR. Nerve injury about the shoulder in athletes, part 1: suprascapular nerve and axillary nerve. *Am J Sports Med*. 2004;32(3):803–819.
2. Steinmann SP, Moran EA. Axillary nerve injury: diagnosis and treatment. *J Am Acad Orthop Surg*. 2001;9(5):328–335.
3. Galvin JW, Eichinger JK. Outcomes following closed axillary nerve injury: a case report and review of the literature. *Mil Med*. 2016;181(3):e291–e297.
4. Yang X, Xu B, Tong JS, et al. Triceps motor branch transfer for isolated axillary nerve injury: outcomes in 9 patients. *Orthop Traumatol Surg Res*. 2017;103(8):1283–1286.
5. Baltzer HL, Kircher MF, Spinner RJ, et al. A comparison of outcomes of triceps motor branch-to-axillary nerve transfer or sural nerve interpositional grafting for isolated axillary nerve injury. *Plast Reconstr Surg*. 2016;138(2):256e–264e.

CLINICAL PEARLS

Axillary nerve injury should be suspected in individuals with a glenohumeral dislocation or humeral neck fracture who have weakness.

ALERT

Normal sensation of the lateral upper arm does not rule out axillary nerve injury.

- EMG/NCV tests should be performed in a suspected axillary nerve injury but no sooner than 3 weeks postinjury.
- Despite variable recovery rates of the axillary nerve and deltoid muscle, functional recovery of the shoulder is excellent.

BAROTRAUMA

Edgar M. VanHorne, MD • Terrance L. Leighton III, BS, DO • Eric A. Rosson, DO, MBA

BASICS

- Barotrauma is defined as physical damage to the body from the mechanical effects of pressure.
- Can occur due to overpressurization (during ascent) or more commonly underpressurization (during descent)
- Boyle law states that at a constant temperature, pressure (P) is inversely related to volume (V):
  - $PV = K$ (constant) or $P_1V_1 = P_2V_2$
  - Increase in pressure mandates a reduction in volume by same factor.
  - Example: If an average breath-hold diver (lungs contain ~5 L of gas) takes a full breath at the surface and descends to 10 m, the volume of air in his lungs may be reduced from 5 L to 2.5 L.
- Gas-filled cavities in the body are subject to expansion/contraction:
  - Lung
  - Middle ear
  - Sinus
  - Teeth
  - Gastrointestinal (GI) system
- Barotrauma is the most common form of diving-related injury (1).
- There are five requirements for barotrauma to occur and they are commonly remembered with the pneumonic GRAVE: Gas-filled space, Rigid walls, Ambient pressure change, Vascular lined membrane space, Enclosed space.
- Following drowning, pulmonary barotrauma (PBT) is the second leading cause of death in scuba divers (1).
- Pulmonary overinflation syndrome (POIS) is an umbrella term for four distinct conditions with the same etiology of PBT: pneumothorax, mediastinal/subcutaneous (SC) emphysema, and arterial gas embolism (AGE).
- Volume changes experienced during diving are greatest in the few feet nearest the surface.

ALERT

- For barotrauma of descent, unless an air-filled cavity has ruptured, no progression of the disease upon return to normal atmospheric pressure is expected.
- If patient transport requires air evacuation, maintain air cabin pressure at 1 atm or fly below 1,000 feet to avoid aggravating barotrauma.

ETIOLOGY AND PATHOPHYSIOLOGY

- During descent: Increase in pressure with subsequent decrease air volume in a space that also contains tissue can lead to vascular engorgement, mucosal edema, and hemorrhage.
- During ascent: Decrease in pressure with subsequent increase in gas volume in a confined space can result in disruption or rupture of tissue.
- There are several different causes of ear barotrauma; most common etiology is flying.
- Blast injuries as result of combat, terrorist attacks, and working hazards have become more prevalent:
  - Barotrauma results from a rapid air pressure wave generated by an explosion without time to equalize the pressure.
  - Injuries include bruising of the eardrum, bleeding into the drum and middle ear, eardrum rupture, ossicular disruption, and inner ear injury.
- Middle ear:
  - Barotrauma of descent
  - Most common type of barotrauma
  - Seen in 30% of inexperienced divers and 10% of experienced divers
  - Results from inadequate equalization of pressure between the middle ear and the external ear canal
  - Eustachian tube provides the sole route of pressure equalization for the middle ear.
  - Upper respiratory infections may cause dysfunction of the eustachian tube.
  - The resulting tissue damage includes congestion, hemorrhage, outward or inward bulging, and possible rupture of tympanic membrane (TM).
- External ear:
  - Barotrauma of descent or ascent
  - Due to the presence of a tight-fitting hood, ear plugs, a cerumen plug, or bony growths (exostoses)
  - Pressure cannot equalize throughout the canal, and a relative intracanal vacuum is created as the pressure differential across the obstruction increases.
- Inner ear:
  - Barotrauma of descent
  - Infrequent
  - Results from forceful attempts at equalizing middle ear pressure
  - Increased inner ear pressure can raise intracranial pressure and cause rupture of the round or labyrinth windows, allowing perilymph to enter the middle ear.
- Paranasal sinus (2):
  - Barotrauma of descent
  - Relatively common diving injury usually resulting from sinus outflow compromise, such as inflammatory mucosal thickening, polyps, and structural deviations
  - Nasal ostia act as a valve to regulate sinus pressure.
  - If the ostia fail to allow pressure equalization, congestion, edema, and hemorrhage can occur.
  - Frontal sinus most commonly affected
- Teeth (barodontalgia):
  - Barotrauma of ascent
  - Rapid volume change in the air spaces of adjacent fillings or at the roots of infected teeth
  - Common in novice and experienced divers
- GI (aerogastralgia):
  - Barotrauma of ascent
  - Swallowed air in the GI tract expands as external pressure decreases.
  - Risk of stomach rupture, resulting in pneumoperitoneum
- PBT or POIS:
  - Occurs with ascent
  - Lungs expand against a closed glottis.
  - Ascending diver due to inadequate exhalation and overexpansion of the lungs; can occur from depths as shallow as 2 to 4 feet.
  - Can result in pneumomediastinum, pneumothorax; interstitial gas dissecting the esophagus can result in pneumoperitoneum.
  - Most serious complication is AGE.
  - Divers with decrease lung compliance/increased lung volumes at increased risk (chronic obstructive pulmonary disease [COPD], asthma).

GENERAL PREVENTION

- Avoid diving with upper respiratory infection, which may not allow for equalization of pressures across the TM because of eustachian tube dysfunction.
- Pre-dive medical examination can help to identify individuals at increased risk for barotrauma.
- Taking pseudoephedrine 30 minutes prior to diving was shown to decrease the incidence and severity of middle ear barotrauma (3)[C].
- Oxymetazoline is somewhat less effective.
- Attempt to equilibrate pressure in the middle ear to the outside by swallowing to open the eustachian tube or Valsalva maneuver.

DIAGNOSIS

Essential workup:

- Head, eyes, ears, nose, and throat (HEENT) exam with particular attention paid to the TM to determine if rupture has occurred
- Pulmonary exam looking for signs of SC emphysema and pneumothorax
- Neurologic exam looking for signs of inner ear pathology or AGE

PHYSICAL EXAM

Signs and symptoms:

- Middle ear (barotitis media):
  - Begins as a clogged sensation
  - Increasingly painful as the pressure differential across the TM increases
  - When rupture occurs, initial ear pain from pressure will diminish rapidly
  - Associated symptoms include nausea, vertigo, tinnitus, conductive hearing loss, and, occasionally, facial nerve palsy.
  - Progression to rupture of the TM: appearance of TM congestion → TM edema → gross hemorrhage → TM rupture

- External ear: Canal mucosa becomes edematous, then hemorrhagic, and ultimately may tear.
- Inner ear:
  - Sudden severe vertigo
  - Tinnitus
  - Sensorineural hearing loss in the affected ear
  - Symptoms begin or are associated with forceful attempt to equalize pressures of middle ear during descent.
  - Normal external canal and TM exam with isolated inner ear barotrauma
- Paranasal sinuses (2):
  - Sinus congestion
  - Headache
  - Pain
  - Epistaxis
- External objects:
  - Mask: conjunctival hemorrhage, facial edema, diplopia, and swelling
  - Tight-fitting dive suit: edema and erythema of the skin
- Barodontalgia:
  - Severe tooth pain
  - Possible tooth breakdown
- Aerogastralgia:
  - Excessive belching
  - Flatulence
  - Abdominal distension
  - In divers, abdominal pain during ascent increases in severity as depth becomes shallower.
- Pulmonary:
  - Dyspnea
  - Chest pain
  - Cough with a frothy red sputum
  - SC emphysema of the neck and chest
  - Delayed symptoms, including a bull neck appearance, dysphagia, and changes in voice character
  - Hamman sign: crackling sound heard over the heart during systole (crepitation in the neck associated with SC emphysema)
- Sinus imaging:
  - Computed tomography (CT) scan
  - Plain films
- Chest and neck radiographs for pneumothorax, pneumomediastinum
- Abdominal series (upright, decubitus) for free air from a ruptured viscus

DIFFERENTIAL DIAGNOSIS

- Decompression sickness (DCS)
- Otitis media/externa
- Sinusitis
- AGE
- Substance abuse intoxication
- Asthma exacerbation
- Head injury
- Pneumothorax

DIAGNOSTIC TESTS & INTERPRETATION

Arterial blood gas determinations for pulmonary symptoms

TREATMENT

- Hospital admission criterion: PBT, AGE, unstable patients
- Emergency department (ED) treatment:
  - Establish intravenous (IV) access for unstable patients.
  - Intubation in patients with massive SC emphysema of the neck
  - Immediate needle thoracostomy for evidence of tension pneumothorax
  - Control bleeding from the ear or nose.
  - Antibiotics with TM or sinus rupture
  - Analgesics
  - Consult Divers Alert Network (DAN): 1–919–684–4DAN (4326).
- Outpatient considerations:
  - Middle ear barotrauma:
    - Most TM ruptures heal spontaneously (3 to 6 weeks) if infection is controlled and normal eustachian tube function is restored; large or marginal perforations may require surgery.
    - Spontaneous healing less likely with blast injury
    - Avoid all Cortisporin products in TM rupture (3)[C].
    - Antibiotics only with TM rupture in circumstances where exposed to water; ofloxacin otic, ciprofloxacin eye drops (Ciloxan), Ciprodex (cipro with dexamethasone shown to increase healing rate) (4)[C]
    - Decongestants, glucocorticoids, and antihistamines are not proven to expedite recovery.
    - Analgesics as needed
  - Inner ear barotrauma:
    - Complete bed rest with head elevation (avoids increase in cerebrospinal fluid [CSF] pressure, which can lead to perilymph leakage)
    - May require tympanotomy and patching of the round or oval window
    - Permanent inner ear damage possible → persistent vestibular deficits
  - Myringotomy may be considered to prevent and treat barotrauma related to flying.
  - Myringotomy should not be considered for diving; in the event of spontaneous TM rupture, diving should be aborted.
  - Sinus barotrauma:
    - Consider prophylactic antibiotics for meningitis; coverage should be directed at nasopharyngeal flora (penicillin or cephalosporin classes) (2)[C].

ONGOING CARE

- Good prognosis, with most cases being self-limited
- No diving until TM has healed and other symptoms have resolved.
- Pre-dive medical clearance is recommended for anyone with prior PBT or decompression illness.
- Absolute contraindications to diving: acute asthma, spontaneous pneumothorax, cystic/cavitary/obstructive/restrictive lung disease, seizures, atrial septal defect (ASD), symptomatic coronary artery disease (CAD), chronic perforated TM, inability to equalize sinus or middle ear pressure, or intra-orbital gas
- Educate proper scuba technique; divers who hold their breath as they ascend are at increased risk of barotrauma.
- Ear, nose, and throat (ENT) referral for severe TM, inner ear, or sinus pathology
- Modern commercial aircrafts (lowered barometric pressure, ambient oxygen partial pressure, and low humidity) are safe for most healthy individuals; could be potentially dangerous following neurosurgical, plastic, and otolaryngologic procedures (craniotomy, skull base surgery)

REFERENCES

1. Glazer TA, Telian SA. Otologic hazards related to scuba diving. *Sports Health*. 2016;8(2):140–144.
2. Vaezeafshar R, Psaltis AJ, Rao VK, et al. Barosinusitis: comprehensive review and proposed new classification system. *Allergy Rhinol (Providence)*. 2017;8(3):109–117.
3. Livingstone DM, Smith KA, Lange B. Scuba diving and otology: a systematic review with recommendations on diagnosis, treatment, and post-operative care. *Diving Hyperb Med*. 2017;47(2):97–109.
4. Becker GD, Parell GJ. Barotrauma of the ears and sinuses after scuba diving. *Eur Arch Otorhinolaryngol*. 2001;258(4):159–163.

ADDITIONAL READING

- Bove AA. Diving medicine. *Am J Respir Crit Care Med*. 2014;189(12):1479–1486.
- Divers Alert Network: http://www.diversalertnetwork.org
- Lee YI, Ye BJ. Underwater and hyperbaric medicine as a branch of occupational and environmental medicine. *Ann Occup Environ Med*. 2013;25(1):39.
- Navy Department, Defense Department, Naval Sea Systems Command. *U.S. Navy Diving Manual*. Published December 2016. Accessed August 8, 2025. https://www.govinfo.gov/app/details/GOVPUB-D211-PURL-gpo128923
- Schipke JD, Cleveland S, Drees M. Sphenoid sinus barotrauma in diving: case series and review of the literature. *Res Sports Med*. 2018;26(1):124–137.
- van Rijswijk JB, Dubach P. Binaural tympanic-membrane perforations after blast injury. *N Engl J Med*. 2017;376(19):e41.

CLINICAL PEARLS

- Barotrauma is the most common form of diving-related injury; most common is middle ear barotrauma.
- Most serious complication of barotrauma is AGE.
- Divers with lung disease are at high risk for PBT.
- Most TM ruptures heal spontaneously within 4 to 6 weeks; antibiotics *only* needed when the TM is ruptured
- Decongestants, glucocorticoids, and antihistamines are not the standard of care for ear barotrauma.
- Consider prophylactic antibiotics for meningitis for sinus barotrauma.
- Modern commercial aircrafts can be dangerous following neurosurgical, plastic, and otolaryngologic procedures.
- Unstable patients are typically untenable for recompression in a hyperbaric chamber given space restrictions and equipment limitations in this environment—stabilize life-threatening conditions/optimize medically prior to recompression therapy.

BICEPS TENDINOPATHY

Mitchell P. Anderson, MD ▪ Giorgio A. Negron, MD ▪
Daniel C. Herman, MD, PhD, FAAPMR, FACSM, FISBS, CAQSM

BASICS

DESCRIPTION

- Overuse injury of the long head of the biceps muscle
- Initially begins as inflammation in the tendon sheath known as *tenosynovitis* and then progresses to tendon degeneration and disordered arrangement of collagen fibers, otherwise known as *tendinosis* or *biceps tendinopathy*
- Primary biceps tendinitis (inflammation of the tendon) is estimated to represent only 5% of cases (1).
- Biceps tendinopathy commonly occurs in association with rotator cuff pathology with incidence rates as high as 91% in patients with symptomatic rotator cuff tears (2).

EPIDEMIOLOGY

80% of bicep tendinopathy cases are seen in males with peak incidence in the 5th and 6th decade of life (1).

ETIOLOGY AND PATHOPHYSIOLOGY

- Anatomy:
  - The long head of the biceps muscle arises from the superior glenoid labrum and the supraglenoid tubercle of the scapula.
  - It is an intra-articular but extrasynovial structure.
  - Primary blood supply proximally is the anterior humeral circumflex artery.
- Biomechanics:
  - Primary function of the biceps at the elbow is a flexor and supinator.
  - In the shoulder, the biceps tendon may act as a humeral head depressor and a secondary stabilizer of the glenohumeral joint.
  - During throwing, it assists in deceleration of the humerus.

RISK FACTORS

Repetitive use of upper extremities (especially overhead), such as throwing/hitting, swimming, racquet sports, and gymnastics

- Injuries can be caused by the peel-back phenomenon in the late cocking phase and by eccentric contraction during the follow-through phase (3).

COMMONLY ASSOCIATED CONDITIONS

- Rotator cuff pathology (tendinopathy, impingement, tears)
- Glenoid labral tears (superior labrum anterior and posterior [SLAP] lesions)
- Subluxation/dislocation of the long head of the biceps
- Proximal and distal biceps tendon rupture

DIAGNOSIS

HISTORY

- Anterior shoulder pain localized over the bicipital groove, which may radiate distally toward the biceps
- Pain is aggravated by overhead activities or elbow flexion.

PHYSICAL EXAM

- Examination should begin with inspection of both shoulders looking for any asymmetry.
  - A large mass ("Popeye deformity") in the upper arm, ecchymosis, and swelling following a painful audible pop with quick resolution of pain could indicate biceps tendon rupture.
- On palpation, the patient can experience point tenderness over the bicipital groove with the arm in 10 degrees internal rotation (sensitivity: 54%; specificity: 72%) (4).
  - An audible or palpable snap during arc of motion while throwing may indicate instability or subluxation of the biceps tendon.
- Special tests:
  - Uppercut test: With the patient's shoulder in neutral position and forearm supinated, elbow is flexed 90 degrees with hand in a fist. Patient then rapidly brings fist toward chin against resistance. Pain in the shoulder is considered a positive test (sensitivity: 73%; specificity: 78%) (4).
  - Speed test: With the patient's shoulder elevated to 90 degrees of forward flexion, elbow extended and forearm supinated, the patient flexes the shoulder against resistance. Pain in or about the bicipital groove is considered a positive test (sensitivity: 54%; specificity: 81%) (4).
  - Yergason test: With the patient's elbow flexed to 90 degrees, the patient supinates against resistance. Pain over the biceps tendon in the bicipital groove is considered a positive test (sensitivity: 41%; specificity: 79%) (4).
  - Performing the uppercut test and biceps groove tenderness together has the highest sensitivity and specificity to clinically diagnose long head biceps pathology (4)[A].
- Any positive testing for biceps tendon pathology may also signify a glenoid labral tear (SLAP lesion).
- A thorough neurovascular assessment should also be performed.

DIFFERENTIAL DIAGNOSIS

- Rotator cuff tendinopathy
- Impingement syndrome
- Glenoid labral tears
- Biceps tendon subluxation/dislocation
- Subacromial bursitis
- Adhesive capsulitis
- Acromioclavicular joint separation or arthritis
- Pectoralis minor strain
- Glenohumeral joint arthritis
- Thoracic outlet syndrome
- Cervical radiculopathy
- Cervical facet arthropathy
- Brachial plexus injuries
- Rheumatoid arthritis
- Pancoast tumor
- Humeral head osteonecrosis
- Parsonage-Turner syndrome

DIAGNOSTIC TESTS & INTERPRETATION

- Plain-film radiographs are not helpful in the diagnosis of biceps tendon pathology.
- Magnetic resonance imaging (MRI) may show increased signal on T2-weighted images in the area of the biceps tendon and is beneficial for detecting complete tears (sensitivity: ~60%; specificity: ~100%) (5)[B]. Also useful in detecting pathology of the superior labrum and rotator cuff. Magnetic resonance (MR) arthrography may be superior to conventional MRI in diagnosing biceps tendon lesions and SLAP lesions but is invasive (sensitivity: ~90%; specificity: ~50%) (1)[B].
- Dynamic musculoskeletal ultrasound (US) is becoming more popular in diagnosing biceps tendon rupture, subluxation, and dislocation (sensitivity: 49%; specificity: 97%) (1),(5). Studies have shown that it has superior efficacy in detecting normal tendons, full-thickness and partial-thickness tears, and non-tear abnormalities of the biceps tendon when compared to MRI (5). It is not reliable in evaluating intra-articular tears or the glenoid labrum. US is very operator and facility dependent. Advantages include low cost and lack of radiation exposure.

TREATMENT

Acute treatment:

- Rest, ice, nonsteroidal anti-inflammatory drugs (NSAIDs), and/or acetaminophen
- Rest should not include prolonged immobilization because this may lead to adhesive capsulitis (frozen shoulder).
- Gentle stretching and range of motion (ROM) exercises should be initiated early once symptoms begin to improve.
- Consider physical therapy for persistent symptoms.
- Surgery is reserved for refractory cases.

ADDITIONAL THERAPIES

- Physical therapy:
  - Gentle ROM exercises are begun first.
  - Scapulothoracic stabilization exercises
  - Rotator cuff strengthening
  - Biceps strengthening with progression from low to high loading in the more advanced phases of nonoperative or postoperative rehabilitation (3)
- Include:
  - Iontophoresis: uses electric current to drive a corticosteroid into the affected tissue

SURGERY/OTHER PROCEDURES

- Injections:
  - Corticosteroid injection into the biceps tendon sheath may be considered providing short-term pain control up to 6 weeks, but controversy exists regarding the accuracy of such injections; US may increase the accuracy and analgesic effect (1),(2).
  - Injection into the tendon itself has been associated with tendon rupture and should be avoided.
  - Regenerative injection techniques, including platelet-rich plasma (PRP) and prolotherapy, are increasingly being studied in the treatment of various chronic tendinopathies including biceps tendinopathy (5).
- Surgical options may be considered for patients who fail conservative treatment after 3 months or have refractory pain (1),(2):
  - Tenotomy: surgical release of the long head of the biceps tendon at or near its superior glenoid labral origin:
    - Recommended in older patients with low activity requirements
    - Disadvantage includes association with clinically significant "Popeye sign," muscle cramps and strength deficits
    - Minimal rehabilitation is required.
  - Tenodesis: fixation of the long head of the biceps tendon in the bicipital groove.
    - Minimal loss of function compared with tenotomy
    - No cosmetic defect
    - Recommended in younger, more active individuals
    - Disadvantages include a more complex operation, a period of immobilization, and longer postoperative rehabilitation.
  - Both procedures are effective in reducing pain from biceps tendinopathy in the presence of rotator cuff tears (2).
- Proximal rupture of the long head of the biceps typically relieves symptoms of pain without significant loss of function. Surgery may be considered if there is significant loss of strength or function particularly in younger patients.

REFERENCES

1. Varacallo M, Mair SD. *Proximal Biceps Tendinitis and Tendinopathy*. StatPearls. StatPearls Publishing; 2023.
2. Diplock B, Hing W, Marks D. The long head of biceps at the shoulder: a scoping review. *BMC Musculoskelet Disord*. 2023;24(1):232.
3. Borms D, Ackerman I, Smets P, et al. Biceps disorder rehabilitation for the athlete: a continuum of moderate- to high-load exercises. *Am J Sports Med*. 2017;45(3):642–650.
4. Rosas S, Krill MK, Amoo-Achampong K, et al. A practical, evidence-based, comprehensive (PEC) physical examination for diagnosing pathology of the long head of the biceps. *J Shoulder Elbow Surg*. 2017;26(8):1484–1492.
5. Neph A, O'Connell M, Shin JJ, et al. Biceps tendon. In: Onishi K, Fredericson M, Dragoo JL, eds. *Tendinopathy: From Basic Science to Clinical Management*. Springer; 2021:39–54.

ADDITIONAL READING

- Frank RM, Cotter EJ, Strauss EJ, et al. Management of biceps tendon pathology: from the glenoid to the radial tuberosity. *J Am Acad Orthop Surg*. 2018;26(4):e77–e89.
- Friedman DJ, Dunn JC, Higgins LD, et al. Proximal biceps tendon: injuries and management. *Sports Med Arthrosc Rev*. 2008;16(3):162–169.
- Nho SJ, Strauss EJ, Lenart BA, et al. Long head of the biceps tendinopathy: diagnosis and management. *J Am Acad Orthop Surg*. 2010;18(11):645–656.

CLINICAL PEARLS

- Primary biceps tendinitis is rare and thought to be ~5% of cases.
- Performing the uppercut test and biceps groove tenderness together has the highest sensitivity and specificity to clinically diagnose long head biceps pathology.
- Imaging should be considered with shoulder radiography to rule out primary causes of impingement followed by advanced imaging with either US and/or MRI.
- Nonsurgical measures include rest, NSAIDs, acetaminophen, and physical therapy. Corticosteroid injection in bicipital tendon sheath may provide short-term alleviation of pain.

BICEPS TENDON RUPTURE

Saif Usman, MD, FAMSSM, FAAFP

BASICS

DESCRIPTION

- Biceps brachii muscle is composed of a long head originating from the apex of the glenoid and a short head originating from the tip of coracoid process.
- Distally both heads insert onto the distal radial tuberosity.
- Complete or partial tear of the long bicipital tendon can occur at a proximal or distal location from repetitive microtrauma or acute traumatic injury.

EPIDEMIOLOGY

- Occurs most commonly in males age 30 to 60 years
- Occurs most commonly concomitantly with supraspinatus and subscapularis tears (1)
- 90–97% of biceps tendon ruptures are proximal, at the intertubercular sulcus.
- 3–10% occur distally at the elbow

RISK FACTORS

- Male
- Age >30 years
- Smoking (7.5 times increased risk of distal biceps rupture)
- Preexisting bicipital tendinopathy
- Rotator cuff tendinopathy or tear (biceps tendon pathologically loaded)
- Overhead athlete (contributes to anterior shoulder stability with repeated abduction/external rotation)
- Prior corticosteroid injection into biceps tendon sheath
- Anabolic steroid use

COMMONLY ASSOCIATED CONDITIONS

- Rotator cuff impingement: Subacromial impingement in combination with repetitive overhead motion, such as with throwing, can lead to proximal biceps tendon degeneration.
- Superior labrum anterior-to-posterior (SLAP) lesions: may involve the biceps anchor (2)
- Supraspinatus rupture/partial rupture
- Subscapularis rupture/partial rupture: Following subscapularis tears, the biceps tendon can sublux medially out of the bicipital groove, causing a painful clicking sensation.
- Rotator interval lesions: The biceps tendon can sublux medially over the lesser tuberosity after tears to the rotator interval, but there usually is an associated subscapularis injury (2).

DIAGNOSIS

HISTORY

- Mechanism is usually forceful eccentric biceps contraction applied to a flexed elbow.
- Pain is usually located more proximal than distal.
- Prior symptoms are indicative of prior rotator cuff or bicipital tendinopathy.
- In some cases of chronic shoulder pain, there may be notable improvement after inflammation subsides.
- Patients with accompanying rotator cuff pathology may complain of overhead pain and weakness and night pain.

PHYSICAL EXAM

- Proximal rupture:
  - Patient may report a sudden tearing or "pop" in the shoulder.
  - Acute pain and later ecchymosis and swelling about the anterior shoulder
  - Visible lump type of deformity in the midupper arm anteriorly, secondary to muscle belly retracting distally ("Popeye sign")
  - Inspect for "Popeye sign" deformity in anterior brachium.
  - Ecchymosis may involve entire anterior biceps.
  - Elbow function generally is preserved. Patient may have mild weakness of elbow flexion and supination.
  - Shoulder function may be diminished, and careful evaluation of rotator cuff integrity is advised.
  - Specialized tests for biceps pathology include the Speed, Yergason, and Ludington tests.
- Distal rupture:
  - History is usually of a sudden eccentric load with elbow at 90 degrees of flexion.
  - Acute tearing sensation with sudden loss of elbow flexion and supination strength
  - Pain, ecchymosis, and swelling localized over the antecubital fossa
  - Variable degree of proximal retraction of muscle belly ("reverse Popeye sign") (3)
  - May visualize absence of distal biceps tendon as it crosses the elbow flexion crease
  - Hook test is useful in differentiating between complete avulsion and sprain or partial tear.
  - Hook test can be nearly 100% sensitive and specific in detecting complete distal ruptures (3).
  - Biceps squeeze test can be very sensitive (96%) in detecting distal biceps ruptures (squeezing biceps should lead to passive supination of elbow).
  - A partial rupture may have many of the same features as a complete rupture, but generally, the tendon still can be palpated in continuity.

DIFFERENTIAL DIAGNOSIS

- Proximal rupture:
  - Superior labral lesion (i.e., SLAP tear)
  - Subscapularis injury
  - Rotator cuff/rotator interval injury
  - Biceps tendon subluxation (rupture of transverse ligament)
  - Long head of biceps tendinitis or tendinosis; onset usually insidious
  - Greater or lesser tuberosity fractures may occur following shoulder dislocation.
- Distal rupture:
  - Distal biceps tendinitis or tendinosis; onset usually insidious
  - Partial distal biceps tendon rupture
  - Anterior capsule strain; occurs with hyperextension injuries and tenderness is more diffuse anteriorly
  - Coronoid process fractures directly tender over coronoid process; no palpable biceps defect
  - Lateral antebrachial cutaneous nerve entrapment syndrome

DIAGNOSTIC TESTS & INTERPRETATION

Initial Tests (lab, imaging)

- Plain films of shoulder are often negative with isolated tendon rupture.
- Standard elbow x-ray series for distal injuries:
  - Check for avulsion fragment of radial tuberosity.
  - Degenerative changes or lipping at the radial tuberosity can be associated with biceps tendinopathy.
- Shoulder ultrasound is reliable for diagnosing complete rupture, subluxation, or dislocation of biceps tendon (4)[C].
- Elbow ultrasound is reliable for detecting complete versus partial distal biceps tendon tears (5)[C].
- Shoulder or elbow magnetic resonance imaging (MRI) confirms diagnosis if clinical exam is not straightforward and if rotator cuff pathology is suspected.
- MRI findings may include absence of the tendon within the intertubercular groove as a result of tendon retraction.

TREATMENT

GENERAL MEASURES

- Proximal rupture:
  - Acute immobilization in posterior elbow splint with the elbow at 90 degrees for comfort and forearm in full supination; add sling for comfort for first 7 to 10 days until pain improves.
  - Younger patients should begin immediate shoulder and elbow passive range of motion (ROM) exercises.
  - Strengthening can begin in 4 to 5 weeks or when there is resolution of pain.
  - Return to unrestricted activities after 2 to 3 months.
  - Patients >50 years of age may require longer period of immobilization prior to strengthening rehab.
  - An injury with minimal symptoms in elderly patients showing acceptable strength may be managed nonsurgically.
  - Most patients are older and will have little to no change in elbow flexion/supination strength; they may opt for surgery, however, if there is additional rotator cuff pathology.
  - Younger patients may prefer surgical treatment (tenodesis vs. tenotomy) for cosmetic reasons or to return to their previous level of functioning, especially if overhead athletes (2).
- Distal rupture:
  - Acute management is the same as for proximal injuries.
  - Nonoperative treatment is reserved for older, lower demand patients or those with unacceptably high risk for surgery.
  - Nonoperative management is associated with significant loss of elbow supination endurance and strength as well as elbow flexion weakness (2)[C].
  - Majority of patients require surgical repair as soon as possible after injury.
  - Surgical repair of distal biceps tendon rupture in athletes can result in return to sport of up to 97.5% of patients (6).
  - The main complaint after conservative management of biceps tendon ruptures, especially distal ruptures, is loss of elbow flexion and forearm supination strength, especially endurance.
  - Most young people and athletes require surgical repair of complete biceps tendon injuries. Many advocate surgical repair of partial ruptures in this population, especially if the ruptures are distal.

REFERENCES

1. Kowalczuk M, Kohut K, Sabzevari S, et al. Proximal long head biceps rupture: a predictor of rotator cuff pathology. *Arthroscopy*. 2018;34(4):1166–1170.
2. Burns JP, Bahk M, Snyder SJ. Superior labral tears: repair versus biceps tenodesis. *J Shoulder Elbow Surg*. 2011;20(2 Suppl):S2–8.
3. Schmidt CC, Savoie FH III, Steinmann SP, et al. Distal biceps tendon history, updates, and controversies: from the closed American Shoulder and Elbow Surgeons meeting—2015. *J Shoulder Elbow Surg*. 2016;25(10):1717–1730.
4. Armstrong A, Teefey SA, Wu T, et al. The efficacy of ultrasound in the diagnosis of long head of the biceps tendon pathology. *J Shoulder Elbow Surg*. 2006;15(1):7–11.
5. Al-Ani Z, Lauder J. Ultrasound assessment in distal biceps tendon injuries: techniques, pearls, and pitfalls. *Clin Imaging*. 2021;75:46–54.
6. Pitsilos C, Gigis I, Chitas K, et al. Systematic review of distal biceps tendon rupture in athletes: treatment and rehabilitation. *J Shoulder Elbow Surg*. 2022;31(8):1763–1772.

ADDITIONAL READING

- Ward JP, Shreve MC, Youm T, et al. Ruptures of the distal biceps tendon. *Bull Hosp Jt Dis (2013)*. 2014;72(1):110–119.
- Zappia M, Reginelli A, Russo A, et al. Long head of the biceps tendon and rotator interval. *Musculoskelet Surg*. 2013;97(Suppl 2):S99–108.

CLINICAL PEARLS

- Proximal biceps tendon ruptures occur most commonly concomitantly with supraspinatus and subscapularis tears.
- Popeye sign is highly indicative of proximal biceps tendon rupture.
- Hook test is nearly 100% sensitive and specific for distal biceps rupture.
- Musculoskeletal ultrasound can reliably diagnose proximal and distal biceps tendon ruptures, both partial and complete.
- Most cases of distal biceps tendon rupture will require surgical repair as soon as possible after injury.
- Up to 97% of athletes with traumatic distal biceps tendon rupture can successfully return to sport after surgical repair.

BITES AND STINGS

Steven A. Greer, MD, CAQ, FAAFP

BASICS

Arthropods inoculate poison or invading tissue and transmit diseases. Inoculation of poison may occur as either a bite or a sting. This discussion is limited to the irritative, poisonous, and allergic effects of these pests.

DESCRIPTION

- Harmful arthropods of the United States include (1):
  - Ants: fire ants, harvester ants
  - Bees: bumblebees, sweat bees, honeybees, Africanized (killer) bees
  - Bugs: kissing, bed, wheel
  - Caterpillars: puss, browntail, buck, moth saddleback
  - Centipedes
  - Fleas: human, cat, dog
  - Flies: deer, horse, black, stable, and biting midges
  - Lice: body, head, pubic
  - Mites: itch mite (scabies), red bugs (chiggers)
  - Mosquitoes
  - Scorpions
  - Spiders: brown recluse, black widow, hobo
  - Ticks: deer, lone star
  - Wasps: hornets, wasps
- Characteristic reactions include:
  - Local tissue irritation, inflammation, and destruction
  - Systemic effects related to inoculated poisons
  - Allergic reactions: immediate or delayed
- System(s) affected: skin/exocrine

EPIDEMIOLOGY

- Affects all ages with 0- to 4-year-olds and 20- to 24-year-olds at highest risk for nonfatal bites/stings (2)
- Nonfatal: males = females
- Fatal: 80% male

Incidence

- Common, with >1 million nonfatal and 64 fatal cases/y (2),(3)
- Eighth most common cause of nonfatal injury from 2000 to 2020
- Anaphylaxis is estimated at 3% in adults and 0.4–0.8% in children.
- Individual stings from Africanized (killer) bees are no more potent than other bees; the danger lies in their predilection to swarm, causing death by multiple stings.

Prevalence

Ubiquitous, varies by region and season (2)

ETIOLOGY AND PATHOPHYSIOLOGY

- Local tissue inflammation and destruction from poison (4)
- Allergic reaction from previous sensitization (0.4–3%)
- Toxic reaction from large inoculation of poison

Genetics

No genetic predilection

RISK FACTORS

- Living environment (4),(5),(6)
- Climate
- Season
- Clothing
- Lack of protective measures
- Perfumes, colognes
- Previous sensitization
- Young or elderly at more risk for morbidity/mortality

GENERAL PREVENTION

Prevention/avoidance (4),(5),(6):

- Avoid reexposure in known hypersensitive individuals.
- Prescribe anaphylactic (ANA kit) or self-administered epinephrine (EpiPen), if indicated.
- Educate on risks of increasing anamnestic responses in the future.
- Consider desensitization with immunotherapy in severe cases.
- Cover as much skin as possible.
- Use repellants on uncovered areas.
- Apply sunscreen first, then repellant.
- N,N-Diethyl-meta-toluamide (DEET), picaridin, or other proven insect repellants
- Oil of lemon eucalyptus, p-menthane-3,8-diol (PMD), and IR3535 are considered biopesticides by the Environmental Protection Agency (EPA), but be sure to use EPA-approved products because many versions have not been tested.
- Permethrin applied to clothes is effective through multiple washings.
- Permethrin-infused clothing is commercially available and effective.
- Consider immunization/prophylaxis for travel to endemic areas.

DIAGNOSIS

PHYSICAL EXAM

- Signs and symptoms (4),(5),(6):
  - Erythema
  - Pain
  - Heat
  - Swelling
  - Itching
  - Blisters
  - Secondary infection: cellulitis, abscess
  - Necrosis
  - Ulceration
  - Drainage
- Toxic reactions (nonantigenic):
  - Nausea
  - Vomiting
  - Headache
  - Fever
  - Diarrhea
  - Light-headedness
  - Syncope
  - Drowsiness
  - Muscles spasms
  - Edema
  - Convulsions
- Systemic reactions (allergic):
  - Itching eyes
  - Facial flushing
  - Generalized urticaria
  - Dry cough
  - Chest/throat constriction
  - Wheezing
  - Dyspnea
  - Cyanosis
  - Abdominal cramps
  - Diarrhea
  - Nausea
  - Vomiting
  - Vertigo
  - Chills/fever
  - Stridor
  - Shock
  - Loss of consciousness
  - Involuntary bowel/bladder action
  - Frothy sputum
  - Respiratory failure
  - Cardiovascular collapse
  - Death
- Delayed reaction:
  - Serum-sickness–like reactions
  - Fever
  - Malaise
  - Headache
  - Urticaria
  - Lymphadenopathy
  - Polyarthritis
- Unusual reactions:
  - Encephalopathy
  - Neuritis
  - Vasculitis
  - Nephrosis
  - Extreme fear/anxiety

DIFFERENTIAL DIAGNOSIS

- Local reaction: infection, cellulitis, dermatoses, punctures, foreign bodies
- Toxic reaction: chemical exposure/ingestion, medications, intravenous (IV) drug abuse, environmental, plants
- Allergic reaction: medications, illicit drugs, foods, topical products, environmental, plants, chemicals

DIAGNOSTIC TESTS & INTERPRETATION

- Lab: Leukocytosis, thrombocytopenia, hypofibrinogenemia, abnormal coagulation, disseminated intravascular coagulation, proteinuria, hemoglobinemia, hemoglobinuria, myoglobinemia, myoglobinuria, and azotemia are uncommon but possible manifestations in severe reactions.
- Pathologic findings: inflammation, ulceration, vesiculation, pustulation, rupture, eschar, swelling (4)

TREATMENT

- Long-term treatment (4):
  - Recommended for those with hypersensitivity reaction but may be considered for individuals with large local reactions
  - Self-administered epinephrine device
  - Hypersensitivity identification
  - Venom immunotherapy for 3 to 5 years is up to 98% effective, and remains 90% effective after cessation of treatment.

- Acute treatment (4),(6):
  - Outpatient or inpatient, depending on individual response to injury
  - Hospitalize for severe systemic reactions with threatened airway obstruction, bronchospasm, hypotension, severe angiodermatitis, or pain

GENERAL MEASURES

- First aid measures, local treatment, activate emergency services in severe reactions. If history of allergy or large envenomations, don't wait to seek emergency care (4),(6).
- Use ANA kit and over-the-counter antihistamines, if available and required.
- Local (depending on severity):
  - Remove stinger (scrape it out—don't squeeze with tweezer).
  - Cleanse wound.
  - Ice packs to bite or sting site (alternate 10 minutes on or 10 minutes off)
  - Elevation of affected part
  - Débride ulcers.
  - Drain abscesses.
- Systemic (depending on severity and type of reaction): home use—EpiPen:
  - Adequate airway (intubation, tracheostomy): if needed to bypass obstruction
  - Oxygen (4 to 6 L/min): if needed for respiratory distress
  - Hospitalize and observe 24 to 48 hours.

MEDICATION

First Line

- Local (depending on severity):
  - Analgesics
  - Antihistamines: diphenhydramine (Benadryl) 25 to 50 mg QID
  - Steroids topical or oral: Prednisone 20 to 40 mg/day is unproven but may be helpful for large local reactions.
  - Antibiotics only if there is a secondary infection
- Systemic (depending on severity and reaction type):
  - Epinephrine (1:1,000) subcutaneous (SC): to combat urticaria, wheezing, angioedema—child: 0.01 mL/kg; adult 0.3 to 0.5 mL/kg
  - Diphenhydramine: 25 to 50 mg IV or intramuscular (IM) to combat urticaria, wheezing, angioedema
  - Albuterol 5 mg inhalation and ipratropium bromide 0.5 mg inhalation: bronchospasm
  - IV fluids (Ringer lactate): if needed for hypotension, hypovolemia
  - Dopamine: 200 mg in 250 mL at 5 μg/kg/min to correct vascular collapse
- Titrate to maintain systemic blood pressure (BP) over 90 mm Hg:
  - Hydrocortisone: 100 to 250 mg IV, if needed, for severe urticaria or spider bite
  - Tetanus prophylaxis and antibiotics: only if secondary infection, rarely indicated
  - Diazepam (Valium): 5 to 10 mg, if needed, for severe muscle spasms
  - Morphine or meperidine (Demerol): if needed for pain
- Antivenins may be appropriate based on availability, identification of organism, and previous sensitivity.
- Topical insecticides:
  - Lice: 1% permethrin (Nix, Elimite) is still considered first line, particularly for children 2 to 6 months of age, and during pregnancy, despite up to 75% resistance. 0.5% Ivermectin (Sklice), 0.9% Spinosad (Natroba), or 0.5% malathion (Ovide) may be used as initial choice or for permethrin failure. Pyrethrin (Rid) is also effective.
  - Scabies: 5% permethrin is drug of choice, but 10% crotamiton (Eurax) is also effective.
- Contraindications: Refer to manufacturer's literature.
- Precautions:
  - Dosing appropriate to age
  - If severe reaction, do not delay treatment.
  - Severe vascular collapse may require central pressure monitor.
- Significant possible interactions: Refer to manufacturer's literature.

Second Line

Alternative drugs (6),(7):

- Other H_1 antihistamines (e.g., loratadine [Claritin], fexofenadine [Allegra])
- H_2 blockers (e.g., ranitidine [Zantac], cimetidine [Tagamet], famotidine [Pepcid])
- Oral ivermectin (Mectizan) is effective for lice and scabies. Although only FDA approved for this purpose in adults, it is recommended by the American Academy of Pediatrics (AAP) for topical failure in children weighing 15 kg or more.

SURGERY/OTHER PROCEDURES

Optimal treatment of necrotic spider bites is not well defined. Surgical repair may be required for severe ulcerative lesions but not until primary necrotizing process is complete (5).

COMPLEMENTARY & ALTERNATIVE MEDICINE

- Oil of lemon eucalyptus, PMD, and IR3535 are considered biopesticides by the EPA, but be sure to use EPA-approved products because essential oils have not been tested (6),(8).
- Turmeric has been shown effective for pain.

ONGOING CARE

FOLLOW-UP RECOMMENDATIONS

No activity restrictions

Patient Monitoring

Follow-up wound care

DIET

No special diet; nothing by mouth if severe systemic reaction

PATIENT EDUCATION

- Protective measures, ANA kit/EpiPen use, risks (4),(5),(6)
- Individuals with known sensitivity should wear medical identification (bracelet, tag) or carry a card.

PROGNOSIS

Expected course (4):

- Minor reactions—excellent
- Severe reactions—excellent with early, appropriate treatment

COMPLICATIONS

- Infection (4),(6):
  - Bacterial
  - Arthropod-associated diseases with tick, fly, bug, and mosquito bites (e.g., Lyme borreliosis, rickettsial disease [Rocky Mountain spotted fever], arboviral encephalitis, malaria, leishmaniasis, trypanosomiasis, dengue)
- Scarring
- Drug reactions
- Multisystem failure
- Death

Pediatric Considerations

Not a contraindication to appropriate management

REFERENCES

1. Centers for Disease Control and Prevention. Pictorial keys: arthropods, reptiles, birds, and mammals of public health significance. Published May 22, 2000. Accessed August 8, 2025. https://stacks.cdc.gov/view/cdc/60114
2. Centers for Disease Control and Prevention. All intents all injury deaths and rates per 100,000. Data years: 2023, United States, all ages, all sexes, all races, all ethnicities. Accessed August 8, 2025. https://wisqars.cdc.gov/reports/?o=MORT&y1=2023&y2=2023&t=0&i=0&m=20810&g=00&me=0&s=0&r=0&ry=2&e=0&yp=65&a=ALL&g1=0&g2=199&a1=0&a2=199&r1=INTENT&r2=NONE&r3=NONE&r4=NONE
3. Quickstats: number of deaths from hornet, wasp, and bee stings, among males and females—National Vital Statistics System, United States, 2000–2017. *MMWR Morb Mortal Wkly Rep.* 2019;68(29):649.
4. Golden DBK, Demain J, Freeman T, et al. Stinging insect hypersensitivity: a practice parameter update 2016. *Ann Allergy Asthma Immunol.* 2017;118(1):28–54.
5. Centers for Disease Control and Prevention. *CDC Health Information for International Travel 2016.* Oxford University Press; 2015.
6. Kimberlin DW, Barnett ED, Lynfield R, et al, eds. *Red Book: 2021–2024 Report of the Committee on Infectious Diseases.* 32nd ed. American Academy of Pediatrics; 2021.
7. Nolt D, Moore S, Yan A, et al. Head Lice. *Pediatrics.* 2022;150(4):e2022059282.
8. Daily JW, Yang M, Park S. Efficacy of turmeric extracts and curcumin for alleviating the symptoms of joint arthritis: a systematic review and meta-analysis of randomized clinical trials. *J Med Food.* 2016;19(8):717–729.

CLINICAL PEARLS

- Prevention is often more effective than treatment.
- Vigilant observation for systemic reaction allows for early treatment and better recovery.
- Allergic reactions worsen with each successive exposure.

BRACHIAL PLEXUS INJURIES (BURNERS AND STINGERS)

Nicole Madrilejo, MD

BASICS

DESCRIPTION

- Acute trauma to the neck and shoulder area injuring the brachial plexus
- Typically causes burning or stinging pain in the upper shoulder radiating down the entire upper extremity, hence, the names "burner" and "stinger"
- Most commonly involves the upper trunk of the plexus or cervical nerve roots C5 and C6
- Mechanism of injury:
  - Traction to the plexus when the shoulder is depressed and the head is forced away from the injured side
  - Compression of cervical nerve roots when the head is forced toward the side of injury
  - Direct blow to the brachial plexus at the supraclavicular fossa

EPIDEMIOLOGY

Incidence

- Exact incidence unknown due to underreporting of mild injuries by athletes
- Common in contact sports (football, rugby, wrestling, hockey); football career incidence reported between 26% and 50.3%
- Younger athletes may be more susceptible due to less developed musculature.
- Frequent recurrence, reported as high as 87% (1),(2)

ETIOLOGY AND PATHOPHYSIOLOGY

- Most are limited to neurapraxia, nerve dysfunction with demyelination.
- Minority involve axonotmesis with subsequent wallerian degeneration and eventual regeneration of axons.

RISK FACTORS

- Previous burner
- Limited range of motion of the neck or shoulder
- Cervical canal and foraminal stenosis

GENERAL PREVENTION

- Neck roll, shoulder pad lifter, or rigid collar (e.g., cowboy collar) in football might reduce injury risk.
- Encourage proper tackling in football and neck strengthening exercises for athletes in high-risk sports.

DIAGNOSIS

HISTORY

- Mechanism of injury (Falling on an outstretched arm suggests alternative injury.) (3)
- Details of symptom quality, severity, and location (Bilateral or lower extremity symptoms indicate cervical fracture or cord injury until proven otherwise; symptoms not typical of burners mandate search for an alternative diagnosis.)
- Modifying factors (Limitation or pain with shoulder motion suggests alternative shoulder diagnosis.)
- Initial versus recurrent injury (Recurrence typically requires more aggressive rehabilitation.)

PHYSICAL EXAM

- Signs and symptoms (3):
  - Burning or stinging pain radiating down one arm circumferentially (i.e., nondermatomal pattern)
  - Sometimes numbness, paresthesias, and weakness in the extremity
  - Athlete often immediately holds the arm close to the body or even shakes the upper extremity.
  - Symptoms often last a few minutes but can persist for weeks, particularly in recurrent episodes.
- Physical examination:
  - Inspection (asymmetry or postural abnormality to address in therapy)
  - Palpation (Tenderness suggests alternative diagnosis; spasm is common but nonspecific.)
  - Neurologic examination (strength, sensation, reflexes to localize injury, rule out cord injury)
  - Weakness most common in deltoid, biceps, and rotator cuff (3)
  - Spurling test may be positive.
  - Tinel sign at the supraclavicular fossa (Positive result indicates plexus injury.)
  - After serious cervical injury is ruled out, Spurling neuroforaminal compression test (disk herniation, burner from cervical foraminal stenosis)

DIFFERENTIAL DIAGNOSIS

- Cervical injury (fracture, dislocation, spinal cord injury, disc herniation):
  - Bilateral symptoms, cervical vertebral tenderness, or lower extremity findings indicate cervical fracture or spinal cord injury until proven otherwise.
- Glenohumeral dislocation
- Acromioclavicular separation
- Clavicle fracture
- Thoracic outlet syndrome (when chronic, recurrent):
  - Repetitive athletic movements with pitching or swimming

DIAGNOSTIC TESTS & INTERPRETATION

Initial Tests (lab, imaging)

- Not routine
- Cervical spine x-rays if recurrent injury, findings localizing to one cervical level, symptoms in more than one extremity, to evaluate bony abnormalities (3)

- X-ray cervical spine if fracture, dislocation, or cervical instability suspected:
  - Required if severe nerve pain, focal cervical spine tenderness, limited range of motion, weakness, or recurrence
  - Anteroposterior (AP), lateral, oblique, flexion, extension
- Magnetic resonance imaging (MRI) or computed tomography (CT) cervical spine if x-rays are unrevealing to identify neuroforaminal stenosis, disc herniation, or mass as possible causes of nerve root impingement (3); often not needed for uncomplicated cases and some risk of false positive:
  - Indications:
    - Neurologic symptoms and signs that are not improving daily
    - Bilateral symptoms (burning hands syndrome)
    - Recurrence within 1 year

Diagnostic Procedures/Other

Electromyography/nerve conduction velocity (EMG/NCV) if symptoms last at least 3 weeks for confirmation, localization, and prognosis (EMG normalization lags far behind clinical and neurologic recovery, so follow-up EMG generally not indicated.) (3)

TREATMENT

GENERAL MEASURES

- Stretch tight muscles at neck and shoulder.
- Strengthen neck, shoulder, and muscles weakened by injury.
- These strategies apply, regardless of injury mechanism, to focus on functional recovery.
- Schedule follow-up until symptoms and examination normalize.
- Enhancing protective equipment
- Return to play only when asymptomatic and normal neurologic examination (2),(3).
- Recommend orthopedic or neurosurgical evaluations for possible surgeries for severe cases.

COMPLEMENTARY & ALTERNATIVE MEDICINE

Football players can consider neck roll, shoulder pad lifter, or rigid collar when returning to play.

ONGOING CARE

Prevention:

- Chest-out posture
- Ensure correct playing technique.
- Maintain strength and flexibility of neck and shoulder.

REFERENCES

1. Kuhlman GS, McKeag DB. The "burner": a common nerve injury in contact sports. *Am Fam Physician.* 1999;60(7):2035–2042.
2. Miller TP, Smith JS, Svoboda KJ, et al. Brachial plexus injuries in athletes: epidemiology, mechanisms of injury, and return-to-play considerations. *Am J Sports Med.* 2023;51(1):156–166.
3. Zoch DS, Herring SA, Standaert CJ. Stingers in contact sports: current concepts in etiology, diagnosis, and management. *Clin J Sports Med.* 2018;28(5):407–415.

ADDITIONAL READING

- Aval SM, Durand P Jr, Shankwiler JA. Neurovascular injuries to the athlete's shoulder: part I. *J Am Acad Orthop Surg.* 2007;15(4):249–256.
- Aval SM, Durand P Jr, Shankwiler JA. Neurovascular injuries to the athlete's shoulder: part II. *J Am Acad Orthop Surg.* 2007;15(5):281–289.
- Choi ES, Shin DS, Yoon BB, et al. Management of avulsion injuries of the brachial plexus in athletes: a systematic review. *J Am Acad Orthop Surg.* 2020;28(4):e326–e336.
- Rihn JA, Anderson DT, Lamb K, et al. Cervical spine injuries in American football. *Sports Med.* 2009;39(9):697–708.
- Safran MR. Nerve injury about the shoulder in athletes, part 2: long thoracic nerve, spinal accessory nerve, burners/stingers, thoracic outlet syndrome. *Am J Sports Med.* 2004;32(4):1063–1076.
- Smith JS, Miller TP, Shin AS, et al. Surgical management of brachial plexus injuries in athletes: a comprehensive review. *J Am Acad Orthop Surg.* 2021;29(18):e859–e869.
- Standaert CJ, Herring SA. Expert opinion and controversies in musculoskeletal and sports medicine: stingers. *Arch Phys Med Rehabil.* 2009;90(3):402–406.

CLINICAL PEARLS

- Nerve damage is generally not permanent, but a few patients have symptoms lasting months to years (3).
- Conditioning and rehabilitation should begin immediately. You can return to contact activity when the symptoms are gone and your strength and sensation are back to normal (1).
- Continue stretching and strengthening at least the rest of the season. Continuance of exercises throughout your career will lower the chance of having another burner (1).

BRUGADA SYNDROME

Chau Bui, DO • Paul Meirick, MD

BASICS

DESCRIPTION

- Channelopathies refer to a group of inherited arrhythmogenic diseases caused by mutations in genes encoding for ion channel proteins in cardiomyocytes that disrupt the balance of currents in the cardiac action potential. These disruptions may lead to ventricular arrhythmias and sudden cardiac death (SCD).
- The channelopathies include Brugada syndrome, long QT syndrome (LQTS) (see chapter on QT syndromes), short QT syndrome (SQTS) (see chapter on QT syndromes), and catecholaminergic polymorphic ventricular tachycardia (CPVT) (see supplemental materials for CPVT).
- Brugada syndrome: mostly commonly affects the cardiac sodium channel and is characterized by electrocardiogram (ECG) findings of a pseudo–right bundle branch block (RBBB), ST-segment elevation in leads V_1 to V_3, and an increased risk of SCD.

EPIDEMIOLOGY

- Most commonly presents in the 3rd or 4th decades of life. Average age at diagnosis is 41 years (1).
- Majority of affected individuals are Asian.

Prevalence

- Approximately 1:2,000
- Prevalence higher in South Asia than in Western countries

ETIOLOGY AND PATHOPHYSIOLOGY

- Autosomal dominant inheritance of a mutation affecting the cardiac sodium channel gene
- >12 genes associated with Brugada syndrome

Genetics

The most common cause is the autosomal dominant inheritance of an SCN gene mutation that affects the cardiac sodium channel with variable penetrance (2); clinical penetrance is 8-fold higher in men than women. (3)

RISK FACTORS

The primary risk factor for channelopathies is genetic:

- Risk factors for precipitating a fatal arrhythmia in Brugada syndrome are swimming, fever or any cause of hyperthermia, intake of abundant meals and imbibing excessive alcohol, cocaine use, and overdose of psychotropic drugs (neuroleptics, tricyclic antidepressants).
- Arrhythmic events with Brugada syndrome occur most commonly at rest or during sleep when vagal tone predominates.

GENERAL PREVENTION

- SCD resulting from a Brugada syndrome may be prevented by carefully screening and identifying athletes with the condition. The preparticipation evaluation is the most important tool for identifying athletes with symptoms that may represent an inherited channelopathy. Any athlete with symptoms of palpitations, syncope, presyncope, any collapse, or with a family history of SCD or "accidental" death should be further evaluated with the tools reviewed below.
- Automatic external defibrillators (AEDs) are another important tool in preventing SCD from undiagnosed Brugada syndrome.

DIAGNOSIS

- Brugada pattern is used to describe those with typical ECG features but no other clinical criteria.
- Brugada type 1 is diagnosed on the basis of (4):
  - Type 1 ST-segment elevation (coved type) in >1 right precordial lead (V_1 to V_3) in the presence or absence of a sodium channel blocker plus at least one of the following:
    - Documented ventricular fibrillation (VF)
    - Self-terminating polymorphic ventricular tachycardia (VT)
    - Family history of SCD at <45 years
    - Type 1 ST-segment elevation in family members
    - Electrophysiologic inducibility of VT
    - Unexplained syncope suggestive of a tachyarrhythmia
    - Nocturnal agonal respiration
- Brugada type 2 or 3 is diagnosed on the basis of (4):
  - Type 2 or 3 ST-segment elevation (saddleback type) in >1 right precordial lead under baseline conditions with conversion to type 1 ST-segment elevation following challenge with a sodium channel blocker plus at least one of the following:
    - Documented VF
    - Self-terminating polymorphic VT
    - Family history of SCD at <45 years
    - Type 1 ST-segment elevation in family members
    - Electrophysiologic inducibility of VT
    - Unexplained syncope suggestive of a tachyarrhythmia
    - Nocturnal agonal respiration
- Prehospital:
  - In the case that any patient with a Brugada syndrome converts into a life-threatening arrhythmia in the field, the most useful immediate tool and treatment is an AED.

HISTORY

- Pertinent history in screening athletes: Gathering a detailed and careful history during the preparticipation physical or during the evaluation of an athlete who comes to your attention is critical. The following questions should be included when interviewing an athlete:
  - Have you ever passed out, become dizzy, or had chest pain during or after exercise?
  - Do you get tired more quickly than others during exercise?
  - Has anyone in the family died suddenly and unexpectedly before the age of 50 years? (Remember to ask about family members who died of accidental causes such as sudden infant death syndrome, drownings, and motor vehicle accidents because they may be clues to an undiagnosed family history of channelopathy.)
  - Have you ever had a heart abnormality or murmur diagnosed by a doctor?
  - Have you ever had an abnormal heart rate, palpitations, or irregular heartbeats?
  - Have you had high blood pressure (BP) or high cholesterol?
  - Has a physician ever denied or restricted your participation in sports for heart problems?
  - Have any of your relatives ever had cardiomyopathy, Marfan syndrome, LQTS, SQTS, or significant heart arrhythmias?
- Pertinent history in potentially affected athletes:
  - Most common clinical presentation in Brugada syndrome is life-threatening arrhythmia.
  - More common at night and while sleeping
  - Not usually related to exercise
  - Inquire about a history of syncope, presyncope, past history of sudden cardiac arrest, or a family history of SCD.

PHYSICAL EXAM

- The most important elements of the exam are general (including level of consciousness), cardiac, and pulmonary examinations and, in the case of a patient who has sustained a life-threatening arrhythmia, complete trauma examination.
- Because patients with Brugada syndrome typically have structurally normal hearts, it is not uncommon to observe a completely normal examination when a life-threatening arrhythmia is not present.
- When arrhythmias are present, the examination may be notable for bradycardia or tachycardia, either regular or irregular, depending on the patient's rhythm.

B

DIFFERENTIAL DIAGNOSIS

QT syndromes, CPVT, acquired LQTS with its many reversible metabolic and drug-induced causes, acute coronary syndrome, true RBBB, pericarditis, drug-induced VT or VF

DIAGNOSTIC TESTS & INTERPRETATION

Initial Tests (lab, imaging)

In the setting of a life-threatening arrhythmia, it may be indicated to rule out ischemic or metabolic causes with a basic or comprehensive metabolic panel and cardiac enzymes.

Diagnostic Procedures/Other

ECG is the most important initial diagnostic tool. Holter monitors and echocardiograms may be of use as well:

- Brugada syndrome:
  - Classic Brugada type 1: Elevated ST segment (≥2 mm) descends with an upward convexity to an inverted T wave—"coved type" Brugada pattern.
  - Brugada types 2 and 3:
    - "Saddle back" ST-T wave: Elevated ST segment descends toward the baseline and then rises again to the upright or biphasic T wave.
    - ST segment elevated ≥1 mm in type 2 and <1 mm in type 3
    - Moving the right precordial chest leads up to the 2nd or 3rd intercostal space may increase the sensitivity.
    - The ECG findings may be transient and not present each time an ECG is performed.
    - Electrophysiology testing may be used in evaluating Brugada syndrome but is not heavily relied on.

TREATMENT

The mainstay of treatment in Brugada syndrome is implantable cardioverter defibrillator (ICD), although quinidine has shown promising data as a preventative pharmacotherapy.

MEDICATION

- Adjunctive pharmacotherapy for patients with frequent ICD discharges includes amiodarone and quinidine.
- Electrical storm in Brugada syndrome is treated with isoproterenol or quinidine.

SURGERY/OTHER PROCEDURES

- ICD implantation can prevent SCD in Brugada syndrome (3)[B].
- Selection of patients for ICD is not entirely clear, but ICD may be used in higher risk patients such as those with syncope or with VT without cardiac arrest (3)[C].

ADMISSION, INPATIENT, AND NURSING CONSIDERATIONS

As always, all patients who present with a life-threatening arrhythmia should be treated emergently with cardioversion and/or pharmacotherapy as dictated by standard advanced cardiac life support (ACLS).

ONGOING CARE

All patients with channelopathies should be followed regularly by a cardiologist. Education and restrictions regarding exercise are crucial to survival.

FOLLOW-UP RECOMMENDATIONS

Return-to-play decisions:

- SCD in Brugada syndrome usually is not related to exercise.
- The latest American Heart Association/American College of Cardiology (AHA/ACC) 2015 participation guidelines: In a symptomatic athlete, competitive sports participation may be considered following expert consultation from electrophysiologist and cardiologist, initiation of treatment, appropriate precautionary measures, and the athlete has been asymptomatic for at least 3 months (5)[C].
- Asymptomatic athlete with genotype-positive/phenotype-negative (concealed channelopathy) may participate in all competitive sports with appropriate precautionary measures (avoidance of Brugada exacerbating drugs, appropriate electrolyte/hydration replenishment, avoidance of hyperthermic conditions, acquire personal AED, and establish appropriate emergency action plan) (5)[C].
- Competitive sports participation may be considered for an athlete with either previously symptomatic or electrocardiographically evident Brugada syndrome, assuming appropriate precautionary measures and disease specific treatments are in place, and that the athlete has been asymptomatic on treatment for at least 3 months (5)[C].
- Caution should be used to avoid sports where impaired consciousness would be dangerous or lethal, such as with SCUBA diving, swimming, weight lifting with free weights, and horseback riding.
- The latest European Society of Cardiology (ESC) 2020 guidelines agree with 2015 AHA guidelines above and add prescription drugs that may aggravate Brugada syndrome, electrolyte abnormalities, and increases in core body temperature >39°C are not recommended (6)[C].

REFERENCES

1. Brugada J, Campuzano O, Arbelo E, et al. Present status of Brugada syndrome: JACC state-of-the-art review. *J Am Coll Cardiol.* 2018;72(9):1046–1059.
2. Drezner JA, Ackerman MJ, Cannon BC, et al. Abnormal electrocardiographic findings in athletes: recognising changes suggestive of primary electrical disease. *Br J Sports Med.* 2013;47(3):153–167.
3. Mazzanti A, O'Rourke S, Ng K, et al. The usual suspects in sudden cardiac death of the young: a focus on inherited arrhythmogenic diseases. *Expert Rev Cardiovasc Ther.* 2014;12(4):499–519.
4. Wilde AA, Antzelevitch C, Borggrefe M, et al. Proposed diagnostic criteria for the Brugada syndrome: consensus report. *Circulation.* 2002;106(19):2514–2519.
5. Ackerman MJ, Zipes DP, Kovacs RJ, et al. Eligibility and disqualification recommendations for competitive athletes with cardiovascular abnormalities: task force 10: the cardiac channelopathies: a scientific statement from the American Heart Association and American College of Cardiology. *Circulation.* 2015;132(22):e326–e329.
6. Pelliccia A, Sharma S, Gati S. 2020 ESC guidelines on sports cardiology and exercise in patients with cardiovascular disease. *Eur Heart J.* 2021;42(1):17–96.

ADDITIONAL READING

Priori SG, Wilde AA, Horie M, et al. HRS/EHRA/APHRS expert consensus statement on the diagnosis and management of patients with inherited primary arrhythmia syndromes: document endorsed by HRS, EHRA, and APHRS in May 2013 and by ACCF, AHA, PACES, and AEPC in June 2013. *Heart Rhythm.* 2013;10(12):1932–1963.

CLINICAL PEARLS

- Brugada syndrome most often affects the cardiac sodium channel and is characterized by ECG findings of a pseudo–RBBB, ST-segment elevation in leads V_1 to V_3, and an increased risk of SCD.
- Risk factors for precipitating a fatal arrhythmia in Brugada syndrome are swimming, fever or any cause of hyperthermia, intake of abundant meals and imbibing excessive alcohol, cocaine use, and overdose of psychotropic drugs (neuroleptics, tricyclic antidepressants), although most events occur during sleep or rest.
- Diagnosis of Brugada syndrome is made by ECG.
- The first-line treatment of Brugada syndrome is an ICD.
- Return to play after diagnosis of Brugada syndrome should be a careful conversation between physician and athlete and follow the AHA/ACC 2015 participation guidelines.

BURSITIS

Ziad Fahad Rayes, MBBS, MBA, Ccfp(Sem), Dip Sport Med(Casem) ▪ Muath Alammar, MBBS, SBFM, ABFM, JBFM

BASICS

- Definition: inflammation or irritation of the bursa (fluid-filled sacs located between mobile structures that decrease friction and provide a cushion between bones, tendons, muscles, and skin)
- **Important Consideration: Often a Secondary Problem:** It is crucial to recognize that many bursal swellings are not isolated, independent problems. Instead, they frequently arise as a consequence of, or in conjunction with, underlying pathologies such as **tendonitis (inflammation of a tendon), partial tendon tears, or osteoarthritis (OA)** of the adjacent joint. Therefore, assessment of bursitis should often include an evaluation for these related conditions.
- May be difficult to distinguish from fractures. Suspicious joints should be immobilized, particularly in the setting of trauma. Also, septic joint is a possibility that needs to be excluded. Two types of bursa and potentially either of them may be affected:
  - Deep bursa "commonly seen in clinical practice":
    - Subacromial (subdeltoid) bursa: lies between the acromion and the rotator cuff; overusing their rotator cuff muscles, and doing an overhead lifting and forceful pulling are risk factors for subacromial bursitis.
    - Scapulothoracic bursa: lies between superior-medial angle of the scapula and the adjacent ribs. Scapulothoracic bursitis is mainly caused by overuse and trauma.
    - Iliopsoas bursa: lies between the iliopsoas tendon and the lesser trochanter (largest bursa in the body). Iliopsoas bursitis is mostly caused by trauma, injury or having some sort of arthritis such as rheumatoid arthritis or psoriatic arthritis.
  - Superficial bursa:
    - Olecranon bursa: lies between the olecranon process and the overlying skin. Olecranon bursitis can be caused by trauma or constant pressure on the elbow (for example, repetitive leaning on a hard surface).
    - Prepatellar bursa: lies between the patella and the skin. Trauma and repetitive kneeling increases risk and seen with certain occupations (i.e., carpenters and plumbers).
    - Pes anserine bursa: lies between the tibia and the insertions of the sartorius, gracilis, and semitendinosus tendons. Pes anserine bursitis may be caused by inadequate stretching before exercise, tight hamstring muscles, increase weight, osteoarthritis of the knee, or having genu varum or genu valgus.
- Trochanteric bursa: has superficial and deep components. The superficial bursa lies between the tensor fascia lata and skin; the deep bursa is located between the greater trochanter and the tensor fascia lata. Trochanteric bursitis is often the result of injury, repetitive motions, posture abnormalities, arthritis, or surgery.
- Calcaneal bursitis: two bursae at the level of insertion of the Achilles tendon. The superficial one is located between the skin and the tendon called posterior Achilles tendon bursa. Retrocalcaneal bursa aka posterior Achilles tendon bursa is the deep bursa located between the calcaneus and the tendon. Posterior Achilles tendon bursitis is caused by wearing a shoe that has a rigid back support that presses against the soft heel tissue. Retrocalcaneal bursitis is aggravated by injury or shoes with hard back support.

DESCRIPTION

- Bursae are flattened sacs that serve as a protective buffer between bones and overlapping muscles (deep bursae) or between bones and tendons/skin (superficial bursae). In the normal state, they contain minimal amounts of fluid to reduce friction and facilitate pain-free movement during muscle contraction.
- Bursitis can be acute or chronic. Acute bursitis is result of an injury, infection, or inflammation. Chronic bursitis follows a long period of repetitive use or motion. Chronic bursal swelling is often due to tendinopathy of the underlying tendons.
- Humans have >160 bursae.

ETIOLOGY AND PATHOPHYSIOLOGY

- Trauma (acute and chronic): most common cause
- Prolonged pressure: prolonged kneeling or leaning on an elbow
- Overuse
- Infection (septic bursitis): direct introduction of microorganisms through traumatic injury or hematogenous
- For septic bursitis: *Staphylococcus aureus* causes 80%, followed by *Streptococcus* in acute infections and *mycobacteria* in chronic infections
- Crystal deposition: gout or pseudogout
- Inflammatory arthritis: rheumatoid arthritis, psoriatic arthritis, or spondyloarthritis

RISK FACTORS

- Professions and activities that require repetitive motion or pressure on particular bursae (e.g., carpet laying, tile setting, gardening, bicycling, baseball, ice skating)
- Rheumatoid arthritis
- Osteoarthritis
- Gout
- Thyroid disease
- Diabetes

DIAGNOSIS

- Full assessment of regional musculoskeletal function
- Ultrasonography or magnetic resonance imaging (MRI) for deep bursitis
- Aspiration for suspected infection, hemorrhage (due to trauma or anticoagulants), or crystal-induced bursitis
- Aspiration of hip and other deep bursae should be done by a well-trained physician and may be guided by ultrasound (US).

PHYSICAL EXAM

- Localized tenderness (1)[A]
- Swelling (1)[A]
- Decreased range of motion or pain with movement
- Erythema or edema (seen in superficial bursitis) (1)[A]
- Traumatic bursitis often follows traumatic event or overuse of related joints.
- Muscle atrophy (seen in chronic bursitis related to immobility)

DIFFERENTIAL DIAGNOSIS

- Arthritis: rheumatoid, septic, osteoarthritis
- Cellulitis
- Gout and pseudogout
- Fracture, tendon/ligament tear, contusion, sprain
- Tendonitis

DIAGNOSTIC TESTS & INTERPRETATION

- In cases where there is clinical concern for inflammatory disorders and/or infection, obtain complete blood count (CBC) with differential, erythrocyte sedimentation rate, serum protein electrophoresis, rheumatoid factor, serum uric acid (1)[A],(2)[A].
- Aspiration and analysis of bursa fluid: cell count with differential, glucose and total protein, crystal determination, Gram stain, and culture (1)[A],(2)[A]

- Normal fluid: Fluid is clear yellow with 0 to 200 white blood cells (WBCs), 0 red blood cells (RBCs), low protein, and glucose is same as serum (1)[A],(2)[A].
- Traumatic bursitis: Fluid is bloody/xanthochromic with <2,000 WBCs, many RBCs, high protein, and normal glucose.
- Infective bursitis: Fluid is **cloudy yellow** with >50,000 WBCs, few RBCs, slightly increased protein, and decreased glucose; bacteria on Gram stain (1)[A],(2)[A].
- Rheumatoid and microcrystalline inflammation: Fluid is yellow, can be cloudy, has >2,000 WBCs, few RBCs, slightly increased protein, and variable glucose; use polarizing microscope to identify crystals.
- Chronic or recurrent bursitis should be sent for acid-fast staining and cultured on special media for mycobacteria, *Brucella*, and algae.
- Monosodium urate crystals seen in gout; calcium pyrophosphate crystals seen in pseudogout
- X-rays to exclude other suspected pathologies (i.e., fractures, dislocations, or foreign body) (1)[A]
- X-rays may demonstrate chronic arthritic changes or calcium deposits or rheumatologic features.
- US for both diagnosis and diagnostic aspiration or treatment injections (1)[A]
- MRI helps depict bursa/prebursal fluid, associated abscesses, and adjacent soft tissue structures.

TREATMENT

Acute treatment:

- Shoulders should not be immobilized for >2 to 3 days due to the risk of adhesive capsulitis.
- Aseptic bursitis:
  - First-line treatment:
    - Rest (1)[A],(2)[A],(3)[A]
    - Ice (application of an ice pack for 20 minutes for superficially bursa), compression, elevation (1)[A],(2)[A],(3)[A]
    - Short course 8 to 10 days of nonsteroidal anti-inflammatory drugs (NSAIDs) (1)[A],(2)[A],(3)[A]
    - Physical therapy (stretching, strengthening, and maintaining range of motion) (1)[A],(2)[A],(3)[A],(4)[A].
  - If first-line treatment failed, physician can discuss with patient other modalities of treatment as follows:
    - Bursa aspiration (1)[A],(2)[A],(3)[A]
    - Intrabursal steroid injections (1)[A],(2)[A],(3)[A],(4)[A],(5)[A],(6)[A]
    - Intrabursal platelet-rich plasma (PRP) injection (6)[A]
    - Extracorporeal shock wave therapy (ESWT) (6)[A]
- Septic bursitis: If suspected, treat with antibiotics while awaiting culture results and drain bursae; may require repeat aspiration (6)[A]
- Superficial infected bursitis can be treated with oral therapy (1)[A].
- Septic bursitis with fulminant onset, systemic symptoms, or those who are immunocompromised require hospitalization and/or intravenous (IV) antibiotics (6)[A].
- Crystal-induced: treat underlying etiology.

MEDICATION

- Most patients may be treated as an outpatient.
- NSAIDs

SURGERY/OTHER PROCEDURES

In general, bursitis is not treated surgically. However, bursectomy may be indicated with adhesive bursitis, recurrent refractory bursitis, or severe limitation of joint motion. During surgery, the adhered bursa is removed, and the contiguous tissues are released (1)[A],(2)[A].

ADMISSION, INPATIENT, AND NURSING CONSIDERATIONS

- Immobilize joint if pain is severe.
- Admission criteria: septic bursitis with systemic symptoms, surrounding cellulitis, unable to take oral antibiotics, failed outpatient therapy, or immunocompromised

ONGOING CARE

FOLLOW-UP RECOMMENDATIONS

- Most patients respond to therapy within 1 week.
- Rheumatology or orthopedic referral is recommended for patients with repetitive acute bouts, necessitating repeated joint/bursa aspirations or, eventually, surgical excision of involved bursa.

REFERENCES

1. Baumbach SF, Lobo CM, Badyine I, et al. Prepatellar and olecranon bursitis: literature review and development of a treatment algorithm. *Arch Orthop Trauma Surg*. 2014;134(3):359–370.
2. Nchinda NN, Wolf JM. Clinical management of olecranon bursitis: a review. *J Hand Surg Am*. 2021;46(6):501–506.
3. Lustenberger DP, Ng VY, Best TM, et al. Efficacy of treatment of trochanteric bursitis: a systematic review. *Clin J Sport Med*. 2011;21(5):447–453.
4. Hsieh LF, Kuo YC, Huang YH, et al. Comparison of corticosteroid injection, physiotherapy and combined treatment for patients with chronic subacromial bursitis—a randomised controlled trial. *Clin Rehabil*. 2023;37(9):1189–1200.
5. Sayegh ET, Strauch RJ. Treatment of olecranon bursitis: a systematic review. *Arch Orthop Trauma Surg*. 2014;134(11):1517–1536.
6. Gouda WA, Abbas AS, Abdel-Aziz TM, et al. POS1347 evaluating the efficacy of local corticosteroid injection, platelet-rich plasma, and extracorporeal shockwave therapy in patients with pes anserine bursitis: a pilot randomized, comparative clinical trial. *Annals of the Rheumatic Diseases*. 2023;82(Suppl 1):1024–1028.

ADDITIONAL READING

- Kim JY, Chung SW, Kim JH, et al. A randomized trial among compression plus nonsteroidal anti-inflammatory drugs, aspiration, and aspiration with steroid injection for nonseptic olecranon bursitis. *Clin Orthop Relat Res*. 2016;474(3):776–783.
- Lieber SB, Fowler ML, Zhu C, et al. Clinical characteristics and outcomes of septic bursitis. *Infection*. 2017;45(6):781–786.
- Sayegh ET, Strauch RJ. Treatment of olecranon bursitis: a systematic review. *Arch Orthop Trauma Surg*. 2014;134(11):1517–1536.

CLINICAL PEARLS

- Bursitis can happen in any tendon mobilizing over skin or bone.
- Conservative treatment with ice, NSAIDs, and modifying activity is the treatment in most cases.
- Any suspicion of infection warrants aspiration of bursae (especially superficial bursa).

B

CALCIFIC TENDONITIS

Marcus Anthony, MD • Julia Louisa Iafrate, DO

BASICS

DESCRIPTION

- Calcific tendonitis (CT) is a disorder characterized by the deposition of calcium, most commonly hydroxyapatite, within a tendon.
- Calcium deposition within a tendon can lead to pain and functional impairment as a result of increased intratendinous pressures, inflammation, and/or impingement.
- CT is typically a self-limiting condition with spontaneous resolution of symptoms within 3 to 6 months (1).
- CT can occur in any tendon but most commonly involves the rotator cuff (supraspinatus most commonly affected).
- Synonyms include calcific tendinopathy and CT.
- CT must be differentiated from calcific periarthritis and degenerative enthesophytes.

EPIDEMIOLOGY

- More common in females and individuals between 30 and 60 years of age
- Approximately 50% of calcium deposits are asymptomatic (2).
- Rotator cuff CT, the most common and most studied CT, has an estimated prevalence of roughly 3–40% in individuals with shoulder pain, of which 10% may be bilateral (3),(4).
- The prevalence rates of CT affecting other tendons (gluteus medius, Achilles, hamstring, etc.) have not been well established (5).

ETIOLOGY AND PATHOPHYSIOLOGY

- Although the etiology is not unanimously agreed on, CT is commonly thought to be secondary to chondral metaplasia (transformation of tenocytes to chondrocytes), which may be triggered by hypoxia (2).
- Unlikely related to trauma or overuse
- CT progresses through three stages:
  - Precalcific stage: Fibrocartilaginous transformation occurs, during which time chondrocytes begin to appear in the tendon.
  - Calcific stage:
    - Formative phase: Calcium produced by the chondrocytes is deposited in the tendon. Deposits may be painful. Large deposits may cause mechanical symptoms via impingement.
    - Resorptive phase: An inflammatory reaction occurs with cell-mediated resorption of the calcification; hypothesized to be the most painful phase (2)
  - Postcalcific stage: The deposit is resorbed and fibroblasts reconstitute the normal collagen pattern of tendon.

Genetics

Currently, there is no evidence to support a genetic disposition to CT.

RISK FACTORS

CT is rarely part of a systemic disease but has been associated with diabetes mellitus, nephrolithiasis, and thyroid and estrogen disorders.

DIAGNOSIS

HISTORY

- Pain localized to the affected tendon is the cardinal symptom. The presence and severity of pain can depend on stage.
- Pain is typically atraumatic but can be acute or subacute on chronic.
- Severe acute pain often presents during the resorptive phase due to local inflammation and/or associated leakage of calcium crystals into the overlying bursa. This pain is likely to improve within 1 to 2 weeks.
- Nocturnal pain and inability to sleep on affected area is common.
- Strenuous manual labor and athletic activity do not increase risk.

PHYSICAL EXAM

- Acute pain phase: guarding of affected tendon with tenderness to palpation
- Chronic or subacute phase: Pain increases considerably with active range of motion (ROM) versus minimal symptoms with passive ROM.
- For CT involving the rotator cuff, shoulder impingement tests (Hawkins and Neer) are often positive.

DIFFERENTIAL DIAGNOSIS

- Acute or chronic tendinopathy
- Degenerative enthesophyte
- Calcific periarthritis
- Gout
- For CT involving the rotator cuff:
  - Rotator cuff tendinopathy
  - Adhesive capsulitis
  - Subacromial impingement
  - Osteoarthritis of glenohumeral or acromioclavicular joint
  - Biceps tendonitis
  - Cervical radiculopathy
- Rare: tumoral calcinosis

DIAGNOSTIC TESTS & INTERPRETATION

Initial Tests (lab, imaging)

- Radiographs (x-ray) and ultrasound (US) reveal characteristic calcium deposits.
- X-ray: multiple views required to adequately assess location, size, and morphology
  - X-ray evaluation of the shoulder should include anteroposterior (AP), internal and external rotation, axillary, and outlet views.
- Appearance on x-ray (6)[A]:
  - Formative phase: well-circumscribed lesion with homogenous appearance and high radiodensity
  - Resorptive phase: fluffy lesion with ill-defined borders that may have increased radiodensity at its center
- US: short- and long-axis views required to fully evaluate the lesion
- Appearance on US (6)[A]:
  - Formative phase: well-circumscribed hyperechoic lesions with acoustic shadowing
  - Resorptive phase: fluffy poorly circumscribed lesions that may be fragmented, cystic, or nodular in shape. Power Doppler can reveal increased vascularity around the deposit.
- Tenderness with sonopalpation of deposit can confirm the observed calcium deposit is symptomatic (6)[A].
- Magnetic resonance imaging (MRI) or computed tomography (CT) scan are not indicated in routine evaluation but can be used for surgical planning.

Follow-Up Tests & Special Considerations

Repeat radiographs and/or US may be helpful to assess interval change and guide secondary treatment.

TREATMENT

GENERAL MEASURES

- Expectant management may be offered given often self-limited benign course.
- First-line therapy is conservative and focused on symptom relief.
  - Initial treatment options include oral anti-inflammatories and analgesics, glucocorticoid injections, and physical therapy (PT). Little evidence to suggest one initial treatment is preferred over others.
  - A subacromial bursa (SAB) glucocorticoid injection (e.g., 20 to 40 mg of triamcinolone, methylprednisolone) is effective for acute pain relief and does not impact the resorption of the deposited calcium (7).
- Second-line treatment options include US-guided barbotage (one or two needle approach), extracorporeal shock wave therapy (ESWT), and percutaneous ultrasonic tenotomy.
  - US-guided barbotage with SAB glucocorticoid injections has improved 1 year outcomes in patients with rotator cuff CT when compared to SAB glucocorticoid injection alone, although no difference in outcomes exists at 5 years (8)[A].

- ESWT has been shown to have varying levels of effectiveness for the treatment of CT involving the rotator cuff, although the optimal type (focal vs. radial ESWT) and energy level have yet to be determined.
- Several meta-analyses have demonstrated that US-guided barbotage provides superior improvement in both pain and function when compared ESWT for the treatment of rotator cuff CT (9),(10),(11)[A].
- A collection of case reports and case series have shown benefit of US-guided barbotage for CT outside of the rotator cuff as well (12).
- When compared to US-guided barbotage for the treatment of rotator cuff CT, percutaneous ultrasonic tenotomy may provide equal improvement in pain and less frequent need for a repeat procedure (13)[B].

SURGERY/OTHER PROCEDURES

- Up to 30% of patients may not respond to first- and second-line treatments and could benefit from surgery (11).
- There have been several open and arthroscopic surgical techniques described for the treatment of CT with no existing consensus on the optimal approach (11).

COMPLEMENTARY & ALTERNATIVE MEDICINE

Scant low-level evidence supports the use of acetic acid iontophoresis, therapeutic heat, therapeutic US, and microwave diathermy for the treatment of CT.

ONGOING CARE

FOLLOW-UP RECOMMENDATIONS

- General follow-up considerations:
  - Evaluate for interval changes in severity of reported pain and tenderness to palpation, ROM, and strength.
  - If pain and functional limitations persist despite any combination of off-loading, oral anti-inflammatories, and/or PT, a SAB glucocorticoid injection may be beneficial if not already performed on initial evaluation.
  - Repeat imaging reserved for patients with persistent symptoms to guide treatment plan.
  - Follow-up timeline depends on severity of pain and functional limitation.
- Follow-up for US-guided barbotage, percutaneous ultrasonic tenotomy, or ESWT:
  - Each should occur alongside a 3- to 4-month PT program aimed at restoring strength and ROM.
  - If still symptomatic and calcific deposit visualized on imaging after US-guided barbotage or ESWT, consider percutaneous ultrasonic tenotomy.

PROGNOSIS

- 50% are asymptomatic within 3 months spontaneously or with conservative treatment (1).
- 70% are asymptomatic within 1 year of onset (14).
- 30% have persistent symptoms for several years. Of these, 66% improve with barbotage or ESWT (15).
- Negative prognostic indicators: female, bilateral limbs, dominant limb involvement, and large or multiple calcifications. In these selected patients, more aggressive treatments earlier in the disease course can improve long-term outcomes (16)[B].

COMPLICATIONS

- Acute or degenerative tearing of the affected tendon
- Ossifying tendonitis: very rare and associated with arthroscopic surgical intervention
- Osteonecrosis: extremely rare and related to ESWT
- For CT involving the rotator cuff: adhesive capsulitis Very rarely greater tuberosity osteolysis

REFERENCES

1. Noël E. Treatment of calcific tendinitis and adhesive capsulitis of the shoulder. *Rev Rhum Engl Ed.* 1997;64(11):619–628.
2. Uhthoff HK, Loehr JW. Calcific tendinopathy of the rotator cuff: pathogenesis, diagnosis, and management. *J Am Acad Orthop Surg.* 1997;5(4):183–191.
3. Bosworth BM. Calcium deposits in the shoulder and subacromial bursitis: a survey of 12,122 shoulders. *JAMA.* 1941;116(22):2477–2482.
4. Louwerens JKG, Sierevelt IN, van Hove RP, et al. Prevalence of calcific deposits within the rotator cuff tendons in adults with and without subacromial pain syndrome: clinical and radiologic analysis of 1,219 patients. *J Shoulder Elbow Surg.* 2015;24(10):1588–1593.
5. Draghi F, Cocco G, Lomoro P, et al. Non-rotator cuff calcific tendinopathy: ultrasonographic diagnosis and treatment. *J Ultrasound.* 2020;23(3):301–315.
6. Merolla G, Singh S, Paladini P, et al. Calcific tendinitis of the rotator cuff: state of the art in diagnosis and treatment. *J Orthop Traumatol.* 2016;17(1):7–14.
7. Le Goff B, Berthelot JM, Guillot P, et al. Assessment of calcific tendonitis of rotator cuff by ultrasonography: comparison between symptomatic and asymptomatic shoulders. *Joint Bone Spine.* 2010;77(3):258–263.
8. de Witte PB, Kolk A, Overes F, et al. Rotator cuff calcific tendinitis: ultrasound-guided needling and lavage versus subacromial corticosteroids: five-year outcomes of a randomized controlled trial. *Am J Sports Med.* 2017;45(14):3305–3314.
9. Brindisino F, Marruganti S, Lorusso D, et al. The effectiveness of extracorporeal shock wave therapy for rotator cuff calcific tendinopathy: a systematic review with meta-analysis. *Physiother Res Int.* 2024;29(3):e2106.
10. Arirachakaran A, Boonard M, Yamaphai S, et al. Extracorporeal shock wave therapy, ultrasound-guided percutaneous lavage, corticosteroid injection and combined treatment for the treatment of rotator cuff calcific tendinopathy: a network meta-analysis of RCTs. *Eur J Orthop Surg Traumatol.* 2017;27(3):381–390.
11. Angileri HS, Gohal C, Comeau-Gauthier M, et al. Chronic calcific tendonitis of the rotator cuff: a systematic review and meta-analysis of randomized controlled trials comparing operative and nonoperative interventions. *J Shoulder Elbow Surg.* 2023;32(8):1746–1760.
12. Spinnato P, Ponti F, D'Agostino V, et al. Ultrasound-guided percutaneous irrigation of calcific tendinopathy outside the rotator cuff: short-term evaluation. *Skeletal Radiol.* 2022;51(10):2039–2044.
13. Berrigan W, Olufade O, Negron G, et al. Calcific tendinopathy of the shoulder: a retrospective comparison of traditional barbotage versus percutaneous ultrasonic barbotage. *Clin J Sport Med.* 2022;32(5):458–466.
14. Wölk T, Wittenberg RH. Calcifying subacromial syndrome—clinical and ultrasound outcome of non-surgical therapy. *Z Orthop Ihre Grenzgeb.* 1997;135(5):451–457.
15. Lee SY, Cheng B, Grimmer-Somers K. The midterm effectiveness of extracorporeal shockwave therapy in the management of chronic calcific shoulder tendinitis. *J Shoulder Elbow Surg.* 2011;20(5):845–854.
16. de Witte PB, van Adrichem RA, Selten JW, et al. Radiological and clinical predictors of long-term outcome in rotator cuff calcific tendinitis. *Eur Radiol.* 2016;26(10):3401–3411.

ADDITIONAL READING

Erickson JL, Jagim AR. Ultrasonic tenotomy and débridement for calcific tendinopathy of the shoulder: a pilot case series. *J Prim Care Community Health.* 2020;11:2150132720964665.

CLINICAL PEARLS

- CT is typically a self-limiting disorder with spontaneous resolution of symptoms and resorption of calcium deposits.
- CT is not precipitated by strenuous manual labor or athletic activities and occurs equally among sedentary and active individuals.
- Acute pain from CT often improves within several weeks but may require an SAB glucocorticoid injection for pain management.
- US-guided barbotage, percutaneous ultrasonic tenotomy, and ESWT are three safe, minimally invasive procedures that should be considered for the treatment of CT in individuals that fail to respond to conservative measures.

C

CALCIUM PYROPHOSPHATE DEPOSITION DISEASE (CPPD) (PSEUDOGOUT)

Kenneth M. Bielak, MD, MBA, FAAFP, FACSM

BASICS

DESCRIPTION

- Calcium pyrophosphate deposition disease (CPPD) is a crystal arthropathy characterized by deposition of calcium pyrophosphate (CaPPi) dihydrate crystals in joints.
- Synonym(s):
  - Pseudogout: describes an acute attack of CPPD crystal-induced synovitis (similar to gout) but less intense symptoms
  - Chondrocalcinosis: radiographic calcification but is not absolutely specific for CPPD because it can be caused by other calcific deposits on hyaline cartilage
  - Pyrophosphate arthropathy: specifically associated with inorganic pyrophosphate metabolism as the etiology for CPPD
  - CaPPi dihydrate crystal deposition disease

EPIDEMIOLOGY

- Prevalence of chondrocalcinosis is 5–8% in the general population but 15% by the 9th decade.
- Due to asymptomatic depositions and need for confirmatory aspiration for diagnosis, incidence has not been reliably recorded.
- Female-to-male ratio: 2 to 7:1
- Peak age: 65 to 75 years

ETIOLOGY AND PATHOPHYSIOLOGY

CPPD crystal formation is initiated in cartilage located near the surface of chondrocytes. The CPPD crystal formation may be a combination of elevated levels of either calcium or pyrophosphate and/or matrix changes that enhance local CaPPi supersaturation. Many cases of CPPD deposition are idiopathically sporadic but more commonly are precipitated by trauma or various metabolic disorders.

Genetics

<1% of cases may show an autosomal dominant inheritance pattern.

RISK FACTORS

- Gout (20% may be hyperuricemic)
- Hemochromatosis
- Hypothyroidism
- Trauma
- Osteoarthritis
- Hyperparathyroidism
- Hemosiderosis
- Hypophosphatasia
- Hypomagnesemia
- Aging
- Amyloidosis

GENERAL PREVENTION

- There are no absolute prevention measures, but mainstays include adequate hydration (to prevent crystal precipitation) and decreasing purine-rich foods, such as organ meats, mushrooms, legumes, asparagus, and coffee.
- For three or more attacks per 1 year, colchicine has been found to reduce the recurrence rate (1)[B], (2)[A].

COMMONLY ASSOCIATED CONDITIONS

- Pseudorheumatoid arthritis: a nonerosive, inflammatory arthritis with demonstrable CPPD crystals in the joint fluid. Both are clinically similar with morning stiffness, fatigue, synovial thickening, edema, and loss of motion. Both conditions may coexist but must be differentiated because the treatment options vary.
- Pseudoarthritis: progressive joint degeneration involving multiple joints. CPPD differs by radiographic evidence of calcifications in the absence of a preceding trauma.
- Case reports of CPPD associated with Charcot joints
- Several case reports involving bisphosphonates and CPPD deposition have been reported (3)[C].
- CPPD, especially familial patterns, can be found along the spine and resemble ankylosing spondylitis.

DIAGNOSIS

HISTORY

- Acute joint swelling in one or more joints with previous episodes involving the same joint (characteristic of crystal arthropathies)
- The most common joint is the knee, followed by the wrist, shoulder, and hip.
- May be severe and associated with malaise and fever
- Period of previous episodes (typically several days to weeks)
- Patients often are symptom-free between attacks.

PHYSICAL EXAM

- Involved joint:
  - Warmth
  - Edema/effusion
  - Tender
  - Limited range of motion
- Uncommon presentations include tendinopathy, tenosynovitis, and bursitis.
- Chronic CPPD: symmetrical polyarthritis affecting knees, metacarpophalangeal joints, wrists, ankles, and shoulders:
  - May involve the spine
  - Affected joints show signs of osteoarthritis with varying degrees of synovitis.
  - Predominantly affects women

DIFFERENTIAL DIAGNOSIS

- Gout (can coexist)
- Septic arthritis (can coexist)
- Rheumatoid arthritis
- Osteoarthritis
- Trauma (hemarthrosis)
- Human leukocyte antigen B27–related peripheral arthritis (psoriatic arthritis, ankylosing spondylitis, reactive arthritis)
- Hypertrophic osteoarthropathy
- Pseudorheumatoid arthritis: severe synovitis in rheumatoid pattern

DIAGNOSTIC TESTS & INTERPRETATION

- Initial diagnosis of CPPD should be followed with calcium, magnesium, thyroid-stimulating hormone, ferritin, transferrin, iron, phosphorus, and alkaline phosphatase levels.
- Synovial fluid microscopy with compensated polarized light microscopy showing weakly positive birefringent rhomboidal-shaped crystals is diagnostic; Gram stain and culture should be considered to rule out differential diagnoses. In addition, crystal analysis up to 3 days postaspiration does not adversely affect crystal identification (4)[B].
- Erythrocyte sedimentation rate, C-reactive protein, rheumatoid factor, uric acid, white blood cell count (leukocytosis), and blood cultures may be considered to rule out differential diagnoses.
- Leukocyte concentration typically in the range of 15,000 to 30,000/mm^3 with 90% neutrophils
- Plain radiography to evaluate for calcium crystal deposition (5)[C]
- X-ray: calcification of articular fibrocartilage (chondrocalcinosis) in menisci of the knee, triangular fibrocartilage complex in the wrist. Other sites include glenoid and acetabular labra and symphysis pubis.
- High-resolution ultrasound (US) may improve noninvasive diagnosis of the crystal-induced arthropathies and allow monitoring of intra-articular tophi if radiation is a concern.
- Features may show a homogeneously punctate pattern or sharply defined hyperechoic bands within the articular cartilage (5),(6)[C].
- Optimal imaging is best with computed tomography (CT) for further definition of tophi and bone erosion, and 3D CT assessment of tophus volume is a promising outcome measure in gout.
- Magnetic resonance imaging (MRI) is also a reliable method for assessment of tophus size in gout and has an important role in detection of complications of disease in clinical practice.

TREATMENT

- Acute treatment:
  - Joint aspiration often significantly reduces pain (7)[C].
  - Intra-articular corticosteroid injection can be effective (8)[C].
  - Joint rest and splinting if needed
  - Nonsteroidal anti-inflammatory drugs (NSAIDs) are an effective first-line option both in treatment and prophylaxis of CPPD (9). Early initiation at full doses is more likely to be beneficial in symptom management. However, most CPPD patients are elderly and safety profile should be considered before starting NSAIDs. Celecoxib has a lower risk of major toxicities compared to Naproxen and Ibuprofen and should be preferred in elderly patients (10)[A],(11)[A].
  - Colchicine and systemic corticosteroids can be used if other treatments are contraindicated.

- Some clinical evidence that intraarticular injections of low-dose corticosteroid along with joint aspiration can shorten time to resolution of CPPD pain in attacks (9).
- Colchicine has proven efficacy in the treatment of CPPD through its anti-inflammatory effects and attenuation of IL-1β expression in-vitro. However, it is a CYP3A4 inhibitor and drug-drug interactions can occur (9)[A].
- Synthetic ACTH (Tetracosactide) is an option for patients with contraindications to CS, NSAID or colchicine. Signs of inflammation have been noted to resolve in as little as 24 hours (12)[B],(13)[B].
- Anakinra is an IL-1R antagonist that can be administer by subcutaneous route in patients refractory to standard therapies. Physician reported decreases in visual analog scale (VAS) scores and C-reactive protein (CRP) levels have been noted (9)[A].
- Oral NLRP3 inflammasome inhibitors such as dapansutrile affect IL-1β production by targeting the NLRP3 inflammasome pathway. Early trials have shown acceptable safety profile and efficacy (9)[A],(14)[B],(15)[B],(16)[B].

• Long-term treatment:
- For patients suffering recurrent attacks of pseudogout, oral daily colchicine may be effective as a prophylactic agent at a usual dosage of 0.6 mg BID (1)[B].
- Repeat joint aspiration may be required.
- Once acute attacks have settled, the aims of treatment are to relieve symptoms and regain function.
- No specific treatment exists for chronic CPPD, and no treatments are available that reverse joint damage.
- Methotrexate has been used in the long-term treatment of CPPD due to its established benefits in reduced inflammation, disease activity and progression in the treatment of rheumatoid arthritis. However, there is insufficient evidence to support its use in CPPD at this time (9)[A].
- Tocilizumab is an IL-1β receptor monoclonal antibody that suppresses IL-1β expression and affects CRP levels, resulting in lower VAS pain scores reported. However, its use does carry increased risk of infections, and masks the CRP elevations seen in infections as well (9)[A],(17)[B].
- Hydroxychloroquine: has been studied in a small double-blinded randomized controlled trial (RCT) in 36 patients and showed response rate (at least 30% reduction in number of swollen and tender joints) of 76% compared to 32% in placebo group. However, this was a study performed more than 20 years ago with study population not clearly defined and nonvalidated outcome measures. Further studies are warranted given safety profile of hydroxychloroquine (9)[A],(18)[B].

MEDICATION

NSAIDs are first-line treatment.

ADDITIONAL THERAPIES

Antibiotics if septic arthritis is suspected until joint and blood cultures return negative

SURGERY/OTHER PROCEDURES

Joint arthroplasty may be required for severely damaged joints.

COMPLEMENTARY & ALTERNATIVE MEDICINE

There have been anecdotal reports of cured acute attacks by the consumption of dark cherries or cherry juice or herbs that contain xanthene oxidase inhibitors to decrease urate formation, but none have been well studied.

ONGOING CARE

- Primary metabolic disorders or familial predisposition is uncommon but should be considered if CPPD occurs before 55 years of age or if there is florid polyarticular CPPD.
- After the age of 55 years, hyperparathyroidism should be considered in all patients.

COMPLICATIONS

Although acute pseudogout usually responds well to therapy, chronic CPPD often is progressive and may cause considerable disability.

REFERENCES

1. Alvarellos A, Spilberg I. Colchicine prophylaxis in pseudogout. *J Rheumatol.* 1986;13(4):804–805.
2. Rainer TH, Cheng CH, Janssens HJ, et al. Oral prednisolone in the treatment of acute gout: a pragmatic, multicenter, double-blind, randomized trial. *Ann Intern Med.* 2016;164(7):464–471.
3. Couture G, Delzor F, Bagheri H, et al. First cases of calcium pyrophosphate deposition disease after zoledronic acid therapy. *Joint Bone Spine* 2017;84(2):213–215.
4. Tausche AK, Gehrisch S, Panzner I, et al. A 3-day delay in synovial fluid crystal identification did not hinder the reliable detection of monosodium urate and calcium pyrophosphate crystals. *J Clin Rheumatol.* 2013;19(5):241–245.
5. Ciapetti A, Filippucci E, Gutierrez M, et al. Calcium pyrophosphate dihydrate crystal deposition disease: sonographic findings. *Clin Rheumatol.* 2009;28(3):271–276.
6. Grassi W, Meenagh G, Pascual E, et al. "Crystal clear"-sonographic assessment of gout and calcium pyrophosphate deposition disease. *Semin Arthritis Rheum.* 2006;36(3):197–202.
7. Dalbeth N, McQueen FM. Use of imaging to evaluate gout and other crystal deposition disorders. *Curr Opin Rheumatol.* 2009;21(2):124–131.
8. Announ N, Guerne PA. Treating difficult crystal pyrophosphate dihydrate deposition disease. *Curr Rheumatol Rep.* 2008;10(3):228–234.
9. Andrés M, Sivera F, Pascual E. Therapy for CPPD: options and evidence. *Curr Rheumatol Rep.* 2018;20(6):31.
10. Solomon DH, Husni ME, Libby PA, et al. The risk of major NSAID toxicity with celecoxib, ibuprofen, or naproxen: a secondary analysis of the PRECISION trial. *Am J Med.* 2017;130(12):1415.e4–1422.e4.
11. Stack J, McCarthy G. Calcium pyrophosphate deposition (CPPD) disease—treatment options. *Best Pract Res Clin Rheumatol.* 2021;35(4):101720.
12. Daoussis D, Antonopoulos I, Yiannopoulos G, et al. ACTH as first line treatment for acute calcium pyrophosphate crystal arthritis in 14 hospitalized patients. *Joint Bone Spine.* 2014;81(1):98–100.
13. Parperis K, Papachristodoulou E, Kakoullis L, et al. Management of calcium pyrophosphate crystal deposition disease: a systematic review. *Semin Arthritis Rheum.* 2021;51(1):84–94.
14. Campillo-Gimenez L, Renaudin F, Jalabert M, et al. Inflammatory potential of four different phases of calcium pyrophosphate relies on NF-κB activation and MAPK pathways. *Front Immunol.* 2018;9:2248.
15. Conway R, McCarthy GM. Calcium-containing crystals and osteoarthritis: an unhealthy alliance. *Curr Rheumatol Rep.* 2018;20(3):13.
16. Klück V, Jansen TLTA, Janssen M, et al. Dapansutrile, an oral selective NLRP3 inflammasome inhibitor, for treatment of gout flares: an open-label, dose-adaptive, proof-of-concept, phase 2a trial. *Lancet Rheumatol.* 2020;2(5):e270–e280.
17. Latourte A, Ea HK, Frazier A, et al. Tocilizumab in symptomatic calcium pyrophosphate deposition disease: a pilot study. *Ann Rheum Dis.* 2020;79(8):1126–1128.
18. Rothschild B, Yakubov LE. Prospective 6-month, double-blind trial of hydroxychloroquine treatment of CPPD. *Compr Ther.* 1997;23(5):327–331.

ADDITIONAL READING

- Courtney P, Doherty M. Joint aspiration and injection and synovial fluid analysis. *Best Pract Res Clin Rheumatol.* 2013;27(2):137–169.
- Couto AR, Brown MA. Genetic factors in the pathogenesis of CPPD crystal deposition disease. *Curr Rheumatol Rep.* 2007;9(3):231–236.
- Doherty M. Crystal arthropathies: calcium pyrophosphate dihydrate. In: Klippel JH, Dieppe PA, eds. *Rheumatology.* Mosby-Year Book Europe Limited; 1994:1–7.
- Ea HK, Lioté F. Advances in understanding calcium-containing crystal disease. *Curr Opin Rheumatol.* 2009;21(2):150–157.
- Fodor D, Albu A, Gherman C. Crystal-associated synovitis—ultrasonographic feature and clinical correlation. *Ortop Traumatol Rehabil.* 2008;10(2):90–110.
- Richette P, Bardin T, Doherty M. An update on the epidemiology of calcium pyrophosphate dihydrate crystal deposition disease. *Rheumatology (Oxford).* 2009;48(7):711–715.
- Ryan LM, McCarty DO. Calcium pyrophosphate crystal deposition disease, pseudogout and articular chondrocalcinosis. In: Koopman WJ, ed. *Arthritis and Allied Conditions: A Textbook of Rheumatology.* 13th ed. Williams & Wilkins; 1997:2103–2125.
- Shah K, Spear J, Nathanson LA, et al. Does the presence of crystal arthritis rule out septic arthritis? *J Emerg Med.* 2007;32(1):23–26.

CLINICAL PEARLS

- The cause of CPPD is unknown (unlike gout, in which hyperuricemia leads to precipitation of uric acid crystals into joints).
- Aspiration of joint fluid is key to diagnosis.
- There is no preventive treatment for recurrent attacks, although colchicine may be useful as prophylaxis in those with frequent recurrences (2)[A].

CALLUSES AND CORNS

Kathleen Weber, MD, MS

BASICS

- Calluses and corns are common skin conditions.
- They result from increased pressure or friction over the skin or underlying bony prominence; typically located on the hands and feet
- A callus is an adaptive response to repetitive friction.
- Calluses and corns may lead to considerable discomfort and pain.

DESCRIPTION

- A callus is a plaque of hyperkeratosis of relatively even thickness caused by repetitive friction, pressure, or trauma, and commonly occurs over bony prominences (1),(2).
- A corn is a localized, tender, and sharply defined area of hyperkeratosis found usually on the foot (1).
- A corn has a central core that penetrates the dermis.

EPIDEMIOLOGY

Calluses and corns are common skin conditions.

ETIOLOGY AND PATHOPHYSIOLOGY

- Calluses and corns develop as a result of hyperkeratosis and thickening of the stratum corneum, a normal physiologic response of the skin to chronic friction, pressure, or mechanical trauma and commonly occur over bony prominences (1),(2),(3).
- A callus hyperkeratosis is more diffuse, whereas a corn is a more well-defined focal area of hyperkeratosis.
- Calluses commonly develop overlying bony prominences as a normal adaptation of the body to protect the skin when chronic pressure or friction is encountered (4).
- Abnormal stresses may be either extrinsic (e.g., tight toe box, repetitive movements) or intrinsic (e.g., hallux valgus, hammer toe deformities) or a combination of both (2),(4).

RISK FACTORS

- Activity: occupational (e.g., manual workers); musicians (e.g., guitarists); athletic activities that apply increased stress to the skin (i.e., racquet sports—hands, runners—feet, rowers—hands, sacrum) (5)
- Ill-fitting footwear: tight, loose irregularities in shoe, or not wearing shoes (4)
- Bony prominences
- Faulty foot mechanics or foot structure (4)
- Toe deformities

GENERAL PREVENTION

- Proper footwear (low-heeled, a soft upper portion, and wide toe box) (1),(2),(3)
- Orthotics
- Toe separators (4)
- Place felt pads over bony prominences or areas of increased friction to the skin (2),(3),(4).
- Wear gloves to protect the hands (5).
- Keep the skin of the hands and feet soft by applying a moisturizer.

DIAGNOSIS

- The diagnosis of calluses and corns is based on their clinical appearance.
- Radiographs may be obtained if an underlying bony prominence is suspected as a contributing factor.
- Dermatoscopy can be used to help distinguish a wart from a callus, as it can show areas of hyperkeratosis without vascular or hemorrhagic structures that is mainly seen in warts (6).

HISTORY

- Corns and calluses are typically located at sites of friction, pressure, repetitive trauma, or at bony prominences (3),(4).
- Inquire about factors that typically provoke the formation of corns and calluses:
  - Sports that require cutting, turning, racquets, weightlifting, and sudden stops; callus formation is sometimes desired to allow pain-free play (3).
  - Occupations that are categorized as manual labor requiring the repetitive use of the hands or kneeling, such as a carpenter or landscaper (4)
  - Leisure activity that involves activities that cause repeated friction or pressure
  - Poorly fitting footwear
  - Coexisting illnesses (e.g., diabetes, rheumatoid arthritis)
  - Inherited disposition (autosomal-dominant inheritance)

PHYSICAL EXAM

- Physical examination of the area is typically all that is necessary to make the diagnosis.
- Note the location of the hyperkeratotic lesions:
  - Common sites for corns and calluses on feet: plantar surface (under the metatarsal heads, sides of the arch, and the heel), dorsum of the foot (over the interphalangeal joints), and over bony prominences (4)
  - Common sites for calluses on hands: palmar surface and over metacarpophalangeal joints
  - Calluses may occur anywhere on the skin as a result of friction.
- Note the appearance of the hyperkeratotic lesions:
  - A hard corn, or heloma durum, is a dry horny mass found commonly over the interphalangeal joints (dorsally) or the 5th toe (dorsolaterally) (1).
  - Soft corns, or heloma mole, are extremely painful; occur primarily in the interdigital web spaces; skin appears white and macerated; commonly located between the 4th interdigital space (often mistaken for tinea) (1)
  - Periungual corn occurs near or off the edge of a nail.
  - A callus may be asymptomatic or painful, often appearing as a thick yellowish plaque that retains the natural skin lines (helps distinguish from warts) (5).
  - Corns can be difficult to differentiate from plantar warts. Corns have plantar skin lines. When paring a corn there is no capillary dotting, also known as Auspitz sign, that is present in plantar warts.
  - Observe gait and the alignment of the feet for any faulty mechanics.
- Assess for pain or tenderness.

DIFFERENTIAL DIAGNOSIS

- Verruca vulgaris or plantaris (differentiated by paring the skin; the corn becomes more normal in appearance, and the wart displays the characteristic tiny red dots when pared).
- Tinea pedis (interdigital)
- Psoriatic plaque: hyperkeratosis with a red base

DIAGNOSTIC TESTS & INTERPRETATION

- Imaging usually not necessary
- Radiographs: hands and weight-bearing views of the feet used to identify bony prominences or abnormalities, especially in lesions that are refractory to treatment (4)[C]

TREATMENT

GENERAL MEASURES

Treatment is aimed at providing symptomatic relief and avoiding the underlying mechanical forces that caused the development of the callus or corn (1),(2),(3),(4),(5)[C]:

- Careful and regular paring
- Use an emery board or a pumice stone daily, if necessary, to remove excess thickened skin.
- The pumice stone works best after bathing when the thickened skin has softened.
- Soft corn: toe separator or lamb's wool
- Doughnut-shaped corn pads
- Proper footwear with soft upper and a roomy toe box
- Orthotics can reduce pressure by redistributing forces.
- Use a skin-softening cream to prevent cracking of the callus or corn.

MEDICATION

First Line

- Salicylic acid pads (40%) (2),(5)[C]; salicylic acid solutions are available over the counter and soften hyperkeratotic lesions.
- Can also use salicylic acid gel (10–20%) when pad is too small for lesion
- Careful application of pads containing keratolytic agents; high concentration of salicylic acid (40%) may lead to maceration. Caution in diabetics and peripheral neuropathy. Avoid pads in patients with peripheral neuropathy.

ISSUES FOR REFERRAL

Consider referral to dermatology, podiatry, or orthopedic surgery (foot and ankle) if failed conservative measures or need for surgical intervention.

ADDITIONAL THERAPIES

Antibiotics are only indicated when there is evidence of an infected corn or callus.

SURGERY/OTHER PROCEDURES

- Shaving or sharp débridement can be therapeutic (3)[C].
- Surgery may be required to correct the bony abnormalities or deformities (claw toe, hammer toe, etc.) and is indicated only if all conservative measures have failed (1),(3)[C].
- Laser therapy can be used to pare deep lesions.

ONGOING CARE

FOLLOW-UP RECOMMENDATIONS

Follow-up is needed for ongoing corns and calluses despite conservative management, signs of infection, or severe pain.

Patient Monitoring

- Diabetics, the elderly, and individuals with peripheral arterial disease or peripheral neuropathy should consult with their health care providers before initiating treatment for calluses or corns.
- These individuals should be monitored closely for signs of nonhealing or infection.

COMPLICATIONS

- Recurrence
- Pain from procedure
- Although unlikely, there is potential for nonhealing and/or infection.

REFERENCES

1. Freeman DB. Corns and calluses resulting from mechanical hyperkeratosis. *Am Fam Physician*. 2002;65(11):2277–2280.
2. Becker BA, Childress MA. Common foot problems: over-the-counter treatments and home care. *Am Fam Physician*. 2018;98(5):298–303.
3. Phillips S, Seiverling E, Silvis M. Pressure and friction injuries in primary care. *Prim Care*. 2015;42(4):631–644.
4. Singh D, Bentley G, Trevino SG. Callosities, corns, and calluses. *BMJ*. 1996;312(7043):1403–1406.
5. Cordoro KM, Ganz JE. Training room management of medical conditions: sports dermatology. *Clin Sports Med*. 2005;24(3):565–598.
6. Patil S, Borkar M, Pande S, et al. Dermoscopic findings in clinically diagnosed cases of plantar warts, corns, and calluses: a cross-sectional study. *Cureus*. 2023;15(4):e38093.

ADDITIONAL READING

- Al Aboud AM, Yarrarapu SN. *Corns*. Treasure Island. StatPearls Publishing; 2023.
- Robbins JM. Recognizing, treating, and preventing common foot problems. *Cleve Clin J Med*. 2000;67(1):45–47, 51–52, 55–56.
- Spink MJ, Menz HB, Lord SR. Distribution and correlates of plantar hyperkeratotic lesions in older people. *J Foot Ankle Res*. 2009;2:8.

CLINICAL PEARLS

- Calluses and corns are common skin conditions resulting from repetitive friction or pressure.
- Diagnosis is often clinical, but imaging may be needed to evaluate an underlying bony prominence.
- Treatment is often aimed toward alleviating symptoms and removing contributing mechanical forces.
- First-line medical therapy is use of a salicylic acid pad.
- In some sports, calluses are desired by athletes to allow for pain-free participation.

CARDIAC ARRHYTHMIAS: ATRIAL FIBRILLATION, SVT

Charles W. Webb, DO, FAMSSM, FAAFP, CAQSM • Ricardo Villanueva Alvarez, MD

BASICS

Arrhythmias can stem from irregular impulse initiation, encompassing deviations from the typical sinus rhythm, which are broadly categorized as either bradyarrhythmias (slow) or tachyarrhythmias (fast) (1),(2).

EPIDEMIOLOGY

Incidence

- Bradyarrhythmias (1),(2):
  - Sinus bradycardia and atrioventricular (AV) block are often regarded as physiologic adaptations stemming from prolonged physical activity. This decline in heart rate may arise due to alterations in autonomic regulation, specifically an augmented parasympathetic tone or diminished sympathetic tone, as well as a potential reduction in the intrinsic heart rate.
  - Sinus bradycardia (50–80% of athletes vs. 23% in general population)
  - Sinus arrhythmias (13.5–69% of athletes vs. 2.4–20% in general population)
  - Sinus pause of >2 seconds (37.1% of athletes vs. 5.7% in general population)
  - First-degree AV block (6–33% of athletes vs. 0.65% in general population)
  - Second-degree AV block, Mobitz I (2.4–10% of athletes vs. 0.003% in general population)
  - Third-degree AV block (0.017% in athletes vs. 0.00002% in general population)
  - Junctional rhythms (0.031–7% of athletes vs. 0.06% in general population)
  - These changes are readily reversed in athlete's heart as increased sympathetic drive overcomes resting vagal tone; if presents with symptoms (impaired consciousness or fatigue) or not readily reversed, often associated with underlying cardiac disease
- Tachyarrhythmias (1),(2):
  - Atrial fibrillation (AF) more common in competitive athletes (0.063%) than general population (0.004%)
  - In the general population, the prevalence of supraventricular tachycardia (SVT) stands at 2.25 per 1,000 individuals. Women are at a higher risk of developing SVT, twice as great as men.
  - Wolff-Parkinson-White (WPW) syndrome (electrocardiogram [ECG] showing short PR interval with wide QRS and slurred upstroke or delta wave) equal in athletes and general population (0.15%)
  - Premature ventricular contractions occur at similar rates in athletes versus general population.
  - Complex ventricular arrhythmias are always pathologic and should seek prompt cardiology examination.

ETIOLOGY AND PATHOPHYSIOLOGY

Special considerations (3):

- Regular and long-term exercise (at least 4 h/wk) is linked to distinct electrical changes, indicating enlarged cardiac chambers, and increased vagal tone.
- Systematic training may cause physiologic adaptations, including a variety of abnormal ECG findings, in about 40% of elite athletes, termed the "athlete's heart."
- Increased QRS voltage, incomplete right bundle branch block, early repolarization, and peaked T waves related to increase in overall cardiac mass
- Endurance athletes develop cardiac alterations that are associated with AF in nonathletes including increased vagal tone, bradyarrhythmias, increased atrial pressures during exercise, left atrial enlargement, elevated inflammatory markers, and myocardial remodeling with fibrosis.
- Increased vagal tone in trained athletes favors a reduced refractoriness and enhanced myocardial excitability.

RISK FACTORS

- Structural heart disease (hypertrophic cardiomyopathy, anomalous coronary syndrome, arrhythmogenic right ventricular dysplasia, Marfan syndrome, aortic stenosis, dilated cardiomyopathy) (2)
- Myocarditis
- Atherosclerotic coronary artery disease (especially if >35 years old)
- Drugs (amphetamines, cocaine, ephedrine)
- Electrical disorders of the heart
- Long QT syndrome with QTc >0.46 second (congenital vs. iatrogenic, including medications such as class IA antiarrhythmics, antifungals, nonsedating antihistamines, antibiotics, promotility agents)
- Commotio cordis (direct nonpenetrating trauma to chest wall)
- Metabolic abnormalities (electrolyte disturbances, hyperthyroidism)

DIAGNOSIS

- Wide range of clinical presentations, from occasional palpitations to SCD (3)
- Bradyarrhythmias can present with impaired consciousness or fatigue.
- Tachyarrhythmias can cause palpitations, chest pain, and exertional dyspnea.
- Unstable ventricular tachyarrhythmias may cause lightheadedness or syncope.
- SVT:
  - Evaluation:
    - 12-lead ECG (4)[B]
    - Echocardiogram (5)[B]
    - Ambulatory cardiac/ECG monitoring
    - Identify rate response of SVT during activity or exercise.
    - If unable to induce SVT with exercise, can induce with either atrial/esophageal pacing, then monitor with exercise stress test.
- AF:
  - May be present intermittently or chronically
  - More common with diseases such as coronary artery disease and hypertension
  - Evaluation:
    - 12-lead ECG (2)[B]
    - Echocardiogram (2)[B]
    - Ambulatory cardiac/ECG monitoring (2)[B]
    - Determination of ventricular response with athletic activity

HISTORY

Based on American Heart Association (AHA) consensus panel recommendations for preparticipation athletic screening (1),(2):

- Family history:
  - Premature SCD
  - Heart disease in relatives <50 years old
- Personal history:
  - Heart murmur, fatigue, systemic hypertension, exertional chest pain, syncope/near syncope during or after exercise, unexplained or disproportionate exertional dyspnea
  - Presence of palpitations, chest pain, lightheadedness, syncope, and relation of symptoms to activity or rest
  - Note prescription and over-the-counter (OTC) medications, especially cold or diet remedies (especially those containing ephedra), nutritional supplements, alcohol use, and recreational drugs (especially cocaine).

PHYSICAL EXAM

- Vital signs (pulse, temperature, blood pressure [BP], respiration rate)
- Dynamic heart evaluation looking for heart murmur documented in at least two positions (usually supine and standing) to discern murmurs with outflow obstruction
- Hypertrophic obstructive cardiomyopathy murmur *increases* with maneuvers that decrease venous return (such as Valsalva or moving from squat or stand).
- Aortic stenosis murmur decreases with the same maneuvers.
- Pathologic murmur identified as any systolic murmur graded 3/6 or greater, any diastolic murmur, or any holosystolic murmur
- Palpation of radial and femoral pulses to exclude coarctation of the aorta (3),(4)

DIFFERENTIAL DIAGNOSIS

- Anxiety disorder, panic attacks
- Angina
- Costochondritis
- Neurocardiogenic syncope
- Heat stroke
- Seizure
- Thyroid dysfunction

DIAGNOSTIC TESTS & INTERPRETATION

Workup for athletes with significant arrhythmia includes (5),(6):

- 12-lead ECG (4)[B]
- Echocardiogram (evaluate for hypertrophic cardiomyopathy, dilated cardiomyopathy, and valvular abnormalities) (5)[B]
- Exercise stress test to identify exertional arrhythmias or induced ischemia; may need to be adapted specifically for athlete (i.e., at peak energy for sprinter) as well as sport (maximal ergometer stress test for rower reproducing training conditions that produce symptoms):
  - Nonpathologic bradycardias in athlete usually resolve with exercise testing.
  - Nonpathologic premature ventricular complexes usually resolve with exercise testing.

- Ambulatory cardiac monitoring, if possible during specific type of participation exercise
- Electrophysiologic studies (when ablation is being considered)
- Implanted loop recorder, cardiac magnetic resonance imaging (MRI) rarely required

TREATMENT

- Acute treatment:
  - Symptomatic athletes should initially have airway, breathing, and circulation (ABCs) assessed and stabilized.
  - If athlete is unstable, may require advanced cardiac life support, immediate direct current (DC) cardioversion, and emergent transport to a medical facility (3).
  - Suspected SVT may respond to conventional vagal maneuvers (e.g., Valsalva maneuver, carotid massage, forceful coughing, and ice applied to the face/neck) with reported effectiveness ranging from 19% to 54%. These maneuvers trigger a reflex stimulation of the vagus nerve, leading to the release of acetylcholine increasing parasympathetic tone (4).
- Long-term treatment bradyarrhythmias:
  - Treatment is generally unnecessary for asymptomatic exercise induced bradyarrhythmias, except for severe cases (HR <30 bpm or PR intervals >300 ms), which require further evaluation (3).
  - Symptomatic athletes with exercise-induced bradycardia or AV blocks may benefit from reducing exercise intensity or duration or discontinuing exercise (3).
  - Pacemaker implantation should adhere to guidelines. Pacemaker-dependent patients should avoid contact sports, whereas nondependent patients may consider participation (3).
- Long-term treatment SVT:
  - For SVT associated with hemodynamic instability, electrical cardioversion is the preferred acute treatment (5).
  - Treatment of paroxysmal SVT with β or sodium channel blockers is discouraged in athletes because these drugs may reduce performance during sports and have limited ability to prevent arrhythmia recurrence during sports activity. β-blockers are listed by the World Anti-Doping Agency as prohibited in particular sports (5).
  - If athlete has a short refractory period bypass tract capable of anterograde conduction and a history of AF, they should have ablation of the bypass tract due to risk of life-threatening arrhythmias (6)[B].
- Long-term treatment AF:
  - Treatment of underlying cardiac disease, rate control medications, antiarrhythmic medications
  - β-Adrenergic blocking agents banned in some competitive sports (2)
  - Consider competitive athletic population, curative treatment via ablation should be contemplated, as it offers equally safe outcomes with similar acute success rates in both athletes and nonathletes (3)[B].
  - Competitive sports can typically be resumed within 1 to 3 months following ablation, with additional ECG follow-ups at 6 months and 1 year, considering the minimal risk of late preexcitation recurrence (6).

ONGOING CARE

- Return-to-play guidelines:
  - A comprehensive cardiac examination is crucial to detect underlying structural heart disease, as sudden cardiac death (SCD) ranks as the primary cause of mortality in athletes engaged in sports and exercise (1).
  - Ensuring cardiovascular safety during sports participation is imperative for individuals of all ages and skill levels, as it helps prevent potentially catastrophic and avoidable SCD incidents (1).
  - Athletes with syncope or near syncope should not participate in sports where the likelihood of loss of consciousness could be hazardous until the cause has been determined and treated (2).
  - Athletes with symptoms such as impaired consciousness and fatigue attributed to arrhythmias should be treated and if asymptomatic for 2 to 3 months during treatment may participation in all sports (3).
  - Athletes with symptomatic tachycardia/bradycardia arrhythmias should be treated, if no structural heart disease, for 2 to 3 months and then they can return to sports (3).
- Atrial flutter:
  - Athletes with atrial flutter in the absence of structural heart disease may participate in all sports if without flutter for 2 to 3 months.
  - Athletes with atrial flutter and structural heart disease can participate in sports such as billiards, bowling, cricket, curling, golf, and rifle (Bethesda Guidelines class 1A sports).
  - Athletes without structural heart disease who have had ablation or surgery can participate in all sports after 2 to 4 weeks without recurrence.
  - Athletes who require anticoagulation cannot participate in competitive sports where the chance of collision is present.
- AF:
  - In cases where asymptomatic individuals with atrial fibrillation without underlying heart issues demonstrate sufficient rate control during exercise stress tests or ECG monitoring, in the context of training or competition, they can safely participate in all sports (2)[B],(6)[C].
  - Low- to medium-intensity exercise programs can generally be resumed 1 week after ablation provided there is no specific risk of arrhythmia recurrence (2)[B].
  - Athletes can typically return to competitive sports within 1 to 3 months following ablation, and additional ECG follow-ups at 6 months and 1 year are recommended due to the very low risk of late pre-excitation recurrence (2)[B].
  - Athletes who require anticoagulation cannot participate in competitive sports where the chance of collision is present (2),(6).
  - Athletes with AF and structural heart disease who have rate control can participate to the limits and recommendations of the structural disease. (Use caution because β-blockers are banned in some sports.) (6)
- SVT:
  - Athletes with SVT and symptom-free premature atrial beats and no structural heart disease can engage in all sports (2)[C].
  - Athletes with syncope, near syncope, or significant symptoms due to arrhythmia, or who have structural heart disease may participate in class 1A sports once treated and have no recurrence for 2 to 4 weeks (5).
  - Atrioventricular reentrant tachycardia (AVRT) or AF associated with WPW syndrome, ablation is necessary. Following successful ablation and 1 month without recurrence, athletes can safely resume all sports (5)[B].
  - For SVT associated with hemodynamic instability, electrical cardioversion is the preferred acute treatment (5)[B].
  - Paroxysmal SVT management with β-blockers or calcium channel blockers (CCB) in athletes is discouraged due to their potential to impair sports performance and their limited ability to prevent arrhythmia recurrence during physical activity (5).

REFERENCES

1. Pelliccia A, Zipes DP, Maron BJ. Bethesda conference #36 and the European Society of Cardiology Consensus Recommendations revisited a comparison of U.S. and European criteria for eligibility and disqualification of competitive athletes with cardiovascular abnormalities. *J Am Coll Cardiol*. 2008;52(24):1990–1996.
2. Pelliccia A, Sharma S, Gati S, et al. 2020 ESC Guidelines on sports cardiology and exercise in patients with cardiovascular disease: the task force on sports cardiology and exercise in patients with cardiovascular disease of the European Society of Cardiology (ESC). *Eur Heart J*. 2021;42(1):17–96.
3. Guasch E, Mont L. Diagnosis, pathophysiology, and management of exercise-induced arrhythmias. *Nat Rev Cardiol*. 2017;14(2):88–101.
4. Drezner JA, Sharma S, Baggish A, et al. International criteria for electrocardiographic interpretation in athletes: consensus statement. *Br J Sports Med*. 2017;51(9):704–731.
5. Brugada J, Katritsis D, Arbelo E, et al. 2019 ESC Guidelines for the management of patients with supraventricular tachycardia. The task force for the management of patients with supraventricular tachycardia of the European Society of Cardiology (ESC): developed in collaboration with the Association for European Pediatric and Congenital Cardiology (AEPC). *Eur Heart J*. 2020;41(5): 655–720.
6. Elliott AD, Mahajan R, Lau DH, et al. Atrial fibrillation in endurance athletes: from mechanism to management. *Cardiol Clin*. 2016;34(4):567–578.

CLINICAL PEARLS

- Document pertinent negatives in history.
- Document a dynamic heart exam during physicals and evaluations of symptomatic individuals.
- Consider ECG as first step in evaluation of arrhythmias (4).

CARPAL TUNNEL SYNDROME

Stephen Shaheen, MD, CAQSM, FACEP

BASICS

DESCRIPTION

- Clinical condition caused by entrapment of the median nerve in the carpal tunnel at the wrist
- Classically presents as pain, weakness, and paresthesias on the palmar surface on the radial 3½ digits
- Can be acute or chronic (idiopathic)

EPIDEMIOLOGY

- Carpal tunnel syndrome (CTS) accounts for ~90% of all entrapment neuropathies (1).
- Predominant gender: female > male (from 3:1 to as high as 10:1) (1)
- Predominant age: Peak prevalence is among women aged 55 years and older; prevalence increases with age (2),(3).
- Higher prevalence in the dominant extremity; bilateral up to 50% of the time (2)

Incidence

- Lifetime incidence is ~10% (4).
- Estimated that 1 million adults annually in the United States require medical treatment (4).

Prevalence

Prevalence is 7–16% of the population depending on the criteria for diagnosis (3).

ETIOLOGY AND PATHOPHYSIOLOGY

Exact pathogenesis of CTS is unclear. Most accepted theories are mechanical compression, microvascular insufficiency, and vibration (fibrous hypertrophy of the synovial flexor (5). Pressure in the sheath is typically between 1 and 20 mm Hg but can rise between 8- and 10- with normal activity (3).

- Acute:
  - Acute cases are less common but can be caused by a sudden rise in pressure in the carpal tunnel.
  - Most commonly seen with radial fracture; also associated with burns, coagulopathy, local infection, and injections
- Chronic:
  - Idiopathic: Only 50% of cases have an identifiable cause, which can be local, regional, or systemic in origin (4).
  - Local: inflammation, trauma, tumors, and anatomic anomalies
  - Regional: osteoarthritis, rheumatoid arthritis, amyloidosis, and gout
  - Systemic: diabetes, obesity, hypothyroidism, pregnancy, menopause, systemic lupus erythematosus (SLE), scleroderma, dermatomyositis, renal failure, long-term hemodialysis, acromegaly, multiple myeloma, sarcoidosis, leukemia, alcoholism, and hemophilia (3)

RISK FACTORS

- Repetitive wrist motion is the most widely recognized risk factor for occupational CTS, with correlated increased risks in industrial and office workers (3).
- Narrow bony measurements of the wrist, elevated body mass index, increased age, female gender, and pregnancy are other common risk factors.

Pregnancy Considerations

- Common during pregnancy
- Usually in the 3rd trimester and often bilateral
- Usually, symptoms resolve spontaneously after delivery or with conservative treatment during pregnancy.

COMMONLY ASSOCIATED CONDITIONS

- Activities involving repetitive wrist motion, vibration, and excessive forces through the wrist
- Diabetes, thyroid disease, advancing age, and rheumatoid arthritis all have been associated with the development of CTS.
- Traumatic carpal bone dislocation or wrist fracture can disrupt the median nerve through the carpal tunnel through direct trauma to the nerve or mechanical entrapment secondary to cortical disruption and subsequent compression.
- Lipomas, ganglion cysts, and other anatomic anomalies can grow and directly compress the median nerve.
- Proximal upper extremity nerve entrapment or nerve root compression— "double crush" syndrome

DIAGNOSIS

HISTORY

- Complaints of pain, weakness, and paresthesias on the palmar surface on the first (radial) 3½ digits
- Exacerbated by specific wrist motion (e.g., sports, occupational tasks, sleeping, driving)
- Nighttime symptoms
- Improved with "shaking of the hands" (a.k.a. flick sign)
- Consider cervical root pathology or radiculopathy if complaint of "shooting pain" down arm; consider generalized peripheral polyneuropathy if complaint of "sock and glove" distribution of pain in upper and lower extremities.

PHYSICAL EXAM

- Classically presents as pain, weakness, and paresthesias on the palmar surface on the first 3½ digits; however, there can be variations.
- Nocturnal acroparesthesia (i.e., extremity numbness, tingling, or other abnormal sensation) is the symptom most characteristic of CTS (6).
- Flick sign, in which a patient may demonstrate vigorous shaking of the hand and wrist in order to relieve symptoms, may be present.
- Pain or paresthesia evoked by hand grip
- Observe and palpate the region of the thenar muscle mass for atrophy (late finding).
- Usually, normal hand and wrist range of motion
- Strength testing of the abductor pollicis brevis muscle, which can reveal weakness
- Sensory evaluation, especially in the median nerve distribution, using a variety of testing dependent on resources and experience (e.g., two-point discrimination, vibrometry, monofilaments, graphesthesia)
- Provocative tests:
  - Tinel sign: Percuss over the region of the carpal tunnel at wrist to elicit paresthesias in the distribution of the nerve; 38–100% sensitive and 80% specific (6)[A]
  - Phalen test: Position wrists adjacent to each other in complete flexion for at least 60 seconds to elicit paresthesias; 42–85% sensitive and 80% specific (6)[A]
  - Carpal compression test: Press with thumbs over the carpal tunnel for 30 seconds to elicit symptoms; reported 87% sensitivity and 90% specificity for CTS (6)[A]
  - Square wrist sign: Increased wrist ratio (thickness: width) has an increased odds ratio for CTS (5)[A].
  - Tourniquet test: Temporary increase in carpal tunnel pressure and symptoms can be elicited by blood pressure cuff application to arm or forearm.
  - Diagnosis usually can be made on history and physical examination alone.

DIFFERENTIAL DIAGNOSIS

- de Quervain tenosynovitis
- Cervical radiculopathy, C6–C7
- Proximal median nerve entrapment, pronator teres syndrome, or anterior interosseous syndrome
- Ulnar neuropathy at the elbow or wrist
- Brachial plexus neuropathy
- Wrist arthritis or other lesions in the wrist
- Colles fracture, lunate dislocation
- Generalized peripheral polyneuropathy
- Angina pectoris
- Upper motor neuron pathology
- Syringomyelia
- Mononeuritis multiplex
- Multiple sclerosis
- Space occupying lesion, mass, lipoma, ganglion

DIAGNOSTIC TESTS & INTERPRETATION

Initial Tests (lab, imaging)

- Indicated when the classic defining features of CTS are not present:
  - Plain films generally are normal. Occasionally, carpal tunnel views may be helpful to rule out anatomic variants, fractures with trauma, and narrowing or calcification in the carpal tunnel.
  - Ultrasound (US) of the wrist may show structural abnormalities with nerve swelling. Cross-sectional area of the median nerve is significantly greater in patients with CTS than healthy controls (7).
  - Sensitivity of diagnosis with US of median nerve enlargement can be up to 97.9% (7).
- Magnetic resonance imaging (MRI) has been used to visualize structural abnormalities in and around the nerve:
  - There are limited studies examining the sensitivity and specificity of MRI for this purpose.
  - One small study showed no difference in diagnostic accuracy between MRI and US.
  - MRI is costly and cumbersome and cannot assess the physiologic integrity of the median nerve across the carpal tunnel segment.

Diagnostic Procedures/Other

- Electrodiagnostic examinations can confirm and/or support the diagnosis of CTS.
- Nerve conduction studies provide a highly sensitive (>85%) and specific (>95%) means for assessing the physiologic integrity of the median nerve across the carpal tunnel segment (6)[A].
- Can be used to classify severity of CTS and to monitor progression of median nerve entrapment
- Needle electromyography is useful for documenting the presence of axonal loss to intrinsic hand muscles innervated by the median nerve distal to the carpal tunnel segment and if the study includes structures proximal to the carpal tunnel, and also in identifying other or coexisting neuromuscular pathology (e.g., cervical radiculopathy).

TREATMENT

- Conservative treatment:
  - Restriction of precipitating activities may relieve symptoms.
  - Wait and see (8)[A]:
    - Can be considered in patients with mild symptoms
    - Improvement in 23–40%, although symptoms often recur
  - Splinting:
    - Splinting the wrist at a neutral angle helps to decrease repetitive flexion and rotation, thus relieving mild soft tissue swelling or flexor tenosynovitis.
    - Compared with nighttime-only splint use, full-time use has been shown to provide greater improvement of symptoms and electrophysiologic measures; however, compliance with full-time use is more difficult (9)[B].
  - Corticosteroids:
    - With regard to symptom management, oral corticosteroids have shown efficacy for up to 8 weeks. Nonsteroidal anti-inflammatory drugs (NSAIDs) or diuretics are not effective in short-term treatment (9)[A].
    - Corticosteroid injection into or proximal to the carpal tunnel provides greater clinical improvement at 10 weeks than placebo (9).
    - Surgery should be considered if patient needs more than two injections.
  - Platelet Rich Plasma (PRP) (8):
    - Evidence is extremely limited.
    - Doses, preparation methods are heterogenous between kits and production companies
    - Possible small improvement at 3 months compared to control in very small study
  - Gabapentin (8):
    - Literature is limited but does *not* support the use.
    - Placebo-control study showed no benefit at 2 and 8 weeks.
    - Small randomized controlled trial (RCT) found a limited, nonclinically relevant benefit for the medication but was unblinded.
  - Median nerve hydrodissection:
    - Increasing trials have shown this as an emerging treatment option.
    - Optimal technique and injectate solution/quantity debatable in literature
  - Other conservative treatments and their evidence:
    - Level 1 (strong evidence of efficacy): local and oral steroids
    - Level 2 (moderate evidence of efficacy): Splints and therapeutic US are effective; NSAIDs, diuretics, and vitamin B_6 are ineffective (7),(9).
    - Level 3 (limited/conflicting evidence of efficacy): Yoga, laser, and nerve glide exercises are effective short-term (7). Wait and see and platelet-rich plasma (PRP) can be considered but are variable, inconsistent, and have limited or poor data.
- Surgical treatment:
  - Patients who fail conservative therapy or who have severe symptoms (e.g., nerve entrapment on nerve conduction studies, thenar atrophy, or motor weakness)
  - Surgical decompression of the carpal tunnel segment by sectioning of the transverse carpal ligament has been reported to result in good symptomatic improvement in 70–90% of patients and may prevent further median nerve axon loss.
  - Slightly quicker return to work noted in endoscopic repair versus open repair (7)
  - Complications of surgery include injury to median nerve, scar tenderness, hypertrophic scarring, loss of grip strength, pillar pain (i.e., tenderness on the base of the palm), reflex sympathetic dystrophy/complex regional pain syndrome, and bow stringing of flexor tendons.

Geriatric Considerations

Surgery has been found to provide better symptom relief, functional status, and general satisfaction than nonoperative therapy. However, advancing age at initial surgery may see decreasing returns in symptom improvement (1).

ONGOING CARE

PATIENT EDUCATION

- Use of wrist wraps, and taping may minimize forces through the carpal tunnel by limiting excessive motion through the wrist in upper extremity weight-bearing sports such as gymnastics and weightlifting.
- Improvements in wrist pain and paresthesias may be noted within a few weeks after CTS surgery, but maximal improvements in thenar strength and numbness may take as long as 9 months.
- Diagnosis often can be made based on history and physical examination findings alone.
- Corticosteroids (oral and injection), splinting, and surgery have the best evidence for treatment.

REFERENCES

1. Jackson R, Beckman J, Frederick M, et al. Rates of carpal tunnel syndrome in a state workers' compensation information system, by industry and occupation—California, 2007–2014. *MMWR Morb Mortal Wkly Rep*. 2018;67:1094–1097.
2. Bland JDP, Rudolfer SM. Clinical surveillance of carpal tunnel syndrome in two areas of the United Kingdom, 1991–2001. *J Neurol Neurosurg* Psychiatry. 2003;74(12):1674–1679.
3. Malakootian M, Soveizi M, Gholipour A, et al. Pathophysiology, diagnosis, treatment, and genetics of carpal tunnel syndrome: a review. *Cell Mol Neurobiol*. 2023;43(5):1817–1831.
4. Aroori S, Spence RA. Carpal tunnel syndrome. *Ulster Med J*. 2008;77(1):6–17.
5. Aboonq MS. Pathophysiology of carpal tunnel syndrome. *Neurosciences (Riyadh)*. 2015;20(1):4–9.
6. Wilder-Smith EP, Seet RCS, Lim ECH. Diagnosing carpal tunnel syndrome—clinical criteria and ancillary tests. *Nat Clin Pract Neurol*. 2006;2(7):366–374.
7. Wipperman J, Goerl K. Carpal tunnel syndrome: diagnosis and management. *Am Fam Physician*. 2016;94(12):993–999.
8. Karjalanen T, Raatikainen S, Jaatinen K, et al. Update on efficacy of conservative treatments for carpal tunnel syndrome. *J Clin Med*. 2022;11(4):950.
9. Graham B, Peljovich AE, Afra R, et al. The American Academy of Orthopaedic Surgeons evidence-based clinical practice guideline on: management of carpal tunnel syndrome. *J Bone Joint Surg Am*. 2016;98(20):1750–1754.

ADDITIONAL READING

- Gerritsen AAM, de Vet HCW, Scholten RJPM, et al. Splinting vs surgery in the treatment of carpal tunnel syndrome: a randomized controlled trial. *JAMA*. 2002;288(10):1245–1251.
- McDonagh C, Alexander M, Kane D. The role of ultrasound in the diagnosis and management of carpal tunnel syndrome: a new paradigm. *Rheumatology (Oxford)*. 2015;54(1):9–19.
- Shiri R. A square-shaped wrist as a predictor of carpal tunnel syndrome: a meta-analysis. *Muscle Nerve*. 2015;52(5):709–713.
- Wainner RS, Fritz JM, Irrgang JJ, et al. Development of a clinical prediction rule for the diagnosis of carpal tunnel syndrome. *Arch Phys Med Rehabil*. 2005;86(4):609–618.

CLINICAL PEARLS

- CTS is a very common compressive neuropathy of the upper extremity.
- It classically presents as pain, weakness, and paresthesias on the palmar surface on the first 3½ digits.
- Patients also complain of nighttime symptoms and needing to shake their hands to help the pain.
- The vast majority of patients respond initially to conservative management (80%)—although the recurrence rate (80%) after 1 year is high.

CATECHOLAMINERGIC POLYMORPHIC VENTRICULAR TACHYCARDIA (CPVT)

Chau Bui, DO • Paul Meirick, MD

BASICS

DESCRIPTION

- Channelopathies refer to a group of inherited arrhythmogenic diseases caused by mutations in genes encoding for ion channel proteins in cardiomyocytes that disrupt the balance of currents in the cardiac action potential. These disruptions may lead to ventricular arrhythmias and sudden cardiac death (SCD).
- The channelopathies include catecholaminergic polymorphic ventricular tachycardia (CPVT), long QT syndrome (LQTS) (see chapter on "Congenital QT Syndromes"), short QT syndrome (SQTS) (see chapter on "Congenital QT Syndromes"), and Brugada syndrome (see chapter on "Brugada Syndrome").
- CPVT: characterized by exercise or catecholamine-induced biventricular tachycardia, polymorphic ventricular premature beats, or ventricular tachycardia (VT) in young individuals with a structurally normal heart

EPIDEMIOLOGY

CPVT often presents with symptoms in 1st decade of life, but cases have been reported to present in the 4th decade (1),(2).

Prevalence

Prevalence is generally unknown but estimated at ~1/10,000.

ETIOLOGY AND PATHOPHYSIOLOGY

- Sporadic or inherited mutations in the cardiac ryanodine receptor or calsequestrin (2)
- Genetic defects in *RyR2* and *CASQ2* genes alter calcium homeostasis in cardiac myocytes and lead to delayed after repolarizations that may precipitate supraventricular and ventricular arrhythmias (2).

Genetics

Two genetic variants known: autosomal dominant related to mutations in the *RyR2* gene encoding for the cardiac ryanodine receptor and an autosomal recessive form, resulting from mutations in *CASQ2* gene encoding for cardiac calsequestrin (2)

RISK FACTORS

The primary risk factor for most channelopathies is genetic:

- Physical effort (including swimming) and emotional stress are the most common precipitants of VT or ventricular fibrillation (VF).
- Strong association between arrhythmic events and exercise or catecholamine stimulation

GENERAL PREVENTION

- SCD resulting from channelopathies may be prevented by carefully screening and identifying athletes with the condition, although CPVT generally first presents with life-threatening arrhythmia. The preparticipation evaluation is the most important tool for identifying athletes with symptoms that may represent an inherited channelopathy. Any athlete with symptoms of palpitations, syncope, presyncope, any collapse, or with a family history of SCD or "accidental" death should be further evaluated with the tools reviewed below.
- Automatic external defibrillators (AEDs) are another important tool in preventing SCD from undiagnosed CPVT.

DIAGNOSIS

- Most patients present only after experiencing life-threatening VT or VF.
- Prehospital:
  - In the case that any patient with a CPVT converts into a life-threatening arrhythmia in the field, the most useful immediate tool and treatment is an AED.

HISTORY

- Pertinent history in screening athletes: Gathering a detailed and careful history during the preparticipation physical or during the evaluation of an athlete who comes to your attention is critical. The following questions should be included when interviewing an athlete:
  - Have you ever passed out, become dizzy, or had chest pain during or after exercise?
  - Do you get tired more quickly than others during exercise?
  - Has anyone in the family died suddenly and unexpectedly before the age of 50 years? (Remember to ask about family members who died of accidental causes such as sudden infant death syndrome, drownings, and motor vehicle accidents because they may be clues to an undiagnosed family history of channelopathy.)
  - Have you ever had a heart abnormality or murmur diagnosed by a doctor?
  - Have you ever had an abnormal heart rate, palpitations, or irregular heartbeats?
  - Have you had high blood pressure (BP) or high cholesterol?
  - Has a physician ever denied or restricted your participation in sports for heart problems?
  - Have any of your relatives ever had cardiomyopathy, Marfan syndrome, LQTS, SQTS, or significant heart arrhythmias?
- Pertinent history in potentially affected athletes:
  - CPVT is most commonly asymptomatic until initial presentation with syncope or life-threatening VT or VF.
  - May have a family history of sudden cardiac arrest or SCD

PHYSICAL EXAM

- The most important elements of the exam are general (including level of consciousness), cardiac, and pulmonary examinations and, in the case of a patient who has sustained a life-threatening arrhythmia, complete trauma examination.
- Because patients with CPVT typically have structurally normal hearts, it is not uncommon to observe a completely normal examination when a life-threatening arrhythmia is not present.
- When arrhythmias are present, the examination may be notable for bradycardia or tachycardia, either regular or irregular, depending on the patient's rhythm.

DIFFERENTIAL DIAGNOSIS

QT syndromes, acquired LQTS with its many reversible metabolic and drug-induced causes, Brugada syndrome, acute coronary syndrome, true right bundle branch block (RBBB), pericarditis, drug-induced VT or VF

DIAGNOSTIC TESTS & INTERPRETATION

Initial Tests (lab, imaging)

In the setting of a life-threatening arrhythmia, it may be indicated to rule out ischemic or metabolic causes with a basic or comprehensive metabolic panel and cardiac enzymes.

Diagnostic Procedures/Other

Electrocardiogram (ECG) is the most important initial diagnostic tool. Holter monitors and echocardiograms may be of use as well:

- No distinguishing ECG diagnostic markers; resting ECG is usually normal until a life-threatening ECG pattern of VT or VF develops.
- Reported findings include sinus bradycardia, U waves, or a short PR interval.
- Exercise stress testing or strong emotions can elicit a pathognomonic bidirectional or polymorphic VT. Exercise-induced supraventricular tachyarrhythmias are common.

TREATMENT

The primary treatment is implantable cardioverter defibrillator (ICD) placement with careful programming and β-blockers.

MEDICATION

- β-Blockers are the cornerstone of CPVT therapy.
- Flecainide also has been shown to be effective.

SURGERY/OTHER PROCEDURES

- ICD is recommended for patients who continue to experience syncope and/or documented VT despite treatment with β-blockers (3)[C].
- ICD should be programmed with long delays before shock delivery and high cutoff rates due to inappropriate shocks that may lead to proarrhythmic effect (3),(4).
- Left cardiac sympathetic denervation considered when β-blockers are ineffective (3)[C].

ADMISSION, INPATIENT, AND NURSING CONSIDERATIONS

As always, all patients who present with a life-threatening arrhythmia should be treated emergently with cardioversion and/or pharmacotherapy as dictated by standard advanced cardiovascular life support (ACLS).

ONGOING CARE

All patients with CPVT should be followed regularly by a cardiologist. Education and restrictions regarding exercise are crucial to survival.

FOLLOW-UP RECOMMENDATIONS

Return-to-play decisions:

- Participation in all competitive sports except those of very low intensity is not advised for symptomatic athletes or asymptomatic athletes with exercise-induced premature ventricular contractions in bigeminy, couplets, or nonsustained VT (5)[C].
- Exceptions should only be made after consultation with a CPVT specialist.
- Early data suggests recurrent events may be less frequent than previously reported. One CPVT specialist center reports similar recurrence rates between patients who return to sport and those who choose not to return to sport (6).

REFERENCES

1. Cheung CC, Laksman ZWM, Mellor G, et al. Exercise and inherited arrhythmias. *Can J Cardiol*. 2016;32(4):452–458.
2. Priori SG, Napolitano C, Memmi M, et al. Clinical and molecular characterization of patients with catecholaminergic polymorphic ventricular tachycardia. *Circulation*. 2002;106(1):69–74.
3. Mazzanti A, O'Rourke S, Ng K, et al. The usual suspects in sudden cardiac death of the young: a focus on inherited arrhythmogenic diseases. *Expert Rev Cardiovasc Ther*. 2014;12(4):499–519.
4. Roston TM, Jones K, Hawkins NM, et al. Implantable cardioverter-defibrillator use in catecholaminergic polymorphic ventricular tachycardia: a systematic review. *Heart Rhythm*. 2018;15(12):1791–1799.
5. Ackerman MJ, Zipes DP, Kovacs RJ, et al. Eligibility and disqualification recommendations for competitive athletes with cardiovascular abnormalities: task force 10: the cardiac channelopathies: a scientific statement from the American Heart Association and American College of Cardiology. *Circulation*. 2015;132(22):e326–e329.
6. Ostby SA, Bos JM, Owen HJ, et al. Competitive sports participation in patients with catecholaminergic polymorphic ventricular tachycardia: a single center's early experience. *JACC Clin Electrophysiol*. 2016;2(3):253–262.

CLINICAL PEARLS

- CPVT is a channelopathy that can be induced by physical or emotional stress in a structurally normal heart.
- CPVT generally first presents with life-threatening arrhythmia, therefore the preparticipation evaluation is the most important tool for identifying athletes with symptoms that may represent an inherited channelopathy.
- Resting ECG is usually normal until a life-threatening ECG pattern of VT or VF develops.
- The primary treatment is placement of an ICD with careful programming and β-blockers.
- Symptomatic athletes or asymptomatic athletes with exercise-induced premature ventricular contractions in bigeminy, couplets, or nonsustained VT are not advised to return to play in competitive sports, except those sports with very low intensity, without CPVT specialist consultation.

CAUDA EQUINA SYNDROME

Suraj A. Achar, MD, FAAFP, CAQSM • Jarrod Yamanaka, MD, CAQSM

BASICS

- Cauda equina syndrome (CES) is a rare condition associated with mechanical compression caused by an intraspinal lesion caudal to the conus that injures ≥2 of the 18 nerve roots constituting the cauda equina within the lumbar spinal canal.
- The CES is typically associated with marked neurologic disability.
- It is characterized by a variable combination of symptoms and signs that can include back pain, bowel and bladder dysfunction, saddle anesthesia, and varying degrees of loss of lower extremity sensory and motor function.
- When diagnosed, the treatment is urgent surgical decompression.

DESCRIPTION

- CES can have an acute or chronic presentation with "saddle anesthesia" (sensory changes in the groin and perineal area); bladder, rectal, and/or sexual dysfunction with back pain; and often with radicular symptoms and signs.
- CES can be classified into:
  - Incomplete syndrome (CES-I): Patients present with motor and sensory changes, including saddle anesthesia but have yet to develop full retention or incontinence of either bowel or bladder. Instead, symptoms include altered urinary sensation, loss of urgency, poor urinary stream, and straining to urinate. Saddle and genital area sensory deficits are usually unilateral or partial.
  - Complete syndrome with true retention (CES-R): characterized by painless urinary retention and overflow incontinence; similarly, either retention or incontinence of the bowel may be experienced. This is usually concurrent with extensive or complete saddle and genital sensory deficit along with inability to detect bladder fullness.

EPIDEMIOLOGY

Incidence

- CES is a relatively uncommon condition with an estimated incidence in the population ranging between 1 in 33,000 and 1 in 100,000 (1).
- CES is reported in approximately 0.04% of all patients presenting with low back pain (LBP).
- Peak incidence is in the 4th and 5th decades.
- It is estimated that CES occurs in approximately 0.12–2% of cases of lumbar herniated disks (1),(2).
- 50–70% of patients with CES have urinary retention (CES-R) on presentation and 30–50% have CES-I (1).
- Men and women are affected equally.

ETIOLOGY AND PATHOPHYSIOLOGY

- The most common cause of CES is mechanical compression arising from a large central lumbar disk herniation.
- Other etiologies include:
  - Mass effect, where something new grows or collects in the spinal canal, such as tumors, an epidural abscess (a collection of pus), or an epidural hematoma (a bleed)
  - Structural and traumatic issues can also be the cause, including severe vertebral fractures or lumbar stenosis, which is a degenerative narrowing of the canal.
  - Various inflammatory and infectious conditions can lead to severe swelling of the nerves or surrounding tissues, including ankylosing spondylitis, spinal arachnoiditis (scarring of nerve membranes), or infections like tuberculosis and Lyme disease.
- Nerve root injury may be due to compression, ischemia, venous congestion, or inflammation.
- Interruption of the sympathetic and parasympathetic bladder reflex arcs by the lower motor neuron lesion of CES results in loss of sensory and motor innervation to the bladder with subsequent urinary retention and overflow incontinence.

RISK FACTORS

- A congenitally stenotic spinal canal or acquired spinal narrowing can predispose to the development of CES.
- History of trauma, including falls, motor vehicle accident (MVA), weightlifting, and chiropractic manipulation
- Previous spine surgery
- Anticoagulation
- Spine infections

ALERT
High index of suspicion with trauma and anticoagulation

COMMONLY ASSOCIATED CONDITIONS

- Bladder dysfunction
- Lumbar spondylolisthesis and stenosis
- Motor weakness

DIAGNOSIS

ALERT
- Early identification of the patient's neurologic deficits and prompt surgical intervention reduces the likelihood of permanent neurologic sequelae.
- The widely varying clinical presentation of CES is a major cause of delayed recognition.

- CES must be considered in the presence of:
  - Severe LBP
  - Sciatica: often bilateral, sometimes absent
  - Saddle and/or genital sensory disturbance
  - Bladder, bowel, and sexual dysfunction

HISTORY

- Most cases are of sudden onset and progress rapidly within hours or days.
- Less frequently, CES can evolve slowly.
- Pain often described as progressively worsening
- Acute severe or sudden increase in LBP with or without radicular symptoms
- Patients do not always complain of pain or can have chronic, intermittent LBP with gradually worsening sciatica over weeks to months with incomplete deficits of bowel/bladder function.
- Inquire about changes in bowel and bladder habits and sexual function.
- Bowel disturbance may include fecal incontinence or constipation.
- Inquire about saddle and perianal area sensory changes.
- Unilateral or bilateral sensory changes or numb sensation in the lower limbs

PHYSICAL EXAM

- Motor exam:
  - Most patients have ≥4/5 strength in ≥1 spinal nerve distributions often manifesting as:
    - Gait difficulties
    - Difficulty with heel/toe walking
    - Difficulty with sit-to-stand test
    - Foot drop
- Sensory exam must include comparison of pinprick to light touch testing:
  - Most patients present with an objective sensory deficit in the lower extremities.
  - 76% of patients have decreased perianal, perineum, buttock sensation, and posterior thigh sensation to pinprick (2).
- Rectal exam to evaluate for decreased tone, often an early sign of CES
- Reflexes: absent or diminished bulbocavernosus, anal, and lower limb reflexes

DIFFERENTIAL DIAGNOSIS

- Conus medullaris syndrome
- Herniated nucleus pulposus
- Spine injuries
- Guillain-Barré syndrome
- Multiple sclerosis
- Peripheral neuropathy
- Lumbosacral plexopathy
- Polyradiculopathy
- Spinal tumor

DIAGNOSTIC TESTS & INTERPRETATION

Initial Tests (lab, imaging)

- Urgent magnetic resonance imaging (MRI) of the lumbosacral spine is essential in the setting of neurologic compromise to confirm the diagnosis (3)[B].
- If MRI contraindicated, computed tomography (CT) scan and myelography indicated
- Spine radiographs useful to evaluate spine trauma, listhesis, and disk degeneration in suspected cases
- Urodynamic studies useful in bladder function assessment subacutely

Follow-Up Tests & Special Considerations

Clinical diagnosis of CES is difficult and has a 43% false-positive rate, so accurate confirmatory imaging is important (3)[B].

TREATMENT

GENERAL MEASURES

- Immediate surgical consultation
- Although not always reversible, surgical decompression may be the only chance to reverse the neurologic deficits.
- Surgical decompression is necessary within 48 hours after the onset of symptoms and preferably performed within 6 hours of injury (4),(5)[B].

ISSUES FOR REFERRAL

- Recent bowel or bladder changes
- Sexual dysfunction
- Saddle anesthesia
- Lower extremity weakness or paralysis
- Sensory loss in a nerve root distribution
- Muscle atrophy
- Absent bulbocavernosus, anal, patellar, Achilles, and plantar reflexes
- Gait disturbance
- Upper motor neuron (UMN) signs such as clonus, spasticity, hyperreflexia, or Babinski sign

SURGERY/OTHER PROCEDURES

- The timing of surgical intervention is controversial, with immediate, early, and late surgical decompression showing varying results (1)[C].
- It is well established that the outcome for patients with CES-I at the time of surgery is generally favorable, whereas those who have deteriorated to CES-R when the compression is relieved have a poorer outcome (4),(5)[B],(6)[C].
- The surgery as an emergency situation is recommended in the first 48 hours of onset of symptoms. Any delay in diagnosis and treatment leads to a poor prognosis of CES (7).
- Surgical technique is often wide laminectomy and extensive decompression with foraminotomies if needed for stenosis (2)[C].
- Surgical treatment might also include instrumentation/fusion for stabilization or discectomy.

ADMISSION, INPATIENT, AND NURSING CONSIDERATIONS

- Malignant disease that is considered inoperable may be treated with radiation therapy and chemotherapy.
- Glucocorticoids indicated in CES cases associated with spinal cord compression or other conditions amenable to steroids
- Pain management as needed
- Antibiotic treatment if infection is suspected
- Establishment of a bowel and bladder program

ONGOING CARE

FOLLOW-UP RECOMMENDATIONS

- Early involvement of rehabilitation team, including a spinal cord injury rehabilitation physician, physical therapist, and occupational therapist to identify and monitor community and home integration issues and other issues associated with deficits in toileting, strength, coordination, transfers, activities of daily living, and ambulation
- Primary care physician follow-up to monitor post-hospital medications and other laboratory tests
- Regular follow-up for patients with renal or bladder complications and impotence due to the increased tendency for recurrent urinary tract infection and calculi
- Regular follow-up urodynamic studies, renal ultrasound, and general cancer screening should be performed.

PROGNOSIS

- Time since symptom onset inversely correlates with chances of return of function (2)[C].
- Patients have a significantly better chance of improvement in retention than in incontinence.
- Onset of erectile dysfunction is an uncommon but prognostically poor symptom.
- Although most presenting symptoms improve significantly after surgery, urinary and bowel incontinence, and sexual dysfunction might persist with sexual dysfunction being the most prevalent (5)[B].

REFERENCES

1. Gardner A, Gardner E, Morley T. Cauda equina syndrome: a review of the current clinical and medico-legal position. *Eur Spine J*. 2011;20(5):690–697.
2. Gitelman A, Hishmeh S, Morelli BN, et al. Cauda equina syndrome: a comprehensive review. *Am J Orthop (Belle Mead NJ)*. 2008;37(11):556–562.
3. Bell DA, Collie D, Statham PF. Cauda equina syndrome: what is the correlation between clinical assessment and MRI scanning? *Br J Neurosurg*. 2007;21(2):201–203.
4. Srikandarajah N, Boissaud-Cooke MA, Clark S, et al. Does early surgical decompression in cauda equina syndrome improve bladder outcome? *Spine (Phila Pa 1976)*. 2015;40(8):580–583.
5. Venkatesan M, Nasto L, Haddad S, et al. Cauda equina syndrome: a single centre review of 147 operated cases. *Spine J*. 2017;17(3):S6.
6. Todd NV, Dickson RA. Standards of care in cauda equina syndrome. *Br J Neurosurg*. 2016;30(5):518–522.
7. Kapetanakis S, Chaniotakis C, Kazakos C, et al. Cauda equina syndrome due to lumbar disc herniation: a review of literature. *Folia Med (Plovdiv)*. 2017;59(4):377–386.

ADDITIONAL READING

- Kim JS, Seong JH. Endoscope-assisted oblique lumbar interbody fusion for the treatment of cauda equina syndrome: a technical note. *Eur Spine J*. 2017;26(2):397–403.
- Lavy C, James A, Wilson-MacDonald J, et al. Cauda equina syndrome. *BMJ*. 2009;338:b936.
- Small SA, Perron AD, Brady WJ. Orthopedic pitfalls: cauda equina syndrome. *Am J Emerg Med*. 2005;23(2):159–163.
- Spector LR, Madigan L, Rhyne A, et al. Cauda equina syndrome. *J Am Acad Orthop Surg*. 2008;16(8):471–479.
- Tan KA, Sewell MD, Markmann Y, et al. Anterior lumbar discectomy and fusion for acute cauda equina syndrome caused by recurrent disc prolapse: report of 3 cases. *J Neurosurg Spine*. 2017;27(4):352–356.

CLINICAL PEARLS

- CES should be considered in all patients with severe LBP from any cause.
- It is a rare disorder that is usually a surgical emergency.
- It is important to try to prevent CES-I, with its more favorable prognosis, from progressing to CES-R.

CELLULITIS IN SPORTS

Shane Hudnall, MD, CAQSM ▪ Kenneth P. Barnes, MD, MSc, CAQSM, FACP, FACSM, FAMSSM

BASICS

An inflammation of the skin and underlying subcutaneous tissues (specifically the dermal and subcutaneous fat layers) caused by a spreading infiltration of bacteria through the skin surface

DESCRIPTION

- Typically results from entry of bacteria through a break in the skin, from contiguous foci (abscess), or from metastatic dissemination via bacteremia
- Can be classified into purulent and nonpurulent cellulitis
- Most commonly involves the lower extremities
- Can occur anywhere on the body, including periorbital area, upper extremities, and abdominal wall
- *Streptococcus pyogenes* is the most common cause of nonpurulent cellulitis.
- *Staphylococcus aureus* is the most common cause of purulent cellulitis.
- Methicillin-resistant *S. aureus* (MRSA) is a concern due to increasing prevalence in the community setting.

EPIDEMIOLOGY

Incidence

One case per 500 patient-years

RISK FACTORS

- Previous cellulitis
- Disruption of skin from trauma or scratching
- Wounds (including human and animal bites)
- Edema
- Venous stasis
- Eczema or other inflammation
- Underlying skin infections (i.e., tinea pedis)
- Obesity
- Elderly
- Intravenous (IV) drug use
- Surgeries
- MRSA risk factors:
  - Recent antibiotics
  - Recent hospitalization
  - Residence in long-term care facility
  - Homelessness
  - Previous MRSA infection
  - IV drug abuse
  - Immunocompromised
  - Prisoners
  - Military recruits
  - Contact sports

COMMONLY ASSOCIATED CONDITIONS

Consider treating for the specific organisms identified in these populations:

- Diabetes: anaerobes and gram negatives
- Neutropenia: *Pseudomonas*
- Human bite: *Eikenella corrodens, Fusobacterium* species, viridans *Streptococci*
- Cat bite: *Pasteurella multocida*
- Dog bite: *Pasteurella multocida, Capnocytophaga canimorsus*
- Hot tub: *Pseudomonas*
- Fresh water: *Aeromonas hydrophila*
- Salt water: *Vibrio* species
- IV drug abuse: MRSA, *Pseudomonas*
- Immunocompromised: *Cryptococcus neoformans*

DIAGNOSIS

HISTORY

- Breakdown in normal skin barriers almost always precedes this infection.
- Preexisting venous stasis alone may predispose to cellulitis.
- Bilateral presentation is rare and should raise suspicion of alternate diagnosis.

PHYSICAL EXAM

- Area of involvement denoted by spreading erythema, warmth, and swelling with ill-defined margins
- Associated pain and tenderness
- Streaks of erythema and tenderness indicative of lymphatic spread
- Bullae may develop but, generally, rash is not raised.
- Fever, sweats, shaking chills common but bacteremia infrequent
- Regional lymphadenopathy
- Look for evidence of predisposing factors: lower extremity venous stasis, tinea infection, IV drug abuse track marks, eczema, radiation (irritation and thinning of skin)
- Use of pen/marker to demarcate the leading edge of cellulitis is helpful in monitoring during follow-up.

DIFFERENTIAL DIAGNOSIS

Approximately 41% of cases are misdiagnosed as cellulitis when they are due to other conditions listed in the differential (1).

- Erysipelas (infection of the superficial layers of the skin, usually caused by group A streptococci)
- Fasciitis/necrotizing fasciitis
- Myonecrosis/gas gangrene
- Toxic epidermal necrolysis
- Osteomyelitis
- Cutaneous candidal infection
- Septic arthritis
- Gout
- Herpes zoster
- Erythema migrans
- Contact dermatitis
- Eczema
- Stasis dermatitis
- Deep venous thrombosis
- Thrombophlebitis
- Ruptured Baker cyst
- Drug rash
- Insect bite

ALERT

Necrotizing fasciitis

- Pain: intense, severe pain, often out of proportion to the visible skin changes; described as deep, aching, and unrelenting
- Swelling: rapidly spreading swelling and redness beyond the initial wound site
- Skin changes:
  - Skin may appear pale, dusky, or even purplish-black.
  - Blisters or bullae (large fluid-filled blisters) may form, often with a dark, foul-smelling fluid.
  - Skin may feel unusually tight or "crackly" (crepitus) due to gas produced by the bacteria.
- Systemic symptoms: High fever, chills, rapid heart rate (HR), low blood pressure, confusion, and even shock can occur as the infection spreads.
- Progression: The infection progresses very quickly, with noticeable changes within hours.

DIAGNOSTIC TESTS & INTERPRETATION

- Blood testing nonspecific and typically not (may include increased white blood cell [WBC] count, erythrocyte sedimentation rate [ESR], C-reactive protein [CRP])
- Wound culture for bacterial identification and anti-microbial sensitivity in abscesses unless <2 cm and uncomplicated
- Blood cultures rarely helpful (<10% positive) (2)[C]
- Needle aspiration of abscess or bullae most likely to be helpful if present
- Culture of overlying intact skin is not helpful and recommended against.
- Imaging not recommended unless concerned about osteomyelitis (magnetic resonance imaging [MRI]), underlying abscess (ultrasound), or other conditions in differential (i.e., deep vein thrombosis).

TREATMENT

If staph is isolated, consider treating for MRSA if patient has MRSA risk factors and/or if local prevalence of MRSA is high.

GENERAL MEASURES

- If abscess present, incision and drainage required
- If underlying venous stasis noted, elevation of affected limb and, if possible, compression stockings (not over area of skin involvement) recommended.

MEDICATION

- Treat presumptively with close follow-up
- Duration of therapy 5 to 14 days total
- Improvement anticipated in 1 to 2 days
- If no improvement or clinical deterioration, admit for parenteral antibiotics and broaden differential diagnosis to include possibility of potentially fatal infections such as necrotizing fasciitis.
- Should admit for parenteral antibiotics and monitoring if two or more of the following are also present: temp >38°C or <36°C, HR >90/min, respiratory rate (RR) >20/min, WBC count >12,000 or <4,000/mm^3 (3)[C].
- In nonpurulent cellulitis without MRSA risk factors, addition of antibiotics targeting MRSA does not improve outcomes.
- Treatment recommendations (2)[C],(4)[A]:
  - Outpatient for nonpurulent cellulitis: dicloxacillin 500 mg PO QID, cephalexin 500 mg PO QID, or penicillin VK 250 to 500 mg q6h; may use clindamycin 300 to 450 mg PO q6–8h if allergic to penicillins
  - Inpatient for nonpurulent cellulitis: nafcillin 1 to 2 g IV q4h, ceftriaxone 1 to 2 g/day IV
  - Outpatient for purulent cellulitis: Bactrim DS 2 tabs PO BID or doxycycline 100 mg PO BID (not recommended for children <8 years old) or clindamycin 300 to 450 mg PO q6–8h (Check local resistance patterns.)
  - Inpatient for purulent cellulitis: vancomycin (15 mg/kg/dose IV q12h), linezolid 600 mg PO or IV BID (expensive and need to monitor for thrombocytopenia)

ISSUES FOR REFERRAL

- If patient not responding to antibiotic treatment in timely manner
- If development of crepitance suggesting a gas-forming organism
- If the cellulitis is on the face, there is a low threshold for referral
- If a high-risk patient or immunocompromised for any reason, have a low threshold for involvement of an infectious disease specialist if not readily responding to treatment.

ADDITIONAL THERAPIES

- Human bites: Augmentin (outpatient), ampicillin/sulbactam (inpatient); penicillin allergy: moxifloxacin + clindamycin or Bactrim + Flagyl
- Animal bites: Augmentin (outpatient), ampicillin/sulbactam (inpatient); penicillin allergy: (doxycycline or moxifloxacin or Bactrim) + (clindamycin or Flagyl)
- Use of cell-wall active antibiotics (i.e., β-lactams) causes an initial worsening prior to improvement due to rapid release of a bolus of exotoxins
- In patients with recurrent cellulitis (3+ episodes per year) underlying factors should be identified and corrected (i.e., obesity, venous stasis). Otherwise, patients may benefit from antibiotic prophylaxis with penicillin VK, erythromycin, or intramuscular penicillin.

ONGOING CARE

PATIENT EDUCATION

- Early identification is important.
- If infection considered contagious, must not participate in contact or collision sports
- MRSA becoming more prevalent in locker rooms as well as in the community
- Do not share towels, razors, and/or other products
- Frequent skin inspections
- Cover all wounds
- Disinfect all shared athletic equipment and whirlpools.
- Education and posters recommended in all training rooms and locker rooms
- Liberal use of antibacterial soap or alcohol-based hand sanitizer

ALERT

Wrestling return to play:

- 72 hours after initiation of antibiotic therapy, with clinical improvement and no new lesions for 48 hours, if new lesions after 72 hours
- No participation with exudative, moist, or draining lesions
- Active lesions should not be covered to allow participation (National Federation of State High School Associations Skin Form Approved April 2024, NCAA Wrestling Kin Evaluation and Participation Status Form) (5)[C]

REFERENCES

1. Nightingale R, Yadav K, Hamill L, et al. Misdiagnosis of uncomplicated cellulitis: a systematic review and meta-analysis. *J Gen Intern Med.* 2023;38(10):2396–2404.
2. Bystritsky RJ. Cellulitis. *Infect Dis Clin North Am.* 2021;35(1):49–60.
3. Rrapi R, Chand S, Kroshinsky D. Cellulitis: a review of pathogenesis, diagnosis, and management. *Med Clin North Am.* 2021;105(4):723–735.
4. Stevens DL, Bisno AL, Chambers HF, et al. Practice guidelines for the diagnosis and management of skin and soft tissue infections: 2014 update by the Infectious Diseases Society of America. *Clin Infect Dis.* 2014;59(2):e10–e52.
5. Zinder SM, Basler RSW, Foley J, et al. National Athletic Trainers' Association position statement: skin diseases. *J Athl Training.* 2010;45(4):411–428.

ADDITIONAL READING

- Benjamin HJ, Nikore V, Takagishi J. Practical management: community-associated methicillin-resistant *Staphylococcus aureus* (CA-MRSA): the latest sports epidemic. *Clin J Sport Med.* 2007;17(5):393–397.
- McNamara DR, Tleyjeh IM, Berbari EF, et al. Incidence of lower-extremity cellulitis: a population-based study in Olmsted county, Minnesota. *Mayo Clin Proc.* 2007;82(7):817–821.
- Moran GJ, Krishnadasan A, Mower WR, et al. Effect of cephalexin plus trimethoprim-sulfamethoxazole vs cephalexin alone on clinical cure of uncomplicated cellulitis: a randomized clinical trial. *JAMA.* 2017;317(20):2088–2096.
- Oh CC, Ko HCH, Lee HY, et al. Antibiotic prophylaxis for preventing recurrent cellulitis: a systematic review and meta-analysis. *J Infect.* 2014;69(1):26–34.
- Pallin DJ, Binder WD, Allen MB, et al. Clinical trial: comparative effectiveness of cephalexin plus trimethoprim-sulfamethoxazole versus cephalexin alone for treatment of uncomplicated cellulitis: a randomized controlled trial. *Clin Infect Dis.* 2013;56(12):1754–1762.
- Quirke M, Ayoub F, McCabe A, et al. Risk factors for nonpurulent leg cellulitis: a systematic review and meta-analysis. *Br J Dermatol.* 2017;177(2):382–394.
- Raff AB, Kroshinsky D. Cellulitis: a review. *JAMA.* 2016;316(3):325–337.

CLINICAL PEARLS

- Admit patients for parenteral antibiotics if they have severe cellulitis or worsen despite oral antibiotics.
- If patient has uncomplicated cellulitis without MRSA risk factors, addition of antibiotics targeting MRSA does not improve outcomes.
- Incision and drainage if abscess is present
- Consider prophylaxis for patients with recurrent cellulitis.

CENTRAL SLIP AVULSION AND PSEUDOBOUTONNIÈRE DEFORMITIES

Jeffrey P. Feden, MD, FACEP, CAQSM • Razib Khaund, MD

BASICS

DESCRIPTION

- Boutonnière deformity describes a characteristic flexion deformity of the proximal interphalangeal (PIP) joint and hyperextension deformity of the distal interphalangeal (DIP) joint resulting from disruption of the central slip at or near its insertion onto the dorsal aspect of the base of the middle phalanx.
- Mechanism of injury is often forced flexion of an extended PIP joint or volar dislocation of the middle phalanx, causing avulsion of the central slip.
- Deformity of the finger may develop several weeks after an untreated injury.
- Pseudoboutonnière deformity results from hyperextension of the PIP joint; the volar plate is ruptured, but the central slip remains intact.

EPIDEMIOLOGY

Unknown incidence but relatively uncommon

ETIOLOGY AND PATHOPHYSIOLOGY

- Boutonnière deformity:
  - Following avulsion of the central slip, the intact lateral bands slowly migrate in a volar direction as the central slip retracts.
  - The head of the proximal phalanx "buttonholes" through the injured extensor mechanism.
  - The lateral bands become flexors of the PIP joint and extenders of the DIP joint.
- Pseudoboutonnière deformity: Contracture and fibrosis of the volar plate following injury leads to a flexion deformity of the PIP joint.

RISK FACTORS

Ball-handling sports

DIAGNOSIS

HISTORY

- Always consider injury to the central slip when an athlete "jams" a finger or following reduction of a PIP joint dislocation.
- Knowledge of the mechanism of injury and/or direction of a PIP joint dislocation may localize the injury and guide treatment:
  - Forced flexion of an extended PIP joint or *volar* dislocation of the middle phalanx may cause *central slip* injury.
  - Hyperextension of the PIP joint or *dorsal* dislocation of the middle phalanx may cause *volar plate* injury.

PHYSICAL EXAM

- Early: swollen PIP joint with dorsal tenderness, weak active extension, full passive extension; classic deformity is rarely seen in the acute setting.
- Late: flexion deformity of the PIP joint with hyperextension of the DIP joint
- Positive Elson test: With a flexed PIP joint at 90 degrees at edge of table, the patient attempts to extend the middle phalanx against resistance; if the central slip is disrupted, there is weak PIP extension with a rigidly extended DIP (normal: DIP remains lax) (1),(2)[C].
- Unlike a true boutonnière deformity, pseudoboutonnière deformity is characterized by a *fixed* flexion contracture of the PIP joint, inability to achieve passive extension, and mild or absent DIP joint hyperextension.

DIFFERENTIAL DIAGNOSIS

- Fracture
- PIP joint dislocation
- Volar plate disruption
- Collateral ligament tears

DIAGNOSTIC TESTS & INTERPRETATION

- Plain radiographs (especially a true lateral view) to evaluate for fracture and/or dislocation
- Role of ultrasound in boutonnière deformity diagnosis:
  - Direct visualization:
    - Early detection of central slip rupture or even subtle injuries (primary injury)
    - Assesses tendon retraction and gap
    - Detects lateral band subluxation.
    - Helps distinguish from other conditions by showing tendon pathology
  - Dynamic assessment:
    - Real-time observation of tendon and joint movement
    - Confirms lack of active PIP extension
    - Reveals extensor tendon subluxation/dislocation

TREATMENT

GENERAL MEASURES

- Boutonnière deformity:
  - Strict immobilization of the PIP joint in continuous extension for 4 to 6 weeks; nighttime splinting for another 2 to 3 weeks (3),(4),(5)[C]
  - Allow active and passive flexion of the DIP joint without immobilization (3),(4),(5)[C].
  - Gentle active and passive range of motion after splinting is completed (3),(4),(5)[C]
  - Splinting is appropriate initial treatment even for chronic deformity (5)[C].
- Pseudoboutonnière deformity:
  - May be treated with progressive extension splinting if the flexion contracture is <45 degrees; otherwise, surgical release should be considered (6)[C].
  - Acute volar plate injuries should be treated initially with an extension block splint and active flexion for 3 weeks, followed by gradual extension (6)[C].

ISSUES FOR REFERRAL

Referral is recommended for:

- Inability to reduce a PIP joint dislocation or a large, displaced intra-articular PIP joint fracture
- Failure of nonoperative treatment with splinting
- Chronic flexion contractures of >45 degrees

SURGERY/OTHER PROCEDURES

Consider surgical management for:

- Interposed soft tissue preventing congruent reduction of a volar PIP dislocation
- Large, displaced intra-articular PIP fracture at the base of the middle phalanx
- Flexion contractures of >45 degrees
- Symptomatic, chronic deformities

ONGOING CARE

The athlete's sport and position will dictate his or her ability to participate with the injured finger immobilized.

REFERENCES

1. Carruthers KH, Skie M, Jain M. Jam injuries of the finger: diagnosis and management of injuries to the inter-phalangeal joints across multiple sports and levels of experience. *Sports Health*. 2016;8(5):469–478.
2. Chauhan A, Jacobs B, Andoga A, et al. Extensor tendon injuries in athletes. *Sports Med Arthrosc Rev*. 2014;22(1):45–55.
3. Hong E. Hand injuries in sports medicine. *Prim Care*. 2005;32(1):91–103.
4. Peterson JJ, Bancroft LW. Injuries of the fingers and thumb in the athlete. *Clin Sports Med*. 2006;25(3):527–542.
5. Lee SJ, Montgomery K. Athletic hand injuries. *Orthop Clin North Am*. 2002;33(3):547–554.
6. Rettig AC. Athletic injuries of the wrist and hand: part II: overuse injuries of the wrist and traumatic injuries to the hand. *Am J Sports Med*. 2004;32(1):262–273.

ADDITIONAL READING

- Aronowitz ER, Leddy JP. Closed tendon injuries of the hand and wrist in athletes. *Clin Sports Med*. 1998;17(3):449–467.
- Hogan CJ, Nunley JA. Posttraumatic proximal interphalangeal joint flexion contractures. *J Am Acad Orthop Surg*. 2006;14(9):524–533.

CLINICAL PEARLS

- Central slip injury may not be immediately recognized; careful history, examination, and suspicion are essential in addition to close follow-up.
- An acutely injured PIP joint with dorsal tenderness and weak active extension should be treated empirically even in the absence of a classic boutonnière deformity.
- Accidental flexion of the PIP joint during the treatment period must be avoided to prevent disruption of the healing process.
- Most central slip injuries can be treated nonoperatively with satisfactory results.
- The mechanism and direction of injury at the PIP joint may help to differentiate boutonnière from pseudoboutonnière deformities.

CERVICAL DISC DISEASE

Sara L. Neal, MD, MA, CAQSM

BASICS

DESCRIPTION

- Cervical radiculopathy is a syndrome of pain and/or sensorimotor deficits resulting from compression and inflammation of a cervical nerve root at or near the neural foramen.
- The most common causes of nerve root compression and irritation are herniated cervical discs and spondylosis.
- Spondylosis describes the degenerative aging process of the intervertebral discs, ligaments, facet joints, and vertebral bodies.
- Mechanical compression can be a result of facet and uncovertebral joint hypertrophy, vertebral body osteophytes, disc protrusion, or some combination of all three.

EPIDEMIOLOGY

- Peak age for cervical radiculopathy is 50 to 54 years.
- Male > female with ratio 1.7:1

Incidence

Annual incidence rates of cervical radiculopathy:

- 85 cases per 100,000 people (1)

ETIOLOGY AND PATHOPHYSIOLOGY

- Cervical radiculopathy occurs when the nerve root becomes dysfunctional from compression, stretch, and/or irritation.
- Radiculopathy can also be a result of infection (herpes zoster, Lyme disease), granulomatous infiltration (sarcoid), vasculitis, or tumor.
- Causes of nerve root dysfunction: spondylosis > disc herniation > infection > granulomatous > tumor
- Pathophysiology of spondylosis:
  - As discs age, they undergo desiccation, loss of compressibility, and bulging with result of loss in disc height.
  - As the bony spine ages, osteophytes form at the uncovertebral and facet joints.
  - The ligamentum flavum undergoes hypertrophy.
  - These changes can cause narrowing of the neural foramen, impinging the nerve as it exits the cord.
- Pathophysiology of disc herniation:
  - Disc herniation is more common in the older age group. It can occur in adults <45 years old, but more force generally is needed to cause herniation because the discs are more resilient in the younger population.
  - With progressive age, the annular fibers surrounding the nucleus pulposus degenerate.
  - Under certain conditions such as mechanical force, the nucleus pulposus can herniate through the annular fibers.
  - Herniated disc material impacts and compresses the nerve root.
  - Herniation also incites inflammatory cytokines causing irritation of the nerve.
- Pathoanatomy:
  - Cervical nerve roots exit above their correspondingly numbered pedicles.
  - C6 nerve root exits between C5 and C6.
  - C7 nerve root exits between C6 and C7.
  - C8 nerve root exits between C7 and T1
  - Most common level: The C7 nerve root (>50%) and second most common is the C6 nerve root (25%) (1).
  - Disc herniations can prolapse laterally into the neural foramen (common) or can be directed posteriorly, impacting the spinal cord; posterior herniation is less common and may cause cord compression and bilateral symptoms including myelopathy.

DIAGNOSIS

HISTORY

- If the radiculopathy is from a herniated disc, symptoms are usually acute; symptoms from spondylosis are typically more insidious.
- Acute symptoms from herniation may be from trauma to the spine such as axial loading and/or hyperflexion.
- Symptoms are typically unilateral and can include neck, shoulder, or arm pain; paresthesias; numbness; muscle weakness; and/or diminished deep tendon reflexes.
- Classically, pain in the limb is in the distribution of the cervical nerve myotome.
- If present, numbness and paresthesia occur in a dermatomal distribution; however, due to overlap of dermatomes, this may not be clinically evident or follow the classic dermatomal pattern.
- The patient may report relief of symptoms by abducting the upper limb because this maneuver decreases the amount of stretch on the nerve root.
- Weakness can develop in the muscles supplied by the nerve.
- Red flags:
  - Symptoms indicating a myelopathy (cord compression) rather than a radiculopathy include gait disturbance, bowel/bladder dysfunction, hand clumsiness or loss of manual dexterity, hyperreflexia, and/or clonus.
  - Fever, chills, unexplained weight loss
  - Constant and progressive symptoms
  - Bilateral symptoms
  - Unremitting night pain
  - Immunosuppression
  - History of cancer
  - Intravenous (IV) drug abuse

PHYSICAL EXAM

- Evaluate neck range of motion (ROM) with attention to any movement that worsens or alleviates symptoms.
- Motor testing of shoulders, arms, forearm/wrist, hand, and finger; evaluating for weakness/asymmetry
- Deep tendon reflexes should be symmetrical.
- Test sensation of dermatomes evaluating for asymmetry or abnormality.
- Spurling maneuver may be positive:
  - This position increases foraminal narrowing/compression and may reproduce symptoms.
  - To perform, extend the neck, rotate the head toward the side of symptoms, and apply downward pressure to the head. It is positive if symptoms are reproduced or increased.
  - Specificity of this test is moderate to high, whereas the sensitivity is moderate (2).
- Red flags: physical exam findings that may suggest myelopathy rather than radiculopathy:
  - Hyperreflexia
  - Note that a classic pattern of myelopathy at the C5–C6 interspace is suggested by hyperreflexia at the triceps reflex (C7) with diminished bicep and supinator reflexes (C5 and C6).
  - Babinski sign
  - Ankle clonus
  - Lhermitte sign: shock-like sensation radiating down the spine with neck flexion
  - Lower extremity weakness
  - Muscle atrophy in bilateral hands
  - Gait disturbance

DIFFERENTIAL DIAGNOSIS

- Peripheral nerve entrapment
- Myelopathy (from central disc herniation)
- Brachial plexus lesion, inflammation, or injury
- Thoracic outlet syndrome
- Spinal tumor
- Spinal infection/discitis
- Complex regional pain syndrome
- Herpes zoster
- Rotator cuff disorders
- Pancoast tumor

DIAGNOSTIC TESTS & INTERPRETATION

Initial Tests (lab, imaging)

- X-rays:
  - Obtain on initial visit if red flags; otherwise, optional
  - Anteroposterior, lateral, and oblique views
  - Spondylosis is a common finding, not diagnostic of radiculopathy.
- Magnetic resonance imaging (MRI; noncontrast): reveals good soft tissue detail of discs and nerves:
  - Indications:
    - Symptoms or signs of myelopathy
    - Red flags suggestive of tumor or infection (Get contrast MRI.)
    - Progressive or disabling neurologic deficit
    - Consider MRI if no improvement after 6 to 8 weeks of conservative treatment.
  - Disc herniation seen best on T2 images
  - Caution should be used when interpreting MRIs because findings *must* correspond with symptoms to be clinically significant.
- Computed tomography (CT) myelogram:
  - Useful if patient has metallic surgical hardware in the neck because there can be distortion of MRI images
  - May offer better analysis of bony impingement on foramina
  - Disadvantages: It is invasive and uses radiation.

Diagnostic Procedures/Other

Electrodiagnostic studies (nerve conduction study with electromyogram):

- Obtain only if diagnosis is unclear.
- Can help differentiate from peripheral nerve entrapment
- False-negative results common if test performed too early in workup (must wait at least 3 weeks minimum)

TREATMENT

- Optimal treatment is controversial. Most recognize conservative therapy as the initial treatment choice.
- Subsequent options include physical therapy, epidural steroid injections, and surgical procedures. The data for each of these treatment options is limited to relatively small studies. No large well-controlled studies have shown clear evidence of improved outcome for any specific treatment versus conservative treatment alone (3)[A].
- Because of a relatively high rate of spontaneous resolution, initial treatment is usually nonoperative. Exceptions that may require further workup and subspecialty consultation include:
  - Progressive neurologic deficit
  - Disabling weakness
  - Infection or tumor
  - Vertebral fracture or subluxation from trauma (3)[A].
- Traditionally, conservative therapy has included some combination of the following modalities: oral analgesics, avoidance of provocative activities, short-term neck immobilization with soft collar, cervical traction, a short course of oral steroids, and physical therapy. Recent guidelines call into question the appropriateness of oral glucocorticoids and benzodiazepines given their unfavorable risk/benefit ratio (4)[C].
- Patients should be reevaluated at regular intervals during the treatment process so that worsening symptoms can be identified promptly.

C

MEDICATION

First Line

- Nonsteroidal anti-inflammatory drugs (NSAIDs):
  - Use at anti-inflammatory doses (e.g., ibuprofen 600 mg QID).
  - Block formation of inflammatory mediators at the site of the disc herniation.
  - Use cautiously if:
    - Risk factors for gastrointestinal (GI) bleeding.
    - Risk factors for renal disease.
    - In older patients (>65 years old)
- Oral steroids:
  - More potent anti-inflammatory agents than NSAIDs, although greater potential side effects
  - May consider using if:
    - Not responding to NSAIDs
    - Severe pain
    - Weakness
    - Renal insufficiency
  - Avoid using with NSAIDs.
  - Dose:
    - Typical regimen: Start with 50 to 70 mg/day of prednisone; taper over next 10 days (3)[A].
  - Side effects: have not been shown to alter the natural history of cervical radiculopathy, and risk/benefit ratio is unfavorable (4)[C]

Second Line

- Narcotics:
  - May be considered for short-term use if pain is severe and not controlled by other medications and modalities (5)[C]
  - Have additive effect with NSAIDs on pain relief
  - Typical prescription: hydrocodone/acetaminophen—5/325 mg q4–6h PRN for pain
  - Potential side effects: drowsiness, vomiting, constipation, dependency
- Antispasmodic agents (muscle relaxants):
  - Consider using if muscle spasm is prominent.
  - Additive effect on pain relief when used with a NSAIDs or narcotic; drowsiness when combined with a narcotic may be intolerable.
  - Typical prescription: cyclobenzaprine—10 mg TID
  - Avoid using for >2 to 3 weeks.
  - Potential side effects: sedation, dependency

ADDITIONAL THERAPIES

- Rest and avoidance of provocative activities:
  - "Relative rest" is typically recommended. Patient is encouraged to be as active as the pain allows.
- Cervical collar to limit motion:
  - Limited data on efficacy
  - May consider initially if severe pain when moving head
  - Limit use to <1 to 2 weeks (to avoid weakness and stiffness).
  - Come out of the collar several times per day for ROM exercises within limits of pain.
- Formal physical therapy or home exercise program:
  - Start ROM exercises as early as possible within limits of pain.
  - Heat/cold, active ROM, isometric strengthening as tolerated
  - Add resistive exercises as tolerated.
  - May add nonimpact aerobic exercise; gear toward an activity that allows the neck to remain in neutral position (e.g., walking, stationary bike)
  - Postural education
  - Ergonomic adjustments
- Traction:
  - Limited reliable data
- Spinal manipulation (chiropractic treatment):
  - No consistent data showing benefit. Possible complications include spinal cord and vertebral artery injury if done improperly.
- Fluoroscopically guided epidural steroid injections:
  - May be effective in reducing pain and reducing need for surgery, but evidence of effectiveness is of low quality and serious complications are possible (6)[B]
  - Specific risks of procedure:
    - Dural puncture
    - Nerve damage
    - Spinal cord and brain stem infarction

SURGERY/OTHER PROCEDURES

- Consider referring to spine surgeon if:
  - Progressive or severe neurologic deficit
  - Recalcitrant radicular pain or numbness despite nonoperative treatment for 6 to 12 weeks; no data on the optimal timing
  - Instability of the spine with radicular symptoms
  - Moderate to severe myelopathy
  - Muscle atrophy
- Surgical outcomes for relief of arm pain range from 80% to 90% (2)[C].
- Typical procedure for cervical radiculopathy:
  - Anterior cervical discectomy and fusion (ACDF): allows removal of the disc and uncovertebral spur without neural retraction. Bone graft or plate is placed anteriorly to vertebral body.
- Total disc arthroplasty (experimental):
  - Diseased disc is removed, and an artificial disc is placed.

ONGOING CARE

PATIENT EDUCATION

In attempts to decrease recurrence of symptoms:

- Keep the neck and shoulder girdle muscles strong.
- Use correct posture when sitting (head centered over shoulders).
- Set up workstations ergonomically.
- Avoid forcing the neck into extremes of motion.
- Regular aerobic exercise

PROGNOSIS

- Resolution of all or most symptoms occurs within 6 to 12 weeks in most patients.
- Acute cervical radiculopathy has up to a 75% rate of spontaneous improvement (3)[A].

COMPLICATIONS

Delayed treatment: If weakness is present for too long, patient may never regain full strength and function.

REFERENCES

1. Magnus W, Viswanath O, Viswanathan VK, et al. *Cervical Radiculopathy*. StatPearls Publishing; 2023. Updated January 31, 2024. https://www.ncbi.nlm.nih.gov/books/NBK441828/
2. Thoomes EJ, van Geest S, van der Windt DA, et al. Value of physical tests in diagnosing cervical radiculopathy: a systematic review. *Spine J*. 2018;18(1):179–189.
3. Taso M, Sommernes JH, Kolstad F, et al. A randomised controlled trial comparing the effectiveness of surgical and nonsurgical treatment for cervical radiculopathy. *BMC Musculoskelet Disord*. 2020;21(1):171.
4. Chou R, Côte P, Randhawa K, et al. The global spine care initiative: applying evidence-based guidelines on the non-invasive management of back and neck pain to low- and middle-income communities. *Eur Spine J*. 2018;27(Suppl 6):851–860.
5. Dowell D, Ragan KR, Jones CM, et al. CDC clinical practice guideline for prescribing opioids for pain—United States, 2022. *MMWR Recomm Rep*. 2022;71(3):1–95.
6. Borton ZM, Oakley BJ, Clamp JA, et al. Cervical transforaminal epidural steroid injections for radicular pain: a systematic review. *Bone Joint J*. 2022;104-B(5):567–574.

ADDITIONAL READING

- Kang KC, Lee HS, Lee JH. Cervical radiculopathy focus on characteristics and differential diagnosis. *Asian Spine J*. 2020;14(6):921–930.
- MacDowall A, Moreira NC, Marques C, et al. Artificial disc replacement versus fusion in patients with cervical degenerative disc disease and radiculopathy: a randomized controlled trial with 5-year outcomes. *J Neurosurg Spine*. 2019;30(3):323–331.
- Zhang Y, Lv N, He F, et al. Comparison of cervical disc arthroplasty and anterior cervical discectomy and fusion for the treatment of cervical disc degenerative diseases on the basis of more than 60 months of follow-up: a systematic review and meta-analysis. *BMC Neurol*. 2020;20(1):143.

CLINICAL PEARLS

- Distinguish radiculopathy from myelopathy.
- Weakness is the most serious complication of cervical radiculopathy and should be followed closely.
- MRI is the test of choice for imaging the discs and nerves.
- Treatment in most patients is nonoperative.
- The timing of surgical intervention for cervical radiculopathy has not been established, but surgery should be considered if there is significant weakness or symptoms that are refractory to nonoperative treatment.
- Do not miss the red flags: cervical myelopathy, tumor, and infection.

CERVICAL STENOSIS/MYELOPATHY

Julio A. Martinez-Silvestrini, MD, FAAPMR, CAQSM • Roman Zolotoy, DO

BASICS

DESCRIPTION

- Cervical spondylosis is a congenital or progressive disease defined by changes affecting the vertebrae, intervertebral disks, facets, and associated ligaments (1).
- Functional spinal stenosis manifests by loss of the cerebrospinal fluid (CSF) around the spinal cord or a clear deformation of the cord demonstrated by computed tomography (CT) scan, magnetic resonance imaging (MRI), or myelography (2).
- Degenerative disk disease, spondylosis, and/or other degenerative pathology can progressively narrow the cervical spinal canal and can result in neurologic impairment due to compression of the cervical spinal cord and/or surrounding blood vessels (1).
- Compression of the cervical spinal cord can produce a syndrome of spinal cord dysfunction known as cervical spondylotic myelopathy (CSM).
- CSM is the most common cause of spinal cord injury and the incidence increases with age, affecting men more often than women.
- CSM accounts for 54% of spinal cord injuries in North America (1).
- Other potential sequelae include functional decline, progressive disability, reduction of quality of life, compromise of independence, and ability to perform activities of daily living.
- Synonym(s): cervical cord neurapraxia (CCN); CSM; degenerative cervical myelopathy (DCM)

EPIDEMIOLOGY

Incidence

- The incidence of cervical stenosis is unknown; the incidence of hospitalizations for this condition is 4.04 per 100,000 person-years (1).
- The incidence of spinal cord injuries in the United States is 40 cases per million, with 8.9% related to sporting events (2).
- DCM is accepted as the most common cause of spinal cord injury in developed countries (3),(4).

Prevalence

- Cervical stenosis prevalence increased with age as it is predisposed by degenerative spine changes.
- MRI evidence of spinal cord compression found to be as high as 31.6% in the 5th decade and 66.8% in the 8th decade (4).
- 22.6% of patients with evidence of cervical cord compression go on to develop cervical myelopathy, approximately 8% within the 1st year (1).
- CSM occurs in 5–10% of patients with symptomatic cervical spondylosis (1).

ETIOLOGY AND PATHOPHYSIOLOGY

- Narrowing of the cervical spinal canal is often incited by degeneration of intervertebral discs resulting in disc bulging or herniation. This causes the spinal column to shorten and alters cervical spine biomechanics. These changes lead to buckling and/or hypertrophy of the ligamentum flavum, hypertrophy of the facet joints, facet cysts, uncovertebral degeneration, vertebral body osteophyte formation and ossification of the posterior longitudinal ligament (OPLL).
- These changes cause direct compromise to the spinal canal and decrease range of motion (ROM) at the affected level. Consequently, the adjacent levels can become hypermobile (3).
- Flexion and extension of the neck may exacerbate compression and cause further neurologic deficits (2).
- Cervical hyperextension can predispose collapse of the ligamentum flavum dorsally into the spina canal and flexion could potentiate exacerbation of anterolisthesis leading to compressive lesion (1).
- Combination of mechanical compression of neural elements, spinal cord ischemia due to compression of the arterial, and/or venous blood supply to the cord can cause dysfunction of the spinal cord.
- Chronic compression of the spinal cord can also result in spinal cord vascular disruption, loss of blood-spinal cord barrier integrity, glutamate excitotoxicity, microglia activation, apoptosis, demyelination, astrogliosis, and axonal degeneration, all contributing to deterioration (3).

RISK FACTORS

- Congenital or acquired defects, which include bulging disk, hypertrophied or unstable ligaments, and degenerative changes.
- Congenital spinal stenosis or instability secondary to Down syndrome, Klippel-Feil syndrome, Ehlers-Danlos syndrome, odontoid abnormality, atlantooccipital fusion
- Progressive cervical kyphosis has been linked with CSM.
- Involvement in sports that engage in potential axial loading, such as football, ice hockey, diving, headfirst sliding in baseball, wrestling, soccer, gymnastics, and rugby.
- Potential hereditary component of OPLL, ossification of ligamentum flavum, and degenerative disk disease
- Athletes who participate in sports with excessive forces to cervical spine such as football and rugby
- High-performance athletes such as cyclists and triathletes have also been found to have a higher incidence of cervical spine degenerative conditions.
- Men more than women; labor-intensive employment (1)

DIAGNOSIS

HISTORY

- During preparticipation physical examination, determination of any prior history of neurologic events, such as burners/stingers or transient neurologic events, is critical.
- If the athlete gives a positive response, all data from previous evaluations must be reviewed. If no workup has been done, then consider imaging before allowing the athlete to begin contact/collision sports.
- Some athletes experience a slow and stepwise deterioration, whereas others experience prolonged periods of stability. Abrupt worsening can occur, often following minor neck injuries (2)[C].
- If the athlete has risk factors predisposing to cervical stenosis, the athlete must be further evaluated.

PHYSICAL EXAM

- Cervical stenosis may be asymptomatic until forced hyperflexion or hyperextension occurs with an axial load, which causes CCN.
- The patient may develop acute transient sensory paresthesia and/or motor paresis.
- Gait dysfunction (slower speed, decreased step length, longer stride time, increased step width) and difficulty with fine hand dexterity are the most common initial symptoms of CSM (1)[C].
- Other CSM symptoms can include upper and/or lower extremity weakness; neck pain and/or stiffness; numbness and/or paresthesia in the upper extremities; urinary and/or rectal sphincter dysfunction; Lhermitte phenomenon; Hoffmann reflex; inverted radial reflex; hyperactive pectoralis reflex.
- Presence of upper motor neuron characteristics (Hoffman sign, hyperreflexia, increased tone) Babinski sign and clonus have low sensitivity and high specificity (1)[C].
- Findings are usually bilateral.
- Paresthesia is described as burning pain, numbness, or tingling of the affected region.
- Motor changes can range from weakness to complete paralysis.
- Neurapraxia can take more than 24 hours to resolve (2)[C].
- During the preparticipation physical examination, the Spurling foraminal compression test can be done. If symptoms are elicited, further workup can be started. The yield is very low unless the patient already has stenosis. It should be done on any athlete who has a history of neurologic events.
- If the initial event occurs on the field, start with assessment of the athlete's level of consciousness. If unconscious, immobilize and transport. If conscious, proceed to assess neck pain. If neck pain is present or absent and the athlete has neurologic symptoms, immobilize and transport for further workup.
- Common grading system used to gauge for level injury related to CSM is the modified Japanese Orthopaedic Association Myelopathy Evaluation Questionnaire. This questionnaire evaluates motor function of upper limbs, motor dysfunction of the lower extremity, sensory dysfunction of upper extremity and sphincter dysfunction on zero-to-17-point scale (1)[C],(4)[C],(5)[C].

DIFFERENTIAL DIAGNOSIS

- Stable spinal fracture
- Any cause of permanent spinal cord injury
- Spear tackler's spine
- Unstable fracture
- Spinal fracture with dislocation
- Ligamentous injury
- Herniated cervical disk.
- Amyotrophic lateral sclerosis
- Guillain-Barré syndrome
- Normal pressure hydrocephalus
- Multiple sclerosis
- Peripheral nerve entrapment
- Syringomyelia
- Primary cord tumors
- Metastatic tumors
- Hereditary spastic paraplegia
- Normal pressure hydrocephalus
- Spinal cord infarction

DIAGNOSTIC TESTS & INTERPRETATION

- The initial radiographic examination should start with cervical spine x-rays, which can be used to evaluate for gross fracture or dislocation.
- On the lateral x-ray, the Torg-Pavlov ratio can be calculated. Measure (in millimeters) the distance from the posterior aspect of the vertebral body to the spinolaminar line (*a*) and the width of the vertebral body (*b*) and then calculate the ratio *a*/*b*.
- The normal canal measures >15 mm; <12 mm correlates with cord compression and <8 mm is considered spinal stenosis (1)[C].
- A large vertebral body can result in a false-positive result; the false-positive rate has been reported as high as 88%. If the patient has spinal stenosis, the ratio is almost always abnormal.
- Cervical x-ray limitations include the failure of roentgenography to appraise the width of the cord and an inability to appreciate stenosis resulting from ligamentous hypertrophy, ligamentous laxity, or disk protrusion.
  - Therefore, the next step is to use MRI or CT myelography.
- MRI is considered the gold standard for CSM confirmation. Increased signal intensity on T2 weighted imaging (especially with low signal intensity on T1 weighted imaging) is a poor prognosticating factor for future outcome (1)[C].
- MRI is superior in providing intramedullary detail of spinal cord pathology. It is not as effective e as CT myelography in evaluating bone and calcified tissues.

TREATMENT

Conservative treatment:

- Cervical immobilization
- Restriction of high-risk activities, including avoidance of collision sports and sports with high potential for cervical load
- Physical therapy
- Pain management with analgesics, muscle relaxants, antidepressants, or anticonvulsants
- Overall, patients with moderate to severe SCM have a poor prognosis with nonoperative treatments, with up to 54% of patients treated conservatively requiring surgery (1)[C],(4)[C].

ADDITIONAL THERAPIES

- After the first episode of neurapraxia, if the initial workup is negative for stenosis, a generalized neck strengthening program should be started.
- Athletes involved in collision sports should be able to support their body weight with the cervical spine in neutral and in all directions when positioned at a 45-degree angle.

SURGERY/OTHER PROCEDURES

- If an acquired cause for spinal stenosis is detected, consultation with a neurosurgeon or orthopedic spine surgeon for consideration of surgery can be undertaken.
- Surgery should also be considered in athletes with progressive deterioration and/or myelopathy causing neurologic deficits. However, after surgery, the athlete is unlikely to participate in contact or collision sports (2)[C].
- 20–60% of patients with CSM will deteriorate neurologically over time without surgical intervention, thus CSM is generally considered to be a surgical disease. Surgical patients have better outcomes with respect to functional status, pain, neurologic, and symptoms (1)[C].
- Factors that predict worse outcomes include longer duration of symptoms, advanced age, smoking, gait dysfunction, and more severe preoperative degree of CSM (1)[C],(3)[C].
- Surgical interventions involve anterior, posterior, or combined approaches. Anterior approach (anterior cervical discectomy and fusion (ACDF), anterior corpectomy) is preferred for anterior cord compression and cervical kyphosis, whereas congenital stenosis, posterior cord compression, multilevel compression and OPLL can be addressed via the posterior surgical approach (laminectomy, posterior fusion) (1)[C]. Most severe cases may require a combined approach (3)[C].

ONGOING CARE

FOLLOW-UP RECOMMENDATIONS

- Team physicians should be mindful of functional spinal stenosis. If present, and the athlete incurs spinal cord symptoms, the athlete should not continue in contact/collision sports because such activities predispose athletes to a worse neurologic outcome and future disability in the context of cervical spine injuries.
- Data collected by the National Center for Catastrophic Sport Injury Research (NCCSIR) from 1977 to 2022 showed a reduction in spinal cord injuries from 2018 to 2022, but the low sports participation during the COVID-19 pandemic may have influenced this data (6)[B].
  - Between 2018 and 2022, most patients with spinal cord injuries had incomplete recovery (6)[B].
  - Most of the injuries were cervical spine fractures (45.0%) followed by cervical cord/nerve injuries (35.0%), cervical cord contusions (10.0%), or unspecified cervical spine injuries (7.5%) (6)[B].
- Quadriplegia without spine fracture has been seen only when functional spinal stenosis is present (2)[C].
- Given the excellent sensitivity of the Torg ratio, any athlete with an abnormal ratio along with spinal cord symptomatology should undergo MRI, as it is considered the gold standard. If contraindicated, CT should be considered.
- If surgery is deferred in milder cases, close neurologic follow-up is recommended.
- Return-to-play (RTP) considerations: (2)[C]
  - Athletes may return to contact sports after cervical spine injury if they are asymptomatic with full ROM, normal neurologic examination, and their imaging shows no evidence of "functional" spinal stenosis, no evidence of disc disease or instability.
  - Relative contraindication to RTP:
    - Symptomatic burner/stinger or transient quadriparesis lasting >24 hours.
    - Three or more stingers or two episodes of transient quadriparesis.
    - One- or two-level cervical fusion.
  - Absolute contraindication to RTP:
    - Previous transient quadriparesis with a history or exam findings of cervical myelopathy
    - Neck discomfort, reduced ROM, or neurologic deficit from baseline after spine injury.
    - Cervical ligamentous laxity, C1–C2 hypermobility or other medical conditions that cause cervical instability
    - Symptomatic cervical disc herniation.

REFERENCES

1. McCormick JR, Sama AJ, Schiller NC, et al. Cervical spondylotic myelopathy: a guide to diagnosis and management. *J Am Board Fam Med*. 2020;33(2):303–313.
2. Cantu RC, Li YM, Abdulhamid M, et al. Return to play after cervical spine injury in sports. *Curr Sports Med Rep*. 2013;12(1):14–17.
3. Milligan J, Ryan K, Fehlings MG, et al. Degenerative cervical myelopathy: diagnosis and management in primary care. *Can Fam Physician*. 2019;65(9):619–624.
4. Nouri A, Cheng J, Davies BM, et al. Degenerative cervical myelopathy: a brief review of past perspectives, present developments, and future directions. *J Clin Med*. 2020;9(2):535.
5. Choi SH, Kang CN. Degenerative cervical myelopathy: pathophysiology and current treatment strategies. *Asian Spine J*. 2020;14(5):710–720.
6. Kucera KL, Klossner D, Cantu RC. Annual survey of catastrophic football injuries. National Center for Catastrophic Sport Injury Research. 2023. Accessed March 15, 2025. https://nccsir.unc.edu/wp-content/uploads/sites/5614/2023/07/Annual-Football-Catastrophic-2022-FINAL-web.pdf

CLINICAL PEARLS

- During preparticipation physical examination, it is critical to determine any prior history of spinal cord–related neurologic events and consider imaging before allowing the athlete to begin contact/collision sports.
- Early recognition, prompt medical evaluation and management of cervical cord and spine injuries is critical for preventing permanent disability and death.
- Although subtle gait dysfunction is the most common presentation of CSM, bilateral upper motor neuron findings are common.
- Cervical spine x-rays are the initial radiographic modality, which can be used to evaluate for gross fracture or dislocation, whereas MRI/CT myelography provide a more accurate measure of spinal cord pathology.
- MRI is the gold standard for imaging in patients with cervical stenosis or CSM.
- Cervical immobilization, restriction of high-risk activities, physical therapy, and pain management are the initial treatment steps.
- Surgical intervention is considered for acquired causes of spinal stenosis, failure to respond to conservative care, or progressive deterioration and/or myelopathy.
- Absolute contraindications for RTP include transient quadriparesis in patients with known cervical myelopathy, cervical spine instability or symptomatic disc herniations.

CERVICAL STRAINS

Jeffrey M. Mjaanes, MD, CAQSM, FAAP, FACSM • Elizabeth E. Brown, MD

BASICS

DESCRIPTION

- Cervical strain refers to a stretch-type injury within the muscle substance or at the myotendinous junction of the cervical and upper back muscles. In addition to the muscle and tendons, injury may involve the ligamentous structures of the cervical spine.
- Synonym(s): cervical sprain; whiplash (whiplash-associated disorders)

EPIDEMIOLOGY

- Most frequently caused by whiplash injury, that is, hyperextension, then hyperflexion, of the cervical spine from a rear-end motor vehicle collision
- >1 million cases per year are reported in the United States.
- Higher incidence seen in females
- More common in adults than children
- In general, collision sports are responsible for a high number of injuries to the head and neck.
- In NCAA football over two seasons, the rate of cervical strain was 0.96 per 10,000 athlete exposures and 57.1% of these led to time lost from play. Injuries more commonly occurred during competition and in the setting of a contact mechanism (1). A similar study found Division I athletes to have the highest rate of cervical injury as compared to other divisions. Cervical strains were most common in the cornerback or safety positions for American football (2).
- Cervical muscle injury has been cited as the most common injury overall as studied in multiple high school sports over a 10-year period (3).

ETIOLOGY AND PATHOPHYSIOLOGY

- In sports, cervical strain often occurs as the result of a blow to the head or neck during muscular contraction. In motor vehicle accidents, the causative force is usually a rear-end collision leading to a hyperextension then hyperflexion of the neck. The applied force often creates an eccentric contraction causing microscopic or gross tensile failure, most often at the myotendinous junction and in ligamentous structures.
- Muscles with high ratios of type II or fast-twitch muscle fibers demonstrate a higher risk for strains or shearing-type injuries.
- Cervical strains can also be chronic in nature and related to repetitive stress or abnormal postural biomechanics.

RISK FACTORS

Speculated: age, level of conditioning, prior history of neck injury, cervical degenerative disk disease, head position at time of impact, mechanism of injury, personality traits, and psychosocial factors

DIAGNOSIS

HISTORY

- When taking the history, it is essential to determine the mechanism of injury. For example, if the injury is the result of a motor vehicle accident, important information includes the approximate speed of the vehicles, the location of the patient within the vehicle, and whether the patient was restrained.
- Onset, time course, and location of symptoms
- Activities and head positions that aggravate or alleviate symptoms
- Presence of any neurologic symptoms and course: upper or lower extremity sensory changes, pain radiating into the arms past the elbows, or weakness in upper extremities
- Previous treatment, including modalities, medications, physical therapy, traction, manipulation, injection, and surgical treatments
- Prior episodes of similar symptoms, previous neck injury or surgery
- Social history, including level of physical activity, occupation, job satisfaction, ongoing litigation, and use of nicotine, alcohol, and/or other substances
- Pain is the most common presenting complaint in cervical strains. Frequently, patients may have minimal pain immediately after the injury but have increasing pain severity several hours to days later. Pain may be referred to the shoulder, upper limb, and occipital or temporal regions of the head. Neuropathic pain and peripheral nerve pathology is not uncommon in patients with whiplash-associated disorder (WAD).
- Soft tissue swelling may be present; muscle spasm or tightness is common, stiffness, pain at rest and/or with movement.
- Limitation in range of motion at the neck
- Other symptoms may include unusual skin sensations at head/face, dizziness, light-headedness, concentration and memory deficits, tinnitus, blurred vision, hearing difficulties, and other cranial nerve deficit complaints.

PHYSICAL EXAM

- Observation: head and neck posture, movement during normal conversation, weak or stiff movement
- Range of motion: active range of motion, usually reduced, particularly in directions stretching the injured muscles
- Palpation: tenderness, usually noted along the cervical paraspinal muscles; may be present along muscles where symptoms are referred, muscles with associated hypertonicity, or "spasm"
- Generally normal neurologic examination, although subjective sensory deficits may be present
- A thorough neurologic exam should be completed, including sensory examination for dermatomal deficits, deep tendon reflexes/muscle stretch reflexes, manual muscle testing for deficits in myotomal distribution, and Hoffman or Babinski signs (helpful in identifying upper motor neuron issues).
- Provocative tests are negative in an isolated soft tissue strain.
- Spurling test is performed by extending the neck and rotating the head and then applying downward pressure on the head; considered positive if pain radiates into the ipsilateral limb; specific but not sensitive in diagnosing acute radiculopathy
- Lhermitte sign is performed by passively flexing the neck; considered positive if "electric-like" sensation radiates down the spine; positive with cervical stenosis, myelopathy, spinal cord injury due to tumor, multiple sclerosis, and other conditions
- Axial compression test is performed by gently applying an axially directed pressure on top of the seated patient's head. The patient's neck is in neutral. Pain radiating distal to the elbow is considered positive for likely radicular origin. Manual distraction often greatly reduces neck and limb symptoms in patients with radiculopathy.

DIFFERENTIAL DIAGNOSIS

- In evaluation of the patient with acute and subacute neck pain, it is essential to rule out more serious conditions, such as fractures, dislocations, instability, and spinal cord injury. In chronic neck pain, other diagnoses, such as neoplasia, must be considered.
- Differential diagnosis includes:
  - Cervical fracture
  - Cervical instability, subluxation, or dislocation
  - Disk annulus fibrosis injury
  - Facet joint injury
  - Myofascial pain
  - Cervical radiculopathy
  - Myelopathy
  - Brachial plexus injury
  - Thoracic outlet syndrome
  - Peripheral nerve entrapment (e.g., suprascapular nerve)

DIAGNOSTIC TESTS & INTERPRETATION

Initial Tests (lab, imaging)

- In the management of cervical strain, radiographs are usually not necessary. In trauma patients, however, plain radiographs are used to rule out other potentially serious conditions, such as fractures or dislocations.
- Minimum views include anteroposterior, lateral, and oblique cervical spine views for evidence of acute fracture or subluxation with trauma, and open mouth view for evidence of atlantoaxial instability and odontoid fractures. Flexion and extension lateral views are helpful to look for evidence of spinal instability.
- Any victim of blunt cervical trauma who is unconscious or conscious and complaining of neck pain or extremity paresthesias/paralysis should be assumed to have a cervical spine injury, spine must be stabilized, and the patient transported to the local hospital. All posttrauma patients with cervical pain should be evaluated using National Emergency X-radiography Utilization Study (NEXUS) low-risk criteria or the Canadian C-spine rule to guide the use of cervical spine radiography.
- Computed tomography (CT) offers superior sensitivity for detection of acute fractures than plain radiographs. When combined with myelography, CT has significant sensitivity and specificity for radiculopathy and stenosis.
- Magnetic resonance imaging (MRI) is the study of choice to detect soft tissue pathology including disk or ligament disruption, nerve root or spinal cord compression/injury. MRI is also indicated for patients with deterioration in neurologic findings to detect spinal cord changes.
- Research exists exploring the role of muscle fat infiltration (MFI) in cervical musculature in people who have had whiplash injuries. Studies have shown higher cervical muscle MFI in those with severe symptoms after whiplash injury (4)[B]. Whether MFI was present before the injury and is a risk factor for cervical injury remains unclear.

Diagnostic Procedures/Other

- Electrodiagnostic studies are used to diagnose nerve root dysfunction when the diagnosis is uncertain or to distinguish a cervical radiculopathy from other lesions that are unclear on physical examination.
- Ideally performed 3 or more weeks after injury because diagnostic abnormalities will first be seen 18 to 21 days after the onset of radiculopathy.

TREATMENT

- Early discussion involving reassurance, treatment, recovery, and maintaining daily activity as tolerated is important in the initial management.
- A multimodal treatment approach (medications, soft tissue treatment, stretching, exercises as tolerated) has been shown to be superior to a minimal intervention approach (advice and medications only).

- **Acute treatment** directed at reducing pain and inflammation. Therapies include local icing and avoidance of positions that increase symptoms. Patient should be encouraged to be as active as pain allows; bed rest is discouraged.
- Nonsteroidal anti-inflammatory drugs (NSAIDs) are often used. Other pharmacologic therapies include muscle relaxants to decrease spasm and tonicity and other analgesics such as acetaminophen. Narcotic analgesics are often used for pain relief, but in general, their use should be limited due to the potential of opioid-associated side effects.
- Consider myofascial trigger point injections or modalities such as electrical stimulation if pain not controlled by initial therapies in the acute phase.
- Gentle stretching: first passive then active mobilization to reestablish nonpainful range of motion
- Gentle strengthening: isometric cervical strengthening in a single plane (flexion, extension, lateral flexion, rotation), scapular stabilization, and cervicothoracic stabilization programs. All exercises should be performed without pain.
- If unable to engage cervicothoracic region due to persistent pain, consider isometric strengthening of uninvolved musculature (i.e., quadriceps), which may help decrease pain in chronic WADs.
- Low-level aerobic cross-training (e.g., stationary bike, stair stepper, treadmill, aquatic running) begun as soon as tolerated to avoid deconditioning.
- Use of soft and rigid collars for cervical strain management is controversial and has not been proven effective. Several randomized studies show no significant difference in outcomes (headache and neck pain intensity, disability, and work capability) between those treated with immobilization and those treated with an "act-as-usual" approach. An updated systematic review on the use of soft collars in cervical strain favors active rehabilitation compared to use of soft collars; however, more research is needed (5)[A].
- **Recovery phase** directed toward normalizing active range of motion, neuromuscular control, strength, and posture; progressive passive and active stretching, mobilization, and manipulation as appropriate; progressive strengthening (isometric to isotonic) with independent single-plane and complex multiple-plane coordinated motions to include cervicothoracic, scapulothoracic, and scapulohumeral stabilization activities
- **Maintenance phase** directed toward sport/activity-specific training
- Guidelines for returning to competition: no pain at rest, full pain-free range of motion, normal posture, normal strength, and normal physical examination; athletes should not return to competition until they can perform at the level of their preinjury abilities.

MEDICATION

- Analgesics, such as acetaminophen, can be used in the acute phase for pain relief.
- NSAIDs, such as ibuprofen and naproxen, have anti-inflammatory as well as analgesic effects and are often used successfully in the management of cervicalgia.
- Muscle relaxants are often prescribed acutely as adjunct therapy to decrease the spasm and hypertonicity experienced in acute muscle strain.

ADDITIONAL THERAPIES

- Follow-up is recommended to ensure there has been no deterioration in symptoms or exam findings. Ideally, patients should follow up with their primary care physician within 1 week.
- Often, referral to physical therapy may be necessary, especially in patients who have significant spasm and decreased cervical motion.
- Therapy focusing on progressive motion, stretching, and finally strengthening is often beneficial. Vassiliou et al. demonstrated in a randomized controlled trial involving 200 patients with whiplash injury that those who participated in a consistent physical therapy regimen had decreased pain intensity scores after 6 weeks and 6 months compared to controls (6).
- Patients with chronic pain often benefit from a multidisciplinary approach to rehabilitation and recovery. A study looking at an 8-week multidisciplinary rehabilitation program for patients with whiplash injury showed that positive expectations regarding recovery were related to pain reduction at the time of discharge from the program. Additionally, decreased fear of movement and reinjury as well as pain catastrophizing was significantly associated with increased recovery expectation (7)[B]. Despite these findings, more research is needed to truly establish the relationship between kinesiophobia and pain catastrophizing and how this affects pain and disability after whiplash injury.
- Osteopathic manipulation may be helpful in treating cervical strains. Avoid manipulation in the following scenarios: focal neurologic deficits, severe cervical spasm or pain, advanced age, rheumatoid arthritis, point tenderness over bone, cervical fusion or fracture, osteoporosis, and cervical laxity.
- Other potential treatments could include acupuncture, therapeutic ultrasound, and topical analgesic creams. For chronic pain, consider adding supervised exercise programs such as tai chi, qigong, or yoga.

ONGOING CARE

COMPLICATIONS

Neck strain can result in stiffening in the cervical region with resultant decreased motion. The prolonged muscle spasm itself can become a source of long-term pain and disability. Morbidity from cervical strains comes from disuse, weakness, and spasm. Cervical strain can lead to chronic pain syndromes in certain patients.

REFERENCES

1. Lee KM, Kay MC, Kucera KL, et al. Epidemiology of cervical muscle strains in collegiate and high school football athletes, 2011–2012 through 2013–2014 academic years. *J Athl Train.* 2019;54(7):780–786.
2. Chung AS, Makovicka JL, Hassebrock JD, et al. Epidemiology of cervical injuries in NCAA football players. *Spine (Phila Pa 1976).* 2019;44(12):848–854.
3. Meron A, McMullen C, Laker SR, et al. Epidemiology of cervical spine injuries in high school athletes over a ten-year period. *PM R.* 2018;10(4):365–372.
4. Elliot JM, Courtney M, Rademaker A, et al. The rapid and progressive degeneration of the cervical multifidus in whiplash: an MRI study of fatty infiltration. *Spine (Phila Pa 1976).* 2015;40(12):e694–e700.
5. Christianson SWM, Rasmussen MB, Jespersen CL, et al. Soft-collar use in rehabilitation of whiplash-associated disorders—a systematic review and meta-analysis. *Musculoskelet Sci Pract.* 2021;55:102426.
6. Vassiliou T, Kaluza G, Putzke C, et al. Physical therapy and active exercises—an adequate treatment for prevention of late whiplash syndrome? Randomized controlled trial in 200 patients. *Pain.* 2006;124(1–2):69–76.
7. Elphinston RA, Thibault P, Carriere JS, et al. Cross-sectional and prospective correlates of recovery expectancies in the rehabilitation of whiplash injury. *Clin J Pain.* 2018;34(4):306–312.

ADDITIONAL READING

- Al-Khazali HM, Ashina H, Iljazi A, et al. Systematic review and meta-analysis neck pain and headache after whiplash injury: a systematic review and meta-analysis. *Pain.* 2020;161(5):880–888.
- Brinkman JC, Tummala SV, McQuivey KS, et al. Epidemiology of spine injuries in National Collegiate Athletic Association Men's Wrestling Athletes. *Ortho J Sports Med.* 2021;9(9):23259671211032007.
- Dorshimer GW, Kelly M. Cervical pain in the athlete: common conditions and treatment. *Prim Care.* 2005;32(1):231–243.
- Elliot JM, Walton DM, Albin SR, et al. Biopsychosocial sequelae and recovery trajectories from whiplash injury following a motor vehicle collision. *Spine J.* 2023;23(7):1028–1036.
- Eyre A. Overview and comparison of NEXUS and Canadian C-spine rules. *Am J Med.* 2006;3(4):12–15.
- Fundaun J, Kolski M, Baskozos G, et al. Nerve pathology and neuropathic pain after whiplash injury: a systematic review and meta-analysis. *Pain.* 2022;163(7):e789–e811.
- Kongsted A, Qerama E, Kasch H, et al. Neck collar, "act-as-usual" or active mobilization for whiplash injury? A randomized parallel-group trial. *Spine (Phila Pa 1976).* 2007;32(6):618–626.
- Luque-Suarez A, Falla D, Morales-Asencio JM, et al. Is kinesiophobia and pain catastrophizing at baseline associated with chronic pain and disability in whiplash-associated disorders? A systematic review. *Br J Sports Med.* 2020;54(15):892–897.
- Maujean A, Sterling J, Sterling M. What information do patients need following a whiplash injury? The perspectives of patients and physiotherapists. *Disabil Rehabil.* 2018;40(10):1135–1141.
- Michaleff ZA, Maher CG, Verhagen AP, et al. Accuracy of the Canadian C-spine rule and NEXUS to screen for clinically important cervical spine injury in patients following blunt trauma: a systematic review. *CMAJ.* 2012;184(16):E867–E876.
- Smith A, Ritchie C, Pedler A, et al. Exercise induced hypoalgesia is elicited by isometric, but not aerobic exercise in individuals with chronic whiplash associated disorders. *Scand J Pain.* 2017;15:14–21.
- Southerst D, Nordin MC, Côté P, et al. Is exercise effective for the management of neck pain and associated disorders or whiplash-associated disorders? A systematic review by the Ontario Protocol for Traffic Injury Management (OPTIMa) collaboration. *Spine J.* 2016;16(12):1503–1523.
- Sutton DA, Côté P, Wong JJ, et al. Is multimodal care effective for the management of patients with whiplash-associated disorders or neck pain and associated disorders? A systematic review by the Ontario Protocol for Traffic Injury Management (OPTIMa) collaboration. *Spine J.* 2016;16(12):1541–1565.

CLINICAL PEARLS

- Cervical strain is common and is usually a benign, self-limited condition.
- Management should be multimodal including analgesics, muscle relaxers, soft tissue massage/mobilization, and various exercises.
- Care must be taken not to miss more serious conditions such as fractures or dislocations, especially in patients with acute neck pain.
- Victims of trauma with neck pain or tenderness and unconscious victims need to be treated with cervical stabilization until the spine can be fully evaluated with imaging.

CHRONIC EXERTIONAL COMPARTMENT SYNDROME

Brian Lowell, MD, CAQSM

BASICS

DESCRIPTION

- Chronic exertional compartment syndrome (CECS) is a rare condition that can cause significant pain localized to the affected compartment.
- Cases have been reported in the forearm, thigh, and foot, but the majority are reported in the lower leg.
- CECS is caused by an increase in interstitial pressure in a closed fascial compartment, which leads to ischemic pain that may be associated with paresthesias and muscular dysfunction.
- CECS can be easily misdiagnosed due to the vague nature of symptoms experienced by the patient. Delayed diagnosis can increase severity of condition.
- It is seen in a variety of sports, but most often those associated with lower extremity stresses:
  - Runners
  - Dancers
  - Soccer players
  - Speed skaters
  - Military populations (marching)
- The anterior compartment is most commonly affected and consists of the tibialis anterior, extensor hallucis longus, extensor digitorum longus, peroneus tertius, and deep peroneal nerve. The other compartments of the lower extremity include the lateral (peroneal longus, peroneus brevis, and superficial peroneal nerve), the superficial posterior (gastrocnemius, soleus, plantaris, and tibial nerve), and the deep posterior (tibialis posterior, flexor hallucis longus, flexor digitorum longus, popliteus, and the tibial nerve).
- CECS of the forearm, although much less common, has been observed in motorcycle racers, climbers, and rowers (1).

EPIDEMIOLOGY

Incidence

- CECS has an incidence reported at up to 27–33% in competitive athletes with pain related to exercise.
- Described in athletic populations at a rate of approximately 0.49 cases per 1,000 person-years.
- Younger patients more likely to develop CECS. Mean age of presentation is in the late 20s.

Prevalence

- The prevalence of CECS decreases with age.
- Gender prevalence data has been conflicting (2).

ETIOLOGY AND PATHOPHYSIOLOGY

The etiology of CECS is multifactorial. The most described theory involves transient ischemia during exercise caused by an increase in intramuscular pressure which compromises blood supply to the affected compartment. Factors which lead to compartmental pressure include trauma (repetitive activities), and genetic (predisposition to hypertrophic musculature or poor elasticity of fascia).

RISK FACTORS

- Rapid increase in repetitive activity
- Participation in high-risk sport activities
- Significant musculature of the lower extremity
- Diabetes mellitus

DIAGNOSIS

HISTORY

- Typically, no associated trauma or injury
- Pain is described as fullness, cramp-like, or tightness.
- Pain reoccurs consistently with specific amounts of exertion (time, distance, or intensity).
- Pain is typically bilateral in nature.
- Pain generally associated with neurologic abnormalities that include paresthesia or weakness (e.g., foot drop).
- Symptoms generally resolve <30 minutes after cessation of inciting activity.

PHYSICAL EXAM

- Exam is usually normal at rest. A physical exam without abnormal findings largely assists in narrowing the differential.
- Postexertional examination can greatly assist with diagnosis of CECS. Following exertion, pain may become present, muscle/facial tightness may be palpable, and neurovascular abnormalities may become present. Passive stretching of the muscles in the affected compartment may also cause pain.

DIFFERENTIAL DIAGNOSIS

- Acute compartment syndrome
- Stress fracture
- Medial tibial stress syndrome
- Fascial hernia
- Tendonitis
- Popliteal artery entrapment syndrome
- Peripheral nerve entrapment
- Thrombosis
- Peripheral vascular disease

DIAGNOSTIC TESTS & INTERPRETATION

Initial Tests (lab, imaging)

- Radiographs, magnetic resonance imaging (MRI), and computed tomography (CT) are used to evaluate for other causes of lower extremity pain, such as stress reactions or tumors.
- MRI/magnetic resonance angiography (MRA) is useful in identifying popliteal artery entrapment.

Diagnostic Procedures/Other

- Needle manometry is currently the gold standard test of choice.
- Intracompartmental pressure measurements before and after exercise are useful in validating the clinical diagnosis of CECS. Although scrutinized, most clinicians use the modified Pedowitz criteria to indicate a positive test (3)[C]:
  - Preexercise pressure ≥15 mm Hg
  - 1-min postexercise pressure ≥30 mm Hg
  - 5-min postexercise pressure ≥20 mm Hg (3)
- T2-weighted MRI comparing water contents in tissue during preexertional and postexertional states has recently been used to aid in supporting the diagnosis of CECS (4).

TREATMENT

GENERAL MEASURES

- Despite great evidence, nonsurgical measures are usually initiated first. These include stretching, prolonged rest, decreasing activity levels, avoiding activities that exacerbate symptoms, taping, and orthoses (3)[C].
- Physical therapy to address any biomechanical predisposition (i.e., foot strike)

MEDICATION

No evidence for benefit with pharmacologic intervention; specifically nonsteroidal anti-inflammatory drugs (NSAIDs) or acetaminophen

ADDITIONAL THERAPIES

Nonsurgical therapeutic modalities have recently been studied in small numbers, some with promising results. These therapies include the following:

- Massage: no change in postexercise compartment pressure, but decrease in postexercise pain (5)[C]
- Gait training: Forefoot gait led to a significant change in compartment pressure postintervention (5)[C].
- Chemodenervation: treatment via botulinum toxin A assisted with pain relief; however, there were concerns with lower extremity weakness associated with such therapies (5)[C].
- Ultrasound-guided fascial fenestration: no significant surgical risks; full return to sport without reoccurring pain; case report: further research needed (5)[C]

SURGERY/OTHER PROCEDURES

- Surgery is the definitive treatment. The gold standard is decompressive fasciotomy (6)[C].
- Surgery consists of a fasciotomy of the affected compartment or compartments; open or endoscopic
- Endoscopic release is hypothesized to decrease surgical healing time and minimize risk for dehiscence. There is no evidence for improvement in postsurgical fibrosis formation.
- Studies report satisfactory results in 60–80% of patients. Greater successes were seen with anterior compartment intervention, whereas less favorable outcomes were seen with intervention to the other three compartments.
- Common surgical complications include infection, wound dehiscence, bleeding, hematoma, nerve injury (peroneal neuritis), venous injury (saphenous), and inadequate release of fascia during initial surgical intervention and postsurgical fibrosis.
- Reoccurring symptoms are seen in approximately 20–30% of postsurgical patients and typically occur from localized muscle constrictions secondary to fibrosis (6).
- Special considerations:
  - Acute compartment syndrome and acute exertional compartment syndrome are different from CECS:
    - Acute compartment syndrome: typically associated with fracture or crush injury
    - Acute exertional compartment syndrome: nontraumatic, unilateral, commonly associated with significant increase in activity, symptoms do not resolve with rest
  - Remember pain out of proportion to physical exam along with neurovascular abnormalities on physical exam at rest.
  - The acute compartment syndromes are surgical emergencies that must be treated with emergent fasciotomy to avoid muscle necrosis (7).

ONGOING CARE

- Very little literature on rehabilitation after fasciotomy
- Small study rehabilitation protocol includes:
  - Crutches for ambulation immediately postfasciotomy
  - Remove crutches when one can bear weight without significant limp.
  - Control swelling with ice, elevation, and compression.
  - Gait training and progression to full weight-bearing
  - Progressive strengthening of the lower extremity with goal of sport-specific training between 6 and 8 weeks (8)
- >80% of elite athletes return to previous sports participation in 8 to 12 weeks.

REFERENCES

1. Smeraglia F, Tamborini F, Garutti L, et al. Chronic exertional compartment syndrome of the forearm: a systematic review. *EFORT Open Rev.* 2021;6(2):101–106.
2. de Bruijn JA, van Zantvoort APM, van Klaveren D, et al. Factors predicting lower leg chronic exertional compartment syndrome in a large population. *Int J Sports Med.* 2018;39(1):58–66.
3. Vajapey S, Miller TL. Evaluation, diagnosis, and treatment of chronic exertional compartment syndrome: a review of current literature. *Phys Sportsmed.* 2017;45(4):391–398.
4. Velasco TO, Leggit JC. Chronic exertional compartment syndrome: a clinical update. *Curr Sports Med Rep.* 2020;19(9):347–352.
5. Rajasekaran S, Hall MM. Nonoperative management of chronic exertional compartment syndrome: a systematic review. *Curr Sports Med Rep.* 2016;15(3):191–198.
6. Campano D, Robaina JA, Kusnezov N, et al. Surgical management for chronic exertional compartment syndrome of the leg: a systematic review of the literature. *Arthroscopy.* 2016;32(7):1478–1486.
7. Livingston KS, Meehan WP III, Hresko MT, et al. Acute exertional compartment syndrome in young athletes: a descriptive case series and review of the literature. *Pediatr Emerg Care.* 2018;34(2):76–80.
8. Irion V, Magnussen RA, Miller TL, et al. Return to activity following fasciotomy for chronic exertional compartment syndrome. *Eur J Orthop Surg Traumatol.* 2014;24(7):1223–1228.

ADDITIONAL READING

Roscoe D, Roberts AJ, Hulse D. Intramuscular compartment pressure measurement in chronic exertional compartment syndrome: new and improved diagnostic criteria. *Am J Sports Med.* 2015;43(2):392–398.

CLINICAL PEARLS

- Typical presentation is a young athlete who has recurrent lower extremity pain that is aggravated with repetitive activity and alleviated with rest.
- A high index of suspicion if athletes endorse symptoms, but physical exam findings on exam are benign.
- The diagnosis of CECS is clinical. Needle manometry assists with diagnosis.
- Surgical treatment via fasciotomy is the gold standard, but successful treatment of pain may be achieved with nonsurgical interventions.
- Surgical treatment success rates are high, but complications and postsurgical reoccurrences are seen.

CLIMBING INJURIES

Ilona Barash, MD, PhD, CAQSM

BASICS

DESCRIPTION

- Rock climbing is becoming more mainstream, especially after its inclusion in the 2020 summer Olympic Games. There are multiple climbing activities/styles that can be broadly separated into outdoor climbing pursuits such as mountaineering, traditional and big wall climbing, and more indoor focused climbing such as sport climbing, bouldering, and speed climbing. Sport climbing and bouldering are often also done outdoors, but it is estimated that there are almost twice as many exclusively indoor climbers compared to those who also climb outdoors in the US (1).
- Climbing-related injuries are categorized as:
  - Impact injury from either the climber falling or something falling onto the climber
  - nonimpact acute injury
  - chronic overuse injuries
- Focus will be on finger injuries because these are fairly climbing specific and common among climbers, but wrist, elbow, shoulder, and lower extremity injuries are also seen.

EPIDEMIOLOGY

Incidence

- Estimates vary but approximately 4.2 injuries per 1,000 participation hours (1).
- Career incidence 1.5 to 4.2 injuries per subject
- Most common overall: lower extremity injury from falls (1)
- Most common nontraumatic injury: finger injuries (1)

Prevalence

Estimates vary, approximately:

- 10–81% irrespective of cause
- 10–50% impact injuries
- 28–81% nonimpact acute injury
- 33–44% chronic overuse injury

ETIOLOGY AND PATHOPHYSIOLOGY

- Finger injuries represent 33–52% of all injuries:
  - Most commonly middle and ring fingers
  - Annular pulleys most commonly injured:
    - Five pulleys per finger: A1, A2, A3, A4, A5
    - A2 (proximal phalanges) and A4 (distal phalanges) directly attached to underlying bone
  - Holds: the parts of the rock that climbers grip or stand on to ascend the rock. Large holds (jugs) are easier to hold onto compared to the small holds (crimps), and less likely to cause injury. Slopers are rounded and do not have a distinct edge. Pinches must be gripped between the thumb and other fingers, and pockets can often only accommodate 1 to 3 fingers.
- Grip: method by which climber uses a hold:
  - Crimp: proximal interphalangeal joint (PIPJ) flexed to 100 degrees, distal interphalangeal (DIP) hyperextended to 120 degrees; thumb over index finger; highest force and also highest likelihood of injury to A2 pulley
  - Half crimp: PIPJ flexed to 90 degrees, DIP fully extended, thumb is not over index finger; slightly less force than full crimp
  - Open handed: thumb not in contact with index finger, PIPJ not as flexed, DIP somewhat flexed; less force on A2, more on A4; more common with jugs or slopers.

RISK FACTORS

Inconsistent data, but the following factors may affect risk of injury:

- Intrinsic: sex, age, skill level, experience, body mass index (BMI), grip strength
- Extrinsic: type of climbing (indoor vs. outdoor, lead climbing vs. top roping vs. bouldering), climbing volume, climbing intensity, drugs/alcohol

GENERAL PREVENTION

- No consistent proven reduction in injury with warm-up or stretching but still generally recommended (2)[C]
- Taping fingers/wrists and weight training may help, especially if recovering from injury.
- Avoid sudden increases in load or training intensity.
- Avoid full crimp if possible. Most acute injuries occur in full crimp and with sudden eccentric force such as a foot slip or dynamic (jumping) movement
- Warming up the fingers does increase physiologic bowstringing of the tendons by up to 30%. Theoretically, this also evens out the forces across the tendons and decreases peak force at the tendon sheath (2).
- Recommendation: warm up 50 moves per hand before full activity (2)[C]

COMMONLY ASSOCIATED CONDITIONS

- Impact: fractures (usually lower extremity), abrasions/lacerations, head injuries, ankle sprains, knee ligament injuries, spinal fractures
- Nonimpact: finger pulley injury, strain finger flexor tendon or joint capsule, capsulitis, superior labrum anterior and posterior (SLAP) tear
- Overuse: tenosynovitis, epicondylitis, shoulder impingement, Dupuytren disease, ganglion cyst

Pregnancy Considerations

- Data are very limited on the safety of climbing while pregnant.
- One study showed no difference in preterm birth in women who climbed (3).
- Generally recommended to limit lead climbing and fall potential (even while bouldering) during pregnancy, but no evidence that top roping in itself is harmful (3)[B].

ALERT

The incidence of relative energy deficiency in sport/female and male athlete triad and other eating disorders in competitive climbers may be elevated, similar to other sports reliant on high strength/weight ratios (4). Be aware of this and screen and treat appropriately.

DIAGNOSIS

HISTORY

- Sudden versus gradual onset
- May report hearing or feeling a "pop" if finger pulley rupture with sudden pain and reduced grip strength, sometimes swelling over the involved joint
- Often report weakness and/or pain when gripping, even door handles

PHYSICAL EXAM

- Pain and tenderness palmar aspect of pulley site
- Often accompanied by swelling +/− bruising
- Pain with grip testing, reduced grip strength
- Sometimes reduced range of motion of fingers or chronic PIPJ flexion contracture
- Grade 4: may have palpable or visible bowstringing

DIFFERENTIAL DIAGNOSIS

- Other relatively climbing-specific upper extremity injuries include:
  - Hamate fractures
  - Epiphyseal overuse fractures in fingers
  - Third or fourth lumbrical tear
  - Brachialis injury "climber's elbow:" strain/tear of brachialis muscle at the musculotendinous junction due to overload of brachialis while pronated. Pain at anterior elbow worsened by flexion and pronation (1)
- Common upper extremity/hand injuries in climbers, not climbing specific, but often present due to hypertrophy of climbing specific muscles and use patterns:
  - Flexor tendinopathies
  - Capsular inflammation
  - Extensor hood rupture
  - Collateral ligament damage
  - Osteoarthritis
  - Medial > lateral epicondylitis
  - de Quervain tenosynovitis
  - Intersection syndrome
  - Rotator cuff injuries
  - Shoulder impingement syndrome
  - SLAP tears
  - Biceps tendinopathy
  - Nerve entrapment syndromes
  - Neurogenic and venous thoracic outlet syndrome
  - Scapular dyskinesis

DIAGNOSTIC TESTS & INTERPRETATION

Initial Tests (lab, imaging)

- X-rays to rule out fracture
- Ultrasound:
  - A2 pulley rupture will show >2 mm of dehiscence between tendon and bone, also known as bowstringing.
  - Pulley strain if <2 mm dehiscence
  - Can have chronic dehiscence without acute rupture
- Magnetic resonance imaging (MRI):
  - Sagittal MRI with fingers flexed may show the 2 mm dehiscence.
- Grading:
  - Grade 1: pulley strain
  - Grade 2: rupture of A4 or partial rupture of A2 or A3
  - Grade 3: complete rupture of A2 or A3
  - Grade 4: multiple pulley ruptures (A2/A3, A2/A3/A4) or A2 or A3 plus collateral ligament or lumbrical rupture

Pediatric Considerations

- Epiphyseal fractures of the 3rd and 4th finger PIPJ in adolescent sport climbers are common
- Average age 13 to 15 years old, peak growth spurt combined with intense load on fingers
- Increased risk with dynamic finger training such as use of a campus board
- Epiphyseal fractures much more common than pulley injuries in children

- Usually diagnosed with history and exam, but x-ray (including oblique) can be diagnostic, and CT and MRI are more sensitive (4)
- Often can have delay in diagnosis due to low level of suspicion of injury (2- to 360-day delay seen), and this can delay recovery (4)
- Treatment: complete climbing cessation vs decreased loading and splinting/casting, sometimes with some percutaneous spot-drilling epiphysiodesis; time after diagnosis to return to climbing: 82 ± 66 days in one center (4)[C]

ALERT

Pain and/or tenderness of dorsal aspect of the PIPJ, usually in the middle or ring finger in an adolescent climber must be recognized and treated as a growth plate fracture to avoid premature growth plate closure and allow timely return to sport

TREATMENT

GENERAL MEASURES

- Nonsurgical measures usually work.
- Relative rest
- Taping (see below)
- Progressive resistance training
- Climber's media (magazines and web sites) and climbers are possible sources of rehabilitation advice.
- Common home directed therapy incudes tendon glides and rice bucket exercises.

MEDICATION

First Line

Medications for climbing related injuries in general should only be used in conjunction with rest and/or splinting (see below). Nonsteroidal anti-inflammatory drugs (NSAIDs), topical or systemic, can help with symptom control.

Second Line

Corticosteroid injections (1)[C]:

- Only for chronic tendinitis or tenosynovitis who have failed other treatments
- Great caution needed to avoid causing tendon rupture
- Generally not indicated
- Treatment protocols/return to sport
  - Grade 1 injuries (2)[C]:
    - Stop climbing, functional therapy with pulley protection H-tape or thermoplastic pulley protection splint) for 2 to 4 weeks
    - Resume light climbing after 4 weeks.
    - Resume full climbing after 6 weeks.
    - H-Tape fingers for 3 months
  - Grade 2 injuries (2)[C]:
    - Optional Immobilization <5 days in palmar splint with metacarpophalangeal joint in flexion, interphalangeal joints in extension or slight flexion
    - 6 weeks pulley protection splint plus rehab
    - Light climbing: 6 weeks
    - Full climbing: 8 to 10 weeks
    - H-tape for 3 months
  - Grade 3 injuries (2)[C]:
    - Optional immobilization <5 days
    - 6 to 8 weeks pulley protection splint plus functional therapy
    - Resume easy sport-specific activity (light climbing) after 8 weeks.
    - Resume full climbing after 3 months.
    - Consider pulley protection with tape or ring for 3 to 6 months after injury.
  - Grade 4 injury: high-grade pulley injury associated with ligamentous or lumbrical injury. Refer for possible surgery (2)[C].
    - Grade 4A: multiple ruptures, but no major bowstringing, + ultrasound proven reposition, and no delay in therapy: may possibly be treated nonsurgically; follow grade 3 protocol but with a few extra weeks at each step.
    - Grade 4B: multiple ruptures with significant bowstring, contractures, therapy resistant tenosynovitis, other complication—likely surgical intervention
  - Taping (2)[C]:
    - Does not help prophylactically
    - H-tape figure-of-8 technique resulting in slight PIPJ flexion decreases tendon to bone distance and increases strength of injured finger.
    - Thermoplastic pulley protection splint likely somewhat more effective

ISSUES FOR REFERRAL

- Grade 4 injury as noted above
- Failure of non-surgical treatment

Treatment course

- Time for full return to climbing:
  - Pulley strain: 6 weeks
  - Pulley rupture: 6 to 12 weeks
  - High-grade injury: 6 months
  - A4 generally heals faster than A2.

SURGERY/OTHER PROCEDURES

Palmaris longus tendon graft or extensor retinaculum in a loop:

- Allows early active motion
- Multiple methods reconstruct the pulley.
- Most climbers can return to previous level of climbing after surgery.

ADMISSION, INPATIENT, AND NURSING CONSIDERATIONS

Not routine

ONGOING CARE

FOLLOW-UP RECOMMENDATIONS

- Consider taping for prolonged period after injury.
- Physical therapy and strengthening exercises can continue indefinitely:
  - Finger tendon glides (gradual flexion of all finger joints from distal to proximal and then reverse this)
  - Strengthening: rubber bands, putty, grip balls, fingers moving in rice

Patient Monitoring

Worsening pain/symptoms should prompt further assessment.

PATIENT EDUCATION

- Appropriate rest and rehab is key.
- Consider H-taping—the climbing literature has good resources for how to do this effectively.
- The climbing literature and community is very proactive with self-treatment plans and diagnoses, and climbers can be resistant to medical recommendations. It is important to maintain a collaborative approach to recovery and rehabilitation, especially if the clinician is not well versed in climbing specifics, in order to promote positive therapeutic relationships
- Familiarity with different hold/grip types can be helpful, as open-handed jugs are much less stressful on the finger pulleys then full crimps (for example), and may allow patients to continue some activity but at a lower risk level.

PROGNOSIS

Most climbers will recover from pulley and other overuse injury with minimal complications, if they follow sufficient treatment time and rehabilitation.

COMPLICATIONS

- Chronic stiffness
- Further injury

REFERENCES

1. Leung J. A guide to indoor rock climbing injuries. *Curr Sports Med Rep*. 2023;22(2):55–60.
2. Miro PH, vanSonnenberg E, Sabb DM, et al. Finger flexor pulley injuries in rock climbers. *Wilderness Environ Med*. 2021;32(2):247–258.
3. Drastig J, Hillebrandt D, Rath W, et al. Pregnant women in sport climbing—is there a higher risk for preterm birth? *Z Geburtshilfe Neonatol*. 2017;221(1):25–29.
4. Joubert LM, Gonzalez GB, Larson AJ. Prevalence of disordered eating among international sport lead rock climbers. *Front Sports Act Living*. 2020;2:86.

ADDITIONAL READING

- Gnecchi S, Moutet F. *Hand and Finger Injuries in Rock Climbers*. Springer; 2015.
- Schöffl V, Schöffl I, Flohé S, et al. Evaluation of a diagnostic-therapeutic algorithm for finger epiphyseal growth plate stress injuries in adolescent climbers. *Am J Sports Med*. 2022;50(1):229–237.

CLINICAL PEARLS

- Finger pulley injuries are a relatively common, climbing-specific injury.
- Most will respond well to conservative therapy.
- Refer the high-grade/grade 4 injuries to a hand surgeon for evaluation.
- Be aware of increasing incidence of disordered eating among competitive climbers.
- Finger pain among young/adolescent climbers will often be from growth plate fractures rather than pulley injuries.
- The high forces and unique stresses imposed by climbing result in some unique injuries, both from acute trauma and from overuse.

COMPLEX REGIONAL PAIN SYNDROME

Nandakumar Ponnusamy, MBBS, MD, FASA • Julio A. Martinez-Silvestrini, MD, FAAPMR, CAQSM

BASICS

DESCRIPTION

- Severe, continuing pain, disproportionate to any inciting event and duration
- Manifested by four clinical characteristics based on Budapest criteria:
  - Intense pain
  - Vasomotor disturbances
  - Sudomotor (sweat glands) disturbances, as increased sweating or clammy skin
  - Various associated motor or trophic changes
- Functional recovery delay may be observed if the patient is not treated properly.
- A consensus statement grouped several previously identified syndromes as "complex regional pain syndrome" (CRPS):
  - CRPS type I
  - Not related to a nerve injury
  - 90% of CRPS cases
  - CRPS type II ("causalgia")
  - Directly related to a nerve injury
  - The clinical syndrome is diffuse and not following the usual nerve injury distribution of pain and muscle dysfunction.
- Also known as:
  - Reflex sympathetic dystrophy
  - Shoulder-hand syndrome
  - Sudeck atrophy

EPIDEMIOLOGY

- Adult:
  - Female:male = 4:1
  - Median age at onset: 46 years (1)[C]; incidence may vary (40 to 70 years). This large variability has been attributed to differences in ethnic and socioeconomic background of the cohorts as well as the application of the diagnostic criteria (2)[C].
  - Upper limb twice as common as lower limb
  - Most report a triggering event
  - Most common trigger: fracture (46%)
  - Most common triggering fracture: distal radius:
    - Only 1% of radius fractures develop CRPS.
  - Incidence following peripheral nerve injury: 2–14%
- Children:
  - Majority are female (67–86%).
  - Symptoms typically start just prior to puberty.
  - Lower limb more likely to be involved than upper limb (5:1)
  - Often less clear inciting event
  - Higher recurrence rate
  - More responsive to treatment than adults

Incidence

5.46 per 100,000 person-years at risk (1)[C],(2)[C]

Prevalence

20.57 per 100,000 person-years

ETIOLOGY AND PATHOPHYSIOLOGY

Pathogenesis is unclear, but several theories exist:

- Reflex arc following inciting event
- Sympathetic nerve reflex arc causes central sympathetic dysfunction, causing peripheral vascular dysfunction.
- Increased sensitivity of injured nerves to endocrine and paracrine substances
- Inappropriate inflammatory mediator control (especially interleukin [IL]-6, IL-1β, tumor necrosis factor [TNF]-α, substance P, neuropeptide, and calcitonin gene-related peptide)
- Several studies have demonstrated central nervous system (CNS) modulation as cause of CRPS.
- A model of "neurogenic inflammation" attempts to tie the above theories together into a unifying theory of pathogenesis.

Genetics

Human leukocyte antigen (HLA) type:

- Increased incidence in those with HLA-A3, B7, and DR2 (15)
- HLA-DR2 (15) may predict poor treatment outcome.
- HLA testing has no role in clinical management of CRPS.
- No specific single-gene polymorphisms have been clearly linked to CRPS.

RISK FACTORS

- Precipitating event (adults):
  - Fracture
  - Surgery (especially arthroscopic procedures)
  - Sprain
  - Myocardial infarction
  - Hemiplegia
  - Immobilization (bracing, casting, stroke)
  - Placement of arteriovenous graft for hemodialysis
  - Peripheral nerve injury
  - May be observed in the absence of a precipitating event
- Precipitating event (children):
  - 50% have a vague, minor, or no precipitating event:
    - Sprains
    - Strains
    - Minor contusions
  - Surgery (especially arthroscopic procedures of the knee)
  - Henoch-Schönlein purpura
  - Emotional stress
  - Injections or vaccination
- Constitutional or psychiatric predisposition (2)[C]:
  - Underlying anxiety and depression in these patients may play a role.
  - Suspected by many clinicians but no conclusive evidence to support

GENERAL PREVENTION

- Stroke:
  - Early mobilization following stroke decreases risk of CRPS.
  - Limited evidence supports early mobilization following injury and myocardial infarction.
- Fracture:
  - Recent studies suggest that vitamin C supplementation is not effective in preventing CRPS (3)[A].
- Regional anesthesia:
  - Intravenous regional anesthesia (IVRA) is commonly used to provide anesthesia during extremity surgery.
  - IVRA with or without clonidine may decrease the chance of developing postsurgical CRPS (1)[C].

COMMONLY ASSOCIATED CONDITIONS

- Precipitating injury or event
- Possible psychiatric or personality disorders
- Other pain syndromes have been reported as associated conditions:
  - May represent heterogeneity of a single disease or susceptible phenotype

DIAGNOSIS

- Clinical diagnosis
- Positive response to sympathetic block confirms the presence of sympathetically mediated pain
- Laboratory and imaging studies are only indicated if diagnosis is uncertain.

HISTORY

- Stage 1: early disease following inciting event or spontaneous initiation:
  - Nondermatomal progressive limb pain
  - Burning pain
  - Occasional throbbing
  - Diffuse aching
  - Sensitivity to cold and/or touch
  - Localized edema
- Stage 2: progressive physical changes (see "Physical Exam"):
  - Progressive functional limitation
- Stage 3: severe disease:
  - Worsening pain
  - Permanent functional limitation
  - Increasingly dramatic physical findings (see "Physical Exam")
- Other symptoms (not stage specific): urinary urgency, frequency, and/or incontinence

PHYSICAL EXAM

- Stage 1:
  - Allodynia
  - Localized edema
  - Vasomotor disturbances:
    - Color changes
    - Temperature changes (usually cool but can be warm)
- Stage 2:
  - Progressively worsening soft tissue edema
  - Thickening of the skin
  - Muscle wasting
  - Dystonia
- Stage 3:
  - Joint contractures
  - Waxy appearance to skin
  - Brittle nails
- Other findings (not stage specific):
  - Hyperhidrosis
  - Abnormal hair growth (patchy, sparse, or excessive hair)
  - Urinary retention
- Budapest criteria (3)[A]
  - Must report at least one symptom in three of the four following categories:
    - Sensory: hyperalgesia and/or allodynia
    - Vasomotor: temperature asymmetry and/or skin color changes
    - Sudomotor/edema: edema and/or sweating changes and/or sweating asymmetry
    - Motor/trophic: decreased range of motion and/or motor dysfunction (weakness, tremor, dystonia) and/or trophic changes (hair, nails, skin)
  - Must display at least one sign at time of evaluation in two or more of the following categories:
    - Sensory: hyperalgesia (to pinprick) and/or allodynia (severe pain with light skin stroking, touch, local temperature changes, or joint movement):
      - Vasomotor: temperature asymmetry and/or skin color changes
      - Sudomotor/edema: edema and/or sweating changes
      - Motor/trophic: decreased range of motion and/or motor dysfunction
  - There is no other diagnosis that better explains the signs and symptoms.

DIFFERENTIAL DIAGNOSIS

- Fracture/stress fracture
- Infection
- Tumor (especially Pancoast syndrome)
- Nerve root impingement
- Vasculitis
- Rheumatoid arthritis
- Peripheral neuropathy
- Deep vein thrombosis
- Angioedema
- Other pain syndromes

DIAGNOSTIC TESTS & INTERPRETATION

Initial Tests (lab, imaging)

- Tests to exclude other systemic causes of pain:
  - Complete blood count (CBC)
  - Erythrocyte sedimentation rate (ESR)
  - Fasting blood glucose
  - Serum ionized calcium level
  - Thyroid-stimulating hormone and free thyroxine (T_4) levels

C

- Bone scan (triple-phase technetium-99m bone scintigraphy):
  - Increased uptake in 2/3 of adult patients with reflex sympathetic dystrophy
  - Findings vary by phase:
    - 30 seconds: increased flow but decreased tracer uptake in affected limb
    - 3 minutes: capillary leak around affected joint
    - 3 hours: increased uptake of tracer at periarticular bone of affected joint
  - Findings less reliable in pediatric patients:
    - 1/3 exhibit increased uptake (usually in late stages of disease).
    - 1/3 exhibit normal findings.
    - 1/3 exhibit decreased uptake (usually in early stages).
  - Can also be used to help rule out other diagnoses, such as stress fracture or tumor
- Plain radiography:
  - Initially normal
  - After 3 months, may show patchy subchondral osteopenia
  - Late stages show profound bone demineralization.
  - Radiographic findings are less common in children.
- Magnetic resonance imaging (MRI):
  - Multiple nonspecific changes (edema, skin thickening)
  - Useful to rule out constant stimulants (such as meniscal tear or loose body)
- Thermography:
  - Significant skin temperature asymmetry
  - Cold challenge may increase sensitivity and specificity.
- Computed tomography (CT) scan:
  - Focal areas of osteoporosis
  - "Swiss cheese" appearance of bone in stage 3 CRPS can be dramatic.
  - Costs, radiation dose, and poor sensitivity and specificity limit use.

Diagnostic Procedures/Other

- Autonomic testing:
  - Resting sweat output (RSO)
  - Resting skin temperature (RST)
  - Quantitative sudomotor axon reflex test (QSART)
  - Abnormal RSO and QSART are highly sensitive for CRPS.
  - Use of these tests should be limited to patients with uncertain diagnosis.
- Sympathetic blockade:
  - Typically causes abrupt improvement in symptoms
  - Those with cool affected limbs typically have increase of 1–3°C in skin temperature.
  - Lack of response has high negative predictive value.
  - Relief is typically transient.
  - Stellate or lumbar sympathetic blocks are more diagnostically useful than regional blocks(4)][B].
- Usually more effective early in disease (5)[B]
- Follow a stepwise approach, starting with least risky/invasive and progressing to more invasive as needed (1)[C].
- An interdisciplinary program seems to be the most effective approach to CRPS (1)[C]:
  - Physical therapy
  - Occupational therapy
  - Psychotherapy
  - Medications
  - Interventional procedures

TREATMENT

Functional rehabilitation:

- Physical therapy is the mainstay of CRPS treatment.
- Tactile desensitization is most effective if used early.
- Joint mobilization, progressive weight bearing, strengthening, and return to daily activities are important aspects of care directed by physical therapy.
- Transcutaneous electrical nerve stimulation can be beneficial.
- Behavioral management
- Relaxation techniques
- Stress management
- Mirror therapy
- Aerobic exercise
- Somatosensory rehabilitation (6)[B]

MEDICATION

First Line

- Bisphosphonates and short course of steroids are recommended early in the disease (1)[B],(7)[A]:
  - Pamidronate, alendronate, and clodronate have been the most studied.
- Tricyclic antidepressants have been shown to decrease pain in multiple studies and should be considered (1)[C].

Second Line

- Antiepileptic drugs:
  - Thoroughly tested for other pain syndromes but cannot extrapolate results to CRPS
  - Gabapentin most widely used, but studies have demonstrated variable efficacy.
  - Pregabalin is also widely used but has not been studied for treatment of CRPS.
- Selective serotonin and norepinephrine reuptake inhibitors have not been studied for treatment of CRPS.
- Topical capsaicin cream is effective in other types of neuropathic pain. It is generally safe and may be a useful adjuvant treatment for CRPS (1)[C].
- Ketamine may decrease pain immediately with effects lasting up to 3 months (3)[A].
- Opioid use should be limited (5)[C].
- Several other medications have been reported to be effective in small trials but are rarely used (2)[C], (4)[C],(7)[A]:
  - Free radical scavengers (dimethyl sulfoxide and *N*-acetylcysteine)
  - Intrathecal agents
  - Memantine
  - Botulism toxin
  - Plasma exchange
  - Chemotherapeutic agents
  - Sulfonamides are promising in the future (4).

SURGERY/OTHER PROCEDURES

- Nerve blockade:
  - Sympathetic nerve blockade can be both therapeutic and diagnostic:
    - Lumbar sympathetic block for lower extremity
    - Stellate ganglion block for upper extremity
  - Unclear which patients are good candidates for sympathetic blocks
  - Unpredictable response to repeated sympathetic blocks
- Neuromodulation:
  - Dorsal root ganglion (DRG) stimulator improves pain and quality of life than conventional spinal cord stimulation (SCS) (6).
- Other interventional procedures:
  - Peripheral nerve stimulation
  - Chemical and surgical sympathectomy
  - Implanted spinal infusion pumps and/or intrathecal injections:
    - Baclofen may be useful if significant dystonia.
  - Deep brain stimulation

COMPLEMENTARY & ALTERNATIVE MEDICINE

Acupuncture:

- Popular complementary therapy
- High patient satisfaction
- Well-designed studies have shown no difference when compared to placebo (5)[C].
- May have a role as part of an interdisciplinary approach to CRPS

ONGOING CARE

FOLLOW-UP RECOMMENDATIONS

A strong partnership with the patient and all participating caregivers is essential, including pain management specialists, physiatrists, psychiatrists, and other behavioral health specialists, and physical and occupational therapists.

Patient Monitoring

- Weekly or biweekly follow-up is appropriate.
- Have a flexible treatment plan:
  - Stepwise approach to care
  - Therapeutic trials of only 1 to 2 weeks before moving on to the next treatment modality.

PROGNOSIS

- Early diagnosis and treatment can lead to resolution by 6 to 12 months.
- Late diagnosis is associated with permanent residual symptoms.
- Children are more likely to relapse than adults.
- Three distinct phases (described above):
  - Patients in stage 1 and 2 respond better to therapy.
  - Stage 3 disease is often more refractory to treatment.

REFERENCES

1. Limerick G, Christo DK, Tram J, et al. Complex regional pain syndrome: evidence-based advances in concepts and treatments. *Curr Pain Headache Rep.* 2023;27(9):269–298.
2. Goh EL, Chidambaram S, Ma D. Complex regional pain syndrome: a recent update. *Burns Trauma.* 2017;5:2.
3. Urits I, Shen AH, Jones MR, et al. Complex regional pain syndrome, current concepts and treatment options. *Curr Pain Headache Rep.* 2018;22(2):10.
4. Culletta G, Almerico AM, Tutone M. Treatment of complex regional pain syndrome (CRPS): new perspectives in the use of sulfonamides as modulators of P2X receptors. *Recent Adv Inflamm Allergy Drug Discov.* 2023;17(2):88–95.
5. Dowd GSE, Hussein R, Khanduja V, et al. Complex regional pain syndrome with special emphasis on the knee. *J Bone Joint Surg Br.* 2007;89(3):285–290.
6. Pinckard-Dover H, Palmer A, Petersen EA. A review of neuromodulation for treatment of complex regional pain syndrome in pediatric patients and novel use of dorsal root ganglion stimulation in an adolescent patient with 30-month follow-up. *Neuromodulation.* 2021;24(4):634–638.
7. Duong S, Bravo D, Todd KJ, et al. Treatment of complex regional pain syndrome: an updated systematic review and narrative synthesis. *Can J Anaesth.* 2018;65(6):658–684.

ADDITIONAL READING

- American Academy of Orthopaedic Surgeons. Complex regional pain syndrome. In: Armstrong AD, Hubbard MC, eds. *Essentials of Musculoskeletal Care.* 5th ed. American Academy of Orthopaedic Surgeons; 2016:65–71.
- Tran J, Ramachandran VS, Altschuler EL. Complex regional pain syndrome. In: Frontera WR, Silver JK, Rizzo TD, eds. *Essentials of Physical Medicine and Rehabilitation.* 4th ed. Elsevier; 2019:543–548.

CLINICAL PEARLS

- Clinical diagnosis of an exaggerated response to injury of a limb with intense prolonged pain, vasomotor disturbances, delayed functional recovery, and trophic changes
- Pathology is unclear, but there is central sympathetic dysregulation that causes or modulates peripheral symptoms.
- Diagnostic tests should be reserved for unclear cases and to rule out other diagnoses.
- Treatment should be initiated immediately at diagnosis and follow a rapid stepwise approach from least to most invasive.
- In patients with an unclear but high level of suspicion of CRPS, an oral steroid taper and gabapentin can be used safely with minimal adverse effects, if not contraindicated. In some instances, early intervention may prevent the development of the syndrome.

CONCUSSION, PEDIATRIC

Jeremy Swisher, MD • Matthew Waldrop, MD • Daryl Rosenbaum, MD

BASICS

DESCRIPTION

- Pediatric concussion refers to a mild traumatic brain injury (TBI) typically resulting from a blow or jolt to the head or body, causing the brain to move rapidly within the skull.
- Signs and symptoms of a concussion cannot be explained by outside factors, including but not limited to drugs, alcohol, distracting injuries, or other comorbid conditions.

EPIDEMIOLOGY

- In 2020, almost 7% of children aged 0 to 17 years at some point have had symptoms of a concussion (1).
- 3.9% of children are diagnosed with a concussion by a health care professional (1).
- Boys are more likely to report symptoms and be diagnosed of a concussion than girls (1).
- Children aged >12 years are at significantly increased risk for symptoms of concussion and diagnosis of concussion than ages ≤11 years (1).
- Non-Hispanic white children are more likely than all other races to report symptoms of concussion and be diagnosed with a concussion (1).
- Sport-related concussions account for 9% of high school athletic injuries (2).
- Football and girls soccer produce the highest rates of concussions (2).

ETIOLOGY AND PATHOPHYSIOLOGY

- Concussions result from biomechanical forces transmitted to the brain, leading to neuronal injury and functional disturbances.
- Pathophysiology mechanisms include rapid acceleration-deceleration forces, rotational forces, and shearing strains on brain tissue.

Genetics

Genetics may play a role in risk, symptoms, and recovery from concussion, but no direct links have been found yet (3).

RISK FACTORS

- Traumatic injury to the head or neck
- Prior concussion
- History of migraine headaches
- History of attention deficit hyperactivity disorder (ADHD)
- History of mood disorder
- Participation in a contact sport

GENERAL PREVENTION

- Strategies for preventing pediatric concussion in sport involve education, rule enforcement, proper technique instruction, and the use of appropriate protective equipment.
- Implementing concussion protocols, including preseason baseline testing and gradual return-to-play guidelines can help mitigate the risk of recurrent injury and guide treatment plans.

DIAGNOSIS

HISTORY

- Mechanism of injury (e.g., direct blow, collision)
- Context (sports, recreational activity)
- Symptoms at time of injury:
  - Headache
  - Dizziness
  - Confusion
  - Visual disturbances
  - Nausea/vomiting
  - Loss of consciousness (LOC)
- Delayed symptoms
- Evolution of symptoms over hours, days, and weeks
- Previous concussion history:
  - Number, severity, and outcomes of prior concussions
  - Cumulative effect on symptomatology
- Medical and psychosocial history:
  - Preexisting medical conditions
  - Medications, allergies
  - Previous head/neck injuries
  - History of mental health concerns
  - History of learning disabilities
  - Psychosocial factors impacting recovery
- Return-to-play considerations:
  - Involvement in sports/physical activities
  - Aspirations regarding return to play
  - Importance of following return-to-play guidelines
- Return-to-learn considerations:
  - Current school-based workload
  - Accommodations needed
  - Importance of following return-to-learn guidelines

PHYSICAL EXAM

- Immediate exam:
  - Pediatric Glasgow coma scale (GCS)
  - Cervical spine assessment
- Sideline exam:
  - Orientation assessment
  - Immediate memory testing
  - Concentration (months in reverse, digits backwards)
  - Delayed recall
  - Balance testing
  - Tandem gait
  - Finger-to-nose
  - Pupillary exam
  - Extraocular movements, tracking
  - +/− additional neurologic testing
- In-office exam:
  - Consider repeating sideline exam and comparing.

DIFFERENTIAL DIAGNOSIS

- Differential diagnosis of pediatric concussion includes other causes of head injury such as skull fracture, intracranial hemorrhage, cervical spine injury, and TBI with more severe symptoms.
- Nontraumatic conditions such as migraine, vestibular dysfunction, cervical spine pathology, heat exhaustion, and psychological factors may also present with symptoms overlapping those of concussion and require consideration during evaluation.
- Red flag symptoms such as LOC >30 minutes, worsening headache, focal neurologic deficits, repeated vomiting, numbness or weakness in extremities, and GCS score <15 should prompt emergency medical services (EMS) transport and emergent evaluation.

DIAGNOSTIC TESTS & INTERPRETATION

- Sport concussion assessment tool 6 (SCAT-6): a tool intended to aid in the evaluation of sport-related concussions in the acute phase; most effective in the first 72 hours after injury with diminishing results, thereafter, up to 7 days; concussed individuals can still perform within normal ranges on the SCAT-6 (false negative); for use in children ≥13 years old, and in adults. Baseline testing can be considered when resources allow, but there is not great evidence for it. SCAT-6 should not be used alone when deciding on return to sport (4)[C].
- Child SCAT-6: a tool intended to aid in the evaluation of sport-related concussions in the acute phase; most effective in the first 72 hours after injury with diminishing results, thereafter, up to 7 days; for use in children 8 to 12 years old; used the same way as the SCAT-6 (5)[C]
- Sports concussion office assessment tool 6 (SCOAT-6): a tool intended to aid in the evaluation of sport-related concussions in the subacute phase; most effective at 3 to 30 days postinjury. Some of the key differences in this tool include orthostatic vitals, a timed tandem gait, and moving to a 10-word immediate recall to limit the ceiling effect; for use in children ≥13 years old, and adults. This is a newer tool that requires more flexibility in a clinical office-based setting (6).
- Child SCOAT-6: a tool intended to aid in the evaluation of sport-related concussion in the subacute phase; most effective at 3 to 30 days postinjury; for use in children 8 to 12 years old. This is a newer tool that requires more flexibility in a clinical office-based setting (6)[C].
- Pediatric Emergency Care Applied Research Network (PECARN) head trauma algorithm: a tool used to aid in ruling out severe acute TBIs that would require further evaluation with a computed tomography (CT) scan and potential surgical evaluation; for use in children of all ages

Initial Tests (lab, imaging)

Imaging is usually not necessary in the evaluation of a concussion unless red flag symptoms are present, suggesting an alternative or additional diagnosis. Such symptoms include LOC, persistent vomiting, visual disturbances, ongoing confusion, neurologic deficits, or concerns when calculating the GCS and cervical spine assessment.

TREATMENT

GENERAL MEASURES

- Whereas prior recommendations included an emphasis on complete physical and mental rest in the acute recovery phase of concussion, more recent data suggests initiation of light aerobic exercise and mental stimulation below the symptom threshold in the first 48 hours of injury can promote recovery.
- Avoiding screen time in the first 48 hours after injury has shown to shorten recovery time significantly.
- A return-to-learn protocol should be in place with the patient's school to ensure a gradual return to schoolwork without exacerbation of concussion symptoms.
- Formal school testing and quizzes should not occur while recovering from concussion as it is likely not a true reflection of their understanding of the material.
- A return-to-play protocol should also be in place with the patient's physician and school medical staff to ensure a gradual stepwise return to full activity while staying under the concussion symptom threshold.
- Any return in concussion symptoms should result in a return to the prior step in the stepwise sequence in any return-to-learn or return-to-play protocol.
- Patients should *not* be cleared to play on the same day they are diagnosed, or if they are still experiencing symptoms to decrease the risk of severe injury, such as second-impact syndrome.
- Early aerobic activity has been shown to shorten recovery time in adolescent patients, and this involves reaching a target heart rate of approximately 80% of the heart rate that causes symptom exacerbation. For example, if a heart rate of 150 beats/min worsens concussion symptoms initially, a target heart rate for aerobic exercise would be 120 beats/min.

MEDICATION

- Medication management of pediatric concussion focuses primarily on symptomatic relief and addressing associated conditions.
- Pharmacologic interventions may be considered for headache, nausea, sleep disturbances, and mood-related symptoms, depending on the individual's presentation and severity of symptoms.

ONGOING CARE

FOLLOW-UP RECOMMENDATIONS

Close follow-up until symptom resolution and full return to play and return to learn have been achieved is advised.

Patient Monitoring

Patients should be monitored for subsequent head or neck injuries as they are at increased risk for more concussions with each subsequent concussion injury.

DIET

- Although no specific dietary restrictions are typically recommended for pediatric concussion, maintaining a well-balanced diet is important to support overall health and recovery.
- Encourage adequate hydration, balanced nutrition, and avoidance of excessive caffeine or alcohol consumption, which may exacerbate symptoms or interfere with recovery.

PATIENT EDUCATION

- Patient education plays a central role in the management of pediatric concussion, empowering patients and caregivers with knowledge about the injury, recovery process, and strategies for symptom management.
- Provide information on concussion symptoms, potential complications, return-to-play guidelines, academic accommodations, and strategies for coping with cognitive and emotional challenges. It is also important for them to understand how they can incorporate aerobic exercise early and limit screen time to enhance their recovery.

PROGNOSIS

- The prognosis for pediatric concussion is generally favorable, with most individuals experiencing complete recovery within a few weeks to months following injury.
- Factors influencing prognosis include the severity of initial symptoms, history of previous concussions, adherence to recovery guidelines, presence of coexisting medical or psychosocial conditions, and access to supportive resources.
- Studies have shown that pediatric concussion does not lower IQ scores in the weeks to months following the injury.

COMPLICATIONS

- Second-impact syndrome is a life-threatening emergency stemming from a second TBI prior to the resolution of a first TBI, resulting in a massive amount of brain swelling. This risk underscores the importance of taking the proper precautions when evaluating for concussions and deciding when to allow an athlete to return to play.
- Postconcussion syndrome is a condition where symptoms can last for >1 month after a concussion. Most people recover completely but can experience severe symptoms for extended periods. Symptoms include, but are not limited to, headache, dizziness, concentration difficulty, depression, anxiety, insomnia, and vision disturbances.

REFERENCES

1. Black LI, Zablotsky B. Concussions and brain injuries in children: United States, 2020. *NCHS Data Brief.* 2021;(423):1–8.
2. Jinguji TM, Krabak BJ, Satchell EK. Epidemiology of youth sports concussion. *Phys Med Rehabil Clin N Am.* 2011;22(4):565–575,vii.
3. Guth T, Ketcham CJ, Hall EE. Influence of concussion history and genetics on event-related potentials in athletes: potential use in concussion management. *Sports (Basel).* 2018;6(1):5.
4. Echemendia RJ, Brett BL, Broglio S, et al. Introducing the sport concussion assessment tool 6 (SCAT6). *Br J Sports Med.* 2023;57(11):619–621.
5. Davis GA, Echemendia RJ, Ahmed OH, et al. Introducing the child sport concussion assessment tool 6 (Child SCAT6). *Br J Sports Med.* 2023;57(11):632–635.
6. Patricios JS, Davis GA, Ahmed OH, et al. Introducing the sport concussion office assessment tool 6 (SCOAT6). *Br J Sports Med.* 2023;57(11):648–650.

ADDITIONAL READING

- Leddy JJ, Haider MN, Ellis MJ, et al. Early subthreshold aerobic exercise for sport-related concussion: a randomized clinical trial. *JAMA Pediatr.* 2019;173(4):319–325.
- Macnow T, Curran T, Tolliday C, et al. Effect of screen time on recovery from concussion: a randomized clinical trial. *JAMA Pediatr.* 2021;175(11):1124–1131.

CLINICAL PEARLS

- Do *not* clear athletes to return to play while still symptomatic.
- Do *not* clear them to return to play the same day the concussion occurred.
- Avoid second-impact syndrome—even a minor second blow to the head can lead to this condition, causing severe complications and even death.
- Return to school and return to play should be done in a gradual stepwise fashion but should not be delayed if at all possible.
- More concussions are associated with a higher risk of consequences, including general injuries, mental health concerns, substance abuse, and early Alzheimer disease.
- Emphasize reasonably limiting screen time in the first 48 hours after concussion and emphasize sub-symptom aerobic exercise to enhance recovery in patients.

CONCUSSION, SPORTS-RELATED

Alan Shahtaji, DO, CAQSM • Priya Sharma, DO • Kenneth S. Taylor, MD, FAAFP, CAQSM

BASICS

DESCRIPTION

- Sport-related concussion (SRC) is a traumatic brain injury (TBI) induced by biomechanical forces.
- The clinical signs and symptoms cannot solely be explained by drug, alcohol, or medication use; other injuries (e.g., cervical injuries, peripheral vestibular dysfunction); or other comorbidities (e.g., psychological factors or coexisting medical conditions) (1).
- Several common features that may be used in clinically defining the nature of a concussive head injury include:
  - SRC may be caused either by a direct blow to the head, face, neck, or elsewhere on the body with an impulsive force transmitted to the head (2),(3).
  - SRC typically results in the rapid onset of short-lived impairment of neurologic function that resolves spontaneously. However, in some cases, signs and symptoms evolve over a number of minutes to hours.
  - SRC may result in neuropathologic changes involving neurotransmitters, metabolic dysfunction, and possible axonal injury with blood flow and inflammatory changes. These disruptions are a functional rather than a structural injury, and as such, no abnormality is seen on standard structural neuroimaging studies.
  - SRC results in a range of clinical signs and symptoms that may or may not involve loss of consciousness (LOC). Resolution of the clinical and cognitive features typically occurs within days. However, in some cases, symptoms may be prolonged (2).
  - Synonym(s): mild TBI (mTBI); minor head trauma; commotio cerebri

EPIDEMIOLOGY

- Globally, concussion or mTBI affects about 42 million people per year with 1.6 to 3.8 million SRC in the United State. (4)
- Annually, an estimated 1.1 to 1.9 million SRCs occur in US children aged ≤18 years, with 1 to 1.8 million cases identified from emergency and office visits, and approximately 400,000 among high school athletes (3).
- Many cases are not captured in health care settings; up to 45–65% of pediatric concussions may go unreported (1).
- Before age 10 years, children tend to sustain concussions primarily from non–sports-related falls and then transition to sports-related injuries after age 10 years (5),(6),(7),(8).
- The incidence may be higher because athletes, coaches, or medical providers may fail to recognize the signs and symptoms of a concussion or symptoms are underreported (1),(6),(9),(10).
- Self-reported concussion rates have not changed significantly, but the rate at which athletes report suspected concussions has increased significantly (78.6% in 2013 vs. 47.3% in 1999 to 2002) (11).
- Rugby, American football, ice hockey, wrestling, soccer, and lacrosse are the sports at highest risk for SRC with female athletes having a higher reported incidence than males (3),(6),(11)(12).
- 2–15% of athletes participating in organized sports will suffer a concussion during one season (1).

ETIOLOGY AND PATHOPHYSIOLOGY

- Complicated pathophysiology that is incompletely understood (10),(13),(14).
- Impact and resulting forces create shear injury to vessels and neurons (10),(14).
- Biochemical chain reactions are set in place, some of which may involve the release of excitatory amino acids (1),(2),(3),(10),(14),(15).
- Resulting decrease in cerebral metabolism occurs (1),(2),(3),(10),(14),(15).
- Temporarily decreased cerebral blood flow
- Alternatively, the blow may create immediate neuronal depolarization followed by a refractory period where neural transmission does not happen (1),(2),(3),(14).

RISK FACTORS

- The most consistent risk predictor of slower recovery is the severity of the acute and subacute symptoms. The systematic review of return-to-learn (RTL) and return-to-sport (RTS) within the sixth consensus statement found that continuing to play and delayed access to health care professionals after concussion are associated with longer recovery.
- An athlete with >1 previous concussion may be more likely to have a repeat concussion or any other injury than an athlete without a history of a concussion (9),(10).
- Additional risk factors include type of sport, athlete exposure, certain techniques (e.g., leading with the head, or "spearing" in football or body checking in hockey), certain comorbidities (such as migraines, learning disabilities, mental health problems) (2),(3),(4),(16).

GENERAL PREVENTION

- Prevention was the second priority for future research identified at the Berlin Consensus Conference.
- Most effective prevention strategies have centered around policy change (2):

Policy	Outcome
Disallowing body checking in child or adolescent ice hockey	58% reduction of concussion in games
Decreasing contact practices, limiting amount/intensity of contact and reducing collision time in American football	64% reduction in practice-related concussion

- Protective equipment:
  - Mouthguards were associated with a 28% reduced concussion rate across all age groups in ice hockey (2).
- Training strategies:
  - Neuromuscular training (NMT) warm-up programs completed at least 3 times a week are associated with lower rates of concussion across all age groups in rugby. No specific data exists for other sports.
- Concussion management:
  - Implementation and enforcement of laws and protocols for removal from play; health care provider–driven return-to-play (RTP) progression; and education for athletes, coaches and parents are associated with reduction in *recurrent* concussion rates (17).
- Helmets are not designed to prevent concussions but instead, to prevent skull fractures.
- Guardian caps are soft-shell helmet covers designed to reduce head impact forces in American football.
  - Associated with a reduction in practice concussion rates in the National Football League (NFL).
- There is not a reduction in concussion rates in college or high school football. A large prospective cohort study in high school football showed no decreased risk of SRC (18).

DIAGNOSIS

SRC is an mTBI induced by biomechanical forces. It is a clinical diagnosis.

HISTORY

- Direct blow to the head, sudden rotational or acceleration–deceleration force to the head in the absence of direct trauma, or transmitted force to the head from a blow to other body parts (2),(3),(6),(19)
- Athletes often fail to recognize or report their symptoms. Concussion should be considered in anyone demonstrating signs of a concussion (2),(10).
- Standardized symptom checklists such as the one found in the Sport Concussion Assessment Tool 6 (SCAT6) (SCAT6, Child SCAT6, or SCOAT6) that allow the athlete to score his or her complaints on a scale of 0 to 6 may be useful when evaluating the concussed athlete (2),(13).
  - The SCAT6 is designed to be used as a sideline tool and within the first 72 hours (and up to 1 week). The SCOAT6 is appropriate for office assessments after 72 hours.
- Symptoms are the most sensitive indicator of concussion, but may be underreported (1).
- Athletes may complain of any of the following: headache (HA) or neck pain; feeling off-balance or dizzy; nausea or vomiting; problems with vision or hearing including ringing in the ears; confusion; slowness, fatigue, or sleepiness; irritability or other emotional problems; concentration difficulty; memory problems; dinged; dazed; in a fog; or don't feel right (4),(6),(9).

- Prospectively validated symptoms include HA, dizziness, blurred vision, attention deficit, memory problems, and nausea (9).
  - LOC is uncommon and typically brief (<1 minute) (4).
  - Conscious athletes in whom C-spine trauma is not suspected may exit the field and undergo a more thorough exam (6),(19).
  - Immediately transfer athletes with prolonged LOC, focal neurologic deficits, including asymmetric pupils and declining Glasgow Coma Scale (GCS), worsening symptoms, concern for unstable C-spine injury, athletes with comorbidities (e.g., hemophiliacs), and those with persistent vomiting (1),(6),(9).

PHYSICAL EXAM

- The suspected diagnosis of SRC can include ≥1 of the following clinical domains:
  - Symptoms: somatic (e.g., HA), cognitive (e.g., feeling like in a fog), and/or emotional symptoms (e.g., lability)
  - Physical signs (e.g., LOC, amnesia, neurologic deficit)
  - Balance impairment (e.g., gait unsteadiness)
  - Behavioral changes (e.g., irritability)
  - Cognitive impairment (e.g., slowed reaction times)
  - Sleep/wake disturbance (e.g., somnolence, drowsiness)
- Use SCAT6 to provide standardized on- and off-field assessment of SRC.
- Address airway, breathing, and circulation and assess level of consciousness with Glasgow Coma Scale (GCS) assessment.
- Consider cervical spine (C-spine) immobilization if concern for neck injury (all unconscious athletes should have C-spine immobilization) (6),(10). In general, do not remove the helmet in football or ice hockey players if C-spine injury is suspected (19). The facemask may be removed to allow for airway access.
- Thorough trauma and neurologic assessments are warranted to rule out more serious injury.
- Remove a player who shows any signs or symptoms of an SRC:
  - The player should be evaluated by a physician or other licensed health care provider on site using standard emergency management principles, and particular attention should be given to exclude a C-spine injury:
    - The appropriate disposition of the player must be determined by the treating health care provider in a timely manner. If no health care provider is available, the player should be safely removed from practice or play and an urgent referral to a physician arranged.
      - Once the first aid issues are addressed, an assessment of the concussive injury should be made using the SCAT6 or other sideline assessment tools, with evaluation ideally occurring in a safe, quiet, and distraction-free location.
      - The player should not be left alone after the injury, and serial monitoring for deterioration is essential over the initial few hours after injury.
      - A player with diagnosed SRC should not be allowed to RTP on the day of injury (2).
- The SCAT6 (and the child SCAT6 for patients age 8 to 12 years) was developed by the Concussion in Sport Group and was finalized following the 6th International Conference on Concussion in Sport in Amsterdam, providing important updates to the previously used SCAT5. It has optimum utility in the first 72 hours and up to a week after injury (2).
- The SCAT5 incorporated two prospectively validated tests, the Maddocks score and the standardized assessment of concussion (SAC), into a comprehensive tool (9),(13),(20).
  - The on-field includes a C-spine assessment, GCS, Maddocks, and observable signs.
  - The off-field includes history, GCS, SAC, the modified balance error scoring system (m-BESS) and a new neurologic screening exam, as well as disposition recommendations (2).
- The SCAT6 built on the SCAT5 following a systematic review and expert panel discussion to provide the following modifications (2):
  - Added a more robust set of visible signs and emphasis on cervical assessment
  - Longer word and digit recall lists as well as timed months-in-reverse to improve sensitivity for cognitive deficits
  - Addition of timed dual task gait assessment to evaluate functional balance and cognitive-motor integration
  - Addition of the SCOAT6 to address the need for a standardized office-based assessment allowing for serial evaluations in the subacute and chronic phase (72 hours to weeks from initial injury)
- The SCAT6 should not be used as the only tool to diagnose concussions, to determine whether recovery has occurred, or to decide when to allow an athlete to RTP (1),(2),(13),(20).

DIFFERENTIAL DIAGNOSIS

- Intracranial hemorrhage:
  - Subdural hematoma (acute or subacute)
  - Epidural hematoma, which can result in rapid deterioration after a "lucid interval" (21)
  - Intraparenchymal hemorrhage
- Subarachnoid hemorrhage
- Diffuse axonal injury (DAI) or shear injury to white matter that leads to prolonged LOC and often causes residual deficits (21)
- Other medical conditions, including trauma-induced migraine, peripheral vestibular dysfunction, C-spine injury, skull fracture, medical or psychological comorbidities

DIAGNOSTIC TESTS & INTERPRETATION

Initial Tests (lab, imaging)

- SCAT6 and SCOAT6 for initial evaluation as noted above
- Research conducted on more severe head injury suggests that many genetic and cytokine factors are induced (22).
- As yet, the significance of these factors in concussion is not fully known and no routine laboratory testing is recommended (1),(22).
- Cranial computed tomography (CT) scan: useful in acute imaging to rule out intracranial bleed; consider if prolonged LOC or if symptoms are worsening or failing to resolve in a timely manner (1),(9),(13)
- The Centers for Disease Control and Prevention (CDC) recommends against routine CT scans (in pediatric patients) (23).
- Magnetic resonance imaging (MRI) modalities such as gradient echo and perfusion and diffusion imaging may diagnose structural lesions better than CT scan, but use of MRI does not add to routine concussion evaluation. It may be valuable in cases with atypical or prolonged recovery (1),(13).
- Functional MRI (fMRI) may illustrate the degree of symptoms and their resolution but is not yet part of standard concussion management (1),(13).
- Experimental imaging technology includes positron emission tomography (PET), diffusion tensor imaging, MRI spectroscopy, magnetoencephalography (MEG), and functional connectivity (1),(13).

Diagnostic Procedures/Other

- Clinicians are encouraged to screen for mood symptoms, which may be associated with or exacerbated by concussion, using validated mental health screening instruments such as those included in the Sport Mental Health Assessment Tool (SMHAT) (2).
- Neuropsychological (NP) testing, where accessible, can be used to assess SRC and its sequelae, although there is insufficient evidence to support its use in identification of concussion in preadolescent age groups (2),(16).
- NP testing is not mandatory, nor necessary, for concussion diagnosis or management. When available, it may add value but is never to be used in isolation (2),(6).

- Orthostatic vital signs are an easy and cheap way to assess orthostatic tolerance. It is part of the SCOAT6. The blood pressure and heart rate are measured after 2 minutes lying supine and then the standing blood pressure is measured after 1 minute. Assess for dizziness or light-headedness immediately upon standing and after standing for 1 minute (2).
- The vestibular oculomotor screen (VOMS) is included in the SCOAT6. This can be done on the sideline but validation studies are lacking. There are U.S. Food and Drug Administration (FDA)-approved devices for more objective testing but these are not necessary (2),(3),(13).
- The balance error scoring system (BESS) is a clinical tool for assessing postural stability that has low to moderate diagnostic accuracy in identifying concussion (sensitivity 34–64%, specificity 91%) (16).
  - BESS evaluates the ability of a person to hold without "error" three positions (legs together, single-leg stance, and tandem stance) with eyes closed and hands on the hips. The test is conducted on a firm and a foam surface and can be performed on the sideline or in the training room (9).
  - It has been prospectively validated (9) and has demonstrated practice effect.
  - An m-BESS is one component of the SCAT6.
- The buffalo treadmill test is a validated and effective tool to determine exercise tolerance and/or to prescribe a heart rate-based protocol for exercise recovery (1). A buffalo bike test has been described for those patients who cannot do the treadmill test.

TREATMENT

- Treatment should be on an individual basis according to the burden, nature, and duration of symptoms and other individual factors (e.g., other preexisting medical and psychological factors, sport, position).
- Patient monitoring:
  - A patient should not be left unsupervised following a concussion until a disposition is made (3),(13). There is no indication for the need to wake the patient from sleep.
  - A patient should be monitored for the following: focal neurologic deficit, declining mental status or LOC, and uncontrolled vomiting.
  - Emergent medical care should be sought if any of the preceding occur (1),(6),(9).
- Prior recommendations for strict cognitive and physical rest did not show improved outcomes and management now focuses on early cognitive and physical activity and graduated aerobic exercise initiated within 24 to 72 hours after injury (1),(2),(3),(4). Subthreshold aerobic exercise reduces the risk of persisting symptoms.
- Reduce screen time in the first 48 hours but beyond that the evidence is lacking (2).
- Activity progression should follow a graded and stepwise protocol and is tailored to symptoms and heart rate if available. Athletes should be allowed to progress provided no new symptoms and only mild (increase of no more than 2 points of the preexercise value) and brief (<1 hour) symptom exacerbation is noted (2),(3),(4).
  - The athlete should be fully recovered prior to returning to activities that increase the risk of concussion (i.e., contact practice).
  - RTL typically precedes RTS.
  - Furthermore, there are definitions that aid the clinician (2):
    - *Symptom resolution at rest*: resolution of symptoms associated with the current concussion at rest
    - *Complete symptom resolution*: resolution of symptoms associated with the current concussion at rest with no return of symptoms during or after maximal physical and cognitive exertion
    - *RTL*: return to preinjury learning activities with no new academic support, including school accommodations or learning adjustments
    - *RTS*: completion of the RTS strategy with no symptoms and no clinical findings associated with the current concussion at rest and with maximal physical exertion
- Good sleep hygiene should be encouraged to facilitate recovery as sleep disturbance is associated with increased risk of persisting symptoms (2),(4).
- Address and treat premorbid and comorbid conditions.
- Currently, no medication exists for the treatment of concussion (6).
- Symptom management for HAs and pain can be considered with acetaminophen (but nonsteroidal anti-inflammatory drugs (NSAIDs) and aspirin should be avoided initially) and is not recommended long-term to avoid medication-overuse HAs (3),(6).
- Use of nutraceuticals has high interest in recovery and prevention but evidence is limited and additional research is needed to guide practice recommendations (1).
- Athletes should avoid sedating medicines or substances such as alcohol that may affect cognitive function.

ONGOING CARE

FOLLOW-UP RECOMMENDATIONS

- After sustaining a concussion, an athlete should be evaluated and followed by a medical professional prior to RTL and RTP (1),(2),(3),(19). Depending on the setting and resources, weekly appointments are a reasonable cadence for follow-up visits in the outpatient setting.
- Discussion of the potential risks and harms of driving is recommended but currently no widely accepted return to driving protocol exist (1),(3).
- With both physical and cognitive activity, the absolute avoidance of symptoms in the subacute time period is not recommended. For example, prolonged absences from school are associated with delayed recovery (1),(4).
- Cervicovestibular and/or vestibular rehabilitation is recommended if dizziness, neck pain, and/or HA are present >10 days (1),(4).
- Recovery should be a clinical determination based on individualized assessment of the athlete and their progression (taking into consideration symptoms, physical exam, additional testing as appropriate, etc.) (1),(2).

PROGNOSIS

- Most athletes recover within days to a few weeks after an SRC (4).
- For most athletes, cognitive deficits, balance, and symptoms improve rapidly during the first 2 weeks after injury. There is a sizable minority of youth, high school, and collegiate athletes who take much >10 days to clinically recover and RTS.

COMPLICATIONS

- Previously, "post-concussion syndrome" was diagnosed in athletes who had a prolonged recovery. This is no longer used. Although not currently an ICD-10 diagnosis, the favored terminology is "persisting symptoms after concussion" (PSaC). PSaC is used when symptoms last >4 weeks in all cohorts (children, adolescents, and adults), and are not necessarily representative of ongoing concussive injury to the brain (1),(2).
  - When resources are available, it is generally recommended to refer to concussion clinicians/clinics to address complicated cases and/or persistent symptoms.
  - A multimodal approach by a multidisciplinary team is helpful to address different phenotypical presentations.
- There has been notable interest, and many studies have been conducted to evaluate for association between concussion and future sequelae such as mental health problems, cognitive impairment, and neurologic diseases. The studies conducted to date are methodologically limited as they are unable to examine or account for confounding factors that may affect the development of these issues. As a result, additional research is needed to establish any clear association (1),(2),(4),(6).

- Chronic traumatic encephalopathy (CTE) is more recently identified as a neuropathologic entity suspected to be secondary to repetitive brain trauma (1),(2),(3).
  - It has been shown to be more common in the brains of former professional athletes who donated their brains postmortem (2),(24).
  - A causal relationship between postmortem CTE changes and premortem cognitive and behavioral changes has not been demonstrated and additional research is necessary (1),(6).
- Second impact syndrome is a rare and catastrophic brain injury that occurs when a second injury is sustained in the context of an existing unresolved concussion. The syndrome is controversial with supporting evidence consisting of case series. All cases have been in male athletes aged 13 to 23 years. The pathophysiology appears to be diffuse cerebral edema with resultant increased intracranial pressure and brain herniation (3),(9),(25).
- No evidenced-based guidelines exist for temporary or permanent disqualification after concussion (1),(6),(20).
- Retirement from sports participation is a complex and multifaceted decision and must be individualized. The discussion should be thorough, incorporating a comprehensive clinical evaluation, and should ideally involve a multidisciplinary team (2).

ALERT

Para sport:

- The consensus guidelines produced an expert opinion summary given the complexity and nuance with this population (2):
  - Athletes may benefit from baseline testing.
  - Athletes with a history of CNS injury may require an extended period of initial rest.
  - Recovery testing may require modifications (i.e., arm ergometer instead of bike/treadmill).
  - RTS protocols must encompass the athlete's personal adaptive equipment and guides, when applicable.

REFERENCES

1. Harmon KG, Clugston JR, Dec K, et al. American Medical Society for Sports Medicine position statement on concussion in sport. *Br J Sports Med*. 2019;53(4):213–225.
2. Patricios JS, Schneider KJ, Dvorak J, et al. Consensus statement on concussion in sport: the 6th International Conference on Concussion in Sport–Amsterdam, October 2022. *Br J Sports Med*. 2023;57(11):695–711.
3. Herring S, Kibler WB, Putukian M, et al. Selected issues in sport-related concussion (SRC|mild traumatic brain injury) for the team physician: a consensus statement. *Br J Sports Med*. 2021;55(22):1251–1261.
4. Leddy JJ. Sport-related concussion. *N Engl J Med*. 2025;392(5):483–493.
5. Bakhos LL, Lockhart GR, Myers R, et al. Emergency department visits for concussion in young child athletes. *Pediatrics*. 2010;126(3):e550–e556.
6. Halstead ME, Walter KD, Moffatt K, et al; Council on Sports Medicine and Fitness. Sport-related concussion in children and adolescents. *Pediatrics*. 2018;142(6):e20183074.
7. Karlin AM. Concussion in the pediatric and adolescent population: "different population, different concerns." *PM R*. 2011;3(10 Suppl 2): S369–S379.
8. Meehan WP III, Bachur RG. Sport-related concussion. *Pediatrics*. 2009;123(1):114–123.
9. McCrea M, Hammeke T, Olsen G, et al. Unreported concussion in high school football players: implications for prevention. *Clin J Sport Med*. 2004;14(1):13–17.
10. LaRoche AA, Nelson LD, Connelly PK, et al. Sport-related concussion reporting and state legislative effects. *Clin J Sport Med*. 2016;26(1):33–39.
11. Hootman JM, Dick R, Agel J. Epidemiology of collegiate injuries for 15 sports: summary and recommendations for injury prevention initiatives. *J Athl Train*. 2007;42(2):311–319.
12. Van Pelt KL, Puetz T, Swallow J, et al. Data-driven risk classification of concussion rates: a systematic review and meta-analysis. *Sports Med*. 2021;51(6):1227–1244.
13. McIntosh AS, McCrory P, Finch CF, et al. Does padded headgear prevent head injury in rugby union football? *Med Sci Sports Exerc*. 2009;41(2):306–313.
14. Aubry M, Cantu R, Dvorak J, et al. Summary and agreement statement of the First International Conference on Concussion in Sport, Vienna 2001. Recommendations for the improvement of safety and health of athletes who may suffer concussive injuries. *Br J Sports Med*. 2002;36(1):6–10.
15. Iverson GL, Gardner AJ, Terry DP, et al. Predictors of clinical recovery from concussion: a systematic review. *Br J Sports Med*. 2017;51(12):941–948.
16. Giza CC, Kutcher JS, Ashwal S, et al. Summary of evidence-based guideline update: evaluation and management of concussion in sports: report of the Guideline Development Subcommittee of the American Academy of Neurology. *Neurology*. 2013;80(24):2250–2257.
17. Eliason PH, Galarneau JM, Kolstad AT, et al. Prevention strategies and modifiable risk factors for sport-related concussions and head impacts: a systematic review and meta-analysis. *Br J Sports Med*. 2023;57(12):749–761.
18. Hammer E, Mosiman S, Joachim MR, et al. The association between Guardian Cap use during practices and sport-related concussion risk in high school American football players. *Br J Sports Med*. 2025;59(4):257–262.
19. Inter-Association Task Force for the Appropriate Care of the Spine-Injured Athlete. Prehospital care of the spine-injured athlete. Accessed October 3, 2025. http://www.nata.org/statements/consensus/NATAPreHospital.pdf
20. Guskiewicz KM, Marshall SW, Bailes J, et al. Association between recurrent concussion and late-life cognitive impairment in retired professional football players. *Neurosurgery*. 2005;57(4):719–726.
21. McCrea M, Meier T, Huber D, et al. Role of advanced neuroimaging, fluid biomarkers and genetic testing in the assessment of sport-related concussion: a systematic review. *Br J Sports Med*. 2017;51(12):919–929.
22. Lumba-Brown A, Yeates KO, Sarmiento K, et al. Centers for Disease Control and Prevention guideline on the diagnosis and management of mild traumatic brain injury among children. *JAMA Pediatr*. 2018;172(11):e182853.
23. Bailes JE, Cantu RC. Head injury in athletes. *Neurosurgery*. 2001;48(1):26–45.
24. Ryan LM, Warden DL. Post concussion syndrome. *Int Rev Psychiatry*. 2003;15(4):310–316.
25. McLendon LA, Kralik SF, Grayson PA, et al. The controversial second impact syndrome: a review of the literature. *Pediatr Neurol*. 2016;62:9–17.

ADDITIONAL READING

- Dick RW. Is there a gender difference in concussion incidence and outcomes? *Br J Sports Med*. 2009;43(Suppl 1):i46–i50.
- Echemendia RJ, Brett BL, Broglio S, et al. Sport concussion assessment tool 6 (SCAT6). *Br J Sports Med*. 2023;57(11):622–631.
- Patricios J, Schneider GM, van Ierssel J, et al. Sport concussion office assessment tool 6 (SCOAT6). *Br J Sports Med*. 2023;57(11):651–667.

CLINICAL PEARLS

- No RTS the same day in any suspected concussion
- Recognition and treatment of SRC reduces the risk of prolonged recovery and persistent symptoms.
- Early mild cognitive and physical activity (within 24 to 72 hours) is now recommended for initial management.
- A stepwise and gradual return to academic and physical activities should occur, using symptoms (and heart rate if accessible) to guide progression.
- Persistent symptoms after concussion is the preferred nomenclature for symptoms >4 weeks after concussion. A multimodal and multidisciplinary approach is recommended for treatment.
- Policy changes and rule changes in contact sports have reduced the rate of concussion and decreased subconcussive head trauma.

CONGENITAL CERVICAL SPINE ANOMALIES

Sara L. Neal, MD, MA, CAQSM

BASICS

- Congenital cervical spine anomalies (CCSA) are not common.
- They can exist in isolation or as part of a syndrome; 50% are part of the Klippel-Feil syndrome.
- Many anomalies are asymptomatic.
- CCSA can predispose to neurologic injury of the spinal cord during sporting activities.
- CCSA are frequently divided into (i) upper (C1–C3, including the craniovertebral junction and the atlantoaxial interface) and (ii) lower cervical spine abnormalities.

DESCRIPTION

- CCSA can increase risk for myelopathy from cervical stenosis or instability.
- Specific abnormalities are characterized by cervical spine level include craniovertebral junction.
- Upper cervical anomalies: present at a younger age, usually as instability and neurologic problems after minor trauma
- Lower cervical anomalies: commonly present in adults, usually as advanced degenerative changes in hypermobile segments adjacent to fused segments

EPIDEMIOLOGY

- Congenital cervical spine abnormalities are rare but can predispose to myelopathy.
- Often discovered incidentally
- Frequently associated with other congenital defects such as cardiac, retinal, or renal abnormalities

Prevalence

- Unknown because many are asymptomatic
- Prevalence within certain syndromes may be high (e.g., Klippel-Feil, Morquio, and trisomy 21 [Down] syndromes).
- Estimated incidence of CCSA is approximately 0.29% of live births (1).
- Lower cervical spine fusion is associated with some syndromes (most common is Klippel-Feil syndrome).

ETIOLOGY AND PATHOPHYSIOLOGY

- Many abnormalities arise due to failure of formation or segmentation of the spine during embryologic development (1).
- Five patterns of CCSA carry especially high risk for neurologic injury, even with minor trauma: (i) fusion of the occiput to C1, (ii) fusion of C1–C2, (iii) fusion of C2–C3, (iv) long cervical fusion (more than three segments fused) plus abnormal junction of the occiput with C1, and (v) two fused segments with a single open interface (two vertebra fused adjacent to one normal vertebra which is then adjacent to two more fused) (2).
- Abnormalities in the cervical spine cause altered mechanical transfer of axial loading forces, predisposing to neurologic injury.

Genetics

Teratologic insults (i.e., maternal smoking, alcohol) and mutations in the homeobox (Hox) genes may play a role.

RISK FACTORS

Increased incidence in Klippel-Feil, trisomy 21 (Down), and Morquio syndromes

COMMONLY ASSOCIATED CONDITIONS

- CCSA may be isolated or part of a genetic syndrome.
- Discovery of a cervical spine abnormality should alert the physician to look for associated pathology.
- Klippel-Feil syndrome is defined by the congenital fusion of two or more cervical spine vertebral bodies. Associated abnormalities include:
  - Scoliosis/kyphosis/lordosis (>50%)
  - Hearing impairment (30%)
  - Congenital elevation of the scapula (25–35%)
  - Genitourinary anomalies
  - Cardiovascular anomalies (more common in females), ventricular septal defect most common
  - Rib abnormalities
  - Omovertebral bone (3)
- Lower cervical spine fusion is also seen in fetal alcohol syndrome, Alport syndrome, Crouzon syndrome, and Goldenhar syndrome.
- C1–C2 instability is common in trisomy 21 (Down), Marfan, and Morquio syndromes; juvenile rheumatoid arthritis; and rickets.
- Basilar invagination (narrowing of the foramen magnum) is frequent in achondroplasia.
- Occipitocervical junction anomalies are common in trisomy 21 (Down) syndrome, familial cervical dysplasia, and hyperlaxity syndromes (Ehlers-Danlos and Marfan syndrome).

DIAGNOSIS

HISTORY

CCSA may present with an episode of transient paresis after trauma; more commonly, they are asymptomatic or present with nondescript symptoms such as neck pain or stiffness, headaches, syncope, weakness, numbness, and torticollis.

- Occasionally: symptoms consistent with pyramidal tract or vertebrobasilar insufficiency
- Rarely: cranial nerve or posterior column disturbance
- Those with occipitoatlantal fusion may remain asymptomatic throughout life or present with symptoms after mild trauma; common symptoms (in decreasing frequency): pain in occiput/neck, vertigo, weakness, and ataxia in the lower (and occasionally upper) limbs; occasionally: paresis, paresthesias, hoarseness, dysphagia
- Those with basilar impression and invagination (narrowed foramen magnum) may not have symptoms present until 2nd to 3rd decade.
- Those with occipitoatlantal instability may be symptomatic even in absence of trauma: neck pain, headache, torticollis, weakness, and vertebrobasilar symptoms.
- Those with odontoid anomalies: asymptomatic 50% of the time and average age at diagnosis 19 to 30 years

PHYSICAL EXAM

- Loss of range of motion (ROM), especially lateral bending, is considered a red flag.
- Syndromic clinical signs that may be associated with CCSA include:
  - Pterygium colli (webbed neck), shortened neck, torticollis, low posterior hairline
  - Other anomalies that can be associated with CCSA include dwarfism, funnel chest, pes cavus, syndactylies, jaw anomalies, cleft palate, congenital ear deformities, hypospadias, other genitourinary tract defects, and scoliosis (present in 60% of Klippel-Feil syndrome patients) (2).
- Symptoms prompting further evaluation:
  - Radiculopathy: concerning for nerve root irritation from osteophytes at hypermobile segments adjacent to fused vertebrae
  - Upper extremity weakness, numbness, or pain
  - Long-tract signs (spasticity, hyperreflexia, abnormal reflexes) due to pyramidal compression
  - Posterior column signs (altered sensation to deep touch, vibration, and proprioception)
  - Nystagmus, ataxia, and imbalance from cerebellar herniation

DIFFERENTIAL DIAGNOSIS

- Neurologic abnormalities: extensive but include cervical disk disease, congenital spinal stenosis, vascular disease, Arnold-Chiari malformation, and odontoid nonunion
- Torticollis: congenital muscular torticollis (sternocleidomastoid tumor [SMT], muscular torticollis, postural torticollis without SMT mass or tightness), ocular deficiency, hearing deficit, Grisel and Sandifer syndromes, tumor of posterior fossa, syringomyelia/Arnold-Chiari malformation, rotatory cervical instability, infection, and cervicothoracic scoliosis
- Basilar impression:
  - Secondary basilar impression (owing to softening of osseous skull base): not congenital disease
  - Occasionally, secondary to rickets, osteomalacia, osteogenesis imperfecta, Paget disease, neurofibromatosis, skeletal dysplasia, ankylosing spondylitis, and rheumatoid arthritis
  - Occasionally, erroneously diagnosed as multiple sclerosis, posterior fossa tumors, amyotrophic lateral sclerosis, or traumatic injury

DIAGNOSTIC TESTS & INTERPRETATION

Initial Tests (lab, imaging)

- X-rays: cervical spine anteroposterior (AP) view; open-mouth odontoid view; lateral views in neutral, flexion, and extension ± thoracolumbar posteroanterior and lateral views; abnormalities seen include:
  - AP views: Look for vertebral fusion of facets and spinous processes; AP narrowing of the vertebral bodies (wasp-waist sign); presence of hemivertebrae, omovertebral bone, or spina bifida; condylar dysplasia.
  - On flexion/extension views: Look for decreased movement between fused segments and increased movement between adjacent, nonfused portions.
  - Open-mouth view: odontoid anomalies
  - Lateral flexion/extension: Evaluate translational instability (anterior or posterior translation >5 mm) or fusion.
  - Basilar impression is difficult to see on x-ray.
  - Computed tomography (CT) scan useful for suspected atlanto-occipital fusion, basilar invagination, canal stenosis, and odontoid abnormalities
- Magnetic resonance imaging (MRI): indicated in patients with neurologic deficits; excellent for evaluation of canal stenosis, cord compression, disk bulge/herniation, and craniovertebral junction narrowing; evaluates for associated conditions such as myelomalacia, syringohydromyelia, diastematomyelia, diplomyelia, and Chiari I malformation:
  - Obtain for full evaluation of atlantoaxial instability, basilar invagination, and canal stenosis.

Diagnostic Procedures/Other

Arteriography (or magnetic resonance angiography) if surgery planned or if symptoms warrant (basilar impression, occipitoatlantal fusion, atlas aplasia) because there is increased incidence of vertebral artery anomalies with CCSA

TREATMENT

- Conservative treatment (e.g., activity modification, bracing, and traction) may reduce symptoms. Indications for and timing of surgical stabilization are not clearly defined; consider for significant pain despite conservative measures.
- Spinal stabilization recommended in presence of a neurologic lesion or instability
- If a neurologic process occurs in presence of known canal stenosis, decompression ± stabilization should be considered.

MEDICATION

Analgesics (i.e., acetaminophen, nonsteroidal anti-inflammatory drugs [NSAIDs]) for headache

ISSUES FOR REFERRAL

Generally, all congenital cervical disease should be referred to neurosurgeon and/or neurologist for concurrent observation and management.

SURGERY/OTHER PROCEDURES

- Surgical indication: Posterior column signs and symptoms (most common indication for surgery) require decompression of posterior elements.
- Procedures:
  - Posterior fusion of occiput-atlas complex in occipitoatlantal fusion
  - Suboccipital decompression with decompressive laminectomies of atlas and axis with posterior fusion in basilar impression
- Surgical indication: odontoid abnormalities with any of the following coexisting:
  - Myelopathy, instability of ≥10 mm in flexion and extension, progressive instability, or persistent neck pain with C1–C2 instability
  - Procedure: atlantoaxial arthrodesis (± excision of odontoid)
- Surgical indication: occipitoatlantal instability:
  - Procedure: arthrodesis
- Surgical indication (rarely required): familial cervical dysplasia; procedure: posterior fusion of C1–C2

ONGOING CARE

FOLLOW-UP RECOMMENDATIONS

Patient Monitoring

Return-to-play recommendations are primarily expert opinions.

- Absolute contraindications to contact/collision sports: odontoid abnormalities, occipitoatlantal fusion, Klippel-Feil syndrome with fusions above C3, and atlantoaxial instability (2),(3)[C]
- Caution but no absolute contraindication for Klippel-Feil syndrome with fusion of one or two interspaces below C3; full cervical ROM; and absence of occipital cervical anomalies, instability, disk disease, or degenerative changes (2),(3)[C]

PATIENT EDUCATION

- All congenital cervical diseases: Trauma can be catastrophic (more often with translational instability and with stenotic cervical canal).
- CCSA that carry especially high risk for neurologic injury, even with minor trauma: (i) fusion of the occiput to C1 or C2, (ii) fusion of C2–C3, (iii) long cervical fusion (more than three segments fused) plus abnormal junction of the occiput with C1, and (iv) two fused segments with a single open interface (Two vertebra fused adjacent to one normal vertebra which is then adjacent to two more fused.)

PROGNOSIS

Klippel-Feil syndrome:

- Hypermobility of upper cervical spine: increased risk for neurologic issues
- Lower cervical spine involvement: increased risk for degenerative disease
- Overall prognosis is good, with most patients remaining relatively asymptomatic with occasional mild complaints of headaches, nonradicular weakness, and numbness.

COMPLICATIONS

CCSA may be asymptomatic but can predispose to catastrophic outcomes with minor trauma, including paresis or sudden death.

REFERENCES

1. Passias PG, Poorman GW, Jalai CM, et al. Incidence of congenital spinal abnormalities among pediatric patients and their association with scoliosis and systemic anomalies. *J Pediatr Orthop.* 2019;39(8):e608–e613.
2. Litrenta J, Bi AS, Dryer JW. Klippel-Feil syndrome: pathogenesis, diagnosis, and management. *J Am Acad Orthop Surg.* 2021;29(22):951–960.
3. Frikha R. Klippel-Feil syndrome: a review of the literature. *Clin Dysmorphol.* 2020;29(1):35–37.

ADDITIONAL READING

- Babcock L, Olsen CS, Jaffe DM, et al. Cervical spine injuries in children associated with sports and recreational activities. *Pediatr Emerg Care.* 2018;34(10):677–686.
- Bouchard M, Bauer JM, Bompadre V, et al. An updated algorithm for radiographic screening of upper cervical instability in patients with Down syndrome. *Spine Deform.* 2019;7(6):950–956.
- Courvoisier A. Congenital cervical spinal deformities. *Orthop Traumatol Surg Res.* 2023;109(1 Suppl):103459.

CLINICAL PEARLS

- Discovery of a cervical spine abnormality should alert the physician to look for associated pathology, especially in cardiovascular, renal, and retinal systems.
- Absolute contraindications to contact/collision sports: odontoid abnormalities, occipitoatlantal fusion, Klippel-Feil syndrome with fusions above C3, and atlantoaxial instability (2),(3)[C]
- Caution but no absolute contraindication for Klippel-Feil syndrome with fusion of one or two interspaces below C3; full cervical ROM; and absence of occipital cervical anomalies, instability, disk disease, or degenerative changes (2)[C]
- X-rays: basic: cervical spine AP view and open-mouth odontoid view; consider lateral views in neutral, flexion, and extension.
- CT scan useful for suspected atlanto-occipital fusion, basilar invagination, and canal stenosis; also used for flexion/extension evaluation of odontoid abnormalities
- MRI: indicated in patients with neurologic deficits; excellent for evaluation canal stenosis, cord compression, disk bulge/herniation, and craniovertebral junction narrowing; evaluates for associated conditions

C

CONGENITAL QT SYNDROMES

Chau Bui, DO ▪ Paul Meirick, MD ▪ Suraj A. Achar, MD, FAAFP, CAQSM

BASICS

DESCRIPTION

- Channelopathies refer to a group of inherited arrhythmogenic diseases caused by mutations in genes encoding for ion channel proteins in cardiomyocytes that disrupt the balance of currents in the cardiac action potential. These disruptions may lead to ventricular arrhythmias and sudden cardiac death (SCD).
- The channelopathies include long QT syndrome (LQTS), short QT syndrome (SQTS), Brugada syndrome (see chapter on Brugada Syndrome), and catecholaminergic polymorphic ventricular tachycardia (CPVT) (see supplemental materials for CPVT).
- Congenital QT syndromes:
  - LQTS is a collection of disorders of prolonged myocardial repolarization characterized by a long QT interval:
    - There are two clinical phenotypes of inherited LQTS.
    - Romano-Ward syndrome (autosomal dominant):
      - Characterized by LQTS without other cardiac abnormalities or deafness
      - Most common phenotype
    - Jervell and Lange-Nielsen syndrome (autosomal recessive):
      - Characterized by LQTS and sensorineural deafness
      - Typically has a more malignant course
  - SQTS is a disorder of accelerated myocardial repolarization characterized by a short QT interval:
    - Mutations of potassium channel genes and loss of function of calcium channel genes
    - Associated with malignant atrial and ventricular arrhythmias and SCD

EPIDEMIOLOGY

Often presents in childhood (mean onset age 14 years) but may be as early as the newborn period or go undiagnosed into middle age.

Prevalence

- Congenital LQTS:
  - Incidence estimated at 1:2,000 to 3,000; however, the true incidence of mutations in the population is likely much higher.
  - Congenital LQTS is associated with 3,000 to 4,000 sudden deaths in childhood in the United States per year.
- Congenital SQTS: 1:10,000—uncommon (1)

ETIOLOGY AND PATHOPHYSIOLOGY

- LQTS: >13 genes have been identified that encode for subunits of the potassium, sodium, or calcium voltage-dependent ion channels.
- SQTS: Seven genes that encode potassium and calcium channels have been identified.

Genetics

- LQTS: >13 genes identified, with mutations of *KCNQ1* (LQTS1), *KCNH2* (LQTS2), *SCN5A* (LQTS3) accounting for over 90% of cases
- SQTS: Gain of function mutations in potassium channel encoding genes *KCNH2* (SQTS1), *KCNQ1* (SQTS2), *KCNJ2* (SQTS3) (2) and loss of function mutations in several calcium channel encoding genes result in accelerated repolarization.

RISK FACTORS

The primary risk factor for most channelopathies is genetic:

- LQTS:
  - Acquired LQTS can be caused by medications and metabolic or electrolyte abnormalities, particularly hypokalemia and hypomagnesemia.
  - Family history of SCD: First-degree relatives had greater cardiac events than second-degree relatives (26% vs. 10%).
  - Risk factors for precipitating a fatal arrhythmia in a patient with LQTS include swimming (primarily LQTS1) and any strenuous exercise.
  - A corrected QT interval (QTc) >0.46 second
  - Female gender
- SQTS:
  - SCD most often occurs during rest or sleep (83%), whereas minority occurred during emotional stress or physical effort (3).

GENERAL PREVENTION

SCD resulting from QT syndromes may be prevented by carefully screening and identifying athletes with the condition.

- The preparticipation evaluation is the most important tool for identifying athletes with symptoms that may represent an inherited channelopathy.
- Any athlete with symptoms of palpitations, syncope, presyncope, any collapse, or with a family history of SCD or "accidental" death should be further evaluated with the tools reviewed below.
- Automatic external defibrillators (AEDs) are another important tool in preventing SCD from undiagnosed QT syndrome.

COMMONLY ASSOCIATED CONDITIONS

For certain patients with LQTS only, sensorineural hearing loss is associated.

DIAGNOSIS

Diagnosis is based mostly on electrocardiogram (ECG) pattern because patients may be symptomatic or asymptomatic.

HISTORY

- Pertinent history in screening athletes:
  - Have you ever passed out, become dizzy, or had chest pain during or after exercise?
  - Do you get tired more quickly than others during exercise?

Meds Associated with QT Prolongation

Antiarrhythmic Drugs

Quinidine
Procainamide
Disopyramide
Amiodarone
Sotalol
Dofetilide, ibutilide, azimilide, sematilide

Antimicrobial Drugs

Macrolide antibiotics: erythromycin, telithromycin, clarithromycin, azithromycin (minor)
Pentamidine
Fluoroquinolone: moxifloxacin, gatifloxacin, levofloxacin, sparfloxacin
Spiramycin
Chloroquine, halofantrine, mefloquine

Psychotropic Drugs

Thioridazine
Phenothiazines
Tricyclic antidepressants
Haloperidol
Selective serotonin reuptake inhibitors (SSRIs)
Risperidone
Methadone

Antihistamines

Terfenadine
Astemizole

Other Drugs

Diuretics
Motility drugs: cisapride, domperidone
Droperidol
HIV protease inhibitors
Vasodilators: prenylamine, bepridil, mibefradil
Ketanserin
Ranolazine
Organophosphate insecticides
Cocaine
Papaverine
Chloral hydrate
Arsenic trioxide
Some Chinese Herbs

ALERT

Has anyone in the family died suddenly and unexpectedly before the age of 50 years? (*Remember to ask about family members who died of accidental causes such as sudden infant death syndrome, drownings, and motor vehicle accidents because they may be clues to an undiagnosed family history of channelopathy.*)

  - Have you ever had a heart abnormality diagnosed by a doctor?
  - Have you ever had an abnormal heart rate (HR), palpitations, or irregular heartbeats?
  - Has a physician ever denied or restricted your participation in sports for heart problems?
  - Have any of your relatives ever had cardiomyopathy, Marfan syndrome, LQTS, SQTS, or significant heart arrhythmias?
- Pertinent history in potentially affected athletes:
  - LQTS:
    - Most commonly asymptomatic
    - Common symptoms include palpitations, syncope, presyncope, seizures, and cardiac arrest.
    - Hearing loss (occurs in Jervell and Lange-Nielsen phenotype patients only)
    - Arrhythmias are most commonly precipitated by exercise, followed by exercise and emotion together, emotion alone, and less commonly, loud noise or anesthesia.
    - Use of any medications that may cause LQTS or torsade de pointes
    - LQTS1: susceptible to cardiac events with physical exertion (62%) and emotional stress (26%), especially prone during swimming (4)
    - LQTS2: emotional triggers and events occurring during sleep without arousal; auditory events (alarm clocks)
    - LQTS3: susceptible during sleep without arousal
  - SQTS:
    - Most common clinical presentations are cardiac arrest followed by palpitations, syncope, and atrial fibrillation (2).
    - No pattern or association with onset as it has been reported at rest, after startle, and during daily activities
    - Strong family history component

PHYSICAL EXAM

- Because patients with QT syndrome typically have structurally normal hearts, it is not uncommon to observe a completely normal examination when a life-threatening arrhythmia is not present.

- When arrhythmias are present, the examination may be notable for bradycardia or tachycardia, either regular or irregular, depending on the patient's rhythm.

DIFFERENTIAL DIAGNOSIS

Brugada syndrome, CPVT, acquired LQTS with its many reversible metabolic and drug-induced causes, acute coronary syndrome, true right bundle branch block (RBBB), pericarditis, drug-induced ventricular tachycardia (VT) or ventricular fibrillation (VF)

DIAGNOSTIC TESTS & INTERPRETATION

Initial Tests (lab, imaging)

- Genetic testing for identifying the type of LQTS is available:
  - Indications for testing include family history of unexplained early cardiac death, family members with history of LQTS, or clinical suspicion based on patient's personal history.
- In the setting of a life-threatening arrhythmia, it may be indicated to evaluate ischemic or metabolic causes with a basic or comprehensive metabolic panel and cardiac enzymes:
  - Hypomagnesemia, hypocalcemia, and hypokalemia may precipitate torsade de pointes in those with a given mutation.

Diagnostic Procedures/Other

ECG is the most important initial diagnostic tool. Holter monitors and echocardiograms may be of use as well. Recently, exercise testing (treadmill or bicycle) has become part of the diagnostic workup (5).

ALERT

Prolonged QTc: 440 to 460 milliseconds represent 90 to 95th percentile in general population (>470 ms in men or >480 milliseconds in women (99th percentile) should prompt further evaluation (4).
- Confirm QTc using Bazett formula ($QTc = QT / \sqrt{RR}$; QT in millisecond, RR in seconds)—although Bazett correction decreases in accuracy with extremes in HR (ensure HR >50 bpm) (4).
- Common potential ventricular arrhythmias are torsade de pointes (type of polymorphic VT), multiform ventricular premature beats, uniform ventricular premature beats, and monomorphic VT.

ALERT

Note: Degree of LQTS penetrance is variable, so some patients may have normal or borderline QTc.
- SQTS: QTc <360 milliseconds in symptomatic patient or with familial history of sudden death at young age. 240 to 330 milliseconds is generally considered affected even if asymptomatic and requires further workup usually with genetic testing (6).

TREATMENT

- Prehospital:
  - In the case that any patient with a QT syndrome converts into a life-threatening arrhythmia in the field, the most useful immediate tool and treatment is an AED.
- Congenital LQTS:
  - All patients with congenital or acquired QT syndrome should be referred to an electrophysiologist or cardiologist.

ALERT

All symptomatic patients should be treated owing to the high risk for SCD. This risk may be up to 50–60% in 10 years.

  - Treatment of asymptomatic individuals is less clear but may be strongly considered in the following asymptomatic patients: newborns and infants, patients with sensorineural hearing loss, patients with siblings with LQTS and SCD, patients with QTc >0.60 second.
  - Treatment includes lifestyle modification, medical therapy with β-blockers or other agents, avoidance of QT prolonging medications, and may include surgical options such as an implantable cardioverter-defibrillator (ICD).
- Congenital SQTS: Mainstay of treatment is ICD, consider medical therapy as adjunct to ICD or if there is a contraindication to ICD placement.

MEDICATION

- LQTS:
  - β-Blockers reduce the risk of syncope and SCD (4) [B]; first-line therapy unless contraindicated
  - Propranolol (2 to 3 mg/kg/day) or nadolol (1 to 1.5 mg/kg/day); atenolol and metoprolol are associated with more clinical failures (4).
  - Efficacy of β-blockers varies by LQTS genotype (maximally effective in LQTS1).
  - Adjunctive treatments include potassium, flecainide, mexiletine, or ranolazine.
- SQTS: Quinidine is effective in prolonging the QT interval (3).

SURGERY/OTHER PROCEDURES

- LQTS:
  - ICD placement or left cardiac sympathetic denervation
    Recommended for patients who fail β-blockers (syncope or VT), have survived cardiac arrest, or have risk factors for SCD (4)[B]
  - Left cardiac sympathetic denervation:
    - Removal of the first four thoracic ganglia
    - Reserved for patients who fail other treatments or ICD contraindicated (4)[C]
- SQTS:
  - ICD placement is first-line treatment (6).
  - Medication is only an adjunct or to be used if contraindication to ICD placement.

ADMISSION, INPATIENT, AND NURSING CONSIDERATIONS

As always, all patients who present with a life-threatening arrhythmia should be treated emergently with cardioversion and/or pharmacotherapy as dictated by standard advanced cardiac life support (ACLS).

ONGOING CARE

All patients with channelopathies should be followed regularly by a cardiologist or electrophysiologist. Education and restrictions regarding exercise are crucial to survival.

FOLLOW-UP RECOMMENDATIONS

Return-to-play decisions:

- Previously, athletes were limited to class IA sports (low static and low dynamic stresses): billiards, bowling, cricket, curling, golf, or riflery.
- The latest American Heart Association/American College of Cardiology (AHA/ACC) 2015 participation guidelines: In a symptomatic athlete, competitive sports participation may be considered following expert consultation from electrophysiologist and cardiologist, initiation of treatment, appropriate precautionary measures, and the athlete has been asymptomatic for at least 3 months.

ALERT

Asymptomatic athlete with genotype-positive/phenotype-negative (concealed channelopathy) may participate in all competitive sports with appropriate precautionary measures (avoidance of QT-prolonging drugs, appropriate electrolyte/hydration replenishment, avoidance of hyperthermic conditions, acquire personal AED, and establish appropriate emergency action plan).

- Athlete with an ICD may be permitted to participate in sports if there have been no shocks for 3 months.
- Recreational swimming should be avoided by all patients unless proven to be a genotype other than LQTS1.

ALERT

Caution should be used to avoid sports where impaired consciousness would be dangerous or lethal, such as with SCUBA diving, swimming, weight lifting with free weights, and horseback riding.

- Avoid medications that may cause QT prolongation (as listed in table).

REFERENCES

1. Drezner JA, Ackerman MJ, Cannon BC, et al. Abnormal electrocardiographic findings in athletes: recognizing changes suggestive of primary electrical disease. *Br J Sports Med*. 2013;47(3):153–167.
2. Brugada R, Hong K, Dumaine R, et al. Sudden death associated with short-QT syndrome linked to mutations in HERG. *Circulation*. 2004;109(1):30–35.
3. Hammond-Haley M, Patel R, Providência R, et al. Exercise restrictions for patients with inherited cardiac conditions: current guidelines, challenges, and limitations. *Int J Cardiol*. 2016;209:234–241.
4. Gomez AT, Prutkin JM, Rao AL. Evaluation and management of athletes with long QT syndrome: an evolved paradigm. *Sports Health*. 2016;8(6):527–535.
5. Yee LA, Han HC, Davies B, et al. Sex differences and utility of treadmill testing in long-QT syndrome. *J Am Heart Assoc*. 2022;11(18):e025108.
6. Mareddy C, Thomas MT, McDaniel G, et al. Exercise in the genetic arrhythmia syndromes—a review. *Clin Sports Med*. 2022;41(3):485–510.

ADDITIONAL READING

Ackerman MJ, Zipes DP, Kovacs RJ, et al. Eligibility and disqualification recommendations for competitive athletes with cardiovascular abnormalities: Task Force 10: the cardiac channelopathies: a scientific statement from the American Heart Association and American College of Cardiology. *Circulation*. 2015;132(22):e326–e329.

CLINICAL PEARLS

- Any athlete with symptoms of palpitations, syncope, presyncope, any collapse, or with a family history of SCD or "accidental" death should be further evaluated with the tools reviewed.
- Asymptomatic athlete with genotype-positive/phenotype-negative (concealed channelopathy) may participate in all competitive sports with appropriate precautionary measures (avoidance of QT-prolonging drugs, appropriate electrolyte/hydration replenishment, avoidance of hyperthermic conditions, acquire personal AED, and establish appropriate emergency action plan).
- Caution should be used to avoid sports where impaired consciousness would be dangerous or lethal, such as with SCUBA diving, swimming, weight lifting with free weights, and horseback riding.
- Treatment of asymptomatic individuals is less clear but may be strongly considered in the following asymptomatic patients: with sensorineural hearing loss, patients with siblings with LQTS and SCD, and patients with QTc >0.60 second.

CORNEAL ABRASIONS

Nilesh Shah, MD, FAAFP, CAQSM • Brandon Arehart, DO

BASICS

DESCRIPTION

- Removal or scraping away of the superficial layers of the cornea (stratified squamous epithelium) without penetration of Bowman membrane
- In the general population, injury usually results from contact lenses misuse but also can be attributed to foreign bodies, tangential shearing injuries, and contusion to the globe.
- In the workplace, both physical trauma and chemical trauma may be an etiology for corneal abrasions.
- In sports, the mechanism is more commonly direct trauma.
- Severe corneal injuries also can involve the deeper, thicker stromal layer; in this situation, the term *corneal ulcer* may be used.

EPIDEMIOLOGY

- Most common eye injury after soft tissue injuries
- More common in sports with projectiles/balls
- More common in collision sports

RISK FACTORS

- Collision/contact/combat sports
- Sports with projectiles/balls
- Contact lens use
- Failure to wear eye protection: There were reportedly a 26% decrease in pediatric ocular injuries between 2006 and 2014 that may be attributed to preventative eyewear precautions (1)[B].

GENERAL PREVENTION

- Single-piece construction protective eyewear with 3-mm polycarbonate lenses will likely reduce the risk of eye injuries.
- Mandatory protective eyewear rules in sports such as field hockey, women's lacrosse, and hockey have demonstrated significantly fewer eye injuries in these sports (1)[A].

COMMONLY ASSOCIATED CONDITIONS

- Hyphema: blood in the anterior chamber
- Hypopyon: pus in anterior chamber
- Globe perforation/rupture: Look for vitreous leak.
- Intraocular foreign body
- Rust ring: metal object injury
- Orbital fracture
- Iridodialysis: defect of the iris caused by its separation from the scleral spur
- Corneal ulcer: penetrating superficial cornea, often superimposed infection
- Recurrent erosion syndrome

DIAGNOSIS

HISTORY

- Mechanism of injury guides physical exam for associated injuries and delineates the need for further studies.
- History of previous injuries: possible viral keratitis or recurrent erosion syndrome
- Contact lenses history (hard, soft, overuse): Symptoms are usually better with contact in place, acting as a bandage.
- Risk of foreign body: particular sports (dirt, rocks, artificial grass fields, etc.), windy conditions, etc.

PHYSICAL EXAM

- Signs and symptoms include:
  - Pain
  - Redness
  - Lacrimation
  - Foreign-body sensation
  - Photophobia
  - Blepharospasm
  - Possibly decreased visual acuity depending size and central location over the pupil
- Physical examination includes:
  - General bony orbital exam
  - Cranial nerve assessment
  - Ocular movements
  - Visual fields
  - Visual acuity
  - Topical anesthetic and/or cycloplegic agents: may be needed to decrease pain and photophobia for optimal exam
  - Loupe with good light or slit lamp (preferable)
  - Fluorescein dye drops/strips: sharply demarcate defects in corneal epithelium and help to differentiate traumatic abrasion (linear or geographic pattern) from herpes keratitis (dendritic pattern with terminal bulbs). Abrasion will appear yellow under normal light and green under cobalt blue light.
  - Seidel sign: Evidence of vitreous fluid leak under cobalt blue light indicates globe rupture or penetration.
  - Anterior chamber and corneal exam: slit lamp preferred to rule out associated injuries (hyphema, perforation)
  - Eversion of upper and lower lids: Identify any foreign bodies under tarsal plate. If discovered, it must be removed by trained individual.

ALERT

- Intraocular pressure (IOP) is considered a vital part of the ocular exam *unless* perforation or rupture is suspected.
- Performing IOP in setting of globe rupture risks worsening extravasation of intraocular contents when pressure is applied to diagnose.

DIFFERENTIAL DIAGNOSIS

- Foreign body
- Corneal laceration
- Perforation/ruptured globe
- Corneal ulcer
- Acute angle closure glaucoma
- Infectious keratitis: herpetic, bacterial, fungal
- Photokeratitis/retinitis
- Conjunctivitis: infectious/allergic
- Iridocyclitis
- Iritis
- Scleritis/episcleritis
- Optic neuritis
- Retinal detachment
- Vitreous detachment
- Blepharitis
- Trichiasis
- Canaliculitis
- Periorbital cellulitis
- Orbital fracture
- Dry eye syndrome

DIAGNOSTIC TESTS & INTERPRETATION

- Imaging is typically not necessary for simple corneal abrasions. A detailed ocular physical exam is usually enough.
- One should consider imaging if there are concerns for other diagnoses such as orbital fractures, metallic foreign body, or other intraocular or soft tissue injuries.
  - Computed tomography (CT) scan is the gold standard imaging of choice for any concern of orbital trauma, fractures, soft tissue injuries, intraocular injuries, and foreign bodies (2)[B]. These can frequently be 3-D reconstructed as well for surgical planning.
  - Orbital series radiographs, ultrasound (US) (brightness [B]-scan), magnetic resonance imaging (MRI) can all be considered depending on resources available but are believed to be less sensitive and specific than CT scans.
  - Avoid MRI if suspected metal fragment.
  - Avoid US/B-scan if suspected ruptured globe.

TREATMENT

GENERAL MEASURES

The goal of treatment is to prevent bacterial superinfection, speed healing, and provide symptomatic relief to patients.

ALERT

- For initial pain control and immediate diagnostics, topical ocular anesthetics (i.e., proparacaine, tetracaine) can provide temporary relief and aid in completing a full physical exam (3)[A],(4)[A].
- However, improper prolonged use of ocular anesthetics has feared complications of corneal melting and persistent corneal defects as they may block protective corneal reflexes and sensation, potentially increasing the risk of further ocular injury (3)[B].
- This being said, there are studies that have found no differences in healing at 72 hours between topical anesthetics and control groups (3)[B],(4)[B]. If there are any considerations for prescribing topical anesthetics, it is advocated for dilute proparacaine formularies as opposed to full dose tetracaine, but there is fear of prolonged complications (5)[C].

MEDICATION

- Tetanus vaccination prophylaxis should be considered in individuals who are not up-to-date.
- Antibiotics:
  - General population: broad-spectrum topical antibiotic ointments or drops: aid with lubrication and infection prophylaxis (e.g., erythromycin, sulfacetamide, fluoroquinolones)
  - Contact lens associated: often colonized with *Pseudomonas aeruginosa* and other gram-negative organisms. Consider a *fluoroquinolone* or *aminoglycoside* (e.g., ciprofloxacin, ofloxacin, gentamicin).
  - Water sport associated: pseudomonal coverage (e.g., fluoroquinolones/aminoglycosides)
- Pain control:
  - Topical nonsteroidal anti-inflammatory drugs (NSAIDs): In the past have lacked evidence to support their use. However, a more recent systematic review and meta-analysis from 2021, has demonstrated strong evidence to suggest reduced pain in the first 48 hours and need for oral analgesics when compared to controls and against other medications (5)[A].

- Cycloplegic anticholinergic agents: Historically have been used for pain control in corneal abrasions. More recent studies have shown they do not significantly reduce pain scores. They may be considered for relief of ciliary muscle spasm–related pain if present. Caution should be used in patients with narrow angles because mydriatic medications can lead to acute angle–closure glaucoma (4)[A].
- Preservative-free artificial tears can aid in topical lubrication and decrease irritation.
- Oral analgesics: Oral anti-inflammatory medications and narcotic pain medications may be used for pain control. These may be cheaper than topical NSAIDs and can be taken into consideration. One must weigh the risks of systemic toxicities and narcotic abuse versus financial costs when deciding what to prescribe.

ISSUES FOR REFERRAL

- Immediate ophthalmology referral if significant vision loss or diplopia, corneal infiltrate/ulcer, hypopyon, hyphema, dilated/nonreactive/irregular pupil, or evidence of penetrating eye injury
- Urgent referral for recurrent abrasions, erosions, larger abrasions, rust rings, infections, corneal ulcers, or failure to improve 24 to 48 hours after initial treatment

ADDITIONAL THERAPIES

- Topical antibiotics are typically continued for 4 times per day until asymptomatic for 24 hours or 3 to 5 days after reepithelialization.
- Watch for recurrent erosion syndrome—sudden pain, redness, and tearing after initial improvement—possibly requiring débridement and further specialized treatment.
- Pressure patch: Once a traditional standard of treatment, eye patching is no longer recommended treatment as multiple studies have shown no difference in pain control when compared to controls and a trend toward increased complications (5)[A],(6)[A].
- Bandage contact lenses: Soft lenses that are placed day and night and thought to enhance comfort and healing. However, there is insufficient evidence to support or refute their efficacy or safety (5)[A].

ONGOING CARE

FOLLOW-UP RECOMMENDATIONS

- Most uncomplicated corneal abrasions heal in 24 to 48 hours. Daily monitoring until reepithelialization and symptom resolution is recommended.
- If the abrasion is small (4 mm or less), vision is normal, and symptoms are improving, referral is not necessarily needed.
- Follow-up within 24 hours is recommended for those with large abrasions (>4 mm), contact lenses–related abrasions, and for those whose visual acuity is affected.
- Contact lenses wearers: Recommend daily monitoring until abrasion is healed. Discard old contact lenses. New lenses should not be worn until abrasion is healed and symptoms have resolved.

PATIENT EDUCATION

- Eye protection during the healing process is important, especially in patients whose jobs put them at increased risk of corneal abrasions or ultraviolet (UV) exposure.
- Educate about proper use of contact lens wearing and prevention of future injuries.
- Eye rest (i.e., minimize reading or heavy computer work that requires substantial eye movement): This helps to minimize irritation and interference with reepithelialization.
- Avoid light or wear sunglasses for comfort if significant photophobia is present.
- If the patient is unconscious or cannot voluntarily close his or her eyelids (e.g., Bell palsy or other neuropathies), eyelids may be taped closed and/or use of lubrication and artificial tears should be considered.

PROGNOSIS

- The prognosis is usually good, with healing and full recovery of vision if prompt evaluation and treatment are initiated.
- Some deep abrasions heal with a scar. If this occurs in the central visual axis (area of the cornea directly over the pupil), visual acuity may be permanently lost. Deep abrasions within the central visual axis should be considered for ophthalmologic referral.
- Healing of minor abrasions is expected within 24 to 48 hours. Extensive or deep abrasions may require a week to heal.

COMPLICATIONS

- Deep corneal involvement may result in facet formation in the epithelium or scar formation in the stroma.
- Central, large abrasions can result in at least temporary loss of visual acuity.
- Progression of abrasions into corneal ulcers may lead to devastating outcomes.
- Abrasions involving exposure to vegetable matter are at risk of fungal ulcers.
- Sight-threatening infections
- Abrasions from contact lenses use are at risk for *Pseudomonas* and amoebic keratitis.
- Recurrent erosion syndrome
- Allergic reactions to treatment medications
- Loss of school and work time/productivity
- Use of mydriatics may lead to systemic anticholinergic symptoms or can induce acute angle closure glaucoma in narrow anterior chamber individuals.
- Chronic use of topical anesthetics run the risk of corneal ulcers.

REFERENCES

1. Matsa E, Shi J, Wheeler KK, et al. Trends in US emergency department visits for pediatric acute ocular injury. *JAMA Ophthalmol*. 2018;136(8):895–903.
2. Cellina M, Cè M, Marziali S, et al. Computed tomography in traumatic orbital emergencies: a pictorial essay-imaging findings, tips, and report flowchart. *Insights Imaging*. 2022;13(1):4.
3. Puls HA, Cabrera D, Murad MH, et al. Safety and effectiveness of topical anesthetics in corneal abrasions: systematic review and meta-analysis. *J Emerg Med*. 2015;49(5):816–824.
4. Thiel B, Sarau A, Ng D. Efficacy of topical analgesics in pain control for corneal abrasions: a systematic review. *Cureus*. 2017;9(3):e1121.
5. Yu CW, Kirubarajan A, Yau M, et al. Topical pain control for corneal abrasions: a systematic review and meta-analysis. *Acad Emerg Med*. 2021;28(8):890–908.
6. Lim CH, Turner A, Lim BX. Patching for corneal abrasion. *Cochrane Database Syst Rev*. 2016;7(7):CD004764.

ADDITIONAL READING

- Ahmed F, House RJ, Feldman BH. Corneal abrasions and corneal foreign bodies. *Prim Care*. 2015;42(3):363–375.
- American Academy of Pediatrics Committee on Sports Medicine and Fitness. Protective eyewear for young athletes. *Pediatrics*. 2004;113(3):619–622.
- Aslam SA, Sheth HG, Vaughan AJ. Emergency management of corneal injuries. *Injury*. 2007;38(5):594–597.
- Calder LA, Balasubramanian S, Fergusson D. Topical nonsteroidal anti-inflammatory drugs for corneal abrasions: meta-analysis of randomized trials. *Acad Emerg Med*. 2005;12(5):467–473.
- Heimmel MR, Murphy MA. Ocular injuries in basketball and baseball: what are the risks and how can we prevent them? *Curr Sports Med Rep*. 2008;7(5):284–288.
- Lincoln AE, Caswell SV, Almquist JL, et al. Effectiveness of the women's lacrosse protective eyewear mandate in the reduction of eye injuries. *Am J Sports Med*. 2012;40(3):611–614.
- Menghini M, Knecht PB, Kaufmann C, et al. Treatment of traumatic corneal abrasions: a three-arm, prospective, randomized study. *Ophthalmic Res*. 2013;50(1):13–18.
- Shipman S, Painter K, Keuchel M, et al. Short-term topical tetracaine is high efficacious for the treatment of pain caused by corneal abrasions: a double-blind, randomized clinical trial. *Ann Emerg Med*. 2021;77(3): 338–344.
- Toldi JP, Thomas JL. Evaluation and management of sports-related eye injuries. *Curr Sports Med Rep*. 2020;19(1):29–34.
- Wakai A, Lawrenson JG, Lawrenson AL, et al. Topical non-steroidal anti-inflammatory drugs for analgesia in traumatic corneal abrasions. *Cochrane Database Syst Rev*. 2017;5(5):CD009781.
- Watson SL, Barker NH. Interventions for recurrent corneal erosions. *Cochrane Database Syst Rev*. 2007;(4):CD001861.
- Wilson SA, Last A. Management of corneal abrasions. *Am Fam Physician*. 2004;70(1):123–128.
- Wipperman JL, Dorsch JN. Evaluation and management of corneal abrasions. *Am Fam Physician*. 2013;87(2):114–120.

CLINICAL PEARLS

- Simple corneal abrasions are often self-limiting and can be followed closely with quick return to play once symptoms resolve and no visual difficulties. However, providers must maintain a high index of suspicion for other, more complicated injuries.
- Early treatment goals are prevention of superimposed infection, pain control, monitoring appropriately, and prevention of future complications. Pain control is debatable. More recent evidence suggests the use of topical NSAIDs to be more effective and safest short-term treatment. However, providers must weigh the appropriate evidence before choosing an individualized treatment plan.
- Patients may wear their contact lenses again when the abrasion has healed fully (usually 3 to 5 days). Furthermore, contact lenses should be replaced and new ones not started until complete healing of the abrasion has occurred.
- Different sports have differing regulations for certain eyewear. It appears that optimal protective eyewear is made of a sturdy frame single-piece construction that will not allow posterior dislocation of the lenses of the eyewear. The lenses should have a 2- to 3-mm center thickness and be made of polycarbonate.

CORNEAL AND INTRAOCULAR FOREIGN BODIES

Kevin Waninger, MD, MS, FAAFP, FACEP, FACSM, FAMSSM, CAQSM

BASICS

The cornea is the entry point to the eye and is commonly exposed to foreign bodies (FB). Eyelids protect the eye, and any FB that is not removed by spontaneously blinking may need to be removed. Particles such as glass, metal, sand, wood, plastic, or plant matter may become embedded in the corneal surface from activities including hobbies, work, or play. Corneal foreign bodies (CFB) should be removed to prevent eye infection, inflammation, and to prevent central corneal scar formation. When a CFB penetrates the cornea, it is referred to as an intraocular foreign body (IOFB). Depending on the type and location, the presence of an IOFB can cause pain and serious visual problems if not surgically removed.

EPIDEMIOLOGY

- *Adults*: often the result of work-related accidents (high-risk mechanisms include hammering, chiseling, or grinding, especially metal-on-metal contact; machine-yard work such as lawn mowing; exposure to explosives or blast injuries; high-speed machines like drills, saws; windy environments); sports injuries
- *Children*: often with explosives, weapons (toys that shoot projectiles), sports, windy weather
- Like most other traumatic injuries, CFBs and IOFBs are seen mostly in 25- to 40-year-old males (1),(2),(3).

GENERAL PREVENTION

- Protective eyewear of appropriate quality (3 mm of polycarbonate) prevents virtually all injuries from CFB/IOFBs. Patients should be instructed to wear appropriate protective eyewear in any situation that may lead to a risk of particles or objects getting into the eyes (sports; play activities with toys that shoot projectiles, like BB guns and air rifles; construction; workshops; explosives; machine-yard work).
- The eyes should not be rubbed if you suspect a possible CFB/IOFB. No attempt should be made by the patient to remove the FB if perforation of the eye is suspected. If perforation is not suspected, eye irrigation may be attempted to wash out any potential foreign materials.

DIAGNOSIS

- Superficial CFBs that are removed after the injury typically leave no permanent sequelae. However, corneal scarring, cataracts, and infection may occur, and the longer the time interval between the eye injury and treatment, the greater the likelihood that complications may occur (1).
- Morbidity increases if the FB penetrates the anterior or posterior chambers of the eye, as damage to the iris, lens, and retina may occur and severely affect visual acuity. Any IOFB may lead to infection if not managed appropriately and can result in glaucoma, synechia, iritis, uveitis, cataract formation, endophthalmitis, or retinal detachment (2),(3).

HISTORY

- The activities of the patient and their surroundings at the time of the injury are important and should lead to a high index of suspicion for CFB/IOFB. A focused history includes presenting symptoms, type of FB, penetrability, entry velocity, duration since injury, concurrent contact lens usage, and ocular history.
- Patients frequently feel something entering their eye with no obvious external changes; hence, the incident is often dismissed quickly. Sometimes, patients may not complain of vision loss or severe pain.
- Past medical history should be obtained, including prior surgeries, medications, allergies, tetanus status, and last meal (if surgery is a possibility).
- Does the patient wear contacts (daily or extended wear) or glasses? Document if patient was wearing contacts or glasses at the time of the accident.
- Inquire whether the patient was wearing eye protection at the time of injury and whether the eyewear was still intact. Most FB eye injuries occur in patients who lack appropriate eye protection.
- The usual CFB/IOFB is a very small (<2 mm) sharp-edged object that enters the eye at high speed.
- Symptoms are usually unilateral; explosives may cause binocular injuries with multiple FBs.
- What type of material is suspected as an FB?
  - *Organic* (high incidence of infection): wood, soil, plants, insect parts
  - *Inorganic*: oxidizing metals (e.g., iron, copper). Iron can cause long-term toxicity; *siderosis bulbi* refers to the pigmentary degenerative process of the eye following chronic retention of an iron-containing FB. Copper FBs are very irritating and cause a marked inflammatory response that can cause progressive diminution of vision, defects in the visual field, and impaired color vision. Rust rings can progress to reactive iritis, causing significant pain and vision loss and putting the patient at risk for secondary infection or keratitis.
  - *Inert material*: paint, glass, plastic, gold, fiberglass, nonoxidizing metals, sand. Inert materials can be left in the eye for longer periods of time because they usually do not cause an immediate inflammatory response.

PHYSICAL EXAM

- Note that CFBs/IOFBs can be deceptively subtle on initial presentation. The symptoms of an ocular FB may range from irritation to intense, excruciating pain. This is dependent on the size, location, material, and injury pattern.
- Note that high-speed projectiles may not produce pain or visual acuity problems initially because the FB may be located below the epithelial or conjunctival surface.
- In 20–40% of cases, penetrating IOFBs are in the anterior chamber, allowing identification with slit-lamp exam alone. However, most IOFBs are in the posterior chamber of the eye and will require a fully dilated pupil examination to identify accurately (2),(3).
- Seidel sign is used to look for globe penetration that is not obvious on initial examination. A penetrated globe can be identified by an oozing aqueous humor at the site of the corneal penetration that appears under ultraviolet or blue light as a "dark waterfall," clearing away excess fluorescein as it flows over the cornea. However, the streak may be absent when penetrating injuries are self-sealing.
- If an IOFB is suspected, orbital computed tomography (CT) scanning should be reviewed, and urgent referral to Ophthalmology is recommended.
- Eye pain and FB sensation may be relieved significantly by topical anesthesia.
- Eye redness and tearing are common complaints, and light sensitivity (photophobia) may be present.
- Although patients may present with blurred/decreased vision, vision problems are not a reliable indicator of a FB because visual acuity may not be affected as long as the visual axis is not involved.
- A complete examination of both eyes should be documented, including visual acuity and visual field examination, with lid eversion to check for retained FB. Pupil size, shape, and reactivity should be documented; any pupillary irregularities like a peaked pupil shape should alert of the possibility of a corneal perforation. Carefully access the pupillary direct reflex and look for an abnormal afferent pupillary defect.
- Note the wound location and size if visible, depth of the anterior chamber (compared to other side), iris and lens condition, blood in the anterior chamber (hyphema), or vitreous humor leakage. Document any cataracts, conjunctiva chemosis, or hemorrhage.
- Slit lamp, fluorescein, and funduscopic examinations should all be performed as soon as possible. Perform intraocular pressures if there is no suspicion or evidence of perforation.
- Minimize manipulation of the globe and exercise caution during examination if perforation is suspected to prevent prolapse of ocular contents.
- Note normal or decreased visual acuity, any conjunctival injection, ciliary injection, any visible FB, any visible rust ring (especially if a metallic FB has been embedded for at least several hours), any epithelial defect that stains with fluorescein, any corneal edema, and any anterior chamber floating cells and flare reaction from protein in the aqueous humor.
- If a corneal infiltrate is present, an infectious cause needs to be considered.
- History, physical, and imaging studies should be used to access the number, size, shape, location, composition, visibility, trajectory, and accessibility of any identified IOFBs.

DIFFERENTIAL DIAGNOSIS

- Corneal abrasion/corneal ulcer
- Conjunctival and CFBs/IOFB
- Keratitis, bacterial and/or fungal
- Corneal perforation/ruptured globe
- Other trauma without retained IOFBs

DIAGNOSTIC TESTS & INTERPRETATION

- Unless an infectious corneal infiltrate, corneal ulcer, or IOFB is suspected, no laboratory work is indicated.
- Infectious corneal infiltrates and corneal ulcers generally require scrapings for smears and cultures.
- Plain radiographs, with Caldwell or Water projections, may demonstrate the presence of metallic or glass (lead content), but radiographs have low sensitivity for small and nonmetallic objects (like wood or plant material). The Sweet localization techniques using frontal and lateral projections can be used if necessary to help localize IOFB locations when CT scanning is not available.
- If a retained IOFB is suspected, orbital CT scanning should be immediately performed with 0.5-mm cuts in both the axial and coronal planes to allow the most precise and accurate identification and localization of IOFBs (2),(3).
- Ocular ultrasound is also excellent for identifying and localizing IOFBs, but it must be performed with caution to avoid placing too much pressure on the globe and causing vitreous prolapse.
- Magnetic resonance imaging (MRI) is initially contraindicated due to the risk of magnetized IOFBs, but may be used to localize small nonmetallic IOFBs after metallic IOFBs have been ruled out by CT scanning.

TREATMENT

- No topical medications or ointments should be administered if globe perforation is suspected.
- Topical anesthetics (proparacaine/tetracaine) may be used to assist with the examination and decrease discomfort unless globe perforation is suspected.
- Try to minimize patient nausea and vomiting to prevent the resultant increase in intraocular pressure.
- Pediatric patients may require sedation to facilitate examination and FB removal.

- If an IOFB is suspected, place a hard shield over the injured eye to protect the eye and avoid any pressure on the globe. Both eyes should be shielded to prevent contralateral eye movement/tracking if IOFB with globe perforation is suspected. Instruct the patient not to squeeze the affected eye. Position the patient sitting upright to decrease intraocular pressure.
- Topical antibiotics may be started after CFB removal to prevent infection until any epithelial defect heals. If perforation is suspected, systemic antibiotics may be started prior to surgical intervention. Endophthalmitis rates have been shown to decrease with early antibiotic administration.
- Topical corticosteroids may be used to decrease inflammation, but such intervention should only be started after consultation with an ophthalmologist and a slit-lamp examination to rule out herpetic infection.
- Topical cycloplegic agents may be initiated to relieve pain and photophobia.
- Tetanus should be updated if indicated.
- Liberal use of opioid and other pain meds should be given because these injuries are extremely painful.
- Corneal patching is no longer recommended.
- ED treatment:
  - For CFBs, manual removal may be attempted if trained in the technique. Topical anesthetic ophthalmic solution is necessary to facilitate the exam and CFB removal. Procedure risks, benefits, and complications must be discussed, with signed informed consent. If globe perforation is suspected, this procedure should not be attempted, and the patient should be referred directly to ophthalmology for management.
  - If the CFB is superficial, the eye should be irrigated to moisten the cornea. Removal of the CFB can be attempted by using a gentle rolling motion with a wet cotton-tipped applicator. Pressure should not be applied, as this may push the FB deeper into the cornea or even create a corneal abrasion. An attempt to wash the CFB off the cornea may be attempted with sterile normal saline directed at an oblique angle off the cornea.
  - An embedded CFB cannot be removed with irrigation or a cotton-tipped applicator. An embedded FB can be removed by using a gentle flicking motion with an eye spud, if available, or with a 25-gauge or 27-gauge sterile needle. Using a slit lamp to immobilize the patient's head and visualize the FB, the hub of the needle may be placed on a 3-mL syringe for easier control. The cornea should be approached from the side with the needle in a plane tangent to the cornea and the bevel away from the corneal surface to minimize the chance of corneal perforation. Good anesthesia of the corneal surface is required. Once dislodged from its embedded position in the cornea, remaining FB debris can be removed with a wet cotton-tipped applicator.
  - Within 3 hours, iron-containing CFBs oxidize, leaving a rust ring/stain on adjacent epithelial cells, which can delay healing and act as an irritant focus. Removal of a rust ring at the time of FB removal may be attempted with a small-gauge needle or a pothook burr, but a rust ring often seems to be easier to remove 24 hours after the CFB is initially removed, when the cells around the ring have loosened and can be readily lifted off and removed with a small burr instrument (1),(4),(5),(6).
  - Documenting a negative Seidel sign after removal of a corneal FB is good practice to confirm no iatrogenic penetration of the cornea occurred.

MEDICATION

- Topical antibiotics are recommended to reduce infection rates until the epithelial defect heals.
- Systemic penicillins, vancomycin, cephalosporins, and fluoroquinolones are commonly administered orally or intravenously for IOFBs. The fluoroquinolones have been shown to have excellent intraocular penetration after administration, but are often avoided in active individuals due to the association with tendon rupture.
- Topical anesthetics may prolong epithelial healing and are not routinely prescribed for home pain relief.
- Ophthalmic nonsteroidal medications appear to be useful for decreasing pain with corneal injury.

ISSUES FOR REFERRAL

- Penetrating injuries require urgent referral to an ophthalmologist because endophthalmitis and permanent scarring may occur, and delayed surgical removal of IOFBs has been associated with significantly worse outcomes.
- Patients who present to the ED with emergent conditions should be discussed and/or referred to an ophthalmologist on the day of presentation. Patients with urgent conditions can be seen the following day.
- Emergent conditions:
  - Hyphema (blood in the anterior chamber) associated with a suspected IOFB
  - Diffuse corneal defect or opacity
  - Laceration of the cornea or sclera
  - Single dilated pupil or an abnormally shaped pupil
  - A deep or shallow anterior chamber (when compared to the contralateral eye)
  - Suspected penetration of the globe
  - Positive Seidel sign
  - Multiple eye FBs
  - Uncooperative patient (e.g., young child, intoxicated patient, patient with mental disability)
- Urgent conditions:
  - Significant lid edema
  - Large corneal abrasion
  - Corneal ulceration

ADMISSION, INPATIENT, AND NURSING CONSIDERATIONS

- Patients with a history of assault, gunshot wound, explosive injury, or an inability to communicate an effective history need a systemic comprehensive examination with vital signs.
- If the examination in the office or the ED is not sufficient to rule out ocular perforation, then an examination under anesthesia should be considered. This is especially true for children, where there should be a low threshold to examine the child in the operating room.
- FBs that present any potential for intraocular penetration must be explored in the operating room within 24 hours of initial examination.
- All CFBs, corneal ulcers, and corneal abrasions require close follow-up in 24 to 48 hours for reexamination. If rust rings are not completely removed, follow-up should be made within 24 hours for rust ring removal.

ONGOING CARE

FOLLOW-UP RECOMMENDATIONS

Patient Monitoring

- Follow-up every 1 to 2 days until all epithelial defects are well healed, and all corneal infiltrates have resolved.
- No activity or body position restrictions are necessary once the corneal wound heals.
- Gonioscopy should be performed by ophthalmologist after resolution and improvement. Annual follow-up care for intraocular pressure should be planned if the severity of trauma raises a suspicion of angle closure glaucoma in later life.
- A dilated fundus examination should be performed on a routine basis after any injury severe enough to potentially damage the retina.

PATIENT EDUCATION

Eye protection when taking part in risky activities (e.g., hammering, mowing the lawn) is strongly recommended.

PROGNOSIS

Prognosis is good unless a rust ring or scarring involves the visual axis. If infection develops, prognosis is more guarded. Globe-penetrating injuries and IOFB have much worse prognoses, but reading vision is usually retained/regained, if properly treated.

COMPLICATIONS

Endophthalmitis, corneal scarring, elevated intraocular pressure, cataract, retinal detachment, proliferative vitreoretinopathy, and metallosis (e.g., chalcosis, siderosis) are all possible complications.

REFERENCES

1. Fraenkel A, Lee LR, Lee GA. Managing corneal foreign bodies in office space general practice. *Aust Fam Physician*. 2011;46(3):89–93.
2. Jung HC, Lee SY, Yoon CK, et al. Intraocular foreign body: diagnostic protocols and treatment strategies in ocular trauma patients. *J Clin Med* 2021;10(9):1861–1878.
3. Loporchio D, Mukkamala L, Gorukanti K, et al. Interocular foreign bodies: a review. *Surv Ophthalmol*. 2016;61(5):582–596.
4. Guier CP, Stokkermans TJ. *Corneal Foreign Body Removal*. StatPearls Publishing; 2023.
5. Koetting C. Foreign body removal start to finish. Review of Optometry. Published April 15, 2020. https://www.reviewofoptometry.com/article/foreign-body-removal-start-to-finish
6. Mendelsohn A, Pokeza N. Removal of corneal foreign bodies. EyeWiki. Updated January 27, 2025. https://eyewiki.org/Removal_of_Corneal_Foreign_Bodies

CLINICAL PEARLS

- Accurate history-taking that involves attention to the mechanism of ocular injury should be obtained; clinical presentation of CFB/IOFB can initially be subtle.
- Make sure you have good pain relief for your patient, so that you can get an adequate examination.
- Do not limit your clinical focus to the eye injury and forget to do a complete exam to rule out other systemic injury beyond that of the eye injury.
- Discuss any ocular pathology with an ophthalmologist, and plan adequate referral.
- Protective eyewear of appropriate quality prevents virtually all injuries from CFB/IOFB.
- Penetrating injuries require urgent referral to an ophthalmologist.

COVID-19

Michelle Doscas, MD, CAQSM • Alexandra Tee, MD, CAQSM

BASICS

DESCRIPTION

- COVID-19 is an infectious disease caused by the SARS-CoV-2 virus.
- Infection may affect the cardiopulmonary system.

EPIDEMIOLOGY

In March 2020, World Health Organization (WHO) declared COVID-19 a pandemic.

ETIOLOGY AND PATHOPHYSIOLOGY

- Transmission through close range contact via respiratory particles
- Contaminated surfaces are not considered a major source of transmission.
- A person is most likely to be contagious in the first 7 to 10 days of infection.

RISK FACTORS

- Exposure risks include length of time exposed, physical distance, cough or heavy breathing of infected person, symptoms of infected person, mask use, vaccination status, and ventilation of shared space.
- Physical activity is a protective factor in COVID-19 adverse outcomes (1).

DIAGNOSIS

HISTORY

- Most common symptoms include fever, chills, and sore throat.
- Less common symptoms include muscle aches, fatigue, runny nose or congestion, sneezing, headache, dizziness, new and persistent cough, shortness of breath, appetite loss, nausea, vomiting, abdominal pain, diarrhea, loss or change of sense of taste or smell, difficulty sleeping.
- Identifying the first day of symptoms is important for return-to-play protocols.

PHYSICAL EXAM

- Objective temperature, respiratory rate, oxygen saturation, heart rate
- Pulmonary exam
- Cardiovascular (CV) exam

DIFFERENTIAL DIAGNOSIS

- Other viral upper respiratory illness
- Pneumonia
- Asthma
- Costochondritis

DIAGNOSTIC TESTS & INTERPRETATION

- COVID-19 antigen test
- There is no evidence to use advanced CV tests such as cardiac magnetic resonance imaging (MRI) or echocardiogram (ECHO) to screen for CV dysfunction in athletes with COVID-19 (2).
- Consider a chest radiograph if there is clinical suspicion for pneumonia (i.e., low oxygen saturation, prolonged fever, or worsening productive cough).
- Blood tests are not regularly used in diagnosing COVID-19.

TREATMENT

GENERAL MEASURES

- Supportive care including rest, hydration, over-the-counter (OTC) medications such as acetaminophen and ibuprofen to control fever and body aches
- Isolation from others for at least 5 days from the onset of symptoms

- If symptoms are mild, the athlete may stop isolation after day 5 if their symptoms are improving and they have been fever free for 24 hours. They must wear a high-quality mask when around others for 5 additional days.
- If symptoms are moderate (i.e., shortness of breath or difficulty breathing), they must isolate for 10 days.
- The athlete may stop wearing a mask around others on day 11.
- An antiviral medication, nirmatrelvir-ritonavir (Paxlovid), may be considered in athletes at high risk for progressing to severe COVID-19 (e.g., those with severe symptoms or older athletes with comorbidities). For optimal effectiveness, treatment with Paxlovid must be initiated as soon as possible after diagnosis of COVID-19 and within 5 days of symptom onset. Attention to kidney function and potential drug-drug interactions with other medications is necessary when using Paxlovid, requiring careful review by a health care provider.
- Return to play:
  - If the athlete has mild symptoms, consider 3 days of no exercise followed by a light individual exercise program prior to the end of isolation.
  - If the athlete has moderate symptoms, there should be complete rest from exercise for 5 days, followed by a medical evaluation prior to returning to sport.
  - If there are cardiopulmonary symptoms present, consider electrocardiogram (ECG), ECHO, and troponin testing.
  - If any positive findings on cardiac screening, consider cardiac MRI and consultation with a cardiologist before returning to any exercise.
  - Generally, cardiac screening before returning to sport is not necessary (2).

ONGOING CARE

FOLLOW-UP RECOMMENDATIONS

- The athlete should be followed closely during their return-to-play protocol by an athletic trainer.
- If there are any cardiopulmonary symptoms noted during the return to play, medical evaluation should occur and CV screening tests should be considered.

REFERENCES

1. Young DR, Sallis JF, Baecker A, et al. Associations of physical inactivity and COVID-19 outcomes among subgroups. *Am J Prevent Med.* 2023;64(4):492–502.
2. Hédon C, Schnell F, Sosner P, et al. Cardiac screening before returning to elite sport after SARS-CoV-2 infection. *Arch Cardiovasc Dis.* 2022;115(11):562–570.

ADDITIONAL READING

Elliott N, Martin R, Heron N, et al. Infographic: graduated return to play guidance following COVID-19 infection. *Br J Sports Med.* 2020;54(19):1174–1175.

CLINICAL PEARLS

- Treatment of COVID-19 infection in athletes is supportive care.
- Isolation is recommended from others for at least 5 days since onset of symptoms.
- Symptom severity can help guide return-to-play timeline.
- Moderate-to-severe cardiopulmonary symptoms may warrant further cardiac screening.

CUBITAL TUNNEL SYNDROME

Connor Farrell, DO ▪ Denice Praxidio, DO ▪ Michael Prestgard-Duke, MD

BASICS

DESCRIPTION

- Compression, traction, or irritation of the ulnar nerve as it passes through the cubital tunnel of the medial elbow.
- The cubital tunnel is bounded by the medial trochlea, the medial epicondylar groove, and the posterior portion of the ulnar collateral ligament and is roofed by the triangular arcuate ligament.
- Primary complaints are medial elbow and forearm pain exacerbated by elbow flexion.
- Additional complaints are paresthesias in the ring/little finger, and the dorsoulnar hand.
- May result in motor symptoms such as loss of strength in power grip as well as fine motor skill such as pinch grip and delicate finger control.
- Synonym(s): ulnar tunnel syndrome, ulnar nerve entrapment

EPIDEMIOLOGY

Incidence

- The second most common compressive neuropathy (after carpal tunnel syndrome).
- Affects 2–6% of the population
- Male > female (~2:1)

ETIOLOGY AND PATHOPHYSIOLOGY

The medial elbow is the most common site of ulnar nerve compression/irritation. Possible causes include:

- Prolonged pressure on the cubital tunnel
- Subluxation of the ulnar nerve over the medial epicondyle
- Osteophytes
- Ganglia, lipomas, other soft tissue tumors/masses
- Cubitus valgus
- Enlarged medial head of the triceps muscle
- Ulnar collateral ligament instability/tears
- Triangular arcuate ligament tears in baseball pitchers
- Repetitive elbow flexion and extension
- Anconeus epitrochlearis: anomalous muscle in 70% of the population

RISK FACTORS

- Male gender (1)
- Overhead-throwing athletes
- Repetitive upper extremity activities (either professional or recreational)
- Smoking (1)
- Thyroid disease (1)

GENERAL PREVENTION

- Avoid prolonged pressure on the medial elbow and repetitive work or overuse.
- Tobacco avoidance/cessation

COMMONLY ASSOCIATED CONDITIONS

- Ulnar collateral ligament instability
- Osteoarthritis
- Thyroid disease (hypothyroidism or hyperthyroidism)

DIAGNOSIS

HISTORY

- Early symptoms include paresthesias, numbness/tingling, and electric shocks or burning sensations over the 4th and 5th digits.
- Late symptoms include weakness of interosseous and abductor digiti minimi muscles of the hand, weakened grip, hypothenar atrophy, loss of dexterity, and clumsiness.
- Elbow symptoms include vague, aching pain in the region of the elbow, worsening with overhead activities, snapping, or popping sensation of medial elbow.
- Overhead throwing athletes will complain of loss of control of the ball with activity.

PHYSICAL EXAM

- Pain with palpation of cubital tunnel of affected elbow
- Positive Tinel sign: Tapping over the ulnar nerve at the elbow will reproduce symptoms.
- Elbow flexion test: Placing the elbow in full flexion and the wrist in maximal extension will cause pain or paresthesias after 1 minute (2).
- Scratch test: Patient faces examiner with arms adducted, elbows flexed, and hands outstretched with wrists in a neutral position. Patient resists adduction/internal rotation to the forearms applied by the examiner. The examiner scratches or wipes fingertips over the cubital tunnel, and resistance to adduction/internal rotation is again applied. In a positive test, the patient has immediate and temporary loss of external resistance tone, which resolves within 5 seconds (2)[B].
- Sensory changes in ulnar nerve distribution can be detected with Semmes-Weinstein monofilament testing and two-point discrimination tests.
- Chronic changes: asymmetric hypothenar atrophy, decreased pinch and grip strength, abducted little finger, or severe claw deformity of little finger only (Wartenberg sign, intrinsic muscle weakness and wasting of the flexor carpi ulnaris, ulnar flexor digitorum profundus, and 1st dorsal interosseous muscle)

DIFFERENTIAL DIAGNOSIS

Systemic: diabetes (peripheral neuropathy), renal disease uremic neuropathy), multiple myeloma (direct nerve compression), amyloidosis, chronic alcoholism (direct toxic effects of alcohol and its metabolites on nerve tissue), nutritional deficiencies particularly of B vitamins (like thiamine—B_1), malnutrition

- Compression: postoperative occupational or recreational activities requiring repetitive flexion and extension, supracondylar process, ligament of Struthers, medial head of triceps, ulnar nerve compression at Guyon canal
- Medial epicondylitis which can coexist with cubital tunnel syndrome
- Ulnar collateral ligament injury
- Cervical radiculopathy
- Brachial plexus injury or nerve compression at the shoulder
- Thoracic outlet syndrome
- Carpal tunnel syndrome

DIAGNOSTIC TESTS & INTERPRETATION

- Radiograph of elbow to evaluate for cortical changes or osteophytes
- Magnetic resonance imaging (MRI) of elbow to evaluate cubital tunnel for soft tissue masses, nerve enlargement, nerve compression, and continuity of ulnar collateral ligament (3),(4)
- Nerve conduction velocity (NCV) to evaluate how fast neurologic signals travel down the nerve to detect the site of compression or constriction. Studies must be performed with elbow at 45 degrees of flexion to lessen chance of erroneous results (5)[C] per the American Association of Neuromuscular & Electrodiagnostic Medicine, greatest strength of evidence is conduction velocity <50 m/s across the elbow (3)[C].
- Electromyogram (EMG) may be negative early in the disease but progresses to reduced recruitment of motor units and then motor axon loss and denervation (3).
- Advanced diagnostic testing will show a progression from ischemia to demyelination to axonal loss (3).
- Diagnostic ultrasound (US) has been shown to have a sensitivity of 93% and specificity of 85% (4).
- Diagnostic US will show hypoechoic swelling of the ulnar nerve with loss of the fascicular pattern is a sonographic sign of cubital tunnel (6)[B].
- Subluxation, tumors, or ganglia of the ulnar nerve may be seen with dynamic US (4).
- A cross-sectional area (CSA) of 10 mm^2 as a diagnostic cutoff for ulnar entrapment at the elbow (7)[B]
- Pathologic findings:
  - At decompression, specific sites of nerve compression can usually be found.
  - Inspect the arcade of Struthers, intermuscular septum, cubital tunnel, and Osborne fascia (between two heads of flexor carpi ulnaris).

TREATMENT

- Conservative treatment is considered first line for mild to moderate symptoms with the goal of symptom control and prevention of progression.
- The most effective treatment is activity modification and cessation of activity that is causing the problem (8).
- Wearing a splint to limit movement and reduce irritation or an elbow pad to protect against chronic irritation from hard surface may have some benefit.
- A systematic review by Kooner et al. recommends activity modification and an elbow flexion splint to limit range of motion for a period of 6 to 12 weeks (8)[B].
- Topical or oral nonsteroidal anti-inflammatory drugs (NSAIDs) PRN
- Physical therapy modalities such as nerve mobilization/gliding, pulsed US, and laser therapy have been used but currently have weak evidence (8)[B].
- Perineural dextrose (D5W) and corticosteroid injections have been shown to decrease pain and ulnar nerve CSA (8),(9).

SURGERY/OTHER PROCEDURES

- Consider surgery if symptoms continue after 3 months of conservative therapy or multiple recurrences in a throwing athlete (10)[C]:
  - Address ulnar collateral ligament instability if coexisting.
  - Decompression (open vs. endoscopic) of the nerve in the canal, especially in the setting of bone spurs.
  - Transposition of the nerve (submuscular vs. subcutaneous) out of the canal in an anterior direction
- There have been no statistically significant differences between the types of surgery and response to treatment, return to work, and reoperation rate (11)[A].
- No clinical or NCV differences between decompression and ulnar nerve transposition have been noted either.
- Endoscopic decompression showed higher rates of complication, but lower postoperative chronic pain compared to open in situ decompression.
- Hypermobile nerve is most frequently treated with epicondylectomy or transposition (12)[B].
- Preference for overhead athlete is transposition of the ulnar nerve to allow for improved movement of the nerve throughout the range of motion (13)[C]:
  - Subcutaneous technique: anterior transposition of nerve without detachment of flexor mass; fascial sling used to prevent subluxation of nerve
  - Submuscular technique: allows inspection and treatment of ligament and osseous pathology; nerve stabilized deep to flexor-pronator muscles but more morbidity and potential for deep scarring

Pediatric Considerations

- Dominant arms of young throwing athletes (12)
- Nonsurgical management only relieves symptoms roughly ~45% of the time (12).
- Anterior transposition should be considered due to the substantial revision rate after decompression (12).

REFERENCES

1. Uzunkulaoğlu A, Afsar SI, Karataş M. Association between gender, body mass index, and ulnar nerve entrapment at the elbow: a retrospective study. *J Clin Neurophysiol*. 2016;33(6):545–548.
2. Cheng CJ, Mackinnon-Patterson B, Beck JL, et al. Scratch collapse test for evaluation of carpal and cubital tunnel syndrome. *J Hand Surg Am*. 2008;33(9):1518–1524.
3. Nakashian MN, Ireland D, Kane PM. Cubital tunnel syndrome: current concepts. *Curr Rev Musculoskelet Med*. 2020;13(4):520–524.
4. Burahee AS, Sanders AD, Shirley C, et al. Cubital tunnel syndrome. *EFORT Open Rev*. 2021;6(9):743–750.
5. Sattari S, Emad M. Changes in ulnar nerve conduction velocity across the elbow in different angles of elbow flexion. *Electromyogr Clin Neurophysiol*. 2007;47(7–8):373–376.
6. Draghi F, Bortolotto C. Importance of the ultrasound in cubital tunnel syndrome. *Surg Radiol Anat*. 2016;38(2):265–268.
7. Chang KV, Wu WT, Han DS, et al. Ulnar nerve cross-sectional area for the diagnosis of cubital tunnel syndrome: a meta-analysis of ultrasonographic measurements. *Arch Phys Med Rehabil*. 2018;99(4):743–757.
8. Kooner S, Cinats D, Kwong C, et al. Conservative treatment of cubital tunnel syndrome: a systematic review. *Orthop Rev (Pavia)*. 2019;11(2):7955.
9. Chen LC, Ho TY, Shen YP, et al. Perineural dextrose and corticosteroid injections for ulnar neuropathy at the elbow: a randomized double-blind trial. *Arch Phys Med Rehabil*. 2020;101(8):1296–1303.
10. Charles YP, Coulet B, Rouzaud JC, et al. Comparative clinical outcomes of submuscular and subcutaneous transposition of the ulnar nerve for cubital tunnel syndrome. *J Hand Surg Am*. 2009;34(5):866–874.
11. Abourisha E, Srinivasan AS, Barakat A, et al. Surgical management of cubital tunnel syndrome: a systematic review and meta-analysis of randomised trials. *J Orthop*. 2024;53:41–48.
12. Boone S, Gelberman RH, Calfee RP. The management of cubital tunnel syndrome. *J Hand Surg Am*. 2015;40(9):1897–1904.
13. Bencardino JT, Rosenberg ZS. Entrapment neuropathies of the shoulder and elbow in the athlete. *Clin Sports Med*. 2006;25(3):465–487.

ADDITIONAL READING

- Cutts S. Cubital tunnel syndrome. *Postgrad Med J*. 2007;83(975):28–31.
- Keefe DT, Lintner DM. Nerve injuries in the throwing elbow. *Clin Sports Med*. 2004;23(4):723–742.

CLINICAL PEARLS

- Hallmark classic early symptoms include: paresthesias and numbness/tingling over the 4th and 5th digits.
- Hallmark late symptoms include hypothenar atrophy and weakness.
- Diagnostic US and EMG/nerve conduction studies (NCS) are sufficient enough to provide a diagnosis.
- Activity modification and bracing are first-line treatments for mild and moderate symptoms.
- For severe and recalcitrant cases, surgical options include open versus endoscopic decompression or submuscular versus subcutaneous nerve transposition.

CUBOID SUBLUXATION AND FRACTURE

Dana W. Brooks, DO, CAQSM • Karl B. Fields, MD, CAQSM, FAMSSM

BASICS

DESCRIPTION

- Fracture: can be avulsion fractures, intra-articular, or extra-articular. The majority (48%) are avulsion fractures (1).
- The cuboid is the cornerstone of the lateral column allowing motion and stabilization for the midtarsal (Chopart) and tarsometatarsal (Lisfranc) joints (2).
- Frequently associated with other fractures, dislocations, or ligamentous injuries
- A "nutcracker" fracture occurs when an axial load is placed on an abducted plantarflexed fixed foot crushing the cuboid between the calcaneus and the 4th and 5th metatarsals bases. Ballet dancers are a special group at risk for this type of injury (3).
- Subluxation: poorly understood; can occur as a result of acute ankle inversion injury or as an overuse syndrome; noted in patients with hypermobility; most commonly reported in ballet dancers (4)
- Isolated dislocation is extremely rare; usually associated with concomitant fractures of the midfoot
- Cuboid stress fractures are extremely rare (5).
- Synonym(s):
  - Subluxation and dislocation: cuboid syndrome; locked cuboid; dropped cuboid; calcaneal cuboid fault syndrome; lateral plantar neuritis
  - Fracture: nutcracker fracture

EPIDEMIOLOGY

Incidence

- Subluxation: Subluxation is considered rare, but some propose that it is underdiagnosed.
- Dislocation: rare
- Fracture: relatively uncommon with estimated annual incidence of <2 per 100,000 individuals (2)

RISK FACTORS

- Subluxation:
  - Pronated feet
  - Tight peroneus longus tendon
  - Ballet dancing—due to en pointe foot position (4)
  - Trail running or running on uneven surfaces
  - Hypermobility syndrome
- Fracture and dislocation:
  - Activities at high risk for foot trauma (e.g., motor vehicle accident [MVA], motorsports, equestrian)
  - Long-distance running (stress fracture)

DIAGNOSIS

HISTORY

- Subluxation:
  - May follow inversion ankle injury
  - Subluxation may be precipitated by increased activity, training on uneven terrain, or initiation of new activity, especially in patients with excess pronation.
  - Pain in lateral midfoot proximal to and involving the base of the 4th and/or 5th metatarsal, exacerbated with activity
  - Often with symptom-free intervals
  - Associated with foot weakness or difficulty with ambulation
- Fracture and dislocation:
  - Substantial traumatic force is required due to stable ligamentous attachments.
  - Three common mechanisms of injury:
    - Eversion injury with compression ("cracking") of the cuboid
    - Direct crush injury
    - Avulsion injury (See Figure 75) in Appendix A:
  - Most patients with fractures have difficulty bearing weight, especially walking on their tiptoes.
  - Dislocations often are associated with severe weakness and markedly antalgic gait or the inability to weight bear.
  - Midfoot deformity or localized swelling may be present with fracture or dislocation.
  - Stress fractures generally present with an insidious onset of lateral midfoot pain.

PHYSICAL EXAM

- Subluxation:
  - Tenderness to palpation over cuboid (dorsal and/or plantar surface)
  - Increased mobility to manipulation of the cuboid at the Lisfranc joint
  - Midtarsal adduction test causes pain.
- Dislocation and fracture:
  - Midfoot swelling
  - Tenderness to palpation over cuboid (dorsal and/or plantar surface)
  - With dislocation, abnormal indentation in lateral midfoot may be noted with concomitant fullness in the plantar surface.
  - May be unable to bear weight
  - When fracture is suspected, the foot, ankle, and lower leg need to be carefully inspected because concomitant injury is common.

DIFFERENTIAL DIAGNOSIS

- Peroneus longus tear or tenosynovitis
- Base of 4th and 5th metatarsal fracture
- Calcaneonavicular tarsal coalition
- Peroneus longus tendon subluxation
- Os peroneum fracture
- Other midfoot fractures

DIAGNOSTIC TESTS & INTERPRETATION

- Radiographs: Recommend anteroposterior, lateral, and 45 degrees oblique views. Weight-bearing films should be obtained when possible because subtle injuries to the midtarsal joint complex (i.e., Lisfranc) are often missed on non–weight-bearing views:
  - Oblique view usually demonstrates a cuboid fracture, and dislocation can be seen if medial border of 4th metatarsal is not aligned to medial border of the cuboid.
  - Subluxation is often not seen.

- Computed tomography (CT) scan is gold standard for diagnosis and is often beneficial if fracture is present.
- Magnetic resonance imaging (MRI) is the most sensitive test for stress fracture.

TREATMENT

- Subluxation:
  - Manipulate cuboid back into place.
  - Patient stands with support, affected leg with knee bent to 90 degrees. Examiner grasps forefoot with fingers and places thumbs (one over the other) on plantar aspect of cuboid. Cuboid is manipulated with a quick downward thrust of the thumbs in a dorsal and lateral direction.
  - Alternative: Cuboid whip midfoot manipulation, which involves having the athlete lie prone with the knee flexed to 90 degrees, and the examiner "whips" the cuboid back into place with rapid ankle dorsiflexion and plantar flexion (6)[C].
  - Orthotics, use of cuboid pad, and arch straps/ taping recommended
  - Strength and proprioception rehabilitation (3)[C]
- Dislocation:
  - No consensus in current literature regarding optimal treatment, but open reduction is most commonly required
- Fracture:
  - Avulsion fractures can be managed symptomatically (1); short leg weight bearing (SLWB) or air splint often used
  - Isolated extra-articular fractures can be treated in a controlled ankle motion (CAM) walker boot or short leg walking cast for 6 to 8 weeks.
  - Surgery is indicated for compressed cuboid fractures with ≥1 mm of articular displacement or >3 mm of lateral column shortening (2).
  - Most intra-articular fractures require open reduction and internal fixation (ORIF) and should be referred to a surgeon (1).
  - Remember that most cuboid fractures have an association with other more complex foot injuries.
  - Stress fractures heal well with activity modification. Patient may need to be non–weight-bearing or partial weight-bearing on crutches for a few weeks if they have pain with walking. A progressive walk to cross-train to running program requires 6 to 12 weeks. Ensure proper arch support and correct underlying gait insufficiencies, such as excessive supination or pronation.

ONGOING CARE

FOLLOW-UP RECOMMENDATIONS

- Subluxation:
  - Return to play depends on the severity of the athlete's symptoms.
  - Most athletes should be able to return to play almost immediately given proper treatment with orthotics/cuboid pad/arch supports.
  - Some patients may need a period of relative rest with return to play after physical therapy and symptom improvement.
  - Some patients also learn to self-treat in the field after instruction in self-administration of the cuboid whip maneuver.
- Fracture/dislocation:
  - Return to play for cuboid stress fractures is similar to other foot stress fractures.
  - Athletes should follow a slow, incremental, symptom-free return-to-play protocol with rest and regression of intensity if symptoms develop.
  - Return to play for most fractures and dislocations should proceed only after clearance by the orthopedic surgeon and would be slow and incremental.
  - Depending on the severity of the injury, there may be chronic damage ultimately limiting return to play.

COMPLICATIONS

- Subluxation and dislocation: Chronic instability can be a problem for both dislocation and subluxation.
- Fracture: arthritis and shortening of the lateral column leading to pes planovalgus
- Cuboid vascularization is abundant for bone consolidation in cases of fracture; nonunion and osteonecrosis are extremely rare, unless diagnosis/ treatment is delayed (2).

REFERENCES

1. Fenton P, Al-Nammari S, Blundell C, et al. The patterns of injury and management of cuboid fractures: a retrospective case series. *Bone Joint J*. 2016;98-B(7):1003–1008.
2. Engelmann EWM, Rammelt S, Schepers T. Fractures of the cuboid bone: a critical analysis review. *JBJS Rev*. 2020;8(4):e0173.
3. Carsen S, Quinn BJ, Beck E, et al. "Nutcracker fracture" in a ballet dancer performing in The Nutcracker. *J Dance Med Sci*. 2015;19(3):124–127.
4. Macintyre J, Joy E. Foot and ankle injuries in dance. *Clin Sports Med*. 2000;19(2):351–368.
5. Mandell JC, Khurana B, Smith SE. Stress fractures of the foot and ankle, part 2: site-specific etiology, imaging, and treatment, and differential diagnosis. *Skeletal Radiol*. 2017;46(9):1165–1186.
6. Patterson SM. Cuboid syndrome: a review of the literature. *J Sports Sci Med*. 2006;5(4):597–606.

ADDITIONAL READING

- Clements JR, Dijour F, Leong W. Surgical management navicular and cuboid fractures. *Clin Podiatr Med Surg*. 2018;35(2):145–159.
- Hunter JC, Sangeorzan BJ. A nutcracker fracture: cuboid fracture with an associated avulsion fracture of the tarsal navicular. *AJR Am J Roentgenol*. 1996;166(4):888.
- Main BJ, Jowett RL. Injuries of the midtarsal joint. *J Bone Joint Surg Br*. 1975;57(1):89–97.
- Omey ML, Micheli LJ. Foot and ankle problems in the young athlete. *Med Sci Sports Exerc*. 1999;31(Suppl 7):S470–S486.

CLINICAL PEARLS

- Frequently associated with other fractures and midfoot injuries
- Weight-bearing foot x-rays should be done if possible because subtle associated injuries to the Lisfranc joint may be missed on non–weight-bearing views. CT scan is gold standard.
- Avulsion fractures and isolated extra-articular fractures can be managed conservatively.
- Intra-articular fractures should be referred to an orthopedist for definitive treatment.
- Stress fractures heal well with activity modification.

DE QUERVAIN TENOSYNOVITIS

David A. Wang, MD ▪ Ryan J. Lingor, MD, AT-C, RD, CSCS

BASICS

DESCRIPTION

- First described by Swiss physician Fritz de Quervain in 1895
- de Quervain tenosynovitis is a stenosing tenosynovitis of the 1st dorsal compartment of the wrist.
- The abductor pollicis longus (APL) and extensor pollicis brevis (EPB) tendons course through this compartment.

ALERT
About 40% of cadavers demonstrate an intracompartmental septum between the APL and EPB tendons, with a higher incidence noted in those who have failed injections or required surgical intervention.

- It is the most frequently encountered tendinosis on the dorsal side of the wrist.
- de Quervain tenosynovitis is typically an overuse injury but may result from direct trauma.
- **Synonym(s)**: de Quervain disease; 1st dorsal compartment tenosynovitis; stenosing tenosynovitis; stenosing tendinitis; peritendinitis; styloid tenovaginitis; stenosing tendovaginitis; texting tenosynovitis; mommy thumb

EPIDEMIOLOGY

- Usually seen in adults aged 30 to 50 years
- More common in females than males

ETIOLOGY AND PATHOPHYSIOLOGY

- Repetitive or sustained tension on tendons of the 1st dorsal compartment causes an inflammatory and then fibroblastic response.
- There is thickening and swelling of the extensor tendons and retinaculum.
- Pain is produced from resisted gliding of the APL and EPB tendons in the narrowed fibroosseous canal.
- Histopathology is consistent with collagen disorientation and mucoid changes (tendinosis), not inflammation.

RISK FACTORS

- Activities requiring forceful grasp with excessive ulnar wrist deviation or repetitive use of the thumb (e.g., golfing, bowling, wrestling, fly fishing, racquet sports [squash, badminton, tennis pickleball], javelin or discus throwing).
- Direct trauma with associated scarring
- Can be seen as systemic component of conditions such as diabetes mellitus, hypothyroidism, rheumatoid arthritis, and systemic lupus erythematosus
- Pregnancy, postpartum mothers, and caretakers of young infants
- Frequent use of electronic devices (e.g., texting, tablets, cell phones)

DIAGNOSIS

Clinical diagnosis based on history and physical exam findings

HISTORY

- Gradual onset of pain along the radial styloid of the wrist for several weeks to months
- Acute onset of pain over the radial styloid after trauma
- Pain is aggravated by repetitive motions of the wrist or thumb.
- Pain may radiate to the thumb or up the dorsoradial aspect of the forearm.

PHYSICAL EXAM

- Swelling, tenderness, and/or crepitus to palpation of the APL and EPB tendons near the radial styloid process.
- Positive Finkelstein test is pathognomonic and the most commonly used test (1)[C].

ALERT
To perform the Finkelstein test, the examining physician grasps the thumb of the patient, and the hand is ulnar deviated sharply. A positive test produces sharp pain along the distal radius.

- A similar test that is often confused with the Finkelstein test was previously described by Eichhoff, in which the thumb is placed in the palm of the hand and held with the fingers; the hand is then ulnar deviated, causing intense pain over the radial styloid.
- Other tests:
  - Brunelli test (abducting the thumb with the wrist in radial deviation) and wrist hyperflexion and abduction of the thumb (WHAT) test (wrist fully flexed with thumb fully extended and abducted while examiner applies a gradually increasing abduction resistance to the thumb)
- Usually, no imaging is necessary for diagnosis.
- Obtain x-rays if patient has history of trauma or to rule out other bone pathology such as osteoarthritis (OA).
- Ultrasound (US) can be helpful as a diagnostic tool:
  - Can demonstrate fluid surrounding the tendons or thickened retinaculum
  - Can identify anatomical variant with intracompartmental septum
- Magnetic resonance imaging (MRI) is often unnecessary but may be used to rule out concomitant pathologies if considering surgery.

DIFFERENTIAL DIAGNOSIS

- Thumb carpometacarpal joint arthritis
- Intersection syndrome
- Radial styloid fracture
- Scaphoid fracture
- Radial neuritis
- Wartenberg syndrome
- Trigger thumb
- Flexor carpi radialis tendonitis
- Ganglia

TREATMENT

GENERAL MEASURES

- Rest from offending activity.
- Ice massage may be beneficial when used early.

MEDICATION

Topical and oral anti-inflammatory agents may benefit some patients especially during an acute onset of symptoms when used in conjunction with rest (2)[C].

ALERT
Corticosteroid injection is an effective treatment:

- Place a rolled-up towel under the wrist to position it in slight ulnar deviation.
- Use a 2-mL mixture of analgesic (lidocaine 1%) and corticosteroid (triamcinolone 10 mg/mL or dexamethasone 10 mg).
- Water-soluble corticosteroid decreases local complications, including subcutaneous atrophy and hypopigmentation.
- Inject into the 1st dorsal compartment at the radial styloid through a 25- or 27-gauge needle at a 45-degree angle to the skin.

- Inject along the axis of the sheath.
- Infiltrate the sheath from distal to proximal.
- Fusiform swelling occurs in the 1st dorsal compartment if properly placed.
- Pain relief is often immediate.
- Patient must be cautioned against overuse following an injection.
- Palpation-guided injection have demonstrated success of at least 52% (3)[B].

ALERT

Failure of palpation-guided injection is typically due to an anatomic variant with two tendon sheaths, a septation in the 1st dorsal compartment, or the presence of a ganglion in the 1st compartment. In addition, there can be multiple slips of the APL or EPB tendon. Anatomic variants may be seen in as many as 40–60% of patients who fail injections.

- If palpation-guided injection fails, consider repeat injection under US guidance.
- US-guided injection may help confirm the diagnosis, and ensure proper placement of medication, which may increase efficacy and decrease complications and possibly recurrences.
- US guided cortisone injections have shown success rates of at least 76% (4)[B].
- Immobilization after cortisone injection may or may not provide additional benefit than cortisone injection alone.
- Consider surgical referral if second injection fails.

ADDITIONAL THERAPIES

- Using a thumb spica splint alone may relieve pain in patients with mild or early symptoms. There is little research supporting other therapeutic modalities, including stretching, strengthening, iontophoresis, acupuncture, laser therapy, extracorporeal shock-wave therapy, Kinesio tape, prolotherapy, ketorolac injections, and therapeutic US.
- There is a growing body of evidence to support platelet-rich plasma (PRP) of the first dorsal compartment, but further research is still needed (5)[B].

SURGERY/OTHER PROCEDURES

- If conservative therapy is ineffective with persistent symptoms longer than 3 months after corticosteroid injection, surgical release of the fibrous first dorsal compartment may be considered.
- Surgical intervention has demonstrated >90% cure rate with relatively low risk for complication (6)[B].

ONGOING CARE

PATIENT EDUCATION

Discussion of the risk factors can lead to insight into what caused the problem and can help reduce recurrence.

PROGNOSIS

Most patients have a very good prognosis; however, recurrence is common, so modification of activities must be a part of the treatment plan.

COMPLICATIONS

ALERT

Complications of injection:

- SC fat atrophy
- Hypopigmentation
- Pain
- Neuritis
- Fat necrosis
- Tendon rupture
- Postinjection flare
- Local infection

Complications of surgery:

- Radial sensory nerve injury
- Incomplete decompression
- Volar subluxation of the APL and EPB tendons

REFERENCES

1. Huisstede BM, Coert JH, Fridén J, et al. Consensus on a multidisciplinary treatment guideline for de Quervain disease: results from the European HANDGUIDE study. *Phys Ther*. 2014;94(8):1095–1110.
2. Lane LB, Boretz RS, Stuchin SA. Treatment of de Quervain's disease: role of conservative management. *J Hand Surg*. 2001;26(3):258–260.
3. Oh JK, Messing S, Hyrien O, et al. Effectiveness of corticosteroid injections for treatment of de Quervain's Tenosynovitis. *Hand (N Y)*. 2017;12(4):357–361.
4. De Keating-Hart E, Touchais S, Kerjean Y, et al. Presence of an intracompartmental septum detected by ultrasound is associated with the failure of ultrasound-guided steroid injection in de Quervain's syndrome. *J Hand Surg Eur Vol*. 2016;41(2):212–219.
5. Kumar V, Talwar J, Rustagi A, et al. Comparison of clinical and functional outcomes after platelet-rich plasma injection and corticosteroid injection for the treatment of de Quervain's Tenosynovitis. *J Wrist Surg*. 2022;12(2):135–142.
6. Garçon JJ, Charruau B, Marteau E, et al. Results of surgical treatment of de Quervain's tenosynovitis: 80 cases with a mean follow-up of 9.5 years. *Orthop Traumatol Surg Res*. 2018;104(6):893–896.

ADDITIONAL READING

- Earp BE, Han CH, Floyd WE, et al. de Quervain tendinopathy: survivorship and prognostic indicators of recurrence following a single corticosteroid injection. *J Hand Surg*. 2015;40(6):1161–1165.
- Larsen CG, Fitzgerald MJ, Nellans KW, et al. Management of de Quervain Tenosynovitis: a critical analysis review. *JBJS Rev*. 2021;9(9).
- Peters-Veluthamaningal C, van der Windt DA, Winters JC, et al. Corticosteroid injection for de Quervain's tenosynovitis. *Cochrane Database Syst Rev*. 2009;(3):CD005616.
- Richie CA III, Briner WW Jr. Corticosteroid injection for treatment of de Quervain's tenosynovitis: a pooled quantitative literature evaluation. *J Am Board Fam Pract*. 2003;16(2):102–106.

CLINICAL PEARLS

- First-line treatment typically involves activity modification, splinting, ice massage, and a topical or oral anti-inflammatory.
- Corticosteroid injection can improve symptoms in a large percentage of patients and can be considered first-line therapy in those with severe or limiting symptoms.
- If a palpation-guided corticosteroid injection fails, consider an anatomical variant and repeating the injection under US guidance.

DENTOALVEOLAR TRAUMA

Tyson A. Jackson, MD • Christopher S. Bossart, MD • Christopher McGrew, MD, FACSM, CAQSM • Jaison Medayil, DO

BASICS

DESCRIPTION

Dentoalveolar injuries include dental avulsion, dental luxation, extrusion and intrusion, enamel and crown fractures, root fracture, and alveolar bone fracture.

EPIDEMIOLOGY

- 25% of all respondents in the United States between the ages of 6 and 50 years reported suffering at least one traumatic dental injury (TDI) to their anterior teeth (1).
- The worldwide prevalence is ~15% (2).
- About 1/3 of children of toddlers and 1/4 of adolescents and adults have had a TDI (3).
- The peak period for trauma to the primary teeth is 2 to 6 years of age because this is a time of increased mobility for the relatively uncoordinated toddler (4). Injuries to primary teeth usually result from falls and collisions as the child learns to walk and run (2).
- With regard to permanent teeth, school-aged boys suffer trauma almost twice as frequently as girls.
- Sports accidents and fights are the most common cause of dental trauma in teenagers.
- In adult patients, cycling (42.2%), baseball (15.3%), and football (10.6%) were the most common orofacial traumatic injury. In children, kickboard (12%), baseball (8.3%), martial arts (6.5%), and football (4.6%) were the most common. A large retrospective study shows that 79.5% of the injuries were incurred by males. The age group between 10 and 19 years was the most commonly affected (4).
- 90.3% of crown fractures or crown-root fractures occur from direct trauma (3).
- The most commonly involved teeth were the central maxillary incisors (42%), and the second most were the maxillary lateral incisors (4.9%) (5).
- There seems to be a seasonal variation in incidence of orofacial trauma. Many studies demonstrate the probable correlation between outdoor activities and predominance of dental trauma during warmer times of the year (in the northern hemisphere) (1),(4).
- Predominant gender: male-to-female ratio ranging from 1.3 to 2.5:1 for trauma to permanent teeth (6). Higher rates sometimes reported for females than males when corrected for exposure rates.

ETIOLOGY AND PATHOPHYSIOLOGY

- Etiology (2):
  - Fall or collision while walking is considered as the most common etiology ranging from 37.7% to 44.8% (7).
  - TDIs account for 18–30% of all oral injuries (8).
  - Sports-related injuries occurred in 18% of cases.
  - Bicycle and scooter accidents accounted for 13% of cases.
  - Assaults made up 7% of cases.
  - Road traffic accidents resulted in 1% of cases.
  - All others 12% (9)
- Pathophysiology (5):
  - Enamel fracture only (Ellis class I), 74.9%:
    - Uncomplicated crown fracture
    - Roughness of chipped tooth on tongue
    - May go unnoticed by athlete
    - Not a dental emergency
  - Enamel and dentin fracture (Ellis class II), 17.8%:
    - Uncomplicated crown fracture
    - Exposure of yellow dentin
    - Pain with dentin exposure to air, cold drinks, or touch
    - Pulp sensibility tests are unreliable in primary teeth and are therefore not recommended (10).
    - Not a dental emergency
  - Enamel, dentin, pulp exposed (Ellis class III), 0.97%:
    - Complicated crown fracture
    - Dental emergency (within 3 hours)
    - Exposure of red-pink dental pulp
    - Vital with closed root apex: less complex treatment
    - Vital pulp with open root apex: more complex but viable
    - Dental pulp opening appears dry or oozes putrescent exudates and no pain:
      - Nonviable
  - Root fractures (Ellis class IV), 3.4%:
    - Dental emergency (within 3 hours)
    - Middle (1/3) root fractures
      - Good prognosis with timely evaluation and treatment
      - Identified by longer visible coronal segment, partially extruded, and bleeding from gingival sulcus
      - If tooth not markedly loose, athlete can finish sporting event with mouth guard and seek follow-up in 24 hours (11),(12).
    - Cervical third fracture (worst prognosis)
    - Apical root fractures (best prognosis) (12)
  - Extrusion, intrusion, lateral luxations:
    - Displacement (not fracture) involving periodontal ligament (i.e., stretch, compress, rupture ligament)
    - Lateral luxation involves movement of tooth in any plane but axial: Follow up with dentist within 24 hours for splinting or immediately if tooth cannot be repositioned.
    - Intrusion involves movement of tooth inward:
      - May be extremely painful, painless, or numb depending on the extent of nerve root injury
      - Dental emergency (within 3 hours)
    - Extrusion is movement of the tooth out of the socket: Follow up with dentist within 24 hours for splinting or immediately if tooth cannot be repositioned.
  - Avulsion (tooth exarticulation): dental emergency (immediate): Time to definitive treatment is inversely related to viability.
  - Associated soft tissue injury (4):
    - Contusion: 3.7%
    - Abrasions: 3.7%
    - Lacerations: 72.4%

RISK FACTORS

- Protection: Large meta-analysis showed that athletes are 1.6 to 1.9 times more likely to have orofacial injuries playing sports not traditionally associated with mouth guard use compared to those sports mandating mouth guards (13).
- Male gender, age, greater overjet, lip coverage, anterior open bite, caries, overweight, a previous history of TDI, tongue piercing, alcohol, and sports were all associated with higher TDI rates (14).

GENERAL PREVENTION

- Face masks, in sports such as hockey and football, provide protection against facial trauma.
- Mouth guards reduce oral injuries and cushion impact.
- Stock mouth guards are inexpensive but lack custom fit and may pose danger if patient becomes unconscious.
- Mouth-formed or boil-and-bite mouth guards offer better fit but still have inconsistency in retention fit and quality.
- Custom-fitted mouth guards are fitted by a dentist to increase comfort, compliance, and protection.
- High cost of custom mouth guards can be justified compared to cost of cosmetic or restorative dentistry.

COMMONLY ASSOCIATED CONDITIONS

- Facial contusion, laceration, fracture
- Mandible fracture
- Intraoral laceration (tongue, buccal mucosa, gingiva)
- Concussion

DIAGNOSIS

HISTORY

- Mechanism of injury and associated injuries (15)
- Force and vector of injury: This is paramount to identify all injuries visible or potentially concealed by soft tissue injury and swelling.
- Time since injury, time tooth was out of mouth, method of storage and transport
- Past dental history, past general medical and surgical history
- Medications and allergies
- Last tetanus shot

PHYSICAL EXAM

- Signs and symptoms include:
  - Pain and tenderness to percussion or palpation
  - Temperature sensitivity
  - Color changes
  - Tooth loosening
- Physical examination:
  - Assess consciousness and airway, breathing, and circulation (ABCs).
  - General examination of head, face, and neck
  - Extra oral exam:
    - Palpate mandible, zygoma, TMJ, and mastoid region.
    - Check for mandibular or maxillary fractures, focusing on the lower border of the mandible.
    - Examine for extraoral lacerations, bruises, or swelling.
    - Inspect upper or lower lip lacerations for foreign bodies.
    - Careful palpation of mandibular condyles and maxilla
    - Check jaw movement for normal range.
    - Confirm condylar fractures with panoramic radiograph.
  - Intraoral exam:
    - Examine oral cavity for dental and oral mucosa damage.
    - Account for missing teeth.
    - Check labial and buccal mucosa, maxillary frenum, gingival tissues, and tongue for bruising or lacerations.
    - Palpate alveolus for fractures.
    - Evaluate dental occlusions by having the patient clench teeth.
    - Examine each tooth for damage or mobility, suspecting multiple type of injuries per tooth.
    - Excess mobility suggests root and alveolar fractures, or luxation injuries to a lesser extent.
    - Malalignment may indicate luxation injuries or fractures.
    - Modular movement of adjacent teeth suggests alveolar fractures.

DIFFERENTIAL DIAGNOSIS

- Dental fracture, subluxation, luxation, concussion
- Facial bone fracture
- Mandibular dislocation
- Soft tissue injury

DIAGNOSTIC TESTS & INTERPRETATION

- Radiographic examination: For evaluating injuries of permanent teeth with uncomplicated or complicated crown fractures, or concussion injury, one parallel periapical radiograph is recommended.
- For uncomplicated and complicated crown-root and root, alveolar fractures, subluxation, luxation (extrusive, intrusive, lateral), additional radiographs are needed including two additional radiographs of the tooth taken with different vertical and/or horizontal angulations and an occlusal radiograph with consideration of cone beam computed tomography (CBCT), if radiographs are insufficient (10)[A].
- For primary teeth with enamel fracture or concussion injury, no radiograph is recommended.
- For enamel and dentin fracture, a radiograph is optional.
- For complicated crown fracture, crown-root fracture, root fracture, alveolar fracture, subluxation, luxation (extrusive, intrusive, lateral), or avulsion, a periapical or occlusive radiograph is recommended (3)[A]. Fractures may not be evident initially; negative films may be repeated 1 to 2 days after injury.
- Postreduction views are needed to rule out root or alveolar fractures and confirm placement after reimplantation or splinting of an avulsed tooth.
- Photographic documentation: The use of preoperative and postoperative photography may be useful for documentation purposes.

TREATMENT

- Initial stabilization:
  - Establish ABCs.
  - Control soft tissue bleeding with pressure.
  - Provide analgesics with lidocaine (regional or local).
  - Orthodontic wax for exposed pulp, dentin, or sharp edges
  - Oral pain medications are not recommended initially due to partial ingestion of debris.
- Tooth avulsions (16):
  - Avulsed primary teeth should not be replaced.
  - Obtain imaging of soft tissue if unable to find lost tooth fragment (10).
  - Handle tooth by crown only.
  - Flush tooth and socket with sterile solution or milk. Do not brush.
  - Replant as soon as possible (ASAP).
  - Firmly reinsert tooth.
    - Have patient gently bite on gauze to seat tooth.
    - Ensure anatomic alignment with adjacent tooth.
    - Immediately transfer to dentistry or emergency room (ER) with on call dentistry.
  - For avulsed tooth/fragment not implantable store in:
    - Milk or sterile balanced salt solution (Hank solution)
    - Can store in milk for 3 to 6 hours and longer in balanced solution; only store up to 2 hours in saliva
    - Avoid storing in water.
  - Dentist treatment:
    - Prescribe 5 to 10 days of antibiotics (penicillin V, amoxicillin, or clindamycin) (17).
    - Use short-term, passive, and flexible splint along labial side for 2 weeks.
- Concussion:
  - Tooth is tender, no bleeding, or movement.
  - Follow up with dentist in 4 weeks if pain persists.
- Subluxation:
  - Slight tooth movement, not displaced from normal position with possible gingival bleeding.
  - Splint and follow up with dentist in 2 weeks (17) [C].
- Tooth fractures (18):
  - Can evaluate with illumination to assist in visualization of fine fracture lines
  - Enamel only (Ellis class I):
    - Locate fragment if possible.
    - If unable to reattach, place in balanced salt solution
    - May be reattached within 48 hours by dentist with resin or bonding
    - Can also non-urgently refer for smoothing edge or cosmetic repair 4 to 8 weeks later if needed
  - Enamel and dentin (Ellis class II):
    - Fragment may be reattached with bonding agent or composite resin.
    - Arrange dental referral ASAP (same day).
    - Seal exposed dentin to prevent bacterial contamination ASAP.

D

- Enamel, dentin, and pulp (Ellis class III):
  - Emergent evaluation within 3 hours by a dentist
  - Treatment based on pulp status and dental age
  - Direct pulp capping or partial pulpotomy may be indicated.
  - Root canal treatment for teeth with moderate pulp exposure and closed apices
- Crown-root fractures (cleave fractures):
  - Fractures near the alveolar crest rarely heal without root canal therapy and post/crown placement or extraction and prosthodontics treatment.
- Root fracture (Ellis class IV):
  - Reposition coronal portion and confirm with x-rays.
  - Splint with passive and flexible splint for 1 to 4 months (19),(20)
  - Prognosis poorer with greater distance from apical segment
- Middle third fractures:
  - Require urgent care.
  - Sterile gauze and gentle pressure after repositioning.
  - Subsequent dental evaluation and possible root canal over 6 to 8 weeks

• Luxation:
- For lateral luxation (subluxation of the dentoalveolar joint), if minor, it may be appropriate to attempt reduction if possible.
- If reduction is possible and successful, provider may approximate and suture any gingival injury; passive and flexible splint for 2 to 4 weeks, and follow up with pulp vitality testing, local anesthesia, firm repositioning, and splinting with close follow-up.
- Urgent referral (same day) only if repositioning cannot be done
- Extrusion injuries: repositioning and splinting with anesthesia as needed
- Intrusion injuries are dental emergencies. Record the distance of intrusion. Do not splint. Allow re-eruption without intervention initially (19)[C]. For intrusive and lateral luxation injuries, it was previously recommended to extract the primary tooth. That is no longer advised as research has shown that these teeth can re-erupt spontaneously (10)[C].
- Urgent dental follow-up in 24 to 48 hours

• Alveolar fractures:
- Immediate reduction with manual pressure after clinical diagnosis followed by radiographs and rigid splinting for 1 to 2 months reduces pulp necrosis.
- Empirical antibiotic therapy against oral flora is recommended to reduce contamination.
- Suture gingival lacerations if present (19)[C].

MEDICATION

• Immunizations: tetanus; consider if open wound
• Antibiotic therapy: Consider prophylactic antibiotics in cases of exposed pulp or avulsion. Penicillin V potassium or clindamycin may be used (20). There is limited evidence for the use of systemic antibiotics in the emergency management of luxation injuries and no evidence that antibiotics improve the outcomes for root-fractured teeth (19)[C].
• Pain medications

ISSUES FOR REFERRAL

• Patients should be advised to see their dentist in the time frame outlined earlier.
• Parents/patients should clean the affected area with a soft brush or cotton swab and use alcohol-free chlorhexidine gluconate 0.12% mouth rinse applied topically twice a day for one week (10)[A].
• Urgent oral surgical referral may be necessary owing to associated injuries.

ADDITIONAL THERAPIES

• Photographs and meticulous documentation are particularly important in cases of assault or motor vehicle accidents.
• Aspiration: If an avulsed tooth is not accounted for, a chest film or soft tissue film may be indicated. Swallowed teeth rarely require treatment and should not be retrieved unless there is concern for gastrointestinal (GI) obstruction.
• Damage to primary teeth may result in damage to permanent teeth in 25–70% of injuries.

SURGERY/OTHER PROCEDURES

• Dental splinting is used as an initial treatment for subluxed or avulsed teeth that are replaced.
• Root canal might be considered as delayed treatment in cases of injury resulting in damage to the root.

ADMISSION, INPATIENT, AND NURSING CONSIDERATIONS

Hospital admission or observation is rarely required. Criteria may include:

• Multiple, complicated trauma
• Vital signs instability
• Abuse or violence is suspected in injury history.
• Concern for aspirated tooth

ONGOING CARE

• Tooth avulsion:
- Endodontic treatment is usually required at 1 to 2 weeks in teeth with a closed apex.
- Teeth with open apex may reestablish blood supply, thermal sensitivity testing is performed every 3 to 4 weeks, with root canal treatment delayed until clinical or x-ray signs of disease.
- Must follow up with dentistry every 6 months for years.

• Tooth fractures:
- Crown fractures: Definitive restoration should be performed ASAP, especially if the arch is crowded, because delay may allow encroachment of adjacent teeth and necessitate orthodontic treatment before restoration. Root canal treatment may be required in 1 to 2 weeks in cases of pulp exposure.
- Root fractures: Monthly clinical and radiographic evaluation should be performed during splinting and then every 3 to 6 months for at least 2 years; 20–45% have pulpal necrosis and require pulpotomy, root canal treatment, or prosthesis. Hard tissue union is more likely with pulpal vitality, younger patients, closer fragment opposition, and increased root diameter.

- Tooth luxation:
  - Intrusion: Radiographic monitoring for pulp necrosis or root resorption should occur every 3 weeks. Orthodontic extrusion is required if re-eruption is not satisfactory after 3 months. Root canal treatment is required in 2 to 3 weeks for 95% of teeth with mature roots and 65% of teeth with immature roots owing to pulp necrosis.
  - Lateral luxation requires follow-up with radiographs every 3 months for 2 years to ensure that root resorption or loss of pulp vitality is not evident.

DIET

Soft or liquid diet may be necessary for a time to further protect teeth and allow for healing.

REFERENCES

1. Ranalli DN. Sports dentistry and dental traumatology. *Dent Traumatol.* 2002;18(5):231–236.
2. Petti S. Over two hundred million injuries to anterior teeth attributable to large overjet: a meta-analysis. *Dent Traumatol.* 2015;31(1):1–8.
3. Cagetti MG, Marcoli PA, Berengo M, et al. Italian guidelines for the prevention and management of dental trauma in children. *Ital J Pediatr.* 2019;45(1):157.
4. Park HK, Park JY, Choi NR, et al. Sports-related oral and maxillofacial injuries: a 5-year retrospective study, Pusan National University Dental Hospital. *J Oral and Maxillofacial Surg.* 2021;79(1):203.e1–203.e8.
5. Dighe K, Kakade A, Takate V, et al. Prevalence of traumatic injuries to anterior teeth in 9–14 year school-going children in Mumbai, India. *J Contemp Dent Pract.* 2019;20(5):622–630.
6. Lam R. Epidemiology and outcomes of traumatic dental injuries: a review of the literature. *Aust Dent J.* 2016;16(Suppl 1):4–20.
7. Goswami M, Rahman B, Singh S. Outcomes of luxation injuries to primary teeth—a systematic review. *J Oral Biol Craniofac Res.* 2020;10(2):227–232.
8. Spinas E, Mameli A, Giannetti L. Traumatic dental injuries resulting from sports activities; immediate treatment and five years follow-up: an observational study. *Open Dent J.* 2018;12:1–10.
9. Wright G, Bell A, McGlashan G, et al. Dentoalveolar trauma in Glasgow: an audit of mechanism of injury. *Dent Traumatol.* 2007;23(4):226–231.
10. Day PF, Flores MT, O'Connell AC. International Association of Dental Traumatology guidelines for the management of traumatic dental injuries: 3. Injuries in the primary dentition. *Dent Traumatol.* 2020;36(4):343–359.
11. Gould TE, Piland SG, Caswell SV, et al. National Athletic Trainers' Association position statement: preventing and managing sport-related dental and oral injuries. *J Athl Train.* 2016;51(10):821–839.
12. Babu AN. Common dental injuries in athletes—a review. 2020;7(5):1436–1440.
13. Knapik JJ, Marshall SW, Lee RB, et al. Mouthguards in sport activities: history, physical properties, and injury prevention effectiveness. *Sports Med.* 2007;37(2):117 144.
14. Magno MB, Nadelman P, de França Leite KL, et al. Associations and risk factors for dental trauma: a systematic review of systematic reviews. *Community Dent Oral Epidemiol.* 2020, 48(6).447–463.
15. Greenberg MS, Springer PS. Diagnosis and management of oral injuries. In: Torg JS, ed. *Athletic Injuries to the Head, Neck, and Face.* 2nd ed. Mosby-Year Book; 1991:635–649.
16. Dewhurst SN, Mason C, Roberts GJ. Emergency treatment of orodental injuries: a review. *Br J Oral Maxillofac Surg.* 1998;36(3):165–175.
17. Fouad AF, Abbott PV, Tsilingaridis G, et al. International Association of Dental Traumatology guidelines for the management of traumatic dental injuries: 2. Avulsion of permanent teeth. *Dent Traumatol.* 2020,36(4):331–342.
18. Camp JH. Management of sports-related root fractures. *Dent Clin North Am.* 2000;44(1):95–109, vi–vii.
19. Bourguignon C, Cohenca N, Lauridsen E, et al. International Association of Dental Traumatology guidelines for the management of traumatic dental injuries: 1. Fractures and luxations. 2020;36(4):314–330.
20. Mark DG, Granquist EJ. Are prophylactic oral antibiotics indicated for the treatment of intraoral wounds? *Ann Emerg Med.* 2008;52(4):368–372.

ADDITIONAL READING

- American Academy of Pediatric Dentistry. Guideline of Management of Acute Dental Trauma. AAPD. Accessed February 1, 2025. https://www.aapd.org/assets/1/7/g_trauma.pdf
- Inouye J, McGrew C. Dental problems in athletes. *Curr Sports Med Rep.* 2015;14(1):27–33.
- Trope M. Clinical management of the avulsed tooth. *Dent Clin North Am.* 1995;39(1):93–112.

D

DEVELOPMENTAL DYSPLASIA OF THE HIP

Sunny Gupta, DO

BASICS

Developmental dysplasia of the hip (DDH) is the most common hip disorder in children.

DESCRIPTION

- *Dysplasia* refers to an acetabulum that is shallow or underdeveloped.
- *Subluxation* refers to a femoral head that is not centered within the acetabulum.
- *Dislocation* refers to a femoral head that is completely out of the acetabulum.
- *Teratologic* dislocation refers to a femoral head that is in a fixed dislocated position usually associated with a genetic, developmental, or neuromuscular disorder.
- An *unstable hip* refers to a femoral head that can be subluxed or dislocated on physical examination.
- DDH refers to a wide spectrum of hip disorders from mild underdevelopment of the acetabulum to frank teratologic dislocation of the femoral head from the acetabulum.

EPIDEMIOLOGY

Incidence

- Incidence varies with gender, age, and race.
- Incidence of hip dysplasia is 0.5–2% of live births; however, true dislocation occurs in 0.1–0.2% of live births (1).
- Late dysplasia, subluxation, and dislocation occur in 0.04% of children (2).

ETIOLOGY AND PATHOPHYSIOLOGY

- Caused by any mechanism that prevents femoral head from being positioned correctly within the acetabulum, resulting in a shallow acetabulum
- Firstborn
- Intrauterine factors:
  - Abnormal intrauterine positioning: Breech presentation positions hip in such a way that the femoral head is forced out of the acetabulum.
  - Oligohydramnios
- Underlying ligamentous laxity
- Collagen vascular disorders
- Infection
- Environmental: culture-associated neonatal swaddling
- Congenital:
  - Arthrogryposis
  - Lumbosacral agenesis
  - Spina bifida
  - Neonatal Marfan syndrome
  - Fetal hydantoin syndrome
  - Larsen syndrome

RISK FACTORS

- Predominant race: more common in Caucasians of European descent; rare in African Americans
- Predominant gender: females > males (6:1)
- Birth order: increased risk with firstborns
- Family history: very strong risk factor
- Risk ~13% with one parent with hip dysplasia and 35% with affected parent and sibling
- Intrauterine factors: increased risk with breech presentation and oligohydramnios

GENERAL PREVENTION

- There is no true way to prevent occurrence.
- Early diagnosis is key to management.
- Thorough examination of hips of newborns and infants is the mainstay of early diagnosis.

COMMONLY ASSOCIATED CONDITIONS

Commonly associated with torticollis (20% coexistence) and metatarsus adductus (10% coexistence)

DIAGNOSIS

HISTORY

- Determine risk:
  - Breech delivery or position in 3rd trimester?
  - Female?
  - Firstborn?
  - Family history?
  - Race?
- Is the baby moving both lower extremities symmetrically or if bilateral DDH are they moving lower extremities proportionally to upper extremities?
- Any abnormal position of lower extremities noticed by parents?
- Delay in crawling, cruising or standing

PHYSICAL EXAM

- All infants require clinical screening by a primary care provider who has experience in examining the hip at every well child visit until infant or toddler is walking normally.
- Examine patient in supine position.
- Every attempt should be made to examine the infant when he or she is not crying to avoid tensing of lower extremity muscles.
- Ortolani test:
  - Abduction and external rotation of hip with examiner's middle finger over greater trochanter
  - Palpable clunk is positive sign produced by reduction of dislocated hip.
- Barlow test:
  - Adduction and internal rotation of hip
  - Palpable clunk is positive sign as hip dislocates.
- Observe for signs of asymmetries:
  - Decrease in abduction of hip with adduction contracture (best test >3 months)
  - Asymmetric gluteal, anterior upper thigh and popliteal skin folds
  - Galeazzi sign: apparent femoral shortening with hips and knees flexed together
- Examination may be normal initially despite the presence of hip dysplasia. Consequently, hip evaluation should be performed as part of neonatal physical examination through 4 months of age (1).
- For the older infant or child, Barlow and Ortolani examination is of limited utility due to development of contractures (3).

DIAGNOSTIC TESTS & INTERPRETATION

- False-positive results: Hip clicks will be present in 10% of infants; only a small percentage will have hip dysplasia.
- Overdiagnosis can rarely be a problem because avascular necrosis of femur can occur (rarely) as a result of therapeutic interventions (4).
- X-rays:
  - Not useful prior to 3 to 4 months, when the femoral head epiphysis ossifies and acetabular parameters are better defined
  - Various reference lines (Hilgenreiner, Shenton, and Perkin) and angles (acetabular index) are useful to detect frank dislocation (1).

- Ultrasound (US):
  - Most sensitive and effective form of screening
  - Recommended to evaluate with US starting at age 4 to 6 weeks in patients with risk factors, any abnormal history or abnormal or asymmetric hip exam (4)
  - Static and dynamic imaging (with Barlow and Ortolani maneuvers) to assess femoral head displacement
  - Useful in monitoring progress of therapy
  - Requires experienced ultrasonographer
  - Cost-effective (5)[A]
- Computed tomography (CT) scan and magnetic resonance imaging (MRI) are not useful in diagnosis.

TREATMENT

- Subluxation at birth often resolves spontaneously and therefore may be observed for 3 weeks.
- Indication for treatment: Subluxation of hip persists beyond 3 weeks, confirmed on physical exam or US. Refer to a pediatric orthopedist (2).
- Pavlik harness:
  - Indicated for infants from ages 3 weeks to 6 months
  - Applied by orthopedist; hips positioned in flexion and abduction
  - Requires weekly evaluation of straps and radiologic confirmation of hip reduction; if hip is stable at 2 weeks, reevaluation every 2 weeks
  - Gradually weaned as hip stability continues
  - Duration of treatment: 3 months after hip stability achieved (1)[A]
  - 70–95% success rate (6)[A]
- Hip spica cast:
  - Indicated for children from ages 6 to 18 months
  - Applied by orthopedist under general anesthesia; hips positioned in flexion and abduction with cutouts for perineal care
  - Cast changes every 6 weeks
  - Duration of treatment: 3 to 4 months (1)[A]
- Open reduction:
  - Indicated if closed reduction fails or excess abduction (>60 degrees) required for concentric reduction
  - Corrects barriers to reduction and safely increases stability (1)[A]
- Femoral/pelvic osteotomies:
  - Indicated if all prior closed and open reductions fail
  - Usually considered in children from ages 18 to 36 months (1)[A]

ONGOING CARE

PROGNOSIS

If diagnosed early, prognosis is uniformly excellent.

COMPLICATIONS

- Missed early diagnosis can result in more complicated management and less favorable outcome.
- Failed reduction and redislocation
- Osteonecrosis of femoral head
- Hip labral pathology in adolescence or adulthood
- Osteoarthritis in adulthood

REFERENCES

1. Schwend RM, Shaw BA, Segal LS. Evaluation and treatment of developmental hip dysplasia in the newborn and infant. *Pediatr Clin North Am*. 2014;61(6):1095–1107.
2. Tomlinson J, O'Dowd D, Fernandes JA. Managing developmental dysplasia of the hip. *Indian J Pediatr*. 2016;83(11):1275–1279.
3. Yang S, Zusman N, Leiberman E, et al. Developmental dysplasia of the hip. *Pediatrics*. 2019;143(1):e20181147.
4. Kotlarsky P, Haber R, Bialik V, et al. Developmental dysplasia of the hip: what has changed in the last 20 years? *World J Orthop*. 2015;6(11):886–901.
5. Pandey RA, Johari AN. Screening of newborns and infants for developmental dysplasia of the hip: a systematic review. *Indian J Orthop*. 2021;55:1388–1401.
6. Swarup I, Penny CL, Dodwell ER. Developmental dysplasia of the hip: an update on diagnosis and management from birth to 6 months. *Curr Opin Pediatr*. 2018;30(1):84–92.

ADDITIONAL READING

- Beaty JH. Congenital and developmental anomalies of hip and pelvis. In: Canale ST, ed. *Campbell's Operative Orthopaedics*. 10th ed. Mosby; 2003:1079–1117.
- Guille JT, Pizzutillo PD, MacEwen GD. Development dysplasia of the hip from birth to six months. *J Am Acad Orthop Surg*. 2000;8(4):232–242.
- Vitale MG, Skaggs DL. Developmental dysplasia of the hip from six months to four years of age. *J Am Acad Orthop Surg*. 2001;9(6):401–411.

CLINICAL PEARLS

- DDH is the most common hip disorder in children.
- Early diagnosis is key to management. This is accomplished with a thorough examination of hips of newborns and infants. Delay in diagnosis can lead to significantly worse outcomes.
- US is the most sensitive and effective form of screening; start screening with US at age 4 to 6 weeks in patients with risk factors, persistent clunk on hip exam or asymmetric hip exam.
- Refer to pediatric orthopedist for treatment if subluxation of hip persists beyond 3 weeks, confirmed on physical exam or US.

DIABETES IN SPORTS

Andrew Nobe, MD, CAQSM • Samuel Bell, MD

BASICS

DESCRIPTION

Diabetes mellitus (DM) is a chronic disease caused by a genetic and/or acquired deficiency of insulin production due to destruction of the islet cells of the pancreas (type 1) or due to ineffectiveness of the insulin produced (type 2) resulting in elevated blood glucose levels.

EPIDEMIOLOGY

Incidence

The incidence of diabetes in the United States in 2021 was 1.2 million for adults. The incidence of diabetes in the United States in 2017–2018 was 23,362 for children and adolescents.

Prevalence

In 2021, an estimated 38.4 million people or 11.6% of the U.S. population had diabetes.

RISK FACTORS

- Type 2 DM: obesity, family history, cardiovascular disease, physical inactivity, glucose intolerance, gestational diabetes, and older age
- Type 1 DM: family history, environmental triggers, and younger age

GENERAL PREVENTION

- Lifestyle and behavioral interventions in combination with an individualized reduced-calorie meal plan has been shown to prevent and delay type 2 DM in randomized controlled trials:
  - In the Diabetes Prevention Program, goal-based interventions of 7% weight loss and 150 minutes of moderate-intensity physical activity per week reduced the incidence of type 2 DM.
- Pharmacologic intervention with metformin or weight loss drugs may considered to prevent type 2 DM in those with high risk:
  - Aged 25 to 59 years
  - BMI ≥35 kg/m^2
  - Fasting blood glucose >110 mg/dL
  - A1C ≥6%
  - History of gestational diabetes
- For type 1 DM, lack of physical activity and higher dietary glycemic index intake has been associated with increased risk of progression to clinical DM, and increased physical activity has been associated with reduced risk of progression to clinical DM.
- Infusions of teplizumab can be considered to delay onset of symptomatic type 1 DM in certain patients.

DIAGNOSIS

HISTORY

Known case of diabetes type 1 or type 2. Assess for symptoms of hyperglycemia (e.g., polydipsia, polyphagia, polyuria, weight loss, blurry vision) or hypoglycemia (e.g., dizziness, weakness, tremor, palpitations).

PHYSICAL EXAM

- Body mass index (BMI)
- Vital signs, in particular blood pressure
- Skin and foot examination to assess for skin breakdown, deformities, and skin infection
- Peripheral pulses to assess for peripheral arterial disease
- Neurologic examination of sensation (i.e., monofilament) to assess for neuropathy
- Eye examination to assess for retinopathy and visual loss

DIAGNOSTIC TESTS & INTERPRETATION

Initial Tests (lab, imaging)

A person can be diagnosed with diabetes if blood tests show the following results:

- A1C ≥6.5% (48 mmol/mol)
- Fasting plasma glucose ≥126 mg/dL (7 mmol/L)
- 2-hour plasma glucose ≥200 mg/dL (11.1 mmol/L) during OGTT
- In a patient with classic symptoms of hyperglycemia or hyperglycemic crisis, a random plasma glucose of ≥200 mg/dL (11.1 mmol/L) (1)[A]

Follow-Up Tests & Special Considerations

- A second confirmatory test is required, unless there is a clear clinical diagnosis (e.g., patient in a hyperglycemic crisis or with classic symptoms of hyperglycemia and a random plasma glucose 200 mg/dL).
- It is recommended that the same test be repeated, or a different test be performed, without delay using a new blood sample for confirmation.
- If clinical suspicion is high for type 1 DM (e.g., young onset, early insulin dependence, lack of metabolic risk factors for type 2 DM), the presence of autoantibodies against glutamic acid decarboxylase (GAD), islet antigen 2 (IA2), zinc-transporter 8 (ZnT8), and fasting C-peptide may be considered to assess for type 1 DM (1).

Diagnostic Procedures/Other

Additional testing/procedures are targeted on assessing for comorbidities and surveillance and prevention of complications.

- Fasting lipid profile, liver function tests, spot urinary albumin-to-creatinine ratio, serum creatinine and estimated glomerular filtration rate, thyroid-stimulating hormone, complete blood count, electrolytes
- Team-based management with ophthalmology, nutritionist, diabetes educator, podiatry, dental
- Ankle-brachial index to screen for peripheral artery disease in patients ≥50 years old, known microvascular disease, foot complications, or end-organ damage
- Consider cardiac stress testing in patients with cardiac symptoms, signs or symptoms of vascular disease, or abdominal resting electrocardiogram.

TREATMENT

GENERAL MEASURES

Therapeutic lifestyle changes including exercise, healthy diet, weight control, and tobacco cessation are recommended.

- Exercise/physical activity risks and benefits:
  - Benefits of exercise include improved insulin sensitivity and decreased insulin dosage, weight loss, improvements in blood pressure, lipid profiles, cardiovascular health, mental health, bone mineral density, and overall mortality (2)[A].
  - Risks of exercise include hypoglycemia and hyperglycemia; heat-related illness; or complications from autonomic neuropathy, cardiovascular, or pulmonary.
- Exercise/physical activity guideline recommendations:
  - Most adults with type 1 or type 2 DM should engage in 150 minutes or more of moderate- to vigorous-intensity aerobic activity weekly, spread over at least 3 days/wk, with no more than 2 consecutive days without activity. Shorter durations (minimum 75 minutes/wk) of vigorous-intensity or interval training may be sufficient for younger and more physically fit individuals (3)[B]. Also, 2 to 3 sessions of resistance exercise on nonconsecutive days are recommended (3)[B]. Flexibility and balance training are recommended 2 to 3 times/wk for older adults. Yoga and tai chi may be included based on individual preferences to increase flexibility, muscular strength, and balance (3)[C]. Children and adolescents with type 1 or type 2 DM should engage in 60 minutes/d or more of moderate- or vigorous-intensity aerobic activity, with vigorous, muscle-strengthening, and bone-strengthening activities included at least 3 days/wk (3)[C].
- Preexercise considerations:
  - Preexercise medical clearance is generally unnecessary for asymptomatic individuals prior to beginning low- or moderate-intensity physical activity not exceeding the demands of brisk walking or everyday living.
  - Indications for preexercise medical screening include patients with symptoms of cardiovascular disease, attempting to begin a vigorous exercise program, or individuals who are increasing from a sedentary lifestyle to a more vigorous level of exercise.
  - A medical screening examination should carefully screen for the presence of macrovascular and microvascular complications that may be worsened by the exercise program and review the risk of both hypoglycemic and hyperglycemic events within the context of the athlete's intended activity.
  - Athletes should check blood glucose levels before engaging in moderate- to high-intensity exercise.
  - Avoid exercise if fasting glucose levels are >250 mg/dL and ketosis is present and use caution if glucose levels are >350 mg/dL and no ketosis is present.
  - Insulin regimen and carbohydrate intake changes should be used to prevent exercise-related hypoglycemia and hyperglycemia. Other strategies involve including short sprints, performing resistance exercise before aerobic exercise in the same session, and activity timing (3)[B].
  - Risk of nocturnal hypoglycemia following physical activity may be mitigated with reductions in basal insulin doses, inclusion of bedtime snacks, and/or use of continuous glucose monitoring (CGM) (3)[C].
  - Physical activity done with peripheral neuropathy necessitates proper foot care to prevent and detect problems early to avoid ulceration and amputation (3)[B].

MEDICATION

- Type 1 DM: insulin which can be delivered via an insulin pump/continuous subcutaneous insulin infusion (CSII) or multiple daily injections (MDI). Management strategies to address exercise related hypoglycemia, postexercise hyperglycemia, and nocturnal hypoglycemia are complex:
  - For athletes with CSII, basal insulin rate can be reduced by 50–80% 90 minutes prior to exercise, temporary increase in insulin rate post exercise, and decrease in insulin rate overnight (4).
  - For athletes with MDI, the basal insulin dose can be reduced by 20–50% before exercise and reduction in evening bolus insulin by 50% (4).
- Type 2 DM: Metformin is the first drug to be initiated (1)[A]. If glycemic goals are not achieved, subsequent glucose-lowering agents should be considered and individualized to each patient (1)[A]. Options include (preferred) SGLT2 inhibitor, GLP-1 receptor agonist (RA) (or dual GIP/GLP-1), DPP-4 inhibitor, insulin, and (not preferred) sulfonylureas, thiazolidinediones.

ALERT
Athletes should be aware that insulin and sulfonylureas have hypoglycemia risk. Glucagon hormone should be given to unconscious or semiconscious diabetic patients in acute hypoglycemic state. It can be administered as subcutaneous or intramuscular injection.

ALERT
SGLT2 inhibitors act as a modest diuretic, so athletes may be prone to dehydration.

ALERT
GLP-1 RAs can slow gut transit and could delay absorption of nutrients and affect circulating glucose levels.

ISSUES FOR REFERRAL

- Disease complications: Consider annual review—more frequent if disease complications not well managed (1)[B].
- Endocrinologist in cases where management is difficult
- Consider cardiology, nephrology, neurology, ophthalmology, and podiatry/vascular surgery referrals for organ-specific complications.

ADDITIONAL THERAPIES

- Moderate-intensity statin therapy recommended patients with diabetes ages 40 to 75 years. If high cardiovascular risk, high-intensity statin therapy recommended (1)[A]. Use American College of Cardiology (ACC) 10 year atherosclerotic cardiovascular disease (ASCVD) risk calculator to determine risk.
- Aspirin 75 to 162 mg daily in patient with high cardiovascular risk (1)[A]
- Angiotensin-converting enzyme (ACE) inhibitors/angiotensin II receptor blockers (ARBs) for hypertension and diabetic nephropathy (1)[A]
- Gabapentin, pregabalin, or duloxetine oral for neuropathic pain (1)[A]
- SGLT2 inhibitor or GLP-1 RA recommended for patients with diabetes and known cardiovascular disease (3)[A]

ADMISSION, INPATIENT, AND NURSING CONSIDERATIONS

- Perform HbA1C for all patients admitted, if not checked in last 3 months (1)[B].
- Insulin therapy should be initiated for treatment of persistent hyperglycemia starting at a threshold ≥180 mg/dL (10 mmol/L) (1)[A].
- A target glucose range of 140 to 180 mg/dL (7.8 to 10 mmol/L) is recommended for the majority of critically ill patients (1)[A] and noncritically ill patients (1)[C].

ONGOING CARE

FOLLOW-UP RECOMMENDATIONS

- A1C every 3 to 6 months with a target goal of <7% to prevent microvascular complications (1)[A]
- Dilated eye exam, comprehensive foot exam, dental exam annually
- Comprehensive metabolic panel, fasting lipid profile, urinary albumin-to-creatinine ratio, complete blood count at least annually
- Self-monitoring of blood glucose (SMBG) (e.g., CGM) may be a useful adjunct in selected patients, particularly those with MDI.
- Most patients using intensive insulin regimens (multiple-dose insulin or insulin pump therapy) should perform SMBG prior to meals and snacks, at bedtime, occasionally postprandially, prior to exercise, when they suspect low blood glucose, after treating low blood glucose until they are normoglycemic, and prior to critical tasks such as driving (1)[B].

DIET

- Athletes with diabetes should strive for a healthy diet individualized to achieve glycemic and body weight goals and delay or prevent diabetic complications.
- Food-based dietary patterns should be emphasized more than specific macronutrient patterns.
- Avoid added sugars, processed foods, and alcohol.
- Additional carbohydrates may be needed before, during, and after exercise to maintain blood glucose in a normal range (consider 0.4 to 1.3 g carbohydrate per kilogram of body mass per hour while exercising).
- Having diabetes does not change the necessary protein intake for athletes.
- Comanagement with nutritionist is encouraged.

PATIENT EDUCATION

- It is essential that athletes with DM be educated on signs, symptoms, prevention, and treatment of both hypoglycemia and hyperglycemia.
- It is recommended for diabetic patients to obtain the approval of a doctor before starting a new sport.
- Athletes with diabetes should have on hand at least 15 g of sugar, such as 1 1/2 cup of fruit juice or five candy bars or glucose cubes and/or glucagon injection, to treat hypoglycemia.
- If shivering, anxiousness, dizziness, excessive sweating, or any unusual changes in heart rate develop while exercising, the athlete should stop exercising and immediately check a blood sugar level. If low, treat with carbohydrates or glucagon.
- Diabetic patients should have identification and a health alert bracelet or necklace when going out to exercise, in case of needing medical assistance.
- Blood sugar levels should be checked before and after exercise. It is advisable to determine a safe blood glucose range prior to exercise in conjunction with a physician. This is especially important for people who use insulin.
- Start each exercise session with 5 to 10 minutes of warm-ups, so that the body is ready for sport and is not surprised by difficult and intensive exercise which could cause transient hyperglycemia.
- For individuals with diabetes, a variety of aerobic exercises are recommended. These can include activities like walking, light jogging, swimming, cycling, and kayaking. Other beneficial options are dancing, jumping rope, and playing sports such as tennis or basketball.
- Resistance exercises are also recommended for patients with DM as they will improve muscle mass and strength, body composition, physical function, bone mineral density, mental well-being, insulin sensitivity, lipid profile, blood pressure, and cardiovascular health. All these lead to better control of HbA1C (3)[A].

PROGNOSIS

- DM patients are at 2 to 5 times increased risk for ischemic heart disease and 2 to 3 times increased risk for stroke and peripheral vascular disease. The protective effect of female sex is lost.
- Atherosclerotic disease accounts for most of the excess mortality due to DM.
- Diabetic nephropathy, renal failure, and dialysis are large sources of morbidity and mortality as diabetes progresses.

COMPLICATIONS

- Acute hypoglycemic and/or hyperglycemic events
- Autonomic dysfunction
- Retinopathy
- Cardiovascular disease
- Renal disease
- Foot problems, including ulcers, deformities, and infections, can manifest from neurologic and microvascular complications.

REFERENCES

1. American Diabetes Association. Standards of care in diabetes—2024. *Diabetes Care*. 2024;47(Suppl 1):S5–S244.
2. Trojian T, Colberg S, Harris G, et al. American Medical Society for Sports Medicine position statement on the care of the athlete and athletic person with diabetes. *Clin J Sport Med*. 2022;32(1):8–20.
3. Colberg SR, Sigal RJ, Yardley JE, et al. Physical activity/exercise and diabetes: a position statement of the American Diabetes Association. *Diabetes Care*. 2016;39(11):2065–2079.
4. Riddell MC, Scott SN, Fournier PA, et al. The competitive athlete with type 1 diabetes. *Diabetologia*. 2020;63(8):1475–1490.

ADDITIONAL READING

- Butler AE, Misselbrook D. Distinguishing between type 1 and type 2 diabetes. *BMJ*. 2020;370:m2998.
- Campbell MD, Walker M, Bracken RM, et al. Insulin therapy and dietary adjustments to normalize glycemia and prevent nocturnal hypoglycemia after evening exercise in type 1 diabetes: a randomized controlled trial. *BMJ Open Diabetes Res Care*. 2015;3(1):e000085.
- Cannataro R, Cione E, Cerullo G, et al. Type 1 diabetes management in a competitive athlete: a five-year case report. *Physiol Rep*. 2023;11(13):e15740.
- Centers for Disease Control and Prevention. National diabetes statistics report. Accessed August 6, 2025. https://www.cdc.gov/diabetes/php/data-research/index.html/

CLINICAL PEARLS

- Patients with DM should be strongly advised to obtain regular exercise or physical activity as part of their management plan for glycemic control, overall health, and prevention of diabetic complications.
- Physical activity does carry risk of hypoglycemia and hyperglycemia, notably for patients on insulin or insulin secretagogue therapy. Most hypoglycemic events occur during, immediately after, or 6 to 15 hours after exercise.
- Exercise plans should be tailored according to the individual's specific needs. Moreover, all diabetic adults should be encouraged indulge in regular frequent spells of activity.
- Blood glucose monitoring is an essential tool for diabetic patients to regulate the intensity and duration of their exercise and sports activities.
- Hyperglycemia and hypoglycemia are the greatest risks to exercising for the diabetic athletes, in particular those with type 1 DM and those on insulin. Diabetic patients should be educated regarding the symptoms and signs of hypoglycemia. Hypoglycemia can be avoided through reducing the insulin doses and/or increasing consumption of carbohydrates along with having an available source of sugar (15 g) in case of developing hypoglycemia during exercising.

DIP DISLOCATION

Rukmini Yakkanti, DO ▪ Tenley Murphy, MD, FAAFP, CAQSM ▪ Patrick Jenkins III, MD

BASICS

DESCRIPTION

- Dislocations of distal interphalangeal (DIP) or 1st interphalangeal (IP) joints
- Mechanism is typically a hyperextension injury of the DIP joint.
- Synonym(s): jammed finger

EPIDEMIOLOGY

Incidence

- Pure DIP dislocations are uncommon due to the stability of the joint from the surrounding soft tissue structures (1).
- Mallet finger is commonly associated with DIP dislocations (1).
- DIP dislocations are less common than proximal interphalangeal (PIP) dislocations.
- Most dislocations occur dorsally, especially when associated with injuries during athletic events. These injuries can lead to volar plate injury.
- DIP dislocations are common in basketball and American football (2).

ALERT
Volar dislocations are often associated with crush or twist injuries and with disruption of the terminal extensor tendon at its insertion point, making management more difficult.

- Simultaneous DIP and PIP dislocations are rare but occur most commonly in the small fingers due to exposure (3).

DIAGNOSIS

HISTORY

- Mechanism of injury (i.e., hyperextension, crush injury)
- Presence of an obvious deformity (i.e., distal phalanx positioned above or below the plane of the middle phalanx)
- Often self-reduced by the patient on the playing field or before presentation

PHYSICAL EXAM

- Obvious deformity if not already reduced: distal phalanx sitting above (dorsal dislocation) or below (volar dislocation) the plane of the middle phalanx
- Careful examination: With the PIP joint held in extension, check flexor digitorum profundus (FDP) and terminal extensor function and sensation at the tip of the finger.
- Check collateral ligament: Place radial and ulnar stress across DIP joint with joint in full extension and 30 degrees flexion looking for increased laxity compared to the contralateral side.
- Check volar plate: Increased hyperextension of the joint is indicative of a volar plate injury.
- Evaluate skin for any signs of open injury. This is most commonly seen on palmar surface.
- Evaluate neurovascular status.

DIFFERENTIAL DIAGNOSIS

- Fracture of distal (tuft fracture) or middle phalanx
- FDP rupture (i.e., jersey finger)
- Extensor mechanism rupture (i.e., mallet finger)
- Bony mallet finger (bony avulsion of the insertion of the extensor mechanism at the dorsal base of the distal phalanx)
- Fracture-dislocation
- Collateral ligament disruption
- Chronic instability

DIAGNOSTIC TESTS & INTERPRETATION

- Radiographs: three views preferred (anteroposterior, lateral, and oblique views) pre- and postreduction if it does not significantly delay reduction attempt(s)
- Look carefully for any bony avulsion, especially of the volar plate.
- Other imaging modalities are not typically needed.

TREATMENT

GENERAL MEASURES

- Reduction techniques:
  - On-field reduction should be attempted to reduce pain and usually is easily performed when done immediately.
  - Technique for reduction: Maintaining proximal countertraction to the DIP joint, apply a steady longitudinal traction force of the distal finger (3)[C].
  - Slight hyperextension and volar pressure at the distal phalanx may aid in reduction of dorsal dislocations (4)[C].
  - Sweat can cause the skin to be slick, making reductions attempts difficult. Try using a towel or gauze pad for better grip.
  - Reduction may require a digital ring block if dislocation is prolonged or associated with significant pain (5)[C].

ALERT

Postreduction evaluation:

- Careful examination as discussed above, especially checking FDP/extensor function and for skin injury
- Postreduction radiographs from at least two views to ensure joint congruity (5)[C]

- Complications:
  - Dislocation may be irreducible. This is thought to happen for several reasons:
    - Trapped volar plate
    - FDP entrapment behind a single condyle of middle phalanx
    - P2 buttonholed through the volar plate
    - Extensor tendon displacement around the head of P2
- Immobilization:
  - Dorsal dislocations should be placed in a dorsal extension block (4)[C] or buddy taped (3)[C] for 2 weeks.
  - Volar dislocations should be treated as a mallet finger injury and placed in a splint with the DIP joint in extension for 8 weeks, allowing the extensor tendon to heal.
  - Longer immobilization leads to increased likelihood of long-term joint stiffness
  - When splinting, use caution with regard to the dorsal skin segment between the extensor crease and the nail fold because pressure can cause necrosis.
  - Patient can return to sport once joint stability and range of motion (ROM) are acceptable (3)[C].

ISSUES FOR REFERRAL

- An urgent referral to an orthopedic surgeon or hand specialist should be made when the dislocation is irreducible or an open injury has occurred with joint exposure (6)[B].
- In addition, chronic dislocations, FDP tendon ruptures, fractures involving >30% of the articular surface, and unstable collateral ligaments should be referred to a specialist (4)[C].

ADDITIONAL THERAPIES

- Start ROM exercises immediately after splint removal.
- Use both active and passive ROM initially.
- Start resisted ROM as soon as active and passive motions are pain free (5)[C].
- Swelling control should be quickly initiated because it can block full ROM. This can be achieved with retrograde massage, elevation, ice, and compression.

SURGERY/OTHER PROCEDURES

- Closed reduction and percutaneous pinning (CRPP): Joint instability or associated fracture may require immobilization with use of a Kirschner wire for stabilization.
- Open reduction:
  - May be required in a chronically (>3 weeks) dislocated or subluxated joint to remove scar tissue and release tension to facilitate reduction
  - Use of a Kirschner wire depends on degree of stability.

REFERENCES

1. De Jonge MC, Assink J, Vanhoenacker FM. Acute bony injuries of hand and wrist. *Semin Musculoskelet Radiol.* 2021;25(2):277–293.
2. Meixner C, Loder RT. The demographics of fractures and dislocations across the entire United States due to common sports and recreational activities. *Sports Health* 2020;12(2):159–169.
3. Vasiliadis AV, Maris A, Tsatlidou M, et al. Double interphalangeal joint dislocation of the finger in adolescent athletes: a review of two cases and the relevant literature. *Case Rep Orthop.* 2021:6684553.
4. Childress MA, Olivas J, Crutchfield A. Common finger fractures and dislocations. *Am Fam Physician* 2022;105(6):631–639.
5. Clesham K, Piggott RP, Sheehan E. High-energy traumatic proximal and distal interphalangeal joint dislocation in the same finger. *BMJ Case Rep* 2020;13(6):e235426.
6. Jerome TJ. Open dorsal distal interphalangeal joint dislocations: a report of 20 cases. *Orthop Traumatol Surg Res.* 2021;107(5):102852.

CLINICAL PEARLS

- Athletes can return to play immediately if dislocation is uncomplicated, successfully reduced, and the athlete is allowed to play in a splint or cast.
- Thumb IP dislocations should be treated exactly the same as DIP dislocations.

D

DISCOID MENISCUS

Melissa Nayak, MD, CAQSM

BASICS

DESCRIPTION

- Menisci are semilunar fibrocartilaginous structures located between the femoral condyles and tibial plateaus, composed mainly of type I collagen.
- A discoid meniscus lacks C-shaped configuration:
  - Completely filled in center or small void in center with thicker outer rim (disc or saucer-shaped)
  - Abnormal vascularity and microarchitecture (disorganization of collagen orientation, decreased collagen fibers, mucoid degeneration)
  - Anatomic variation alters normal mechanics and predisposes to tearing.
- Predominantly lateral; may be medial or bilateral
- May be asymptomatic until adolescence or adulthood
- Watanabe classification
  - Most widely accepted classification system
  - Type I (complete):
    - Most common
    - Disc-shaped, thickened meniscus with thin center, complete tibial plateau coverage, and normal posterior attachment
  - Type II (incomplete): semilunar-shaped meniscus with partial tibial plateau coverage and normal posterior attachment
  - Type III (Wrisberg type):
    - Least common
    - Hypermobile meniscus resulting from deficient posterior tibial plateau attachment (missing coronary ligament)
    - Wrisberg ligament present (from posterior horn lateral meniscus to posterior aspect medial femoral condyle)
    - Unstable and may displace

EPIDEMIOLOGY

Incidence

- 3–5% in U.S. population (discoid lateral meniscus)
- 0.1–0.3% (discoid medial meniscus)
- 25% of discoid meniscus cases are bilateral.
- Increased incidence in Asian populations
- ~13% in Japan (discoid lateral meniscus)
- True incidence unknown (due to asymptomatic cases)

ETIOLOGY AND PATHOPHYSIOLOGY

- Exact cause unknown
- May be congenital anomaly or morphologic variant

Genetics

Genetic or familial transmission may play a role.

RISK FACTORS

Asian ancestry

COMMONLY ASSOCIATED CONDITIONS

- Meniscal tears (increased incidence related to structural abnormality, decreased vascularity, and biomechanical stress)
  - Horizontal cleavage tear (most common)
- Osteochondritis dissecans of ipsilateral lateral femoral condyle: likely due to the abnormal biomechanics and increased stress placed on the joint surfaces in the presence of a discoid meniscus
- High fibular head
- Hypoplasia of lateral femoral condyle with lateral joint space widening
- Hypoplasia of lateral tibial spine
- Abnormal shape of lateral malleolus
- Enlarged inferior lateral geniculate artery

DIAGNOSIS

HISTORY

- Patients may be asymptomatic.
- Signs and symptoms (in absence of trauma):
  - Pain
  - Clicking
  - Giving way
  - Popping
  - Snapping
  - Swelling
  - Locking
  - Limited knee extension

PHYSICAL EXAM

- Varies based on patient age, type, and location of the discoid meniscus and if there is a meniscus tear.
- Palpable click near complete extension
- Quadriceps atrophy
- Lack of full extension
- Joint line tenderness
- Effusion
- Positive McMurray Thessaly testing (with associated meniscal tears)

DIFFERENTIAL DIAGNOSIS

- Meniscal tear
- Osteochondritis dissecans
- Loose body
- Patellar instability
- Snapping of extra-articular knee tendons
- Medial plica syndrome

DIAGNOSTIC TESTS & INTERPRETATION

- Radiographs:
  - May be normal
  - Widened lateral joint space
  - Squared-off appearance of lateral femoral condyle

- Cupping of lateral tibial plateau (abnormal shape alters the biomechanics of the knee joint, leading to abnormal stress distribution on the tibial plateau)
- Hypoplasia of lateral tibial eminence
- Elevation of fibular head
- Magnetic resonance imaging (MRI):
  - Test of choice
  - May not show abnormal signal intensity
  - Lateral meniscal height greater than medial, with high intrameniscal signal
  - Abnormal, thickened "bow-tie" appearance of meniscus

TREATMENT

No treatment or surgical indications for asymptomatic patients (1),(2),(3),(4)[C]

ISSUES FOR REFERRAL

Orthopedic surgical consultation is indicated in symptomatic discoid meniscus causing pain and/or mechanical symptoms.

SURGERY/OTHER PROCEDURES

- Goal is meniscal preservation (1),(2),(3),(4)[C].
- Arthroscopic saucerization (partial meniscectomy), with or without meniscal repair, and repair of peripheral rim attachments to the capsule (1),(2),(3),(4)[C]
- Arthroscopic total meniscectomy not recommended because it leads to osteoarthrosis; reserved for large or complex tears not amenable to saucerization or repair.

ONGOING CARE

Postoperative physical therapy for knee range of motion, quadriceps strengthening, hamstring stretching, and gait training

PATIENT EDUCATION

- Asymptomatic discoid meniscus needs no treatment.
- Surgery is recommended if mechanical symptoms present: pain, locking, swelling, giving way, functional limitations, and inability to participate in sports.

PROGNOSIS

- Good prognosis when asymptomatic
- Better prognosis in younger patients
- Poorer prognosis when osteochondritis dissecans present, higher age at presentation, and in patients undergoing total meniscectomy

COMPLICATIONS

- Osteochondritis dissecans of lateral femoral condyle
- Postoperative complications:
  - Cartilage remains thickened and more susceptible to developing tear.
  - Osteochondritis dissecans (if saucerization done)
  - Osteoarthrosis

REFERENCES

1. Tapasvi S, Shekhar A, Eriksson K. Discoid lateral meniscus: current concepts. *J ISAKOS*. 2021;6(1):14–21.
2. Kim JH, Ahn JH, Kim JH, et al. Discoid lateral meniscus: importance, diagnosis, and treatment. *J Exp Orthop*. 2020;7(1):81.
3. Birchard Z, Herron T, Tuck JA. *Discoid Meniscus*. StatPearls Publishing; 2023.
4. Trisolino G, Stallone S, Grassi A, et al. The discoid lateral meniscus in children: a narrative review of pathology, diagnosis, and treatment. *Ann Jt*. 2022;7:38.

CLINICAL PEARLS

- A discoid meniscus involves both morphologic and structural deformation.
- Isolated atraumatic lateral meniscal tear in a child <10 years of age should raise suspicion of a discoid meniscus.
- Horizontal tear is the most common tear pattern associated with a discoid meniscus.
- Discoid meniscus can be asymptomatic.

DISLOCATION, HIP, POSTERIOR

Greg Nakamoto, MD, FACP

BASICS

DESCRIPTION

- Hip dislocations can be congenital or traumatic and can occur in native hips or after total hip arthroplasty.
- A simple dislocation refers to a dislocation without an accompanying fracture. A complex fracture-dislocation refers to a dislocation associated with a fracture.
- The remainder of this topic is dedicated to the evaluation and management of traumatic (posterior) hip dislocations in native hips (a few special considerations in the case of dislocation after total hip replacement are noted in "Additional Therapies"):
  - Posterior hip dislocation is an **orthopedic emergency** in which the femoral head is displaced posteriorly relative to the acetabulum.

ALERT
Primary concerns when evaluating the patient with a posterior hip dislocation are the attainment of early reduction (within 6 hours) to prevent long-term sequelae (avascular necrosis [AVN]) and the search for additional injuries (often life-threatening or limb-threatening due to the high forces necessary to create this injury).

EPIDEMIOLOGY

- 62–93% of hip dislocations occur secondary to traffic accidents (1). The remainders are usually caused by falls, industrial accidents, or high-energy sports injuries (2).
- Posterior dislocations account for ~90% of all hip dislocations, and 70% have an associated acetabular fracture (1).
- Age: Major trauma (such as motor vehicle accident) is a more common cause in patients <35 years. Falls are more common cause in those >65 years.

RISK FACTORS

- High-energy trauma
- Mechanism is a posteriorly directed force against a flexed knee, with the hip flexed and adducted (3).
- Most common cause is knee striking the dashboard in a head-on motor vehicle accident.
- In athletic competition, mechanisms of injury include a forward fall onto the knee with a flexed hip or a blow from behind while down on all four limbs. Noncontact injuries are rare but have been reported (1).

COMMONLY ASSOCIATED CONDITIONS

- Life-threatening internal organ damage, bleeding, and shock reflect the high energy of the trauma typically required to dislocate a hip.
- Fractures of the acetabulum, pelvis, femoral head, femoral neck, and femoral shaft

ALERT
Ipsilateral **sciatic nerve** injury in 10–14% of cases; this changes a posterior hip dislocation from an orthopedic urgency to a true surgical emergency.

DIAGNOSIS

HISTORY

- Mechanism: can help guide the search for associated visceral and orthopedic injuries
- Position at time of injury: Simple posterior dislocation most commonly occurs with force on a flexed knee with the hip in varying degrees of flexion and adduction. Addition of hip abduction increases the risk of associated acetabular fracture or anterior dislocation.

PHYSICAL EXAM

- Immediate severe pain and disability
- Limb shortening with hip flexion, internal rotation, and adduction (2)
- Classic position may be absent if there is an associated femoral shaft fracture.
- Vital signs and complete trauma evaluation are essential because of the high association with life-threatening injuries.
- Pelvic rocking and pubic compression tests to examine for associated pelvic rim fractures
- Distal neurovascular examination to assess for sciatic nerve or vascular injures which merit more urgent reduction

DIFFERENTIAL DIAGNOSIS

- Anterior dislocation of the hip
- Complex fracture–dislocation of the hip
- Isolated fracture of the pelvis, acetabulum, or femur
- Traumatic hip subluxation
- Hip pointer
- Gastrointestinal or genitoureteral visceral injury

DIAGNOSTIC TESTS & INTERPRETATION

- Lab studies, blood type, and cross as needed on the basis of the trauma assessment and for preoperative planning
- Initial x-rays: anteroposterior (AP) and lateral views of the pelvis. AP pelvis often reveals the dislocation, but a true lateral may be needed to confirm the direction.
- Search for associated pelvic rim, acetabular, femoral head, femoral neck, and femoral shaft fractures may merit additional x-rays (including 3/4 internal and external obliques of the pelvis as well as femur films).
- **Role of computed tomography (CT) in the unreduced hip dislocation**:
  - In the case of **suspected nondisplaced femoral neck fracture**, obtain CT before attempted reduction maneuvers so as not to displace an unidentified femoral neck fracture (the presence of a **femoral neck fracture is a contraindication to attempts at closed reduction**; such patients should undergo open surgical reduction) (2),(3)[C].
  - In the case of **irreducible dislocations**, obtain CT prior to open surgical reduction (2),(3)[C].

TREATMENT

- Prehospital: Patients suffering a high-energy trauma sufficient to cause a hip dislocation commonly have associated injuries that take precedence for overall patient stabilization.
  - Establish airway, breathing, and circulation (ABCs). Evaluate and stabilize the spine appropriately.
  - Patients with a hip dislocation can be placed on a backboard and allowed to assume the leg position of maximal comfort (i.e., slight hip flexion with leg adducted).
  - Transport to trauma center appropriate for patient's overall clinical status.
  - An experienced operator might consider attempts at early reduction in the field if conventional treatment is unavailable in a timely manner (e.g., wilderness or backcountry situations).
- Emergency department (ED) treatment: Rule out and/or stabilize life-threatening injuries. Neurovascular examination to determine if coexisting neurovascular injuries; x-rays to confirm the dislocation and evaluate for coexisting fractures.

ALERT
Fracture-dislocations merit urgent orthopedic evaluation. Any dislocation with associated sciatic nerve injury merits **emergent** orthopedic consultation.

- **Indications for primary operative (open) reduction**: Dislocations with associated femoral head or shaft fractures, open traumatic hip dislocations, as well as apparently simple dislocations that otherwise defy closed reduction with the methods described below ("irreducible dislocations") are generally treated initially with open reduction (2),(3)[C].
- **Closed reduction in the ED may be considered in patients without the above contraindications.** Administer analgesics, muscle relaxants, and/or sedation to overcome severe pain and muscular spasm. Some cases may require spinal or general anesthesia to achieve closed reduction.
- Reduction of a simple posterior dislocation (i.e., without fracture, or with an insignificant acetabular fracture) is typically treated with closed reduction only (3)[C].
  - Consider orthopedic consultation prior to attempts at closed reduction if it will not delay reduction beyond a reasonable amount of time, usually within 6 hours, because **reduction under 6 hours reduces the rate of AVN** (4)[A].
  - Some authors advise orthopedic consultation for any hip dislocation, with an orthopedist present when attempting closed reduction.
- For the experienced treating physician, two to three attempts at reduction of a simple dislocation might be reasonable. However, urgent orthopedic consultation should be obtained for simple dislocations that are not easily reducible because **multiple attempts at closed reduction are associated with poorer outcomes** (4)[A].
- For posterior dislocations, closed reduction is attempted through hip flexion, internal rotation, and adduction. Numerous methods of reduction have been described, with no one method proven superior.
- Four of the more common closed reduction methods are described below (5):
  - **Allis method**: An assistant stabilizes the pelvis of the supine patient with downward pressure on the anterior superior iliac spine. The operator applies axial traction in line with the deformity by pulling with his or her hands from behind the flexed knee. While maintaining this traction, the hip is gently flexed to 90 degrees and then gently, internally, and externally rotated until reduction occurs; requires two operators
  - **Stimson method**: Patient placed prone, with affected hip hanging down over edge of bed. Downward traction is applied to the leg while an assistant applies stabilizing pressure to the pelvis. Requires two operators; might be difficult to move multiple-injury patient into proper position and difficult to monitor the airway in the prone position.

- **Tulsa/Rochester/Whistler method**: Patient supine with unaffected knee flexed to 120 degrees such that the unaffected foot is placed firmly on the bed. Standing on the affected side, the operator reaches his hand under the affected knee and places his hand onto the unaffected flexed knee. By straightening his arm and lifting his shoulder, the operator adducts the patient's leg and applies traction until the hip reduces; requires only one operator and airway easily monitored in supine position
- **Waddell method**: Patient supine, with an assistant stabilizing the patient's pelvis. The operator hovers over the patient and places his forearm behind the knee of the affected hip, which is flexed between 60 and 90 degrees. Keeping the back straight, the operator hugs the knee to his chest, and gently leans back, pulling traction through the femur with minimal strain on the operator's back. The operator can then adduct and internally rotate the leg by leaning and rotating as needed; requires two operators, but with less strain on the operator's back than in some other methods

- **If closed reduction cannot be accomplished**, the dislocated hip should be held in a position of relative extension with the ipsilateral knee in flexion until open reduction can be performed. This position puts the least strain on the sciatic nerve.
- In the case of complex fracture-dislocations, success of closed reduction in the emergency room (ER) decreases after 3.5 hours from the time of injury. In such cases, reduction in the operating room should be anticipated (6).

ADDITIONAL THERAPIES

- Postreduction considerations include the following:
  - Repeat neurovascular examination of the injured limb.
  - Examine passive range of motion of the hip to assess clinical stability of the reduction.
  - Repeat x-rays, including AP and lateral views, immediately to confirm reduction (2).
  - **After postreduction x-rays confirm a stable and concentric reduction, obtaining CT scan with fine cuts (2 to 3 mm) through the hips should be part of the standard postreduction evaluation of a traumatic posterior hip dislocation** (2),(3),(4)[A]:
    - To evaluate for presence of osteochondral or intra-articular fragments, femoral head injuries, and acetabular fractures (any of which might make the reduction unstable)
    - Essential in assigning proper classification of posterior fracture-dislocations of the hip, which in turn determines optimal definitive treatment
  - Magnetic resonance imaging (MRI): In children and adolescents, postreduction hip MRI may be better than CT for detecting structural injuries.
  - After successful closed reduction, the leg should be extended and externally rotated until further radiographic and orthopedic evaluation is completed; placing the leg in a knee immobilizer helps prevent inadvertent flexion at the hip.
  - **Operative versus nonoperative treatment of the reduced hip dislocation (based on postreduction physical examination and CT)**:
    - Patients with clinically and radiographically stable, concentric reductions without associated significant fractures may be treated nonoperatively (4)[A].
    - Patients with unstable reductions, displaced fractures, or acetabular fractures that would likely compromise stability are generally treated operatively (4)[A]. Neurovascular deficit that occurs after closed reduction is also an indication for operative management.

- **Dislocation of the prosthetic hip is a special concern**:
  - Prostheses are most susceptible to dislocation at 3 to 4 months after initial surgery.
  - Hip prostheses can also deteriorate over time and subsequently dislocate late with minimal force (e.g., crossing of legs, standing up).
  - Reduction of a prosthetic hip dislocation is less urgent than for a native hip if neurovascular status is intact because concern for AVN or posttraumatic osteoarthritis is nonexistent.
  - Reduction is accomplished with the same maneuvers as for the native hip; however, less force is used so as to avoid iatrogenic fracture.

SURGERY/OTHER PROCEDURES

- Given this injury often occurs in the setting of high-energy trauma, orthopedic evaluation usually occurs in conjunction with the initial trauma evaluation.
- In the absence of contraindications to closed reduction, limited attempts at reduction may be performed if orthopedic consultation is delayed. However, urgent orthopedic referral should be made for any patient in whom closed reduction does not result in easy reduction. Emergent surgical consultation is needed if there is associated neurovascular compromise.
- Postreduction, further orthopedic and radiographic evaluations as above are needed to guide subsequent definitive surgical decision-making.

ONGOING CARE

FOLLOW-UP RECOMMENDATIONS

- Given the high-energy mechanism of injury, most patients require admission for continued evaluation and treatment of associated injuries.
- The duration of non-weight-bearing immobilization after reduction of uncomplicated simple hip dislocation is controversial (see Foulk and Mullis in "Additional Reading"):
  - Many suggest a short period of traction until pain is improved, followed by early gentle range of motion.
  - Recommended period of non-weight-bearing status varies from days to months; prolonged non-weight-bearing has not been shown to influence the incidence of AVN.
  - Physical therapy (PT) often starts with range-of-motion exercises and progresses to include muscle rehabilitation and strengthening; timing of PT might be influenced by coexisting injuries/fractures at the hip or elsewhere.

COMPLICATIONS

- Complication rate increases directly with time elapsed before hip relocation.
- **AVN risk appears to increase with time to reduction, multiple attempts at reduction, or need for open reduction**:
  - In one study, 4% of patients reduced within 6 hours developed AVN, whereas 58% of patients reduced later than 6 hours developed AVN.
  - Early weight-bearing after reduction does not appear to increase the incidence of AVN.
- **Posttraumatic osteoarthritis** affects 16–24% of patients and up to 89% of patients with an associated femoral head or neck fracture (2),(3).
- **Sciatic nerve injury** occurs in up to 10% of adult dislocations (3), either during the initial trauma or during relocation:
  - New neurologic deficits that occur **postreduction** warrant immediate surgical intervention; the importance of a complete neurovascular exam before and after reduction is stressed.
- **Myositis ossificans**, **recurrent instability**, and **labral tears** are also noted as late complications of posterior hip dislocations.

REFERENCES

1. Nowell JA, Coombs S, Tippabhatla A, et al. Posterior hip fracture dislocation from a non-contact injury while playing soccer. "A case report." *Trauma Case Rep*. 2023;47:100885.
2. Beebe MJ, Bauer JM, Mir HR. Treatment of hip dislocations and associated injuries: current state of care. *Orthop Clin North Am*. 2016;47(3):527–549.
3. Mandell JC, Marshall RA, Weaver MJ, et al. Traumatic hip dislocation: what the orthopedic surgeon wants to know. *Radiographics*. 2017;37(7):2181–2201.
4. Yang EC, Cornwall R. Initial treatment of traumatic hip dislocations in the adult. *Clin Orthop Relat Res*. 2000;(337):24–31.
5. Dawson-Amoah K, Raszewski J, Duplantier N, et al. Dislocation of the hip: a review of types, causes, and treatment. *Oschner J*. 2018;18(3):242–252.
6. Lai PJ, Lai CY, Tseng IC, et al. A retrospective study of hip posterior fracture-dislocation: closed reduction at the emergency department or in the operation theater? *J Orhop Traumatol*. 2022;23(1):55.

ADDITIONAL READING

- Dumont GD. Hip instability: current concepts and treatment options. *Clin Sports Med*. 2016;35(3):435–447.
- Foulk DM, Mullis BH. Hip dislocation: evaluation and management. *J Am Acad Orthop Surg*. 2010;18(4):199–209.
- Stein MJ, Kang C, Ball V. Emergency department evaluation and treatment of acute hip and thigh pain. *Emerg Med Clin North Am*. 2015;33(2):327–343.
- Thanacharoenpanich S, Bixby S, Breen MA, et al. MRI is better than CT scan for detection of structural pathologies after traumatic posterior hip dislocations in children and adolescents. *J Pediatr Orthop*. 2020;40(2):86–92.
- Waddell BS, Mohamed S, Glomset JT, et al. A detailed review of hip reduction maneuvers: a focus on physician safety and introduction of the Waddell technique. *Orthop Rev (Pavia)*. 2016;8(1):6253.

CLINICAL PEARLS

- Primary concerns when evaluating the patient with a posterior hip dislocation is the attainment of early reduction (within 6 hours) to prevent long-term sequelae; and the search for additional life- or limb-threatening injury.
- In the case of posterior dislocation without fracture, the experienced physician may perform limited attempts at closed reduction. If reduction is not accomplished with ease, or if there is an associated fracture of the hip, then urgent orthopedic consultation is warranted.
- Even postreduction, further orthopedic and radiographic evaluations are needed to guide surgical decision-making. CT scan should be part of the standard postreduction evaluation.
- Whereas a significant delay between dislocation and reduction may increase the risk of AVN, the overall long-term prognosis is often most dependent on the severity of the initial trauma.

DISTAL CLAVICULAR OSTEOLYSIS

Ryan C. Fowler, MD, CAQSM • Keith A. Stuessi, MD, CAQSM

BASICS

DESCRIPTION

- A loss of subchondral bone detail with osteoporosis, cystic changes, osteolysis, and osteophyte formation of the distal clavicle while sparing the acromion
- Most commonly associated with atraumatic mechanism but can be trauma related

EPIDEMIOLOGY

Incidence

- True incidence of distal clavicular osteolysis (DCO) is unknown.
- In teenage population, about 6.5% who present with shoulder pain may have DCO (1)[B].
- In teenage patients, overhead sports were a risk factor for DCO. Weight lifting and overhead sports conferred the biggest risk (1)[C].
- Also in teenage patients, females were affected at 24% (1)[B]. In adult literature, the vast majority of cases are male.
- Associated with repetitive heavy lifting (particularly heavy bench or military presses) and occasionally as a result of trauma

ETIOLOGY AND PATHOPHYSIOLOGY

- Although the specific pathophysiologic cause has not been determined, atraumatic osteolysis is thought to start as a stress fracture of the distal clavicle from repetitive microtrauma (2).
- Common magnetic resonance imaging (MRI) findings include bone edema and evidence of subchondral injury (2).
- The pathophysiologic process in traumatic injuries is unknown.

RISK FACTORS

- Any activity putting excessive, repetitive force on the acromioclavicular (AC) joint may increase risk.
- Weight lifting appears to be a significant risk factor in nontraumatic cases (3)[B].
- Highest risk factor seen in bench press with high frequency (more than once a week), high duration (>5 years), and with one repetition maximum of >1.5 times the body weight (3)[B].
- Occasionally will result from blunt trauma to the shoulder
- Traumatic injuries include AC joint dislocation and separation as well as clavicle fractures.

GENERAL PREVENTION

- Atraumatic causes are potentially prevented by limiting repetitive lifting, but no studies address this issue.
- Athletes generally are reluctant to decrease training.

DIAGNOSIS

HISTORY

- Insidious onset of aching in the AC joint
- Athletes may have a history of remote trauma.
- Activities placing repetitive stress to the joint may increase the risk.
- In weight lifters, bench press, military press, shoulder shrugs, push-ups, and clean and jerk may cause pain.

PHYSICAL EXAM

- Signs and symptoms:
  - Patient complains of a dull ache over the AC joint.
  - Mild swelling of the joint may be present.
  - Pain usually is worse at the beginning of the exercise period.
  - Any movement of the arm requiring 90 degrees or more of abduction causes pain.
  - Pain can radiate to the adjacent superior trapezius border and deltoid muscles.
- Physical examination:
  - Tenderness over the AC joint
  - Positive cross-arm test: Forward flexion to 90 degrees and adduction of the arm cause pain. This compresses the AC joint.
  - Paxinos test: patient's arm at side resting against chest and hand over top of shoulder; examiner's thumb on acromion and fingers on clavicle and compressing them together; pain is a positive test.
  - O'Brian active compression test:
    - Part 1—patient's arm in 90 degrees of shoulder flexion and elbow fully extended adduction of arm 10 to 15 degrees with forearm pronated. The examiner pushes against resistance.
    - Part 2—same position as above, but the forearm is supinated, and the examiner again pushes against resistance.
    - Pain on top of the shoulder suggests AC joint pathology; if the test elicits a painful "click" in the shoulder joint, this suggests labral pathology.
  - Because it is common to have other shoulder pathology in conjunction with DCO, a local anesthetic injection to the AC joint can be helpful in achieving an accurate diagnosis (4)[C].

DIFFERENTIAL DIAGNOSIS

- AC joint trauma, osteoarthritis
- Other shoulder pathology should be considered (e.g., instability, impingement, rotator cuff tears, tendinitis, and labral disease).
- Also includes hyperparathyroidism, rheumatoid arthritis, multiple myeloma, scleroderma, infection (septic arthritis, tuberculosis), rickets, eosinophilic granuloma, and other, more rare diseases including cleidocranial dysplasia.

DIAGNOSTIC TESTS & INTERPRETATION

Initial Tests (lab, imaging)

- Clavicular or Zanca view: 10 to 35 degrees of cephalic tilt; distal clavicular end will appear frayed; will see bony osteolysis, cystic changes, and translucency of the bone; bilateral Zanca views are helpful in comparing the involved and uninvolved sides.
- Diagnostic ultrasound (US) has the benefit of immediate diagnosis, cost effective, and dynamic. US can assess joint widening, cortical irregularities, joint effusion, edema, and power doppler hyperemia/neovascularization (5)
- MRI can be used to rule out other pathology and often shows bone edema and evidence of subchondral fracture in the distal clavicle (2)[C].
- MRI is useful, as early plain films may appear normal. Majority of cases, 74–86% had evidence of subchondral fracture (1),(2).

Diagnostic Procedures/Other

Diagnostic injection into the AC joint with local anesthetic can be helpful in differentiating the cause of pain (4)[C].

TREATMENT

- Acute treatment:
  - Nonsteroidal anti-inflammatory drugs (NSAIDs) or other pain medications can be used as needed.
  - Cessation of offending activity is often very effective in reducing pain (4),(6)[C].
  - Therapeutic corticosteroid injection to the AC joint is often effective at reducing painful symptoms (4),(7)[C]. This can also be a predictor of successful distal clavicle resection but may only last 20 days (5).
  - US guidance is more effective than palpation-guided injection in both accuracy and symptoms/function up to 6 months postinjection (6),(8)
  - Other symptomatic treatment such as ice can be helpful.
- Long-term treatment:
  - Activity modification (4),(7)[C]
  - Specific activity modifications are to narrow the hand spacing on the barbell (<1.5 times the biacromial width) and controlling the descent phase to end approximately 4 to 6 cm above the chest (4)[B].
  - Often difficult in athletes
  - Activity modification by weight lifters should include decreased weight with increased repetitions or substitution of exercises.
  - In the teenage population, 93% responded to conservative therapy (1)[B].
  - Physical therapy should be instituted if there is evidence of other shoulder pathology. Rehabilitation also should include range of motion (ROM) therapy and strengthening exercises for the rotator cuff and scapulothoracic stabilizer muscles (7)[C].
  - Surgical resection may be considered for those not responding to conservative therapy.

SURGERY/OTHER PROCEDURES

- Surgery consisting of distal clavicle resection, is recommended for those who fail conservative treatment (4),(7)[C].
- Surgery may be performed open or arthroscopic.
- Arthroscopic surgery involves less tissue dissection and faster rehabilitation times (2)[C].
- Arthroscopic surgery can be completed directly through the AC joint or indirectly through the subacromial space. It can give the ability to assess for other concomitant conditions. There is controversy as to the best surgical management.

ONGOING CARE

FOLLOW-UP RECOMMENDATIONS

- Referral to an orthopedic surgeon for failure of nonoperative treatment
- Postoperative physical therapy:
  - Active ROM as tolerated
  - Shoulder strengthening
  - Return to sports as soon as symptoms allow; time frame depends on surgical approach.

REFERENCES

1. Roedl JB, Nevalainen M, Gonzalez FM, et al. Frequency, imaging findings, risk factors, and long-term sequelae of distal clavicular osteolysis in young patients. *Skeletal Radiol*. 2015;44(5):659–666.
2. Kassarjian A, Llopis E, Palmer WE. Distal clavicular osteolysis: MR evidence for subchondral fracture. *Skeletal Radiol*. 2007;36(1):17–22.
3. Nevalainen MT, Ciccotti MG, Morrison WB, et al. Distal clavicular osteolysis in adults: association with bench pressing intensity. *Skeletal Radiol*. 2016;45(11):1473–1479.
4. Schwarzkopf R, Ishak C, Elman M, et al. Distal clavicular osteolysis: a review of the literature. *Bull NYU Hosp Jt Dis*. 2008;66(2):94–101.
5. Singh M, Soo Hoo J. A sports medicine clinician's guide to the diagnosis and management of distal clavicular osteolysis. *Curr Sports Med Rep*. 2023;22(6):230–237.
6. Park KD, Kim TK, Lee J, et al. Palpation versus ultrasound-guided acromioclavicular joint intra-articular corticosteroid injections: a retrospective comparative clinical study. *Pain Physician*. 2015;18(4):333–341.
7. DeFroda SF, Nacca C, Waryasz GR, et al. Diagnosis and management of distal clavicle osteolysis. *Orthopedics*. 2017;40(2):119–124.
8. Sabeti-Aschraf M, Lemmerhofer B, Lang S, et al. Ultrasound guidance improves the accuracy of the acromioclavicular joint infiltration: a prospective randomized study. *Knee Surg Sports Traumaol Arthosc*. 2011;19(2):292–295.

CLINICAL PEARLS

- Can resolve without surgery, but only a minority of cases produce satisfactory results, particularly when the athlete does not stop training long enough for the AC joint to heal
- Athletes can return to their former level of competition after surgical resection.

DROWNING

Kevin Waninger, MD, MS, FAAFP, FACEP, FACSM, FAMSSM, CAQSM

BASICS

- Drowning is the process of experiencing respiratory impairment from submersion (airway goes below the surface of the liquid)/immersion (water splashed over the face) in water (1),(2),(3),(4).
- The terms "drowned" and "near-drowned" have been used to describe the outcomes dead or alive, respectively. The term "near-drowned" has also been used to describe patients who subsequently died from drowning. This usage has led to uncertainty about the meaning of the term. Therefore, the term "near-drowning" has lost favor. The term "drowned" will continue to refer to a person who died or suffered injury from drowning (2),(3).
- Near-drowning, dry drowning, wet drowning, delayed drowning, and secondary drowning are all terms that are not medically accepted diagnosis. These terms should be abandoned in favor of understanding and communicating drowning as a process that is mild, moderate, and severe with fatal or nonfatal outcomes. Someone who drowns has three outcomes: (i) fatal, (ii) nonfatal with injury/illness, and (iii) nonfatal without injury/illness. A person either drowns or does not drown; one cannot be "near drowned." A person can drown and survive, just as a person can have cardiac arrest and survive.
- Dry drowning has been used in cases when no water was found in the lungs at autopsy in persons who were found dead in the water. However, whether this is caused by the victim suffering sudden cardiac death before the drowning or laryngospasm preventing water into the lungs, the management is essentially the same, and no clinical management distinction is made between wet or dry drowning (2),(3).

DESCRIPTION

- Drowning is a process resulting in primary respiratory impairment from submersion or immersion in a liquid medium. The pathophysiology is primarily related to abnormal gas exchange, with resultant hypoxia. The process that contributes to hypoxia includes airway obstruction, surfactant washout, atelectasis, ventilation/perfusion (V/Q) mismatch, and pulmonary edema (1),(2),(3),(4).
- Hypoxia may result from laryngospasm causing no pulmonary gas exchange or the aspiration of fluids causing pulmonary injury and subsequent disruption of productive gas exchange.
- The drowning process is a continuum that begins when the victim's airway lies below the surface of a liquid, usually water, at which time the victim voluntarily holds their breath (submersion or immersion).
- Breath holding is usually followed by an involuntary period of laryngospasm secondary to the presence of liquid in the oropharynx or larynx, resulting in hypoxemia, hypercarbia, and acidosis.
- During this laryngospasm, there is no exchange of air, and the victim may swallow large quantities of water. As arterial oxygen tension drops further, laryngospasm abates and the victim actively breathes liquid. The amount of liquid inhaled varies considerably from victim to victim.
- Changes occur in the lungs, body fluids, blood-gas tensions, acid–base balance, and electrolyte concentrations, which are dependent on the composition and volume of the liquid aspirated and the duration of submersion. Surfactant washout, pulmonary hypertension, and shunting also contribute to the development of hypoxemia.
- The clinical presentation and prognosis vary due to different water temperatures, different fluid properties (fresh water, seawater, Dead Sea water, water contaminated with chemicals and bacteria), and the variety of environments (from toilets to hurricane sea conditions) in which drowning occurs.
- The heart and brain are the organs at greatest risk for permanent, detrimental changes from relatively brief periods of hypoxia. Posthypoxic encephalopathy, with or without cerebral edema, is the most common cause of death in hospitalized drowning victims.
- Reinstitution of adequate ventilation and oxygenation before the occurrence of circulatory arrest and irreversible nervous system damage may result in complete and dramatic restoration of function (if aspiration does not occur). If the person is rescued early, the clinical picture is determined by the reactivity of the airway and the amount of water that has been aspirated.
- When aspiration occurs, due to V/Q mismatch and shunting, prolonged hypoxemia and subsequent complications are more likely to occur.

EPIDEMIOLOGY

- Drowning incidents occur in swimming pools, lakes, rivers, streams, storm drains, hot tubs, bathtubs, and even toilets and buckets in toddlers.
- A swimming pool is 14 times more likely than a motor vehicle to be involved in the death of a child age ≤4 years (5).
- 80% of drowning victims age >1 year are males.
- Although drowning rates have slowly declined, fatal drowning remains the second leading cause of unintentional injury-related death for children ages 1 to 14 years (5).
- 19% of drowning deaths involving children occur in public pools with certified lifeguards present. Of all preschoolers who drown, 70% are in the care of one or both parents at the time of the drowning, and 75% are missing from sight for <5 minutes. 10% of drownings are observed by an adult who does not realize that the child is drowning (5).
- Most children who survive without sequelae are discovered within 2 minutes following submersion, and most children who die are found after 10 minutes (5).
- In areas where lifeguards operate, <6% of rescued persons require medical attention and <0.5% require CPR in their resuscitation (5).

Incidence

- From 2005 to 2014, fatal unintentional drownings in the United States averaged about 10 deaths per day (6).
- Among those 1 to 14 years old, fatal drowning remains the second leading cause of unintentional injury-related death behind motor vehicle accidents (2),(7).
- For every child who died from drowning, another five children received emergency department (ED) care for nonfatal submersion injuries.
- Children (age <5 years) and adolescents (ages 15 to 24 years) have the highest drowning rates.

Prevalence

- Rates of fatal drowning are notably higher among African Americans (1.3 times) and American Indians and Alaskan Natives (1.8 times) compared to Caucasians (5).
- For children ages 5 to 14 years, the fatal drowning rate of African American children (3.2 times) and American Indian and Alaskan Native children (2.4 times) is higher than for Caucasian children (5).

ETIOLOGY AND PATHOPHYSIOLOGY

- Unexpected submersion. Struggle does not always occur. Splashing, waving, and calls for help rarely occur during actual drowning events. Drowning does not look like drowning as often portrayed in the media. People in distress can keep afloat and may signal for help, but drowning patients are suffocating and often unable to signal distress; they are in imminent danger of death within seconds. The mouths of drowning victims are often not above the surface of the water long enough for them to exhale, inhale, and then call out for help. Drowning people cannot voluntarily control their arm movements, and they instinctively extend their arms laterally, pressing down on the water surface to allow their body leverage to lift their mouths out of the water to breathe. This instinctive drowning response is an instinctive reaction that occurs in humans, particularly in nonswimmers, when close to drowning, preventing drowning individuals from performing voluntary movements such as waving for help, moving toward a rescuer, or reaching out for a piece of rescue equipment.
- Aspiration of variable amounts of water. Grossly contaminated water poses a risk of pulmonary infection. Both fresh water and saltwater cause similar surfactant destruction and washout with disruption of the alveolar-capillary membrane (1),(2),(3),(4).
- Laryngospasm
- Hypoxia
- Metabolic acidosis
- Myocardial dysfunction
- Coagulation abnormalities
- Multisystem organ dysfunction with renal failure
- Central nervous system (CNS) dysfunction (posthypoxic encephalopathy)

RISK FACTORS

- Unattended children at water sites; inadequate adult supervision
- Alcohol and/or drug abuse (50% cases involving adolescents and adults)
- Limited swimming ability and exhaustion
- Trauma (6),(7)
- Risky behavior in the water; rough play
- SCUBA: contamination of air supply with toxic gases (i.e., carbon monoxide), running out of air at depth
- Oxygen-induced seizures in divers using oxygen-enriched air mixtures

- Shallow water blackout is the deliberate prolonged submersion with intentional hyperventilation after breath-hold diving or swimming, with no warning felt prior to sudden loss of consciousness from hypoxia.
- Ascent "deep water" blackout caused by latent hypoxia during ascent from depth due to changes in lung partial pressure of oxygen.
- Exacerbation of existing medical problems (seizure disorder, cardiac disease, diabetes, syncope, cerebrovascular accident)
- Cold-water immersion or hypothermia; cold shock response; young children are more susceptible due to larger body surface-to-mass ratio; decreases the metabolic rate, survival to full recovery possible
- Panic/anxiety
- Improper fencing of pools (at least 5 feet high with self-closing latches should be required) (2),(5)

GENERAL PREVENTION

Drowning is preventable! Prevention is the key:

- Parental supervision of children around water; watch empty pails, buckets, and toddlers around toilets.
- Carefully watching children while they bathe
- Swimming lessons: Children 1 to 4 years old who drowned were significantly less likely to have attended swimming classes than matched controls.
- The American Academy of Pediatrics recommends that all children be taught water survival skills training and swim lessons after age 1 year (5).
- Adequate pool fencing; wearing properly sized life jackets; improved pool design preventing children from being trapped when submerged
- Poor pool maintenance resulting in murky or cloudy water, where children cannot be adequately visualized
- Instruction/supervision of lifeguards in methods of waterfront surveillance and resuscitation techniques
- Education of public in prudent consumption of alcoholic beverages; impose severe sanctions against boaters who are intoxicated.
- Encourage people to learn to swim, understand the limits of their swimming ability, and never swim alone.
- Restricted swimming areas; post proper signage in areas of dangerous underwater tow; pay attention to the weather, tides and water conditions, and especially currents. Currents are usually perceived from the outside as weaker than they are.
- Understand the water environment where you are swimming, diving, or boating.
- Instruct greater numbers of the public in basic life support (BLS) and proper cardiopulmonary resuscitation (CPR) techniques.
- Bring a cordless telephone to the pool so children are not left unsupervised while answering a phone call. Avoid distracting phone calls completely while watching children in the water.

DIAGNOSIS

Pediatric Considerations

- Hypothermia may be protective, as the rate of cerebral oxygen consumption is reduced.
- Diving reflex in young children is triggered by submersion of face in cold water, with bradycardia and redistribution of blood flow to the heart and brain.
- Family history of sudden death by drowning may suggest a genetic cause for syncope, such as prolonged QT syndrome (LQT1), because swimming can trigger arrhythmias that cause unexplained drowning in these patients.

HISTORY

- See "Risk Factors."
- Information from witnesses or emergency medical services personnel at the scene

PHYSICAL EXAM

- Cardiac presentation depends on severity of exposure, ranging from sinus tachycardia to cardiac arrest and apnea. It is not uncommon for these patients to respond to prolonged CPR. Children who still require CPR at the time they arrive at the ED have a poor prognosis, with at least half of survivors suffering significant neurologic impairment.
- The process of drowning is characterized by a gradual decrease in arterial oxygen saturation with a simultaneous decrease in cardiac output. Cardiac arrest is, therefore, not sudden but is preceded by a brief period of tachycardia and hypertension, followed by bradycardia with hypotension and electromechanical dissociation (pulseless electrical activity).
- Ventricular fibrillation is rare after submersion, unless resulting from acute hypothermia and/or triggered by mechanical irritation. The sequence of cardiac rhythm deterioration is usually tachycardia followed by bradycardia, pulseless electrical activity, and finally asystole. Drowning victims in cardiac arrest may not respond to defibrillation. The automated external defibrillator may not play a major role in improving the success of resuscitation after drowning (2),(3).
- Whether the drowning event occurs in fresh water or seawater, the result is pulmonary edema, a decrease in pulmonary compliance, and an increase in the V/Q mismatch. In both cases, the primary goals of resuscitation are to restore oxygenation and circulation (1),(2),(3),(4).
- Patients with water aspiration may present with minimal symptoms, severe bloodstained pulmonary edema, or frank cardiopulmonary arrest. Cyanosis, dyspnea, and/or copious pulmonary secretions may be present.
- Cerebral edema/injury
- Look for evidence of trauma/cervical spine injury (6),(7).
- Look for hypothermia; full vital signs with rectal temperature required

DIFFERENTIAL DIAGNOSIS

- Consider a potential underlying cause of submersion injury, such as alcohol or drug intoxication, myocardial infarction, syncope (prolonged QT syndrome), seizure (including O_2 induced), stroke, hypoglycemia, or trauma.
- Head or spinal cord injury/trauma (accidents involving diving, waterskiing, surfing, or watercraft). $<$0.5% of drownings involve cervical spine injuries. Drowning resuscitation with aggressive airway management takes precedence in patients with severe respiratory disease with a possible mechanism that may cause cervical spine injury (3),(6).
- Venomous stings by aquatic animals
- Decompression sickness or arterial gas embolism, nitrogen narcosis from scuba diving
- Consider child abuse/neglect.

DIAGNOSTIC TESTS & INTERPRETATION

- Most drowning victims do not aspirate enough fluid to cause life-threatening changes in electrolytes or blood volume.
- Rarely is there a need for emergent treatment of electrolyte abnormalities unless very large volumes of water are aspirated, or the drowning event occurs in a highly concentrated liquid medium such as the Dead Sea.
- Arterial blood gases should be obtained.
- Complete blood count (CBC); significant changes of hemoglobin and hematocrit are seldom seen in human drowning victims.
- Chemistry panels usually normal, but rule out hyperkalemia, hypernatremia, hyponatremia, or signs of renal failure.
- Urinalysis
- Coagulation panel with prothrombin time (PT)/international normalized ratio (INR)
- Alcohol and toxicology screen
- Chest x-rays may be normal initially or show infiltrates ranging from a patchy distribution to global pulmonary edema.
- Computed tomography (CT) scan of head may be needed to rule out acute or chronic intracranial process in unconscious patients (7).
- Obtain cervical spine films if you suspect head/neck trauma (6).

TREATMENT

- Prehospital:
  - Airway, breathing (give supplemental oxygen), and circulation (ABCs), remove wet clothing, initiate rewarming as soon as possible, intravenous (IV) with 0.9% normal saline (Watch fluids in patients with pulmonary edema, salt-water drowning.)
  - Insert gastric tube as soon as possible for stomach decompression.
  - Thermal insulation to decrease heat loss during transport, if possible
  - Initiate CPR as soon as possible if indicated; begin in the water if can be done without putting rescuer at risk; in-water resuscitation consists of ventilation alone because attempts at chest compression are futile if the rescuer and drowning patient are in deep water. Assessment of a pulse serves no purpose until the rescuer and patient are out of the water and on some solid space (1),(3),(4).
  - BLS, and sometimes rescue breathing alone, performed by laypersons, play a key role in the survival of the drowning victim (1),(3),(4). Drowning patients with only respiratory arrest may respond after a few rescue breaths.
  - CPR with chest compression only is not recommended in management of drowned patients (3),(4),(8). Most drowning victims will have sustained cardiac arrest secondary to hypoxia. Rescue breaths as well as chest compressions are critical for successful resuscitation of these victims. In these patients, compression-only CPR is likely to be ineffective and should be avoided (8). The first and most important treatment of the drowning victim is the immediate provision of ventilation.

- The blood-tinged frothy discharge from drowning victims is a result of hemolysis and lung surfactant and is typically observed during resuscitation attempts in drowning victims who have been submerged for >15 minutes; in <15 minutes, it is typically a whitish froth. Do not attempt to expel or drain clear water or frothy fluid that may accumulate in the upper airway during resuscitation. All attempts to suction or clear this foam from the airway only delay the needed delivery of oxygenation, and prehospital providers should focus on oxygenating and ventilating the patient and not on aggressive suctioning. If there is vomit, blood, sand, or mud blocking the airway, it must be cleared.
- The management of drowning resuscitation can vary depending on whether the drowning occurred in saltwater or freshwater due to some differences in physiology and potential complications. In general, the technique for resuscitation and CPR is the same regardless of the type of water involved. In both cases, the primary goals of resuscitation are to restore oxygenation and circulation. In freshwater drowning cases, the emphasis is on addressing the dilution of surfactant and potential electrolyte imbalances. Freshwater is hypotonic, and inhaling freshwater can lead to the dilution of surfactant and interference with lung function. Freshwater drowning can also lead to electrolyte imbalances due to the dilution of the body's electrolytes. Management involves supportive care, oxygen administration, mechanical ventilation, and electrolyte monitoring and correction as necessary. When a person inhales saltwater, the high salt concentration in seawater can cause increased pulmonary edema, as well as disrupting the pulmonary surfactant. Supportive care and mechanical ventilation may be necessary to manage the pulmonary edema. The patient may also require treatment for hypernatremia if present.
- Endotracheal administration of drugs is not recommended in drowning patients (3),(4).
- Although unusual, recovery with normal neurologic function has been reported even after prolonged cardiac arrest.
- Avoid further aspiration; apply cricoid pressure during bag-valve-mask ventilation. Secure airway if needed and protect against aspiration of stomach contents; intubation with 100% oxygen
- Cervical spine precautions; however, do not delay respiratory resuscitation if not possible (6).
- The subdiaphragmatic thrust (Heimlich) maneuver to remove water from the abdomen is not recommended unless a foreign body is suspected of obstructing the airway (3).

- ED treatment:
  - Correct hypoxia; titrate to oxygen saturation; intubation with positive end-expiratory pressure (PEEP) can be effective in reversing the abnormal V/Q relationships. In patients who are alert, nasal continuous positive airway pressure (CPAP) may be used for ventilation support.
  - The risk for aspiration from water and stomach contents is still present, so aspiration precautions with elevation of head of bed if possible are recommended.
  - If bronchospasm is present or suspected, give nebulized β_2-agonist treatments.
  - Evaluate and treat traumatic injuries.
  - If in cardiopulmonary arrest, initiate advanced cardiac life support measures; continue resuscitation until core temperature >32°C or until spontaneous pulse and respirations return.
  - Follow temperature and continue rewarming efforts if indicated. Implement thermal insulation methods to decrease heat loss.
  - If not already done in prehospital setting, insert a nasogastric tube to decompress the stomach. The most frequent complication during a resuscitation attempt is regurgitation of stomach contents.
  - Insert Foley catheter, if needed, to follow urine output.
  - Check and correct severe electrolyte abnormalities and monitor acid–base balance. Note that routine CBC and electrolytes are usually normal in the initial stages of the drowning workup. If the patient is altered, consider glucose and toxicology screen with an alcohol level (3).
  - Antibiotics are needed only in those patients who become febrile, develop new pulmonary infiltrates, or have purulent secretions. Prophylactic antibiotics do not improve morbidity or mortality. Only 12% of drowning rescues have true pneumonia and require antibiotics. Pneumonia is more likely if aspiration occurs in the setting of polluted water, endogenous flora, and aspirated gastric contents (3).
  - Obtain chest radiographs (CXR). Note that the initial CXR does not correlate well with outcome or disposition. CXRs are usually abnormal within a few hours of presentation if the patient subsequently progresses to acute lung injury (3).
- There is very little evidence to support the use of steroids for reducing pulmonary injury (3),(4).
- Management of patients with suspected hypoxic brain injury includes hyperventilation (maintain $PaCO_2$ at 25 to 30 mm Hg), head elevation (if no C-spine injury is present), diuretics, and muscle relaxants. There is no evidence for clinical benefit of prophylactic diuretics unless there is suspected hypoxic brain injury.
- It appears that in the absence of hypothermia that may have occurred during the drowning process, aggressive brain resuscitation in the neurologically impaired drowning patient, using current techniques, is of limited benefit in returning patients to normal neurologic function.
- Ventilator settings for hospitalized drowning patients should be tailored to the individual patient's condition and needs. Drowning victims may have varying degrees of respiratory distress and lung injury, so the ventilator settings should be adjusted accordingly. Before setting ventilator parameters, the patient's condition should be reassessed comprehensively, including the severity of lung injury, oxygenation, and ventilation requirements (1),(3).
- Begin with a relatively high FiO_2 (100%) to ensure adequate oxygenation and titrate it downward as the patient's oxygen saturation improves. Use low tidal volumes (6 to 8 mL/kg of predicted body weight) to reduce the risk of ventilator-induced lung injury. Adjust the respiratory rate to maintain a target $PaCO_2$ and to provide adequate ventilation. This may vary depending on the patient's condition.
- PEEP is important to improve oxygenation and reduce atelectasis in drowning victims. Start with a low PEEP (e.g., 5 cm H_2O) and adjust based on the patient's response.
- Monitor peak inspiratory pressure to avoid barotrauma. It should be kept as low as possible to protect against ventilator-induced lung injury while still maintaining adequate ventilation. In some cases, noninvasive ventilation (e.g., CPAP or BiPAP) may be considered before invasive mechanical ventilation or as a weaning strategy.
- Continuously monitor the patient's oxygen saturation, arterial blood gases, and ventilator waveforms. Adjust settings as needed to maintain adequate oxygenation and ventilation while minimizing lung injury. Continuous suctioning of the airway as necessary to clear secretions and prevent mucus plugging.
- Ventilator management in drowning patients can be complex due to the potential for lung injury and the need for individualized care. It is essential for a skilled health care team, including respiratory therapists and intensivists, to closely monitor the patient's progress and adjust ventilator settings as needed to support the patient's respiratory recovery (1),(3).

ADMISSION, INPATIENT, AND NURSING CONSIDERATIONS

- Admission criteria:
  - Intensive care unit (ICU):
    - Patients who required CPR or artificial resuscitation
    - Abnormal chest x-ray
    - Arterial blood gas abnormalities
    - Glasgow Coma Scale (GCS) <13
  - Admit observation:
    - Submersion unknown or >1 minute
    - History of cyanosis or apnea
    - Required brief assisted ventilation
    - GCS >13

  - Delayed pulmonary edema (up to 12 hours)
  - Delayed neurologic abnormalities
  - Abnormal vital signs
- Discharge criteria:
  - Questionable history of submersion, after observation in ED for 6 to 8 hours
  - Normal chest x-ray
  - No respiratory distress
  - No neurologic deterioration
  - Discharge to reliable home, with instructions to return for shortness of breath or mental status changes.
  - Pediatric submersion score: safe discharge at 8 hours with (i) normal mentation; (ii) normal respiratory rate; (iii) absence of dyspnea; (iv) absence of airway support; (v) absence of systolic hypertension (9)

ONGOING CARE

PROGNOSIS

- Prognosis of resuscitated drowning victim is related to degree of damage secondary to the anoxic episode and the duration of immersion and pulmonary insult.
- Residual complications of drowning may include intellectual impairment, convulsive disorders, and pulmonary or cardiac complications.

REFERENCES

1. Bierens J, Abelaires-Gomez C, Furelos RB, et al. Resuscitation and emergency care in drowning: a scoping review. *Resuscitation*. 2021;162:205–217.
2. Bierens JJ, Lunetta P, Tipton M, et al. Physiology of drowning: a review. *Physiology (Bethesda)*. 2016;31(2):147–166.
3. Schmidt AC, Sempsrott JR, Hawkins SC, et al. Wilderness Medical Society clinical practice guidelines for the treatment and prevention of drowning: 2019 update. *Wilderness Environ Med*. 2019;30(4S):S70–S86.
4. Szpilman D, Bierens JJ, Handley AJ, et al. Drowning. *N Engl J Med*. 2012;366(22):2102–2010.
5. Centers for Disease Control and Prevention. Drowning prevention. Accessed May 16, 2024. https://www.cdc.gov/drowning/about/index.html
6. Jones T, Rennie A. BET 1: cervical spine immobilization in the management of drowning victims. *Emerg Med J*. 2019;36(12):766–767.
7. Jones T, Rennie A. BET 2: CT head in investigation of near drowning. *Emerg Med J*. 2019;36(12):767–768.
8. Schmidt A, Szpilman D, Berg I, et al. A call for the proper action on drowning resuscitation. *Resuscitation*. 2016;105:e9–e10.
9. Shenoi RP, Allahabadi S, Rubalcava DM, et al. The pediatric submersion score predicts children at low risk for injury following submersions. *Acad Emerg Med*. 2017;24(12):1491–1500.

ADDITIONAL READING

- Boyd C, Levy A, McProud T, et al. Fatal and nonfatal drowning outcomes related to dangerous underwater breath-holding behaviors—New York State, 1988–2011. *MMWR Morb Mortal Wkly Rep*. 2015;64(19):518–521.
- Brenner RA, Taneja GS, Haynie DL, et al. Association between swimming lessons and drowning in childhood: a case-control study. *Arch Pediatr Adolesc Med*. 2009;163(3):203–210.
- Girasek DC, Hargarten S. Prevention of and emergency response to drowning. *N Engl J Med*. 2022;387(14):1303–1308.
- Ho BJ, Crowe JE, Dorfman SR, et al. Correlation of clinical and chest radiograph findings in pediatric submersion cases. *Pediatr Radiol*. 2020;50(4):492–500.
- Idris AH, Berg RA, Bierens J, et al. Recommended guidelines for uniform reporting of data from drowning: the "Utstein style." *Circulation*. 2003;108(20):2565–2574.
- Myers SL, Cuesta AM, Lai Y. Competitive swimming and racial disparities in drowning. *Rev Black Polit Econ*. 2017;44(1–2):77–97.
- Papa L, Hoelle R, Idris A. Systematic review of definitions for drowning incidents. *Resuscitation*. 2005;65(3):255–264.
- Quang CY, Kennedy RO, Blair SG, et al. Is there a clinical difference between salt water and freshwater drowning? *Open J Trauma*. 2017;1:001–002.
- Schmidt AC, Sempsrott JR, Szpilman D, et al. The use of non-uniform drowning terminology: a follow-up study. *Scand J Trauma Resusc Emerg Med*. 2017;25(1):72.
- Szpilman D, Sempsrott J, Webber J, et al. 'Dry drowning' and other myths. *Cleve Clin J Med*. 2018;85(7):529–535.

CLINICAL PEARLS

- Medical authorities traditionally made a great distinction between salt water and freshwater drowning. The theory was that because of its high salt content, seawater in the lungs would affect the body very differently from fresh water in a variety of ways. Although this is true in theory, very few survivors of drowning ingest enough water to make a difference, and this rarely becomes an issue in treating patients who arrive at the hospital. In practice, water temperature and the presence of any contaminants are much more important considerations.
- Hypoxia is the main threat in drowning victims, and resuscitation efforts should be directed toward restoration of optimal oxygenation.
- Key risk factors include male sex, age <14 years, alcohol/drug use, low income, poor education, rural residency, aquatic exposure, risky behavior, and lack of supervision and swimming lessons.
- Prevention is the key to saving lives.
- Sometimes respiratory symptoms and hypoxia are delayed for up to 6 hours after submersion or immersion.
- People who have drowned and have minimal symptoms will usually either get better or get worse within 6 hours. There has never been a case published in the medical literature of a patient who received an adequate clinical assessment, was initially without symptoms at 6 to 8 hours, and who later deteriorated and died. People who have drowned and have minimal symptoms will usually either get better or get worse within a 6-hour observation period.
- It is important to note that the neurologic outcome of a drowning victim depends on various factors, including the duration of submersion, water temperature, the age and overall health of the victim, and the quality of care received. Slow cooling of the patient over minutes to hours before actually drowning can be neuroprotective in some patients and increase survival rates and improved neurologic outcome.
- Near drowning: A person either drowns or does not drown; one cannot be "near-drowned."
- Dry drowning: 10–15% of deaths occur with no water aspiration, due to laryngospasm. These cases may also be due to sudden cardiac death that occurred as a preceding cause of the drowning episode.
- Secondary delayed drowning: Mild symptoms usually resolve by 8 hours without complications. No one drowns, presents without symptoms after 8-hour observation period and then subsequently dies from drowning. Delayed secondary drowning is due to other diagnosis, such as (i) spontaneous pneumothorax; (ii) chemical pneumonitis; (iii) pneumonia; (iv) head injury; (v) asthma; (vi) acute coronary syndrome; (vii) myocarditis; and (viii) chest trauma.

DUPUYTREN CONTRACTURE

Alec Wilhelmi, MD, CAQSM

BASICS

DESCRIPTION

- Progressive hand condition characterized by the thickening and shortening of the palmar fascia secondary to fibrous proliferation
- Results in flexion deformities and loss of function of the fingers; similar changes rarely may occur in plantar fascia.
- Its progression can impair daily activities such as gripping, grooming, and typing.
- Also referred to as Dupuytren disease
- Abbreviations: metacarpophalangeal (MCP), proximal interphalangeal (PIP)

EPIDEMIOLOGY

Incidence

- Predominant age: 50 years for males; 60 years for females
- Predominant gender: male > female (ranges from 2:1 to 10:1)

Prevalence

- Prevalence is estimated at 3–6% of the general population and increases with advancing age.
- Disease prevalence varies from 2% to 42% depending on population and risk factors.
- Overall prevalence is 8.8% in Northern European population.
- African Americans are less likely to get the disease.
- Japanese and Taiwanese have a prevalence equal to that in Northern Europe. These patients usually present with a less severe form of the disease (1).

ETIOLOGY AND PATHOPHYSIOLOGY

- Unknown
- Ischemia to the fascia with oxygen free radical formation
- Possibly related to release of angiogenic basic fibroblast growth factor
- Related to microhemorrhage and release of growth factors

Genetics

- Autosomal dominant with variable penetrance; in one family, the gene has been mapped to chromosome 16q.
- There is a strong genetic association, with up to 80% heritability in studies.
- >30 unique genes were upregulated, and 6 unique genes were downregulated by 4-fold or greater.
- Upregulated genes include ones that code for fibronectin, tenascin C, transforming growth factor β2 (TGF-β2), collagen III, collagen IV, and collagen VI.
- All three forms of TGF-β are upregulated. TGF-β2 is upregulated 10 to 20 times. As in tendinopathy, it may be a TGF receptor lack of response, so TGF continues to be made.
- Musculoaponeurotic fibrosarcoma oncogene homolog B, or *MafB*, in the family of oncogenes is found in the cord but not paracord fascia of normal control individuals.

RISK FACTORS

- Smoking (mean 16 pack-years; odds ratio = 2.8)
- Alcohol intake
- Using both alcohol and cigarettes combined has a higher risk than individual use alone.
- Increasing age (>40 years of age)
- Male (increase in androgen receptors in nodules)
- Northern European, Japanese, Taiwanese
- Diabetes mellitus (1/3 affected, increases with time, usually mild; middle and ring fingers involved)
- Epilepsy (may be medications or disease)
- HIV infection (may or may not be associated)
- Vibration work exposure (Some studies show increased risk, whereas other studies show no risk.)
- Rheumatoid arthritis (lower risk) (2)

GENERAL PREVENTION

None known; avoid risk factors when possible.

COMMONLY ASSOCIATED CONDITIONS

- Alcoholism
- Smoking
- Epilepsy
- Diabetes mellitus
- Occupational hand trauma (manual labor involving vibration tools)

DIAGNOSIS

PHYSICAL EXAM

- Signs and symptoms (2):
  - Typical:
    - Caucasian male aged 50 to 60 years
    - Bilateral, with greater involvement in one hand
    - Family history positive
    - Unilateral or bilateral (50%)
    - Right hand more frequent
    - Ring finger more frequent
    - Ulnar digits more affected than radial
    - Mild pain early
    - Later painless plaques or nodules in palmar fascia
    - Extends into a cordlike band in the palmar fascia
    - Skin adheres to fascia and becomes puckered.
    - Nodules can be palpated under the skin.
    - Digital fascia becomes involved as disease progresses.
    - Web space contractures
    - Dupuytren diathesis can involve plantar (Ledderhose 10%) and penile (Peyronie 2%) fascia.
    - Knuckle pads
  - Atypical:
    - No age, gender differences
    - No family history
    - May have systemic disease (See "Risk Factors")
    - May have a history of trauma
    - More common unilateral
    - No ectopic manifestations (Ledderhose or Peyronie)
    - Nonprogressive
- Physical examination:
  - A firm, painless nodule in the palm of the hand proximal to the MCP joint
  - Palmar pits and grooves
  - Hueston tabletop test, with positive test if patient is unable to flatten his or her hand on the table
  - Evaluate for bilateral and plantar fascia involvement which can indicate more aggressive form.

DIFFERENTIAL DIAGNOSIS

- Callus formation
- Locked trigger finger
- Pulley rupture with bowstringing
- Nodule on flexor tendon
- Camptodactyly—can occur in early teens, tight facial bands on the ulnar side of small finger
- Soft tissue tumor

DIAGNOSTIC TESTS & INTERPRETATION

Initial Tests (lab, imaging)

- Not usually needed except in rare cases; most diagnosed by history and physical examination alone
- Ultrasound (US) can demonstrate thickening of the palmar fascia as well as the presence of a nodule.
- Magnetic resonance imaging (MRI) can assess cellularity of lesions, which correlate with higher recurrence after surgery.

Diagnostic Procedures/Other

Rarely is a biopsy needed to differentiate Dupuytren nodule from a soft tissue tumor:

- Pathologic findings:
  - Myofibroblasts
  - First stage (proliferative): increased myofibroblasts
  - Second stage (residual): dense fibroblast network
  - Third stage (involutional): Myofibroblasts disappear.

TREATMENT

GENERAL MEASURES

- ~10% of patients will have disease regression without treatment; therefore, observation remains a first-line treatment for mild cases.
- Intralesional steroid injection (triamcinolone) has been shown to reduce the need for surgery.
- With a thickened cord, it may be useful to US prior to intralesional injections to identify the underlying tendon and thus avoid the tendon during the injection.
- Although surgical intervention has been shown to be very helpful in cases of advanced DC, there are inherent risks to surgery, such as nerve injury, hematoma, skin necrosis, and infection.
- Although partial fasciectomy has long been the mainstay of treatment for patients with advanced DC, office procedures such as percutaneous needle aponeurotomy and collagenase injections may represent alternatives to surgery in certain patients.
- Whatever the method selected to treat the contracture, each technique carries a significant risk of recurrence.

MEDICATION

First Line

- Collagenase *Clostridium histolyticum* (CCH) at a dose of 0.58 mg per injection for the treatment of DC in a single digit during a 30-day treatment cycle. The collagenase weakens and dissolves the Dupuytren cord. Many patients have a short-term adverse reaction. Treatment is very successful (3)[A].
- Steroid injection (triamcinolone) for an acute tender nodule, painful knuckle pad (3)[B]

Second Line

Radiation therapy, 5-fluorouracil, and hyperbaric oxygen have been used (2)[B].

ADDITIONAL THERAPIES

- Steroid injection for acute tender nodule
- Collagenase injections can be used in two nodules at a time.
- Physiotherapy is ineffective alone, especially for more advanced cases.
- Nonoperative care with observation and hand therapy can be considered if there are nodules alone without functional impairment. Adalimumab (tumor necrosis factor [TNF] blocker injection) shows promise as a potential early-stage treatment for DC but is still undergoing clinical trials (4).

SURGERY/OTHER PROCEDURES

- Surgery: partial fasciectomy (2)[A]:
  - Surgical referral should be made when MCP joint contractures reach 30 degrees, or any degree of PIP joint contracture develops.
  - May require skin grafts for wound closure with severe cutaneous shrinkage
  - 80% have full range of movement if operated on early.
  - Continuous elongation technique is useful to prepare a severely contracted PIP joint for surgery. The digit frequently can be completely extended but will relapse if surgery is not performed.
  - Amputation of little finger, if severe and deforming (rare)
- Needle aponeurotomy, also called percutaneous needle fasciotomy (PNF), is a minimal invasive technique (3),(4)[A]:
  - Done under local anesthetic
  - Type I DC
  - Done through the skin usually blind with 18-gauge needle or special tool
  - US may be beneficial.
  - Recurrence rates can be high, but recovery is faster, and procedure is inexpensive.

ONGOING CARE

FOLLOW-UP RECOMMENDATIONS

- No activity restrictions
- Regularly assess the impact of DC on activities of daily living (ADLs), work, hobbies, personal grooming (5).
- Physical therapy after surgery: started 3 to 5 days after surgery (passive and active exercises, posterior dynamic extension splints)
- Regular follow-up by physician every 6 months to 1 year

Patient Monitoring

Observation is appropriate in early stages of disease. Indications for surgical referral and consideration of operative treatment include MCP flexion contractures >30 degrees or PIP flexion contractures (5).

DIET

No special diet

PATIENT EDUCATION

Avoid risk factors, especially with a strong family history.

PROGNOSIS

- Typical:
  - Unpredictable but usually slowly progressive
  - Patients likely to have aggressive disease (one or more): age 40 years at onset, knuckle pads, positive family history, bilateral disease involving radial side of hand, ectopic involvement (plantar)
  - Reports of clinical regression with continuous passive skeletal traction in extension and under a skin graft
  - Recurrence rate after surgery is 10–34%.
  - Prognosis better for MCP joint versus PIP joint after surgery
  - Most patients with a diagnosis do not require any surgical intervention (5).
- Atypical:
  - Nonprogressive
  - Recurrence unlikely if surgery performed

COMPLICATIONS

- Postoperative stiffness (common)
- Postoperative recurrence or extension 46–80% (common)
- Postoperative development of reflex sympathetic dystrophy (uncommon)
- Postoperative hematoma or infection (rare)
- Intraoperative neurovascular injury (rare)
- Digital infarction (rare)

REFERENCES

1. Lanting R, Broekstra DC, Werker PMN, et al. A systematic review and meta-analysis on the prevalence of Dupuytren disease in the general population of Western countries. *Plast Reconstr Surg*. 2014;133(3):593–603.
2. Rodner CM. Dupuytren's contracture. BMJ Best Practice. Updated July 14, 2023. Accessed September 8, 2025. https://bestpractice.bmj.com/topics/en-gb/983
3. Ball C, Izadi D, Verjee LS, et al. Systematic review of non-surgical treatments for early Dupuytren's disease. *BMC Musculoskelet Disord*. 2016;17(1):345.
4. Hinchliffe RJ, Sanderson RE, Rees KW, et al. Adalimumab as a potential treatment for Dupuytren disease: a cost-effective approach for early stages. *Bone Joint Res*. 2020:690–698.
5. Karbowiak M, Holme T, Khan K, et al. Dupuytren's disease. *BMJ*. 2021;373:n1308.
6. Townley WA, Baker CS, Sheppard K, et al. Dupuytren contracture uncovered: the role of lifestyle, occupation, and genetics. *Br J Plast Surg*. 2019:678–687.

ADDITIONAL READING

- Brazzelli M, Cruickshank M, Tassie E, et al. Collagenase *Clostridium histolyticum* for the treatment of Dupuytren's contracture: systematic review and economic evaluation. *Health Technol Assess*. 2015;19(90):1–202.
- Denkler KA, Vaughn CJ, Dolan EL, et al. Evidence-based medicine: options for Dupuytren's contracture: incise, excise, and dissolve. *Plast Reconstr Surg*. 2017;139(1):240e–255e.
- Hurst L, Hennessey D, Gabbay J. Dupuytren contracture: a systematic review of its pathophysiology, treatment options, and future directions. *Hand Clin*. 2016;32(4):529–534.

CLINICAL PEARLS

- DC is an inherited disease of progressive fibrous tissue contracture of the palmar fascia.
- The disease predominantly affects males of Northern European decent aged >40 years who are smokers, alcohol drinkers, diabetics, or manual labor workers (particularly those who work with vibratory tools) (6).
- Patients present with a small lump or multiple lumps, often painless, with pits in the palm of the hand progressing to contractures of the fingers.
- CCH is an effective injectable treatment option U.S. Food and Drug Administration (FDA) approved in 2010.
- Intralesional steroid injections have been shown to reduce the need for surgery.
- Surgical referral should be made when MCP joint contractures reach 30 degrees or if any degree of PIP joint contracture is present.
- Surgery usually is done in advanced disease to restore function of the hand.
- Percutaneous needle aponeurotomy and collagenase injections are significant therapeutic alternatives to surgery.
- Emerging therapies like adalimumab show promise as cost-effective, minimally invasive treatments (4).

ELBOW DISLOCATION

John Munyak, MD

BASICS

DESCRIPTION

- Separation/disruption of the articulations between distal humerus, proximal radius, and proximal ulna; typically resulting from trauma and injury to the supporting soft tissue structures
- Subtypes: anterior (rare) versus posterior (common) and simple (soft tissue injury) versus complex (fracture-dislocation)
- Complete (dislocation) or partial (subluxation)

EPIDEMIOLOGY

- In adults, the elbow is the second most frequently dislocated major joint after the shoulder.
- In the pediatric population, the elbow is the most common dislocated joint.
- Comprises 10–25% of all elbow injuries
- More frequently seen in wrestling, gymnastics, football, falls, and motor vehicle accidents
- Predominate sex: males > females (1)

Incidence

- Adults: 6 to 8/100,000 (1)
- 10–50% sports related
- Usually on the nondominant side

ETIOLOGY AND PATHOPHYSIOLOGY

- Progression of injury from lateral collateral ligament to capsule to medial collateral ligament in posterior dislocation
- Anterior dislocation from trauma to the posterior portion of a flexed elbow
- Fall on outstretched hand
- Axial loading and rotation upon impact

RISK FACTORS

- Anatomic risk factors include a shallow olecranon fossa and a prominent olecranon tip.
- Age and sports activity
- Fall on an outstretched hand

GENERAL PREVENTION

- Sport protective padding may provide a benefit.
- Injury prevention training modalities
- Avoidance of falls

COMMONLY ASSOCIATED CONDITIONS

- Common: radial head/neck fracture, epicondyle avulsion fracture, soft tissue edema, coronoid process fracture
- Wrist and shoulder injuries, which can occur 10–15% should be ruled out (1)
- Rare: neurovascular injury (brachial artery and median nerve), compartment syndrome

DIAGNOSIS

HISTORY

- Mechanism of fall
- Type of activity leading to injury (sports, fall, work, accident)
- Time since injury
- Reduction attempts

PHYSICAL EXAM

- An obvious visual deformity usually is present.
- Note the condition of the skin: Look for wounds indicating an open dislocation.
- Palpation of deformity and effusion:
  - Prominent olecranon: posterior
  - Long extended forearm: anterior
- Neurovascular evaluation, especially brachial artery and ulnar, interosseous and median nerve function
- Consult orthopedics/vascular surgery urgently for any signs of neurovascular injury.
- Rule out additional injuries, especially in contiguous musculoskeletal structures.
- In reduced elbows: Lateral pivot-shift apprehension test is highly sensitive (2)[C]:
  - Sensation of dislocation is a positive test.

DIFFERENTIAL DIAGNOSIS

- Elbow subluxation
- Spontaneous elbow dislocation and reduction
- Be especially cautious in the pediatric age group because supracondylar fractures are common in 5- to 10-year-olds.
- Nursemaid's elbow (pediatrics)
- Other elbow joint/forearm fracture

DIAGNOSTIC TESTS & INTERPRETATION

Initial Tests (lab, imaging)

- Initial anteroposterior and lateral radiographs: Evaluate relationship between distal humerus and radioulnar complex. Identify associated fracture (1)[C].
- Maintain a high index of suspicion for additional injuries and obtain radiographs of the humerus, forearm, or wrist as indicated.
- Exception: On-field reduction by a medical professional can precede initial films (3)[C].
- Postreduction radiographs: all dislocations (3)[C]
- Computed tomography (CT): reserved for complex fracture-dislocations or reconstruction planning

Diagnostic Procedures/Other

Angiography for suspected arterial injury

TREATMENT

GENERAL MEASURES

- In experienced hands, reduction may be performed on the field without analgesia. Otherwise, transport patient to a medical facility that can treat this injury.
- Appropriate monitoring is required, and proper resuscitation equipment should be available.
- In rare instances, general anesthesia in the operating room may be required.
- Postreduction, check elbow stability with range of motion (ROM).
- Obtain postreduction radiographs.
- Immobilize the elbow in a posterior splint as close to 90 degrees of flexion as possible using avoidance of a diminishing radial pulse as a guide.
- Postreduction position is in pronation; check varus, valgus, and rotatory instability (4)[C].
- Perform a postreduction neurovascular examination.
- Closed reduction of dislocation: Goal is atraumatic reduction with minimal attempts. There are several techniques:
  - Option no. 1: supine patient, forearm traction, humeral counter traction, anterior force on olecranon, and forearm supination (1)[C]
  - Option no. 2: prone patient, apply counter traction while extending the arm at the elbow, manipulate the coronoid process past the trochlea (3)[C]
  - Option no. 3 (one-person reduction): patient's arm across the chest, one hand braces the injured distal arm, the other holds the elbow and olecranon while providing traction to allow the coronoid to pass the trochlea (5)[C]
  - Full passive ROM will signify a successful reduction.
- Postreduction evaluation:
  - Postreduction radiographs to confirm position of radial head and ulna in relation to the capitate and distal humerus; also, to exclude iatrogenic fracture
  - Postreduction lateral radiograph demonstrating "drop sign," which conveys a high risk for recurrent instability (drop sign: ulnohumeral joint is widened >4 mm) (4)[C]
  - Neurovascular reassessment to confirm no nerve impingement
  - Assess joint stability:
    - ROM: no locking or crepitation
    - Joint should be examined under gentle stresses (valgus stress/laxity most common following dislocation) (3)[C].
    - Lateral pivot-shift apprehension test for joint stability (1)[C]
  - Stable joint: arm sling for comfort and early mobilization in 3 to 5 days (4)[C]
  - Unstable joint that stabilizes with pronation: splint in pronation/flexion (1)[C]
  - Joint unstable needs >45 degrees of flexion: Consider surgery (1)[C].
- Issues for referral: initial follow-up with orthopedics/sports medicine for splint removal and early mobilization
- Additional therapies:
  - ROM exercises after initial immobilization for comfort if joint is stable (1)[C].
  - Early mobilization after reduction produces the best overall outcomes: Pooled data show a larger flexion–extension arc with early motion (~137°) versus 1 to 3 weeks of immobilization (~129°); authors give grade B support to early mobilization (<7 days) (6),(7).
  - Unstable joints should have a splint that blocks full extension with encouragement of flexion as tolerated (1)[C].
  - Extended therapy required if ROM not improved by 6 to 8 weeks postinjury (3)[C]
  - Stability should be confirmed prior to full ROM therapy (6),(7)[C].

MEDICATION

- Analgesia:
  - Reduction can be attempted without analgesia (5)[C].
  - Local anesthesia by joint infiltration can reduce needed analgesic doses (1)[C].
  - Nonsteroidal anti-inflammatory drugs (NSAIDs): Heterotopic ossification (HO): A level I randomized controlled trial (RCT) found in indomethacin did not significantly reduce HO versus placebo at 1 year (49% vs. 55%; RR 0.89). Consider risks/benefits rather than routine use solely for HO prevention (8),(9).
- Anxiolysis:
  - Benzodiazepines:
    - Midazolam 1 mg/dose (pediatric 0.05 mg/kg/dose), short acting, rapid onset, preferred for conscious sedation
    - Lorazepam 0.05 mg/kg/dose (pediatrics 0.05 mg/kg/dose), longer duration not ideal for procedural sedation use
- Conscious/procedural sedation (multiple options): goal of adequate pain control and muscle relaxation:
  - Versed/fentanyl: as above
  - Ketamine: pediatric >3 months 1.5 mg/kg IV with 0.5 mg/kg repeat doses (rarely used in adults due to emergence reactions and agitation)
  - Multiple other options, including propofol, barbiturates, and nitrous oxide
- General sedation:
  - Occasionally required for difficult/painful reductions
- Precautions:
  - Be aware of respiratory and airway reflex depression with narcotics and benzodiazepines.
  - Thorough preparation required for procedural sedation, including airway management devices, bag-valve mask for ventilation, reversal agents (naloxone/flumazenil) as appropriate, cardiovascular monitoring equipment

ADDITIONAL THERAPIES

- A follow-up radiograph should be obtained 1 and 2 weeks after injury. A small percentage of patients will develop recurrent instability, which can be due to insufficiency of the lateral ulnar collateral ligament. These patients may require surgical reconstruction to restore stability.
- Rehabilitation after simple elbow dislocation requires 1 to 3 months to return to preinjury status. Typically, the outcome is good, with most athletes experiencing little morbidity or loss of function. The most common problem is loss of extension, which is minimized with an active, aggressive, and early rehabilitation program.

SURGERY/OTHER PROCEDURES

- Surgery is limited to select cases because conservative management is preferred (6)[C].
- Treatment pathway (simple dislocations): Continue to favor conservative care with early functional training; surgery is mainly for moderate to severe or bilateral ligament instability on exam—only about 2.3% of initially conservatively treated patients proceed to surgery (median ~1 month) (8),(10).
- Open dislocation, compartment syndrome, nerve injury/impingement, unstable fractures, and unstable reductions require operative intervention (1)[C].
- Grossly unstable elbows may require acute ligament repair to confer early stability to allow for ROM and enhanced rehabilitation.
- Complex dislocations with fractures, including significant radial head, olecranon, and coronoid fractures, may require surgical stabilization via open reduction and internal fixation (ORIF) of fracture segments (1)[C].
- Isolated lateral collateral ligament repair in recurrent dislocation has shown success (2)[B]. Chronically unstable elbows may require reconstruction of the lateral ulnar collateral ligament.

ADMISSION, INPATIENT, AND NURSING CONSIDERATIONS

- Admission criteria:
  - Fracture-dislocation requiring operative intervention
  - Nonreducible dislocation
  - Neurovascular injury
  - Edema with concern for compartment syndrome development
- Nursing:
  - Providing ordered medications for patient comfort or sedation as necessary
  - Monitoring of vitals for sedation procedures if needed

  Reinforcing discharge instructions/plan
- Discharge criteria:
  - Elbow dislocation confirmed by postreduction radiograph
  - Normal postreduction neurovascular exam documented
  - Supply orthopedic follow-up.
  - Reduced elbow splinted for comfort or to maintain stability as needed

ONGOING CARE

FOLLOW-UP RECOMMENDATIONS

Consultation with an orthopedic surgeon should be obtained in most cases.

PATIENT EDUCATION

Avoid activities that specifically stress the elbow joint (e.g., throwing) until ready upon reevaluation.

PROGNOSIS

- Return to sport (recreational athletes): expect good outcomes with ~82% returning to their preinjury sport and a mean return at ~22 weeks; no major differences in return-to-sport rates between operative and nonoperative groups (9),(10)
- Generally full recovery
- Poor outcome related to stiffness/decreased ROM:
  - Early physical therapy/ROM exercises decrease stiffness.

COMPLICATIONS

- Neurovascular compromise
- Stiffness
- Compartment syndrome
- Recurrent dislocation
- HO

REFERENCES

1. Kuhn MA, Ross G. Acute elbow dislocations. *Orthop Clin North Am*. 2008;39(2):155–161.
2. Burra G, Andrews JR. Acute shoulder and elbow dislocations in the athlete. *Orthop Clin North Am*. 2002;33(3):479–495.
3. O'Driscoll SW. Classification and evaluation of recurrent instability of the elbow. *Clin Orthop Relat Res*. 2000;(370):34–43.
4. Parsons BO, Ramsey ML. Acute elbow dislocations in athletes. *Clin Sports Med*. 2010;29(4):599–609.
5. Mehta JA, Bain GI. Elbow dislocations in adults and children. *Clin Sports Med*. 2004;23(4):609–627.
6. Kumar A, Ahmed M. Closed reduction of posterior dislocation of the elbow: a simple technique. *J Orthop Trauma*. 1999;13(1):58–59.
7. Pott CMJM, de Klerk HH, Priester-Vink S, et al. Treatment outcomes of simple elbow dislocations a systematic review of 1,081 cases. *JBJS Rev*. 2024;12(1).
8. Breulmann FL, Lappen S, Ehmann Y, et al. Treatment strategies for simple elbow dislocation—a systematic review. *BMC Musculoskelet Disord*. 2024;25(1):148.
9. Atwan Y, Abdulla I, Grewal R, et al. Indomethacin for heterotopic ossification prophylaxis following surgical treatment of elbow trauma: a randomized controlled trial. *J Shoulder Elbow Surg*. 2023;32(6):1242–1248.
10. Nolte PC, Walde MV, Elrick BP, et al. High return to sport rate and good patient-reported outcomes in recreational athletes following simple elbow dislocations. *J Orthop Surg Res*. 2023;18(1):453.

ADDITIONAL READING

- Krul M, van der Wouden JC, van Suijlekom-Smit LW, et al. Manipulative interventions for reducing pulled elbow in young children. *Cochrane Database Syst Rev*. 2009;(4):CD007759.
- Taylor F, Sims M, Theis JC, et al. Interventions for treating acute elbow dislocations in adults. *Cochrane Database Syst Rev*. 2012;(4):CD007908.
- Work Loss Data Institute. *Elbow (acute and chronic)*. Work Loss Data Institute; 2008.

CLINICAL PEARLS

- Recognize neurovascular injury early.
- Confirm relocation with a radiograph.
- Early mobilization reduces postreduction stiffness. The elbow is at risk for stiffness, more rapidly and more often than any other joint—can occur as early as 3 days after immobilization.
- Evaluate for other injuries in all traumas.

EPISTAXIS

Alan Shahtaji, DO, CAQSM ▪ Priya Sharma, DO

BASICS

DESCRIPTION

- Bleeding from injured nasal mucosa overlying a blood vessel
- Characterized as either anterior or posterior
- Affected persons usually do not seek medical attention, especially if bleeding is minor or self-limited.
- Synonym(s): nosebleed; nasal bleeding

EPIDEMIOLOGY

- Common problem affecting up to 60% of the general population
- 80–90% of cases occur along the anterior nasal cavity at Kiesselbach plexus (Little area).
- Bimodal age distribution with incidence peaks at ages <10 years and >70 years
- Very common in childhood, with 3 out of 4 children experiencing at least 1 episode of epistaxis, and are most often limited bleeds occurring in anterior nasal cavity
- Severe cases and posterior epistaxis are more common in older adults.
- More frequent in winter months

ETIOLOGY AND PATHOPHYSIOLOGY

- Commonly caused by irritation or trauma to nasal mucosa
- Most common cause is idiopathic followed by trauma.
- Local causes:
  - Local digital trauma
  - Mucosal dryness or lack of humidification
  - Nasal or facial trauma
  - Inflammation (allergic rhinitis)
  - Medications (e.g., intranasal steroids)
  - Infection (rhinitis or sinusitis)
  - Intranasal neoplasm or polyps
  - Chemical irritants (e.g., cigarette smoke)
  - Foreign body
  - Illicit drug use (e.g., cocaine)
  - Aneurysm or other arteriovenous malformations
  - Hereditary hemorrhagic telangiectasia (Osler-Weber-Rendu disease)
  - Iatrogenic instrumentation
- Systemic causes:
  - Coagulopathies (e.g., von Willebrand disease, hemophilia)
  - Renal failure
  - Platelet dysfunction
  - Thrombocytopenia
  - Hematologic malignancies (e.g., leukemia)
  - Alcohol use disorder
  - Hypertension (There is an association between epistaxis and hypertension but no research supporting a causal relationship [1].)
  - Liver disease (e.g., cirrhosis)
  - Medications (e.g., anticoagulants [1],[2],[3]; selective serotonin reuptake inhibitors [SSRIs] [3]; phosphodiesterase-5 [PDE-5] inhibitors [4], controversial data on correlation with aspirin use, no reported association with nonsteroidal anti-inflammatory drugs [NSAIDs])

DIAGNOSIS

HISTORY

- Determine duration, frequency, laterality, and severity of nosebleed.
- Quantify amount of blood loss.
- Presence of nasal obstruction: may indicate a neoplasm, especially with recurrent bleeding from the same side
- Trauma: Consider other associated injuries.
- Other medical conditions that predispose to bleeding:
  - Tumors and coagulation disorders
  - Cirrhosis
  - HIV infection
  - Intranasal cocaine use
- The presence of chronic medical conditions that can be exacerbated by blood loss:
  - Coronary artery disease/atherosclerosis (2)
  - Chronic obstructive pulmonary disease
- Medications:
  - Aspirin
  - Anticoagulants (1),(2)
  - Intranasal steroids
- Use of nasal oxygen or CPAP
- Alcohol and cocaine use
- History of severe nosebleeds, other sites of bleeding or easy bruising
- History of nasal surgery
- Family history of bleeding disorders

PHYSICAL EXAM

Measures to prevent contamination should be observed, and examination should be done with appropriate personal protective equipment.

ALERT

Initial evaluation should focus on airway assessment and cardiovascular stability, looking for signs of airway compromise or hypovolemia.

- Positioning:
  - The examination should take place in a well-lit room, preferably with a headlamp or mirror.
  - The patient should be seated comfortably in an upright position with head movement restricted in a sniffing position.
- Tools:
  - Wear personal protective equipment including eye protection and gloves.
  - A nasal speculum should be used with blades protracting vertically to better view the nasal mucosa.
  - Basin for patient to spit drainage
- Visualize bleeding:
  - Remove clots and foreign bodies in the anterior nasal cavity by blowing nose, with suction (Frazier suction catheter), irrigation, forceps, or cotton-tipped applicators.
  - If no anterior source is identified on inspection, anterior rhinoscopy may be attempted. Ears, nose, and throat (ENT) specialist can perform nasal endoscopy if needed to visualize the remainder of the nasal cavity.
  - Posterior bleeding may be subtle, and the general location of the source of bleeding should be determined (e.g., behind the middle turbinate, roof of the nasal cavity, submucosal masses).
  - Location of bleeding is important because different arteries supply the floor and roof of the posterior nasal cavity.
- Trauma:
  - Assess for deformity with inspection and palpation of bony structures.
  - Evaluate extraocular muscle movements and stability of the teeth to rule out orbital or maxillary fracture. Malocclusion of teeth may indicate maxillary or mandibular fracture.
  - CSF leak should be evaluated for using the ring test, if indicated.

ALERT

In the case of nasal trauma, be sure to evaluate for concussion, facial fractures, and dental injury.

- Recurrent nosebleeds:
  - Evaluate for signs of coagulopathy (e.g., ecchymoses, petechiae, telangiectatic lesions).

DIFFERENTIAL DIAGNOSIS

- Pulmonary hemoptysis
- Upper GI bleed such as bleeding esophageal varices
- Tumor bleeding from the pharynx, larynx, or trachea

DIAGNOSTIC TESTS & INTERPRETATION

Initial tests (lab, imaging)

- Labs are not necessary for the majority of patients with epistaxis.
- For severe bleeding, a complete blood count (CBC) should be performed in addition to blood type and cross-matching for possible transfusion.
- In anticoagulated patients, coagulation studies may be required to determine if anticoagulation levels are supratherapeutic.
- Radiographic studies are usually not helpful unless a facial fracture is suspected.
- Unexplained recurrent unilateral epistaxis should raise suspicion for neoplasm and warrants consideration of computed tomography (CT) scan or magnetic resonance imaging (MRI) and endoscopic evaluation.

TREATMENT

- Anterior bleed:
  - Minor anterior nosebleeds may resolve without intervention prior to clinical evaluation or with initial tamponade.
- Pretreatment/initial tamponade:
  - The patient should blow their nose to remove blood and clots.
  - Local anesthetic and vasoconstrictor should be applied as a topical spray or via saturated cotton pledgets.
    - Drugs commonly used for this purpose are lidocaine with epinephrine and oxymetazoline (Afrin).
    - One small retrospective study found that oxymetazoline spray stopped the bleeding in 65% of consecutive patients with epistaxis presenting to the emergency department (ED) (1).

- The patient should be sitting up and leaning forward to prevent blood from tracking into the pharynx or stomach.
- The patient should tightly pinch the nasal alae (soft cartilaginous part of the nose) against the septum continuously for 10 to 15 minutes.
- A cold compress applied over the bridge of the nose may help with hemostasis. Sucking ice cubes or applying an ice pack to the neck may decrease nasal blood flow (2),(4).
- If an anterior bleeding source is visualized, initial therapy may consist of topical vasoconstrictors or nasal cautery (1)

- Epistaxis that is refractory to pressure and topical vasoconstrictors may require cautery.
  - All cautery may be painful and pretreatment anesthetic is recommended.
    - Chemical cautery is usually performed with silver nitrate.
      - Most useful for minor active bleeds or after active bleeding has stopped and prominent vessels have been identified.
      - Apply the cautery for ~10 seconds.
      - Begin at the periphery of a small area surrounding the bleeding site and move centrally.
      - Exercise caution with silver nitrate because it cauterizes everything that it touches.
    - Electrical cautery is useful for more aggressive bleeding or larger vessels of the anterior nasal septum.
    - The nose must first be anesthetized using local anesthetic because electrical cautery can be extremely painful.
      - Anesthetize bilaterally because the electrical current is transmitted through the septum.
      - Electrocautery must be performed cautiously to avoid excessive destruction of healthy tissue.
      - If cautery is unsuccessful, or if no obvious site of bleeding is seen, nasal packing may be considered to tamponade the epistaxis.

ALERT
Complications from cautery include infection, tissue injury, and possibly septal necrosis and perforation, especially when cautery is used on both sides of the nasal septum.

ALERT
Nasal packing may also be used on the sideline for temporary hemostasis enabling return to play.

- A number of absorbable and nonabsorbable packing materials are available for anterior nasal packing.
- Traditional packing products consist of nondegradable materials that must be removed. It is important to note that removal of packing materials may cause mucosal damage and result in additional bleeding.
  - Gauze impregnated with petroleum jelly (e.g., Xeroform) may be inserted in layers from the floor of the nasal cavity to tamponade the epistaxis.
  - A preformed nasal tampon made of polyvinyl alcohol that expands when wet (e.g., Merocel) will swell and fill the nasal cavity, applying pressure over the bleeding area.
  - An inflatable carboxymethylcellulose pack consisting of a balloon catheter and hydrocolloid coating (e.g., Rapid Rhino) that forms a lubricant on contact with water and remains in contact with mucosa on balloon deflation may cause less discomfort and be easier to insert and remove.
- Absorbable or degradable materials that do not require formal removal are recommended in patients with an increased risk of bleeding (anticoagulation, bleeding disorders, vascular abnormalities) and should be considered in children where removal of packing material may be challenging (1).
  - Oxidized cellulose (e.g., Surgicel) and gelatin foams (e.g., Gelfoam) increase clot formation and provide a degree of tamponade.
  - Bovine-derived thrombin gel (e.g., FloSeal) is conformable to the contours of the nasal cavity, easy to apply, and less painful. Higher costs of its use may be offset by the lack of need for packing removal.
- Packing generally is left in place for 1 to 5 days to ensure adequate clot formation. No benefit has been found with longer duration (1),(5).
- Topical or oral antibiotics may be used with prolonged nasal packing (>24 hours) to limit risk of bacterial infection, although data is mixed (1).
- Other complications of nasal packing include septal hematomas, abscesses, or pressure necrosis from traumatic packing; sinusitis from blockage of sinus drainage; hypoxia from nasal airway blockage or apneic spells; stimulation of the nasovagal reflex causing syncope during packing; and acute airway obstruction from pack displacement into the oropharynx.
- Failure to control anterior bleeding with cautery or packing may necessitate embolization or surgical ligation of the offending vessels (1),(5).
- Referral to an otolaryngologist is appropriate when bleeding is refractory, complications are present, posterior bleed is suspected, or specialized treatment is required.
- Continued bleeding despite an anterior pack may be due to a posterior bleed.

- Posterior bleed:
  - These bleeds can be difficult to treat and may require either balloon insertion or a formal posterior pack.
  - Posterior packing usually necessitates hospitalization out of concern for hypoxic complications, cardiopulmonary events, and the risk of asphyxiation should the packing become dislodged.
  - Posterior packing can be quite uncomfortable and may require significant anesthesia.
  - A posterior pack may be an emergent temporizing measure before surgery or angiographic embolization.

ALERT
Referral to specialist and ED would be appropriate.

ONGOING CARE

- Once epistaxis is controlled, conservative measures may prevent recurrent bleeding owing to local factors.
- Refrain from activities that may stimulate bleeding:
  - Blowing or picking nose
  - Heavy lifting
  - Strenuous activity
- Patients should abstain from alcohol or hot drinks that may cause vasodilation of the nasal vessels.
- Nasal saline washes and water-soluble ointments assist in humidification of the nasal mucosa and promote healing.
- Humidified air, especially for patients using oxygen via nasal canula, may improve local conditions within the nose.

FOLLOW-UP RECOMMENDATIONS

Patients should meet with their primary care physician to investigate for underlying causes and risk factors for epistaxis.

ALERT
All patients with recurrent epistaxis, particularly if unilateral, require formal evaluation with radiographic studies and nasal endoscopy to rule out a neoplastic lesion.

REFERENCES

1. Tunkel DE, Anne S, Payne SC, et al. Clinical practice guideline: nosebleed (epistaxis). *Otolaryngol Head Neck Surg*. 2020;162(1 Suppl):S1–S38.
2. Khan M, Conroy K, Ubayasiri K, et al. Initial assessment in the management of adult epistaxis: systematic review. *J Laryngol Otol*. 2017;131(12):1035–1055.
3. Seidel DU, Jacob L, Kostev K, et al. Risk factors for epistaxis in patients followed in general practices in Germany. *Rhinology*. 2017;55(4):312–318.
4. Beck R, Sorge M, Schneider A, et al. Current approaches to epistaxis treatment in primary and secondary care. *Dtsch Arztebl Int*. 2018;115(1–02):12–22.
5. Shargorodsky J, Bleier BS, Holbrook EH, et al. Outcomes analysis in epistaxis management: development of a therapeutic algorithm. *Otolaryngol Head Neck Surg*. 2013;149(3):390–398.

ADDITIONAL READING

Seikaly H. Epistaxis. *N Engl J Med*. 2021;384(10):944–951.

CLINICAL PEARLS

- Anterior nosebleeds are often controlled with tamponade, topical medications, and cold packs.
- Athletes with an anterior bleed (80–90% of cases) without significant facial trauma, comorbid concussion, and/or underlying condition may return to play during the same event after cessation of bleeding.
- At high-level sports coverage with limited treatment time, consider having topical vasoconstrictors and nasal packing available on the sideline.
- Posterior nosebleeds are more severe and often require specialist involvement and higher level of care.

E

EXERCISE-ASSOCIATED HYPONATREMIA

Alec Wilhelmi, MD, CAQSM

BASICS

DESCRIPTION

- Decrease in serum sodium concentration to <135 mmol/L during or up to 24 hour after physical activity
- Serum sodium concentration and serum osmolarity are maintained by homeostatic mechanisms involving thirst, antidiuretic hormone (ADH), renal handling of filtered sodium, and perhaps sodium loss through sweat.
- Increased serum osmolarity above normal (280 to 300 mOsmol/kg) stimulates hypothalamic osmoreceptors, which then cause increased thirst and circulating levels of ADH.
- Hyponatremia can be associated with hypervolemia, euvolemia, and hypovolemia.
- Most common form is dilutional hyponatremia. This is true in athletes as well as nonathletes:
  - Excess of water in relation to existing sodium stores
  - Sodium stores can be decreased, normal, or increased. However, the serum concentration of sodium is more reflective of fluid balance.

EPIDEMIOLOGY

- Prevalence varies wildly based on sport/event, athlete level, weather, and race time (1),(2).
- Can be seen in up to 51% of ultramarathon participants, 13% of standard marathon finishers, and 25% of Ironman triathletes (1),(2)
- After accounting for race time and body mass index, prevalence is equal between men and women (2)[A].
- Many cases are asymptomatic and may never present for medical care (3).

ETIOLOGY AND PATHOPHYSIOLOGY

- Caused by combination of excessive fluid intake, inadequate sodium replacement, and impaired renal excretion of sodium
- Inappropriate secretion of arginine vasopressin (AVP), also referred to as ADH, despite sodium dilution in plasma leads to impaired water clearance via reduced urine output:
  - Pain, nausea/vomiting, hypoglycemia, and medication use may play a role.
- Interleukin-6 may be elevated after exercise and also stimulate AVP production.
- Rapid absorption of fluid in stomach immediately after exercise

RISK FACTORS

- Excessive fluid intake, above what is dictated by thirst and water/hypotonic drinks (without electrolytes)
- Slower runners and finishers who maintain or increase their prerace body weight due to prolonged fluid consumption
- Excess fluid losses (e.g., excessive sweating, heat stress, vomiting, and diarrhea) that have been replaced primarily by hypotonic fluids
- Inexperienced runner or inadequate training
- Low body weight due to less total body fluid
- Nonsteroidal anti-inflammatory drug (NSAID) medication use before or during activity
- Other disorders that can lead to sodium disturbances:
  - Renal insufficiency, heart failure, cirrhosis, syndrome of inappropriate antidiuretic hormone secretion (SIADH), hypothyroidism, cortisol deficiency, ecstasy use

GENERAL PREVENTION

- Educating participants about dangers of excessive fluid intake
- Instruction to drink as dictated by thirst (rather than perceived exertion, sweating, and distance)
- Reduce availability of fluids along race route.
- Consume fluid at a rate <700 mL/h.
- Monitor body weights before and after events:
  - If weight is gained, reduce fluid and sodium intake postrace.
- Little data to support that sodium ingestion during event is protective (2)

COMMONLY ASSOCIATED CONDITIONS

Few frequently associated conditions, but several conditions have similar symptoms and can co-occur:

- Exercise-associated collapse—common
- Heat stroke—common
- Hypothermia—common
- Hypoglycemia—common
- Rhabdomyolysis—rare

DIAGNOSIS

HISTORY

- Thorough past medical, surgical, and social history
- Ask about previous episodes of sodium problems or post-race medical issues.
- Attempt to estimate water and food intake during race. Inquire about medication use of the following:
  - NSAIDs, selective serotonin reuptake inhibitors (SSRIs), diuretics, antipsychotics, and amiodarone

PHYSICAL EXAM

Signs and symptoms:

- Often asymptomatic
- Mild to moderate: nausea, vomiting, headache, dizziness, fatigue, confusion, muscle cramps
- Severe: seizures, altered mental status, coma, respiratory distress, and even death (due to cerebral edema)
- Vitals signs, including rectal temperature if possible
- Obtain weight and compare to prerace if possible.
- Assess fluid status: blood pressure, skin turgor, edema, pulmonary exam for rales.
- Mental status: confusion, difficulty concentrating, lethargy, lack of responsiveness
- Be cognizant that postrace collapse and dizziness is common and can be associated with other conditions as well.
- Coma, obtundation, seizure activity, decorticate or decerebrate posturing, and respiratory arrest are indications of severe disease and should be treated immediately.

DIFFERENTIAL DIAGNOSIS

- Exercise-associated collapse
- Heat stroke
- Hyperthermia
- Hypothermia
- Hypoglycemia
- Myocardial infarction (MI)
- Stroke
- Adrenal insufficiency and adrenal crisis
- Congestive heart failure and pulmonary edema
- Gastroenteritis

- Hypothyroidism and myxedema coma
- Renal failure, acute
- Renal failure, chronic
- SIADH
- Cirrhosis
- Nephrotic syndrome
- Psychogenic polydipsia
- Medication related

DIAGNOSTIC TESTS & INTERPRETATION
- If possible, measure blood sodium concentration on site.
- Obtain serum glucose; creatinine if available
- An electrocardiogram (ECG) may allow you to rule out MI.
- If serum hyperglycemia is present, then serum sodium must be corrected by a factor of 1.6 mEq/L for each 100 mg/dL increase in serum glucose (4)[A].

TREATMENT

GENERAL MEASURES
- Airway, breathing, and circulation (ABC)
- Obtain rectal temperature (3)[C].
- Consider establishing intravenous (IV) access.
- Place patient in supine position; elevate legs to increase central circulation (1)[A],(3)[C].
- Quickly assess neurologic status (3)[C].
- Assess blood sodium if testing is available (1)[A].
- Consider the differential diagnosis and the possibility of a combination of exercise-associated issues (heat stroke, hypothermia, hyponatremia, collapse, etc.) (3)[C].
- Do not discharge the athlete with suspected exercise-associated hyponatremia until he or she is able to urinate (1)[A],(3)[C].
- For less severe hyponatremia (>130 mEq/L), watchful waiting, with fluid restriction, is appropriate if clinically stable because most will self-correct by diuresis (1)[A],(3)[C]:
  - Fluid restriction would be contraindicated if concerned for comorbid rhabdomyolysis.
  - Oral or IV hypertonic saline would be effective option regardless of fluid status.
- If symptoms do not improve or worsen with the above, IV hypertonic saline would be appropriate.

MEDICATION
- IV and PO hypertonic saline (100 mL 3% saline) have been shown to be equally effective in asymptomatic exercise-associated hyponatremia (5)[A].
- In cases of severe symptomatic exercise-associated hyponatremia, IV hypertonic saline is the best option (6)[A],(7)[A]:
  - Use 100-mL bolus of 3% saline with up to two additional boluses at 10-minute intervals.
  - 50-mL aliquot of 8.4% sodium bicarbonate can provide a similar sodium load (3)[C].
  - Central pontine demyelination is a theoretical concern but has not been reported in athletes receiving hypertonic saline.

ISSUES FOR REFERRAL
Patients with severe exercise-associated hyponatremia requiring IV hypertonic saline should be considered for transfer to a higher level of care, although immediate treatment should still be initiated if possible. This will assure appropriate evaluation for secondary exercise-associated issue through lab work, along with serial lab work to assure resolution of hyponatremia.

ADDITIONAL THERAPIES
Athletes with documented hyponatremia and mild-to-moderate symptoms can be considered good candidates for oral hypertonic solutions (2)[A],(7)[A]:
- 4 bouillon cubes in 125 mL of water
- 100 mL of oral hypertonic saline

ONGOING CARE

PROGNOSIS
- Mild hyponatremia will almost always correct with autodiuresis and has no long-term consequences.
- An episode of exercise-associated hyponatremia may indicate an increase susceptibility to future episodes.
- Untreated severe hyponatremia or hyponatremia worsened with hypotonic saline can lead to cerebral edema, coma, and possibly death.

REFERENCES

1. Urso C, Brucculeri S, Caimi G. Physiopathological, epidemiological, clinical, and therapeutic aspects of exercise-associated hyponatremia. *J Clin Med.* 2014;3(4):1258–1275.
2. Bennett BL, Hew-Butler T, Rosner MH, et al. Wilderness Medical Society clinical practice guidelines for the management of exercise-associated hyponatremia: 2019 update. *Wilderness Environ Med.* 2020;31(1):50–62.
3. Hoffman MD, Joslin J, Rogers IR. Management of suspected fluid balance issues in participants of wilderness endurance events. *Curr Sports Med Rep.* 2017;16(2):98–102.
4. Filippatos TD, Liamis G, Christopoulou F, et al. Ten common pitfalls in the evaluation of patient with hyponatremia. *Eur J Intern Med.* 2016;29:22–25.
5. Owen BE, Rogers IR, Hoffman MD, et al. Efficacy of oral versus intravenous hypertonic saline in runners with hyponatremia. *J Sci Med Sport.* 2014;17(5):457–462.
6. Hew-Butler T. Exercise-associated hyponatremia. *Front Horm Res.* 2019;52:178–189.
7. Buck E, Schwellnus TJ, Derman W, et al. Exercise-associated hyponatremia in athletes: the challenges of prevention, diagnosis, and treatment. *Am J Lifestyle Med.* 2021;15(6):548–556.

ADDITIONAL READING

- Bennett BL, Hew-Butler T, Hoffman MD, et al. Wilderness Medical Society practice guidelines for treatment of exercise-associated hyponatremia: 2014 update. *Wilderness Environ Med.* 2014;25(Suppl 4):S30–S42.
- Krabak BJ, Lipman GS, Waite BL, et al. Exercise-associated hyponatremia, hypernatremia, and hydration status in multistage ultramarathons. *Wilderness Environ Med.* 2017;28(4):291–298.
- Wharam PC, Speedy DB, Noakes TD, et al. NSAID use increases the risk of developing hyponatremia during an Ironman triathlon. *Med Sci Sports Exerc.* 2006;38(4):618–622.

CLINICAL PEARLS
- Exercise-associated hyponatremia is common in long-distance and endurance events.
- Most cases are asymptomatic.
- Excessive fluid intake beyond what is required by thirst is the primary mechanism.
- Exercise-associated hyponatremia can be associated with other exercise-induced conditions and has overlapping symptoms with them as well.
- Oral hypertonic saline is as effective as IV hypertonic saline in mild exercise-associated hyponatremia.
- Proposed regimens include 100-mL hypertonic saline, 3 or 4 broth bouillon cubes in 125 mL water, or a serving of salted pretzels (7).
- When in doubt about hydration status, IV or PO hypertonic saline (100 mL 3% saline) is appropriate.

E

EXERCISE-INDUCED ANAPHYLAXIS

Kimberly Kaiser, MD, CAQSM • Gregory Rubin, DO, CAQSM

BASICS

DESCRIPTION

- Distinct form of physical allergy characterized by a spectrum of exercise-induced symptoms ranging from mild skin symptoms such as pruritus and urticaria to angioedema, hypotension, syncope, and death
- A subgroup may develop food-dependent exercise-induced anaphylaxis (FDEIA).

EPIDEMIOLOGY

Incidence

Unknown

Prevalence

- Lifetime prevalence 0.05–2% (1)
- 0.03% in study of Japanese adolescents (2)
- Occurs in all ages, both sexes (3)
- 2.36–5% of all cases of anaphylaxis (4)

ETIOLOGY AND PATHOPHYSIOLOGY

No single etiology has been agreed upon. Popular theories include (3):

- Release of histamine and tryptase by mast cell degranulation
- Increased gastrointestinal (GI) permeability
- Increased activity of tissue transglutaminase in the gut mucosa
- Increased plasma osmolality causing histamine release by basophils

RISK FACTORS

- Previous episodes
- Vigorous exercise (2)
- Atopic individuals at increased risk (3)
- Associated factors include:
  - Ingestion of certain foods (wheat most common culprit) prior to exercise (5)
  - Ingestion of certain medications (aspirin or nonsteroidal anti-inflammatory drugs [NSAIDs]) before exercise
  - Alcohol consumption (2)
  - Hormonal fluctuations during menstrual cycle may play a role in women (1).
  - Infections or illness
  - Extremes in temperature (1)

GENERAL PREVENTION

Preventive medications include:

- Cromolyn sodium orally 200 mg TID 20 minutes before food ingestion can be useful in FDEIA (4)[C].
- Possible use of oral antihistamines (data conflicting). Some clinicians advocate for avoiding antihistamines because they may block cutaneous manifestations of exercise-induced anaphylaxis (EIA) that often serve as a "warning" of impending anaphylaxis (4).
- Avoid food/medication triggers. Avoid ingestion of food triggers up to 4 to 6 hours before exercise (rarely when ingested shortly after exercise) (4).
- Omalizumab can be helpful in difficult to control and refractory cases (4).

COMMONLY ASSOCIATED CONDITIONS

- Eczema
- Asthma

DIAGNOSIS

HISTORY

- Transient exercise-induced itching and cutaneous erythema ± urticaria
- Other symptoms include generalized itching, dizziness, GI colic, headache, choking sensation, urticaria or angioedema with hypotension or respiratory obstruction, and full anaphylactic shock.
- Occurs within 45 minutes of starting exercise (6)[C]
- History of previous EIA
- Identify possible provocative agent. Diagnosis may require an exercise diary.
- Identify any ingestions prior to exercise. Specific food or medication may be a trigger; most common triggers: wheat, aspirin, alcohol, shellfish, tomato, corn, almond, soybean, rye, bee pollen (4)[C]

PHYSICAL EXAM

Assess circulation, airway, breathing (CAB):

- Hypotension or respiratory difficulty may signify impending anaphylactic shock.
- Dermatologic examination may reveal wheals or angioedema.
- Urticarial lesions are large with diameters measuring 10 to 15 mm as compared to cholinergic urticaria which is 1 to 3 mm punctate wheals (4)[C].

DIFFERENTIAL DIAGNOSIS

- Cholinergic urticaria
- Exercise-induced bronchospasm
- Environmental allergy
- Mastocytosis
- Exercise-associated gastroesophageal reflux

DIAGNOSTIC TESTS & INTERPRETATION

Initial Tests (lab, imaging)

- Serum tryptase levels are not specific to EIA/FDEIA. Elevation at baseline suggests mast cell disorders, kidney failure, and acute myeloid leukemia (2)[A].
- Serum tryptase and histamine levels should be drawn immediately or within 3 hours after the episode and if elevated are suggestive of EIA (5)[A].

Diagnostic Procedures/Other

- Passive warming test (e.g., warm shower or sauna) can be helpful in differentiating cholinergic urticaria from EIA.
- Exercise challenge test using a treadmill or stationary bike can be performed. A positive test (reproduction of symptoms and urticaria) is helpful in diagnosis, but a negative test does not exclude a diagnosis of EIA because reproducibility of symptoms is variable (1)[C],(4)[C]. Emergency equipment should be immediately available if exercise test is performed.
- Allergy testing for potential food and common allergen triggers should be done in all patients with EIA.

TREATMENT

- Prehospital:
  - Assess CAB.
  - Subcutaneous administration of 0.3 to 0.5 mL epinephrine 1:1,000 if systemic symptoms of anaphylaxis are present and then call 911.
  - Trendelenburg position
- Emergency department (ED) treatment:
  - Treat symptoms of anaphylactic shock as necessary in appropriate medical setting (e.g., fluid support for hypotension, assisted ventilation for respiratory obstruction).
  - Epinephrine is first-line treatment (4)[C],(6)[C].
  - Antihistamines may decrease itching and urticaria, but they do not relieve upper and lower airway obstruction or shock.
  - Nebulized albuterol should be given in individuals with severe bronchospasm.

ONGOING CARE

PROGNOSIS

- Generally favorable prognosis for EIA and FDEIA
- Few fatalities have been reported with attacks often becoming less frequent and severe over time.

FOLLOW-UP RECOMMENDATIONS

- Cease physical activity if any symptoms arise.
- Avoid eating 4 to 6 hours before exercise and at least 1 hour after exercise.
- Avoid anti-inflammatory drugs before exercise.
- Avoid exercising in extreme outdoor conditions.
- Allow for a period of gradual warm-up.
- Always exercise with a partner and carry injectable epinephrine.
- Possible role for desensitization to physical activity
- Referral to an allergist for identification of possible associated triggers may be beneficial.
- Follow up to assess recurrence of symptoms and success of drug therapy (1)[C](4)[C].

PATIENT EDUCATION

- Advise patient on epinephrine (EpiPen) use (should have access to one at all times).
- Renew EpiPen annually.
- Advise patient to avoid any known triggers.
- Recommend wearing a medical alert device (1)[C].

REFERENCES

1. Sorace PM, LaFontaine T. Exercise-induced anaphylaxis. *ACSMs Health Fit J*. 2021;25(2):48–50.
2. Feldweg AM. Exercise-induced anaphylaxis. *Immunol Allergy Clin North Am*. 2015;35(2):261–275.
3. Ansley L, Bonini M, Delgado L, et al. Pathophysiological mechanisms of exercise-induced anaphylaxis: an EAACI position statement. *Allergy*. 2015;70(10):1212–1221.
4. Geller M. Clinical management of exercise-induced anaphylaxis and cholinergic urticaria. *J Allergy Clin Immuno Pract*. 2020;8(7):2209–2214.
5. Kulthanan K, Ungprasert P, Jirapongsananuruk O, et al. Food-dependent exercise-induced wheals, angioedema, and anaphylaxis: a systematic review. *J Allergy Immuno Pract*. 2022;10(9):2280–2296.
6. Montgomery SL. Cholinergic urticaria and exercise-induced anaphylaxis. *Curr Sports Med Rep*. 2015;14(1):61–63.

CLINICAL PEARLS

- Epinephrine is first-line treatment.
- Because symptoms may vary significantly from one episode to another and among patients, some patients may not feel comfortable returning to activity knowing that they could have repeat attacks. In addition, patients who have experienced an anaphylactic response to exercise should be cautioned about returning to activity. For those whose symptoms are controlled with medication, it is recommended they continue to carry injectable epinephrine and exercise with a partner.
- EIA can occur with any level of activity and may be precipitated by the ingestion of foods or medications. Unless a specific trigger is identified, there are no restrictions placed on diet or type of activity. A general rule of thumb is to avoid eating for at least 4 hours before exercise.

EXERCISE-INDUCED BRONCHOCONSTRICTION

Irie Paul Padua, MD • Brian Young Kim, MD, MS, CAQSM

BASICS

DESCRIPTION

- A form of airway hyperresponsiveness characterized by a heightened bronchoconstriction response to a variety of stimuli related to exercise
- Characterized by wheezing, coughing, shortness of breath, and/or chest tightness occurring during or after exercise
- Usually within 5 to 15 minutes of the onset of exercise, an acute episode of airway obstruction begins. This is usually followed by recovery within 30 to 90 minutes on completion of the exercise.
- If the athlete has underlying asthma, then it is called *exercise-induced bronchoconstriction (EIB) with asthma*; otherwise, it is *EIB without asthma*.
- Synonym(s): exercise-induced asthma; exercise-induced bronchospasm

EPIDEMIOLOGY

- General population: 5–20% (1)
- Patients with asthma: up to 90% (1)
- Children ≤16 years old: 3–35% (1)
- High performance athletes: 30–70% (1)
- Recreational and elite athletes: 10–50% (2),(3)
- Cold-weather athletes: 20–50% (2),(3)
- A high level of fitness does not confer immunity from either asthma or EIB.
- When controlled, EIB does not restrict exercise performance.

ETIOLOGY AND PATHOPHYSIOLOGY

- The mechanism of EIB has not been established with certainty, however, there are several theories
- The hyperosmolarity theory posits that increased airflow, particularly of dehumidified air, causes water loss from the surface liquid of the airways. This causes a hyperosmolar state in the airways, leading to inflammation and bronchoconstriction (2)[C].
- The thermal theory suggests that an increased respiratory rate cools the cells on the surface of the airways. Once exertion subsides, the airways rewarm, causing dilatation of the airway blood vessels, leading to hyperemia and fluid leakage into the bronchioles. This, in turn, causes inflammation and airway constriction.
- Thermal factors are now thought to be relatively minor compared to hyperosmolarity (2)[C].
- Other theories have associated bronchoconstriction with epithelial cell damage, inflammatory cells, or increased parasympathetic tone.

RISK FACTORS

- Cold-weather sports such as ice hockey, figure skating, and cross-country skiing
- Sports with a long duration of high-intensity exercise such as running, bicycling, swimming, soccer, and rugby
- Environmental factors such as tobacco smoke, chlorine, sulfur dioxide, nitrogen oxide, carbon monoxide, pollens and molds, cold weather, particulate matter, and low humidity

GENERAL PREVENTION

- Nonpharmacologic: preexercise warm-up, use of face mask to promote humidification and prevent water loss, avoidance of inhaling cold air (4)
- Pharmacologic: short-acting $\beta 2$ agonist (SABA) use 15 minutes prior to exercise (4)

COMMONLY ASSOCIATED CONDITIONS

- Asthma (common)
- Allergic rhinitis and hay fever (common)

DIAGNOSIS

HISTORY

- Personal or family history of allergies or asthma
- Symptoms are often a poor predictor of who has EIB.
- Symptoms occur during or after exercise, typically appearing after 5 to 15 minutes of exercise.
- Signs and symptoms include the following:
  - Coughing
  - Wheezing
  - Shortness of breath
  - Chest tightness
  - Headache
  - Fatigue
  - Feeling out of shape
  - Chest pain or discomfort

PHYSICAL EXAM

Physical examination should include the following:

- Look for evidence of allergic disease such as pale nasal mucosa or allergic "shiners."
- Cardiac exam to evaluate for cardiac abnormalities
- Lung examination is typically normal; if wheezing is present, consider chronic asthma.
- On the field or after an exercise challenge, physical examination is more likely to reveal wheezing.

DIFFERENTIAL DIAGNOSIS

- Pulmonary:
  - Asthma with exercise exacerbation
  - Vocal cord dysfunction (VCD)
  - Exercise-induced hyperventilation
  - Restrictive lung disease
  - Cystic fibrosis
- Cardiac:
  - Coronary artery disease
  - Congenital/acquired heart defects
  - Arrhythmias
  - Congestive heart failure
  - Cardiomyopathy
- Ear, nose, and throat (ENT):
  - VCD: This represents a frequently missed cause of dyspnea and throat tightness associated with exercise (particularly in young women). Physicians should consider referral to ENT for evaluation of VCD if the patient is not responding as expected to treatment measures for EIB, or if the patient has atypical clinical features such as inspiratory stridor in the absence of wheezing.
  - Laryngeal prolapse
  - Exercise-induced laryngeal dysfunction
  - Laryngomalacia
  - Chronic sinusitis
- Gastrointestinal (GI): gastroesophageal reflux disease
- Allergic: exercise-induced anaphylaxis/urticaria
- Psych: anxiety disorders, panic attacks
- Other: general state of deconditioning

DIAGNOSTIC TESTS & INTERPRETATION

- Direct testing with pulmonary function tests (PFTs) done before and after albuterol should be performed if asthma is suspected (2),(3)[A].
- If negative, then move on to testing with one of the following indirect tests.
  - PFTs before and after exercise (3)[A]:
    - Spirometry is more accurate than peak expiratory flow rate.
    - 10–15% reduction in preexercise forced expiratory capacity in 1 second (FEV_1) within 30 minutes after activity confirms the diagnosis of EIB.
    - It is best to test athletes during sport-specific exercise or at temperatures of 20–25°C and <50% relative humidity.
    - Exercise at a workload of 80–90% of predicted VO_{2max} for 6 to 8 minutes during testing or workload of 80–90% max heart rate (HR) for 2 to 4 minutes.
  - Eucapnic voluntary hyperventilation (EVH) (2),(5)[A]:
    - Recommended by International Olympic Committee (IOC) Medical Commission for diagnosing athletes, however, this testing is not readily available
    - Hyperventilation of a gas mixture with 21% O_2 and 5% CO_2 for 6 minutes at 85% maximum voluntary ventilation
    - FEV_1 is measured prior to the test and 5, 10, and 15 minutes after the test.
    - Cutoff is 10–15% drop in FEV_1.
  - Inhaled mannitol testing (2)[A]:
    - A fall in FEV_1 >15% from baseline is diagnostic.
    - Allows for a controlled stepwise increase in stimulus
    - Not available in the United States
- Direct testing with methacholine challenge is third line because it is less sensitive and specific for EIB than indirect testing methods including exercise provocation, EVH, or inhaled mannitol testing (2)[B].
- Ideally, testing should be performed during a period of intense training, as airway responsiveness can normalize with de-escalation of exercise.

TREATMENT

GENERAL MEASURES

- Warm-up of 15 minutes at moderate exertion 15 to 30 minutes prior to exercise can induce a refractory period preventing bronchoconstriction (2),(4)[A].
- Avoidance of triggers (cold, dry air; exercise close to busy roads; poorly ventilated chlorinated pool environments), if possible
- In cold weather, a mask can be used to warm the air (3)[B].
- Nose breathing can help to warm and moisturize the air.
- Athletes with underlying asthma should be well controlled before beginning a sport/exercise program.

MEDICATION

- Treat as per asthma guidelines (National Heart, Lung, and Blood Institute) for patients with underlying asthma.
- For elite athletes, check the World Anti-Doping Agency (WADA), United States Anti-Doping Agency (USADA), or National Collegiate Athletic Association (NCAA) list of banned substances to be sure that the medications used are in compliance with their rules.

First Line

Prophylactic (preexercise) medication:

- SABA: 2 to 4 puffs 15 to 30 minutes before exercise; may repeat during exercise as needed (2),(4)[A]. If used on a daily basis, tolerance may develop (2)[A].

Second Line

If not responding adequately to a SABA, or requiring daily SABA use, can add:

- A daily inhaled corticosteroid (6)[A]
- Long-acting β agonists (LABA) may be used in conjunction with inhaled corticosteroids 30 to 60 minutes before exercise (4)[A]. However, daily use can contribute to the development of tolerance toward both SABA and LABA (2)[A]. Avoid using LABA without inhaled corticosteroids due to the increased incidence of asthma-related events when used alone (6)[A].
- Montelukast 10 mg PO 2 hours before exercise (2),(6)[A]
- Cromolyn 4 to 10 puffs 10 to 20 minutes before exercise or nedocromil 2 to 4 puffs 10 to 20 minutes before exercise (4),(6)[A]. Mast cell stabilizing agents are no longer available in the United States but may be prescribed in other countries.
- Short acting muscarinic antagonists may be effective in case of SABA tolerance (4)[C].
- Consider adding an antihistamine for patients who also have allergies (2)[C],(6)[B]. Inhaled anticholinergic agents may be helpful, but evidence is inconsistent (2)[A].

ISSUES FOR REFERRAL

- Consider referral to ENT if high suspicion for VCD, laryngeal prolapse, exercise-induced laryngeal dysfunction, or laryngomalacia.
- If symptoms of EIB are worsening or do not improve with first- and second-line pharmacologic intervention, then can consider referral to pulmonology.

COMPLEMENTARY & ALTERNATIVE MEDICINE

Consider treatment for comorbidities (e.g., treatment as per asthma guidelines for patient with underlying asthma, selective serotonin reuptake inhibitors [SSRI] for anxiety, proton pump inhibitor [PPI] for GERD, antihistamine for allergies).

ONGOING CARE

FOLLOW-UP RECOMMENDATIONS

- Frequent monthly follow-ups after initial diagnosis of EIB to evaluate for possible development of asthma; if no evidence for development of asthma, can consider spacing out follow-up to every 3 to 6 months
- If not responding to an inhaled SABA, consider other diagnoses.
- Have the patient return if their use of SABA increases.
- Must continue to monitor because efficacy of medications can differ over time, particularly in different environments or in response to different types of exercise (2)[A].

DIET

There is low-quality evidence for a diet low in salt, high in fish oils, and high in ascorbic acid (2),(6)[B].

PATIENT EDUCATION

- All athletes with EIB should have a SABA inhaler with them during practices and games.
- All athletes should be taught the proper use of an inhaler.
- Spacers can help to improve delivery of the inhaler medication.
- The athlete should know the difference between his or her controller and as-needed medication.
- Teach patients to avoid triggers.
- Consider allergy testing.

PROGNOSIS

Good so long as patients have close monitoring of possible development of asthma and efficacy of medications.

COMPLICATIONS

Poorly controlled athletes with EIB can progress to airway remodeling that becomes unresponsive to SABA.

REFERENCES

1. Aggarwal B, Mulgirigama A, Berend N. Exercise-induced bronchoconstriction: prevalence, pathophysiology, patient impact, diagnosis and management. *NPJ Prim Care Respir Med*. 2018;28(1):31.
2. Weiler JM, Brannan JD, Randolph CC, et al. Exercise-induced bronchoconstriction update—2016. *J Allergy Clin Immunol*. 2016;138(5):1292.e36–1295.e36.
3. Parsons JP, Mastronarde JG. Exercise-induced bronchoconstriction in athletes. *Chest*. 2005;128(6):3966–3974.
4. Koya T, Ueno H, Hasegawa T, et al. Management of exercise-induced bronchoconstriction in athletes. *J Allergy Clin Immunol Pract*. 2020;8(7):2183–2192.
5. Atchley TJ, Smith DM. Exercise-induced bronchoconstriction in elite or endurance athletes: pathogenesis and diagnostic considerations. *Ann Allergy Asthma Immunol*. 2020;125(1):47–54.
6. Parsons JP, Hallstrand TS, Mastronarde JG, et al. An official American Thoracic Society clinical practice guideline: exercise-induced bronchoconstriction. *Am J Respir Crit Care Med*. 2013;187(9):1016–1027.

ADDITIONAL READING

- Boulet LP, O'Byrne PM. Asthma and exercise-induced bronchoconstriction in athletes. *N Engl J Med*. 2015;372(7):641–648.
- Smoglia JM, Weiss P, Rundell KW. Exercise induced bronchoconstriction in adults: evidence based diagnosis and management. *BMJ*. 2016;352:h6951.
- Weiler JM, Anderson SD, Randolph C, et al. Pathogenesis, prevalence, diagnosis, and management of exercise-induced bronchoconstriction: a practice parameter. *Ann Allergy Asthma Immunol*. 2010;105(Suppl 6):S1–S47.

CLINICAL PEARLS

- First-line treatment is a SABA before exercise.
- Avoid daily use of a SABA because tachyphylaxis may develop. Have the athlete use this during high-intensity practice and competition.
- If an athlete is requiring daily use of a SABA, consider adding a controller medication.
- Warm-up of 15 minutes at moderate exertion 15 to 30 minutes prior to exercise can induce a refractory period preventing bronchoconstriction.
- It is no longer recommended to use LABA without an inhaled corticosteroid.

E

EXERCISE-INDUCED DIARRHEA

Steven K. Poon, MD, CAQSM • Kimberly G. Harmon, MD

BASICS

DESCRIPTION

- Increased stool frequency or volume often accompanied by lower abdominal cramping or urge to defecate associated with strenuous physical activity:
  - Normal physical examination
  - Normal laboratory and diagnostic studies
- Synonym(s): runner's diarrhea; runner's trots

EPIDEMIOLOGY

- Primarily associated with running sports but also common in cycling and reported in swimming, wrestling (1),(2),(3)
- Difficulty with existing research:
  - Difficult to control all variables (diet, exercise intensity, underlying pathology such as irritable bowel syndrome)
  - Studies often lack a denominator, making a true incidence of symptoms difficult to determine.
  - Many studies are surveys with low response rates, which introduce a selection bias.
  - Subject's dietary recall often is inaccurate.

Prevalence

- Prevalence of diarrhea reported from 8% to 60% in athletes
- Prevalence of diarrhea in control subjects reported up to 40%

ETIOLOGY AND PATHOPHYSIOLOGY

Despite prevalence of condition and discomfort experienced by athletes, the exact cause of exercise induced diarrhea is still unclear. Proposed mechanisms (1),(2),(3),(4):

- Mesenteric ischemia:
  - With strenuous exercise, blood is shifted away from the gut and to the working muscle.
  - Exercising at 70% VO_{2max} decreases blood flow to gastrointestinal (GI) tract by 60–70%.
  - May lead to the production of endotoxin
  - Causes a cascade of inflammatory events that can further impair the mucosal integrity
  - Increased activity of the sympathetic nervous system leads to decreased splanchnic blood flow and is caused by:
    - Mental stress
    - Hyperthermia
    - Dehydration
    - Hypoglycemia
- Increased sympathetic nervous system activity:
  - Suppresses parasympathetic activity
  - Decreased gut tone and resistance
  - Increased colonic transit times
  - Secretion of gastroenteropancreatic hormones
- Reduced GI tract perfusion:
  - Gut barrier dysfunction
  - Damage to intestinal tight junction proteins
  - Increased permeability of gut barrier
- Mechanical stimulation of the colon due to intra-abdominal jostling
- Enteric fluid and electrolyte imbalance

RISK FACTORS

- Underlying bowel pathology may worsen with strenuous exercise.
- Dehydration
- Occurs more frequently with increased exercise intensity
- Occurs more frequently in untrained participants
- Type of exercise (running > cycling, swimming, speed skating, cross-country skiing)
- Meals rich in fat, protein, and fiber taken shortly before exercise worsen symptoms.

DIAGNOSIS

HISTORY

- Increased stool frequency or volume, or loose stools after exercise
- Often accompanied by abdominal cramping and urge to defecate
- May occur just with competition and not with training
- Normal bowel function at other times

PHYSICAL EXAM

- Increased stool frequency
- Increased stool volume
- Loose or explosive stools
- Urge to defecate, often necessitating the athlete to cease exercise
- Abdominal cramping
- Unremarkable physical examination
- Exercise-associated diarrhea is a diagnosis of exclusion.
- Workup is used to rule out other causes of diarrhea.

DIFFERENTIAL DIAGNOSIS

- Irritable bowel disease
- Inflammatory bowel disease
- Infection
- Colon cancer
- Superior mesenteric or portal venous thrombosis
- Malabsorption
- Microscopic colitis
- Laxative abuse
- Lactose intolerance
- Hyperthyroidism

DIAGNOSTIC TESTS & INTERPRETATION

Initial Tests (lab, imaging)

- Stool cultures, including *Clostridium difficile*
- Consider immunoglobulin A (IgA) antitissue transglutaminase antibodies to rule out celiac sprue.
- Thyroid-stimulating hormone
- Consider stool osmolar gap if eating disorder and/or laxative abuse is suspected:
  - Increased osmotic gap is suspicious for laxative use.
- Imaging studies should be obtained as clinically indicated:
  - Consider barium enema.
  - Contrast-enhanced computed tomography (CT) scan

Diagnostic Procedures/Other

- Diagnostic procedures such as sigmoidoscopy or colonoscopy may be considered as clinically indicated.
- Hematochezia, melena, abdominal pain, fever, or vomiting are red flags that require a workup.

TREATMENT

GENERAL MEASURES

- Treatment is generally conservative and should include (1)[C],(2)[C],(3)[C]:
  - Training modification:
    - Increase volume and intensity of training slowly.
  - Try to evacuate prior to exercise.
  - Diet modification
- Acute symptoms usually rapidly resolve with cessation of activity.

MEDICATION

- All athletes should consult with the governing bodies of their sports regarding banned substances.
- Because symptoms are generally self-limited and typically cease after end of exercise, medications should be used with caution.

First Line

Antispasmodics may be helpful but have anticholinergic side effects and should be used with caution:

- Dicyclomine (Bentyl) 20 mg PO QID
- Hyoscyamine (Levsin) 0.125 to 0.25 mg PO/SL q4h PRN:
  - Sometimes helpful in stopping abdominal cramping after exercise
  - The athlete should remain well hydrated.
  - Use in hot/humid conditions is not ideal.
- Loperamide (Imodium) 2 to 4 mg 30 minutes before exercise:
  - Decreases intestinal motility and affects water and electrolyte absorption
  - Side effects are rare.

Second Line

- Opiate/atropine combinations (diphenoxylate [Lomotil]) should be used with caution:
  - Opiates are habit forming.
  - May be banned depending on governing body of the sport
  - May adversely affect performance
- Atropine may cause hyperthermia, tachycardia, and heat regulation problems.

ONGOING CARE

DIET

Dietary modification can be helpful (1)[C],(2)[C],(3)[C],(5)[C]:

- Stay well hydrated.
- Avoid caffeine, which is both a diuretic and a cathartic.
- Avoid foods that exacerbate symptoms (e.g., lactose in lactose-intolerant athlete).
- Limit intake of gas-forming foods (broccoli, onions, beans).
- Eat a small, low-fat, and low-fiber meal several hours before competition:
  - Use low-osmolar sports drink between meal and competition or training.
- Avoid large doses of vitamin C, sodium bicarbonate, and carbohydrate drink prior to exercise.
- Avoid high fructose–containing foods.
- Caution against the use of nonsteroidal anti-inflammatory drugs (NSAIDs) in prerace or during race settings
- Avoid sugar substitutes or nonabsorbable sugars such as sorbitol.
- If athlete still has difficulty with diarrhea or urge to defecate while exercising, try complete nutritional liquid that is low in fiber during the day preceding competition.
- Consider meeting with a registered dietitian to discuss appropriate food, sugar, or allergen elimination nutrition plan or a low-fermentable oligo-, di-, mono-saccharides and polyols (FODMAP) diet.
- Probiotics can be considered for appropriate dietary and overall GI health, but there is insufficient evidence to support any meaningful improvements on athletic performance (6)[B].

PROGNOSIS

Most athletes can learn how to manage their symptoms through the use of diet and training.

REFERENCES

1. Casey E, Mistry DJ, MacKnight JM. Training room management of medical conditions: sports gastroenterology. *Clin Sports Med*. 2005;24(3):525–540.
2. Ho GW. Lower gastrointestinal distress in endurance athletes. *Curr Sports Med Rep*. 2009;8(2):85–91.
3. Simons SM, Kennedy RG. Gastrointestinal problems in runners. *Curr Sports Med Rep*. 2004;3(2):112–116.
4. Zuhl M, Schneider S, Lanphere K, et al. Exercise regulation of intestinal tight junction proteins. *Br J Sports Med*. 2014;48(12):980–986.
5. de Oliveira EP, Burini RC, Jeukendrup A. Gastrointestinal complaints during exercise: prevalence, etiology, and nutritional recommendations. *Sports Med*. 2014;44(Suppl 1):S79–S85.
6. de Paiva AKF, de Oliveira EP, Mancini L, et al. Effects of probiotic supplementation on performance of resistance and aerobic exercises: a systematic review. *Nutr Rev*. 2023;81(2):153–167.

ADDITIONAL READING

- Green GA. Gastrointestinal disorders in the athlete. *Clin Sports Med*. 1992;11(2):453–470.
- Swain RA. Exercise-induced diarrhea: when to wonder. *Med Sci Sports Exerc*. 1994;26(5):523–526.

CLINICAL PEARLS

- Exercise-induced diarrhea is associated with strenuous exercise and can worsen with increasing distance or intensity.
- Symptoms are self-limited, and patients are often asymptomatic after cessation of exercise with normal laboratory testing.
- Treatment is usually supportive and focused on dietary modifications, gradual increase in exercise intensity, and managing symptoms.
- The use of antidiarrheals prior to exercise can stop symptoms, making sports participation possible, while dietary modifications are being explored.

E

EXERCISE-INDUCED URTICARIA

Mark E. Halstead, MD

BASICS

DESCRIPTION

- Exercise-induced urticaria is a subtype of cholinergic urticaria which is a subtype of chronic inducible urticaria, which is a subtype of chronic urticaria (1).
- Spectrum of allergic response to exercise ranging from itching, flushing, and cutaneous warmth to development of well-circumscribed wheals (large papular lesions with pale centers and an erythematous ring) and angioedema to severe anaphylactic shock
- Elevation of serum histamine levels with exercise
- Mast cell degranulation seen in skin biopsies suggesting immunoglobulin E–mediated sensitization
- Described with almost any type of physical exercise
- Distinguishable from cholinergic urticaria, which also has exercise as a possible trigger
- Certain foods in combination with exercise may cause symptoms in susceptible individuals.
- Synonym(s): exercise-induced anaphylaxis; hives

EPIDEMIOLOGY

- Very rare (1)
- Predominant gender: male > female
- Predominant age: seen more frequently in young adults but has been described ages 4 to 76 years (2)
- Median age of onset is 23.1 years (3).

RISK FACTORS

- Atopic history (eczema, asthma, allergic rhinitis)
- Other forms of physical allergy
- Food allergy

GENERAL PREVENTION

- Stop exercise with first onset of symptoms.
- Avoid foods 6 to 8 hours before exercise. Exercising first thing in the morning after evening fast is preferable.
- Avoid known problematic food or medication triggers for at least 12 hours before exercise.
- Preventive antihistamine therapy may be useful.
- Patients always should have an epinephrine kit with them while exercising; diphenhydramine (Benadryl) also may be reasonable to have.
- Exercising with a companion knowledgeable in cardiopulmonary resuscitation (CPR) is recommended.
- Recommend wearing medical alert device.

DIAGNOSIS

HISTORY

- Diagnosis usually is made by history.
- Initially, patients describe generalized feeling of tingling, warmth, and itching.
- May start as early as 5 minutes after initiating exercise or can occur after exercise has been completed, usually within 1 hour after exercise.
- May have history of food or medication ingestion within previous 6 to 8 hours before exercise, most often within previous 4 hours.
- Patients often (>50%) have atopic history (i.e., eczema, asthma, allergic rhinitis).
- Foods reported to be associated include wheat (most common reported), alcohol, eggs, lentils, shellfish, peanuts, hazelnuts, tomatoes, peaches, apples, grapes, oranges, celery, cereals, cow's milk, mushrooms, beef, pork, poultry, snails, carrots, and cheese. Cases have been reported with many other foods.
- 90% of patients have only one food culprit that induces reactions.
- Medications: nonsteroidal anti-inflammatory drugs (NSAIDs), aspirin, antibiotics
- Other cofactors reported: menstrual cycle, metal-containing dental amalgams
- Usually resolves within 30 minutes to 4 hours after exercise
- Headaches may continue for up to 3 to 4 days after a severe reaction.
- Running is the most common form of exercise to induce symptoms (3).

PHYSICAL EXAM

- Signs and symptoms:
  - Pruritus
  - Urticaria
  - Wheezing
  - Hypotension
  - Flushing
  - Angioedema
  - Headaches
  - Nausea/vomiting
  - Diarrhea
  - Abdominal pain
  - Choking
  - Profuse sweating
- Physical examination:
  - Generally distinguished from other forms of cholinergic urticaria because larger (>10 mm) wheals are seen in exercise-induced urticaria, whereas fine punctate (<5 mm) lesions are seen in cholinergic urticaria
  - Wheals are not reproducible with generalized heat application or sweating, which is more characteristic of cholinergic urticaria, or cold application (ice cube) common to cold urticaria.
  - Respiratory examination is usually normal unless progressing to exercise induced anaphylaxis then may demonstrate stridor, wheezing, dyspnea, and retractions during acute attack.
  - Angioedema seen in more severe acute attacks

DIFFERENTIAL DIAGNOSIS

- Physical urticarias (cold, dermographic, delayed pressure, solar, aquagenic, vibratory)
- Cholinergic urticaria (induced by increased body temperature)
- Exercise-induced asthma
- Exercise-associated gastrointestinal reflux
- Vocal cord dysfunction
- Insect bites
- Drug eruption
- Urticaria pigmentosa
- Indolent systemic mastocytosis
- Systemic lupus erythematosus
- Erythema multiforme

DIAGNOSTIC TESTS & INTERPRETATION

- Labs not necessary in acute attacks
- May have elevated serum tryptase or histamine following attack but not specific for this disorder
- Allergy testing may be beneficial as an outpatient.
- Best diagnosed with an exercise challenge (progressive increase in activity observing for reproduction of the pruritic and urticarial reaction) (4)
- Emergency resuscitation equipment and medication as well as trained personnel should be present for testing.
- Positive skin testing does not always mean a cause-and-effect relationship. Suspicious positive skin tests may need to be followed by an exercise challenge because patients with positive food skin tests may not always develop urticaria with exercise and consumption of that food.

TREATMENT

MEDICATION

- Epinephrine (EpiPen) 0.2 to 0.5 mg intramuscular (IM) for severe anaphylactic reaction in adults; 0.01 mg/kg in children
- Diphenhydramine (Benadryl) 25 to 50 mg PO q4–6h (children: 5 mg/kg/d divided q6–8h, not exceeding 300 mg/d)
- Hydroxyzine (Atarax) 25 to 100 mg PO q6h (children: 2 mg/kg/d divided q6–8h)
- During exercise, patients should carry an epinephrine kit (EpiPen) with them at all times.
- H_1 antihistamines as prophylaxis have shown mixed results (fexofenadine 60 mg PO BID, loratadine 10 mg PO daily, and cetirizine 10 mg PO daily).
- Cromolyn taken orally has been reported to be of some benefit.
- H_2 antihistamines may be of help (e.g., cimetidine, ranitidine, and famotidine).
- Doxepin, which has both H_1- and H_2-blocking abilities, may be of value.

ADDITIONAL THERAPIES

- Modification of intensity of exercise
- Acutely, care is targeted toward ensuring airway protection if severe anaphylaxis is present.
- Trendelenburg position

ONGOING CARE

FOLLOW-UP RECOMMENDATIONS

- Referral to an allergist may be beneficial for skin testing and controlled exercise challenge testing.
- Because vast majority of patients with food-induced urticaria have only one food trigger, identifying and eliminating that trigger may resolve the issue.
- Preventative medication has been reported to decrease or stabilize attacks in up to 93% of patients (5)[B].

REFERENCES

1. Pozderac I, Lugovic-Mihic L, Artukovic M, et al. Chronic inducible urticaria: classification and prominent features of physical and non-physical types. *Acta Dermatovenerol Alp Pannonica Adriat.* 2020;29(3):141–148.
2. Pravettoni V, Incorvaia C. Diagnosis of exercise-induced anaphylaxis: current insights. *J Asthma Allergy.* 2016;9:191–198.
3. Kulthanan K, Ungprasert P, Jirapongsananuruk O, et al. Food-dependent exercise-induced wheals, angioedema, and anaphylaxis: a systematic review. *J Allergy Clin Immunol Pract.* 2022;10(9):2280–2296.
4. Fukunaga A, Oda Y, Imamura S, et al. Cholinergic urticaria: subtype classification and clinical approach. *Am J Clin Dermatol.* 2023;24(1):41–54.
5. Shadick NA, Liang MH, Partridge AJ, et al. The natural history of exercise-induced anaphylaxis: survey results from a 10-year follow-up study. *J Allergy Clin Immunol.* 1999;104(1):123–127.

ADDITIONAL READING

- Geller M. Clinical management of exercise-induced anaphylaxis and cholinergic urticaria. *J Allergy Clin Immunol Pract.* 2020;8(7):2209–2214.
- Montgomery SL. Cholinergic urticaria and exercise-induced anaphylaxis. *Curr Sports Med Rep.* 2015;14(1):61–63.
- Munoz M, Kiefer LA, Pereira MP, et al. New insights into chronic inducible urticaria. *Curr Allergy Asthma Rep.* 2024;24(8):457–469.
- Sijapati N, Sciturro M, Le M, et al. Exercise-induced urticaria: a rare case report. *Cureus.* 2022;14(3):e23062.

CLINICAL PEARLS

- Exercise may be continued as long as precautions are taken by avoiding all food 6 to 8 hours before exercise and 12 hours after eating food suspected of causing reactions.
- Epinephrine should be carried at all times with the patient when exercising, and a companion who knows CPR ideally would be exercising with the patient.
- Patients who had severe life-threatening reactions likely need counseling to discuss curtailing exercise.
- These reactions are not always preventable. Despite premedication with various antihistamines, patients still can develop urticarial lesions and have anaphylaxis.
- Initiating antihistamine therapy on a daily basis for those who exercise frequently is worthwhile to potentially reduce the number of occurrences of this phenomenon.
- Each individual may react to different foods. Some may react to only a single food but reports of a combination of foods are needed to trigger the reaction.
- It is reasonable to see an allergist for testing and an exercise challenge with suspicious food items.

EXERTIONAL HEADACHE

Nathan Cardoos, MD, CAQSM

BASICS

- There are two types of exertional, or exercise-associated, headaches seen in athletes: (i) primary exercise headache (PEH) and (ii) "weightlifter's headache," a form of primary cough headache.
- These headache syndromes are not associated with intracranial lesions or systemic disorders. They are distinct from migraines, tension headaches, concussion, and cervicogenic headaches—all of which are also seen in athletes—although they may coexist and must be treated accordingly.

DESCRIPTION

- Weightlifter's headache is a short-lasting headache that results abruptly from Valsalva maneuvers, such as with weightlifting, coughing, sneezing, or crying.
- PEH is believed to be distinct from weightlifter's headache because it lasts longer, has a different population profile, results from more sustained intense exercise (such as running, cycling, rowing, swimming, etc.), and is usually not associated with Valsalva maneuvers.

EPIDEMIOLOGY

- PEH occurs typically in younger athletes with an average age of 24 to 40 years, depending on the case series examined (1).
- Weightlifter's headache is more commonly seen in older individuals, with an average age of 55 to 67 years (2).

Prevalence

Lifetime prevalence of PEH is 1% of the general population, based on a Danish study; however, a study of cyclists competing in a strenuous bike race found a prevalence of 26% (3).

ETIOLOGY AND PATHOPHYSIOLOGY

Pathophysiology is largely unknown, but several theories have been postulated:

- Systemic blood pressure (BP) changes or increases in intra-abdominal/intrathoracic pressures during exercise may lead to increased cerebral arterial pressure or cause dilatation of pain-sensitive venous sinuses (2).
- Other theories include inappropriate cerebrovascular dilation with BP changes during exercise or incompetence of the jugular venous valve.

RISK FACTORS

- High altitude (3)
- Hot weather (3)
- Extreme exertion (3)
- Dehydration (3)

GENERAL PREVENTION

Avoidance of physical exertion; it usually takes only a few episodes for the patient to understand what factors precipitate symptoms and to learn to avoid the type of physical exertion that triggers the pain (4).

COMMONLY ASSOCIATED CONDITIONS

- Up to 50% of patients with PEH have a personal or family history of migraine and exercise can be a migraine trigger (3).
- Approximately half of cough headache patients have a space-occupying lesion of the posterior fossa, most commonly a Chiari type I malformation (5).

DIAGNOSIS

HISTORY

- All of the defining features below come from a small number of case series and expert opinion (1),(3).
- PEH:
  - Characterized as bilateral, throbbing, pulsatile
  - Brought on by and occurs only during or after strenuous physical exercise
  - Not associated with head trauma
  - Lasts typically from 5 minutes to 24 hours but can persist up to 48 hours
  - Not associated with nausea or vomiting, although many patients with migraines experience exercise as a trigger and may have these symptoms
  - *The International Classification of Headache Disorders 3rd edition* (ICHD-3) defines PEH as having at least two headache episodes that last <48 hours and are precipitated by or during strenuous exercise, without being better accounted for by another diagnosis (6).
- Weightlifter's headache:
  - Sudden onset brought on by coughing, straining, or other Valsalva maneuver
  - Described as "sharp" or "stabbing"
  - Lasts seconds to minutes
- Thorough history should aim to:
  - Elicit details that may alert to a focal neurologic cause.
  - Rule out history of head trauma.
  - Identify any red flags (SNOOP):
    - S—systemic symptoms/signs/disease: This includes things like fever, weight loss, chills, or a history of cancer or HIV. These could indicate an infection, an autoimmune disease, or a systemic illness causing the headache.
    - N—neurologic symptoms or signs: This refers to any abnormal neurologic findings, such as weakness, confusion, changes in consciousness, seizures, or vision problems. These could be signs of a stroke, a tumor, or other issues in the brain.
    - O—onset: This focuses on the suddenness of the headache. A "thunderclap" headache, which reaches its maximum severity within seconds or minutes, is a significant red flag and can be a sign of a subarachnoid hemorrhage.
    - O—older age of onset: A new headache in a person >50 years old is a concern, as it could indicate conditions like giant cell arteritis.
    - P—progressive or pattern change: This means the headache is getting worse over time, or the headache's characteristics (frequency, severity, location) have changed from the patient's usual pattern. This could signal a progressive neurologic condition.
  - Distinguish exertional headache from migraine or tension headache.
  - Identify personal or family history of migraine disorder or other headache disorders.
  - Identify any past history of bleeding disorders or blood clots.
  - Evaluate for cardiac risk factors.

PHYSICAL EXAM

- Check vital signs.
- Perform complete neurologic examination, including strength, coordination, balance, gait, reflexes, sensation, and cranial nerve function. By definition, the neurologic examination will be normal in PEH.
- Conduct funduscopic exam to look for any papilledema. Test visual fields and pupillary reflex.
- Assess mental status, which is normal in PEH.
- Evaluate for signs of meningismus or neck stiffness.
- The rest of the exam should be determined by any red flags or key components of the history.

DIFFERENTIAL DIAGNOSIS
- Concussion
- Cervicogenic headache
- Tension headache
- Migraine disorder
- Systemic disorder, such as a viral illness
- Drug-induced headache
- Central nervous system (CNS) infection
- Intracranial lesion, such as a brain tumor
- Subarachnoid hemorrhage (SAH)
- Cervical artery dissection
- Reversible cerebral vasoconstriction syndrome
- Cerebral aneurysm or arteriovenous malformation
- Chiari malformation
- Intracranial hypertension
- Cerebral venous thrombosis
- Cardiac cephalgia (cardiac ischemia causing headache without chest pain)
- Pheochromocytoma

DIAGNOSTIC TESTS & INTERPRETATION
Initial Tests (lab, imaging)
If there are any focal neurologic findings or any concern for a structural lesion or a stroke, then neuroimaging, such as computed tomography (CT) or magnetic resonance imaging (MRI), must be done.

ALERT
The ICHD-3 states that it is mandatory to exclude SAH, arterial dissection, and reversible cerebral vasoconstriction syndrome in any initial presentation of PEH (6).

- At younger ages with classic history of PEH, mild symptoms, and normal exam, imaging may not be necessary to make the diagnosis; however, many experts recommend that imaging, including MRI and magnetic resonance angiography (MRA), should be performed for all new or never-evaluated PEH (1),(2),(6)[C].
- The Ottawa SAH Rule for headache evaluation states that patients ≥15 years old with a new, severe, atraumatic headache reaching maximum intensity within 1 hour should be evaluated for SAH if the headache onset occurred with exertion. A patient meeting these criteria should be evaluated acutely for SAH with CT; lumbar puncture should be done if strong suspicion for SAH remains after a normal CT (1)[C].

ALERT
For weightlifter's headache to be considered a benign condition, structural lesions, especially in the cerebral posterior fossa, must be evaluated by neuroimaging (6)[C].

- MRI can better evaluate the posterior fossa than CT scan, but CT more quickly evaluates for hemorrhage.
- Consider evaluating for cardiac ischemia in patients >50 years with known heart disease or risk factors for myocardial infarction.

Diagnostic Procedures/Other
Consider lumbar puncture if there is a suspicion for SAH and the CT scan is normal.

TREATMENT

MEDICATION
- Given the self-limiting nature and short duration of symptoms from weightlifter's headache, avoidance of the provoking activity is the preferred treatment.
- Nonsteroidal anti-inflammatory drugs (NSAIDs) are typically used only for a short course to treat PEH as well as to prevent recurrence.
- Indomethacin (50 to 100 mg PO 30 to 60 minutes prior to the headache-causing physical exertion, or 25 to 50 mg TID for long-term prophylaxis) (4)[C] has been used with some success.
- Ergotamine (unspecified dose prior to exercise) can be used for prophylaxis in cases where NSAIDs are not well tolerated (4)[C], but caution needs to be exercised because of its side effects and drug interaction profile.
- Propranolol (20 to 80 mg TID) is another option for prophylactic therapy (4)[C].

ISSUES FOR REFERRAL
Consider referral to a neurologist if headache symptoms are atypical or recalcitrant to treatment, or if assistance is needed in determining the appropriate diagnostic workup.

ADDITIONAL THERAPIES
- NSAIDs can cause peptic ulcer disease, stomach irritation, nausea, renal dysfunction, and renal failure. They should be taken with food and used sparingly.
- Ergotamine has known complications, including vascular stasis and peripheral vascular constriction, thrombosis, worsening of vascular disease, fibrosis, and increased uterine contractility. It is contraindicated in coronary artery disease, hypertension, liver disease, renal disease, pregnancy, and Raynaud syndrome. It should only be used with caution.

ONGOING CARE

PATIENT EDUCATION
- Patients should be advised to avoid exercising in the heat and to stay hydrated.
- Patients with a history of exertional headache should avoid the type of physical exertion that triggers the pain.
- A sudden, severe headache with exercise should lead to evaluation in an emergency room.

PROGNOSIS
- PEH and weightlifter's headache tend to recur with exercise.
- In a study that followed 93 patients, 32% of patients with PEH sustained complete remission within 5 years, and 78% underwent complete remission or significant improvement in 10 years (3).
- Primary cough headache is generally self-limited, with 50–90% of patients in remission within 2 years (3).

REFERENCES

1. Halker RB, Vargas BB. Primary exertional headache: updates in the literature. *Curr Pain Headache Rep.* 2013;17(6):337.
2. Cutrer FM, DeLange J. Cough, exercise, and sex headaches. *Neurol Clin.* 2014;32(2):433–450.
3. Evans RW. Sports and headaches. *Headache.* 2018;58(3):426–437.
4. Allena M, Rossi P, Tassorelli C, et al. Focus on therapy of the chapter IV headaches provoked by exertional factors: primary cough headache, primary exertional headache and primary headache associated with sexual activity. *J Headache Pain.* 2010;11(6):525–530.
5. Smith JH. Other primary headache disorders. *Continuum (Minneap Minn).* 2021;27(3):652–664.
6. Headache Classification Committee of the International Headache Society (IHS) *The International Classification of Headache Disorders, 3rd edition. Cephalalgia.* 2018;38(1):1–211.

ADDITIONAL READING

Sandoe CH, Kingston W. Exercise headache: a review. *Curr Neurol Neurosci Rep.* 2018;18(6):28.

CLINICAL PEARLS
- PEH occurs during or soon after intense physical activity and can be prevented by avoiding intense exertion. It is typically characterized as bilateral, throbbing, and pulsatile. It lasts 5 minutes to 48 hours, and the average age of onset is 24 years.
- Weightlifter's headache is quick in onset, "stabbing," lasts seconds to minutes, and is associated with the Valsalva maneuver. It more commonly affects older individuals.
- Neuroimaging is generally recommended after the initial presentation of either condition or if there are any signs or symptoms suggestive of intracranial pathology.
- Evidence behind diagnosis and management of exertional headaches is limited.

EXTENSOR CARPI ULNARIS PATHOLOGIES

Joseph Chin, MD, CAQSM • Laura Murphy, DO, CAQSM

BASICS

DESCRIPTION

- This chapter focuses on extensor carpi ulnaris (ECU) overuse pathologies, for which there are two major types: (i) tendinopathy and (ii) tendon subluxation.
- The ECU tendon originates from the lateral epicondyle, comprises the 6th dorsal extensor compartment within the distal ulnar groove, and inserts onto the base of the 5th metacarpal (1).
- The ECU is responsible for ulnar deviation in forearm pronation and wrist extension in forearm supination.
- The ECU tendon is a dynamic stabilizer of the distal radioulnar joint (DRUJ).
- The ECU subsheath is a static stabilizer of the DRUJ, as it is a part of the triangular fibrocartilage complex (TFCC) (2).

EPIDEMIOLOGY

- Precise incidence and prevalence of overuse ECU pathology has not been adequately reported.
- ECU tendinopathy is often associated with racquet sports as well as baseball, rugby, and golf (1).
- ECU pathology has been reported as the most common type of wrist injury in elite golfers and elite tennis players.

ETIOLOGY AND PATHOPHYSIOLOGY

- Repetitive (i) forearm rotational forces with twisting motions or (ii) axial loading of forearm and wrist can chronically stress the tendon and/or subsheath resulting in tendinopathy and instability, respectively.
- Instability is due to chronic tearing of the subsheath resulting in subluxation out of the ulnar groove during supination.
- In athletes, mechanism is often combination of hypersupination and wrist flexion with or without ulnar deviation (2)[C].
- In nonathletes, mechanism is often with repetitive ulnar deviation and wrist extension.
- Chronic DRUJ instability from rheumatoid arthritis has been associated with ECU subluxation or dislocation.

RISK FACTORS

- History of traumatic wrist injury
- Participation in racquet sports, particularly at elite level
- Older age
- Rheumatoid arthritis

COMMONLY ASSOCIATED CONDITIONS

- TFCC injury
- DRUJ instability
- Lunotriquetral injury
- Rheumatoid arthritis

DIAGNOSIS

HISTORY

- Patients report insidious onset dorsal/ulnar-sided wrist pain with repetitive overuse.
- Pain worsens with forearm supination and wrist flexion.
- Patients with instability may mention "popping" with active extension and ulnar deviation.
- Painful snapping or clicking with supination may also be reported in subluxation.

PHYSICAL EXAM

- Swelling and warmth may be present in active tenosynovitis.
- Pain with passive stretching in radial deviation and wrist flexion may be indicative of pathology.
- Palpation may cause tenderness along ECU tendon to the base of the 5th metacarpal.
- Tenderness may be elicited between ulnar styloid and 5th metacarpal base with forearm in pronation and ulnar deviation.
- Assess for pain and weakness in wrist extension and ulnar deviation.
- Ice cream scoop test: wrist extension/pronation/ulnar deviation into supination while maintaining ulnar deviation to test for ECU subluxation or instability (2)

DIFFERENTIAL DIAGNOSIS

- TFCC injury
- DRUJ instability
- Ulnar abutment syndrome

DIAGNOSTIC TESTS & INTERPRETATION

ECU injury in isolation or in conjunction with TFCC

Initial Tests (lab, imaging)

- X-rays
- Diagnostic ultrasound (US): short and long axis of ECU to its insertion on the 5th metacarpal; evaluate for tendinosis, partial-thickness tear, full-thickness tear; light pressure to avoid displacement of intrasheath fluid (3)[B],(4)[B]
  - Dynamic evaluation for subluxation: elbow 90 degrees, transducer in short axis at ulnar groove, passively supinate forearm and allow wrist to drop into flexion and ulnar deviation; normal 0–49% displacement, subluxation 50–99%, dislocation >99%
  - Deviation in supination > neutral > pronation
  - Deviation greater in flexion and ulnar deviation than extension and radial deviation

Follow-Up Tests & Special Considerations

Magnetic resonance imaging (MRI) can assess the tendon, subsheath, and TFCC which is more difficult to differentiate on US (1)[C].

Test Interpretation

- Displacement <50%
- Subluxation 50–99%
- Dislocation >99%

TREATMENT

GENERAL MEASURES

- Acute phase:
  - Rest
  - Immobilization in short arm cast or wrist orthosis in 30 degrees of wrist extension and slight ulnar deviation for 3 weeks for acute tendinosis (2)
  - Oral or topical nonsteroidal anti-inflammatory drugs (NSAIDs)
  - Ice
- Recovery phase:
  - Regain range of motion (ROM)
  - Rehabilitation with isometrics until pain free (usually 5 to 10 days) in acute tendinopathy; progressive loading and grip strengthening exercises (2)
  - For chronic tendinopathy, use load management, eccentrics, isometrics, and strengthening exercise.
  - ECU strengthening in wrist extension and ulnar deviation
  - Medicine ball throws
  - 6 weeks of therapy generally
  - Return to sports: interval sports program for baseball, tennis, golf
- Asymptomatic subluxation does not necessarily require treatment.

MEDICATION

Oral or topical NSAIDs

ADDITIONAL THERAPIES

- CSI to 6th dorsal compartment for pain: US can ensure placement into fibroosseous sheath rather than the tendon to avoid intratendinous rupture (2).
- Platelet-rich plasma (PRP) injection US is also recommended.

SURGERY/OTHER PROCEDURES

- ECU co-compartment release for recalcitrant tenosynovitis: division of septum between 5th and 6th extensor compartment to increase the compartmental volume without removing stability (1)
- ECU tendon and subsheath repair for surgical reconstruction of the 6th extensor compartment (3)
- TFCC repair

COMPLEMENTARY & ALTERNATIVE MEDICINE

- Acupuncture
- Therapeutic US for soft tissue inflammation for 6 to 7 minutes
- Iontophoresis: dexamethasone for anti-inflammatory effect
- Dry needling to stimulate tendon, fascia, and muscle
- Cupping: traction, improve circulation, and healing response (2)

REFERENCES

1. Campbell D, Campbell R, O'Connor P, et al. Sports-related extensor carpi ulnaris pathology: a review of functional anatomy, sports injury and management. *Br J Sports Med.* 2013;47(17):1105–1111.
2. Zarro M, Goel R, Bickhart N, et al. Extensor carpi ulnaris tendinopathy in athletes: a review of conservative and rehabilitative options. *Hand (N Y).* 2024;19(3):407–413.
3. Lee KS, Ablove RH, Singh S, et al. Ultrasound imaging of normal displacement of the extensor carpi ulnaris tendon within the ulnar groove in 12 forearm-wrist positions. *AJR Am J Roentgenol.* 2009;193(3):651–655.
4. Sole JS, Wisniewski SJ, Newcomer KL, et al. Sonographic evaluation of the extensor carpi ulnaris in asymptomatic tennis players. *PM R* 2015;7(3):255–263.

ADDITIONAL READING

- Beutel BG, Konstanty J, Beeker RW, et al. Carpal ligament instability. StatPearls Publishing; 2025. https://www.ncbi.nlm.nih.gov/books/NBK557729/
- Bianchi S, Martinoli C. *Ultrasound of the Musculoskeletal System.* Jaypee Brothers; 2007.
- Graham TJ. Pathologies of the extensor carpi ulnaris (ECU) tendon and its investments in the athlete. *Hand Clin.* 2012;28(3):345–356.
- Kollitz KM, Iorio ML, Huang JI. Assessment and treatment of extensor carpi ulnaris tendon pathology: a critical analysis review. *JBJS Rev.* 2015;3(6):e3.
- Lee YK. Treatment of subacute/chronic ECU tendinopathy using wrist arthroscopy and open surgical repair. *J Orthop Surg (Hong Kong).* 2022;30(1):23094990211067009.
- Romero-Morales C, López-López D, Almazán-Polo J, et al. Prevalence, diagnosis and management of musculoskeletal disorders in elite athletes: a mini-review. *Dis Mon.* 2024;70(1):101629.
- Wu WT, Chang KV, Mezian K, et al. Ulnar wrist pain revisited: ultrasound diagnosis and guided injection for triangular fibrocartilage complex injuries. *J Clin Med.* 2019;8(10):1540.
- Yuine H, Yoshii Y, Iwai K. Assessment of distal radioulnar joint stability in health subjects: changes with dominant hand, sex, and age. *J Orthop Res.* 2021;39(9):2028–2035.

CLINICAL PEARLS

- The primary mechanism of action for the ECU is wrist extension and ulnar deviation.
- Repetitive forearm rotation and wrist twisting increases risk of tendinopathy and, less often, injury of subsheath resulting in subluxation.
- Conservative management with immobilization and rehab is often successful.
- Corticosteroid to the sheath may help with active tenosynovitis where conservative therapy with eccentric exercise has failed; US can avoid tendon injection.
- Surgical compartmental release may be used in refractory tenosynovitis.
- Surgical subsheath repair may be used in chronic, symptomatic subluxers.

EXTERNAL EAR CHONDRITIS/ABSCESS

Arturo J. Aguilar, MD, FAAFP, CAQSM

BASICS

DESCRIPTION

- Inflammation and infection of the pinna (1)
- Commonly a complication of otic trauma (1), burns, or neighboring infection
- It may present as a complication of draining periauricular hematoma (cauliflower ear) in sports such as wrestling and rugby (2)
- Occasionally, chondritis may be a complication of untreated or resistant otitis externa in swimmers (2).
- Cartilage of the external ear is easily damaged and at risk for infection owing to:
  - Lack of overlying subcutaneous tissue
  - Relative avascularity
  - Exposed position

EPIDEMIOLOGY

Incidence is 0.68% among ear, nose, and throat (ENT) causality (3)

- 52% male versus 48% female
- 57% adult versus 43% children
- Mean age 22 years with standard deviation of 16

ETIOLOGY AND PATHOPHYSIOLOGY

- Common causes of chondritis include (1),(2),(3):
  - Chemical or thermal burns
  - Otitis externa
  - Deep abrasions
  - Frostbite
  - High piercing of the earlobe
  - Human bites
  - Iatrogenic from incision and drainage treatment of hematoma
  - Mastoid surgery
- Bacteria involved (3),(4):
  - *Pseudomonas aeruginosa*
  - *Staphylococcus* spp
  - *Streptococcus pyogenes*

RISK FACTORS

- Autoimmune conditions (3)
- Diabetes (3)
- Smokers (3)

DIAGNOSIS

Typical physical findings in combination with preceding causes

PHYSICAL EXAM

- Initially a dull pain that increases in severity
- Pinna (2):
  - Painful
  - Exquisite tenderness
  - Erythematous
  - Warmth
  - Loss of contours caused by edema often with sparing of the lobule
- Increase in the auriculocephalic angle
- Fluctuant areas develop with eventual breakdown and suppuration.
- Entire ear involvement if untreated: Disfigurement can occur (2).
- Tympanic membrane has a normal appearance in the absence of concurrent acute otitis media
- Auditory canal has normal appearance in the absence of concurrent acute otitis externa.
- Fever/chills

DIFFERENTIAL DIAGNOSIS

- Periauricular hematoma: "cauliflower ear" (3),(4)
- Malignant otitis externa (3),(4)
- Keloid (hypertrophic scar) (3),(4)
- Contact dermatitis (3),(4)

DIAGNOSTIC TESTS & INTERPRETATION

- Complete blood count (CBC) with differential for systemic symptoms (2)
- Wound culture for signs of localized infection (2)
- Blood culture if systemic signs of infection (2)

TREATMENT

GENERAL MEASURES

- General postinjury preventive measures:
  - Prevention of chondritis is of the utmost importance (5)[C]:
    - Avoid pressure to the injured ear (unlike the compression treatments used for auricular hematoma).
    - Minimize active débridement of eschars and crusts.
    - Empiric treatment of pinna lacerations with prophylactic antibiotics (6)[B]
  - Gentle washing daily with antibacterial soap and water followed by complete drying and application of topical antibiotics (2)[C]

- Complications: disfiguration of the pinna (3):
  - Occurs without proper treatment
  - Ranges from cauliflower-like ear to complete loss of the external ear and possible stenosis of the auditory meatus
  - Systemic infection
- ENT consult (6)[C]:
  - For treatment of chondritis, abscess, and necrosis of the involved cartilage
  - Early surgical drainage
  - Aggressive early management may prevent gross ear deformity.

MEDICATION

- Oral antibiotics for minor cases:
  - Ciprofloxacin preferred (>18 years old) for pseudomonas coverage (1),(6)[A]
  - 1st generation cephalosporin or clindamycin for staph and strep coverage (1)[B],(4)[C]
  - Intravenous (IV) antibiotics for severe infection (1)[B]
- Medications:
  - Ciprofloxacin: 500 mg PO BID or 750 mg BID (adult)
  - Cephalexin: 500 mg (children: 50 mg/kg/d) PO QID
  - Clindamycin: 150 to 450 mg PO QID (children: 10 to 20 mg/kg/d PO divided TID–QID)

ADMISSION, INPATIENT, AND NURSING CONSIDERATIONS

Admission criteria:

- Parenteral antibiotics and early surgical drainage for patients with complicated chondritis
- Toxic patient with fever and chills
- Immunocompromised patient
- Unreliable patient or caretaker

REFERENCES

1. Fisher C, Kacica M, Bennett N. Risk factors for cartilage infections of the ear. *Am J Prev Med.* 2005;29(3):204–209.
2. Thill M, Horoi M, Ostermann K, et al. Acute external ear lesions: clinical aspects, assessment, and management. *B-ENT.* 2016;(Suppl 26)(1):155–171.
3. Delwar AHM. Perichondritis of the pinna: a real compulsion of hospital linger. *Glob J Med Res.* 2020;(J5):1–10.
4. Kim MM, Goldman RD. Ear-piercing complications in children and adolescents. *Can Fam Physician.* 2022;68(9):661–663.
5. Liu ZW, Chokkalingam P. Piercing associated perichondritis of the pinna: are we treating it correctly? *J. Laryngol Otol.* 2013;127(5):505–508.
6. Namasivaya Navin RB, Prabakaran S, Rajasekaran S, et al. A harrowing experience of pinna lacerations. *J Clin Diagn Res.* 2022;16(8).

CLINICAL PEARLS

- Monitor for signs of external ear chondritis/abscess after draining a periauricular hematoma.
- Symptoms include painful erythematous, warm pinna.
- Most implicated bacteria are *Pseudomonas*, *Staphylococcus*, and *Streptococcus*.
- The preferred antibiotic in adults is ciprofloxacin.
- Preferred antibiotic in children are cephalosporins like cephalexin.

EXTERNAL GENITAL TRAUMA

John C. Walton, MD, MSL • Holly J. Benjamin, MD, FAMSSM, FACSM

BASICS

External genital trauma is an infrequent sports-related injury involving a direct impact to the exposed genitalia. The two most common causes of external genital trauma are straddle injuries, such as those from a bicycle seat, or direct blunt trauma, like a kick to the groin or a ball strike. Because males and females (assigned at birth) have different genital anatomy, when applicable, each section will address males and females separately. Nearly three quarters of genital injuries occur in the pediatric population. Consider nonaccidental trauma or sexual abuse.

- Injuries to female genitalia:
  - Lacerations, hematomas, avulsions
  - Vaginal impalement injuries
  - Vaginal insufflation injuries
  - Urethral injury
  - Anus or rectum injury
  - Genital trauma from sexual or physical abuse
  - Intra-abdominal female organs such as uterus and ovaries are well protected and are unlikely to suffer an injury due to nonpenetrating blunt trauma.
- Injuries to male genitalia:
  - Lacerations, abrasions, hematomas, avulsions of penis/scrotum
  - Penile fracture amputation or penetrating injury
  - Urethral injury
  - Testicular hematoma or rupture
  - Testicular torsion or appendix testis torsion
  - Traumatic hydrocoele or hematocele
  - Anus or rectum injury
  - Genital trauma from sexual or physical abuse (more common in females than males)

DESCRIPTION

- Females:
  - Injuries to the urethra are rare due to the short, unexposed, and mobile urethra. Most occur at the bladder neck.
  - Risk of associated injuries to neighboring organs after blunt trauma is higher than males.
  - Most traumatic injuries are secondary to accidental falls onto objects resulting in impalement or blunt trauma:
    - Blunt trauma:
      - Vulvar lacerations, ecchymosis, hematoma
      - May be associated with voiding problems
      - Can result in crush injury or pelvic fractures
    - Impalement:
      - Physical findings can mimic penetration by blunt forceful trauma; so if suspicious, must consider sexual assault or abuse.
      - Vagina, urethra, bladder, anus, rectum, and peritoneal cavity can be pierced by a sharp object.
  - Insufflation with high-pressure water (e.g., falls off jet skis or water skis) can result in vaginal tears.
- Males:
  - Blunt trauma:
    - Penile/soft tissue:
      - Penile fracture results from rupture of the tunica albuginea.
      - Urethral injuries are more common in the bulbar or penile urethra than the prostatic urethra.
      - ~95% of posterior urethral injuries are caused by pelvic fractures.
      - Anterior urethral injuries are commonly caused by blunt trauma.
      - As many as 25% of pelvic fractures have concomitant urethral injuries (pelvic fracture urethral injury [PFUI]).
      - Laceration, ecchymosis, hematoma, avulsion injuries
    - Scrotal trauma:
      - Most testicular injuries (up to 85%) are from blunt trauma, with the majority occurring during athletic participation.
      - Scrotal ecchymosis, hematoma
      - Hematoceles (blood accumulation in space between tunica albuginea and tunica vaginalis)
      - Testicular rupture: disruption of the tunica albuginea
      - Traumatically induced hydroceles
      - Traumatically induced testicular torsion
      - Not all testicular torsions are caused by trauma but can happen spontaneously; have a high index of suspicion for any acute onset of testicular or groin pain
      - Pelvic fracture with significant blunt trauma
  - Penetrating injury: can cause significant injury to soft tissues and scrotum

GENERAL PREVENTION

- Females:
  - Wearing equipment such as groin protectors especially in ball and contact sports
- Males:
  - Wearing protective equipment such as cups, jock straps, other gear, especially in ball and contact sports
  - Compression shorts can help with extra genital support but are not very effective against blunt trauma injuries.

DIAGNOSIS

HISTORY

- Mechanism of injury
- Prior history of trauma or injury
- Pelvic pain, bleeding, inability to void
- Posttraumatic blood at the urethral meatus or acute hematuria
- Genital pain, swelling, any sign of injury
- Inguinal pain, or lower abdominal pain
- Posttraumatic vaginal pain, bleeding
- Posttraumatic rectal bleeding
- History of possible sexual abuse or assault
- It is important to note that lower abdominal pain or inguinal pain in the absence of genital pain can still be due to a genital injury; therefore, anyone presenting with acute, posttraumatic lower abdominal pain should have a chaperoned, external genital examination performed.

PHYSICAL EXAM

- A genital exam is a sensitive exam for anyone, especially after trauma to the area. It is important to have a chaperone present when performing exams whenever possible to protect the individual patient and the examining health care provider.
- **Females:**
  - External genitourinary (GU) examination to determine extent of injury
  - If injury is minor superficial laceration or hematoma and no history of penetrating injury, external exam may be sufficient.
  - Vaginal lacerations with active bleeding should be packed or repaired by a provider with experience to avoid urethra, bladder, and rectal injury and may require an internal (speculum examination).
  - Vaginal smear to check for spermatozoa and urine and blood analysis may be indicated in certain situations (1),(2).
  - **Indications for exam under anesthesia:**
    - Young or uncooperative patient
    - Transection of the hymen with inability to see the full extent of injury
    - Vaginal hemorrhage
    - Expanding vulvar or vaginal hematoma
    - History of significant blunt, forceful, or penetrating trauma
    - Significant vaginal laceration or soft tissue injury
    - Complex vaginal and perineal lacerations, especially if associated with pelvic fracture or rectal injury
    - Perforation into the peritoneal cavity requires emergent exploratory laparotomy/laparoscopy.
- **Males:**
  - GU examination to determine extent of injury
  - Examine for high-riding prostate, perineal or penile swelling, blood at meatus.
  - Examine testicles for pain or swelling suggestive of rupture, hematocele, and/or torsion.
  - Examine for incarcerated hernia.
  - Examine abdomen to palpate bladder and for other abdominal/intra-abdominal injuries.
  - Evaluate for rectal injuries.

Pediatric Considerations

- If an examination of the genitalia cannot be performed easily, examination under anesthesia should occur.
- An examination in the operating room (OR), in addition to being better tolerated by the patient, can help the physician to determine the true extent of blunt or penetrating genital injuries.

DIFFERENTIAL DIAGNOSIS

- Perineum
- Vagina
- Urethra
- Penis

- Testicle
- Inguinal canal
- Epididymis
- Bladder trauma
- Pelvic fracture
- Physical abuse/assault
- Sexual abuse/assault
- Combination of multiple injuries

DIAGNOSTIC TESTS & INTERPRETATION

- Urinalysis
- Complete blood count
- Blood urea nitrogen (BUN) and creatine (Cr)
- Consider screening for sexually transmitted infections if history or exam is consistent with sexual abuse.
- Scrotal imaging: scrotal ultrasound (SUS):
- Performing an SUS in the setting of suspected external genital trauma is an acute emergency requiring transfer to a center capable of performing imaging or emergency surgical procedures within 30 to 60 minutes of injury.
  - Scrotum exam can be difficult with significant swelling.
  - SUS should be performed because it is sensitive and specific for scrotal injury (1),(2),(3).
  - SUS assesses the integrity and vascularity of the testes.
  - SUS may distinguish testis rupture from hematocele, hydrocele, torsion, and epididymitis (3).
- Urethral injury: retrograde urethrography (RUG):
  - Inability to void, blood at meatus, and any degree of hematuria are absolute indications for RUG (1)[C].
  - Recommended with any penetrating genital injuries (1)[C]
  - Water-soluble contrast material is injected at the urethral meatus.
  - Extravasation of contrast material and location of extravasation can diagnose presence of tear as well as degree of tear.
- Although renal injury is not considered an external genital trauma injury, it is part of the differential diagnosis for acute traumatic hematuria.
- Renal injuries are best visualized by computerized cystography: 40% of urethral injuries have concomitant bladder injuries.
- Proctoscopy: useful when there is a possibility of impalement injury or pelvic fracture (4)

TREATMENT

- Prehospital:
  - Similar considerations as for major trauma victims
- ED treatment:
  - Initial stabilization, control of bleeding, pain control
  - After appropriate evaluation and workup, urologic or gynecologic consult if warranted
  - Urethral contusions, lacerations, and avulsions are best managed by an experienced urologist.
  - Scrotal hematomas, hydroceles, and contusions can be managed with rest, ice, and elevation.
  - Tetanus immunization if warranted for laceration or avulsion

ALERT
It is important after significant blunt trauma without testicular rupture or torsion to have scrotal support with jock strap or support shorts 24/7 for 1 to 2 weeks to assist with pain and swelling.

  - Any suspected acute testicular torsion or penile fracture is a true urologic emergency and must be treated as such with transport to the nearest emergency room or facility with urologic services.
  - In the case of acute testicular torsion and no immediate access to emergency services, a manual detorsion procedure can be attempted.

MEDICATION

Anytime, there is injury to the female mucosal genital surfaces; application of topical estrogen cream may benefit the healing process and decrease scarring (5)[C].

SURGERY/OTHER PROCEDURES

- Females:
  - Simple perineal and vulvar lacerations usually can be repaired in the ED (5).
  - Large hematoma should be incised and drained (4).
  - See "Physical Exam" for indications for exam under anesthesia.
  - Exam under anesthesia, if peritoneal or rectal cavities are determined to be injured, then an exploratory laparotomy is indicated (3).
- Males:
  - Prompt surgical intervention with closure of the tunica albuginea for penile fractures to prevent erectile dysfunction and penile curvature (1)[C], (5)[C]
  - When physical exam findings and mechanism of injury suggest significant testicular injury, operative exploration should be undertaken even with equivocal imaging (2)[C],(3)[C].
  - Prompt drainage of large hematoceles is recommended to prevent secondary infection or pressure atrophy (2)[C].
  - Posttraumatic testicular torsion and testicular dislocation are a urologic surgical emergency.
  - Penetrating trauma to the scrotum or penis warrants prompt surgical exploration (1)[C].
  - Complex avulsions are best managed with initial débridement and delayed reconstruction (3)[C], (5)[C].
  - Minor avulsions are managed as simple lacerations with irrigation and primary closure (3)[C].
  - Complete/obliterated urethral injuries are rare and require urinary diversion, often in the form of suprapubic tube placement for temporary diversion. Urethroplasty for definitive management can be considered in an immediate or delayed fashion, depending on the mechanism of injury (3).

ADMISSION, INPATIENT, AND NURSING CONSIDERATIONS

- Initial stabilization:
  - Airway, breathing, and circulation (ABCs) of trauma care take precedence.
- Admission criteria:
  - Concurrent closed head injury, blunt abdominal trauma, or pelvic fracture
  - Need for operative management of urethral, penile, vaginal, pelvic, or bladder injuries

ONGOING CARE

COMPLICATIONS

- Impotence
- Incontinence
- Strictures
- Infection
- Disfigurement
- Pain
- Scarring
- Infertility
- Erectile dysfunction

REFERENCES

1. Kitrey ND, Campos-Juanatey F, Hallscheidt P, et al. Urological trauma. Accessed August 12, 2025. https://uroweb.org/guideline/urological-trauma/
2. Serafetinidis E, Campos-Janatey F, Hallscheidt P, et al. Summary paper of the updated 2023 European Association of Urology guidelines on urological trauma. *Eur Urol Focus*. 2024;10(3):475–485.
3. Morey AF, Broghammer JA, Hollowell CMP, et al. Urotrauma guideline 2020: AUA guideline. *J Urol*. 2021;205(1):30–35.
4. Bryk DJ, Zhao LC. Guideline of guidelines: a review of urological trauma guidelines. *BJU Int*. 2016;117(2):226–234.
5. Morey AF, Brandes S, Dugi DD III, et al. Urotrauma: AUA guideline. *J Urol*. 2014;192(2):327–335.

ADDITIONAL READING

- Bagga HS, Fisher PB, Tasian GE, et al. Sports-related genitourinary injuries presenting to United States emergency departments. *Urology*. 2015;85(1):239–244.
- Lee SH, Bak CW, Choi MH, et al. Trauma to male genital organs: a 10-year review of 156 patients, including 118 treated by surgery. *BJU Int*. 2008;101(2):211–215.
- McGeady JB, Breyer BN. Current epidemiology of genitourinary trauma. *Urol Clin North Am*. 2013;40(3):323–334.
- Merritt DF. Genital trauma in children and adolescents. *Clin Obstet Gynecol*. 2008;51(2):237–248.

CLINICAL PEARLS

- Must rule out a urethral injury if there is blood at the meatus, inability to void, or hemorrhage.
- Increased risk of injury to neighboring organs in females
- Consider nonaccidental trauma or sexual abuse in pediatrics.
- In the setting of significant testicular or scrotal trauma, surgical referral is necessary even if imaging is inconclusive.

FEMORO-ACETABULAR IMPINGEMENT (FAI)

Uziel Sauceda, MD, CAQSM

BASICS

DESCRIPTION

- Femoro-acetabular impingement (FAI) is a condition resulting from a pathologic malformation of the hip.
- The acetabular rim and the proximal femur have excess contact during the end range of motion (ROM) of the hip.
- Leads to pain and restricted hip motion and can lead to chondral or labral injury
- Synonym: hip impingement

EPIDEMIOLOGY

Incidence

- Unknown in general population; estimated range from 10–15% incidence in adult population
- Cam-type deformity is more common in young active men.
- Pincer lesions are more common in middle-aged women.

Prevalence

- Young patients with hip pain have high prevalence, up to 85% (1).
- Patients may be asymptomatic with radiologic findings: 37% cam, 67% pincer deformity (2).

ETIOLOGY AND PATHOPHYSIOLOGY

Types of FAI:

- Cam type: malformation of the femoral head resulting in neck widening and asphericity
- Pincer type: malformation of the acetabulum that results in over-coverage of the anterosuperior acetabular wall and abnormal retroversion of the acetabulum
- Mixed type: most common type, combination of cam and pincer lesions
- Theory that repetitive injury to proximal femoral physis during adolescence contributes to development of cam deformity.

Genetics

No conclusive evidence FAI is transmitted genetically.

RISK FACTORS

- Idiopathic
- Trauma—malunion of femoral neck fracture, post-traumatic retroversion of the femoral head
- Childhood orthopedic conditions—Legg-Calvé-Perthes disease, slipped capital femoral epiphysis (SCFE), hip dysplasia
- Iatrogenic—femoral osteotomy, overcorrection of retroversion in dysplastic hips
- High-impact sports/activities during bone development (i.e., soccer, basketball, and ice hockey)

GENERAL PREVENTION

Unknown if avoiding high-impact sports during childhood can prevent FAI

DIAGNOSIS

HISTORY

- Anterior or anterolateral hip pain that refers to the groin, associated with activity
- Inability to perform activities such as high hip flexion or internal rotation, including prolonged sitting or squatting
- Painful clicking, locking, or instability from a labral tear secondary to undiagnosed FAI
- Past history of developmental dysplasia, trauma, or predisposing factors of avascular necrosis
- Insidious onset of symptoms in active young and middle-aged adults
- History limited with children, keep FAI in differential with knee or thigh pain, limp after activity
- Adults may describe a stiffness in the hip.

PHYSICAL EXAM

- Reduced ROM: flexion, adduction, and internal rotation (FADDIR)
- FADDIR—positive test if pain elicited with adduction of a flexed, internally rotated hip with the patient supine
- Posterior inferior impingement test—positive test if pain elicited with the hip in hyperextension, passively by hanging the leg over the end of the bed; the affected hip is passively and externally rotated.
- Stinchfield test—resisted straight leg flexion while patient supine; positive if pain elicited on affected hip at groin area
- Flexion, abduction, and external rotation (FABER) test may also produce pain in the affected hip.

DIFFERENTIAL DIAGNOSIS

- Hip dysplasia
- Leg-Calvé-Perthes disease/avascular necrosis femoral head
- SCFE
- Hip subluxation—microinstability
- Labral tear not associated with impingement
- Osteoarthritis
- Muscular pathology of iliopsoas/snapping hip syndrome
- Spinal deformities—scoliosis or kyphosis
- Bone stress injuries
- Prior femoral neck fractures or pelvic osteotomy may also cause impingement.

DIAGNOSTIC TESTS & INTERPRETATION

Initial Tests (lab, imaging)

Laboratory tests only helpful if suspect systemic process (infection, autoimmune):

- *Complete blood count (CBC), chemistries, and liver function tests*
- *Plain radiographs:*
  - Anteroposterior (AP) pelvis view: used to assess cam-type deformity, degenerative changes, and a profunda socket
  - Dunn view: AP of hip in neutral rotation, 45 degrees of flexion, and 20 degrees of abduction
  - Cross-table projection in 15 degrees internal rotation
  - Both Dunn and cross-table projection views assess femoral head neck asphericity.
  - Cross-table view is more practical for routine use as Dunn view requires an assistant to hold the patient's leg.
  - Radiography inadequate to assess for chondral or labral defects
- *Alpha angle usually calculated and helpful to determine amount of cam deformity:*
  - Abnormal if >55 degrees
- *Crossover sign and lateral center edge angle are most commonly used to determine amount of pincer deformity:*
  - Abnormal lateral center edge angle >40 degrees

Follow-Up Tests & Special Considerations

- *Magnetic resonance arthrography (MRA):*
  - Preferred for evaluating labral or chondral pathology
  - May show articular cartilage thinning
- *Position of discomfort (POD) computed tomography (CT) scans:*
  - CT 3D surface reconstruction allows for better mapping of bony pathology, best demonstrating a bony impingement lesion, and helping subsequent planning for surgical resection.

Diagnostic Procedures/Other

- Important to confirm pain origin with a diagnostic hip joint injection
- Can be done under ultrasound guidance in office or with fluoroscopy guidance by interventional radiology

Test Interpretation

If no pain relief from injection, may need to look for alternate etiology of pain

TREATMENT

GENERAL MEASURES

Nonoperative management (3)[C]:

- Modification of activities by avoiding excessive hip end ROM, usually flexion
- Limiting activities and sports are difficult for athletic young individuals.
- Physical therapy with an individualized plan can help with movement pattern retraining, muscle flexibility, and muscle strengthening.
- Current clinical practice recommendations by the American Physical Therapy Association (APTA) suggest benefits for FAI.

MEDICATION

First Line

- Short course of nonsteroidal anti-inflammatory drugs (NSAIDs) can provide symptomatic relief (3)[C].
- Structural defects are not routinely treated with medications.

ISSUES FOR REFERRAL

Best to refer to orthopedic surgeon comfortable with hip arthroscopic or open surgery

SURGERY/OTHER PROCEDURES

- Surgery is the treatment of choice, with the following techniques: arthroscopic, open surgical dislocation (with a trochanteric flip osteotomy), and mini-open (combination of open and arthroscopic procedures) (3)[C],(4)[A],(5)[C],(6)[C].
- Diagnostic imaging was most common criterion in 92% of surgeries reviewed in recent literature, with alpha angle being most commonly reported measure.
- All focus on accessing the area of malformation and correcting the defect.
- Outcomes:
  - Hip arthroscopy was associated with better recovery of function, reduction in nonarthritic hip pain, and a lower reoperation rate.
  - Recent randomized controlled trials (RCTs) and a meta-analysis of these trials show improved validated symptom scores from arthroscopic surgery compared to physical therapy, although both approaches improve symptoms (4)[A].
  - Open surgical dislocation showed more improvement of alpha angle by the Dunn view in patients with cam osteoplasty compared with arthroscopy.

ONGOING CARE

FOLLOW-UP RECOMMENDATIONS

Postoperative care:

- Arthroscopy:
  - Keep patient toe-touch weight-bearing and ambulate with aids for 2 to 4 weeks.
  - After 4 weeks, low-impact active motion may be resumed.
  - Recovery expected at 4 to 6 months back to full activity
- Open surgical dislocation:
  - Restriction to toe-touch weight-bearing for 6 to 8 weeks
  - Prevent falls with walker or crutches
  - Physical therapy starts immediately, working on passive ROM for the first 2 weeks postoperatively.
  - Early ROM prevents adhesions.
- Mini-open:
  - Keeping patients with toe-touch weight-bearing and use of crutches for first 5 days.
  - After 5 days, patients may have full weight-bearing activities without crutches.
  - Patients are also allowed to begin low-impact active exercise, such as cycling.
  - Patients are kept from high-impact or contact sports for a total of 6 months postoperatively.

PATIENT EDUCATION

- Emphasize activity modification if patient is not seeking surgery.
- High-level athletes will likely proceed with surgical consultation.

PROGNOSIS

Common cause for revision surgery is inadequate bony correction of the FAI.

COMPLICATIONS

- Nonsurgical care:
  - Hip degenerative arthritis
  - Labral tears
  - Chondral defects/delamination
- Complications of surgery:
  - Trochanteric nonunion, heterotopic ossification, sciatic nerve palsy, osteonecrosis of the femoral head, femoral neck fracture, injury of the lateral cutaneous femoral nerve, neurapraxia of nerves around the hip joint
  - A meta-analysis by Zhang et al. demonstrated no statistical difference in complications between hip arthroscopy and open surgical dislocation (6).

Geriatric Considerations

Usually, hip pain in elderly is secondary to degenerative arthritis. Insufficiency fractures are possible as well.

Pediatric Considerations

Keep in mind femoral growth plates when evaluating hip pain in pediatric population as well as thinking about SCFE and Legg-Calvé-Perthes disease and bone stress injury.

Pregnancy Considerations

- Hip pain in pregnancy may be due to increased laxity.
- Keep in mind transient osteoporosis of hip in 3rd trimester as well as bone stress injuries.

REFERENCES

1. Ochoa LM, Dawson L, Patzkowski JC, et al. Radiographic prevalence of femoroacetabular impingement in a young population with hip complaints is high. *Clin Orthop Relat Res*. 2010;468(10):2710–2714.
2. Frank JM, Harris JD, Erickson BJ, et al. Prevalence of femoroacetabular impingement imaging findings in asymptomatic volunteers: a systematic review. *Arthroscopy*. 2015;31(6):1199–1204.
3. Griffin DR, Dickenson EJ, O'Donnell J, et al. The Warwick Agreement on femoroacetabular impingement syndrome (FAI syndrome): an international consensus statement. *Br J Sports Med*. 2016;50(19):1169–1176.
4. Gatz M, Driessen A, Eschweiler J, et al. Arthroscopic surgery versus physiotherapy for femoroacetabular impingement: a meta-analysis study. *Eur J Orthop Surg Traumatol*. 2020;30(7):1151–1162.
5. Peters S, Laing A, Emerson C, et al. Surgical criteria for femoroacetabular impingement syndrome: a scoping review. *Br J Sports Med*. 2017;51(22):1605–1610.
6. Zhang D, Chen L, Wang G. Hip arthroscopy versus open surgical dislocation for femoroacetabular impingement: a systematic review and meta-analysis. *Medicine (Baltimore)*. 2016;95(41):e5122.

ADDITIONAL READING

- Griffin DR, Dickenson EJ, Wall PDH, et al. Hip arthroscopy versus best conservative care for the treatment of femoroacetabular impingement syndrome (UK FASHIoN): a multicentre randomised controlled trial. *Lancet*. 2018;391(10136):2225–2235.
- Nepple JJ, Clohisy JC, ANCHOR Study Group Members. Evolution of femoroacetabular impingement treatment: the ANCHOR experience. *Am J Orthop (Belle Mead NJ)*. 2017;46(1):28–34.
- Packer JD, Safran MR. The etiology of primary femoroacetabular impingement: genetics or acquired deformity? *J Hip Preserv Surg*. 2015;2(3):249–257.
- Philippon MJ, Bolia I, Locks R, et al. Treatment of femoroacetabular impingement: labrum, cartilage, osseous deformity, and capsule. *Am J Orthop (Belle Mead NJ)*. 2017;46(1):23–27.
- Rhee C, Le Francois T, Byrd JWT, et al. Radiographic diagnosis of pincer-type femoroacetabular impingement: a systematic review. *Orthop J Sports Med*. 2017;5(5):2325967117708307.
- Wilson AS, Cui Q. Current concepts in management of femoroacetabular impingement. *World J Orthop*. 2012;3(12):204–211.

CLINICAL PEARLS

- Most common type of FAI is combined type.
- Pain at the groin in end ROM is important symptom.
- Surgery is treatment of choice; open surgery may be needed for difficult cases.

FLEXOR CARPI ULNARIS AND RADIALIS TENDONITIS

Surein Theivakumar, DO, CAQSM, RMSK • Elizabeth A. Callahan, DO

BASICS

DESCRIPTION

- Flexor carpi radialis (FCR) and flexor carpi ulnaris (FCU) tendons are located on the radial and ulnar aspects of the wrist, respectively.
- Tendonitis of these tendons may occur from trauma or repetitive use.

EPIDEMIOLOGY

FCU tendonitis is more common than FCR tendonitis.

ETIOLOGY AND PATHOPHYSIOLOGY

- Anatomy and function:
  - FCR inserts on the volar aspects of the trapezium and 2nd and 3rd metacarpal bases:
    - It is difficult to palpate the insertion point owing to overlying thenar muscles.
    - It palmar flexes and radially deviates the wrist.
  - FCU has two heads: The ulnar head originates from the olecranon and posterior border of the ulna, whereas the humeral head originates from the medial epicondyle. Both heads insert at the base of the pisiform, hook of hamate, and base of 5th metacarpal.
    - The pisiform is a sesamoid embedded in the FCU tendon.
    - It palmar flexes and ulnarly deviates the wrist.
- Pathology:
  - With trauma or repetitive use, the tendon can become inflamed.
  - It is important to note that FCR has a tendon sheath, whereas FCU does not. *Tenosynovitis* is the term that describes inflammation of the tendon sheath itself.
  - Long-term repetitive trauma and overuse can cause the tendon architecture to become disrupted and degenerate, a condition called *tendinosis*.
  - *Tendinopathy* is an umbrella term that describes the continuum of tendon injury from tendinitis to tendinosis.
- Etiology of tendonitis:
  - Direct injury can trigger tendonitis.
  - A single macrotraumatic event or repeated microtraumatic events
  - Improper technique

RISK FACTORS

- Diabetes mellitus
- Sports with grip: tennis, racquetball, golf, baseball, cycling, weightlifting, and manual labor
- Frequent typing or computer mouse use

DIAGNOSIS

HISTORY

- Pain and possible swelling on volar aspect of wrist
- Increase in pain with activity and gripping
- Limited motion
- Possible crepitus at the site with movement or palpation
- Acute injury or repeated trauma to the area
- Overuse:
  - Repetitive and forceful activity
  - Sudden increase in activity
  - Change in technique or equipment
- FCR tendonitis: pain with wrist flexion and radial deviation
- FCU tendonitis: pain with wrist flexion and ulnar deviation

PHYSICAL EXAM

- Possible swelling at the volar aspect of wrist
- Tenderness near insertion points:
  - FCR tendonitis:
    - Locate the FCR tendon to the ulnar side of the scaphoid tubercle.
    - Follow the course of tendon about 3 fingerbreadths distally to find the approximate insertion point.
  - FCU tendonitis: tenderness at the pisiform or just distal at the 4th and 5th metacarpal bases
- Provocative tests:
  - FCR tendonitis: resisted wrist flexion with radial deviation. Positive test is elicited pain.
  - FCU tendonitis: resisted wrist flexion with ulnar deviation. Positive test is elicited pain.

DIFFERENTIAL DIAGNOSIS

- Radial aspect of wrist:
  - Fracture of scaphoid, trapezium, or 1st or 2nd metacarpal bases
  - de Quervain tenosynovitis
  - Osteoarthritis at 1st carpometacarpal joint or other joints of the carpus
  - Strain or tendonitis of thenar muscles
  - Ganglion: usually located to the radial side of the FCR tendon
  - Carpal tunnel syndrome
- Ulnar aspect of wrist:
  - Fracture of pisiform, ulnar styloid, hamate hook, or other carpal bone
  - Triangular fibrocartilage complex tear
  - Osteoarthritis of the pisotriquetral joint or other nearby joints
  - Strain or tendonitis of hypothenar muscles
  - Hypothenar hammer syndrome
  - Ulnar nerve entrapment in Guyon canal
- Miscellaneous:
  - FCR/FCU tendinosis
  - FCR/FCU tendon rupture
  - Tenosynovitis from rheumatologic disorder
  - FCR brevis anomaly

DIAGNOSTIC TESTS & INTERPRETATION

Initial Tests (lab, imaging)

- Radiographs:
  - Used to rule out fracture or bony abnormality
  - However, can be used to evaluate for calcified tendonitis, which is the most common presentation of FCU tendonitis
  - Views: posteroanterior, lateral, oblique, and lateral in slight supination of wrist
  - Usually normal but may see:
    - Degenerative changes in the pisotriquetral joint
    - Calcium in the tendon in calcific FCU tendonitis
- Magnetic resonance imaging (MRI):
  - Use when diagnosis is unclear (especially for ulnar-sided wrist pain).
  - Use when not improving with conservative treatment.

- Findings: (best seen on T2 imaging)
  - High fluid signal within the tendon sheath
  - Tendon sheath thickening
  - Tendon may be enlarged.
- Ultrasound (US):
  - FCR tendonitis: fluid distending the synovial sheath
  - FCU calcific tendonitis: calcium deposition in the tendon distal to the ulna, proximal to the pisiform
  - Can visualize FCR brevis (1)[C]
  - FCR/FCU tendinosis:
    - Hypoechoic thickening of tendon
    - May show neovascularization on color flow Doppler

Diagnostic Procedures/Other

Pain relief with lidocaine injection into the tendon sheath aids in diagnosis.

TREATMENT

GENERAL MEASURES

- Initial treatment:
  - Avoiding provocative activities
  - Immobilization with wrist splint in 25 degrees of palmar flexion (2)[C] for 1 to 2 weeks or until symptoms improve
  - Ice
  - Nonsteroidal anti-inflammatory drugs (NSAIDs)
- Subsequent treatment as condition improves:
  - Occupational therapy:
    - Active and passive range of motion exercises, followed by wrist and finger strengthening program
    - Ergonomic improvements
  - Coaching:
    - Improve technique/mechanics.
    - Consider changing racquet grip (3)[C].
- Refractory cases: injection of steroid and local anesthetic in proximity to, but not into, tendon sheath:
  - Resolution of symptoms in 35–40% of patients (4)[C]
  - Calcific tendonitis responds particularly well to steroids.
  - Possibility of tendon rupture after injection (5)[C]
  - Although platelet-rich plasma has growing literature for tendinopathy, there is minimal evidence its use for FCU and/or FCR tendinopathy.

SURGERY/OTHER PROCEDURES

- If symptoms are prominent and not responding to nonoperative treatment, consider surgical consultation.
- Surgical procedure:
  - Surgical release of the tendon
  - Excision of inflamed tenosynovium
  - Tenolysis can be effective (6)[C].
  - Z-plasty lengthening if needed
  - Pisiform excision
- Surgery is usually curative, with return to racquet sports in 6 to 8 weeks (4)[C].

ONGOING CARE

PATIENT EDUCATION

- When introducing a new activity or increasing a current activity, do so slowly to help prevent an overuse injury.
- Allow time for recovery between practices and competition.
- Warm up the area well before playing.
- Maintain proper strength, flexibility, and endurance of the forearms, wrists, and hands.
- Use proper technique.

PROGNOSIS

Usually resolves with conservative treatment within 6 weeks

REFERENCES

1. Budoff JE, Kraushaar BS, Ayala G. Flexor carpi ulnaris tendinopathy. *J Hand Surg Am.* 2005;30(1):125–129.
2. Watanabe A, Souza F, Vezeridis PS, et al. Ulnar sided wrist pain: II clinical imaging and treatment. *Skeletal Radiol.* 2010;39(9):837–857.
3. Smith J, Kakar S. Combined flexor carpi radialis tear and flexor carpi radialis brevis tendinopathy identified by ultrasound: a case report. *PM R.* 2014;6(10):956–959.
4. Rettig AC. Athletic injuries of the wrist and hand: part II: overuse injuries of the wrist and traumatic injuries to the hand. *Am J Sports Med.* 2004;32(1):262–273.
5. Tagliafico AS, Ameri P, Michaud J, et al. Wrist injuries in nonprofessional tennis players: relationships with different grips. *Am J Sports Med.* 2009;37(4):760–767.
6. Palmieri TJ. Pisiform area pain treatment by pisiform excision. *J Hand Surg Am.* 1982;7(5):477–480.

ADDITIONAL READING

- Bencardino JT, Rosenberg ZS. Sports-related injuries of the wrist: an approach to MRI interpretation. *Clin Sports Med.* 2006;25(3):409–432.
- Osterman AL, Moskow L, Low DW. Soft-tissue injuries of the hand and wrist in racquet sports. *Clin Sports Med.* 1988;7(2):329–348.
- Parellada AJ, Morrison WB, Reiter SB, et al. Flexor carpi radialis tendinopathy: spectrum of imaging findings and association with triscaphe arthritis. *Skeletal Radiol.* 2006;35(8):572–578.
- Young D, Papp S, Giachino A. Physical examination of the wrist. *Orthop Clin North Am.* 2007;38(2):149–165.

CLINICAL PEARLS

- FCR and FCU tendonitis usually responds to conservative treatment.
- Steroid/lidocaine injection can be diagnostic as well as therapeutic.
- PRP is used for tendinopathy; however, there is a lack of literature supporting its use for FCU and FCR tendinopathy.
- Surgery is rarely needed.

FLEXOR TENDON AVULSION/JERSEY FINGER

Chau Bui, DO ▪ Suraj A. Achar, MD, FAAFP, CAQSM

BASICS

- An acute injury in which there is an avulsion of the flexor digitorum profundus (FDP) tendon off of the volar aspect of the distal phalanx due to forced hyperextension of the distal interphalangeal (DIP) joint while the finger is actively flexed
- This injury is often missed by players, trainers, and doctors.
  - The Leddy and Packer classification system:
    - Type I: retraction of the tendon into the palm of the hand with nearly complete disruption of the blood supply. The long and short vincula are both ruptured (1).
    - Type II (most common): retraction of the tendon to the proximal interphalangeal (PIP) joint, held in place by the intact vincula longa which helps retain more of its blood supply (1)
    - Type III (unusual): avulsion of a large bony fragment attached to the tendon, remains stuck at the level of the A4 pulley. Both vincula are usually intact maintaining full vascular supply to the tendon (2).
    - Type IV involves a rupture of the FDP tendon insertion with secondary tendon retraction into the finger or palm and a distal phalanx fracture with a large avulsion fragment incarcerated at the A4 pulley (2).

DESCRIPTION

- An avulsion of the FDP tendon from its insertion at the base of the distal phalanx (3)
- Zone I flexor tendon injury (1)
- Synonym(s): jersey finger, rugger finger, FDP avulsion

EPIDEMIOLOGY

- Rare injury seen primarily in contact sports where tackling and grasping of the jersey is probable (rugby, football, hockey, judo)
- Often occurs while grasping the jersey of an opponent who quickly pulls away
- Ring finger is most commonly involved (estimated 75–80% of cases) (4).
- The ring finger is bound on both sides by lumbrical muscles, making it more prone to hyperextension injuries (5).
- May be misdiagnosed as a jammed or strained finger

ETIOLOGY AND PATHOPHYSIOLOGY

The FDP tendon travels along the volar side of the palm and finger. It passes distally through a split in the flexor digitorum superficialis tendon and inserts at the base of the distal phalanx (palmar aspect of P3). Crucial for the tendon health and stability are the mesotendons, also known as vincula. They act like lifelines, providing blood supply to the tendon and tethering it to the underlying phalanx jersey finger injury occurs when the FDP tendon is avulsed from its attachment on the distal phalanx (3).

RISK FACTORS

Participation in contact sports such as rugby and football

DIAGNOSIS

HISTORY

- The mechanism of injury involves a sudden forceful extension of a flexed finger which often occurs while grasping another player's jersey (3)[C].
- Typically seen in football and rugby (1)[C]
- Timing of surgical repair varies based on the level of tendon retraction and the presence of a fracture (1).

PHYSICAL EXAM

- Inspection: Swelling and discoloration may be present along the distal phalanx and DIP joint (3)[C].
- Palpation: Tenderness may be present along the length of the flexor tendon, particularly at the site of FDP tendon insertion. A palpable lump may be present at any point along the proximal digit, frequently at the PIP joint or on the palm of the hand at the A1 pulley (1)[C].
- Range of motion: inability to make a full fist and loss of active DIP joint flexion of the involved digit (pathognomonic finding)

ALERT

- Strength: To assess the integrity of the FDP tendon, hold the PIP joint in full extension and ask the patient to actively flex the DIP joint (2)[C]. Active flexion of the PIP joint and metacarpophalangeal (MCP) joint is preserved in the injured digit.
- Neurovascular exam: should always be assessed and should be normal in jersey finger injuries

DIFFERENTIAL DIAGNOSIS

- DIP joint dislocation
- Distal phalanx fracture
- Flexor digitorum superficialis avulsion

DIAGNOSTIC TESTS & INTERPRETATION

- Three view radiographs (anteroposterior, lateral, and oblique) are necessary to determine the presence and degree of bony avulsion and to potentially assess the level of tendon retraction (6)[C].
- Radiographic findings of jersey finger include mild hyperextension of the DIP and soft-tissue swelling, because most injuries are tendon avulsions without an associated fracture (7).
- Avulsion fractures can be seen on the volar aspect of the distal phalangeal base at the FDP attachment site (3)[C].
- Magnetic resonance imaging (MRI) and ultrasound will show where the tendon has retracted. MRI may show distended tendon "tortuous" or "whirled." Ultrasound offers dynamic imaging to show "asynchrony" movements as well as complete ruptures from focal interruption of fibrillar echo structure of the tendon and posterior acoustic shadowing behind the rupture site.
- Ultrasound is more accurate than physical exam 95% versus 79% (8)[B].

TREATMENT

ALERT
- All FDP avulsion injuries require urgent surgical intervention (3)[C].
- Initial management may include ice, nonsteroidal anti-inflammatory drugs (NSAIDs), and splinting.
- The injured finger should be dorsally splinted to maintain slight flexion at the DIP and PIP joints and avoid DIP extension (1)[C].
- Treatment is influenced by time between injury and treatment, degree of tendon retraction, presence and size of bony avulsion, and level of blood supply to the avulsed tendon (4)[C].

ADDITIONAL THERAPIES
- Treatment options for athletes who present outside the window for primary repair: no treatment, tendon grafting, or terminal interphalangeal joint tenodesis or arthrodesis (3)[C]
- Long palmaris muscle tendon grafting may be offered in certain cases (3)[C].
- Arthrodesis may be offered in cases of DIP instability or articular surface disruption (1)[C].
- Nonoperative treatment generally not recommended unless patient is unable or unwilling to comply with postoperative therapy (4)

SURGERY/OTHER PROCEDURES
- Type I:
  - Surgical repair should be conducted within 7 to 10 days of the injury (4)[C].
- Type II:
  - Early surgical repair within 7 to 10 days is preferred; however, due to the intact vincula longa, surgery can be delayed 6 to 8 weeks (1)[C].
- Type III:
  - Early surgical intervention is preferred, but satisfactory results are possible with delayed repair of 2 weeks, due to an intact blood supply to the tendon (1)[C].
  - Wires can be removed after 3 to 4 weeks postoperatively (4)[C].
- Type IV:
  - The degree of tendon retraction and loss of vascular supply can be similar to a type I injury, requiring surgical intervention within 7 to 10 days (1)[C].

ONGOING CARE
- Following surgery, the affected hand should be placed in a dorsal blocking splint with the wrist in midflexion, the MCP joints at 75 degrees of flexion, and the PIP/DIP joints in extension or near extension (4)[C]. The hand should remain in this splint for 6 weeks (1)[C].
- Passive flexion of the PIP and DIP joints can be started within days of the surgery (4)[C].
- Using an experienced hand therapist early in the postoperative period is recommended (1)[C].
- Strengthening activities can usually begin at 12 weeks postoperatively (1)[C].
- A mitten-type splint/cast that keeps the wrist slightly flexed with the fingers flexed into the palm may allow an athlete to return to play early, provided no grasping of the hand is required (1)[C].
- Return to play with full grasping capabilities usually takes 4 to 6 months and is dependent on sport and position (1)[C].

FOLLOW-UP RECOMMENDATIONS
Immediate referral to an orthopedic/hand surgeon is recommended for all types of FDP avulsion injuries.

REFERENCES

1. Elzinga KE, Chung KC. Finger injuries in football and rugby. *Hand Clin*. 2017;33(1):149–160.
2. Tempelaere C, Brun M, Doursounian L, et al. Traumatic avulsion of the flexor digitorum profundus tendon. Jersey finger: a 29 cases report. *Hand Surg Rehabil*. 2017;36(5):368–372.
3. Lapegue F, Andre A, Brun C, et al. Traumatic flexor tendon injuries. *Diagn Interv Imaging*. 2015;96(12):1279–1292.
4. Bachoura A, Ferikes AJ, Lubahn JD. A review of mallet finger and jersey finger injuries in the athlete. *Curr Rev Musculoskelet Med*. 2017;10(1):1–9.
5. Abrego MO, Shamrock AG. *Jersey Finger*. StatPearls Publishing; 2025. Updated August 7, 2023. Accessed August 11, 2025. https://www.ncbi.nlm.nih.gov/books/NBK545291
6. Cockenpot E, Lefebvre G, Demondion X, et al. Imaging of sports-related hand and wrist injuries: sports imaging series. *Radiology*. 2016;279(3):674–692.
7. Weintraub MD, Hansford BG, Stilwill SE, et al. Avulsion injuries of the hand and wrist. *Radiographics*. 2020;40(1):163–180.
8. Gilleard O, Silver D, Ahmad Z, et al. The accuracy of ultrasound in evaluating closed flexor tendon ruptures. *Eur J Plast Surg*. 2010;33(2):71–74.
9. Kovacic J, Bergfeld J. Return to play issues in upper extremity injuries. *Clin J Sport Med*. 2005;15(6):448–452.

CLINICAL PEARLS
- An acute diagnosis of jersey finger requires urgent surgical treatment (4).
- Return to contact sports may be anticipated 4 to 6 months after surgery (9).
- Depending on the sport, it may be possible for the patient to return to play early provided that a playing splint/cast is worn.
- Delaying surgical treatment, particularly for type I injuries, can result in irreparable scarring of the flexor tendon and permanent loss of flexion at the DIP joint. Although delayed surgical intervention may be offered in certain circumstances, favorable results are not guaranteed. Type II and III injuries frequently can be delayed several weeks without significant changes to surgical outcome, but this is not advised (4).

F

FOLLICULITIS

Timothy Tiu, MD, FAAPMR, CAQSM ▪ Sona Patel, MD, FAAP

BASICS

DESCRIPTION

- Inflammation with infection of hair follicles
- Usually caused by *Staphylococcus aureus* and less commonly by *Streptococcus pyogenes* (1),(2),(3)
- May also be caused by gram-negative organisms (*Pseudomonas*), as in the case of "hot tub" folliculitis (1),(2)

EPIDEMIOLOGY

- Sports-related skin infections account for up to 15% of time-loss injuries in collegiate athletics (3).
- Lesions usually occur on areas of skin traumatized by maceration, such as under shoulder pads or sweaty garments.
- May also develop in areas of occlusion, friction, and perspiration, such as face, neck, scalp, axillae, groin, extremities, and buttocks (4)
- "Hot tub" folliculitis is associated with the use of poorly cleaned hot tubs, whirlpools, jacuzzi, and swimming pools; it can also be spread by sharing sponges or cleaning products (2).

RISK FACTORS

- Poor hygiene (5)
- Improper care of equipment (5)
- Skin breaks associated with turf burns or trauma (football, soccer) (3)
- Contact sports (football, wrestling, rugby) (3)
- Sharing of equipment or clothing (towels) (3)
- Higher body mass index (BMI) (3)
- Anabolic androgenic steroid use (6)

ALERT

Methicillin-resistant *S. aureus* (MRSA) colonization has been documented on wrestling mats, artificial turf, and football training equipment (3).

GENERAL PREVENTION

- Good personal hygiene, wound care (3)[C]
- Avoid sharing equipment (3)[C].
- Refrain from using common tubs and cosmetic shaving (3)[C].
- Cleaning high-touch surfaces (3)[C]

DIAGNOSIS

HISTORY

Maceration caused by sports equipment is a common cause of folliculitis. This knowledge may lead to a definitive diagnosis.

PHYSICAL EXAM

- Erythematous papules and pustules around hair follicles; may progress to nonhealing crusted sores (2)
- Pus limited to epidermis (7)
- Staphylococcal folliculitis: generally pruritic and localized (2)
- Pseudomonas folliculitis: pruritic, urticarial, and erythematous; found as clustered lesions under bathing suits on occluded areas (2),(6)

DIFFERENTIAL DIAGNOSIS

- Furuncles appear as inflammatory nodules with pustules, through which hair emerges (7).
- Carbuncle: infection involving several adjacent follicles; a coalescent inflammatory mass with multiple follicular orifices through which pus drains; larger and deeper than furuncles and found commonly on back of neck (7); often with fever and malaise (4)

- Pityrosporum folliculitis: commonly pruritic lesions, found in setting of warmth and sweating; occurs on chest, back, and proximal extremities (4); appear as 2- to 3-mm papules and pustules, perifollicular, erythematous (4)
- Pseudofolliculitis barbae: ("razor bumps") caused by foreign-body reaction to ingrown hair; not truly a bacterial infection; however, often found to have bacterial superinfection at the site; occurs on any shaved area (2)
- Acne vulgaris

TREATMENT

- Localized folliculitis: daily washes with antibacterial soap and topical antibiotics (mupirocin) (3)[C]
- Resistant or diffuse cases: Treat with oral antibiotics, directed by culture and sensitivities (3)[C]:
  - *S. aureus*: cephalexin, erythromycin, or azithromycin (2),(3)[C]
  - Known MRSA carriers or those at high risk: doxycycline or trimethoprim/sulfamethoxazole (2),(3)[C]
  - *Pseudomonas*: self-limiting in 5 to 7 days; for recalcitrant cases, some recommend quinolone therapy (ciprofloxacin) (2)[C].
- For recurrent or recalcitrant infections, consider chronic *Staphylococcus* colonization, particularly in the nares, on the skin, or in the vagina (3),(7)[C].
- However, there is insufficient evidence to recommend any single oral antibiotic over another in bacterial folliculitis (1)[A].
- Fluctuant folliculitis may be treated with incision and drainage (1)[C].

ALERT
Return to play:

- No new skin lesion for 48 hours (2),(3)[C]
- Completion of 72 hours of antibiotics (2),(3)[C]
- No moist, exudative, or draining lesions (2),(3)[C]
- Active lesions shall not be covered to allow participation (2),(3)[C].

REFERENCES

1. Lin HS, Lin PT, Tsai YS, et al. Interventions for bacterial folliculitis and boils (furuncles and carbuncles). *Cochrane Database Syst Rev*. 2021;2(2):CD013099.
2. Pujalte GGA, Costa LMC, Clapp AD, et al. More than skin deep: dermatologic conditions in athletes. *Sports Health*. 2023;15(1):74–85.
3. Davies HD, Jackson MA, Rice SG, et al. Infectious diseases associated with organized sports and outbreak control. *Pediatrics*. 2017;140(4):e20172477.
4. Cordoro KM, Ganz JE. Training room management of medical conditions: sports dermatology. *Clin Sports Med*. 2005;24(3):565–598.
5. Paradise SL, Hu YW. Infectious dermatoses in sport: a review of diagnosis, management, and return-to-play recommendations. *Curr Sports Med Rep*. 2021;20(2):92–103.
6. Cruz SA, Stein SL. A review of sports-related dermatologic conditions. *Transl Sports Med*. 2020;3(4):300–308.
7. Stevens DL, Bisno AL, Chambers HF, et al. Practice guidelines for the diagnosis and management of skin and soft tissue infections: 2014 update by the Infectious Diseases Society of America. *Clin Infect Dis*. 2014;59(2):e10–e52.

CLINICAL PEARLS

- Personal hygiene and cleaning equipment is important to prevent transmission.
- Consider *S. aureus* colonization in recurrent or recalcitrant infections.

FOOT OSTEOCHONDROSES

Tammy Ng, MD • Kevin J. Burnham, MD, CAQSM •
Daniel C. Herman, MD, PhD, FAAPMR, FACSM, FISBS, CAQSM

BASICS

DESCRIPTION

- Focal disturbance in endochondral ossification due to idiopathic avascular necrosis leading to abnormal bone growth or injury to developing growth plates in children and adolescents (1)
- Examples in the foot:
  - Köhler disease: navicular
  - Freiberg disease: metatarsal head, most commonly 2nd metatarsal head
  - Iselin disease: base of the 5th metatarsal

EPIDEMIOLOGY

- Köhler disease:
  - Seen in children aged 2 to 9 years
  - More common in males than females (6:1)
  - Usually unilateral
- Freiberg disease:
  - Seen in adolescents aged 10 to 18 years
  - More common in females than males (5:1)
  - Usually unilateral
- Iselin disease
  - Seen in physically active children and adolescents aged 8 to 13 years
  - Limited epidemiologic data due to rare occurrence

ETIOLOGY AND PATHOPHYSIOLOGY

- Köhler disease:
  - Associated with delayed ossification of the navicular due to increased risk of ischemia or venous congestion
  - Compression forces between the talus and forefoot make the navicular susceptible to avascular necrosis.
  - May be associated with trauma or recurrent cumulative microtrauma
- Freiberg disease:
  - Frequently affects those with a short 1st metatarsal, leading to 2nd metatarsal overload
  - The 2nd metatarsal is relatively less mobile and thus exposed to greater pressure, which can cause trauma to the surrounding blood vessels, resulting in avascular necrosis.
  - May be associated with systemic conditions (e.g., diabetes mellitus, systemic lupus erythematosus, hypercoagulability)
- Iselin disease:
  - Caused by repetitive traction from fibularis brevis, which inserts into the base of the 5th metatarsal
  - May be associated with sports that involve running, jumping, or lateral pivoting movements (e.g., soccer, basketball, gymnastics, dance)

DIAGNOSIS

HISTORY

- Köhler disease:
  - Gradual onset medial midfoot pain (with or without erythema, warmth, and edema)
  - Pain exacerbated by weight-bearing
- Freiberg disease:
  - Gradual onset pain and edema along the affected metatarsal head region
  - Pain exacerbated by weight-bearing and walking barefoot or in shoes with elevated heels
- Iselin disease:
  - Gradual onset lateral foot pain along the base of the 5th metatarsal
  - Pain exacerbated by weight-bearing, especially with lateral movements, cutting, and jumping

PHYSICAL EXAM

- Köhler disease:
  - Tenderness to palpation of the navicular
  - Pain with resisted plantarflexion and inversion
  - Antalgic gait with shifting of weight to the lateral aspect of the foot
- Freiberg disease:
  - Tenderness to palpation of the affected metatarsophalangeal joint
  - May have edema, crepitus, and decreased range of motion at the metatarsophalangeal joint
  - Mild antalgic gait
- Iselin disease:
  - Tenderness to palpation at the base of the 5th metatarsal (insertion of the fibularis brevis)
  - Pain with resisted eversion and plantar flexion (2)
  - Antalgic gait with shifting of weight to the medial aspect of the foot

DIFFERENTIAL DIAGNOSIS

- Köhler disease:
  - Tarsal coalition
  - Accessory navicular
  - Acute fracture or stress fracture
  - Osteomyelitis
  - Inflammatory arthritis
- Freiberg disease:
  - Idiopathic metatarsophalangeal synovitis or capsulitis
  - Morton neuroma
  - Plantar plate tear
  - Acute fracture or stress fracture
  - Osteomyelitis
  - Inflammatory arthritis
- Iselin disease:
  - Os vesalianum
  - Avulsion fracture of the 5th metatarsal styloid
  - Acute fracture or stress fracture (e.g., Jones fracture)
  - Osteomyelitis
  - Inflammatory arthritis

DIAGNOSTIC TESTS & INTERPRETATION

- Köhler disease:
  - Plain radiographs:
    - Anteroposterior (AP)/lateral views
    - Sclerosis, collapse, and fragmentation of the navicular (1)[C]

- Advanced imaging:
  - Rarely needed for diagnosis
  - Bone scintigraphy may show decreased uptake/"cold area" before changes are seen on plain film (3)[C].
- Frieberg disease:
  - Plain radiographs
    - AP/lateral/oblique views
    - Smillie classification is radiographic classification system that describe five progressive stages of Frieberg disease.
    - Early (Smillie stages I to III): joint space widening due to effusion
    - Late (Smillie stages IV to V): subchondral sclerosis, flattening of the metatarsal head, joint destruction
  - Advanced imaging:
    - May assist in the early detection when radiographs are normal:
      - MRI may show edema during early stages.
      - Bone scintigraphy may show "cold area" surrounded by increased radiotracer uptake.
    - May be used for surgical planning:
      - Hoggett classification system described in 2022 uses sagittal thin slice CT scans to quantify the "zone" of defect (4)[B].
- Iselin disease:
  - Plain radiographs
    - AP/lateral/oblique views
    - Fragmentation, widening of the apophysis, and cystic changes around the apophysis (2)[C]

TREATMENT

GENERAL MEASURES

- Köhler disease:
  - Short leg cast for 4 to 6 weeks
- Freiberg disease:
  - Early (Smillie stages I to III): activity modification, immobilization for 2 to 6 weeks (boot, or cast), or shoe wear modification (stiff sole or rocker bottom)
  - Late (Smillie stages IV to V): surgical management
- Iselin disease:
  - Mild: activity modification, ice, calf stretching
  - Severe: immobilization for 2 to 4 weeks (Aircast, walking cast, or short leg cast with crutches)

MEDICATION

Analgesics (e.g., acetaminophen and nonsteroidal anti-inflammatory drugs [NSAIDs]) for pain

SURGERY/OTHER PROCEDURES

- Köhler disease:
  - Surgical management not indicated
- Freiberg disease:
  - Surgical management for late stages (Smillie stages IV to V) may consist of (5)[A]:
    - Metatarsal osteotomy
    - Interpositional arthroplasty
    - Joint débridement and microfracture
    - Autograft and allograft
    - Metatarsal shortening
    - Hemiarthroplasty or resection arthroplasty
- Iselin disease:
  - Surgery rarely indicated for failure of conservative treatment and symptomatic nonunion:
    - Resection or fixation of symptomatic bone

ONGOING CARE

PROGNOSIS

- Köhler disease:
  - Self-limited with conservative management:
    - Full reconstitution of navicular (6 to 13 months, average 8 months) (6)[B]
    - No evidence of arthritis long term (6)[B]
- Freiberg disease:
  - Early (Smillie stages I to III): responds well to conservative management
  - Late (Smillie stages IV to V): may progress to degenerative joint disease
- Iselin disease:
  - Typically self-limited with conservative management; rarely, may result in nonunion

REFERENCES

1. West EY, Jaramillo D. Imaging of osteochondrosis. *Pediatr Radiol*. 2019;49(12):1610–1616.
2. Forrester RA, Eyre-Brook AI, Mannan K. Iselin's disease: a systematic review. *J Foot Ankle Surg*. 2017;56(5):1065–1069.
3. Khoury J, Jerushalmi J, Loberant N, et al. Kohler disease: diagnoses and assessment by bone scintigraphy. *Clin Nucl Med*. 2007;32(3):179–181.
4. Hoggett L, Nanavati N, Cowden J, et al. A new classification for Freiberg's disease. *Foot (Edinb)*. 2022;51:101901.
5. Alhadhoud MA, Alsiri NF, Daniels TR, et al. Surgical interventions of Freiberg's disease: A systematic review. *Foot Ankle Surg*. 2021;27(6):606–614.
6. Ippolito E, Ricciardi Pollini PT, Falez F. Köhler's disease of the tarsal navicular: long-term follow-up of 12 cases. *J Pediatr Orthop*. 1984;4(4):416–417.

ADDITIONAL READING

Echenique Díaz PJ, Schaufele Muñoz P. Foot osteochondrosis. In: Wagner Hitschfeld E, Wagner Hitschfeld P, eds. *Foot and Ankle Disorders: A Comprehensive Approach in Pediatric and Adult Populations*. Springer International Publishing; 2022:197–212.

CLINICAL PEARLS

- Osteochondrosis is a focal disturbance in endochondral ossification that can affect multiple locations in the foot, notably the navicular, 2nd metatarsal head, and base of the 5th metatarsal.
- Foot osteochondroses typically cause focal, gradual-onset pain.
- Foot osteochondroses typically present with tenderness to palpation and can cause antalgic gait.
- Oblique view radiographs should be obtained if there is a suspicion for Freiberg or Iselin disease, as AP/lateral views may miss the diagnosis.
- Köhler disease and Iselin disease can typically be managed conservatively. Late stages of Freiberg disease may require surgical management.

FRACTURE, CALCANEUS

Greg Nakamoto, MD, FACP

BASICS

DESCRIPTION

Calcaneus fractures can occur secondary to either acute trauma or recurrent stress (i.e., calcaneal stress fracture). The focus here is on the management of acute traumatic calcaneal body fractures. The specific evaluation and management of other types of calcaneal fractures (such as anterior process fracture; extensor digitorum brevis origin avulsion; medial or lateral process fracture; or sustentaculum tali fracture) is beyond the scope of this chapter:

- Of primary concern when evaluating the acute calcaneal body fracture is determining whether the fracture is extra-articular or intra-articular:
  - Most extra-articular fractures can be managed nonsurgically.
  - Current practice is for most intra-articular fractures to be treated surgically. Such fractures should consequently be referred for orthopedic evaluation.
  - Having said that, no universally accepted guidelines exist as to the optimal treatment of displaced intra-articular calcaneal fractures (1),(2),(3).
  - It should be noted that most calcaneal body fractures (other than stress fractures) are intra-articular.
- Secondarily, one should be aware that many patients with acute calcaneus fractures have other coexisting lower extremity or vertebral injuries.
- Synonyms: os calcis fracture; heel bone fracture

EPIDEMIOLOGY

Prevalence

- Most commonly seen in young men, representing ~2% of all fractures seen in adults (1),(3).
- The calcaneus is the most frequently fractured tarsal bone, accounting for 60% of all tarsal fractures (1),(3),(4),(5).
- Approximately 75% of calcaneal fractures are intra-articular (2),(3),(4),(5).
- ~2% are open fractures, approaching 10% if in the setting of high energy trauma (5).

RISK FACTORS

- A fall from a height directly onto the heel is the main cause of calcaneal fractures (3).
- Other mechanisms include a force of impact directly onto the heel (e.g., motor vehicle accident).
- Osteoporosis can predispose to calcaneal fractures despite a seemingly trivial mechanism of injury.
- Extra-articular fractures of the calcaneal body and plantar tuberosity can also be caused by blunt-force trauma or a twisting injury to the hindfoot.
- Avulsion fractures of the calcaneal tuberosity can occur with abrupt contraction of the Achilles.
- Stress fractures of the calcaneus can occur as an overuse injury in athletes.

COMMONLY ASSOCIATED CONDITIONS

- A high-energy mechanism of injury usually is required to cause calcaneal body fractures, resulting in a high incidence of coexisting lower extremity or spinal injury.
- Calcaneal fractures occur bilaterally in 10–15% of patients (3),(5).
- 10% of patients will have sustained a spinal compression fracture as well (5).
- Calcaneal fractures are often associated with significant local soft tissue injury.

ALERT

Acute compartment syndrome of the foot can occur due to a calcaneal fracture and is a surgical emergency.

DIAGNOSIS

HISTORY

Mechanism of injury:

- Extra-articular fractures are more commonly due to an indirect mechanism such as a twisting injury or muscular avulsion.
- Intra-articular fractures are most commonly due to high-energy accidents.
- History of a fall from a height is particularly concerning for additional lower extremity and lumbar spine injury.

PHYSICAL EXAM

- Signs and symptoms include:
  - Heel pain
  - Swelling
  - Ecchymosis
- Physical examination includes the following:
  - **Look for associated soft tissue injury**. Blisters may occur when swelling is substantial. Excessive soft tissue injury will influence duration of splinting before placing into a cast for those being treated nonsurgically or may delay definitive surgical treatment in those being treated operatively.
  - **Assess neurovascular function of the foot**. With significant swelling, pulses may be difficult to assess; check capillary refill of the toes.
  - **Pain elicited with gentle squeeze of the heel** in the palm of the examiner's hand is suggestive of calcaneal fracture.
  - **Ecchymosis that tracks distally to the sole of the foot**, known as the *Mondor sign*, is considered pathognomonic for calcaneal fracture.
  - **Check for evidence of lower extremity compartment syndrome**. Significant swelling in the plantar arch may suggest plantar compartment syndrome. This requires emergent surgical referral even if the fracture itself is nonoperative.
  - **Search for associated lower extremity and vertebral fracture** because of high incidence of coexisting injury.

DIFFERENTIAL DIAGNOSIS

- Fractures of the calcaneus other than the calcaneal body
- Talar fracture
- Cuboid fracture
- Malleolar fracture
- Ankle dislocation
- Ankle sprain

DIAGNOSTIC TESTS & INTERPRETATION

Whereas standard radiographs are often used to make the initial diagnosis, computed tomography (**CT**) **has become the imaging modality of choice** for visualization and staging of calcaneus fractures:

- Standard initial x-rays: anteroposterior, lateral, and axial calcaneus (Harris) views; usually sufficient for diagnosis of calcaneus fracture but often need to be supplemented for full visualization and staging of the injury (4)
- X-ray criteria for diagnosing calcaneal fractures that are not obvious on initial inspection include assessment of the Böhler "tuber-joint" angle (4):
  - A line is drawn between the posterosuperior aspect of the calcaneus and the highest point of the posterior subtalar articular surface; a second line is drawn from the highest point of the anterior process to the posterior margin of the subtalar surface.
  - The angle of intersection of the two lines normally measures between 20 and 40 degrees, with a similar angle found in the two calcanei in any one person.
  - In intra-articular fractures, depression of the subtalar joint results in a decrease in Böhler angle.
- Oblique (Broden) views can be helpful in assessing involvement of the articular surfaces.
- Additional x-rays to consider based on history and physical examination include views of the contralateral foot (because of the significant incidence of bilateral injury and to compare Böhler angle with the injured foot), ipsilateral ankle, and lumbar spine and pelvis (because of high frequency of associated fractures).
- **CT scan is the imaging modality of choice for classification of calcaneus fractures** (4)[A]:
  - In patients in whom x-rays are inconclusive, CT scan is considered the gold standard for confirming the diagnosis of calcaneal fracture.
  - Additionally, if plain films show articular involvement or if suspicion of articular involvement remains high despite equivocal plain films, then a CT scan is essential for a more specific analysis of the subtalar and calcaneocuboid joints because displacement of either will likely require surgical management.
- The **Sanders classification** system is based on axial and coronal CT cuts. It is the classification system most commonly used today in treatment decision making and reporting of results (4):
  - Type 1—nondisplaced fractures
  - Type 2—fractures that are split into two parts
  - Type 3—depressed fractures and/or fractures that are split into three parts
  - Type 4—comminuted fractures
- Magnetic resonance imaging (MRI): Although not generally used for the evaluation of traumatic calcaneus injuries, MRI may be the preferred imaging modality in patients with suspected stress fractures, particularly in patients with severe osteoporosis, in whom a bone scan may appear falsely negative.
- Follow-up and special considerations: For extra-articular fractures being treated nonoperatively, postreduction imaging involves repeating the standard radiographs to assess adequacy of reduction after closed manipulation. Comparison with the opposite foot often is useful.

TREATMENT

- Prehospital: Ice and oral analgesics are useful in the prehospital setting, and oral analgesics may be required for some time after casting.
- Emergency department (ED) treatment: Rule out and/or stabilize life-threatening injuries and evaluate for coexisting lower extremity or spinal injury. Identify indications for immediate surgical intervention (such as open fractures; closed fractures with severe soft tissue pressure from severely displaced fragments; vascular injury; and any fracture which results in compartment syndrome) (5),(6).
- **Nonsurgical treatment of calcaneal body fractures**: Consider for **minimally displaced extra-articular** fractures of the body of the calcaneus which do not change the weight-bearing surface of the foot and do not alter hindfoot mechanics (6)[C]:
  - Reduction techniques: Mediolateral compression of the heel with the palms of the hands can be applied to reduce displaced extra-articular body fractures being treated nonoperatively.

- Postreduction evaluation: Repeat x-rays immediately postreduction and in 1 week in any patient being treated nonoperatively.
- Immobilization: Usually begins with splinting or bulky Jones dressing to accommodate changes in soft tissue swelling.
  - In patients who require casting (see "Ongoing Care"), the splint can be changed to a short leg cast after the initial soft tissue injury has stabilized after ~3 to 5 days.
  - In patients who will require subsequent surgery, splinting is appropriate until the patient can see an orthopedic surgeon.

- **Surgical treatment of calcaneal body fractures**: For other extra-articular fractures (see criteria in "Ongoing Care"), or any intra-articular fracture, obtain urgent orthopedic consultation for consideration of possible surgical treatment.

SURGERY/OTHER PROCEDURES

- In patients who might require operative treatment, referral should be made promptly so that fixation can occur within 5 to 7 days.
- In patients with significant associated soft tissue injury, prompt orthopedic referral allows for early interventions to reduce edema, which can take 7 to 14 days to accomplish. In such cases, operative treatment within the first 2 weeks, before early consolidation of the fracture fragments, is preferred.

ALERT

All cases of open calcaneal body fractures, fracture-dislocations, and fractures resulting in arterial injury or compartment syndrome merit emergent orthopedic evaluation.

ONGOING CARE

Optimal management of calcaneal fractures, particularly of intra-articular fractures, remains controversial (3),(4):

- **Nonoperative treatment of extra-articular calcaneal body fractures:**
  - After closed reduction and a period of splinting or bulky Jones dressing as described above, a reasonable treatment regimen in such cases would include short-leg casting and no weight-bearing for 2 weeks, followed by range of motion exercises. Progressive weight-bearing may start at 8 weeks, with full weight-bearing by 12 weeks.
  - Alternatively, some authors eschew casting for early motion. In such cases, recommendations for duration of initial non–weight-bearing varies, but full radiographic healing and weight-bearing may be anticipated around 12 weeks.
  - Follow-up x-rays at 10 to 12 weeks to confirm healing, longer for persistent symptoms or suspicion of nonunion
- **Operative treatment of extra-articular calcaneal body fractures:**
  - Extra-articular fractures with >10 degrees of varus or valgus malalignment, or broadening or shortening of the heel by >20%, are often best treated surgically. Left uncorrected, such hindfoot deformities may result in functional limitations, ongoing pain, and shoe wear difficulties (6)[B].
  - Displaced tuberosity avulsion fractures, even without an intra-articular component, often cause significant soft tissue compromise and are consequently often treated surgically (6)[C].
- **Operative versus nonoperative treatment of intra-articular fractures:**
  - As a rule, all intra-articular fractures, and the extra-articular fractures as listed earlier, should be referred for orthopedic consultation (3),(4)[B].
  - Completely **nondisplaced** intra-articular fractures (**Sanders type 1**) are still often treated nonoperatively (4)[C].
  - Regarding **displaced** intra-articular fractures (**Sanders types 2, 3, and 4**), there remains a lack of consistent evidence in the literature as to which displaced intra-articular fractures will do best operatively versus nonoperatively; and in the cases of operative treatment, what is the best surgical approach. Having said that, there is a trend in the literature that for most displaced intra-articular fractures, long-term outcomes favor operative treatment, despite possibly having a higher complication rate than nonoperative treatment (1),(2),(3),(4),(6)[B].
  - Risk factors for increased surgical complication rates include severe peripheral vascular disease; poorly controlled diabetes; poor patient compliance; and heavy smoking. The consulting surgeon might take such factors into consideration when deciding whether to operate on a displaced intra-articular fracture (6).

FOLLOW-UP RECOMMENDATIONS

In patients treated nonoperatively, removal from splinting/casting should be followed by referral to physical therapy to restore normal flexibility and strength before allowing return to play.

PATIENT EDUCATION

- Patients should be informed early that treatment can be difficult and that adverse outcomes can be potentially severe and disabling at times, even with optimal treatment.
- Chronic pain and posttraumatic arthritis are not uncommon.

COMPLICATIONS

- In both operatively and nonoperatively treated patients, chronic disability owing to pain from an improperly functioning or arthritic subtalar or calcaneocuboid joint may occur (4).
- Complications specifically seen in patients undergoing open reduction and internal fixation (ORIF) include:
  - Infection
  - Pain
  - Swelling
  - Delayed wound healing
  - Nonunions of the fracture fragments
  - Lateral impingement of the peroneal tendon
  - Sural nerve injury

REFERENCES

1. Selim A, Ponugoti N, Chandrashekar S. Systematic review of operative vs nonoperative treatment of displaced intraarticular calcaneal fractures. *Foot Ankle Orthop*. 2022;7(2):24730114221101609.
2. Kamath KR, Mallya S, Hedge A. A comparative study of operative and conservative treatment of intraarticular displaced calcaneal fractures. *Sci Rep*. 2021;11(1):3946.
3. Wei N, Yuwen P, Liu W, et al. Operative versus nonoperative treatment of displaced intra-articular calcaneal fractures: a meta-analysis of current evidence base. *Medicine (Baltimore)*. 2017;96(49):e9027.
4. Gotha HE, Zide JR. Current controversies in management of calcaneus fractures. *Orthop Clin North Am*. 2017;48(1):91–103.
5. Smitaman EE, Davis M. Hindfoot fractures: injury patterns and relevant imaging findings. *Radiographics*. 2022;42(3):661–682.
6. Rammelt S, Swords MP. Calcaneal fractures—which approach for which fracture? *Orthop Clin North Am*. 2021;52(4):433–450.

ADDITIONAL READING

- Badillo K, Pacheco JA, Padua SO, et al. Multidetector CT evaluation of calcaneal fractures. *Radiographics*. 2011;31(1):81–92.
- Buckley R, Tough S, McCormack R, et al. Operative compared with nonoperative treatment of displaced intra-articular calcaneal fractures: a prospective, randomized, controlled multicenter trial. *J Bone Joint Surg Am*. 2002;84(10):1733–1744.
- Griffin D, Parsons N, Shaw E, et al. Operative versus non-operative treatment for closed, displaced, intra-articular fractures of the calcaneus: randomised controlled trial. *BMJ*. 2014;349:g4483.
- Randle JA, Kreder HJ, Stephen D, et al. Should calcaneal fractures be treated surgically? A meta-analysis. *Clin Orthop Relat Res*. 2000;(377):217–227.
- Renovell-Ferrer P, Bertó-Martí X, Diranzo-García J, et al. Functional outcome after calcaneus fractures: a comparison between polytrauma patients and isolated fractures. *Injury*. 2017;48(Suppl 6):S91–S95.

CLINICAL PEARLS

- Many patients with calcaneus fractures will have a coexisting lower extremity or vertebral fracture. Up to 10% will have coexisting compartment syndrome of the foot, which is a surgical emergency.
- Proper management of calcaneus fractures requires determining if the fracture is intra-articular or extra-articular. Intra-articular fractures generally are best treated surgically, whereas extra-articular fractures (with the exceptions noted under "Ongoing Care") are often treated nonoperatively.
- CT scan is the imaging modality of choice in the evaluation of intra-articular calcaneus fractures.
- Optimal treatment of calcaneal fractures is still controversial, with posttraumatic arthritis being the cause of most cases of chronic disability.
- In nonoperative cases, athletes may be ready to return to play in as little as 8 to 12 weeks depending on the severity of the original injury. In operative cases, the duration of immobilization and recovery is more variable and depends on the particulars of the fracture.
- Consensus suggests that long-term outcome is determined mainly by the degree of joint destruction at the time of injury.
- There seems to be a subset of calcaneal fractures (Sanders type 3 and 4) that often has a poor outcome regardless of treatment (4).

FRACTURE, CARPAL BONE (OTHER)

Dana Hong, DO, CAQSM

BASICS

DESCRIPTION

- Fracture of the carpal bones of the wrist, excluding those of the hamate and scaphoid
- Includes Kienböck disease: a disease of the lunate where the blood supply is compromised and possible osteonecrosis occurs.
- Synonym(s): wrist fracture

EPIDEMIOLOGY

- The carpal bones consist of the scaphoid, lunate, triquetrum (dorsal), and pisiform (volar) in the proximal row and the trapezium, trapezoid, capitate, and hamate in the distal row.
- Hand fractures account for about 18% of all fractures; carpal fractures are 8% of all hand fractures (1).
- Frequency of the eight carpal bone fractures: scaphoid 60%; triquetrum 25%; and hamate, trapezium, pisiform, capitate, lunate, and trapezoid follow ranging from 5.0% to 0.7% (1).
- Carpal fractures are caused by direct or indirect trauma (1). Kienböck disease (osteomalacia of the lunate) is preceded by trauma with the wrist in dorsiflexion in 75% of the cases.

RISK FACTORS

Fractures of the carpal bones other than the scaphoid and lunate bones are often seen in sports using a stick (e.g., hockey, lacrosse).

DIAGNOSIS

HISTORY

- Athletes usually present with a fall on the outstretched hand in the hyperextended position. However, direct trauma or a fall on a flexed wrist can also cause a fracture.
- Pain and restricted motion often are presenting complaints.
- Mechanism of injury can help localize the injury to a specific carpal bone.
- Determine when the wrist began to hurt: Recent versus prolonged is important.
- Determine location of pain: ulnar or radial, and whether it hurts with at rest or with motion
- An occult fracture often will present as a persistent wrist sprain. Carefully examine the patient because Kienböck disease and small chip fractures of the triquetrum can present in this manner (2).

PHYSICAL EXAM

- Pain and tenderness over the dorsum of the wrist
- Localized swelling and limited range of motion (ROM); a prominence may be present.
- Strength testing of the muscles whose tendons insert on or are supported by the injured structure may help localize the injury.
- Neurovascular signs are unusual, except for fracture of the pisiform, which may affect the ulnar nerve and artery.
- Inspect for swelling, deformity, and ecchymosis (the latter usually not seen with carpal fractures).
- Evaluate movement of wrist in flexion, extension, and ulnar and radial deviation.
- Palpate individual carpal bones to determine location of tenderness.
- Test strength of muscles that attach to carpal bones.
- Assess neurovascular integrity (fracture of the pisiform may affect the ulnar nerve, and a lunate dislocation may compress the median nerve.)
- Axial loading of metacarpals above the carpal bones may help in diagnosis.

DIFFERENTIAL DIAGNOSIS

- Sprain of wrist capsule
- Sprain of intercarpal ligaments
- Wrist tendon injury
- Bone contusion
- Soft tissue contusion
- Nerve injuries
- Triangular fibrocartilage complex (TFCC) contusion and tears
- Carpal dislocation
- Metacarpal fracture
- Distal radioulnar fracture
- Osteonecrosis of carpal bones

DIAGNOSTIC TESTS & INTERPRETATION

- Standard wrist radiography series: posteroanterior (PA), radial and ulnar obliques, and true lateral
- Can also obtain views of maximal radial deviation and maximal ulnar deviation; lateral views in maximal flexion and maximal extension
- Additional radiographic views may be needed if a fracture is suspected for certain carpal bones:
  - Hook of hamate: carpal tunnel view
  - Scapholunate instability: PA clenched fist view
  - Trapezium: Bett view (anteroposterior [AP] with approximately 20 degrees of pronation)
- The sensitivity of plain radiographs is <50% for detecting carpal fractures.
- Computed tomography (CT) scanning should be considered if a fracture of the capitate, lunate, pisiform, trapezium, or trapezoid is suspected and negative plain films are seen.
- Cone beam computed tomography (CBCT) has higher resolution, 90% less radiation exposure, and faster scanning time than conventional CT.
- Ultrasonography is a useful adjunct for diagnosing carpal bone fractures.
- Postreduction views should be obtained to confirm reduction and correct anatomical alignment.

TREATMENT

- Immobilization of the wrist; due to soft tissue swelling that may occur from the fracture, initial immobilization is achieved using a removable plaster, fiberglass, or moldable thermoplastic splint. The splint can later be replaced with casting.
- Ice to minimize swelling
- Acetaminophen and rarely opioid analgesics for first 3 to 5 days
- Nonsteroidal anti-inflammatory drugs (NSAIDs) effect on fracture healing remains controversial but may be best avoided with known or suspected acute fractures to minimize the risk of nonunion.
- After wrist immobilization, rehabilitation is extremely important to return to full function and prevent chronic disability (1).
- Open injuries, irreducible dislocations, and injuries with neurovascular compromise should have emergency orthopedic referral.
- All lunate fractures should be referred to a hand surgeon within 72 hours.
- For wrist dislocations, immediate reduction is important to prevent further cartilage damage and relieve pressure on median nerve.
- Generally for fractures and injuries without dislocation, apply a short arm wrist splint, ice, and elevation (1).
- All treatments are for nondisplaced fractures.
- Triquetrum: volar splint with wrist placed in slight extension and metacarpophalangeal (MCP) joints free to prevent joint stiffness; for avulsion fractures, after acute swelling subsides, short arm cast with wrist in slight extension and MCP joints free for 3 to 6 weeks; for nondisplaced, uncomplicated body fractures, short arm cast for 4 to 6 weeks (1)
- Trapezium: short arm thumb spica cast for 4 to 6 weeks (3)[C]

- Pisiform: short arm splint or cast placed in 30 degrees of flexion with slight ulnar deviation; if splint used initially, should be replaced with a cast at 5 to 7 days after injury (1)
- Trapezoid: volar splint for 3 to 5 days if marked swelling and then short arm cast for 4 to 6 weeks (1)
- Capitate: sugar-tong splint for initial immobilization and then a short arm cast once swelling subsides for 4 to 6 weeks. Because usually accompanied by other wrist injuries, referral to hand surgeon is strongly suggested (1).
- Lunate: short arm wrist splint, referral to orthopedic surgeon (1)

ADDITIONAL THERAPIES

ALERT

- Triquetrum:
  - Second most commonly fractured carpal bone
  - Usually ligamentous avulsions fractures
  - Dorsal rim chips of the triquetrum are easily missed on AP view and may be the only sign of a fracture.
  - May have tenderness distal to the ulnar styloid while the hand is in radial deviation
  - Persistent pain after appropriate treatment should alert the treating physician that a concurrent injury (pisiform fracture, TFCC injury, and/or lunate-triquetrum ligament tear) was initially not noticed.
- Capitate:
  - Most often fractured with the scaphoid or metacarpal
  - Largest carpal bone
  - Consider all capitate fractures unstable because of the high likelihood of surrounding carpal instability.
  - Consider serial radiographs in patients with persistent pain.
  - High incidence of delayed nonunion in these fractures
  - Referral to hand specialist is reasonable.
- Trapezium:
  - Easily missed; patients will describe a localized pain at base of the thenar eminence, pain with wrist flexion, and weakness in pinching
  - Missed fractures cause ongoing pain at base of the thumb.
  - Carpal tunnel view demonstrates fracture of the palmar ridge.
  - When displaced, may affect the integrity of the trapeziometacarpal joint, which is responsible for pinch and grasp motions
- Pisiform:
  - Sesamoid bone located within the flexor carpi ulnaris tendon, which can be disrupted if a fracture is present
  - Usually caused by direct blow to hand
  - Can compress the ulnar nerve or artery at Guyon canal
  - The pisiform can be excised in chronically symptomatic cases.
- Trapezoid:
  - Least commonly fractured
  - Patients describe pain at the base of the 2nd metacarpal.
  - Axial compression of 2nd metacarpal will elicit tenderness.
- Lunate:
  - Lunate fractures can be occult.
  - Avascular necrosis (AVN) is seen in 20% of lunate fractures.
  - Kienböck disease may be secondary to lunate injury.
  - Kienböck disease has a high association with ulna-minus variant.
  - In the early stages of Kienböck disease, plain radiographs are usually not diagnostic; magnetic resonance imaging (MRI) is usually needed for definitive diagnosis.
  - Referral to hand specialist is reasonable.
- Initially, while in cast, the athlete may continue fitness training. Constant monitoring of the cast and frequent (weekly) changes may be needed to maintain skin and cast integrity (3)[C].
- Once out of the cast, ROM and then strengthening of the wrist need to be done until restoration of a painless, functional arc of wrist motion and near-normal strength are obtained.

SURGERY/OTHER PROCEDURES

Surgery is needed for displaced fracture(s) through the metacarpo-carpal joint articulation.

ONGOING CARE

FOLLOW-UP RECOMMENDATIONS

- Any displaced fracture of the carpal bones should be referred to an orthopedic surgeon.
- Lunate fractures may develop AVN (Kienböck disease) and should be considered for referral even if not displaced.
- Return to play varies with the degree of injury and casting. In lunate fractures, it is up to 6 months; in triquetrum fractures, it is 4 weeks.
- General requirements for returning to play are complete healing of the fracture and any concurrent soft tissue injuries.
- Thorough rehabilitation with restoration of a painless, functional arc of wrist motion and near-normal strength are essential.
- Wrist stiffness is a common problem after casting, and physical therapy for ROM and strengthening is essential after cast removal.

REFERENCES

1. deWeber K. Overview of carpal fractures. UpToDate. Updated November 11, 2024. Accessed September 1, 2025. https://www.uptodate.com/contents/overview-of-carpal-fractures
2. Suh N, Ek ET, Wolfe SW. Carpal fractures. *J Hand Surg Am*. 2014;39(4):785–791.
3. Rettig ME, Dassa GL, Raskin KB, et al. Wrist fractures in the athlete. Distal radius and carpal fractures. *Clin Sports Med*. 1998;17(3):469–489.

ADDITIONAL READING

- Duckworth AD, Ring D. Carpus fractures and dislocations. In: Court-Brown C, Heckman JD, McKee M, et al, eds. *Rockwood and Green's Fractures in Adults*. 8th ed. Wolters Kluwer Health; 2014: 991–1056.
- Johnson BK, Brou L, Fields SK, et al. Hand and wrist injuries among US high school athletes: 2005/06–2015/16. *Pediatrics*. 2017;140(6):e20171255.
- Klausmeyer MA, Mudgal CS. Hook of hamate fractures. *J Hand Surg Am*. 2013;38(12):2457–2460.
- Papp S. Carpal bone fractures. *Orthop Clin North Am*. 2007;38(2):251–260.
- Rettig AC. Epidemiology of hand and wrist injuries in sports. *Clin Sports Med*. 1998;17(3):401–406.
- Slade JF III, Milewski MD. Management of carpal instability in athletes. *Hand Clin*. 2009;25(3):395–408.
- Vigler M, Aviles A, Lee SK. Carpal fractures excluding the scaphoid. *Hand Clin*. 2006;22(4):501–516.

CLINICAL PEARLS

- Frequency of fracture seen in carpal bones is scaphoid 80%, triquetrum 6%, hamate 5%, trapezium 4%, lunate 3%, capitate 1%, and trapezoid and pisiform, <1% each.
- Dorsal rim chips of the triquetrum are easily missed on AP view and may only be seen on lateral view.
- Trapezium: also easily missed; patients will describe a localized pain at base of the thenar eminence and pain with wrist flexion.
- Pisiform fractures can compress the ulnar nerve or artery at Guyon canal.

FRACTURE, CLAVICLE

Christopher C. Trigger, MD, FACEP, CAQSM

BASICS

- The clavicle is a subcutaneous S-shaped bone.
- First bone to ossify in the human body (5th week of gestation)
- Functionally acts as a strut that connects the shoulder girdle to the axial skeleton

DESCRIPTION

- Allman classification based on fracture site (1),(2)
- Craig further subdivided group II and III fractures:
  - Group I: fracture of the middle third
  - Group II: fracture of the lateral (distal) third:
    - Type I: lateral to coracoclavicular (CC) ligament (typically nondisplaced)
    - Type II: medial to the CC ligaments; causes superior displacement of the medial fragment relative to the lateral fragment
    - Type III: Fracture extends into the acromioclavicular (AC) joint.
    - Type IV: proximal fragment displacement out of periosteal tube (only in children)
    - Type V: comminuted where CC ligaments remain attached to an inferior bone fragment only
  - Group III: fracture of the medial (proximal) third:
    - Type I: nondisplaced
    - Type II: displaced with ligamentous rupture
    - Type III: Fractures extend into the sternoclavicular (SC) joint.
    - Type IV: Fracture causes epiphyseal separation (children and adolescents).
    - Type V: comminuted

EPIDEMIOLOGY

Incidence

- Most commonly fractured bone in children and adolescents
- Bimodal age distribution with peaks <40s and the elderly (>70 years)
- Predominant gender: male > female (2.5:1)
- 70–80% are group I, 15–18% group II, and 3% group III.

RISK FACTORS

- Direct trauma and fall onto the shoulder are the most common mechanisms of injury.
- Highest risk sports in the United States are football, soccer, and snow sports (snowboarding and skiing combined) (2).

COMMONLY ASSOCIATED CONDITIONS

- AC joint injury
- Labral tears
- Rotator cuff injuries
- Proximal humeral fractures
- Rib fractures
- Pneumothorax/hemothorax
- SC joint dislocation
- Brachial plexopathy
- Vascular injuries (uncommon)

DIAGNOSIS

History, physical exam, and appropriate imaging will make the diagnosis.

HISTORY

- Direct trauma or a fall
- Middle-third fractures are frequently seen with fall on an outstretched arm.
- Distal-third fractures most often are associated with loads transmitted to the lateral aspect of the shoulder.

PHYSICAL EXAM

- May have ecchymosis or tenting of the skin over the fracture
- Tenderness to palpation at fracture site
- Pressure along the clavicle may reveal fracture motion or crepitus.
- Careful pulmonary and neurovascular exam must be performed to identify possible associated injury.

DIFFERENTIAL DIAGNOSIS

- AC joint injury
- Glenohumeral dislocation
- Rotator cuff contusion/tear
- Labral injury
- Rib fracture
- Humeral head fracture
- SC joint or physeal injury

DIAGNOSTIC TESTS & INTERPRETATION

Initial Tests (lab, imaging)

- Radiographs:
  - An anteroposterior (AP) view of the clavicle, including the AC and SC joints and the shoulder girdle
  - A 30- to 45-degree cephalic-tilt (Zanca) view is recommended to delineate displacement and comminution in all fracture types.
  - A 40-degree cephalic-tilt view of the SC joint (serendipity view) can rule out SC dislocations.
  - An axillary view can be useful in distal clavicle fractures.
- Computed tomography (CT) scan:
  - Articular fractures of the medial or lateral clavicle may require a CT scan.
  - A CT angiogram or standard angiogram can be used if distal vascular deficit is suspected (1),(3).

Diagnostic Procedures/Other

Special considerations: The proximal clavicular epiphysis is the last growth plate in the body to fuse (approximately age 20 years). Therefore, many injuries involving the SC joint in athletes probably are physeal injuries and are ideally evaluated by thin-cut CT scan (1).

TREATMENT

- Primary goal in treating clavicular fractures is to obtain bony union and restore shoulder function to preinjury level with little or no residual pain, dysfunction, or cosmetic deformity (1),(3).
- Most fractures can be treated nonoperatively (80–90%), but if displaced >2 cm surgical intervention is used more often with lower nonunion rates (2),(4).

- Most clavicle fractures (when treated nonsurgically) will heal clinically in 6 to 8 weeks; radiographic healing takes longer (8 to 12 weeks).
- Arm sling and sling and swathe are the most common forms of immobilization for 2 to 6 weeks based on patient's comfort level (1).
- Figure-of-8 harness is used less frequently because of discomfort, noncompliance, and worse complication rates.
- Range of motion (ROM) and active shoulder flexion (up to 40 degrees) as well as isometric deltoid and rotator cuff strengthening can begin once pain is improved.
- Avoid ROM >45 degrees of forward flexion until clinical evidence of healing is seen.
- As radiographic union progresses, increase ROM and resistive exercises.
- When radiographic union is present, full active use of the arm is allowed.

SURGERY/OTHER PROCEDURES

- Surgery is more commonly performed with varying results.
- Indications for early operative treatment include (1),(3):
  - Displaced or shortened (>2 cm), and comminuted middle-third fractures of the clavicle
  - Type II distal clavicle fractures are typically managed surgically owing to the high rate of nonunion; also, operative treatment is recommended in type IV and V fractures.
  - Neurovascular compromise
  - Any open fractures
  - Tenting of skin over an irreducible fracture
  - Concomitant glenoid neck fracture, also known as *floating shoulder*
  - Posterior fracture dislocations of the medial clavicle should be reduced in the presence of a thoracic surgeon owing to risk of vascular injury.
- Surgical techniques used include open reduction and internal fixation (ORIF) with plates and screws or intramedullary fixation.
- Primary operative fixation is becoming much more common in healthy, young, and professional athletes with a goal of possibly expediting return to play (4).
- Secondary operative treatment is considered for:
  - Persistent (>6 weeks) displacement and shortening despite immobilization
  - Malunion or nonunion

ONGOING CARE

- Follow-up should be scheduled 7 to 10 days after injury to assess clinical symptoms and then every 2 to 4 weeks until clinical and radiographic union occur (1).
- Radiographic union progresses more slowly than clinical union.
- Radiographs should be performed at intervals of 4 to 6 weeks to assess healing.
- A final radiograph to assess callus formation and clinical union can be useful.
- Athletes should not be allowed to return to play until the fracture is clinically and radiographically healed (typically 6 to 8 weeks) (1)[C].
- Noncontact and throwing athletes should have full, painless ROM and at least 90% strength compared with the uninjured arm (usually requires ~6 weeks).
- Return to contact/collision sports may take up to 8 to 12 weeks.

COMPLICATIONS

- Posttraumatic arthritis
- Nonunion:
  - Degree of displacement and comminution most important factors
  - More common in diabetics, smokers, women, and the elderly
  - Recent studies show a 1–3% rate of nonunion in patients managed surgically and 10–16% rate of nonunion in nonoperative patients (5).
  - Rate of nonunion was no different at 6 weeks, but at 9 months, it was significantly reduced with surgical intervention.
- Malunion resulting in angulation, shortening, and a poor cosmetic appearance
- Neurovascular injury (uncommon): medial branch (ulnar nerve) of the brachial plexus most affected
- Hardware removal secondary to pain

REFERENCES

1. Kim W, McKee MD. Management of acute clavicle fractures. *Orthop Clin North Am*. 2008;39(4):491–505.
2. Twomey-Kozak J, Whitlock KG, O'Donnell JA, et al. Epidemiology of sports-related clavicle fractures in the United States: injuries from 2015 to 2019. *Orthop J Sports Med*. 2022;10(10).
3. Moverley R, Little N, Gulihar A, et al. Current concepts in the management of clavicle fractures. *J Clin Orthop Trauma*. 2020;11(Suppl 1):S25–S30.
4. Fanter NJ, Kenny RM, Baker CL III, et al. Surgical treatment of clavicle fractures in the adolescent athlete. *Sports Health*. 2015;7(2):137–141.
5. Ahrens PM, Garlick NI, Barber J, et al. The clavicle trial: a multicenter randomized controlled trial comparing operative with nonoperative treatment of displaced midshaft clavicle fractures. *J Bone Joint Surg Am*. 2017;99(16):1345–1354.

ADDITIONAL READING

- Axelrod DE, Ekhtiari S, Bozzo A, et al. What is the best evidence for management of displaced midshaft clavicle fractures? A systematic review and network meta-analysis of 22 randomized controlled trials. *Clin Orthop Relat Res*. 2020;478(2):392–402.
- Goudie EB, Clement ND, Murray IR, et al. The influence of shortening on clinical outcome in healed displaced midshaft clavicular fractures after nonoperative treatment. *J Bone Joint Surg Am*. 2017;99(14):1166–1172.
- Wiesel B, Nagda S, Mehta S, et al. Management of midshaft clavicle fractures in adults. *J Am Acad Orthop Surg*. 2018;26(22):e468–e476.
- Woltz S, Stegeman SA, Krijnen P, et al. Plate fixation compared with nonoperative treatment for displaced midshaft clavicular fractures: a multicenter randomized controlled trial. *J Bone Joint Surg Am*. 2017;99(2):106–112.

CLINICAL PEARLS

- Most fractures are managed nonoperatively unless displaced and shortened.
- Most patients can return to noncontact sports within 6 to 8 weeks.
- Typical return to contact sports is 8 to 12 weeks.
- Surgical fixation tends to yield sooner return to play and decreased nonunion rates in the appropriate setting.
- Protective donut pads may be useful in protecting the clavicle from reinjury or pain from a direct blow; however, there is no robust evidence that it is beneficial.

FRACTURE, COCCYX

John Munyak, MD

BASICS

- The coccyx is the last bony structure at the caudal end of the vertebral column and is triangular in shape.
- Coccygeal fractures can be caused by trauma such as falling and landing on the buttocks (e.g., during ice skating) or in newborns while passing through the vaginal canal.
- Although the mechanism may be low impact, immobilization should be considered until other spine injuries are properly evaluated.
- Classification: Coccyx fractures are grouped into three types—flexion (type 1), compression (type 2), and extension (type 3) (1),(2).

DESCRIPTION

- Fall landing in sitting position is most common.
- Also can occur during childbirth (1),(3)
- Surgical procedures performed in area of coccyx
- Fractures of the coccyx are usually transverse.
- More common in women

ETIOLOGY AND PATHOPHYSIOLOGY

- The coccyx is made up of three to five fused vertebrae with attachments of several important muscles and ligaments. The muscles include the levator ani group, which supports the pelvic floor and aids in maintaining fecal continence, and the gluteus maximus, which aids in thigh extension.
- The coccyx has limited movement at the sacrococcygeal junction and a curvature such that the tip curves into the pelvis.
- Coccyx injuries are often belittled by physicians, but it should be kept in mind that the pain can be extremely severe and debilitating to the patient. Additionally, the coccyx is a weight-bearing structure in the seated position, and an ill-managed coccyx fracture can cause the patient to apply more weight on the ischial tuberosities, causing bursitis.

RISK FACTORS

- Predominantly occur in females because the female pelvis is broader, and the coccyx is more exposed.
- Advanced age
- Osteoporosis
- Decreased balance causing more falls
- Congenital bone disorder such as osteogenesis imperfecta
- Involvement in activities such as skating or skateboarding

GENERAL PREVENTION

- Calcium and vitamin D supplements to prevent osteoporosis
- Refraining from activities that would predispose to falling on the buttocks, especially if elderly or if underlying medical conditions such as osteogenesis imperfecta are present

DIAGNOSIS

- Mechanism of injury
- Look for ecchymosis and palpate for tenderness in the gluteal fold.
- Prehospital:
  - Evaluate for other associated injuries (other potential life-threatening injuries such as head injuries may be missed if the focus is on the pain from the coccyx injury).

HISTORY

- Mechanism of injury (fall vs. assault vs. childbirth)
- Factors leading up to the fall (mechanical fall vs. syncope)
- Other associated injuries (Other potential life-threatening injuries such as head injuries may be missed if the patient is focusing on the pain from the coccyx injury.)
- Use of blood thinners (for ecchymosis out of proportion to the severity of injury)
- Low back pain, buttock pain, rectal bleeding (if associated rectal tear)
- Pain when sitting or defecating—document the PQRST of pain: *P*alliative or *P*recipitating factors, *Q*uality, *R*egion or *R*adiation, *S*everity (1 to 10), and *T*iming
- Risk for cancer (pathologic fracture): bright red blood per rectum (BRBPR), abnormal vaginal bleeding, weight loss

PHYSICAL EXAM

- Palpation of the sacrococcygeal joint for pain
- Digital rectal examination can be diagnostic with mobility and/or crepitus of the coccyx.
- Assess sacrococcygeal joint mobility by palpating the coccyx anteriorly (digital rectal exam) and posteriorly (externally).
- Anoscopy should be performed if gross blood is present to evaluate for possible rectal perforation (very rare).
- Physical examination of the entire spine is necessary to evaluate for concomitant injury.
- Neurologic exam of the lower extremities to assess radiculopathy

DIFFERENTIAL DIAGNOSIS

- Contusion, hematoma
- Coccyx dislocation or subluxation
- Pilonidal cyst

DIAGNOSTIC TESTS & INTERPRETATION

Initial Tests (lab, imaging)

- Radiographs will identify other suspected spinal injuries.
- Displaced coccyx fractures can be seen best on the lateral coccyx view radiograph.
- Radiographs are not necessary if isolated coccyx fracture is apparent on rectal exam.
- Nondisplaced fractures are difficult to see on x-ray.
- When x-rays are used in the diagnosis, three views needed: anteroposterior (AP), lateral, and cone-down (focused) coccyx view
- More extensive diagnostic imaging is unnecessary in traumatic coccyx injuries (3),(4).

TREATMENT

Emergency department (ED) treatment:

- Symptomatic treatment
- Rarely, bed rest until ambulation can be tolerated
- Oral analgesics are key; may range from over-the-counter (OTC) acetaminophen or ibuprofen to prescription topical agents based on severity of pain
- Aim for conservative management in the pediatric population given high healing rates (4),(5).
- Attempted manipulation and reduction of the displaced fracture by digital rectal approach was originally reported to be not necessary and futile because the coccyx cannot be stabilized.
- Fracture–dislocation treatment: Endorectal manipulative repositioning showed high success in one study (20 cured, 4 remarkable, 4 improved, 1 ineffective out of 29 patients) (6).
- If there is an associated rectal injury, call for a surgical consult immediately. Prescribe antibiotics to cover for enteric pathogens: cefoxitin, cefotetan, and metronidazole.

- Cushions ("doughnuts")
- Sitz baths
- Stool softeners may help to reduce pain during bowel movements.
- Injection therapy: Local anesthetic + glucocorticoid injections are effective in ~60% of patients with sacrococcygeal pain (6).
- Author's anecdotal input—procedural ultrasound guidance enhances the accuracy of the injection as well as putting the patient more at ease with an injection of this anatomical region.
- Healing and aftercare: Recovery is typically 8 to 12 weeks for fractures (~4 weeks for contusions); early management includes icing 20 minutes hourly for 48 hours, then 2 to 3 times/day (7).

MEDICATION

- Cefotetan: adult: 2 g intravenous (IV); children: 80 mg/kg/day divided q6–8h (used with rectal injury)
- Cefoxitin: adult: 2 g IV; children: 80 to 160 mg/kg/day divided q6h (used with rectal injury)
- Metronidazole: adult: 0.5 to 1.0 g IV; children: 30 mg/kg/day divided q12h (used with rectal injury)
- Acetaminophen
- Nonsteroidal anti-inflammatory drugs (NSAIDs)
- Lidoderm 5% patch
- Voltaren 1% gel

ADDITIONAL THERAPIES

Prescription "doughnut pillows" provide comfort until the fracture heals. They are helpful even if only a contusion is present.

SURGERY/OTHER PROCEDURES

Surgery is usually not required. Very rarely, severe trauma results in a comminuted fracture requiring coccygectomy (5).

ADMISSION, INPATIENT, AND NURSING CONSIDERATIONS

- Initial stabilization:
  - Spine immobilization for suspected concomitant cervical, thoracic, or lumbar injuries
  - Pain control with NSAIDs or narcotic analgesics
- Admission criteria:
  - Nearly all patients can be managed on an outpatient basis.
  - Only patients with severe pain, an inability to walk or to take care of themselves, other serious injury, or requiring surgery need to be admitted.
- Discharge criteria:
  - Most patients can be managed as outpatients with appropriate follow-up.
  - The patient is discharged home when other conditions are ruled out, and pain is under control.
  - Pulsed radiofrequency (PRF): Although data are limited for fracture-dislocation, one chronic sacrococcygeal pain series reported ~90% success at 6 months after PRF treatment (6).

ONGOING CARE

FOLLOW-UP RECOMMENDATIONS

- Healing is slow.
- Pain may become chronic.
- Orthopedic consultation and possible coccygectomy may be required in severe cases.

PATIENT EDUCATION

- Avoid activities requiring prolonged sitting such as horseback riding, long travel, biking, and so forth.
- Lean forward while sitting to avoid weight-bearing on the coccyx.

PROGNOSIS

Pain usually resolves about a week after callous forms.

COMPLICATIONS

Rarely, chronic pain or instability may require coccygectomy (5).

REFERENCES

1. Kaushal R, Bhanot A, Luthra S, et al. Intrapartum coccygeal fracture, a cause for postpartum coccydynia: a case report. *J Surg Orthop Adv*. 2005;14(3):136–137.
2. Sukun A, Cankurtaran T, Agildere M, et al. Imaging findings and treatment in coccydynia—update of the recent study findings. Thieme Group; 2024. Accessed October 10, 2025. https://www.thieme-connect.com/products/ejournals/pdf/10.1055/a-2185-8585.pdf
3. Hanna TN, Sadiq M, Ditkofsky N, et al. Sacrum and coccyx radiographs have limited clinical impact in the emergency department. *AJR Am J Roentgenol*. 2016;206(4):681–686.
4. Hamoud K, Abbas J. Fracture dislocation of the sacro-coccygeal joint in a 12-year-old boy. A case report and literature review. *Orthop Traumatol Surg Res*. 2015;101(7):871–873.
5. Ramieri A, Domenicucci M, Cellocco P, et al. Acute traumatic instability of the coccyx: results in 28 consecutive coccygectomies. *Eur Spine J*. 2013;22(Suppl 6):S939–S944.
6. Zhang Y, Gao G. Progress in the diagnosis and treatment of fracture-dislocation of the coccyx (Review). Spandidos Publication. 2025. Accessed October 10, 2025. https://www.spandidos-publications.com/10.3892/etm.2025.12877
7. Mount Sinai Health. Tailbone trauma—aftercare. Accessed October 4, 2025. https://www.mountsinai.org/health-library/selfcare-instructions/tailbone-trauma-aftercare

ADDITIONAL READING

- Rockwood C, Green D, eds. *Fractures in Adults*. 8th ed. Lippincott-Raven; 2014.
- Simon R, Sherman SC. *Emergency Orthopedics: The Extremities*. 6th ed. Appleton & Lange; 2011.
- Tibble CD, Gibbs M. Pelvic fractures. In: Wolfson AB, Cloutier RL, Hendey GW, et al, eds. *Harwood-Nuss' Clinical Practice of Emergency Medicine*. 6th ed. Wolters Kluwer; 2015:277–284.

CLINICAL PEARLS

- More common in women
- May occur owing to falls or during childbirth (1)
- A self-limited condition
- Treatment includes pain management with oral anti-inflammatory medications, topical agents, and doughnut pillows.
- If there is an associated rectal injury, call for a surgical consult immediately. Prescribe antibiotics to cover for enteric pathogens.

FRACTURE, COMPRESSION

Dana Hong, DO, CAQSM • Jun Hwan Park, MD

BASICS

DESCRIPTION

- A compression fracture is defined as failure of the anterior vertebral column of the spine.
- The thoracolumbar spine is divided into three columns:
  - Anterior column (anterior portion of vertebral body, anterior longitudinal ligament, and anterior annulus fibrosus)
  - Middle column (posterior longitudinal ligament, posterior annulus fibrosus, and posterior wall of vertebral body)
  - Posterior column (posterior arch and posterior ligamentous complex)
- Two subtypes: anterior (caused by anterior flexion) and lateral (caused by lateral flexion)
- Three locations: cervical, thoracolumbar (transition between thoracic and lumbar from T10–L2), and lower lumbar vertebrae
- If anterior *and* middle columns are involved, the fracture is termed "burst."
- Synonym(s): wedge fracture

EPIDEMIOLOGY

- Vertebral compression fractures often occur at the midthoracic (T7–T8) spine and the thoracolumbar junction (T12–L1).
- Most common cervical compression fracture is an anterior wedge fracture, usually at C5, from axial loading, as might occur in football or diving.
- ~10% of cervical spine fractures have an associated, noncontiguous spinal column fracture.
- 25% of postmenopausal women >50 years old and 40% by 80 years old will suffer from a vertebral compression fracture (1).

RISK FACTORS

- Cervical spine injuries are most common in diving, American football (poor tackling technique), and wrestling.
- Vertebral compression fractures are the most common type of osteoporotic fracture (1).
- Advanced age, female sex, postmenopausal status, glucocorticoid use, and smoking are potential risk factors for osteoporotic related compression fractures.

DIAGNOSIS

HISTORY

- Hyperflexion and axial loading injuries, such as with "spear tackling" in football or striking the forehead on the bottom of the pool, typically cause cervical compression fractures. Hyperextension mechanism suggests a "teardrop" fracture or defect of posterior spinal elements or pars interarticularis.
- Transient or permanent paralysis and/or sensory deficits can occur with compression fractures but are rare. Neurologic deficits imply spinal cord injury due to retropulsion of disk material or the fracture fragment (i.e., burst fracture).

PHYSICAL EXAM

- Sudden, localized pain immediately following direct trauma or axial loading injury
- Palpate the spinal column for "step-off" defect or tenderness.
- Kyphosis or height loss may be seen.
- Careful neurologic examination, including sensation, motor function, upper motor neuron signs, and reflexes. Should be completely intact, but occasionally transient neurologic symptoms occur in an isolated compression fracture.

DIFFERENTIAL DIAGNOSIS

- Burst fracture (anterior and middle column disrupted, with or without posterior involvement)
- Fracture-dislocation (anterior, middle, and posterior columns disrupted)
- "Teardrop" fracture (triangular fracture of anteroinferior vertebral body)
- Transverse process or spinous process fracture
- Lumbar or cervical strain or sprain
- Spondylolysis and/or spondylolisthesis
- Scheuermann disease: kyphosis >50 degrees, wedging of at least three vertebral bodies by at least 5 degrees, disk space narrowing, and irregularity of endplates
- Spear tackler spine: radiographic evidence of:
  - Developmental narrowing of the cervical spinal canal (<13 mm anteroposterior [AP] diameter of spinal canal on plain film or impedance of contrast medium on myelography)
  - Straightening or reversal of the normal cervical lordotic curve
  - Preexisting minor posttraumatic radiographic evidence of bony or ligamentous injury
  - History of repeated spear tackling; some authors believe that these findings absolutely prohibit return to contact sports. Others believe that if normal cervical lordosis is restored by treatment and the athlete refrains from further spear tackling, and then there is not a high risk of injury in returning to athletic activity.
- Burning hands syndrome: a variant of central cord syndrome with characteristic complaint of burning paresthesia and dysesthesia in both arms or hands and occasionally in legs; associated with bony or ligamentous spine injury in 50% of cases

DIAGNOSTIC TESTS & INTERPRETATION

- The severity of vertebral fractures may be radiographically staged:
  - Grade 1—20–25% height deformity
  - Grade 2—25–40% height deformity
  - Grade 3—>40% height deformity (2)
- AP radiograph: buckling of lateral vertebral cortex next to endplate with decreased interspinous distance; may show lateral wedging with lateral flexion injury
- Lateral radiograph: Height of anterior vertebral body is decreased, whereas posterior height is unchanged, causing increased density of vertebral body from bony impaction and prevertebral swelling; no subluxation of vertebral bodies
- Flexion-extension views: Evaluate cervical ligamentous instability (>3.5 mm horizontal or 11-degree angular displacement between adjacent vertebrae).
- Computed tomography (CT) scan: to confirm intact vertebral ring (posterior wall, pedicles, and lamina); ~25% of compression fractures identified on plain films will be reclassified as burst fractures after CT scanning
- Myelography: rules out osseous protrusion into spinal canal and better evaluates neural compression than CT
- Magnetic resonance imaging (MRI): recommended to evaluate spinal cord or nerve root compression and intrinsic spinal cord abnormalities if neurologic symptoms persist or plain films are abnormal

TREATMENT

- Prehospital:
  - It is estimated that 3–25% of spinal cord injuries may result from improper stabilization of the spinal column during the transportation period.
  - If spinal cord injury is suspected, then management should be with advanced trauma life support procedures: Airway should be established and protected, breathing maintained, and circulation supported.
  - If the player is wearing a helmet, it should *not* be removed. However, the facemask may be removed for airway access.
- Emergency department (ED) treatment:
  - All suspected spinal cord injuries warrant emergency evaluation as soon as possible. Radiographs should be obtained as soon as possible, and full neurologic exam should be documented.

GENERAL MEASURES

- Cervical compression fractures in the absence of subluxation are treated with a rigid brace for 8 to 12 weeks with or without halo.
- Thoracic fractures are relatively stable because of surrounding chest cage and strong costovertebral ligaments and can be treated conservatively with relative rest.
- Thoracolumbar injuries (T10–L2) are inherently more unstable and require a longer recumbency and immobilization in thoracolumbar spinal orthosis.

- Nonoperative treatment of osteoporotic vertebral compression fractures includes pain control, anti-osteoporotic medications, immobilization with an external orthosis, and physiotherapy (3).
- Bracing significantly reduces pain up to 6 months postinjury. No difference in outcomes was observed between soft and rigid braces; therefore, soft braces are recommended due to improved patient comfort (4).

MEDICATION

- Pain control with oral analgesics (e.g., acetaminophen, ibuprofen) with or without intranasal calcitonin are first-line therapy. Immediate-release opioid (e.g., tramadol, tapentadol) can be prescribed for more severe pain.
- Nasal calcitonin 200 units (one spray) once daily alternative nostrils can hasten the relief of pain from vertebral fractures and can be a useful adjunct in the acute setting (5).

ADDITIONAL THERAPIES

- Less severe injuries may be managed with bracing and serial imaging to evaluate healing and alignment.
- Unstable injuries mandate urgent surgical treatment.
- A portion of injuries may require delayed surgical intervention.

SURGERY/OTHER PROCEDURES

- Isolated fractures with <25% anterior compression are considered stable and can be treated with thoracic lumbosacral orthosis brace immobilization.
- A >50% loss of anterior vertebral height, multiple adjacent compression fractures, or angulation >20 degrees at the thoracolumbar junction are associated with segmental instability due to posterior ligamentous injury. This requires surgery to prevent formation of chronic instability and possible further kyphotic deformity. The procedure of choice is usually posterior short-segment pedicle screws or interspinous wiring and fusion.
- Kyphotic deformities may be managed with a posterior approach with osteotomies or a combined anterior approach and posterior procedure, although anterior approaches are associated with higher morbidity and complications.
- Vertebroplasty and kyphoplasty are routinely used for pain associated with osteoporotic and pathologic compression fractures.
- A systematic review and meta-analysis of randomized controlled trials indicate that vertebral augmentation procedures, including vertebroplasty and kyphoplasty, are associated with a lower incidence of adjacent new vertebral fractures compared to conservative treatment (6).

ONGOING CARE

FOLLOW-UP RECOMMENDATIONS

- Any patient with unstable radiographic abnormalities or neurologic deficits should be immediately referred to a neurosurgeon or orthopedic spine surgeon for complete evaluation.
- Always consider an osteoporotic fracture risk assessment and further workup if clinically indicated, including dual-energy x-ray absorptiometry (DEXA) bone density study and laboratory testing for secondary causes of osteoporosis.

REFERENCES

1. Goldstein CL, Chutkan NB, Choma TJ, et al. Management of the elderly with vertebral compression fractures. *Neurosurgery*. 2015;77 (Suppl 4):S33–S45.
2. Genant HK, Wu CY, van Kuijk C, et al. Vertebral fracture assessment using a semiquantitative technique. *J Bone Miner Res*. 1993;8(9):1137–1148.
3. Jang HD, Kim EH, Lee JC, et al. Management of osteoporotic vertebral fracture: review update 2022. *Asian Spine J*. 2022;16(6):934–946.
4. Squires M, Green JH, Patel R, et al. Clinical outcomes after bracing for vertebral compression fractures: a systematic review and meta-analysis of randomized trials. *J Spine Surg*. 2023;9(2):139–148.
5. Boucher E, Rosgen B, Lang E. Efficacy of calcitonin for treating acute pain associated with osteoporotic vertebral compression fracture: an updated systematic review. *CJEM*. 2020;22(3):359–367.
6. Korovessis P, Syrimpeis V, Korovesis A, et al. Incidence of new osteoporotic adjacent vertebral body fractures. A comparison between conservative treatment and vertebral body augmentation (vertebroplasty, kyphoplasty): a systematic review and meta-analysis. *Front Surg*. 2025;12:1594217.

ADDITIONAL READING

- Cantu RC, Bailes JE, Wilberger JE Jr. Guidelines for return to contact or collision sport after a cervical spine injury. *Clin Sports Med*. 1998;17(1):137–146.
- Costa F, Ortolina A, Cardia A, et al. Efficacy of treatment with percutaneous vertebroplasty and kyphoplasty for traumatic fracture of thoracolumbar junction. *J Neurosurg Sci*. 2009;53(1):13–17.
- Denis F. The three column spine and its significance in the classification of acute thoracolumbar spinal injuries. *Spine (Phila Pa 1976)*. 1983;8(8):817–831.
- Khoueir P, Oh BC, Wang MY. Delayed posttraumatic thoracolumbar spinal deformities: diagnosis and management. *Neurosurgery*. 2008;63(Suppl 3):117–124.
- Maroon JC, Bailes JE. Athletes with cervical spine injury. *Spine (Phila Pa 1976)*. 1996;21(19):2294–2299.
- McGirt MJ, Parker SL, Wolinsky JP, et al. Vertebroplasty and kyphoplasty for the treatment of vertebral compression fractures: an evidenced-based review of the literature. *Spine J*. 2009;9(6):501–508.
- Nicholas JA, Herschman EB, eds. Thoracic spine injuries in athletes. In: *The Lower Extremity and Spine in Sports Medicine*. Mosby; 1995.
- Oner FC, Dhert WJA, Verlaan JJ. Less invasive anterior column reconstruction in thoracolumbar fractures. *Injury*. 2005;36(Suppl 2):B82–B89.
- Tatsumi RL, Hart RA. Cervical, thoracic and lumbar fractures. In: Trunkey DD, Asensio JA, eds. *Current Therapy of Trauma and Surgical Critical Care*. Mosby; 2008:513–519.

CLINICAL PEARLS

- Compression fractures without neurologic injuries are considered stable and, once healed completely, should allow the player to return to action when neck pain is gone, range of motion is complete, muscle strength is normal, and fusion is solid (if done).
- Athletes with significant vertebral injury requiring a halo brace or surgical stabilization are considered not to have adequate strength to return to contact sports.

F

FRACTURE, CORONOID

Mary Mitchell, DO • Delmas J. Bolin, MD, PhD, FACSM

BASICS

- The coronoid process:
  - An important stabilizer of the elbow to varus stress and posterior ulnar displacement
  - Part of the sigmoid notch, the portion of the proximal ulna that articulates with the humerus
  - Has several important soft tissue insertions:
    - The brachialis muscle inserts anteriorly, distal to the capsule; the anterior joint capsule inserts very close to the tip of the coronoid; the anterior bundle of the medial collateral ligament (MCL) and the lateral collateral ligament (LCL) complex insert at the base of the coronoid.
- When the coronoid is fractured at the base, the ligament insertion sites are often preserved because failure occurs through bone, not the ligament insertions. Smaller fractures are likely to be associated with ligament injury.
- Unusual to see in isolation; usual mechanism of injury is elbow dislocation as a result of a fall on an outstretched hand.

DESCRIPTION

Coronoid fractures are classified based on anatomic location of the fracture based on lateral radiograph (types 1 to 3) and computed tomography (CT) diagnosis of anteromedial (type 4) and anterolateral (type 5) fractures (1); subclassification according to the associated soft tissue injuries and fractures to determine treatment (2):

- Type 1: fracture of the tip of the coronoid:
  - Tip subtype 1 fractures involve <2 mm of coronoid and may be isolated or associated with a fracture dislocation.
  - Tip subtype 2 fractures involve >2 mm and generally is associated with "terrible triad" injuries (i.e., elbow dislocation, radial head fracture, and coronoid fractures).
- Type 2: fracture of the anteromedial facet:
  - Anteromedial subtype 1 fractures extend from just medial to the tip of the coronoid to the anterior half of the sublime tubercle (the insertion of the medial band of the MCL).
  - Anteromedial subtype 2 fractures extend to the tip of the coronoid.
  - Anteromedial subtype 3 fractures extend to the anteromedial rim and the entire sublime tubercle but do not always extend to the tip of the coronoid.
- Type 3: fracture of the basal aspect of the coronoid involving >50% of the coronoid:
  - Basal subtype 1 fractures involve the basal coronoid alone.
  - Basal subtype 2 fractures are associated with fractures of the olecranon.
- Type 4 or 5: anteromedial or anterolateral fractures

EPIDEMIOLOGY

- Uncommon, rarely occurring as an isolated injury
- In elbow dislocations, 10–15% of cases have coronoid process fractures.

RISK FACTORS

- Displacement of large coronoid process fracture fragments has been associated with recurrent dislocation.
- No known significant risk factors to date

COMMONLY ASSOCIATED CONDITIONS

- Elbow instability
- Radial head fracture
- Olecranon fracture
- Loss of range of motion (ROM)
- Degenerative joint disease (posttraumatic arthritis)
- Ulnar, median, radial, and anterior interosseous nerve injury
- Brachial artery injury
- Heterotopic ossification

DIAGNOSIS

HISTORY

- Common mechanism is fall on outstretched hand.
- Most patients with coronoid fractures present with elbow dislocations.
- Direct impact is a less common cause.

PHYSICAL EXAM

- Diffuse edema within and around the elbow joint
- Tenderness is usually multifocal. Look for radial head tenderness as well as antecubital fossa tenderness.
- ROM is limited, and crepitus on ROM should be noted.
- Evaluate for anterior/posterior and posterolateral rotatory instability.
- Varus posteromedial instability (with anteromedial coronoid fractures) can be assessed by having patient flex and extend elbow with palm down and shoulder in 90 degrees abduction producing mechanical symptoms (3)[B].
- Neurovascular examination is paramount, especially if there is an elbow deformity.
- If elbow is dislocated, perform neurologic and vascular examinations before reduction. Repeat neurovascular examination after elbow dislocation is reduced and assess for elbow instability.
- Palpate radial head and olecranon to look for accompanying fractures.

DIFFERENTIAL DIAGNOSIS

- Elbow subluxation
- Posterior lateral rotatory instability
- Acute ulnar collateral ligament sprain
- Radial head fracture
- Hyperextension injuries to joint capsule

DIAGNOSTIC TESTS & INTERPRETATION

- Initial tests
  - Standard elbow x-ray series (anteroposterior, lateral, and one or both obliques) should be requested at the time of evaluation:
    - Evaluate for comminuted fractures, where reduction may not be advisable.
    - Repeat plain radiographs after elbow relocation.
  - If radial head tenderness is present, radial head view should be added to x-ray series.
  - Advanced imaging: Small coronoid fractures can be difficult to distinguish from radial head fractures, and both CT scanning (1)[B] and magnetic resonance imaging (MRI) should be considered if radiographs are not definitive.
  - Ultrasound imaging, both static and dynamic, can be used to evaluate MCL and LCL structures (4).
- Follow-up tests
  - Radiographs should be repeated after 1 week to ensure continued proper alignment.

TREATMENT

- Acute treatment (1)[B]:
  - Elbow dislocations with coronoid fractures should be evaluated for instability and splinted in position of stability.
  - Tip subtype 1 fractures do not involve the insertion of the anterior capsule and can be treated with immobilization for 1 to 2 weeks or bracing with protected ROM through the stable range.
  - Prolonged immobilization associated with poor outcomes (5)[B]
  - Tip subtype 2 fractures almost always involve the anterior capsule insertion and are often seen in terrible triad injuries. They should be referred to orthopedics; they often will require suture fixation because the fragments are too small to be secured with screws.
  - Anteromedial subtype fractures are associated with incongruent articulation of the ulnohumeral joint and may lead to posttraumatic degenerative joint disease.
  - These fractures require surgical stabilization. In subtypes 1, 2, and 3, the percentages of articular involvement of the sublime tubercle were 0%, 47%, and 79%, and the percentages of articular involvement of the radial notch were 0%, 7%, and 8%, respectively (6).
  - Basal coronoid fractures generally have less soft tissue disruption than tip or anteromedial fractures but require stabilization to prevent recurrent instability and traumatic degenerative joint disease.
- Special considerations:
  - Posttraumatic degenerative joint disease correlates with patient age.
  - Ulnar nerve injuries occur from handling of nerve and do not always resolve.
  - Subluxation or repeat dislocation usually requires repeat surgery.
  - Contractures and heterotopic ossification are common after treatment.
- Rehabilitation:
  - Early mobilization with active and active assistive ROM should begin as soon as comfort allows, generally after 1 week (5)[B].
  - A sling can be used for comfort during the rehabilitation period.
  - A hinged brace generally is prescribed to protect the elbow from varus and valgus stress as well as blocking of the terminal 30 degrees of extension during early rehabilitation is common and continued for the first month.
  - Prophylaxis for heterotopic ossification is not routine (e.g., indomethacin or naproxen).
  - Resistive exercises generally are delayed for 6 weeks.
  - Serial radiographs are commonly obtained to confirm maintenance of concentric reduction.

SURGERY/OTHER PROCEDURES

Surgery to repair soft tissue injuries associated with coronoid fractures is being performed increasingly.

ONGOING CARE

PROGNOSIS

- Joint stiffness and limited ROM are common with prolonged immobilization.
- Presence of posttraumatic arthritis correlates with patient age.
- Pain is a common complaint in at least half of all patients after treatment.

COMPLICATIONS

- Vascular and neurologic injuries associated with elbow dislocations
- Complex dislocations with loss of ROM and stability
- Persistent pain and loss of ROM after treatment

REFERENCES

1. Adams JE, Sanchez-Sotelo J, Kallina CF IV, et al. Fractures of the coronoid: morphology based upon computer tomography scanning. *J Shoulder Elbow Surg*. 2012;21(6):782–788.
2. Ring D. Fractures of the coronoid process of the ulna. *J Hand Surg Am*. 2006;31(10):1679–1689.
3. Ramirez MA, Stein JA, Murthi AM. Varus posteromedial instability. *Hand Clin*. 2015;31(4):557–563.
4. Tagliafico AS, Bignotti B, Martinoli C. Elbow US: anatomy, variants, and scanning technique. *Radiology*. 2015;275(3):636–650.
5. Regan W, Morrey B. Fractures of the coronoid process of the ulna. *J Bone Joint Surg Am*. 1989;71(9):1348–1354.
6. Lee HD, Jung YJ, Oh JK, et al. Morphological characteristics of fractures of the anteromedial facet of the coronoid in posteromedial rotatory instability of the elbow: a three-dimensional CT remodeling study. *J Shoulder Elbow Surg*. 2021;30(7):1527–1536.

CLINICAL PEARLS

- Coronoid fractures can be managed conservatively with meticulous diagnosis.
- Athletes with associated soft tissue injuries or instabilities should be referred early for orthopedic evaluation.
- Athletes return to play when fractures are healed and when they have restored painless ROM with full strength and flexibility.
- Recovery can be prolonged, and careful follow-up is important.
- Patients with type 1 tip fractures generally can return to play within 6 to 8 weeks; surgical patients frequently require longer rehabilitation prior to return to play.
- Lockout elbow bracing should be considered to stabilize the elbow and can be an important adjuvant to healing and rehabilitation.

FRACTURE, DISTAL FEMUR

Rhiannon Ryan, DO ▪ Suraj A. Achar, MD, FAAFP, CAQSM

BASICS

DESCRIPTION

- Fracture involves the distal 15 cm of the femur.
- Fractures may be:
  - Supracondylar: These fractures occur just above the femoral condyles and are often unstable due to the pull of strong thigh muscles
  - Intracondylar and condylar → often are intra-articular

EPIDEMIOLOGY

- Bimodal distribution: young, healthy males, elderly osteopenic females
- Distal femur fractures represent 4–6% of all fractures of the femur (1).
- Predominantly women and in the elderly with >50% of patients who are >65 years old (2)
- No data on the incidence in the athletic population

Pediatric Considerations

- Up to 60% of femoral fractures in children ≤3 years old may be the result of nonaccidental trauma (3).
- Spiral fractures of the femur suggest child abuse (3).

ETIOLOGY AND PATHOPHYSIOLOGY

- Fractures generally occur from significant axial loading with associated varus, valgus, or rotation force.
- May occur from direct trauma as well
- In young adults, fractures are usually associated with high-energy trauma such as:
  - Motor vehicle accidents, falls from heights, direct impact
  - Motor sports, downhill skiing
- In older individuals, especially those with osteoporosis, a slip and fall may be enough force to cause injury.
- Muscle attachments, quadriceps, hamstring, and gastrocnemius cause the observed deformity in distal femur fractures.

RISK FACTORS

- High-energy sports such as motor sports and downhill skiing
- Osteoporosis

COMMONLY ASSOCIATED CONDITIONS

- Fractures are generally from high-energy mechanism, so a full trauma survey should be performed.
- Complications may include:
  - Proximal or shaft fractures of the femur
  - Ligament and cartilage injuries of the knee
  - Proximal tibia fractures
  - Open fractures: 5–10% of all supracondylar fractures
  - Quadriceps tendon injury
  - Vascular injuries are relatively uncommon.

DIAGNOSIS

Pediatric Considerations

- Growth plate vulnerability : The physis (growth plate) is the weakest area of a child's bone. In the distal femur, it's responsible for a significant portion of the bone's growth
- Essential workup:
  - Radiographs
  - Assess distal pulses, palpate compartments, and evaluate sensation and motor function:
    - If pulses are not equal or palpable, bedside Doppler may be necessary.
  - Search for associated injuries.
  - In suspected child abuse, obtain skeletal survey or bone scan.

HISTORY

- History will help to guide examination and workup.
- High-energy injuries require full examination and search for associated injuries.
- Direct trauma and low-energy mechanism do not necessarily require a more comprehensive evaluation.

PHYSICAL EXAM

- Tenderness on examination, deformity, thigh shortening, swelling (secondary to hematoma), and crepitus with movement
- Limited movement of hips and knees
- Commonly presents with associated injuries: chest or abdominal trauma, hip or knee injury, direct blow to the extremity
- Vascular compromise (arterial injury): expanding hematoma, absent or diminished pulses, progressive neurologic deficits in a closed fracture (1)
- Hypotension and tachycardia secondary to significant blood loss
- Radiographs:
  - Anteroposterior (AP) view of pelvis, true lateral of hip, AP and lateral views of femur, and complete knee series
  - Other imaging as indicated by trauma protocols
- Computed tomography (CT) scan: Complex intra-articular injuries generally necessitate CT scan for operative planning:
  - CT scan is recommended because 55% of these fractures are intra-articular (2).
- Arteriography: should be performed for evidence or suspicion of vascular compromise

DIFFERENTIAL DIAGNOSIS

- Hip fracture or dislocation
- Knee dislocation
- Proximal tibia fracture
- Thigh contusion or hematoma

DIAGNOSTIC TESTS & INTERPRETATION

If surgery is planned, complete blood count (CBC), type, and crossmatch

TREATMENT

- Prehospital:
  - Long-leg splint should be applied to the extremity in the position it was found.
  - If signs of neurovascular compromise, reduce limb with in-line traction.
  - Use analgesia when possible.
  - Do not attempt to reduce open fractures in the field.
  - Apply wet sterile dressing over an open fracture.
  - If wound is grossly contaminated, use sterile saline irrigation.

- Emergency department (ED) treatment:
  - Primary and secondary trauma surveys
  - If surgical treatment will be delayed or for selected patients in whom nonoperative management is the treatment of choice, consider fracture reduction.
  - Reduce fractures to near-anatomic alignment by using in-line traction (Hare, Buck, or long posterior splint): reduces pain and helps to prevent hematoma formation
  - Pain management: parenteral or IV opiate-type analgesia
  - Infection prophylaxis: with open fractures, tetanus toxoid if indicated, cefazolin with gentamicin
  - For injuries with highly contaminated wounds, add penicillin G to cover *Clostridium* spp.
  - Emergently consult an orthopedic surgeon.
  - Femur fractures with vascular (expanding hematoma, absent or diminished pulses) or progressing neurologic compromise require immediate angiography or vascular consultation for femoral artery exploration.
  - Consider transferring patients with a femur fracture if:
    - Necessary orthopedic consults are not available.
    - There are associated serious injuries that may require a trauma center for management.

Pediatric Considerations

- Assess markers for nonaccidental trauma:
  - Delay in presentation; history of mechanism inconsistent with the injury
  - Isolated trauma to the thigh; associated burns, bruises, or linear abrasions
  - Younger than walking age
  - Assess for dislocation of the femoral capital epiphysis.
  - Depending on the age of the patient and the fracture type, pediatric femoral fractures may not require operative treatment.
  - Physeal fracture management usually
- **Nonoperative:** considered for nondisplaced or minimally displaced fractures: immobilization with a cast or splint
  - Close monitoring for any displacement
- **Operative:** usually required for displaced fractures

MEDICATION

For open fractures:

- Cefazolin: adult: 2 g IM/IV; children: 20 mg/kg IM/IV
- Gentamicin: 1.5 mg/kg IV
- Penicillin G: adult: 2 million IU IV; children: 25,000 IU/kg/d IV divided q8h

SURGERY/OTHER PROCEDURES

- Surgical reconstruction should be performed as soon as possible (1)[B],(4)[C].
- If surgery will be delayed >24 hours (closed fractures), tibial pin traction should be applied to maintain limb length (5)[C].
- Multiple surgical techniques can be performed to obtain reduction and fixation and depend on both surgeon experience and the specific fracture (2)[C].
- Anatomic reduction of the fracture with particular attention to the articular surface is more closely related to positive outcomes than the actual surgical technique.
- Children aged 6 months to 5 years with a diaphyseal fracture and <2 cm of shortening may be treated with early spica casting or traction and delayed spica casting (6)[B].
- There is unclear benefit of surgery versus casting in fractures with >2 cm shortening or varying degrees or rotation and angulation (6)[C].

ADMISSION, INPATIENT, AND NURSING CONSIDERATIONS

- Monitor heart rate and blood pressure (BP) continuously because large volumes of blood (i.e., 4 to 6 units) may be contained within the thigh.
- Most femur fracture patients should be admitted.
- Conservatively treated fractures in a pediatric patient may not require hospitalization.

ONGOING CARE

PROGNOSIS

- Depends on multiple factors:
  - Fracture type
  - Associated injuries
  - Patient comorbidities
- Fracture with intra-articular involvement carries a high risk of posttraumatic arthritis.

COMPLICATIONS

- Hemorrhagic shock secondary to significant blood loss
- Neurovascular injury
- Compartment syndrome: Swelling within the muscle compartments can compress nerves and blood vessels, requiring emergency surgery
- Growth disturbance: Premature closure of the growth plate can lead to limb length discrepancy or angular deformity.
- Infection secondary to open fractures
- Fat embolism and adult respiratory distress syndrome can cause respiratory failure.
- High mortality rate in elderly populations

REFERENCES

1. Lupescu O, Nagea M, Patru C, et al. Treatment options for distal femoral fractures. *Maedica (Bucur).* 2015;10(2):117–122.
2. Ehlinger M, Ducrot G, Adam P, et al. Distal femur fractures. Surgical techniques and a review of the literature. *Orthop Traumatol Surg Res.* 2013;99(3):353–360.
3. Hui C, Joughin E, Goldstein S, et al. Femoral fractures in children younger than three years: the role of nonaccidental injury. *J Pediatr Orthop.* 2008;28(3):297–302.
4. Bilgehan T. Medial approach for the treatment of femur fractures in association with vascular injury. *Injury.* 2020;51(6):1367–1372.
5. Albert MJ. Supracondylar fractures of the femur. *J Am Acad Orthop Surg.* 1997;5(3):163–171.
6. Kocher MS, Sink EL, Blasier RD, et al. Treatment of pediatric diaphyseal femur fractures. *J Am Acad Orthop Surg.* 2009;17(11):718–725.

ADDITIONAL READING

- Macnicol MF. Fracture of the femur in children. *J Bone Joint Surg Br.* 1997;79(6):891–892.
- Starr AJ, Hunt JL, Reinert CM. Treatment of femur fracture with associated vascular injury. *J Trauma.* 1996;40(1):17–21.

CLINICAL PEARLS

- Be aware of potential associated injuries in all femur fractures.
- Fractures of the distal femur are severe, and medical management and treatment are difficult.
- Evaluate for signs of child abuse in children <3 years.
- It is imperative to achieve anatomical reduction, restoration of functional anatomy, and stable fixation to ensure optimal function and reduce recovery time.

FRACTURE, DISTAL PHALANX

Thomas L. Pommering, DO, FAAFP, FAMSSM • Drew Duerson, MD, RMSK • Jonathan Napolitano, MD, FAAPMR

BASICS

- Fractures of the distal tip (tuft fracture):
  - Open
  - Closed
- Fractures of the shaft (see Fig. 76 in Appendix A):
  - Longitudinal
  - Transverse
- Fractures of the base:
  - Mallet fracture
  - Reverse mallet fracture (jersey finger)
  - Pediatric epiphyseal fractures:
    - Salter-Harris (SH) type I or type II
    - Seymour fracture (pediatric mallet finger)

DESCRIPTION

- *Mallet finger*: a pure tendon injury where there is disruption of the extensor tendon caused by forced flexion of the fingertip while the distal interphalangeal (DIP) joint is in extension. This causes loss of DIP extension, leaving the fingertip in slight flexion.
- *Mallet fracture*: dorsal bony avulsion of the terminal extensor tendon from its insertion onto the proximal aspect of the distal phalanx (see Fig. 77 in Appendix A)
- *Jersey finger*: flexor digitorum profundus (FDP) rupture from its insertion onto the palmar distal phalanx; can be a pure tendinous injury or be a bony avulsion fracture (see Figs. 78 and 79 in Appendix A)
- *Seymour fracture*: extra-articular transverse fracture of the distal phalangeal physis (SH I or II) or can be 1 to 2 mm distal to the physis; this fracture mimics mallet finger deformities but does not involve the articular surface. The FDP tends to pull the distal metaphyseal fragment volarly, whereas the extensor tendon insertion onto the proximal aspect of the distal phalanx pulls the epiphysis dorsally in the opposing direction (see Fig. 80 in Appendix A).
- *Tuft fracture*: a fracture of the distal tip of the distal phalanx; usually from a crush injury and associated with a subungual hematoma and/or a nail bed injury; can be an open or closed injury. This is the most common hand injury in toddlers and preschool-age children.

EPIDEMIOLOGY

Incidence

- Most common peak incidence is during early teenage years, followed by a second peak during toddler years (crush injury in doors).
- In the pediatric population, physeal fractures of the phalanges account for 37% of all physeal fractures, with the small finger being affected most often (30%), followed by the thumb (20%).
- Hand injuries, in general, account for 9% of all sports injuries.
- Seen more often with contact sports, where direct trauma is more likely (e.g., football), or with sports where the hand is exposed to projectiles (e.g., baseball, softball, or basketball).

ETIOLOGY AND PATHOPHYSIOLOGY

- The tip of the distal phalanx ends with broad, spade-like ungual tuberosity that provides a stable and protective base for the distal digital pulp.
- On the palmar surface, the FDP inserts onto the midportion of the distal phalanx.
- On the dorsal side, the terminal extensor tendon attaches to the proximal aspect of the distal phalanx (or the epiphyseal plate in children), blending with the joint capsule and periosteum.
- Collateral ligaments span the DIP joint (or the epiphyseal plate in children) and insert onto the metaphysis of the distal phalanx.
- Lateral interosseous ligaments originate on and span the distance of the distal phalanx, protecting the neurovascular bundle as they pass dorsally from the pulp to the nail bed.

RISK FACTORS

- Crush injury to tip of finger (e.g., getting stepped on by opponent's spiked shoes or finger slammed in a door) results in comminuted fracture or *tuft injury*.
- Acute flexion of an extended DIP joint (e.g., catching a ball on the tip of the finger or striking an object with the finger extended) results in *mallet finger*.
- Forced extension while actively flexing the DIP joint (e.g., grabbing a jersey of a ball carrier in football or catching the rim while dunking a basketball) results in an FDP rupture or *jersey finger*.

GENERAL PREVENTION

- Proper catching technique ("soft hands")
- Buddy taping to the adjacent digit or interphalangeal joint taping for high-risk athletes

DIAGNOSIS

HISTORY

- Crush: *tuft or Seymour fracture*
- Direct trauma, torsional, or hyperflexion/hyperextension mechanism: shaft or base of phalanx fracture
- Blunt trauma or projectile force against the fingertip resulting in forced flexion: *mallet finger/fracture*
- Forced extension on a flexed distal phalanx (e.g., grabbing a jersey during a tackle): *jersey finger*

PHYSICAL EXAM

- Signs and symptoms include:
  - Pain, swelling, and ecchymosis at distal finger
  - Loss of range of motion (ROM), malalignment, or angular deformities
  - Obvious deformity, especially if associated with dislocation
  - Subungual hematomas
  - Traumatic swelling and tenderness over the volar aspect of the distal phalanx with additional palmar pain is a *rupture of the FDP* tendon until proven otherwise.
- Physical examination should include the following:
  - Sites of tenderness, loss of active ROM, evidence of instability, and neurovascular examination
  - Radiographs should be obtained before any manipulative examination.
  - *Mallet finger*: 40- to 45-degree loss of extension at the DIP joint with inability to extend the distal phalanx. There is also pain and swelling over the dorsal aspect of the joint.
  - *Jersey finger*: inability to actively flex the distal phalanx, with tenderness over the volar aspect of the joint; pain in the palm or proximal to the proximal interphalangeal (PIP) could indicate retraction of the tendon proximally.

DIFFERENTIAL DIAGNOSIS

- Fracture
- Sprain
- Volar plate rupture
- Tendon rupture or avulsion
- Interphalangeal dislocations
- Infection

DIAGNOSTIC TESTS & INTERPRETATION

- Imaging should be obtained before any manual reduction attempts.
- Three views of the affected digit: anteroposterior (AP), lateral, and oblique views
- Consider comparison views of the unaffected side if skeletal immaturity and unaccustomed to pediatric radiology.
- Magnetic resonance imaging (MRI), computed tomography (CT) scan, or ultrasound (US) are usually not indicated in the initial evaluation of distal phalanx injuries unless physical exam is equivocal or x-rays are nondiagnostic:
  - MRI and/or US can be used to delineate soft tissue ligamentous or tendon injury.
  - CT scan is occasionally useful to delineate osseous injury for preoperative planning or to evaluate suspicious bone lesions.
  - US can identify some fractures (see Fig. 81 in Appendix A) and also demonstrate dysfunction of a tendon.

TREATMENT

- *Distal phalanx tuft fractures*:
  - *Closed with minimal to no displacement*:
    - Inherently stable
    - Often have an associated subungual hematoma that may need evacuated (see "Surgery/Other Procedures") for pain control
    - Ice for swelling and pain control
    - Protective splint covering the tip of the finger for support and protection; usually not needed for >2 to 3 weeks, leaving the PIP joint free (1),(2)[C]
    - If >50% of nail bed is involved with significant nail bed injury, there is risk for nail bed necrosis (1),(2)[C].
    - Nonunion is rare, but radiographic union can take up to 6 months.
    - The tip of the finger can remain sensitive for up to 6 months after the injury (2)[C].
  - *Open*:
    - Inherently unstable because of disruption of the supporting pulp and nail bed
    - Require careful débridement, irrigation, and soft tissue repair (1),(2)[C]
    - Oral antibiotics and tetanus prophylaxis
    - Consider surgical consultation.
- *Shaft fractures*:
  - *Closed longitudinal or transverse shaft*:
    - Usually inherently stable (1),(2)[C]
    - Longitudinal fractures: heal within 3 to 4 weeks; splint for protection
    - Transverse fractures: take longer to heal, requiring slightly longer support until clinical discomfort abates or radiographic union is evident
  - *Open shaft fractures*:
    - Unstable
    - Proper alignment is necessary.
    - Surgical consultation is recommended.
- *Base-of-phalanx fractures*:
  - Tend to be unstable regardless of the overlying soft tissue involvement owing to the deforming traction of the extensor or flexor tendons (3)[C]
  - Lack of intrinsic support of the overlying nail and nail plate
  - Tend to angulate with the apex pointing dorsally
  - If >1/3 to 1/2 of the articular surface is involved or if displaced, consider surgical consultation.

- *Mallet fracture*:
  - Continue 24-hour splinting with the DIP joint in slight extension using a molded thermoplast splint or other properly fitted splint for 6 to 8 weeks.
  - Splints can be volar bearing, dorsal bearing, or combined (3)[C].
  - An additional 2 to 4 weeks of night splinting is considered if extension lag is still present.
  - Extreme hyperextension (>10 degrees) of the DIP joint should be avoided.
  - PIP joint is always left free.
  - Some extension lag after treatment is common.
  - The goal is to prevent a swan neck deformity.
  - No consensus exists for indications for surgery as outcomes for effective splinting are similar. However, many advocate for operative management for open injuries, those with volar subluxation of the distal phalanx, or if displaced and involving >30% of the joint surface (1),(2)[C],(4)[A].
  - Consider surgery in pediatric patients' due to poor compliance with the strict splinting (5)[C].
  - Surgical consultation is advised for failed conservative treatments and those with subluxation/dislocation complications.
- *Mallet finger*:
  - Pure tendon injury; 7 to 10 weeks of continuous splinting of DIP joint followed by an optional 2 to 4 weeks of night splinting if continued extension lag exists (3)[C],(6)[A].
  - Continuous splinting should be resumed if failed or interrupted treatment because the prognosis for healing is still very good.
  - Chronic mallet fingers (>30 days) should still be considered candidates for conservative treatment because outcomes can be similar to acutely treated injuries (4)[A].
  - Careful follow-up of any injury requiring prolonged splinting because complications of skin breakdown has been reported at 13% (4)[A]
  - Generally, conservative treatment is preferred to surgery owing to similar overall outcomes, extensor lag results (5.7 degrees for surgical and 7.6 degrees for nonsurgical) and complication rates (14.5% for surgical and 12.8% for nonsurgical) (4)[A].

ALERT
When treating a mallet finger injury with prolonged splinting, careful follow-up with skin checks and co-management with a hand therapist is advised.

Pediatric Considerations

Seymour fracture:

- Represents 5% of distal phalanx fractures in children (6)[A]
- Is a displaced distal phalanx fracture with nail bed injury which is often interposed within the fracture (1),(5)[C]
- Caused by a crush injury to the tip of the finger impaction onto another child or moving ball so mimics a mallet injury mechanism
- Mean age of presentation is 9 years with a predilection for males at 70% (6)[A].
- Is usually an open fracture but can be closed (6)[A]
- May clinically present as mallet finger injury with a flexed fingertip but positioning is actually caused by an imbalance between the flexor tendon pulling the distal phalanx volarly versus the intact extensor tendon being unable to extend causing a pseudo mallet appearance (6)[A],(1)[C]
- Radiographic appearance can also mimic a mallet fracture or DIP joint dislocation without close scrutiny which lends to delayed treatment and worse outcomes.
- AP, lateral, and oblique films with attention to the lateral view should provide the diagnosis.
- Most common radiographic appearance is a Salter-Harris II fracture with dorsal displacement of the distal fragment (6)[A].
- Delayed treatment including antibiotic use >24 hours is associated with a 35% increased risk of infection and 16% increased risk of osteomyelitis and risk for nonunion (6)[A].
- Other complications include nonunion, nail dystrophy, and physeal arrest (1),(5)[C],(6)[C].
- This injury is best treated by an experienced surgeon with débridement. Conservative treatment is usually not sufficient due to the nature of the injury.

MEDICATION

First Line

- If reduction is needed or repair of associated soft tissue injuries (e.g., nail bed laceration), a hematoma block, digital block, or wrist block can be used.
- Conscious sedation or reduction under general anesthesia may be needed.

Second Line

Chronic pain control usually can be achieved with splinting alone or with adjunctive nonnarcotic analgesics.

ISSUES FOR REFERRAL

- Displaced fractures not responsive to manual reduction
- Suspected flexor tendon rupture or avulsion fracture
- Open fracture of the shaft or intra-articular fracture
- Open tuft fractures are often unstable and involve complex injuries to the nail bed requiring skilled repair under loop magnification.
- Suspected neurovascular injury or secondary infection
- All Seymour fractures

ADDITIONAL THERAPIES

- Hematoma evacuation from the nail bed when >30–50% of the nail is involved or there is a need for pain control.
- Usually accomplished using either a heated paper clip or electric cautery device. Take care not to damage the nail bed.

ALERT
With fractures associated with subungual hematomas involving >30–50% of the nail, concomitant nail bed lacerations should be suspected and repaired if present. This is usually done using 5 to 0 or 6 to 0 dissolvable sutures and replacing the nail plate if possible. This is treated as an open fracture in the sense that it should be done under sterile conditions followed by antibiotic coverage for 7 to 10 days.

- Physical therapy with a qualified hand therapist is recommended in postoperative cases, after prolonged immobilization, and after splinting mallet finger if return to full ROM is not progressing.

SURGERY/OTHER PROCEDURES

- Reduction of fractures is not amenable to conservative management.
- Tendon repair

ADMISSION, INPATIENT, AND NURSING CONSIDERATIONS

Generally reserved for severe, infected, or complicated injuries requiring surgical intervention.

ONGOING CARE

FOLLOW-UP RECOMMENDATIONS

Repeat radiographs:

- *Mallet fractures*: 1 to 2 weeks to document stability (x-ray in splint) and at 4 to 6 weeks if there is any evidence of extension lag
- *Longitudinal and transverse shaft fractures*: at 2 weeks
- *Pediatric epiphyseal fractures (including Seymour fracture)*: at 1 to 2 weeks to document stability; optional at 4 weeks depending on clinical progress

PROGNOSIS

In general, distal phalanx fractures are usually stable and heal with an uneventful course.

COMPLICATIONS

- Nonunion or malunion
- Infection for open fractures or Seymour fractures
- Joint stiffness or osteoarthritis
- Permanent loss of flexor tendon function or dysfunction with undiagnosed or delayed treatment for flexor tendon avulsions or disruptions
- Physeal arrest in children
- Avascular necrosis with displaced unicondylar fractures, especially in children
- Swan neck deformity especially with mallet finger
- Neurovascular injury
- Skin necrosis from prolonged splinting

REFERENCES

1. Liao JCY, Das De S. Management of tendon and bony injuries of the distal phalanx. *Hand Clin*. 2021;37(1):27–42.
2. Kumar NG, Chung KC. An evidence-based guide for managing phalangeal fractures. *Plast Reconstr Surg*. 2021;147(5):846e–861e.
3. Sivakumar BS, Graham DJ, Ledgard JP, et al. Acute mallet finger injuries—a review. *J Hand Surg Am*. 2023;48(3):283–291.
4. Lin JS, Samora JB. Surgical and nonsurgical management of mallet finger: a systemic review. *J Hand Surg Am*. 2018;43(2):146–163.e2.
5. Loewenstein SN, Adkinson JM. Pediatric fingertip injuries. *Hand Clin*. 2021;37(1):107–116.
6. Kiely AL, Nolan GS, Cooper LRL. Management of Seymour fractures in children and adolescents: a systemic review and meta-analysis. *J Hand Surg Am* 2022;47(12):1223.e1–1223.e20.

CLINICAL PEARLS

- *Mallet finger*: Patients who remove their splint even for a brief moment must start treatment over at day 1. Monitoring of skin care should be a priority because splinting for this injury is continuous and prolonged. Delayed injuries as old as >1 month may be amenable to standard conservative treatment.
- *Tuft fractures and fingertip crush injuries*: Demand careful management of the nail bed and pulp to prevent complications related to nail dystrophy and infection.
- *Seymour fracture*: Pediatric distal phalanx fracture in children mimicking mallet fracture or dislocation injury and whose early treatment directly effects outcomes and demand surgical consultation.
- All open fractures need antibiotic and tetanus prophylaxis.

FRACTURE, DISTAL RADIUS

Amy B. Jones, MD • Haris Vakil, MD

BASICS

DESCRIPTION

- Classically, a Colles fracture involves dorsal displacement and angulation of the fractured distal radius portion, often resulting in a "silver-fork deformity."
- Other variations include:
  - Smith fracture (volar displacement and angulation)
  - Dorsal Barton fracture: dorsal fracture-dislocation involving displacement of carpus with distal fragment
  - Volar Barton (also known as reverse Barton): fracture with volar displacement
  - Hutchinson fracture (also known as chauffeur's fracture): lateral-oriented fracture through radial styloid process extending into radiocarpal articulation
  - Galeazzi fracture-dislocation: fracture of distal third of radius with associated dislocation of distal radioulnar joint
  - Die-punch fracture: a depressed fracture of the lunate fossa on the articular surface of the distal radius
- Synonym(s): Colles fracture; Smith fracture; Barton fracture; dorsal Barton; reverse Barton fracture; volar Barton; Hutchinson fracture; chauffeur's fracture; Galeazzi fracture-dislocation; die-punch fracture

EPIDEMIOLOGY

- Most common fracture of the upper extremity (1)
- Most common fracture in adolescents at the age of puberty (1)
- Incidence also peaks in the 7th to 8th decades of life. A 6-fold higher incidence of Colles fractures occurs in elderly females compared to elderly males (1).
- In one study, an increase in sports-related activities, soccer, and inline skating correlated with an increase in fractures in the pediatric population (1).

ETIOLOGY AND PATHOPHYSIOLOGY

Commonly sustained by falling onto an outstretched hand with the wrist in extension

RISK FACTORS

- In general, decreased bone mineral density and unsteady gait
- In sports activities with high risk of falls and impact: snowboarding, football, ice skating, etc.

COMMONLY ASSOCIATED CONDITIONS

- Arthrosis secondary to poor joint approximation at radioulnar or radiocarpal joint
- Joint stiffness or weakness
- Median nerve dysfunction—the median nerve and flexor tendons run volar to the distal radius.
- Triangular fibrocartilage complex (TFCC) injury

DIAGNOSIS

HISTORY

- Elicit specific details regarding falls or trauma involved in high- or low-energy mechanism.
- Comorbid conditions such as osteoporosis or malignancy

PHYSICAL EXAM

- Key is to always describe fracture location, angulation, displacement, and involvement of either radiocarpal or radioulnar joints.
- Gross visualization of the involved extremity for bony deformity and evidence of open injury
- Pain, swelling, and limitation of movement of distal upper extremity
- Tenderness to the dorsal aspect of the wrist
- Paresthesias, weakness, or coolness to touch (associated neurologic or vascular injury)
- Neurologic evaluation, including radial, median, and ulnar nerve testing
- Vascular evaluation, including capillary refill, radial, and ulnar pulses
- In addition to fracture, one must evaluate for associated injuries at the scapholunate joint, distal radioulnar joint, ulnar styloid, and elbow injuries.
- Multiple classification systems have been described: Fernandez is based on mechanism of injury, Frykman is based on joint involvement, Melone divides intra-articular fractures into four types based on displacement, AO/OTA is a more comprehensive classification system, Lafontaine criteria and the McQueen equation predict secondary displacement after reduction.

DIFFERENTIAL DIAGNOSIS

- Carpal fracture
- Ulnar fracture
- Radiocarpal sprain
- Radioulnar sprain
- Soft tissue/bony contusion

DIAGNOSTIC TESTS & INTERPRETATION

- Consider obtaining bilateral x-rays to compare angulation.
- Anteroposterior (AP)/lateral views of wrist, forearm, and elbow
- AP view of the wrist: measures radial height (normal 13 mm, note shortening >5 mm), radial inclination (normal 22 degrees, note change >5 degrees), articular step-off (note >2 mm step-off), and ulnar variance:
  - Decreased radial height and inclination result in a hand that appears radially deviated with increased prominence of the ulnar head.
- Lateral view of the wrist: measures lateral tilt (normal 11 degrees volar, note dorsal angulation >5 degrees or within 20 degrees of contralateral distal radius):
  - Altered lateral tilt of the articular surface may cause midcarpal instability.
- AP and lateral view of the forearm and elbow: useful for identifying a Galeazzi fracture-dislocation (Loss of radius length producing an ulnar positive wrist increases the chance of symptomatic ulnar impaction syndrome.)
- Computed tomography (CT) scan: important to evaluate intra-articular involvement and for surgical planning
- Magnetic resonance imaging (MRI): useful to evaluate for soft tissue injuries such as TFCC injuries, scapholunate ligament injuries, and lunotriquetral injuries
- In a recent study, sports ultrasound has been found to have a sensitivity of 97.1% specificity of 100%, and a positive predictive value of 100% in diagnosing distal radius fractures in the pediatric population (2)[C].

TREATMENT

Treatment of the fractures may vary significantly based on the type of fracture, patient demands, and physician experience:

- Analgesia:
  - Adequate pain relief using oral and/or intravenous (IV) narcotics
  - Hematoma blocks can provide pain relief for closed reductions (may be less effective than IV regional anesthesia).
- Nondisplaced/minimally displaced fractures:
  - Can be initially immobilized in a sugar tong splint or radial gutter splint until follow-up

- Pediatric torus fracture can be treated safely with a wrist immobilizer. Displaced fractures/unstable fractures warrant orthopedic referral.
- Reduction techniques:
  - Goal is to achieve anatomical alignment to allow proper healing of the fragments and eventual restoration of normal function.
  - Reduction should always be accomplished in a timely manner before soft tissue inflammatory changes progress, especially if signs of neurovascular compromise are present.
  - Finger trap reduction method is most common:
    - Finger traps are applied to thumb, index, and middle fingers with manual traction or by finger traps hanging from an IV pole with the patient's arm at 90 degrees.
    - Reduction may be achieved by distal manual reduction methods or by a weighted stockinette.
  - Multiple attempts at reduction and late remanipulation at >7 days postinjury are known risk factors for physeal arrest (3).
- Postreduction evaluation:
  - Repeat neurovascular examination.
  - Postreduction x-rays (AP and lateral) after application of immobilizing device to assure maintenance of reduction

MEDICATION

Acetaminophen is preferred for mild to moderate pain due to theoretical concern about nonsteroidal anti-inflammatory drugs (NSAIDs) inhibiting bone healing.

ISSUES FOR REFERRAL

- Emergent orthopedic referral:
  - Open fractures
  - Acute neuromuscular compromise
  - Tenting of the skin
  - Compartment syndrome
- Nonemergent orthopedic referral:
  - Unstable fractures
  - Intra-articular involvement
  - Comminution
  - Fractures involving the physis
  - Severe osteoporosis
  - Displacement involving >2/3 the width of the radius
  - Dorsal angulation >5 degrees or >20 degrees of contralateral distal radius
  - >5 mm radial shortening or ulnar variance >5 mm
  - Progressive loss of volar tilt and loss of radial length following closed reduction and casting

ADDITIONAL THERAPIES

There is limited evidence to suggest a short-term benefit of physical therapy after distal radius fracture.

SURGERY/OTHER PROCEDURES

- Operative management is indicated for significantly displaced or unstable fractures.
- Multiple surgical techniques, percutaneous pinning, external fixation, volar or dorsal plating are used in the treatment of distal radius fractures.
- Nonoperative management is generally preferred in the geriatric population in appropriate circumstances.
- In athletes, operative management may allow faster return to play than nonoperative management.
- If athlete performance is not substantially limited by pain or being in a cast, a displaced fracture requiring surgery can be delayed 1 to 2 weeks until the end of the season.

ONGOING CARE

FOLLOW-UP RECOMMENDATIONS

- Most patients should be reexamined and x-rays repeated in 3 to 5 days for nondisplaced, and 2 to 3 days for displaced fractures to ensure fracture stability.
- Splint removed and short-arm cast for 4 to 6 weeks for nondisplaced fractures, and long-arm cast for reduced fractures for 3 to 4 weeks, followed by a short arm cast for a total of 6 to 8 weeks
- Repeat x-rays every 2 to 3 weeks for nondisplaced fractures and every week for reduced fractures.
- Healing time is generally 6 to 8 weeks in adults and 3 to 4 weeks in children.
- Range of motion (ROM) exercises (4)[A]:
  - Whether treated nonoperatively with a cast or operatively, the evidence suggests a home exercise program is sufficient and supervised physical therapy is not routinely required.
- Stepwise return to play can be initiated once at least 80% baseline ROM and strength is achieved.
  - If use of wrist is required, evidence of radiographic healing must be present.
  - If use of wrist is not required, athlete can return to play in a cast.

PROGNOSIS

Generally good, with most patients regaining full function and motion at the wrist

COMPLICATIONS

- Severe acute complications, such as neurovascular injuries and compartment syndrome, are associated with high-energy trauma and are, fortunately, rare.
- TFCC injuries
- Median nerve neuropathy (carpal tunnel syndrome):
  - Most frequent neurologic complication
  - 1–12% in low-energy fractures and 30% in high-energy fractures
  - Prevent by avoiding immobilization in excessive wrist flexion and ulnar deviation (Cotton-Loder position).
- Ulnar nerve neuropathy: seen with distal radioulnar joint injuries
- Extensor pollicis longus tendon rupture (5):
  - Most common in nondisplaced or minimally displaced distal radius fractures (incidence from 0.3–5.0%)
  - Usually between 6.6 weeks after distal radius fracture
- Degenerative changes, stiffness, and pain are more common in intra-articular fractures.
- Malunion and nonunion may occur. Malunion is the most common complication in pediatric patients.

REFERENCES

1. Davis ES, Chung KC. Epidemiology of distal radius fractures. In: Buijze GA, Jupiter J, Chammas M, eds. *Distal Radius Fractures: Evidence-Based Management.* Elsevier; 2021:13–19.
2. Ko C, Baird M, Close M, et al. The diagnostic accuracy of ultrasound in detecting distal radius fractures in a pediatric population. *Clin J Sport Med.* 2019;29(5):426–429.
3. Poublon AR, van der Windt AE, Ploegmakers JJW, et al. Pediatric distal radius fractures. In: Buijze GA, Jupiter J, Chammas M, eds. *Distal Radius Fractures: Evidence-Based Management.* Elsevier; 2021:277–290.
4. Lee HI, Kim JP. Rehabilitation protocols after distal radius fracture. In: Buijze GA, Jupiter J, Chammas M, eds. *Distal Radius Fractures: Evidence- Based Management.* Elsevier; 2021:253–262.
5. Romano N, Fischetti A, Mussetto I, et al. Extensor pollicis longus (EPL) tendon rupture as a complication of distal radius fracture: the role of ultrasound examination. *Med Ultrason.* 2018;1(1):114–115.

ADDITIONAL READING

LaMartina J, Jawa A, Stucken C, et al. Predicting alignment after closed reduction and casting of distal radius fractures. *J Hand Surg Am.* 2015;40(5):934–939.

CLINICAL PEARLS

- Swelling and pain over the physis may indicate a physeal injury even with normal radiographs.
- Physical exam and radiographic analysis are key to determining management of distal radius fractures.

F

FRACTURE, FIBULA

Brian Young Kim, MD, MS, CAQSM • Rachel T. Duong, MD

BASICS

DESCRIPTION

- Isolated fracture of the shaft of the fibula (below the neck of the fibula and proximal to the lateral malleolus) without evidence of associated ligamentous injury
- Synonym(s): fibula shaft fracture; fibula diaphyseal fracture; fibula stress fracture

EPIDEMIOLOGY

- Isolated fibula shaft fractures are rare, and there is limited data on overall incidence and prevalence in the literature.
- A UK trauma study data demonstrated a fibula fracture incidence of 7.57/100,000 per year (1).
- Fibula stress fractures have moderate incidence among stress fractures, 8.6% of all fractures (2).

RISK FACTORS

- Direct blow or trauma to the lateral leg leading to injury of the fibular shaft
- Contact sports or sports that require high repetitive axial loading may make some athletes more susceptible (3),(4).
- Distance running and repetitive jumping on hard surfaces can increase risk of stress fractures (2).
- Independent of trauma, risk factors include low bone density, advanced age, disordered eating, female sex, cigarette smoking (4).

DIAGNOSIS

HISTORY

Patients may describe direct trauma to the lateral leg and complain of pain and swelling in that area. They may be able to bear weight with minimal or no pain.

PHYSICAL EXAM

- Tenderness to palpation over the fracture site with possible swelling and ecchymosis
- It is important to examine the ankle and the knee for concomitant injuries, including proximal fibula fracture, distal fibula or tibia fracture, or injury to the syndesmosis.
- Detailed neurovascular exam with particular attention to the peroneal nerve

DIFFERENTIAL DIAGNOSIS

Fracture or injury to the knee, ankle, tibia, proximal or distal fibula, peroneal nerve, and/or anterior syndesmosis

DIAGNOSTIC TESTS & INTERPRETATION

- Radiographs of the tibia/fibula with anteroposterior, lateral, and mortise views
- Stress views or radiographs of the knee and ankle if suspicion for associated injuries exists
- No further imaging is necessary for isolated fibular shaft fractures.
- High-resolution ultrasound imaging may be useful when radiographs are not immediately available or when evaluating for stress or occult fracture if not seen on initial radiographs (3)[C],(5)[C].

TREATMENT

GENERAL MEASURES

- Treatment is based on patient comfort.
- If patient is having pain with ambulation, then a splint, cast, or walking boot may be used.
- Otherwise, a compression dressing is sufficient.
- Immobilization for 3 to 4 weeks is recommended, followed by graded progression back to sport.
- Healing time usually takes about 6 to 8 weeks but may be prolonged in some athletes (2)[C],(3)[C].

ISSUES FOR REFERRAL

Patient should be referred to an orthopedic surgeon if fracture is comminuted, significantly displaced, there is an associated fracture of the tibia, or there is evidence of neurovascular injury or painful nonunion.

ALERT

Special attention should be given to evaluation of the syndesmosis and peroneal nerve.

REFERENCES

1. Zhang J, Bradshaw F, Hussain I, et al. The epidemiology of lower limb fractures: a major United Kingdom (UK) Trauma Centre study. *Cureus*. 2024;16(34):e56581.
2. Encinas R, Sharpe J, Bakaes Y, et al. Fibula stress fractures: a systematic review. *Foot Ankle Spec*. 2025;18(5):501–507.
3. Canton G, Sborgia A, Maritan G, et al. Fibula fractures management. *World J Orthop*. 2021;12(5):254–269.
4. Graham P. Fibula fracture. *Orthop Nurs*. 2019;38(5):342–345.
5. Smith SE, Chang EY, Ha AS, et al. ACR appropriateness criteria acute trauma to the ankle. *J Am Coll Radiol*. 2020;17(11S):S355–S366.

CLINICAL PEARLS

- Patients should generally be immobilized for 3 to 4 weeks.
- The fracture will heal in 6 to 8 weeks.
- Depending on symptoms, rehabilitation may begin at 4 to 6 weeks and training at 6 to 8 weeks. Return to contact activities may take longer and has increased risk of refracture.
- Usually there are no complications, but a small percentage may result in nonunion, peroneal nerve injury, or associated damage to the interosseus membrane.
- Careful evaluation of the mechanism of injury should be made to avoid missing pronation–external rotation injuries that often have associated ligamentous injury (Weber C fractures). Such fractures may be unstable, and prompt orthopedic referral should be made if they are suspected.

FRACTURE, FIFTH METATARSAL (AVULSION, JONES FRACTURES)

Matthew Wessinger, MD, MPH • Mark E. Lavallee, MD, CSCS, FACSM, FAMSSM

BASICS

DESCRIPTION

- Fractures of the proximal 5th metatarsal occur at different locations, often with different etiologies. Prognosis and treatment differ vastly, and there is potential to have chronic pain and instability of the foot if not treated properly. Proximal 5th metatarsal fractures are classified into three types by region (aka zones), especially in relation to the joint at the base of the 4th/5th metatarsals (1),(2),(3),(4),(5):
  - Avulsion fracture of the tuberosity (zone I):
    - Near splayed insertion of the peroneus brevis tendon (within 0.5 cm from proximal tip of 5th metatarsal)
    - Located extra-articular and do not extend into the joint between the 4th and 5th metatarsal; these fractures intersect cubometatarsal joint.
  - Jones fracture (metaphyseal–diaphyseal junction) (zone II):
    - Fracture line extends into or toward the articulation between the bases of the 4th and 5th metatarsals (measuring usually between 0.5 and 1.5 cm from the proximal tip of the 5th metatarsal).
    - They heal more slowly and are prone to delayed union and nonunion because they have a relatively poor blood supply and have increased stresses across intertarsal ligament and fracture site.
  - Diaphyseal stress fractures (zone III):
    - Most commonly occur just distal to the 4th and 5th intermetatarsal articulation to midshaft
    - Result of chronic, repetitive microtrauma, especially in younger athletes
    - Heal most slowly and have greatest risk of delayed union, nonunion, and recurrence.
  - Torg classification according to healing potential (2):
    - **Type I** (acute): acute without prior fracture. X-rays show clean fracture without sclerosis.
    - **Type II** (delayed union): involves prior symptoms or a known stress fracture. X-rays show medullary sclerosis and a widened fracture line.
    - **Type III** (nonunion): involves prior symptoms or a known stress fracture. X-rays show evidence of repeated trauma, widened fracture line, and exuberant sclerosis (suggesting fracture nonunion).
- Synonym(s): tennis or pseudo-Jones fracture: avulsion fracture of base of the 5th metatarsal

EPIDEMIOLOGY

- 5th metatarsal fractures account for 68% of metatarsal fractures (2).
- **Avulsion fractures** are the most common type of fracture (93% of fractures).
- **Diaphyseal stress fractures** are the least common type of fracture (3% of fractures).

ETIOLOGY AND PATHOPHYSIOLOGY

- Avulsion fracture of the tuberosity: inversion ankle injuries
- Jones fracture: twisting injuries of the forefoot, vertical forces over the lateral aspect of forefoot while foot is plantarflexed, trauma to the area
- Stress fracture: repetitive impact to the lateral foot (3)

RISK FACTORS

- Previous fracture to the proximal 5th metatarsal
- Lateral ankle instability
- Static forefoot adduction
- Genu varum heel
- Tibia vara
- Metatarsus adductus

COMMONLY ASSOCIATED CONDITIONS

Associated injuries and complications:

- Lateral ankle sprain: Tuberosity avulsion fractures are commonly associated with ankle sprains with the foot inverted and plantarflexed. The anterior talofibular and calcaneofibular ligaments often are injured, and there may be swelling and ecchymosis just anterior and distal to the lateral malleolus.
- Proximal 5th metatarsal stress fracture: Patient may have had a previously undiagnosed and slightly symptomatic stress fracture of the proximal 5th metatarsal.
- There is a high incidence of delayed union, nonunion, and refracture with Jones and diaphyseal stress fractures due to retrograde blood supply.

DIAGNOSIS

HISTORY

- Determine mechanism of injury.
- Determine presence of prior injury to the 5th metatarsal.
- Determine history of ankle sprain as this can lead to loss of proprioception and reflex inhibition which predisposes athlete to this injury.
- Determine medical problems predisposing to injury as follows: osteoporosis, multiple prior stress fractures, diabetes, peripheral neuropathy.

PHYSICAL EXAM

- Signs and symptoms:
  - Patient may complain of pain over the lateral aspect of foot, especially when weight-bearing on plantarflexed foot.
  - Patient may note swelling or ecchymosis of the proximal 5th metatarsal and lateral foot.
- Physical examination:
  - Patient is tender to palpation over the proximal 5th metatarsal.
  - Palpate the peroneus brevis tendon to assess its integrity.
  - Vascular status is normally intact, including posterior tibial and dorsalis pedis pulses and capillary refill.
  - Check sensation: If decreased around lateral aspect of foot, the lateral dorsal cutaneous nerve, a branch off the sural nerve, may be injured.
  - Resisted eversion/external rotation of foot activates the peroneus brevis muscle and will typically reproduce pain at fracture site.
  - Full examination of the distal fibular, lateral ligaments, and foot helps identify associated ankle or foot injury.

DIFFERENTIAL DIAGNOSIS

- Peroneus brevis or peroneus longus tendon injury
- Anterior process calcaneus fracture
- Apophysitis (Iselin disease) or apophyseal avulsion fracture. The 5th metatarsal apophysis (secondary ossification center) closes between ages 9 and 11 years in girls, and 11 and 14 years in boys.
- Accessory ossicles
- Hematoma of lateral proximal foot
- Midshaft diaphyseal fracture of the 5th metatarsal
- Sprain of the cubometatarsal joint

DIAGNOSTIC TESTS & INTERPRETATION

- Standard x-ray films: anteroposterior (AP), lateral, and oblique views of the foot. If findings are suggestive of ankle trauma meeting the Ottawa criteria (patient between ages of 15 and 55 years with inability to walk five steps after injury *or* tender over posterior third of distal fibula), ankle films (AP, lateral, and oblique views) should also be taken.
- Acute stress fractures may not be detected on initial radiographs. Repeat radiographs recommended in 10 to 14 days if clinically suspected (2).
- Apophysitis
- Obliquely oriented small bony fleck at the base of the 5th metatarsal which is best seen on oblique radiograph
- Apophyseal irregularity

TREATMENT

Acute treatment:

- **ANALGESIA:**
  - Apply ice, rest, and elevate foot.
  - Oral pain relief (acetaminophen) or topical lidocaine is often sufficient if reduction not necessary.
    - Nonsteroidal anti-inflammatory drugs (NSAIDs) may increase rates of nonunion in acute fractures (6).
  - If reduction is needed, consider performing a hematoma block (2 to 5 mL of 1% lidocaine).
  - Significantly displaced fracture warrants an orthopedic referral for possible surgery.
- **REDUCTION TECHNIQUES:**
  - Generally, not recommended if surgical fixation is an option
  - Distract the 5th toe in the longitudinal plane. Apply plantar or dorsal pressure to the proximal portion of the 5th metatarsal.
- **POSTREDUCTION EVALUATION:**
  - Check alignment via postreduction radiographs.
- **IMMOBILIZATION:**
  - Avulsion fractures (zone I):
    - Place in a hard-soled shoe or postoperative shoe for 3 to 4 weeks (1)[A].
    - Can place in a walking boot or walking cast if cannot ambulate without pain in shoe, or if worried about patient compliance; will reduce plantar flexion thus forefoot load; may weight-bear as tolerated (1),(3)[A]
  - Jones (metaphyseal–diaphyseal) fractures (zone II) and diaphyseal stress fractures (zone III):
    - *Type I* (acute): For nondisplaced or minimally displaced fractures (<2 mm), can place patient in short leg cast and make strict non–weight-bearing for 6 to 8 weeks (or longer). Otherwise, consider surgical fixation (1),(3)[A]. Nonsurgical fracture healing rates approach 75%.
    - *Type II* (delayed union/stress): Consider surgical fixation because of better prognosis and quicker return to activity; occasionally can consider prolonged immobilization (up to 16 weeks) with non–weight-bearing for selective patients (1),(2)[A]
    - *Type III* (nonunion): Consider surgical fixation (1),(3)[A].

ADDITIONAL THERAPIES

- Special considerations: When deciding on treatment for type II fractures, consider the athlete's timetable and previous medical history.
- Operative treatment is preferred for elite athletes who wish to avoid the prolonged immobilization of conservative treatment.
- Occasionally after conservative treatment, a nonunion develops secondary to retrograde vascular supply to the bone.
- Bone stimulation (electrical or ultrasound) has shown in some cases to improve healing for delayed union and nonunion fractures (1)[B]. Progression to surgery may be indicated instead of using bone stimulation or if there is inadequate healing with bone stimulation.
- Faster return to play, shorter time to union, and decrease pain are associated with operative intervention (7)[A].
- **REHABILITATION:**
  - Avulsion fractures: Start with range of motion and progress to strengthening of the peroneus brevis (external rotation and pronation of the foot). Patient may return to play after 3 to 4 weeks and when no longer symptomatic.
  - Jones fractures: Once no longer immobilized, start with range of motion and progress to strengthening. Electrical stimulation may help patient initially learn to reactivate musculature. Resume weight-bearing activities slowly after radiographic and clinical healing progressive rehab for strength and proprioception.

SURGERY/OTHER PROCEDURES

- Avulsion fractures rarely require surgery (4).
- Jones (metaphyseal–diaphyseal) and diaphyseal stress fractures:
  - Type I: Consider surgical fixation (open reduction, internal fixation with a cannulated screw) for athletes and active patients who wish quicker return to play (1),(2),(4),(6).
  - Type II (delayed union) and type III (nonunion): Refer for surgical evaluation (1),(3).

ONGOING CARE

FOLLOW-UP RECOMMENDATIONS

Referral/disposition:

- Orthopedic referral for surgery as indicated above and for avulsion fractures that are displaced (rare), comminuted (rare), or involve >30% of the cubometatarsal articulation.
- Patients not responding to home exercise programs after immobilization is complete may benefit from referral to physical therapy.
- *Type I* Jones or diaphyseal stress fractures should be referred to an orthopedist if patient prefers surgery in order to return to play quicker or the fracture is displaced or comminuted.

REFERENCES

1. Albloushi M, Alshanqiti A, Qasem M, et al. Jones type fifth metatarsal fracture fixation in athletes: a review and current concept. *World J Orthop* 2021;12(9):640–650.
2. Cheung CN, Lui TH. Proximal fifth metatarsal fractures: anatomy, classification, treatment, and complications. *Arch Trauma Res*. 2016;5(4):e33298.
3. Fetzer GB, Wright RW. Metatarsal shaft fractures and fractures of the proximal fifth metatarsal. *Clin Sports Med*. 2006;25(1):139–150.
4. Hatch RL, Alsobrook JA, Clugston JR. Diagnosis and management of metatarsal fractures. *Am Fam Physician*. 2007;76(6):817–826.
5. Wang Y, Gan X, Li K, et al. Comparison of operative and non-operative management of fifth metatarsal base fracture: a meta-analysis. *PLoS ONE*. 2020;15(8):e0237151.
6. Al Farii H, Farahdel L, Frazer A, et al. The effect of NSAIDs on postfracture bone healing: a meta-analysis of randomized controlled trials. *OTA Int*. 2021;4(2):e092.
7. Metzl JA, Bowers MW, Anderson RB. Fifth metatarsal jones fractures: diagnosis and treatment. *J Am Acad Orthop Surg*. 2022;30(4):e470–e479.

ADDITIONAL READING

Porter DA. Fifth metatarsal jones fractures in the athlete. *Foot Ankle Int*. 2018;39(2):250–258.

CLINICAL PEARLS

- Fractures of the 5th metatarsal are classified by location (zones) and by healing potential (types).
- Use physical exam findings or clinical decision tools (i.e., Ottawa Ankle Rules) in conjunction with radiographic imaging to make diagnosis.
- Zone I injuries can typically be managed conservatively. Zone II or III fractures often require operative intervention.
- Operative intervention may be favored in high level athletes to reduce immobilization time from conservative treatment.
- With conservative treatment, clinicians must consider risk of nonunion due to retrograde blood flow of the 5th metatarsal.

FRACTURE, FRONTAL SINUS

Christopher A. Kroner, MD, MPH • Peter Hoang, MD • Anthony Chang, MD

BASICS

Pediatric Considerations

- Frontal sinuses are not present at birth. Although they begin to develop as early as 2 years of age, they are not identifiable by radiology until ages 5 to 7 years and continue developing until puberty (1).
- Ethmoid and maxillary sinuses are present at birth.
- Sphenoid sinuses develop around age 5 years.

DESCRIPTION

- Typically involve high-velocity blunt trauma localized to face/head/frontal sinus area.
- Most common mechanisms of injury are motor vehicle collisions, assaults, falls, sports injuries, and other accidents.
- Because the anterior table is thicker than the more lateral temporal bones, it requires 800 to 2,200 lb of force to cause frontal sinus fracture (twice the force required to fracture other facial bones) (1).
- There is no consensus on classification of frontal sinus fractures. Most common classification identifies involved frontal sinus anatomy:
  - Anterior wall/table
  - Posterior wall/table
  - Anterior and posterior walls/table
  - Nasofrontal duct (NFD) involvement

EPIDEMIOLOGY

- Frontal sinus fractures account for 5–15% of all facial fractures (2).
- 35% have concomitant orbital fractures.
- 17% have zygomatic fractures.
- 15% have nasoorbitoethmoid fractures.
- 0.7–2.1% involve both anterior and posterior walls of the frontal sinus.
- More common in 20 to 40-year-old males.

RISK FACTORS

- High-velocity trauma to the face, especially in presence of other facial bone fractures.
- Motor vehicle collisions, assaults, and falls are the most common causes of mechanisms of injury (3).
- Contact sports, cycling, occupations with fall risk
- Substance abuse
- Lack of protective equipment
- Acromegaly: Size and extension of frontal sinuses are enlarged.

GENERAL PREVENTION

- Proper use of vehicle safety restraints (4)
- Consistent helmet wear and protective equipment
- Fall precautions

COMMONLY ASSOCIATED CONDITIONS

- Laceration of the supraorbital ridge, glabella, or lower forehead
- Frontal ecchymosis
- Disruption of the NFD
- Intracranial injuries in 12–17% of patients with frontal sinus fractures
- Associated cerebrospinal fluid (CSF) leak in 15% of patients with frontal sinus fractures
- Ocular injuries are present in up to 59%.
- Periorbital fractures
- Traumatic subcutaneous emphysema (TSE)
- Pneumothorax is present in up to 24% (5).
- Upper and lower extremity fractures are present in up to 25% (5).
- Concussion

DIAGNOSIS

HISTORY

- Mechanism of injury: victim of motor vehicle collision, assault to head/face, fall, or other high-velocity trauma
- May or may not have loss of consciousness
- Previous facial injuries

PHYSICAL EXAM

Failure to diagnose a frontal sinus fracture can lead to abscess formation, meningitis, mucocele formation, osteomyelitis of the calvarium, or permanent cosmetic deformity.

- Carefully palpate the frontal area for crepitus or depression.
- Lacerations over the frontal sinus area should raise suspicion of frontal sinus fracture and mandate digital palpation for a fracture
- Perform nasal speculum examination looking for blood, septal hematoma, or clear CSF.
- Perform otoscopic exam looking for otorrhea and/or hemotympanum (indicating more serious cranial injury).
- Perform careful neurologic examination to look for central nervous system (CNS) injury, including concussion.
- Perform careful ophthalmologic exam.
- Findings to raise concern for frontal sinus fracture are:
  - Laceration on the supraorbital ridge, glabella, or lower forehead
  - Ecchymosis of periorbital region
  - Periorbital edema
  - Depression or step-off identified on palpation of frontal sinus area that could indicate depressed anterior table fracture.
  - Crepitus over the frontal sinus
  - Periorbital subcutaneous emphysema
  - Associated facial trauma with supraorbital, orbital, nasal, frontonasoethmoid, or maxillary fractures
  - Bloody discharge from the nose without visible nasal source
  - Clear rhinorrhea or otorrhea indicative of CSF leak
  - Diplopia with upward or downward gaze
  - Supraorbital ridge anesthesia
  - Loss of consciousness or altered mental status
  - Facial subcutaneous emphysema following Valsalva maneuver

DIFFERENTIAL DIAGNOSIS

- Frontal bone fractures not involving the frontal sinus (may have a similar presentation)
- Nasofrontoethmoid fractures
- Cribriform plate fractures
- Other facial fractures including orbits, maxilla, nasal, and zygomatic bones
- Temporal bone fracture
- Parietal bone fracture
- Pott puffy tumor

DIAGNOSTIC TESTS & INTERPRETATION

- Double-ring or halo sign test on filter paper to identify CSF leak; confirmatory test for CSF leak is the β_2-transferrin test.
- Requires acute examination and imaging:
  - Computed tomography (CT) scanning is the imaging modality of choice:
    - Serial 1.5 mm cuts in the sagittal, axial, and coronal planes
    - Identification of frontal sinus fractures and concomitant paranasal and facial fractures
    - Anterior table fracture, displaced or nondisplaced; *displacement* is defined as bony displacement more than or equal to the width of the outer table.
    - Posterior table fracture identification: Associated intracranial injuries on CT scan may include subdural hemorrhage or pneumocephalus.
    - Frontonasal duct integrity
  - Caldwell and lateral radiographic views are good for preliminary evaluation, but frontal sinus fractures can be subtle on these films. Sinus pathology is strongly suspected when the x-rays show air-fluid levels, a diffusely cloudy sinus, or pneumocephalus.
  - CSF leaks can be assessed using CT myelogram.

TREATMENT

- Prehospital:
  - Airway, breathing, and circulation (ABCs)
  - Identify concomitant life-threatening injuries (5)[B].
  - Cervical immobilization as needed
- Emergency department (ED):
  - If the patient can taste the irrigating solution or notes the irrigating fluid in the nose during frontal scalp laceration irrigation, the frontal sinus is disrupted.
  - Lacerations overlying frontal sinus fractures involving only the anterior table may be sutured in the ED. Ear, nose, and throat (ENT), plastic surgery, or Oral and maxillofacial surgery (OMFS) should evaluate lacerations associated with more complex sinus injuries.
  - If an isolated simple anterior table fracture is noted without a posterior table fracture and intracranial injuries are ruled out, the presence of a frontonasal duct injury should be evaluated by instilling fluorescein into the frontal sinus. Lack of visualization of the fluorescein in the nose is indicative of disruption of the duct.
  - Perioperative antibiotics are indicated in patients requiring surgical management. The use of antibiotics prophylactically without surgery or postoperatively is not typically recommended (6)[A].
  - Nondisplaced frontal sinus fracture with a patent NFD and *no* neurologic involvement usually can be managed nonsurgically.
  - All displaced anterior wall fractures, all posterior wall fractures, all frontal sinus fractures with involvement/obstruction of the NFD, and all frontal sinus fractures with neurologic involvement require further surgical evaluation and probable surgical repair.

- Surgery/other procedures:
  - Endoscopic surgery (2)[C]
  - Ablation/obliteration
  - Cranialization
  - Open reduction internal fixation (ORIF)

MEDICATION

- Obtain culture if possible.
- Antibiotics
  - Perioperative (<24 hours): For adults, cefazolin 2 g IV q8h (3 g for patients weighing >120 kg); for pediatrics 30 mg/kg
  - Basilar skull fractures with CSF leak: ceftriaxone 2 g IV q8h for better CNS penetration

ADDITIONAL THERAPIES

The approach to each patient should be individualized but, in general, is based on three clinical factors:

- Fracture location and displacement
- Dural and cerebral involvement
- Damage to the frontal sinus drainage system

ADMISSION, INPATIENT, AND NURSING CONSIDERATIONS

- Initial stabilization:
  - ABCs of trauma care: Attend to the airway as the first priority:
    - Rapid sequence intubation (RSI) is the initial airway management of choice.
    - Massive facial injuries may require a surgical airway if RSI is unsuccessful.
  - If associated injuries are present, protect the cervical spine until cleared.
  - Other major injuries and life threats take precedence over the frontal sinus fracture.
- Admission criteria:
  - Patients with other significant associated trauma
  - Patients with posterior table fractures
  - Patients with associated intracranial injuries
  - Patients with CSF leak
- Discharge criteria:
  - Patients with frontal sinus fractures who may be discharged are those with isolated frontal sinus fracture and those who have no involvement of the posterior table or evidence of an intracranial injury on CT scan.
  - Referral to ENT/OMFS in 24 to 36 hours is appropriate.
  - Patients with complex fractures may be discharged when cleared by neurosurgery, ENT, or OMFS.

ONGOING CARE

PATIENT EDUCATION

- Avoid increased sinus pressure (e.g., sneezing, nose blowing, Valsalva) to minimize risk of subcutaneous emphysema.
- Avoid air travel for a period (individualize for each patient) after frontal sinus fracture.
- Long-term use of helmet during sporting activities with high velocity head injury risks

COMPLICATIONS

- Early complications:
  - Postoperative contour deformity
  - Sinusitis
  - Hematoma (1)[C]
  - Wound infection (1)[C]
  - Meningitis
  - Traumatic brain injury (TBI)
  - CSF leak
- Late complications (requires surgical referral for any of these):
  - Cavernous sinus thrombosis
  - Hypoesthesia/anesthesia (1)[C]
  - Encephalitis
  - Mucocele
  - Mucopyocele
  - Osteomyelitis
  - Brain abscess
  - Chronic frontal headaches
  - Diplopia
  - Ophthalmoplegia

REFERENCES

1. Podolsky DJ, Moe KS. Frontal sinus fractures. *Semin Plast Surg.* 2021;35(4):274–283.
2. Vincent A, Wang W, Shokri T, et al. Management of frontal sinus fractures. *Facial Plast Surg.* 2019;35(6):645–650.
3. Fox PM, Garza R, Dusch M, et al. Management of frontal sinus fractures: treatment modality changes at a level 1 trauma center. *J Craniofac Surg.* 2014;25(6):2038–2042.
4. Lopez CD, Colon RR, Lopez J, et al. Frontal sinus fractures: evidence and clinical reflections. *Plast Reconstr Surg Glob Open.* 2022;10(4):e4266.
5. Rodriguez ED, Stanwix MG, Nam AJ, et al. Twenty-six-year experience treating frontal sinus fractures: a novel algorithm based on anatomical fracture pattern and failure of conventional techniques. *Plastic Reconstr Surg.* 2008;122(6):1850–1866.
6. Habib AM, Wong AD, Schreiner GC, et al. Postoperative prophylactic antibiotics for facial fractures: a systemic review and meta-analysis. *Laryngoscope.* 2019;129(1):82–95.

ADDITIONAL READING

- Alon EE, Glikson E, Shoshani Y, et al. Repair of frontal sinus fractures: clinical and radiological long-term outcomes. *J Laryngol Otol.* 2021;135(5):448–451.
- Brasileiro BF, Cortez ALV, Asprino L, et al. Traumatic subcutaneous emphysema of the face associated with paranasal sinus fractures: a prospective study. *J Oral Maxillofac Surg.* 2005;63(8):1080–1087.
- Chouake RJ, Miles BA. Current opinion in otolaryngology and head and neck surgery: frontal sinus fractures. *Curr Opin Otolaryngol Head Neck Surg.* 2017;25(4):326–331.
- Chukwulebe S, Hogrefe C. The diagnosis and management of facial bone fractures. *Emerg Med Clin North Am.* 2019;37(1):137–151.
- Dedhia RD, Morisada MV, Tollefson TT, et al. Contemporary management of frontal sinus fractures. *Curr Opin Otolaryngol Head Neck Surg.* 2019;27(4):253–260.
- Eirale C, Lockhart R, Chalabi H. Conservative treatment in an isolated anterior wall frontal bone fracture in an elite soccer player. *Clin J Sport Med.* 2010;20(2):125–127.
- Hoshal SG, Dedhia RD, Strong EB. Frontal sinus fractures: a contemporary approach in the endoscopic era. *Facial Plast Surg Clin North Am.* 2022;30(1):71–83.
- Jeyaraj P. Frontal bone fractures and frontal sinus injuries: treatment paradigms. *Ann Maxillofac Surg.* 2019;9(2):261–282.
- Jin HR, Shim WS, Jung HJ. Minimally invasive technique to reduce the isolated anterior wall fracture of the frontal sinus. *J Craniofac Surg.* 2019;30(8):2375–2377.
- Jing XL, Luce E. Frontal sinus fractures: management and complications. *Craniomaxillofac Trauma Reconstr.* 2019;12(3):241–248.
- Johnson NR, Roberts MJ. Frontal sinus fracture management: a systematic review and meta-analysis. *Int J Oral Maxillofac Surg.* 2021;50(1):75–82.
- Kaufman BR, Heckler FR. Sports-related facial injuries. *Clin Sports Med.* 1997;16(3):543–562.
- Kim I, Kim JM, Kim J, et al. Management of frontal sinus trauma: a retrospective study of surgical interventions and complications. *Maxillofac Plast Reconstr Surg.* 2024;46(1):4.
- Lofgren DH, McGuire D, Gotlib A. *Frontal Sinus Fractures.* StatPearls Publishing; 2020. Updated June 30, 2023. Accessed October 4, 2025. https://www.ncbi.nlm.nih.gov/books/NBK557519/
- Lopez CD, Colon RR, Lopez J, et al. Frontal sinus fractures: evidence and clinical reflections. *Plast Reconstr Surg Glob Open.* 2022;10(4):e4266.
- Metzinger SE, Metzinger RC. Complications of frontal sinus fractures. *Craniomaxillofac Trauma Reconstr.* 2009;2(1):27–34.
- Schultz JJ, Chen J, Sabharwal S, et al. Management of frontal bone fractures. *J Craniofac Surg.* 2019;30(7):2026–2029.
- Torre DD, Burtscher D, Kloss-Brandstätter A, et al. Management of frontal sinus fractures—treatment decision based on metric dislocation extent. *J Craniomaxillofac Surg.* 2014;42(7):1515–1519.

CLINICAL PEARLS

- Most common etiologies of frontal sinus fracture are motor vehicle accidents, assaults, and falls.
- For lacerations, ecchymosis, and/or edema to frontal sinus region following trauma, consider and evaluate with CT scan for frontal sinus fracture.
- Surgical intervention can vary widely based on injury and include ablation/obliteration, cranialization, and ORIF.
- Trauma patients must be critically evaluated based on advanced trauma life support (ATLS) protocols.

FRACTURE, HAMATE: HOOK, BODY

Mark Stovak, MD • Ryan Muehling, MD, CAQSM

BASICS

DESCRIPTION

A fracture through the hook or the body of the hamate

EPIDEMIOLOGY

Hamate fractures occur in three patterns:

- Type 1: hook
- Type 2a: coronal (dorsal oblique and splitting)
- Type 2b: transverse (1)

Incidence

- Hook fracture:
  - Hook of the hamate fractures account for <2% of all carpal bone fractures (2).
  - The number of hook of the hamate fractures reported in the literature is low because routine x-rays usually are normal, and symptoms are nonspecific. Standard radiographs are often inconclusive and only identify 31% of fractures (2),(3).
  - Delay in diagnosis is common, with time from injury to presentation varying based on activity level of the patient. Although competitive athletes present sooner (4), most patients present to surgeons on average 5.5 to 10.2 months after injury (2).
  - Fractures most commonly occur at the base of the hook (1).
- Body fracture: Body of the hamate fracture is rare and much less common than hook fractures.

ETIOLOGY AND PATHOPHYSIOLOGY

- Acute traumatic injury
- Repetitive stress leads to a stress fracture.

RISK FACTORS

- Hook fracture: sporting activities that involve a bat, club, or racquet (2)
- Body fracture: either an axial load directed through the 4th or 5th metacarpals when a clenched fist strikes an unyielding object (i.e., punching mechanism), or a compressive force to the wrist (5)

GENERAL PREVENTION

Avoid holding the handle end of the bat, club, or stick in the palm to prevent it from creating pressure on the hook of the hamate.

DIAGNOSIS

HISTORY

- Hook fracture:
  - Hook of the hamate fracture occurs in athletes who use equipment with a handle (e.g., golf clubs, baseball bats, and racquets) (2)[C].
  - Athlete grips the handle of the club, bat, or racquet over the distal ulnar aspect of the palm, placing the handle in close proximity to the hook of the hamate (2)[C].
  - In golf, the fracture often occurs when the club head accidentally strikes too much ground and a large divot is taken. In baseball, most fractures occur at the end of forceful check swings as opposed to swings that make contact with the ball (2)[C].
  - A less common mechanism of injury is a fall on an outstretched hand (2)[C].
  - Stress fractures are also possible of the hook and are likely if no traumatic event can be identified in the history (2)[C].
- Body fracture:
  - Body fractures often result from punching a hard, stationary object, such as a wall, with a closed fist (type 2a). The 4th and 5th metacarpals are driven back into the hamate, leading to a fracture. Body fractures may accompany a boxer's fracture (1)[B].
  - 4th and 5th metacarpal dislocations are also common findings with body fractures.
  - They also may occur when the hamate is smashed between two objects in a dorsopalmar fashion (type 2b) (1)[B].
- Stress fractures have been described from repetitive military-style knuckle push-ups (5)[C].

PHYSICAL EXAM

- Point tenderness occurs in the palm over the hook of the hamate. The hook is located by projecting a line from the pisiform to the center of the head of the index metacarpal. Rarely, if the fracture is at the base of the hook, pain may be greater over the dorsal hamate than over the hook in the palm (because the hamate is covered on the volar aspect with thick skin, subcutaneous fibrofatty tissue, and parts of the palmaris brevis muscle and transverse carpal ligament, making palpation difficult) (2)[C].
- Painful and weak grasp (2)[C].
- Positive "pull test" may elicit pain on resisted flexion of the ulnar two digits with the wrist held in ulnar deviation. This test places force against the injured hamate as the flexor tendons lever against it during finger flexion and ulnar deviation (2)[C].
- Check pulses: An Allen test will help to rule out ulnar artery thrombosis (2)[C].
- Signs of partial or complete 4th/5th flexor digitorum profundus (FDP) tendon rupture may be present. Pain with grip; decreased grip strength; crepitance with 4th/5th finger motion; and, eventually, loss of active flexion at the 4th/5th finger distal interphalangeal joints may indicate FDP injury; a small percentage of all hook fractures are correctly diagnosed only after FDP tendon rupture (2)[C],(3)[B].
- Decreased sensation or weakness may be due to ulnar or median nerve injury. The fracture fragments may injure the nerves directly, or swelling and inflammation may injure them indirectly (2)[C].

DIFFERENTIAL DIAGNOSIS

- Flexor/extensor carpi ulnaris tendon injury
- Metacarpal/carpal bone fracture or contusion
- Ulnocarpal ligament sprain
- Triangular fibrocartilaginous complex tear
- Ulnar artery thrombosis
- Ulnar nerve entrapment/neuropathy
- Carpal tunnel syndrome

DIAGNOSTIC TESTS & INTERPRETATION

- Hook fracture:
  - The routine wrist series (anteroposterior [AP], lateral, and oblique views) usually are inconclusive, only identifying 31% of fractures and often delaying diagnosis (2)[C].
  - Ring of the hook can be visualized on AP view; if it is not present, this may be a clue to a hook fracture (3)[B].
  - Carpal tunnel view often will aid in making the diagnosis. However, to obtain this view, the wrist must be forcefully hyperextended. During the acute phase of the injury, pain and limited range of motion may not allow proper positioning to make this x-ray possible. The carpal tunnel view is 40–50% sensitive (2)[C].
  - Another useful view is the supinated oblique thumb–abducted view (2)[C].
  - An additional view is the hamate hook lateral view with the hook in the 1st web space with the wrist ulnar deviated and the thumb opposed (2)[C].
  - Computed tomography (CT) scanning is the gold standard for diagnosis but often is unnecessary if plain films show the fracture. CT scans are useful if plain films are negative and a fracture is highly suspected. CT scanning has the advantage of visualizing both hamates at the same time and can be used to evaluate the extremely rare case of a bipartite hamate, which usually is bilateral and is a normal variant. CT scan is performed with both hands in the praying position (palm to palm). CT scanning has a 100% sensitivity, a 98.4% specificity, and a 97.2% accuracy in the diagnosis of acute fractures (2)[C].
  - Magnetic resonance imaging (MRI) may be useful to evaluate for tendon or nerve injury (2)[C].
- Body fracture:
  - The routine wrist series (AP, lateral, and oblique views) is more useful for the diagnosis of body fractures than for hook fractures. The oblique and lateral views are the most useful. However, many fractures are still missed by plain films (1)[B].
  - CT scan may be needed to delineate further the exact fracture pattern and degree of fragment displacement. CT scan should be considered when routine films are negative, but a fracture is highly suspected (1)[B].

TREATMENT

- Hook fracture:
  - Acute treatment (<2 weeks):
    - *Conservative management:*
      - Conservative option for nondisplaced fractures is a short arm cast. The cast should immobilize the metacarpophalangeal joints of the 4th/5th fingers and be a thumb spica to decrease micromotion at the hook. Cast should be worn for 6 to 12 weeks to prevent nonunion, but nonunion is common with nonoperative management. If pain is still present after cast removal, then excision for nonunion is the treatment of choice (2)[C].
    - Decision between casting and surgery is based on the lifestyle demands of the patient. The athlete who does not want to risk having a nonunion after casting may opt for surgery to minimize the time away from sport. Similarly, a patient with a job that requires repetitive grabbing, gripping, or lifting may elect for excision to reduce the risk of an extended period of time away from work (2)[C].
  - Delayed treatment (>2 weeks):
    - Nonunion of the hook of the hamate is a concern. Nonunion is related to micromotion from the soft tissue attachments to the hook but also may be related to a tenuous blood supply similar to the scaphoid (2)[C].
    - Excision of the hook is the treatment of choice for these injuries. The sooner the fragment is removed and the base smoothed, the less likely is the chance for tendon rupture and/or neurovascular damage. There is a 15–17% incidence of flexor tendon ruptures in untreated hook fractures (2)[C].
    - An alternative approach is open reduction and internal fixation (ORIF); the goal is to maintain maximal grip strength by preserving the pulley system for the 4th/5th FDP tendons. Although this seems logical, the loss of grip strength associated with excision has been minimal, resulting in excision being the most popular surgical treatment method. Owing to the risk of nonunion and the potential for symptomatic hardware, ORIF is not recommended in athletes (2)[C].
    - Treatment for painless nonunion is excision to reduce the risk of tendon rupture and/or neurovascular injury (2)[C].
    - Ultrasound therapy has some reported success. A case study of two baseball players with hook of hamate fracture nonunion 5 and 3.5 months postinjury were successfully treated with ultrasound therapy. The patients received therapy for 20 minutes a day for 4 months and were limited to daily activities during this time. Bone union was confirmed with a CT scan, and neither patient reported any pain nor complications at a 1-year follow-up. However, these athletes were 15 and 16 years of age and began treatment many months after their injury (3)[B].
- Body fracture:
  - Coronal fractures are often associated with 4th and 5th metacarpal dislocations that require reduction. Once reduced, stability must be assessed. If the reduction is stable and the fracture nondisplaced, then a short arm cast can be used for 4 to 6 weeks (1)[C].
  - Transverse fractures, if not displaced, can be treated in a short arm cast for 4 to 6 weeks (1)[C].

SURGERY/OTHER PROCEDURES

- Hook fracture:
  - Acute treatment (<2 weeks):
    - Another option is immediate excision of the hook distal to the fracture rather than conservative treatment. Most patients return to their previous level of functioning in their sport or occupation, and return to activity is symptom dependent (2)[C].
    - Excision has been the favored approach for both displaced and nondisplaced fractures. Immobilization lasts 2 weeks with light motion and throwing at 4 weeks and return to bat or club sports at 6 weeks. The palmar incision may demonstrate prolonged sensitivity for 3 months, but a glove with padding may be used until scar sensitivity resolves (2)[C].
- Body fracture:
  - Acute treatment (<2 weeks):
    - Closed reduction and percutaneous pinning (CRPP) can be employed for coronal fractures associated with hamatometacarpal fracture-dislocations that involve <1/3 of the hamate articular surface, whereas those involving >1/3 of the articular surface require ORIF (5)[C].
    - If the coronal body fracture is displaced, then CRPP or ORIF must be used to obtain congruent joint surfaces to prevent degenerative joint disease (1)[C].
    - For displaced transverse fractures, CRPP or ORIF is recommended (1)[C].
  - Subacute or chronic treatment:
    - For fractures with subacute or chronic presentation and those with extensive articular damage, primary arthrodesis of the 4th or 5th CMC joints may be considered (5)[C].

ONGOING CARE

PROGNOSIS

- Prognosis of hook fractures is generally good if they are diagnosed and treated (cast, excision, ORIF) early before tendon injury/rupture occurs (2).
- Findings of professional baseball players show return to play in 6 to 8 weeks after hook excision. In one cohort study, on average, players began a hitting program at 4.6 weeks after surgery and were released into full baseball activities at 7.1 weeks after surgery (4).
- Prognosis for hamate body fractures is generally good if they are diagnosed and treated (cast, ORIF, closed reduction and pinned) early enough to maintain congruent joint surfaces (5).

COMPLICATIONS

- Complete rupture of the FDP tendon is reported to occur in 15–17% of cases of nonunion. The FDP of the little finger ruptures more commonly than that of the ring finger (2).
- Patients managed nonoperatively showed a nonunion rate of 2%, ulnar neuropathy rate of 1.7%, and tendon rupture rate of 0.2% within 1 year. In distinguishing between hook and body fractures, hook fractures demonstrated a nonunion rate of 2.2%, ulnar neuropathy rate of 2.7%, and tendon rupture rate of 0%, whereas body fractures had a nonunion rate of 1.2%, ulnar neuropathy rate of 1%, and tendon rupture rate of 0% (6).
- Complications associated with hamate body fractures include pain, stiffness, decreased grip strength, carpometacarpal subluxation, arthritis, malunion, nonunion, avascular necrosis, and nerve injury. Among the complications listed, pain, reduced range of motion (stiffness), and decreased grip strength is the most common, occurring in 7.5% of cases. These complications are frequently exacerbated by delayed diagnosis or noncompliance with posttreatment protocols (5).
- Complications postoperatively are variable, with one study finding a 25% incidence, the majority consisting of transient ulnar nerve dysfunction. Complications were more common among nonathletes, those presenting with nonunions, and those experiencing longer intervals between injury and surgery (4).

F

REFERENCES

1. Hirano K, Inoue G. Classification and treatment of hamate fractures. *Hand Surg.* 2005;10(2–3):151–157.
2. Ivy A, Stern P. Hamate hook and pisiform fractures. *Oper Tech Sports Med.* 2016;24(2):94–99.
3. Bachoura A, Wroblewski A, Jacoby SM, et al. Hook of hamate fractures in competitive baseball players. *Hand (N Y).* 2013;8(3):302–307.
4. Sheridan J, Sheridan D, Sheridan D. Hook of hamate fractures in major and minor league baseball players. *J Hand Surg Am.* 2021;46(8):653–659.
5. Price MB, Vanorny D, Mitchell S, et al. Hamate body fractures: a comprehensive review of the literature. *Curr Rev Musculoskelet Med.* 2021;14(6):475–484.
6. Ta CN, Finley Z, Medvedev GA. Complications after nonoperative management of hamate fractures. *Plast Reconstr Surg Glob Open.* 2022;10(5):e4352.

CLINICAL PEARLS

- The treatment option that will allow the quickest return to play with the least residual symptoms is excision of the hook of the hamate.
- Routine plain-film radiographs are not sensitive for identifying hook of the hamate fractures. A specialized view (e.g., carpal tunnel; radial-deviated, supinated oblique with thumb abduction; or hamate hook lateral) or a CT scan is usually needed for identification.
- Surgery is recommended to prevent tendon rupture even in the absence of pain related to fracture.

FRACTURE, HUMERAL SHAFT

Julie Chuan, MD, FAAFP, CAQSM

BASICS

DESCRIPTION

- Direct trauma from a fall on elbow or outstretched hand (FOOSH)
- Direct blow to the upper arm from motor vehicle or industrial accident
- Severe twisting injury from pitching a ball, arm wrestling
- Bone malignancy (pathologic fracture) (4%)
- Most commonly associated with radial nerve injury

Pediatric Considerations

Spiral fractures in children are concerning for child abuse.

EPIDEMIOLOGY

- 3% of all fractures, 14% of all humeral fractures
- Bimodal distribution in the 3rd and 7th decades
- 3rd decade male predominance owing to sports and vehicular trauma
- 7th decade female predominance owing to simple falls (1)
- 90% are due to trauma, low energy (82%) versus high energy (14%) (2)
- Risk factors include trauma, increasing age, and osteoporosis.
- Types:
  - Midshaft: 60%
  - Proximal shaft: 25%
  - Distal shaft: 10% (3)

DIAGNOSIS

- History and physical examination with special attention to a thorough neurovascular and skin examination
- Consider associated injuries such as ipsilateral shoulder, elbow, wrist, or hand fractures, or dislocations.
- Diagnosis is confirmed by x-ray.
- Prehospital:
  - Immobilize with sling and swath for transport.
  - Evaluate for open fracture.
  - Evaluate for distal neurologic and vascular deficit.
  - Rapid transport in presence of neurologic or vascular deficits.

HISTORY

- History of fall: Simple trip and fall, a low-impact force, is often associated with older (70+ years), osteoporotic women.
- Collision or direct blow: higher impact, occurring more commonly in younger men
- Pain after throwing or pitching
- History of malignancy
- *Consider as pathologic fracture for any humerus fracture produced by low-energy mechanism; the humerus can be a common site of metastatic disease.*

Pediatric Considerations

- "Falls" in toddlers or infants are concerning for abuse.
- Check for other bruises and injuries suggesting abuse.
- Examine the elbow in children who are guarding their arm.
- Elbow dislocations are more common in toddlers (nursemaid's elbow).
- Supracondylar fractures are more common in children when they sustain a fall.
- 4% have associated radial nerve palsy.

PHYSICAL EXAM

- Pain and swelling over the area of the humeral shaft
- Shortening, deformity, or decreased mobility
- Crepitus on gentle passive range of motion (ROM)
- Neurologic deficit (2)[C],(3)[B]:
  - Radial nerve is most commonly injured, occurring in 15% of humeral shaft fractures:
    - It runs along the posterior aspect of the humerus within the spiral groove. It is tethered down and emerges through the intermuscular septum at the middle to distal shaft.
    - Injury will affect active extension in the wrist, hand, and fingers.
    - Motor function can be tested by giving the "thumbs-up" sign.
    - Occurs most frequently in middle and distal shaft fractures and spiral fractures
    - Usually a neurapraxia or axonotmesis (perineurium and epineurium intact)
  - Ulnar nerve injury will affect finger abduction (spreading the fingers apart).
  - Median nerve injury will affect thumb opposition (thumb and small finger pinch), loss of sensation on the palmar surface of the thumb, and the index and middle fingers.
  - Injury to the largest branch of the median nerve is the anterior interosseous nerve. Damage will result in loss of hand and finger flexion.
- Vascular injury: presenting as decreased pulse, slow distal capillary refill, and/or cool extremity:
  - Brachial artery
  - Cephalic and basilic veins
- Open fracture: If the skin is disrupted over the site of the fracture, there is a high risk of infection and need for surgical evaluation.

DIFFERENTIAL DIAGNOSIS

- Bone contusion
- Muscle contusion: primarily the biceps, triceps, or deltoid
- Hematoma
- Tendon rupture: primarily the biceps
- Neurapraxia: primarily the radial nerve
- Abscess
- Bone malignancy

DIAGNOSTIC TESTS & INTERPRETATION

- Anteroposterior (AP) and lateral views of the entire humerus are mandatory to assess for fracture pattern:
  - Displacement, including angulation and shortening type of fracture: transverse, spiral, oblique
  - Location of the fracture on the humeral shaft in relation to muscle attachments
  - Number of fracture segments (butterfly fragments) and comminution.
- Include shoulder and elbow views to exclude associated joint involvement.
- The AO/ASIF system defines humeral shaft fractures as follows (3)[B]:
  - Type A (48%): simple fractures:
    - A1: simple spiral
    - A2: simple short oblique
    - A3: simple transverse
  - Type B (36%): wedge fractures:
    - B1: spiral wedge
    - B2: bending wedge
    - B3: fragmented wedge
  - Type C (9%): complex pattern fractures:
    - C1: complex spiral
    - C2: segmental fracture
    - C3: irregular comminuted fracture
- Pathologic findings:
  - Pathologic fractures of the humeral shaft are associated with the following malignancies (1)[B]:
    - Women: breast 40%, myeloma 23%, lung 9%, kidney 9%
    - Men: prostate 33%, kidney 25%, myeloma 8%, lung 8%

TREATMENT

GENERAL MEASURES

- These fractures usually do not require elaborate reduction or immobilization.
- Immobilize for 4 to 6 weeks until clinically and radiographically healed.
- Fractures without neurovascular compromise can be treated conservatively; see immobilization options below.
- Sugar tong splint or hanging casts are used for shortened displaced fractures. It is a full arm plaster cast from the proximal humerus to the wrist with elbow at 90 degrees used for 7 to 10 days to reduce the fracture before bracing.
- Functional bracing—applied after pain and swelling subsided. Brace is clamshell style, removable, and extends from just below the shoulder to above the elbow covering the humeral shaft but leaving the shoulder and elbow to free for full ROM.
- With cast and bracing, healing was average 9.5 weeks to heal closed fractures, and 14 weeks for open fractures; nonunion rate of 2.6% (3)[B]
- Prehospital:
  - With the introduction of functional (Sarmiento) bracing, conservative treatment has become more popular and can be managed in the office.
  - Conservative care can be undertaken with 80% healing rates for adults with low to moderate functional demands.
  - The degree of displacement accepted in these studies was up to 30 degrees rotation, 2 to 3 cm shortening, 20 degrees anteroposterior angulation, or 30 degrees varus or valgus angulation (4)[C].
    - Fractures can displace further after injury owing to contraction of the surrounding muscles (see below).
    - No randomized controlled trials support these recommendations, so they are class C recommendations.
  - Open fractures or fractures associated with neurovascular compromise require immediate orthopedic consultation.
  - Children remodel well and usually are able to compensate with overgrowth for fractures up to 1.5 cm shortening and 20 degrees of angulation.
    - Supracondylar fractures should be considered as different entity.
  - Anyone with high functional demands such as elite athletes, mechanics, and carpenters should be considered for surgical fixation for optimal anatomic alignment.
  - Of the nonunions, 90% ultimately heal with surgical intervention.
  - The carrying angle (valgus angle at the elbow when the arm is fully extended) is most often affected in displaced humeral shaft fractures (4)[C].

MEDICATION

- Immobilization: Immobilize to limit movement at the site of the fracture, which is one of the most effective methods of pain control.
- Ice: Icing the fracture site intermittently (15 minutes QID) for the first few days will reduce swelling and help to control pain.
- Elevation: After immobilization, try to elevate the arm above the level of the heart as much as possible to minimize swelling.
- Open fractures: empiric antibiotics and emergent washout
- Analgesic medications:
  - Narcotic analgesics: initially may be needed for adequate pain control
  - Nonnarcotic analgesics: After the fracture stabilizes (about 1 week), nonsteroidal anti-inflammatory drugs (NSAIDs) and/or acetaminophen should provide sufficient pain relief.

ISSUES FOR REFERRAL

Surgical indications (3)(4)[B]:

- Unacceptable alignment after closed reduction
- Multiple injuries
- Bilateral fractures
- Floating elbow
- Intra-articular extension of the fracture
- Progressive nerve palsy or palsy after reduction
- Significant vascular injury
- Neurologic injury after penetrating injury
- Nonunion/infected nonunion
- Pathologic fractures
- Higher risk fracture patterns with comminution, segmental and butterfly fractures
- Vascular injury: Refer for urgent vascular surgery evaluation.
- Pediatric surgical considerations

ADDITIONAL THERAPIES

Consider displacing forces of the contracted muscles around the site of fracture when immobilizing the injury:

- Supraspinatus, infraspinatus, and teres minor externally rotate the humeral head.
- Subscapularis internally rotates the humeral head.
- Pectoralis pulls fragments toward the chest (medially) and forward (anteriorly).
- Latissimus and teres major pull fragments inward toward the chest.
- Deltoid displaces the fracture outward (abducts) away from the chest.

SURGERY/OTHER PROCEDURES

- Surgical options:
  - Intermedullary nailing
  - External fixation
  - Plate fixation
- Immobilization options for conservative management (1)[C]:
  - Sling and swathe: best for nondisplaced fractures that do not need distraction but can predispose to further shortening
  - Sugar-tong, coaptation, or U-shaped splint: best for limitation of transverse fracture displacement; limits shoulder and elbow motion, predisposing to stiffness after prolonged immobilization
  - Hanging cast: better for displaced or comminuted fractures needing passive distraction:
    - Elbow is placed in 90 degrees of flexion and the forearm in a neutral position.
    - Needs closer follow-up after injury to evaluate for signs of compartment syndrome
    - Cannot keep arm elevated to minimize swelling because gravity aids with distraction of the fracture
  - Functional bracing:
    - Preferred definitive treatment of transverse humerus shaft fractures and most other mid-shaft fractures
    - Allows for elbow flexion, extension, and arm abduction to 60 degrees; applied after initial swelling subsides and fracture starts to stabilize, usually 2 weeks after injury
    - Motion generates compression to help maintain alignment.
  - *Always repeat the vascular and neurologic examination after splint or cast application.*
- Surgical treatment:
  - Benefits:
    - More predictable alignment
    - Immediate stability
    - Open reduction and internal fixation (ORIF) has ≥95% rate of union.
    - Number needed to treat (NNT)-7 to avoid nonunion (5)[A]
    - Radial nerve paralysis is *not* an absolute contraindication for surgery.
  - Risks:
    - Radial nerve palsy: 2–5%; surgery associated with higher risk of transient radial nerve palsy with odds ratio (OR) 8.23 (5)[A]
    - Infection: 1–2% for closed fracture and 2–5% for open fracture
    - Nonunion
    - Anesthesia risks
- Conservative treatment (6)[B]:
  - Benefits:
    - Functional bracing usually allows for full or nearly full shoulder and elbow mobility.
    - Less infection and neurovascular injury risk
  - Risks:
    - Skin breakdown
    - Angular or translational malalignment/deformity
    - Nonunion (higher in simple fractures or type 1)
    - Shoulder or elbow stiffness

ONGOING CARE

- Immobilize until clinical healing and pain free, with bony callus on radiographs, usually 4 to 6 weeks.
- Begin pendulum exercises within 1 week.
- Start passive ROM after 2 weeks to minimize shoulder and elbow stiffness.

FOLLOW-UP RECOMMENDATIONS

Nonunion risk factors:

- Open fracture
- Segmental (more than two fragments)
- Transverse (tend to displace into varus owing to displacing forces)
- Highly comminuted (unable to hold alignment)
- Associations: smoking, use of NSAIDs
- Obesity, large breasts
- Increased fracture gap or no callus at 6 weeks
- Comorbidities: diabetes, hypothyroid, infection, metabolic bone disease (2)[C]

Patient Monitoring

- Coaptation splint, hanging cast or sugar tong at 90 degrees elbow flexion and sling for initial injury.
- Functional bracing at 1 to 2 weeks, adjusting fitness ongoing
- Weekly follow-up: initially, every week to assess for displacement of the fracture
- Every other week: Once the fracture is stable on consecutive radiographs (usually 2 to 3 weeks after injury), follow up every 2 weeks:
  - Once callus is noted on radiograph and no pain on examination, splint can be removed, and shoulder and elbow should be mobilized with gentle ROM exercises.
  - Continue to follow clinically until ROM is restored and healing noted on radiographs (usually 8 to 12 weeks).
- At 6 weeks if no signs of union, unacceptable alignment, or if increased fracture gap occurs during monitoring, refer to surgery.
- At 12 to 14 weeks, if union is not complete clinically and radiographically, consider referral to surgery for intervention.
- Usually regain full resistance capability in 4 to 5 months.
- 85% return to full shoulder and elbow function

PATIENT EDUCATION

- Compartment syndrome signs and symptoms if casted
- Monitor for new neurologic deficit.
- Monitor for new vascular deficit.
- Encourage wrist, hand, and shoulder ROM exercises.
- Sleep upright (recliner) if in a hanging cast until fracture is stable to minimize displacement.

COMPLICATIONS

- The most common complications are neurovascular compromise and nonunion.
- Neurovascular; radial nerve injury
- 11% have associated radial nerve injury with the injury (2% proximal, 15% middle, 24% distal 1/3)
- 90% of radial nerve palsies recovered by 4 months.
- Consider electromyography (EMG) if nerve palsy persists.
- If radial nerve palsy persists after 4 to 6 months, consider surgical exploration for primary nerve repair, grafting, or tendon transfer.
- Nonunion; occurring in 2–10% of all humeral shaft fractures treated nonoperatively
- Varus angulation is most common in transverse fractures.
- Compartment syndrome

REFERENCES

1. Ekholm R, Adami J, Tidermark J, et al. Fractures of the shaft of the humerus: an epidemiological study of 401 fractures. *J Bone Joint Surg Br.* 2006;88(11):1469–1473.
2. Mattila H, Keskitalo T, Simons T, et al. Epidemiology of 936 humeral shaft fractures in a large Finnish trauma center. *J Shoulder Elbow Surg.* 2023;32(5):e206–e215.
3. Wijesekera M, Cowling P. Update on management options for the humeral shaft. *Orthop Trauma.* 2023;37(5):303–313.
4. Orapiriyakul W, Apivatthakakul V, Theppariyapol B, et al. Humerus shaft fractures, approaches and management. *J Clin Orthop Trauma.* 2023;43:102230.
5. Oliver WM, Bell KR, Molyneux SG, et al. Surgical versus nonsurgical management of humeral shaft fractures: a systematic review and meta-analysis of randomized trials. *J Am Acad Orthop Surg.* 2023;31(2):e82–e93.
6. Jawa A, McCarty P, Doornberg J, et al. Extra-articular distal-third diaphyseal fractures of the humerus: a comparison of functional bracing and plate fixation. *J Bone Joint Surg Am.* 2006;88(11):2343–2347.

ADDITIONAL READING

Simon R, Koenigsknecht S. *Emergency Orthopedics: The Extremities.* 3rd ed. Appleton & Lange; 1995.

CLINICAL PEARLS

- Radial nerve injury is the most common neurovascular injury, occurring in about 15% of humeral shaft fractures.
- 10 to 20 degrees of angulation and 1 to 2 cm of shortening generally are well tolerated owing to compensated overgrowth and the surrounding muscles. >30 degrees angulation or >3 cm shortening should be considered for surgical reduction.
- Contraction of the muscles around the humerus can displace the fracture after the initial injury and should be considered when immobilizing the fracture.
- Consider close weekly follow-up after immobilization to monitor for fracture displacement.

FRACTURE, LATERAL AND MEDIAL MALLEOLI

Kathryn M. Alfonso, DO ▪ Aimee Madsen, MD ▪ Daniel Kiehl, DO

BASICS

DESCRIPTION

- Any fracture involving the most distal portions of the fibula or tibia, commonly known as the lateral and medial malleoli, respectively
- Synonyms: ankle fracture

EPIDEMIOLOGY

- Very common: ~4.22 ankle fractures per 10,000 people each year (1)
- Most common mechanisms: falls, sports, exercise (1)
- Fractures to ankle or midfoot occur in <15% of ankle sprains.
- Most ankle fractures are malleolar fractures: 70% are unimalleolar (lateral being most common), 20% are bimalleolar, and 10% are trimalleolar (medial, lateral, and posterior malleoli) (2).

RISK FACTORS

- History of prior ankle injury
- Inadequate rehabilitation of injury
- Skeletal immaturity
- Weakness in dynamic (muscles) and/or static (ligamentous) stabilizers of the ankle
- Abnormal gait and/or foot biomechanics
- Foot and ankle proprioceptive dysfunction (dysfunction in the ability of the foot and ankle to adapt to uneven terrain)
- Cigarette smoking
- Obesity

COMMONLY ASSOCIATED CONDITIONS

- Pilon fracture
- Maisonneuve fracture

DIAGNOSIS

HISTORY

- Mechanism of injury: supination or pronation of the foot with associated force of external versus internal rotation, adduction, or abduction of the ankle joint
- Most frequent mechanism of injury is inversion.
- Occasionally caused by direct blow to the affected malleolus
- Patient may hear or feel a "pop."
- Immediate, disabling pain and difficulty bearing weight
- Acute onset of swelling
- Development of ecchymosis
- Possible neurovascular changes such as paresthesias or dusky appearance of foot

PHYSICAL EXAM

- Swelling (most common) and/or ankle deformity
- Ecchymosis
- Limited range of motion of the ankle
- Tenderness to palpation over the affected malleolus
- Difficulty or inability to bear weight and/or ambulate
- May note instability of the ankle joint on examination
- Check for signs of neurovascular compromise (pulses/sensation in the foot).

DIFFERENTIAL DIAGNOSIS

- Contusion
- Ankle sprain
- Tear of ankle retinacular structures
- Syndesmosis injury ("high ankle sprain")
- Foot fracture
- Posttraumatic subluxation of peroneal or tibialis posterior tendons

DIAGNOSTIC TESTS & INTERPRETATION

- Ottawa Ankle Rules are used to determine whether x-rays are necessary. Obtain x-rays for pain in the malleolar zone associated with any of the following:
  - Bony tenderness along distal 6 cm of posterior tibia or fibula or at medial or lateral malleolar tip
  - Inability to bear weight (four steps) on ankle immediately after injury and at time of evaluation
- The Ottawa Ankle Rules have a high sensitivity for fracture and a modest specificity (3)[A].
- X-rays: anteroposterior (AP), lateral, and mortise (AP with foot in 15 degrees of adduction)
- On the mortise view, the joint space between the talus and lateral malleolus and the distal tibia and medial malleolus should be equal. Inequality should raise suspicion of an unstable ankle injury.
- Computed tomography (CT) is not indicated in most ankle fractures; however, it should be used for malleolar fractures with an unstable syndesmosis fractures involving the posterior malleolus, supination-adduction–type fractures with suspected medial plafond impaction (pilon fracture), spiral fractures of the distal part of the tibial shaft, and transitional ankle fractures in adolescents (2)[B].
- When performed, order thin-cut CT in case coronal or sagittal reconstructions are required.
- Intra-articular displacement of >2 mm on imaging should prompt consideration for surgical referral due to inferior short- and long-term outcomes (2)[B].

TREATMENT

GENERAL MEASURES

- Acetaminophen at recommended age- or weight-based dosages every 6 to 8 hours as needed
- Consider nonsteroidal anti-inflammatory drugs (NSAIDs), although controversy exists as to their effect on bone healing.

- Narcotics as needed for severe pain only
- Cryotherapy applied for 20 to 30 minutes every 2 to 4 hours for the first 24 to 48 hours after injury; use caution to avoid thermal injury to the skin.
- Relative rest and elevation of affected limb for first 48 to 72 hours
- Isolated lateral malleolar fractures with ≤2 mm of displacement do not need reduction. Refer to orthopedist for >2 mm displacement or medial clear space >4 mm in AP mortise view (4)[B].
- Isolated medial malleolar fractures with any displacement other than small avulsion injuries should be referred to an orthopedist. Do not attempt to reduce.
- Check neurovascular status of foot post reduction.
- Postreduction x-rays with same views as initial films
- Initial management should include non–weight-bearing in stirrup or posterior splint, with ankle in neutral position, with follow-up in 3 to 5 days for definitive treatment.
- Isolated, minimally displaced lateral malleolar fracture: short leg walking cast with ankle in a neutral position or fracture boot with (e.g., controlled ankle motion [CAM] walker) or without adjustable ankle range of motion for 4 to 6 weeks
- Isolated simple avulsion fracture of the medial malleolus: Stirrup splint or CAM walker can be used short term for comfort, typically 2 to 4 weeks.
- Recent studies show a 3-week immobilization period for Weber B fracture is noninferior to 6 weeks of immobilization (5)[A].

ISSUES FOR REFERRAL

- Any open fracture or fracture associated with neurologic or vascular deficits requires emergent surgical evaluation.
- Ankle injuries that are unstable or incongruent warrants orthopedic surgery evaluation.

ADDITIONAL THERAPIES

- Patients should seek attention immediately for increasing pain, new or worsening numbness, or skin pallor/duskiness distal to the fracture or splint/cast.
- Repeat x-rays at 2 weeks to ensure maintained alignment and at 6 weeks to assess bony healing (6)[C].
- Repeat x-rays every 2 weeks if not healing.
- Total healing time: 6 to 8 weeks; may take months to see complete radiographic healing
- Athletes should cross-train while healing to maintain fitness.
- Proper rehabilitation of these injuries with a home instructional program or with formal physical therapy guidance is crucial to successful healing and return to full function.
- After a period of immobilization is complete, start standard ankle rehabilitation range of motion exercises, strengthening exercises, and proprioceptive training.
- Shorter periods of immobilization decrease difficulty in regaining ankle motion and strength (4)[B].
- Follow up every 2 to 3 weeks to assess progress of rehabilitation.

SURGERY/OTHER PROCEDURES

The following injuries are frequently managed with surgical intervention:

- Disrupted mortise join
- Bimalleolar fractures
- Trimalleolar fractures
- Unimalleolar fracture with contralateral ligament rupture
- Medial and lateral malleolar fractures with >2 mm displacement (4)[B]
- Lateral malleolar fractures above the tibiotalar joint line (as they are frequently associated with syndesmotic disruption) (2)[B]
- Medial instability with medial clear space >4 mm on AP or mortise view (4)[B]
- Weber C fracture with any displacement (4)[B]

Pediatric Considerations

- 5% of all fractures in pediatrics with a higher incidence in obese children (6)
- Physes are vulnerable, and ligamentous structures are robust (6).
- Salter-Harris (SH) type II is the most common (6).
- SH III and IV may damage the reserve zone and are at a higher risk for causing physeal growth disturbance (6).
- Long-term treatment is to minimize angular deformity and leg length discrepancy, to achieve normal ankle function, and to avoid posttraumatic arthritis (6).

ADMISSION, INPATIENT, AND NURSING CONSIDERATIONS

Admission criteria:

- Open fracture
- Fracture-dislocations in which adequate reduction is not achieved with manual manipulation
- Evidence of or concern for neurovascular compromise (severely comminuted pilon fracture, compartment syndrome)

REFERENCES

1. Scheer RC, Newman JM, Zhou JJ, et al. Ankle fracture epidemiology in the United States: patient-related trends and mechanisms of injury. *J Foot Ankle Surg*. 2020;59(3):479–483.
2. Rammelt S, Boszczyk A. Computed tomography in the diagnosis and treatment of ankle fractures: a critical analysis review. *JBJS Rev*. 2018;6(12):e7.
3. Gomes YE, Chau M, Banwell HA, et al. Diagnostic accuracy of the Ottawa Ankle Rule to exclude fractures in acute ankle injuries in adults: a systematic review and meta-analysis. *BMC Musculoskelet Disord*. 2022;23(1):885.
4. Canton G, Sborgia A, Maritan G, et al. Fibula fractures management. *World J Orthop*. 2021;12(5):254–269.
5. Kortekangas T, Haapasalo H, Flinkkilä T, et al. Three-week versus six-week immobilisation for stable Weber B type ankle fractures: randomised, multicentre, non-inferiority clinical trial. *BMJ*. 2019;364:k5432.
6. Su AW, Larson AN. Pediatric ankle fractures: concepts and treatment principles. *Foot Ankle Clin*. 2015;20(4):705–719.

ADDITIONAL READING

- Eiff MP, Hatch RL. *Fracture Management for Primary Care*. 4th ed. Elsevier; 2020.
- Tornetta P, Ricci WM, Ostrum Rf, et al, eds. *Rockwood and Green's Fractures in Adults*. 9th ed. Wolters Kluwer; 2019.

CLINICAL PEARLS

- 70% are unimalleolar with lateral being the most common.
- Consider Ottawa Ankle Rules with patients who possess adequate communication skills.
- Obtain the following x-rays: AP, lateral, and mortise.
- Any open fracture or fracture with neurologic or vascular compromise requires emergent surgical evaluation.
- In pediatrics, ligamentous structures are more robust than the physis.

FRACTURE, LE FORT

Amy Leu, DO, FAAFP, CAQSM

BASICS

Le Fort fractures are midface maxillary fractures involving the maxilla; the maxilla, orbital bones, and nasal bones; or the maxilla, orbital bones, nasal bones, and zygoma.

Pediatric Considerations

- Maxillofacial fractures occur less frequently in children:
  - Because of the smaller facial skeleton, there is a higher incidence of skull fractures and head trauma compared with midface injuries.
  - Le Fort fractures are particularly uncommon in young children. By ages 10 to 12 years, as facial morphology becomes adult-like, more midfacial and lower facial fractures are seen.
  - Be suspicious of child abuse or family violence as possible causes of midfacial injuries, especially in children aged <6 years.
- Cautions:
  - Airway management:
    - Airway compromise is common.
    - Bag-valve-mask (BVM) ventilation may be difficult.
    - Avoid nasotracheal intubation.
  - Strict cervical spine precautions
  - Multisystem injury is likely with high-energy trauma.

DESCRIPTION

- Maxillofacial fractures caused by high-energy blunt trauma to the midface: The most common causes include motor vehicle accidents (including motorcycle accidents and all-terrain vehicles), physical assault, sports injuries (mountain biking, skiing/snow sports, football, baseball, hockey, soccer among others), and domestic violence. Head and cervical spine injuries are commonly seen in patients with high-velocity facial trauma. Midface fractures are the most common type of maxillofacial trauma, comprising up to 70% of all maxillofacial injuries. There has been a rise in recent years of craniofacial injuries with the introduction of motorized scooters, and midface injury comprising a large percentage of them (1).
- Le Fort fractures are separated into three categories based on the facial bones that are involved. Identification can be made with the initial physical exam. On forward traction of the maxillary arch/hard palate, you should find:
  - Le Fort I (horizontal): movement of the hard palate and maxillary dentition only; can arise from a blow low on the maxillary alveolar rim; involves only the maxillary bone
  - Le Fort II (pyramidal): movement of the hard palate, maxillary dentition, and the nose; can arise from a blow to the lower to middle maxilla; involves the maxilla and nasal bones
  - Le Fort III (transverse): movement of the entire midface, including orbital rims (inferior and lateral aspects); can arise from a blow to the nasal bridge or upper maxilla; involves the maxilla, nasal bones, and zygoma
  - Note that if the patient is intubated, the airway devices may be indirectly stabilizing the teeth and the fracture fragments.

EPIDEMIOLOGY

Prevalence

Midface fractures have been reported to make up ~70% of all facial fractures.

GENERAL PREVENTION

Use of protective equipment including helmets, facemasks, and mouthguards has been shown to significantly reduce the number of craniofacial injuries. This includes but is not limited to helmets with an extension to cover the lower jaw (such as the C-flap on baseball helmets) (2).

COMMONLY ASSOCIATED CONDITIONS

- Higher velocity injuries are commonly associated with head and cervical spine injuries.
- Le Fort III fractures are commonly associated with lateral rim and zygomatic fractures.
- Visual changes may signify a disturbance of the optic canal, problems within the globe or retina, or other neurologic lesions.
- Disturbances of extraocular motion or enophthalmos may signify a blowout in the orbital floor.
- Le Fort III fractures also can extend to the base of the sphenoid and can result in a cerebrospinal fluid (CSF) leak.

DIAGNOSIS

Pediatric Considerations

- Young children are often frightened and in pain. Through kindness, patience, and distraction, cooperation can be gained.
- Sedation may be required to perform a thorough exam after evaluating for head injury.
- Incomplete (greenstick) fractures with minimal or no displacement can occur.
- Be cognizant of possible child abuse and evaluate for prior nonaccidental trauma, if appropriate.
- Evaluate the patency of the airway and need for immediate airway control.
- There is a high incidence of cervical spine injuries associated with facial trauma; thus, cervical spine precautions always must be taken (3)[C].
- Le Fort fractures can be diagnosed by careful intraoral examination and the pattern of facial movement:
  - If fracture fragments are impacted, there may be little or no midface mobility.
  - Carefully evaluate the patient for CSF rhinorrhea and malocclusion.
  - If any disturbance of vision or extraocular motion is suspected, consider the presence of a blowout fracture and/or ophthalmologic involvement.
- Prehospital:
  - Establishing airway patency is of utmost importance. Orotracheal intubation is preferred over blind nasotracheal intubation.
  - Bleeding from facial wounds may complicate endotracheal intubation.
  - If a ruptured globe is suspected, an eye cup or noncontact shielding should be used to prevent compression of the eye while establishing an airway.
  - Avulsed tissue (ears, skin flaps) should be transported with the patient in saline-soaked gauze.
  - Avulsed teeth should also be transported with the patient in their mouth (in between the buccal mucosal and gum) if they have normal mental status and can protect their airway. If they are intoxicated, have altered mental status, are immobilized and cannot sit upright, or are complaining of nausea or vomiting, their teeth should be transported in sterile saline.
  - In severe Le Fort II and III cases, the maxillary plate can be displaced posteriorly and inferiorly, possibly occluding the airway.
  - There is a high incidence of cervical spine injuries associated with facial trauma; thus, cervical spine precautions always must be taken (3)[C].

HISTORY

History may be difficult to obtain directly from the patient, but these types of fractures typically arise from a high-energy force directed at different aspects of the face. Situations can include motor vehicle accidents, altercations, sports injuries, and falls.

PHYSICAL EXAM

- Facial injury with massive swelling and ecchymosis
- Facial hemorrhage/epistaxis
- Airway obstruction may be present.
- Dyspnea (especially when supine)
- Malocclusion
- Vision disturbance (diplopia)
- Facial lengthening or flattening, periorbital ecchymosis (raccoon's eyes), periorbital swelling
- CSF rhinorrhea
- Facial anesthesia, midface mobility on traction, open bite
- Frequently associated with multisystem injury (especially head and cervical spine)

DIFFERENTIAL DIAGNOSIS

- Le Fort fracture classification:
  - Le Fort I: transverse (horizontal) through the maxilla above the roots of the teeth; can be unilateral or bilateral; disjunction of the maxilla from the pterygoid plate
  - Le Fort II: pyramidal; disjunction, including the nasal bridge, maxilla, lacrimal bones, and orbital floor and rim; typically, bilateral
  - Le Fort III: complete disjunction of the maxilla from the skull base; transverse fracture extending from the pterygoid plate up to the zygomaticofrontal suture and horizontally through the orbit to the nasofrontal suture; rare
- Different grade Le Fort fractures may be found on opposite sides of the face.

DIAGNOSTIC TESTS & INTERPRETATION

- Facial imaging may be delayed for 24 to 72 hours in patients requiring care of other life-threatening conditions.
- Computed tomography (CT) scanning with 3D reconstruction if available is the diagnostic standard for defining midface fractures with thin (1 mm) cuts in the coronal and axial planes.
- Conventional radiographs may be used as a screening test. The occipitomental (Waters) and lateral views of the skull may reveal bony fracture/asymmetry, subcutaneous emphysema, or layering of blood in the maxillary sinuses. Sinus films and cervical spine films usually are included as part of the screening examination.
- Ultrasound of the eye can be used in patients with suspected ocular injuries for the detection of vitreous hemorrhage, retinal detachment, and globe rupture if urgent operative management of nonfacial injuries is planned and there is no time for a facial CT.
- Ultrasound has recently been shown to be useful in the detection and measurement of displacement of midface fractures compared to CT. This could be an alternative for qualitative and quantitative assessment for fractures if radiation exposure is a concern.

TREATMENT

Pediatric Considerations

- Surgical cricothyroidotomy should not be considered in children aged <10 years.
- Needle cricothyroidotomy with jet ventilation may be attempted if intubation attempts fail.
- There is a higher incidence of multiple injuries in children, especially head trauma, skull fractures, and orthopedic injuries.
- Cervical spine injuries tend to involve upper levels more commonly in children. Also, spinal cord injury without radiographic abnormality (SCIWORA) syndrome may be seen.
- Definitive repair of pediatric facial fractures should not be delayed for >3 to 4 days. The facial bones heal rapidly, and delayed repair may result in malunion and cosmetic deformity.

GENERAL MEASURES

Emergency department (ED) treatment:

- Cervical spine: Owing to the risk of cervical spine injury in patients with head and maxillofacial trauma, it is imperative that radiographic clearance of the cervical spine is obtained.
- Hemorrhage control: Direct pressure should be applied to areas of bleeding, and nasal packing (anterior and posterior) may be necessary for epistaxis. In some cases, manual reduction of the midface may be required to control intractable hemorrhage. Although blood loss from facial bleeding may be significant, it is rarely a primary cause of hemorrhagic shock.
- Early consultation with oral maxillofacial, ENT, or plastic surgeon
- Analgesics, antibiotics, and tetanus prophylaxis

MEDICATION

	Adult Dose (mg/kg IV)	Pediatric Dose (mg/kg IV)
Sedative/analgesics[a]		
Diazepam	0.1–0.2	0.1–0.2
Droperidol	2.5-mg aliquots	1- to 1.5-mg aliquots
Etomidate	0.2–0.3	0.2–0.3
Fentanyl	2–10 μg	2–3 μg
Ketamine	2	1–2
Meperidine	1–2	1–2
Midazolam	0.1	0.15
Morphine sulfate	0.1–0.2	0.1–0.2
Defasciculating drug		
Vecuronium	0.01	0.01
Paralytic agents		
Pancuronium	0.1–0.15	0.1–0.15
Rocuronium	0.6	0.6
Succinylcholine	1.5	1.5–2
Vecuronium	0.1–0.3	0.1–0.3

[a]All these sedatives/analgesics should be titrated to effect.
IV, intravenous.

SURGERY/OTHER PROCEDURES

- Often, maxillomandibular fixation (MMF) is used in conjunction with open reduction and internal fixation (ORIF) of maxillofacial injuries to maintain optimal immobilization.
- In the pediatric population, several considerations are taken into account, including duration of MMF, use of smaller hardware, and avoiding injury to developing teeth.
- Consultation with an ophthalmologist is appropriate when extensive involvement of the orbit or globe is suspected.

ADMISSION, INPATIENT, AND NURSING CONSIDERATIONS

- Initial stabilization:
  - Aggressive airway control is paramount. Orally suction patients to minimize aspiration of blood, saliva, and stomach contents.
  - Remove any foreign matter or teeth from the airway.
  - After cervical spine clearance, stable and alert patients may be allowed to sit up and suction themselves.
  - When airway management is needed, rapid-sequence induction is recommended to maximize airway control and minimize rise of intracranial pressure (ICP) in patients with head injuries (4)[B].
  - If there is concern that paralysis will result in loss of airway tone and inability to intubate because of subsequent distortion of airway anatomy in patients with severe facial injuries, oral intubation under sedation with midazolam, etomidate, droperidol, or ketamine is an option.
  - Emergency cricothyroidotomy may be necessary if orotracheal intubation is unsuccessful. Recall that BVM ventilation may be difficult owing to loss of bony support and altered anatomy.
  - Nasotracheal intubation is not recommended in patients with midface trauma because of the lack of success and danger of intracranial placement (1)[B],(4)[B],(5)[C].
- Admission criteria:
  - All patients are admitted for ORIF of maxillofacial injuries.
  - Patients should be admitted to an intensive care unit (ICU) setting.

ONGOING CARE

COMPLICATIONS

- Infection can emerge from multiple stages during the treatment process, particularly if there is extensive soft tissue involvement.
- Scarring can occur depending on the suturing technique used as well as the patient's ability to keep the repaired area immobilized.
- Nerve damage can arise from the original trauma as well as a result of the type of surgery used to repair the fractures.
- LeFort III fractures carry a risk of blindness secondary to the fracture extending near the optic nerve.
- Malunion and, less commonly, nonunion also can result if adequate immobilization is not achieved.

REFERENCES

1. Kim JJ, Huoh K. Maxillofacial (midface) fractures. *Neuroimaging Clin N Am*. 2010;20(4):581–596.
2. Larrabee KA, Kao AS, Barbetta BT, et al. Midface including Le Fort level injuries. *Facial Plast Surg Clin North Am*. 2022;30(1):63–70.
3. Rajkumar GC, Ashwin DP, Singh R, et al. Ocular injuries associated with midface fractures: a 5 year survey. *J Maxillofac Oral Surg*. 2015;14(4):925–929.
4. Septa D, Newaskar VP, Agrawal D, et al. Etiology, incidence and patterns of mid-face fractures and associated ocular injuries. *J Maxillofac Oral Surg*. 2014;13(2):115–119.
5. American Academy of Otolaryngology—Head and Neck Surgery. Upper facial trauma. In: *Resident Manual of Trauma to the Face, Head, and Neck*. American Academy of Otolaryngology—Head and Neck Surgery; 2012:41–73.

ADDITIONAL READING

- Lentge F, Jehn P, Zeller AN, et al. Quantitative ultrasonographic diagnostics for midface and mandible fractures. *J Stomatol Oral Maxillofac Surg*. 2022;123(5):e588–e592.
- Shimoyama T, Kaneko T, Horie N. Initial management of massive oral bleeding after midfacial fracture. *J Trauma*. 2003;54(2):332–336.
- Subhashraj K, Nandakumar N, Ravindran C. Review of maxillofacial injuries in Chennai, India: a study of 2748 cases. *Br J Oral Maxillofac Surg*. 2007;45(8):637–639.

CLINICAL PEARLS

- Le Fort fractures are typically the result of high-velocity blunt force trauma to the midface; thus, evaluation for concurrent cervical spine injury and intracranial trauma must be considered.
- True Le Fort fractures rarely happen in children aged <12 years given their smaller facial skeleton. Head trauma and skull fractures are more likely.
- Be suspicious for child abuse/family violence for pediatric patients who present with a midface fracture, especially in those <6 years of age.
- Airway management is of utmost importance during evaluation, and if an airway is needed, orotracheal intubation is preferred over blind nasotracheal intubation due to risk of intracranial displacement.

F

FRACTURE, LISFRANC

William H. West, MD, CAQSM • Kenneth M. Bielak, MD, MBA, FAAFP, FACSM

BASICS

DESCRIPTION

- Injury to the forefoot complex. Tarsometatarsal (TMT) complex includes the three cuneiforms, cuboid, and five metatarsals. Injury can occur from direct or indirect mechanisms and may include damage to ligaments, bones, or both.
- Direct injury occurs with traumatic crush injury to the TMT joint.
- Causes of indirect injury:
  - Hindfoot placed in a fixed position with forefoot forcefully abducted in sports such as equestrian and windsurfing produces lateral displacement of the metatarsals with associated fracture of 2nd metatarsal base.
  - An axially applied force to a plantarflexed foot, causing disruption of the dorsal ligament complex
  - A force applied to the heel and the axis of the foot with the toes fixed in plantar position
- Synonyms: Lisfranc injury; TMT fracture; 1st and 2nd metatarsal–cuneiform fracture

EPIDEMIOLOGY

- 1 case/50,000 to 60,000 patients/y
- American football study showed that 90% of injuries occurred while player was engaged with another player. Injury occurred most with the foot plantarflexed and toes dorsiflexed. The majority of these injuries were due to external rotation of the midfoot (1).
- A review of 2,000 reported cases reported that 43% occurred from motor vehicle accident; 10% during sport activity; 13% due to crush injuries; 24% from falls, jumps, and twisting injuries; and 9.7% were due to sports injuries (2).
- 0.2% of all fractures per year
- Estimated that 20% are missed on initial presentation.

ALERT

- Males 4 times more likely than females due to high impact sports
- Majority are closed (87.6%).
- 2nd TMT joint is most frequently injured.

RISK FACTORS

- Slips, falls, motor vehicle accidents, high-energy sports
- Positional injury may also occur by using high heels because foot is continually plantarflexed.
- Horseback riding also common source of injury in the event of a fall due to foot being plantarflexed in a stirrup

COMMONLY ASSOCIATED CONDITIONS

- Cuneiform and cuboid fracture dislocations
- Compartment syndrome of the foot
- Ankle sprain/fracture
- Metatarsal fractures

DIAGNOSIS

HISTORY

- Determine the mechanism of injury as outlined above.
- History of previous foot injury/fracture
- May present with diffuse foot pain:
  - High index of suspicion needed. Up to 20% of subtle injuries may be missed on initial exam.
- Was the injury associated with a low- or high-velocity trauma?
  - High velocity, usually has an obvious deformity, whereas low velocity may cause only minor discomfort in the midfoot.
  - Low velocity, usually trips, falls, slips

PHYSICAL EXAM

- Signs and symptoms:
  - Midfoot pain and swelling
  - Evident change compared to contralateral foot possible
  - Plantar ecchymosis common
  - Instability with palpation, ambulation, and/or weight-bearing

ALERT

Pain with or inability to bear weight, particularly with walking on tiptoes

  - Plantar ecchymosis
  - Possible deformity of foot if injury was sustained due to high energy trauma
  - Gap sign between the 1st and 2nd metatarsals.
- Physical examination should include:
  - Evaluation of the integrity of the soft tissue and performing a neurovascular examination
  - Palpation of each articulation for tenderness and swelling. Medial cuneiform and 1st metatarsal joint are the most frequent sites of pain and swelling.
  - Piano key test: stressing 2nd metatarsal joint by elevating and depressing the 2nd metatarsal head relative to the 1st metatarsal head; elicits pain in Lisfranc joint
  - Compression of midfoot from side to side reproduces pain in interval between the bases of the 1st and 2nd metatarsals.
  - Flexion at Lisfranc joint may demonstrate instability and dorsal subluxation of the metatarsals.
  - Marked swelling, redness, and deformity may indicate complete dislocation and risk for compartment syndrome; may be misdiagnosed as cellulitis
  - Medial or lateral stress force applied to the metatarsals may reveal more specifically which part of the joint is unstable.

DIFFERENTIAL DIAGNOSIS

- Lisfranc fracture/dislocation
- TMT sprain
- Metatarsal fracture
- Cuboid fracture
- Cuneiform fracture
- Plantar fascia tear
- Contusion

DIAGNOSTIC TESTS & INTERPRETATION

Initial Tests (lab, imaging)

Plain radiograph:

- Unilateral non–weight-bearing radiograph may be the initial study:
  - Anteroposterior (AP), internal oblique, and lateral views should be taken.
  - This is often sufficient to see *obvious* Lisfranc injuries but may miss up to 50% of subtle injuries. Therefore, weight-bearing radiograph should be performed next. Also consider weight-bearing images of the contralateral foot for comparison.

ALERT

- Bilateral weight-bearing radiograph:
  - AP, internal oblique, and lateral views should be taken.
  - Subtle differences between the feet may be more easily seen if bilateral.
  - May be too painful. If that is the case, regional anesthesia with ankle block or general anesthesia may be necessary.
  - Craniocaudal angulation during AP view can give very good visualization of Lisfranc joint.
  - Look for the following relationships (3)[C]:
    - Good alignment of medial margins of 2nd metatarsal and middle cuneiform
    - Lateral margin of 1st metatarsal should be aligned with lateral margin of medial cuneiform.
    - Medial margins of 4th metatarsal and cuboid should be well aligned (oblique view).
    - Any malalignment indicates Lisfranc dislocation.

- Any small fractures in and around the Lisfranc joint should cause suspicion of significant injury in that area.
- Diastasis >1 to 2 mm between 1st and 2nd metatarsal bases indicates rupture of Lisfranc ligament (best seen in AP view).
- "Fleck sign" avulsion fracture in medial cuneiform 2nd metatarsal space represents rupture of Lisfranc ligament.
- Compression fracture of cuboid ("nutcracker injury") may be apparent.

- Computed tomography (CT) scan
  - Used to help identify subtle injuries, especially superimposed bone fragments and tendon damage
  - A good modality overall for verifying radiographic findings and locating subtle fractures
- Magnetic resonance imaging (MRI):
  - Allows optimal evaluation of malalignment of the midfoot and is superior modality to detect injury to ligaments
  - T1- and T2-weighted sequences most helpful in detection
  - Expensive and may result in higher rate of false positives
  - Most helpful when index of suspicion is high, but there is an equivocal exam (4)[C]
- Ultrasound:
  - In office testing available
  - Can distract and look for abnormal motion
  - Can see small fleck avulsions and can see ligament tears
- Bone scintigraphy:
  - Most helpful for diagnosis of low-grade injuries when other imaging modalities do not depict abnormalities (5)

Test Interpretation

Multiple classification systems used describe level of diastasis as well as dislocation of metatarsals.

TREATMENT

- Nonoperative management for those with stable injury with no diastasis (3):
  - Immobilization in short walker boot with protected weight-bearing for 2 weeks and then reexamination:
    - If tenderness has resolved and no evidence of diastasis on repeat imaging, weight-bearing as tolerated in boot
    - Weight-bearing out of boot after 6 weeks
    - No high-impact activity for first 3 to 4 months after injury; return to sports in 3 to 6 months after injury.
    - If pain with weight-bearing after 2 weeks, advanced imaging indicated for further evaluation
    - Multiple studies to determine outcomes of nonoperative management have different primary and secondary outcomes, as well as criteria to determine conservative versus operative treatment.
  - Resulted in some studies recommending operative treatment due to conservative failure (6)[A]
- Single leg hop test pain-free before activity permitted
- Any evidence of dynamic instability or clear diastasis at Lisfranc joint complex requires operative management:
  - Returning to sport is variable. Studies have shown a range of 3 to 8 weeks of non–weight-bearing and a range of 9 to 12 months before returning to sport.
  - Open reduction and internal fixation (ORIF) and primary arthrodesis are usually successful and have high likelihood for successful return to play, although some may experience a decrease in level of performance, and residual pain is not uncommon in some.
- Prehospital: Immobilize with posterior splint, non–weight-bearing, elevation, and ice/compression.

SURGERY/OTHER PROCEDURES

ALERT

Any diastasis (>1 mm) or fracture may require surgical intervention:

- Unfortunately, no clear consensus on surgical intervention and optimal treatment due to multiple classification systems.
- Primary treatment by ORIF is the most common surgical intervention for athletes, although arthrodesis may be another option.
- Functional improvement and earlier return to work and activity have been seen with ORIF; however, some injury patterns have shown to improve better with primary arthrodesis.

ONGOING CARE

FOLLOW-UP RECOMMENDATIONS

Early orthopedic referral is indicated for any fracture, dislocation, or instability of the Lisfranc joint.

REFERENCES

1. Kent RW, Lievers WB, Riley PO, et al. Etiology and biomechanics of tarsometatarsal injuries in professional football players: a video analysis. *Orthop J Sports Med.* 2014;2(3):2325967114525347.
2. Lievers WB, Frimenko RE, Crandall JR, et al. Age, sex, causal, and injury patterns in tarsometatarsal dislocations: a literature review of over 2000 cases. *Foot (Edinb).* 2012;22(3):117–124.
3. Yan A, Chen SR, Ma X, et al. Updates on Lisfranc complex injuries. *Foot Ankle Orthop.* 2021;6(1):2473011420982275.
4. Chen J, Sagoo N, Panchbhavi VK. The Lisfranc injury: a literature review of anatomy, etiology, evaluation, and management. *Foot Ankle Spec.* 2021;14(5):458–467.
5. Siddiqui NA, Galizia MS, Almusa E, et al. Evaluation of the tarsometatarsal joint using conventional radiography, CT, and MR imaging. *Radiographics.* 2014;34(2):514–531.
6. Guerreiro F, Abdelaziz A, Ponugoti N, et al. Nonoperative management of Lisfranc injuries—a systematic review of outcomes. *Foot (Edinb).* 2023;54:101977.

ADDITIONAL READING

- Coetzee JC. Making sense of Lisfranc injuries. *Foot Ankle Clin.* 2008;13(4):695–704.
- Eleftheriou K, Rosenfeld P. Lisfranc injury in the athlete: evidence supporting management from sprain to fracture dislocation. *Foot Ankle Clin.* 2013;18(2):219–236.
- Lau S, Bozin M, Thillainadesan T. Lisfranc fracture dislocation: a review of a commonly missed injury of the midfoot. *Emerg Med J.* 2017;34(1):52–56.

CLINICAL PEARLS

- Have high index of suspicion for Lisfranc injuries with high-energy trauma, plantar ecchymosis, or inability to bear weight.
- Bilateral weight-bearing radiographs are important to help determine any subtle changes in structure. If equivocal with symptoms, consider MRI/CT for further evaluation.
- Late recognition and treatment: posttraumatic arthritis with resulting pes planus and forefoot abduction, which may require tarsometatarsal arthrodesis
- Instability requires prompt referral to orthopedic surgeon for evaluation.
- Postsurgical recovery includes non–weight-bearing cast for 6 weeks, followed by progressive weight-bearing in a cast or range of motion boot for 3 to 6 weeks. Return to sport is estimated at 9 to 12 months.

FRACTURE, LUNATE/KIENBÖCK DISEASE

Michael Troy, DO ▪ Catherine Carragee, MD ▪ Kenneth S. Taylor, MD, FAAFP, CAQSM

BASICS

DESCRIPTION

- Kienböck (pronounced "Keen-bock") disease, or lunatomalacia, is a painful disorder of the wrist, characterized by histologic and radiologic evidence of avascular necrosis (osteonecrosis) of the lunate.
- First described in 1910 by Robert Kienböck
- **Synonym(s):** lunatomalacia; lunate avascular necrosis

EPIDEMIOLOGY

- Most commonly occurs between ages 20 and 40 years
- More prevalent in the dominant hand, especially in manual laborers
- Bilateral involvement is rare.
- Incidental asymptomatic findings may occur in up to 2% of screened populations (1).
- Slight male predominance

ETIOLOGY AND PATHOPHYSIOLOGY

- The precise cause of Kienböck disease remains unknown. The final common pathway involves lunate osteonecrosis, often progressing to collapse and wrist arthropathy.
- Essentially, two theories exist: vascular and mechanical (2).
- Increased intraosseous pressures have been recorded in Kienböck disease, supporting impaired venous outflow as a potential etiology.
- Vascular: Compromised blood flow (especially venous outflow) causes ischemia. Vascularized bone graft success and dynamic Magnetic resonance imaging (MRI) perfusion studies support this mechanism.
- Mechanical theory describes necrosis secondary to progressive trabecular collapse of the lunate owing to excessive loads and repetitive microfractures. Anatomic factors that would lead to abnormal pressure on the lunate would include:
  - Negative ulnar variance
  - Trapezoidal lunate shape
  - Radial inclination
  - Midcarpal facet contact with the hamate (3)

RISK FACTORS

- Previous wrist trauma including lunate fracture
- Negative ulnar variance
- Repetitive trauma (manual labor)
- Anatomic and biomechanical features, including vulnerable blood supply or fixed position of the wrist (loss of range of motion)

DIAGNOSIS

Lichtman classification of staging for Kienböck disease (via x-ray) (1):

- Stage I: normal architecture and bone density; may be either a linear or a compression fracture
- Stage II: definite density changes, but size, shape, and anatomic relationship of the bones not altered; later in this stage, anteroposterior (AP) view shows loss of height on radial side of lunate.
- Stage IIIA: Entire lunate collapses, but the carpal height is relatively unchanged.
- Stage IIIB: There is additionally proximal migration of the capitate and disruption of the carpal architecture, including a fixed hyperflexion of the scaphoid (cortical ring sign). On lateral view, a dorsovolar ribbon-like elongation of the lunate is seen.
- Stage IV: in addition to stage III changes, generalized degenerative changes in the carpus
- Note: Recent literature emphasizes MRI-based staging to capture early disease (4).

HISTORY

- Dull, aching wrist pain worsened with activity
- May follow trauma or arise insidiously
- Symptoms often present >1 month before
- Weak grip strength or stiffness may be reported

PHYSICAL EXAM

- Painful, stiff, and often swollen wrist joint
- Pain most often mild to moderate in severity
- Asymptomatic presentation can occur
- Look for swelling, erythema, and warmth at the radioulnar joint. Erythema and warmth are *not* associated with Kienböck disease.
- Evaluate range of motion; decreased in Kienböck disease, especially dorsiflexion
- Tenderness over the dorsal lunate
- Grip strength may be diminished.

DIFFERENTIAL DIAGNOSIS

- On physical examination:
- Triangular fibrocartilage complex tear (more ulnar)
  - Scapholunate ligament instability
  - Distal radioulnar joint complex ligament instability
  - Monoarticular arthritides (multiple)
  - Intraosseous cyst
  - Ulnar impaction syndrome
- On x-ray:
  - Lunate fracture
  - Ulnar abutment
  - Degenerative joint disease carpals

DIAGNOSTIC TESTS & INTERPRETATION

Initial Tests (lab, imaging)

- Laboratory tests for the diagnosis of inflammatory and erosive arthritides (i.e., sedimentation rate, C-reactive protein, rheumatoid factor, anti–cyclic citrullinated peptide [CCP] antibodies, etc.) can be used in those with wrist symptoms to evaluate for other conditions.
- Standard AP, lateral and oblique radiographs with attention to changes in lunate morphology and density
- Initially, the lunate may have normal architecture and density.
- Subsequently, there is increasing density of the lunate and then altered shape and diminished size.
- Adjacent arthritic changes and carpal row collapse can ultimately occur.
- Computed tomography (CT) scan may be useful to detect early changes, including fracture lines.
- Radiographic measures such as a smaller lunate diameter and height, a more radially inclined lunate tilting angle, and a flatter radial inclination have been shown in those with Kienböck disease (5)[B].
- MRI:
  - T1: hypointensity in lunate (early sign of avascular necrosis [AVN])
  - T2: may show hyperintensity in early stages; late stages often hypointense
  - Dynamic contrast-enhanced MRI may help assess vascularity.
  - If negative, unlikely Kienböck disease in a patient with wrist symptoms; may show alternative diagnosis better than plain films

Diagnostic Procedures/Other

- Wrist arthroscopy has been used to assess and classify Kienböck disease.
- Assessment of the surfaces of the lunate is used to stage disease and plan appropriate surgical interventions.

TREATMENT

Acute treatment

ALERT

Immobilization:
- Initial wrist splinting or casting may be considered in early disease (stage I) for up to 6 to 12 weeks.
- Immobilization helps reduce synovitis but does not prevent progression of osteonecrosis.
- Patients should be reevaluated with repeat imaging to assess response.

ADDITIONAL THERAPIES

Over time, it has become evident that immobilization will not prevent long-term collapse of the lunate. Some studies showed similar pain relief in conservative versus surgical treatment.

SURGERY/OTHER PROCEDURES

- If the patient still has pain after conservative measures or has more advanced disease, there are a few other options.
- Hand therapy with fluidotherapy and ultrasound protocol to unload wrist and increase blood flow supply to lunate (6)[C]
- In stages II and IIIA: Revascularization procedure can be considered. One such procedure is called a keyhole vascularization, where a vascularized bone graft from the distal radius employing the 4th and 5th extracompartmental artery pedicles is used as a mechanical support to enable fracture union (7)[C].
- In stage II or IIIA *with positive ulnar variance*: direct revascularization plus external fixation or temporary scaphotrapeziotrapezoid pinning (stage II only), radial wedge or dome osteotomy, capitate shortening with or without capitohamate fusion, combination of joint leveling, and direct revascularization procedures
- In stages II and IIIA with *negative or neutral ulnar variance*: radius-shortening osteotomy, ulnar lengthening, capitate shortening
- In stage IIIA: distal radius metaphyseal core decompression with cancellous bone impaction without shortening procedure leading to improved vascularization (6)[B]
- In stages II, IIIA, IIIB: bone marrow transfusion, low intensity pulsed ultrasound, and external fixation (8)[B]
- In stages IIIA, IIIB, IV: tendon ball arthroplasty using a palmaris longus tendon to fill the defect (9)[B]
- In stage IIIB: scaphotrapeziotrapezoid or scaphocapitate fusion with or without lunate excision with palmaris longus autograft, radius-shortening osteotomy, proximal row carpectomy
- In stage IV: proximal row carpectomy, wrist arthrodesis, wrist denervation (10)
- Lunate excision can reduce symptoms but does not prevent carpal collapse.

ONGOING CARE

FOLLOW-UP RECOMMENDATIONS

Prompt referral to an orthopedist after detection to evaluate, accurately stage, and discuss with the patient available current treatments.

COMPLICATIONS

- A continuum from wrist stiffness to a fused and immovable wrist
- Persistent pain
- Nonunion in attempted arthrodesis

REFERENCES

1. Allan CH, Shoji M, White DM, et al. Kienböck disease: a review of management strategies. *J Am Acad Orthop Surg*. 2020;28(7):e315–e324.
2. van Leeuwen WF, Kalichman L, Porsius JT, et al. Vascularized bone grafting for Kienböck disease: a systematic review. *Clin Orthop Relat Res*. 2016;474(3):808–813.
3. Chang J, Chia CP, Yin J, et al. The role of mechanical factors in the pathophysiology of Kienböck disease. *J Hand Surg Am*. 2019;44(6):486–494.
4. Takemura Y, Okada T, Nakamura R, et al. MRI findings and early-stage Kienböck disease. *J Wrist Surg*. 2022;11(2):123–131.
5. Schreiber JJ, Bednar MS, Linscheid RL, et al. Risk factors for Kienböck disease: a comprehensive review of the literature. *JAAOS*. 2021;29(14):e706–e715.
6. Wollstein R, Wollstein A, Rodgers J, et al. A hand therapy protocol for the treatment of lunate overload or early Kienbock's disease. *J Hand Ther*. 2013;26(3):255–259.
7. Havulinna J, Jokihaara J, Paavilainen P, et al. Keyhole revascularization for treatment of coronal plane fracture of the lunate in Kienböck disease. *J Hand Surg Am*. 2016;41(11):e441–e445.
8. De Carli P, Zaidenberg EE, Alfie V, et al. Radius core decompression for Kienböck disease stage IIIA: outcomes at 13 years follow-up. *J Hand Surg Am*. 2017;42(9):752.e1–752.e6.
9. De Smet L, Malghem J, Fabry G, et al. Long-term outcomes of scaphoid excision and tendon interposition for Kienböck disease. *J Hand Surg Eur Vol*. 2023;48(3):260–267.
10. Mariconda M, Soscia E, Sirignano C, et al. Long-term clinical results and MRI changes after tendon ball arthroplasty for advanced Kienböck's disease. *J Hand Surg Eur Vol*. 2013;38(5):508–514.

ADDITIONAL READING

- Bain GI, Begg M. Arthroscopic assessment and classification of Kienböck's disease. *Tech Hand Up Extrem Surg*. 2006;10(1):8–13.
- Bonzar M, Firrell JC, Hainer M, et al. Kienböck disease and negative ulnar variance. *J Bone Joint Surg Am*. 1998;80(8):1154–1157.
- Calfee RP, DeFranco MJ, Baumgarten KM, et al. Treatment of Kienböck disease with biologic therapies. *JBJS Rev*. 2023;11(1):e21.00045.
- Luo J, Diao E. Kienböck's disease: an approach to treatment. *Hand Clin*. 2006;22(4):465–473.
- Mennen U, Sithebe H. The incidence of asymptomatic Kienböck's disease. *J Hand Surg Eur Vol*. 2009;34(3):348–350.
- Ogawa T, Ochiai N, Nishiura Y, et al. A new treatment strategy for Kienböck's disease: combination of bone marrow transfusion, low-intensity pulsed ultrasound therapy, and external fixation. *J Ortho Sci*. 2013;18(2):230–237.
- Schuind F, Eslami S, Ledoux P. Kienböck's disease. *J Bone Joint Surg Br*. 2008;90(2):133–139.
- Wolfe SW, Hotchkiss RN, Pederson WC, et al. *Green's Operative Hand Surgery*. 8th ed. Elsevier; 2022.

CLINICAL PEARLS

- Most commonly seen in ages 20 to 40 years with a predilection to the dominant
- Previous wrist trauma, repetitive trauma, and negative ulnar variance are predisposing factors.
- X-ray shows sclerosis initially and then lucency, but MRI can show changes at an earlier stage.
- Casting for immobilization is the initial therapy and then orthopedic referral for other treatment considerations.

FRACTURE, MANDIBULAR

Hernan Goldsztein, MD

BASICS

DESCRIPTION

- Fracture of the mandible is usually due to a direct blunt force.
- The most commonly fractured sites vary slightly by study but generally include the angle, condyle, symphysis/parasymphysis, body, and ramus.
- Mandibular fractures frequently occur at >1 site simultaneously.

EPIDEMIOLOGY

Mandibular fractures are the second most common facial fracture after nasal fractures. They account for approximately 36–70% of maxillofacial fractures, depending on the population studied. In pediatric populations, mandibular fractures comprise up to 40% of facial fractures, particularly in older children. Incidence is highest in males in their 20s and lowest in children age >5 years.

ETIOLOGY AND PATHOPHYSIOLOGY

- Leading cause of mandible fractures in the Western Hemisphere is interpersonal violence, whereas vehicular accidents are primary etiology in Africa and Asia.
- Additional etiologies include contact sports, falls, work accidents, and pathologic/iatrogenic factors.

RISK FACTORS

- Drug and alcohol use
- Male between the ages of 21 and 30 years

COMMONLY ASSOCIATED CONDITIONS

- Additional traumatic facial fractures, other facial injuries, and dentoalveolar trauma
- Patients may be intoxicated and unable to give a complete history of the injury complicating diagnosis and delaying treatment.

DIAGNOSIS

- The first priority in evaluating a possible mandible fracture is to protect the airway. Severe fractures of facial structures may result in airway obstruction from lack of glossal supporting structures, soft tissue swelling, blood clots in the airway, loose teeth, dentures, or bony fragments.
- Depending on the trauma, C-spine stabilization may be required during the evaluation process.

HISTORY

- The source, size, and direction of traumatic force are helpful in diagnosis.
- Patients involved in motor vehicle accidents tend to sustain complex often comminuted fractures.
- Localized trauma (e.g., pipe, stick, hammer, fist) tends to cause a single linear or localized fractures because the force is concentrated in a small area.
- Blunt trauma with broader distribution commonly results in multiple fractures (e.g., symphysis and condyle) secondary to shape of the mandible and the distribution of the force throughout the mandible.
- Direction of the force can help in making the diagnosis of concomitant fractures. Trauma directed to the chin often results in a symphyseal fracture with concomitant unilateral or bilateral condylar fractures.
- Patient complaints include:
  - Facial asymmetry, deformity, dysphagia, and mandibular pain
  - Malocclusion, decreased range of motion of the temporomandibular joint (TMJ), or a grating sound conducted to the ear with movement of the mandible

PHYSICAL EXAM

- Inspect the maxillofacial area for obvious deformity:
  - Note facial lacerations, swelling, and hematomas.
  - A common site for a laceration is under the chin and is associated with subcondylar or symphysis fracture.
- Look for loose, fractured, or missing teeth; gross malalignment of teeth; separation of tooth interspaces; and ecchymosis or hematoma of the floor of the mouth suggesting a mandibular body or symphyseal fracture.
- Palpate the inferior border of the mandible from the symphysis to the angle on each side. Note areas of swelling, step-off deformity, or tenderness.
- Palpate the movement of the condyle through the external auditory meatus. Pain elicited through palpation of the preauricular region should alert the clinician to a possible condylar fracture.
- Observe any deviation on opening of the mouth or for an inability to chew or open mouth:
  - Deviation with opening commonly occurs towards the side of the mandibular condyle fracture.
  - Note any limited opening and trismus, temporomandibular effusion, or mechanical obstruction to the coronoid process resulting from depression of the zygomatic bone or arch.
- Evaluate for protrusion or lateral excursion of the jaw and any interference with normal mandibular function, including decreased range of motion or deviation of the mandible with opening:
  - The examiner should be able to insert three fingers between the mandible and maxilla.
- Changes in occlusion with early contact of the teeth are highly suggestive of a fracture due to loss of mandibular height.
- Paresthesia of the lower lip or gums strongly indicates a damage to the inferior alveolar nerve.

DIFFERENTIAL DIAGNOSIS

- Dislocation of the mandible
- Contusions
- Isolated dental trauma

DIAGNOSTIC TESTS & INTERPRETATION

- Computed tomography (CT) scan has become the primary modality for diagnosis of mandibular fracture with 3D digitally reconstructed views helping to best visualize complex mandibular fracture (1)[A].
- CT scan, however, may not be adequate in characterizing dental trauma, and a Panorex view may still be needed in the case of dental concerns.
- Additional radiographs potentially helpful in diagnosis of mandibular fractures:
  - Panoramic radiograph
  - Bilateral oblique radiographs
  - Posteroanterior mandibular view
  - Reverse Towne view
  - Mandibular occlusal view

TREATMENT

GENERAL MEASURES

- Up to 40% of patients have associated injuries and treatment should address the most lethal concerns from airway obstruction, aspiration, major hemorrhage, cervical spine or cord injury, and/or intracranial injury.
- Airway compromise can occur due to intraoral edema and hematoma, bony fragments, loose teeth, and loss of tongue support.
- Always maintain C-spine precautions until cleared.
- If intubation is needed, an oral intubation can be attempted.
- Nasotracheal or cricothyrotomy may be indicated, depending on the extent of the injuries and surgical planning.

MEDICATION

- Use of preoperative and perioperative antibiotics in mandible fractures with dentate involvement is well established to reduce the risk of infection. Evidence for prolonged postsurgical antibiotics shows no improvement in infection rates (2),(3)[A].
- Clindamycin: adult: 600 to 900 mg IV; pediatrics: 20 mg/kg 30 to 60 minutes prior to procedure
- Cefazolin: adult: 1 g IV; pediatrics: 50 mg/kg 30 to 60 minutes prior to procedure
- Metronidazole: adult: 500 mg IV; pediatrics: 15 mg/kg IV 30 to 60 minutes prior to procedure

SURGERY/OTHER PROCEDURES

- Linear, nondisplaced, or greenstick fractures may be treated with a soft/liquid diet without wiring.
- Maxillomandibular fixation by wiring upper and lower teeth in occlusion for 4 to 6 weeks in cases with (1) [C]:
  - Nondisplaced or minimally displaced fractures
  - Favorable angle fractures
  - Clinically unstable patients
- Open reduction and internal fixation (ORIF) is indicated in (1)[C]:
  - Displaced fractures (>2 mm)
  - Unstable or comminuted
  - Open or infected fractures (3)[C]
  - Bilateral mandibular body or angle fractures
- With the exception of condylar fractures, many mandibular fractures are associated with mucosal, gingival, or tooth socket disruption and should be treated as open fractures.
- Patients should have their tetanus updated if needed.
- If mandible dislocation is present, reduction may be necessary to free the condyle from its anterior position to the eminence:
  - The operator's thumbs are placed on the external oblique line of the mandible (lateral to the 3rd molar area) or, after wrapping the thumbs in gauze, on the occlusal surface of the lower molars. The other fingers are curled under the mandible.
  - The patient is asked to open wide, as if yawning, and the operator then applies downward force on the molars while applying upward force over the chin until the mandible reduces.
  - Once reduced, the patient should be placed in a Barton bandage for temporary immobilization until he or she receives definitive care.
  - Reduction is facilitated by muscle relaxants (diazepam or midazolam) or anesthetic injection of mastication muscles.
  - A bite block should be used or examiner's fingers should be wrapped in gauze to prevent injury to the treating provider.

Pediatric Considerations

Mandibular fractures are uncommon in children <5 years of age. When they do occur, they are usually greenstick fractures and can be managed with soft diet alone. Parents should be informed that any fracture of the mandible has the potential to damage permanent teeth and cause facial asymmetry; long-term follow-up with a specialist is advisable.

ADMISSION, INPATIENT, AND NURSING CONSIDERATIONS

- Those fractures in which there is significant displacement or associated dental trauma, or those fractures that are thought to be open, require urgent specialty consultation for admission.
- The severity of associated trauma may indicate admission.
- Any patient with the potential for airway compromise, including oropharyngeal edema or bilateral mandibular body fractures, should be admitted after securing the airway.
- Patients unable to follow instructions or at risk for airway compromise should be admitted for definitive fixation.
- In pediatric cases with concern for inconsistent trauma history, consider nonaccidental trauma and report accordingly.
- Consider the possibility of substance abuse and withdrawal particularly if patient is admitted and is to undergo bimaxillary fixation.

ONGOING CARE

PATIENT EDUCATION

- Smokers and patients with systemic medical conditions may have higher rates of complications, including nonunion and infection.
- Evaluate for possible substance use disorder.
- Parents of children should be informed that any fracture of the mandible has the potential to damage permanent teeth and cause facial asymmetry; long-term specialist follow-up should be recommended.

PROGNOSIS

- Patients will usually be immobilized for 4 to 6 weeks and can resume contact sports within 1 to 2 months after treatment with appropriate protective equipment (e.g., customized headgear to provide protection).
- A better prognosis is achieved with removal of grossly diseased teeth.
- Physical therapy is also recommended to improve jaw opening.

COMPLICATIONS

- Prolonged delay in treatment increases the risk of infection.
- Adequate reduction and immobilization are critical in avoiding delayed union, nonunion, and infection.
- Potential complications include malocclusion, infection, nonunion, chronic pain, neurosensory disturbances, TMJ dysfunction, tooth loss, and inability to chew hard food.

REFERENCES

1. Pickrell BB, Hollier LH Jr. Evidence-based medicine: mandibular fractures. *Plast Reconstr Surg*. 2017;140(1):192e–200e.
2. Adalarasan S, Mohan A, Pasupathy S. Prophylactic antibiotics in maxillofacial fractures: a requisite? *J Craniofac Surg*. 2010;21(4):1009–1011.
3. Morris LM, Kellman RM. Are prophylactic antibiotics useful in the management of facial fractures? *Laryngoscope*. 2014;124(6):1282–1284.

ADDITIONAL READING

- Fonseca RJ. *Oral and Maxillofacial Surgery*. 3rd ed. Elsevier; 2018.
- Koshy JC, Feldman EM, Chike-Obi CJ, et al. Pearls of mandibular trauma management. *Semin Plast Surg*. 2010;24(4):357–374.
- Pickrell BB, Serebrakian AT, Maricevich RS. Mandible fractures. *Semin Plast Surg*. 2017;31(2):100–107.
- Purnell CA, Ettinger RE. Mandible fractures: consensus and controversy. *Plast Reconstr Surg*. 2025;156(1):132e–146e.
- Shorey CW, Campbell JH. Dislocation of the temporomandibular joint. *Oral Surg Oral Med Oral Pathol Oral Radiol Endod*. 2000;89(6):662–668.
- Singleton C, Manchella S, Nastri A, et al. Mandibular fractures—what a difference 30 years has made. *Br J Oral Maxillofac Surg*. 2022;60(9):1202–1208.
- World Health Organization. Global Health Observatory. Accessed October 2, 2025. https://www.who.int/data/gho

CLINICAL PEARLS

- Consider a mandibular fracture for any athlete that has facial deformity, dysphagia, and mandibular pain after direct trauma to the face.
- The first priority is to maintain the airway and the C-spine.

FRACTURE, METACARPAL BASE/SHAFT: II–V

Tara Robbins, MD

BASICS

DESCRIPTION

- Metacarpal shaft and base fractures are defined by their location, pattern, and displacement:
  - Three types of metacarpal shaft fractures: transverse, oblique or spiral, and comminuted
  - Two types of metacarpal base fractures: intra-articular and extra-articular
- Metacarpal fractures involving the 1st metacarpal (thumb) are considered separately from those involving the 2nd to 5th metacarpals.
- Two intra-articular fractures of the thumb deserve special mention:
  - Bennett fracture: fracture combined with a subluxation or dislocation of the metacarpal joint
  - Rolando fracture: T- or Y-shaped fracture involving the joint surface

EPIDEMIOLOGY

- Metacarpal fractures account for up to 50% of all hand fractures.
- Small finger is the most commonly injured (50%), followed by the thumb, index, long finger, and ring finger.
- Fractures of metacarpal base occur most commonly in the 4th and 5th metacarpals.
- Metacarpal fractures account for 10–39% of pediatric hand injuries.

Incidence

Lifetime incidence of metacarpal fracture is 2.5%.

ETIOLOGY AND PATHOPHYSIOLOGY

- Transverse and comminuted metacarpal shaft fractures usually result from a direct blow:
  - Dorsal angulation is common.
- Spiral metacarpal fractures result from indirect trauma or rotational torque applied to a digit:
  - Fracture fragments tend to shorten and rotate, especially in the index and small fingers.
- Intra-articular metacarpal base fractures are high-energy injuries and usually result from a direct blow over the base of the metacarpal or a significant axial force or torque applied to the digit:
  - Associated with carpometacarpal (CMC) dislocations
  - Most frequently occur in ring and small fingers
  - Uncommon in index and middle fingers
  - Avulsion fractures usually occur due to tractional forces from tendons that insert into the base of the metacarpals.
- Extra-articular metacarpal base fractures occur from same forces as intra-articular metacarpal base fractures:
  - Most are stabilized by intermetacarpal ligament, resulting in only minimal displacement.
  - Can be associated with CMC dislocation of adjacent digit

RISK FACTORS

Gymnastics, contact sports, racquet sports, boxing, karate

DIAGNOSIS

HISTORY

- Direct blow versus indirect blow with rotational torque: Rotational torque often leads to spiral fractures.
- Nerve injury or damage to the extensor tendon frequently is associated with crush injuries.

PHYSICAL EXAM

- Tenderness and swelling over the dorsal hand
- Pain with motion
- Inability to make a fist
- All patients require a thorough neurovascular examination distal to the fracture site. 4th and 5th metacarpal base fractures may cause injury to the motor branch of the ulnar nerve, resulting in paralysis of the intrinsic hand muscles.

ALERT

Evaluate for rotational malalignment:

- All the fingers of a semi-clenched fist should point to the scaphoid tubercle.
- In comparison to the asymptomatic hand, no crowding or digital overlap should be present when the digits are fully flexed.
- With metacarpophalangeal (MCP) at 90 degrees flexion and digits in extension, the plane of the fingernails should be parallel on the injured and normal hand.

- Function of each flexor and extensor tendon must be documented.

DIFFERENTIAL DIAGNOSIS

- Metacarpal head and neck fractures
- MCP collateral ligament injuries
- CMC fracture dislocation

DIAGNOSTIC TESTS & INTERPRETATION

- Radiographic evaluation with three views is mandatory because many fractures are overlooked or misinterpreted.
- Standard anteroposterior and lateral views: Pronation of 10 to 30 degrees in lateral view facilitates visualization of the 2nd and 3rd metacarpals; supination of 10 to 30 degrees in lateral view aids in viewing the ring and small fingers.
- Oblique views allow better visualization of intra-articular fractures, spiral fractures, and epiphyseal plate injuries.
- Robert view with the hand in maximal pronation is helpful for differentiating between intra-articular and extra-articular fractures of the thumb because it allows for visualizing intra-articular extension of an epibasal fracture.
- Tomograms or computed axial tomographic scans help define CMC relationships and are of benefit for defining comminuted intra-articular fractures (1)[B].

ALERT

Malrotation should be suspected if there is metacarpal shortening or a discrepancy in the shaft diameter.

TREATMENT

GENERAL MEASURES

- Once thorough neurovascular examination is complete, wrist or hematoma block may facilitate reduction if necessary.
- Impaction fractures of the metacarpal bases that are not significantly displaced can be treated with splinting, followed by early mobilization.
- Fractures amenable to closed manipulative reduction are transverse fractures, isolated spiral/oblique fractures with <3 mm of shortening, and extra-articular fractures of the thumb.
- Closed reduction of metacarpal shaft fractures is performed with longitudinal traction, dorsal pressure at the fracture site, and rotation as needed.
- Closed reduction of extra-articular base fractures typically requires only longitudinal traction.
- Postreduction films are mandatory. Limits of angular deformity depend on mobility of different metacarpals at base.
  - The index and long fingers are limited in motion relative to the ulnar most digits due to their attachment to the trapezoid and capitate and can only tolerate 10 to 15 degrees of angulation (2)[B].
  - The ring and small finger articulation at the hamate permit a greater range of motion (ROM) and, therefore, may tolerate more angulation of 30 to 45 degrees in the ring and up to 50 degrees in the small finger (2)[B].
- Orthopedic referral is required if satisfactory reduction cannot be performed or maintained.
- Radiographs should be repeated 1 week after injury to reevaluate for angulation, rotation, and shortening.
- Dorsal and volar splints must include all metacarpal shafts and wrist while avoiding immobilization of the interphalangeal joint. Splint should be left in place for 3 to 4 weeks (1)[B].
- Ulnar gutter splint for 3 to 4 weeks for extra-articular metacarpal base fractures if ring and/or little finger(s) are involved.
- Volar or radial gutter for 3 to 4 weeks for extra-articular metacarpal base fractures of index and long finger
- Functional brace (Galveston) if fracture requires significant reduction
- Thumb spica cast for extra-articular fractures of the thumb for 4 to 6 weeks
- Bulky compressive dressing for unstable fractures
- The index and long fingers are limited in motion relative to the ulnar most digits due to their attachment to the trapezoid and capitate and can only tolerate 10 to 15 degrees of angulation. However, the ring and small finger articulation at the hamate permit a greater ROM and, therefore, may tolerate more angulation of 30 to 45 degrees in the ring and up to 50 degrees in the small finger.
- For angulated fractures, closed reduction with local block or conscious sedation and immobilization is generally effective for children (1)[B].

- Referral is needed for unstable or unsatisfactory reductions in children.
- Long oblique and spiral fractures typically require closed reduction and percutaneous pinning in children (1)[B].
- Fractures involving the physis and epiphysis are uncommon in children:
  - Usually Salter-Harris type II, which almost always are treatable with closed reduction and immobilization.
  - Salter-Harris type III fractures are rare. These require open reduction because osteonecrosis of the metacarpal head can result if inadequately reduced.
- Children can be immobilized longer due to additional flexibility.

ISSUES FOR REFERRAL

ALERT

- Any rotational deformity
- >5 mm of shortening
- >10 degrees angulation for 2nd and 3rd metacarpals, >30 degrees angulation for 4th and 5th metacarpals, >25 degrees angulation of the thumb
- >25% articular surface involvement, >1 mm step-off
- Intra-articular base fractures
- Inability to perform or maintain satisfactory closed reduction
- All surgical cases, including special situations such as multiple fractures, nerve or tendon injury, and open fractures

ADDITIONAL THERAPIES

- Field management: Splint immobilization provides comfort and minimizes soft tissue injury.
- Ice packs should be used proximal to the metacarpals to prevent digital injuries.
- Buddy taping may provide stability when mobilization begins.
- Clinical union is manifested by absence of tenderness at the fracture site with palpation and ROM. Radiographic union will lag behind clinical union by several weeks.

SURGERY/OTHER PROCEDURES

- Open reduction and internal fixation or closed reduction with percutaneous pinning is advocated for patients with malunion or unstable fractures (Bennett, Rolando, comminuted, intra-articular, spiral/oblique with shortening, and rotation).
- Recently, a novel intraoperative kickstand technique has been reported to reduce angulated metacarpal neck fractures before retrograde headless intramedullary screw fixation (3)[C].
- For oblique and spiral fractures, lag screws can be applied with neutralization plating, although transverse fractures should have plates used in compression mode. This approach allows for more inherent stability and earlier ROM exercises in the postoperative period with favorable outcomes in ROM and a return to activity (2)[B].

ONGOING CARE

FOLLOW-UP RECOMMENDATIONS

- Follow up 1 week after injury with radiographs to evaluate for angulation, rotation, and shortening.
- Splint or cast should remain in place for 3 to 4 weeks minimum.
- For those patients who undergo percutaneous fixation, early ROM can be difficult due to soft tissue adhesions to the K-wire but should require implementation once a clinical union is obtained, commonly at 3 to 6 weeks (4)[B].
- Those with plate fixation can be exercised immediately upon the removal of the sutures, which commonly occurs at the first postoperative visit (2)[B].
- Rehabilitation should be delayed until 3 to 4 weeks postinjury for distal metacarpal shaft fractures (5)[C].
- Both active and passive ROM at interphalangeal joints can be started immediately for metacarpal base and proximal shaft fractures (5)[C].
- Gentle active ROM at the MCP joint is allowed in most proximal stable shaft fractures 3 to 4 weeks after injury (5)[C].
- Passive ROM at MCP joint can be added when there are signs of clinical union, usually 5 to 6 weeks after the injury (5)[C].
- Strengthening exercises should be added at 8 weeks (5)[C].

COMPLICATIONS

- Stiffness can develop after prolonged immobilization or delayed rehabilitation.
- Chronic CMC joint stiffness is associated with intra-articular fractures.
- Malunion usually manifests as malrotation or dorsal angulation, so confirm that the patient's fingertips point toward the scaphoid tuberosity in flexion at each visit:
  - 5 degrees of malrotation can result in 1.5 cm of digital overlap and cause a decrease in grip strength.
  - Function is more likely to be affected if the malunion is proximal, involves either the 2nd or the 3rd metacarpal, or is rotational.
- Nonunion is uncommon in metacarpal fractures.
- Surgical complications can also arise. Plates and other prominent hardware frequently cause tendon adhesions and stiffness. Metal may become tender to palpation. Treatment includes hardware removal and extensor tendon tenolysis (6)[C].

REFERENCES

1. Chin SH, Vedder NB. MOC-PSSM CME article: metacarpal fractures. *Plast Reconstr Surg*. 2008;121(Suppl 1):1–13.
2. Kozin SH, Thoder JJ, Lieberman G. Operative treatment of metacarpal and phalangeal shaft fractures. *J Am Acad Orthop Surg*. 2000;8(2):111–121.
3. Braig ZV, Kakar S. Kickstand technique for intraoperative reduction of fifth metacarpal neck fractures. *J Hand Surg Am*. 2022;47(8):799.e1–799.e7.
4. Guldagger KVS, Dahlin LB, Brogren E, et al. Metacarpal fractures. Article in Danish. *Ugeskr Laeger*. 2020;182(47):V08190477.
5. Weinstein LP, Hanel DP. Metacarpal fractures. *J Am Soc Surg Hand*. 2002;2(4):168–180.
6. Kollitz KM, Hammert WC, Vedder NB, et al. Metacarpal fractures: treatment and complications. *Hand (N Y)*. 2014;9(1):16–23.
7. Peyronson F, Ostwald CS, Hailer NP, et al. Nonoperative versus operative treatment for displaced finger metacarpal shaft fractures: a prospective, noninferiority, randomized controlled trial. *J Bone Joint Surg Am*. 2023;105(2):98–106.

ADDITIONAL READING

- Antosia RE, Lyn E. Hand. In: Marx JA, Hockberger R, Walls RM, et al, eds. *Marx: Rosen's Emergency Medicine: Concepts and Clinical Practice*. 6th ed. Mosby; 2006.
- Ben-Amotz O, Sammer DM. Practical management of metacarpal fractures. *Plast Reconstr Surg*. 2015;136(3):370e–379e.
- Capo JT, Hastings H II. Metacarpal and phalangeal fractures in athletes. *Clin Sports Med*. 1998;17(3):491–511.
- Diaz-Garcia R, Waljee JF. Current management of metacarpal fractures. *Hand Clin*. 2013;29(4):507–518.
- Harrison BP, Hilliard MW. Emergency department evaluation and treatment of hand injuries. *Emerg Med Clin North Am*. 1999;17(4):793–822.
- Mastey RD, Weiss AP, Akelman E. Primary care of hand and wrist athletic injuries. *Clin Sports Med*. 1997;16(4):705–724.
- Peterson JJ, Bancroft LW. Injuries of the fingers and thumb in the athlete. *Clin Sports Med*. 2006;25(3):527–542.
- Simon RR, Koenigsknecht SJ, eds. *Emergency Orthopedics*. Appleton & Lange; 1996.
- Wong VW, Higgins JP. Evidence-based medicine: management of metacarpal fractures. *Plast Reconstr Surg*. 2017;140(1):140e–151e.

CLINICAL PEARLS

- Metacarpal fractures that are more distal and ulnar are better tolerated and are more amendable to nonoperative treatment.
- Boxer's fractures are metacarpal neck fractures involving the small finger.
- Return to play needs to be individualized, depending on the type of fracture, mobility, and clinical healing.
- For some displaced fractures without other complicating features, nonoperative management may lead to comparable functional outcomes. A randomized trial of displaced oblique or spiral metacarpal shaft fractures (n = 42) reported comparable or better results with nonsurgical management compared with surgical fixation in the primary outcome (grip strength at 1 year) and in several secondary outcomes (e.g., complications, duration of absence from work, and patient satisfaction) despite significantly worse bone shortening in the nonoperative group (5.3 mm vs. 2.3 mm for surgery group) (7)[B].

FRACTURE, METACARPAL NECK: I–V

Chris Koutures, MD, FAAP

BASICS

DESCRIPTION

- The metacarpal neck (distal metaphysis) is the aspect of the metacarpal shaft immediately underneath the metacarpal head.
- The weakest point of the metacarpal is located at the distal metaphysis, so metacarpal fractures frequently involve the neck (1).
- The mechanism of injury is usually an axial load on the metacarpophalangeal (MCP) joint while in a flexed position, such as when throwing a punch.
- Fractures about the metacarpal neck must be scrutinized for malrotation and angulation.
- As 2nd and 3rd metacarpals are necessary for handgrip power, much less angulation is tolerated in these injuries.
- Synonym(s): boxer's fracture; 5th metacarpal neck fracture

EPIDEMIOLOGY

- 5th metacarpal neck fractures (boxer's fractures) are the most common hand fracture, accounting for 20% of all hand fractures (1).
- Fractures of the 1st metacarpal neck are uncommon.

ETIOLOGY AND PATHOPHYSIOLOGY

- Due to the action of the interosseous muscles, the distal fracture fragment (metacarpal head) displaces volarly, resulting in an apex dorsal angulation.
- The index and long fingers cannot tolerate angulation deformities given their relatively fixed articulations with the distal carpal bones.
- The ring and small fingers, however, have limited flexion and extension, so angular deformities are better tolerated and they heal with minimal loss of function.

RISK FACTORS

"Out-of-control tempers": Boxer's fractures usually are due to striking an opponent or a wall with a clenched fist.

DIAGNOSIS

HISTORY

- Axial load or direct trauma, often to clenched fist or dorsum of the hand
- Immediate pain and swelling noted

PHYSICAL EXAM

- Swelling and tenderness on the dorsum of the hand, often accompanied by MCP joint depression
- Extreme angulation may lead to pseudoclawing, which is hyperextension of the MCP joint along with proximal interphalangeal (PIP) joint flexion as the patient attempts to extend the finger.
- Tenderness and swelling about the dorsal aspect of the distal metacarpals. Examine skin closely for teeth marks, redness, warmth, or streaking suggesting infection or other injuries.
- Evaluate the digits for malrotation, which occurs more in 4th and 5th metacarpal neck fractures. Have the patient bring all the fingernails into the palm and compare with the noninjured hand. All the nails should point toward the base of the 1st metacarpal. If the injured finger is out of this alignment, strongly suspect significant fracture malrotation.

DIFFERENTIAL DIAGNOSIS

- Metacarpal head fracture
- Metacarpal shaft fracture
- Open fracture
- MCP joint dislocation
- MCP joint sprain

DIAGNOSTIC TESTS & INTERPRETATION

- Anteroposterior, oblique, and true lateral radiographic views of the hand usually are sufficient.
- Normally, the metacarpal neck is situated with a baseline of 15 degrees of volar angulation. Ensure adequate visualization on the lateral view to evaluate the degree of fracture angulation.
- A conservative rule for limits of acceptable angulation of the 2nd through 5th digits is 10 to 30. Thus, the 2nd digit can only tolerate 10 degrees of angulation (in addition to the baseline 15 degrees); the 5th metacarpal can accept 30 degrees above the baseline. Many other experts will tolerate a greater degree of angulation of the 5th metacarpal; this decision often is influenced by the particular activity profile, hobbies, work requirements, or sport of the patient.
- Degrees of acceptable angulation vary in current literature. For the index or long finger, some authors report that angulation of >15 degrees above baseline is not tolerated due to the lack of carpal metacarpal motion (1)[C]. Others report that for the ring finger, up to 30 degrees of excessive angulation (above baseline) at the metacarpal neck is acceptable, and for the small finger, up to 40 degrees of excessive angulation (above baseline) at the 5th metacarpal neck is acceptable (2)[B],(3)[C].

TREATMENT

GENERAL MEASURES

- Nonsteroidal anti-inflammatory drugs (NSAIDs) can be used along with ice for immediate analgesia.
- Teeth marks can represent entry pathway for infection, especially if noted adjacent to MCP joint. Any sign of deeper infection (including fever, redness, streaking, or focal discharge) requires immediate evaluation by a hand surgical specialist.
- Closed reduction is considered in cases of significant angulation of 4th (>20 degrees above baseline) and 5th (>30 degrees above baseline) metacarpal neck fractures.
- Anesthesia can be obtained by hematoma block or ulnar nerve block.
- Flex the MCP, PIP, and distal PIP joints all to 90 degrees. Apply dorsally directed pressure along the proximal phalanx shaft through the flexed PIP joint while simultaneously applying volarly directed pressure over the proximal fracture fragment (3)[C].
- Obtain a postreduction lateral view of the hand to ensure adequate reduction and immobilization.
- Nondisplaced and nonangulated fractures of the 2nd or 3rd metacarpal necks can be immobilized in a radial gutter splint with the wrist in 30 degrees extension, MCP joint in 70 to 90 degrees of flexion, and PIP/distal interphalangeal (DIP) joints near full extension.
- Mildly angulated 4th (<20 degrees above baseline) and 5th (<30 degrees above baseline) metacarpal neck fractures can be immobilized in ulnar gutter splints with the same positions.
- Alternatively, some literature recommends functional treatment by casting (glove cast) or by taping with pressure bandage (2)[B],(3)[C]. For functional casting, the cast is applied circularly around the metacarpals and it starts distal to the palmar crease of the wrist and ends just proximal to the MCP joint. This allows maximal range of motion of the finger and wrist while providing immobilization and protection of the fracture fragment.
- Elevate the hand and consider application of ice for 20 minutes intervals on a regular basis over the first 24 to 48 hours after injury.
- Splints should be applied to injuries requiring orthopedic referral (see below) unless that consultant is immediately available.
- There are variable recommendations regarding the optimal management for metacarpal neck fractures, particularly for fracture of the 5th metacarpal neck.

- Points of discussion include:
  - How much angulation is acceptable (recommendations in literature vary from 20 to 70 degrees for the 5th metacarpal)?
  - Which splinting method is most optimal, and if splinting is absolutely necessary?
  - What length of immobilization is optimal (literature varies anywhere from no immobilization to 1 week of immobilization followed by functional treatment to pure immobilization ranging from 2 to 4 weeks)?
- No differences in functional outcome were found between boxer's fractures treated with immobilization in an ulnar gutter cast for 3 weeks and those treated with functional taping for 1 week. Furthermore, range of motion of the 5th MCP joint was not affected in fractures with angulation <70 degrees that were not reduced (2)[B].
- A randomized controlled trial supported the use of soft wrap and buddy taping for treatment of boxer's fracture with palmar angulation ≤70 degrees and no rotational deformity. Although there was no statistical difference in satisfaction with the aesthetic appearance, the patient must be willing to accept the loss of the "knuckle" with this treatment method (4)[B].
- A 2005 Cochrane Review concluded that there is no single nonsurgical treatment method that can be recommended as superior to another (5)[B].
- Management of fractures associated with bite wounds:
  - Key principles:
    - **Thorough irrigation and débridement:** The wound must be meticulously cleaned and any devitalized tissue removed to reduce the bacterial load and prevent infection.
    - **Antibiotic prophylaxis and close monitoring:** Broad-spectrum antibiotics are crucial to combat the polymicrobial nature of bite wound infections. Close follow-up is necessary to identify any signs of infection early.
    - **Fracture stabilization:** The fracture should be adequately stabilized to allow for proper healing and minimize the risk of complications like malunion or nonunion.
    - **Tetanus prophylaxis:** Ensure the patient's tetanus immunization is up-to-date.

ISSUES FOR REFERRAL

Open reduction and internal fixation is indicated for:

- Significant angulation of 2nd (>10 degrees above baseline) and 3rd (>10 degrees above baseline) metacarpal neck fractures or those with any displacement
- Failure to achieve acceptable angles after reduction of the 4th and 5th metacarpals
- A retrospective study found that closed reduction and splint immobilization of 5th metacarpal neck fractures was not an effective means of maintaining a significant improvement in fracture alignment upon healing. Other means, such as closed reduction with pin fixation or open reduction internal fixation, should be considered when maintenance of reduction is desired (6)[B].
- Any metacarpal neck fracture with rotational malalignment or comminution
- Any potential open fracture → including bite wounds
- Degree of residual angulation that is unacceptable to the patient
- Inability to hold reduction position
- Athlete who desires immediate return to play in cast orthosis
- Surgical techniques include: closed reduction and pinning, pinning (cross, crucifix, and bouquet), plate and screw fixation, and intramedullary fixation
- There is no consensus among hand surgeons as to the single most effective technique. As such, multiple fixation constructs exist with various risks and benefits. The lack of an ideal surgical fixation technique necessitates further investigation of current treatment strategies as well as the development of further novel techniques that may lead to improved outcomes (7)[A].

ONGOING CARE

- If splint used, fractures should remain splinted for a minimum of 3 to 4 weeks.
- Clinical healing is defined as no tenderness with palpation of the fracture site.
- Once the splints are removed, begin range of motion work with emphasis on handgrip and manipulation strength: key to prevent stiffness of the MCP joint.

FOLLOW-UP RECOMMENDATIONS

- Follow-up radiographs may not be indicated for most 5th metacarpal base and neck fractures. Follow-up radiographs should be performed at the discretion of the treating physician on an as-needed basis for fractures at risk for displacement (8).
- For 2nd and 3rd metacarpal neck fractures, follow-up radiographs should be obtained in 5 to 7 days to monitor fracture alignment.
- For 4th and 5th metacarpal neck fractures, follow-up radiographs should be considered at 7 to 10 days.
- Perform follow-up visits at 2-week intervals to monitor for malalignment, rotational deformity, angulation, and progress of healing.

Patient Monitoring

- Return to sports participation recommended when there is pain-free range of motion and when strength approaches that of the contralateral hand.
- In general, conservative guideline for return to contact sports with splint/orthotic protection is after 2 to 4 weeks of immobilization. Some experts may allow immediate return to play with a protective cast or splint.
- Use of orthotic protection during contact sports should continue for 8 to 10 weeks after the initial injury.

PATIENT EDUCATION

- Patients should be warned that despite reduction and splinting, loss of knuckle prominence may result.
- After splint removal, educate patient on range-of-motion exercises to prevent MCP joint stiffness.

COMPLICATIONS

- MCP joint stiffness due to prolonged immobilization, interosseous muscle contractures, or tendon adhesions
- Cosmetic deformity without functional loss still may ensue.
- Although uncommon, delayed union or nonunion of the fracture site may occur.
- Pseudoclawing

REFERENCES

1. Capo JT, Hastings H II. Metacarpal and phalangeal fractures in athletes. *Clin Sports Med.* 1998;17(3):491–511.
2. Statius Muller MG, Poolman RW, van Hoogstraten MJ, et al. Immediate mobilization gives good results in boxer's fractures with volar angulation up to 70 degrees: a prospective randomized trial comparing immediate mobilization with cast immobilization. *Arch Orthop Trauma Surg.* 2003;123(10):534–537.
3. Leggit JC, Meko CJ. Acute finger injuries: part II. Fractures, dislocations, and thumb injuries. *Am Fam Physician.* 2006;73(5):827–834.
4. van Aaken J, Fusetti C, Luchina S, et al. Fifth metacarpal neck fractures treated with soft wrap/buddy taping compared to reduction and casting: results of a prospective, multicenter, randomized trial. *Arch Orthop Trauma Surg.* 2016;136(1):135–142.
5. Poolman RW, Goslings JC, Lee JB, et al. Conservative treatment for closed fifth (small finger) metacarpal neck fractures. *Cochrane Database Syst Rev.* 2005;(3):CD003210.
6. Pace GI, Gendelberg D, Taylor KF. The effect of closed reduction of small finger metacarpal neck fractures on the ultimate angular deformity. *J Hand Surg Am.* 2015;40(8):1582–1585.
7. Padegimas EM, Warrender WJ, Jones CM, et al. Metacarpal neck fractures: a review of surgical indications and techniques. *Arch Trauma Res.* 2016;5(3):e32933.
8. Heckmann N, Dusch MN, Pannell WC, et al. The utility of plain films for nonoperative fifth metacarpal fractures: are follow-up radiographs necessary? *Hand (N Y).* 2018;13(6):646–651.

CLINICAL PEARLS

- Must consider metacarpal neck fractures in any punching, striking, or axial load injury mechanism.
- Common complications include open bite wounds, malrotation, and significant fracture angulation.
- Patient's opinion may help dictate treatment in cases of angulation that may result in cosmetic concerns or functional impact on sport choice (using racquets, ball placement in hand).

FRACTURE, METATARSAL

Adam T. Chrusch, MD, CAQSM

BASICS

The anatomy of the foot is divided into the hindfoot, the midfoot, and the forefoot:
- The hindfoot includes the calcaneus and talus.
- The midfoot includes the navicular, cuboid, and cuneiform bones.
- The forefoot includes the metatarsals and phalanges:
  - The forefoot functions to transmit ground reaction forces to the midfoot with weight-bearing activities.
  - Fractures in the forefoot can alter the normal distribution of weight and lead to secondary metatarsalgia (pain) as well as transfer lesions such as plantar calluses and stress lesions.

DESCRIPTION
- A metatarsal fracture can be described as being extra-articular, partial intra-articular, or articular, depending on where on the metatarsal the fracture occurs. Extra-articular fractures may be transverse (straight across the long axis), oblique, or spiral. An articular or partial intra-articular may be a simple isolated fracture extending into the joint, comminuted, or an avulsion fracture.
- A stress injury with normal radiographs but a positive exam (pain to palpation) may be categorized as macrotrabecular (visible fracture lines on magnetic resonance imaging [MRI], usually T1) or stress reaction (T2 signal change on MRI without visible fracture lines).

EPIDEMIOLOGY
- Metatarsal fractures are likely more common in athletes involved in weight-bearing exercise.
- Any direct trauma, however, can cause a fracture.

Incidence
- Metatarsal fractures are common with the 5th metatarsal constituting 80% (1)[B].
- Single metatarsal fractures are predominately 5th metatarsal, seasonally dependent (spring/summer), whereas multiple metatarsal fractures have a more homogenous incidence (1)[B].

ETIOLOGY AND PATHOPHYSIOLOGY
- When the cortical bone's mechanical strength is exceeded acutely by direct trauma it will fracture.
- A fracture may also occur when the bone-tendon interface is acutely stressed past its mechanical failure point (avulsion fracture).
- An additional mechanism for fracture occurs when repetitive subthreshold forces are incompletely healed, and the additive damage eventually causes an overt fracture (completion of a stress fracture).

RISK FACTORS
- Those with osteopenia or osteoporosis have a greater risk.
- Any activity that increases the likelihood of direct trauma to the foot increases the risk of metatarsal injury.
- Twisting mechanism is associated with 5th metatarsal fractures (1)[B].
- Excessively rapid progression of training volume increases the risk of metatarsal stress injury.

GENERAL PREVENTION
- Gradual increases in workload allow a bone to adapt to mechanical stress and become stronger.
- Balance and slow progression allow a bone to remodel and adapt to stress.

COMMONLY ASSOCIATED CONDITIONS
- Other injuries to consider:
  - Midtarsal joint injury (calcaneocuboid or talonavicular): can include lateral process of talus or anterior process of calcaneus
  - Navicular or cuboid contusion/fracture
  - Metatarsocuneiform (MTC)/cuboid injury: Lisfranc joint injury may include ligamentous disruption and/or fracture of surrounding bone.
  - MTP injury: can include capsular or ligamentous sprain (turf toe) or fracture of adjacent bone
- Predisposing conditions:
  - Hallux valgus/hallux rigidus: Altered mechanics at the 1st MTP joint leads body weight shifting laterally over the lesser caliber 2nd metatarsal.
  - Osteopenia/osteoporosis: Decreased mechanical strength of the bone increases susceptibility to stress fracture and acute fracture.

DIAGNOSIS

- Diagnosis of overt metatarsal fracture is by radiograph.
- Standard views include the anteroposterior (AP), lateral, and oblique views.
- Weight-bearing with comparison views of the opposite foot help identify subtle lesions as well as Lisfranc injuries.
- Diagnosis of radiographically negative stress injury is via a technetium-99 bone scan or MRI.

HISTORY
- Direct trauma to the foot or a twisting injury
- More subtle stress injuries will typically have a history of recent increases in training volume or impact load and possibly a prior history of other stress fractures, disordered eating, or menstrual irregularities.

PHYSICAL EXAM
- Point-tenderness directly over the metatarsal
- Foot swelling in comparison to the unaffected foot and possibly bruising.
- Gross displacement is not common.

DIFFERENTIAL DIAGNOSIS
- MTP joint synovitis: inflammation of the joint rather than stress reaction in the bone itself. Bone scan will show distal uptake around the MTP joint. MRI is diagnostic. Claw toe may also cause synovitis with plantar displacement of metatarsal head or a metatarsal stress reaction.
- MTP capsular strain and/or chip fracture of 1st metatarsal head (turf toe)
- Lisfranc sprain/fracture: injury to the 2nd MTC articulation. Any pain at the proximal 2nd metatarsal in association with a twisting injury in plantar flexion should raise concern for this injury.
- Midfoot sprain: injury to MTC ligamentous structures
- Forefoot mass (ganglion or tumor)
- Morton neuroma (interdigital neuroma)
- Freiberg infarction: osteonecrosis of 2nd metatarsal head; more common in adolescent athletes with unilateral (usually) pain in 2nd metatarsal head

DIAGNOSTIC TESTS & INTERPRETATION
- Plain radiographs will show cortical disruption if a significant fracture has occurred.
- The findings may be subtle with mild injury.
- A stress fracture may show subtle sclerotic borders/periosteal elevation or be entirely normal.
- Plain films only become positive once healing has progressed enough to produce visible bony callus. In the interim, an MRI should show changes on T2 images and a bone scan should be positive for focal uptake over the painful area.
- A computed tomography (CT) scan may be indicated for an intra-articular fracture to delineate any articular step-off.

TREATMENT

The goal of treatment is to stabilize the fracture such that normal length, rotation, and declination of the metatarsal is maintained, and the area is protected from further injury until healing has occurred:
- Prehospital:
  - If possible, the foot should be elevated and cooled with ice as soon as possible after injury.
  - Limited or crutch-assist weight-bearing is advisable until emergency department (ED) or physician evaluation has occurred.
  - Chronic complaints can be evaluated in a physician's office rather than an ED.
- ED treatment:
  - Evaluation of acute injury to the foot in the ED includes AP, lateral, and oblique plain radiographs. neurovascular status must be verified, as compartment syndrome can occur. Closed or open reduction is then assessed. Multiple metatarsal fractures with >4 mm of displacement or an apical angulation of the metatarsal head of >10 degrees on the lateral view could require open/closed reduction.

- Open reduction of metatarsal, phalangeal, and MTP joint injuries can cause scarring and stiffness. It is used to maintain a plantigrade foot for normal weight-bearing. Open fractures require surgical intervention.
- Nondisplaced fractures of the metatarsal neck and shaft may be treated with a short leg cast, fracture brace, or a cast shoe. Weight-bearing is permitted as tolerated on discharge from ED. The minimum amount of immobilization necessary for comfort should be used. Fractures at the base of the 5th metatarsal may be treated with an ankle stirrup brace, cast shoe, or fracture brace to maintain comfort.
- Treatment of two or more fractures should involve CT imaging for surgical planning and it is preferable to use rigid fixation with plates/screws as it yields better functional outcomes (2)[B]

MEDICATION

- Nonsteroidal anti-inflammatory drugs (NSAIDs) short course only <10 days
- Acetaminophen

ISSUES FOR REFERRAL

- Multiple/open metatarsal fractures
- Single metatarsal fracture with >4 mm of displacement
- Single metatarsal fracture with >10 degrees of dorsal angulation of distal segment
- Possible compartment syndrome
- Displaced/comminuted fracture of the 1st metatarsal
- Proximal 5th metatarsal fracture nonunion after 12 weeks of conservative care
- Lisfranc fracture dislocation—even subtle injuries have long term implications (3)[B].

ADDITIONAL THERAPIES

- Proximal 5th metatarsal avulsion fracture (pseudo-Jones fracture):
  - Mechanism:
    - Acute inversion injury to the ankle in plantar flexion
    - Avulsion of the peroneus brevis or lateral plantar aponeurosis at the metatarsal tuberosity
    - Tend to be nondisplaced and experience relatively rapid union with conservative care
    - More distal injuries (without being a Jones fracture) may require short leg casting with non–weight-bearing (NWB) status for up to 6 to 8 weeks.
    - Open reduction and internal fixation (ORIF) for delayed union or nonunion, significant displacement
- Jones fracture (proximal shaft of 5th metatarsal):
  - The metaphyseal/diaphyseal junction is a watershed zone for blood flow and is susceptible to delayed union or nonunion. Consider ORIF in higher level athletes primarily and if nonunion occurs as well as displaced acute Jones fractures. Treat initially with short leg cast/fracture brace with no weight-bearing until evidence of bony callus formation is seen. Progress to weight-bearing at that point; may present with pre-injury symptoms similar to stress fracture exacerbated by inversion injury
- Spiral fracture of 5th metatarsal (dancer's fracture):
  - This is typically treated nonsurgically with a fracture brace or cast shoe. Weight-bearing is allowed as tolerated. Radiographic healing may take up to 12 weeks.

SURGERY/OTHER PROCEDURES

- Proximal 5th metatarsal fracture/Jones fracture: ORIF with malleolar screw Kirschner wires
- Bone grafting may be required with a nonunion.
- Lisfranc fracture/dislocation: involves 2nd through 5th MTC joints; ORIF with cortical screws and Kirschner wires

ONGOING CARE

- Follow up should be within 1 to 2 weeks for repeat x-ray and examination.
- The least-limiting form of immobilization should be considered. With the exception of a Jones fracture, most metatarsal fractures tolerate weight-bearing with use of a cast shoe/wooden-soled shoe fairly quickly, if not at the time of diagnosis. If fracture brace/controlled ankle motion (CAM) boot use is required initially, transition to a stiff-soled or cast shoe should be considered when tolerated. A steel shank insert into a gym shoe may also be used.
- Restriction from full weight-bearing stress without protection should continue for at least 4 weeks for a stress fracture and for 4 to 6 weeks for a nondisplaced metatarsal fracture. Evidence for radiographic healing, resolution of edema, and pain-free direct palpation are needed for return to sports.
- Jones fracture:
  - Once diagnosis is made, an NWB fracture brace/cast is used for 6 weeks to allow for healing to occur. Repeat radiographs are done at this point to assess progress, but up to 12 weeks may be needed. Nonunion at 12 weeks may require ORIF.
  - The decision to pursue ORIF for a Jones fracture in a competitive athlete may occur at the time of initial diagnosis although current literature is mixed on primary surgical fixation in elite athletes. (4)[B]

PATIENT EDUCATION

- Elevate the leg frequently to minimize forefoot edema.
- Notify the physician if there is any significant increase in pain/swelling during the recovery process.
- Reduce activity level to remain pain free and use stiff-soled shoe for all weight-bearing activity until healing is complete.

PROGNOSIS

Good

COMPLICATIONS

- Nonunion
- Malunion with painful plantar calluses under the metatarsal head
- Dorsal corns secondary to friction over prominent metatarsal head

REFERENCES

1. Herterich V, Hofmann L, Böcker W, et al. Acute, isolated fractures of the metatarsal bones: an epidemiologic study. *Arch Orthop Trauma Surg*. 2023;143(4):1939–1945.
2. Egrise F, Bernard E, Galliot F, et al. Treatment of two or more metatarsal fractures. *Orthop Traumatol Surg Res*. 2022;110(1):103285.
3. Garriguez-Perez D, Puerto-Vazquez M, Delgado JLT, et al. Impact of the subtle Lisfranc injury on foot structure and function. *Foot Ankle Int*. 2021;42(10):1303–1310.
4. Goodloe JB, Cregar WM, Caughman A, et al. Surgical management of proximal fifth metatarsal fractures in elite athletes: a systematic review. *Orthop J Sports Med*. 2021;9(9):23259671211037647.

ADDITIONAL READING

Jin J. Risks of codeine and tramadol in children. *JAMA*. 2017;318(15):1514.

CLINICAL PEARLS

- The 1st metatarsal carries a large amount of load, and fractures of it are often surgical.
- Fracture-dislocations involving the Lisfranc joint are often missed on NWB films and routinely need surgery to prevent long term pain. Careful evaluation should be used to avoid missing this diagnosis.
- Dancer's fractures, even displaced, will usually heal with conservative nonoperative management, whereas Jones fracture has a higher rate of nonunion and more often needs surgical fixation in elite athletes.
- Multiple metatarsal fractures are more likely to cause chronic issues therefore more likely to require initial surgical intervention (2)[A].

FRACTURE, MIDDLE PHALANX

Mitchell P. Anderson, MD • Daniel C. Herman, MD, PhD, FAAPMR, FACSM, FISBS, CAQSM • Brandon Hassid, MD

BASICS

DESCRIPTION

- Phalangeal fractures account for 23% of below-elbow fractures in the United States and are the most common injuries of the upper extremity (1).
- Each phalanx consists of a proximal base, a central diaphysis, and a distal head (2).
- The middle phalanx head is formed by two condyles separated by an intercondylar groove.
- The shaft is the most common location for fractures, except in the pediatric population (3).
- Physeal fractures often occur in skeletally immature individuals.
- Collateral ligaments lie on the radial and ulnar borders of the proximal interphalangeal (PIP) and distal interphalangeal (DIP) (4).
- A single digital nerve and artery lie on both the radial and ulnar aspects of each ray.

ETIOLOGY AND PATHOPHYSIOLOGY

- Middle phalanx fractures can be classified into extra-articular and intra-articular occurring along the base, shaft, and condyle.
- For extra-articular fractures, bending forces usually produce transverse fractures, torsional or angular forces create oblique fractures, and crushing injuries result in comminuted fractures (2).
- Intra-articular fractures are most commonly produced by an axial loading injury.
- The flexor digitorum superficialis (FDS) and the central extensor slip (CES) insert onto the middle phalanx and account for the primary deforming forces on shaft fractures.
- Fractures proximal to the insertion of the FDS result in flexion of the distal fragment (leading to apex dorsal angulation of the fracture).
- Fractures distal to the insertion of the FDS will result in flexion of the proximal fragment (and apex volar angulation of the fracture).
- Midshaft fractures of the middle phalanx typically present with a dorsal angulation deformity and can be associated with a mallet deformity of the DIP joint (5).
- Interphalangeal collateral ligament injuries may result in avulsion fractures affecting articular surfaces.

COMMONLY ASSOCIATED CONDITIONS

- DIP or PIP joint dislocations
- Digital artery or nerve injury
- Extensor mechanism injuries
- Volar plate injuries and resulting swan neck deformity
- Mallet deformity
- Skin lacerations

DIAGNOSIS

HISTORY

- Mechanism of injury:
  - Grabbing a jersey, jammed finger (axial load), crush, traction, twisting, or contact with sporting equipment or playing surface
- Document occupation and hand dominance.
- Consideration must be made to the specific sport being played (1)[C].

PHYSICAL EXAM

- Inspect for deformity, ecchymosis, swelling, and open wound.
- Assess joint range of motion proximal and distal to the bony injury.
- Assess integrity of all joint structures.
- Assess rotational alignment (all digits should point to scaphoid tuberosity when flexed) (2)[C].
- The motor and sensory function of the radial, median, and ulnar nerves should be assessed with a phalanx injury (6)[C].
- Specific to phalanx fractures, the integrity of the flexor and extensor mechanisms of the PIP and DIP joints must be assessed (2)[C].
- Assess capillary refill.
- Compare with the uninjured hand.
- Assess stability of the PIP and DIP joint.

DIFFERENTIAL DIAGNOSIS

- PIP joint dislocation
- DIP joint dislocation
- Flexor or extensor tendon rupture
- Volar plate disruption
- CES separation
- Bone or soft tissue contusion
- Capsular or ligament sprain
- Finger infection
- Gout
- Neoplasm

DIAGNOSTIC TESTS & INTERPRETATION

ALERT

All fractures require anteroposterior (AP), true lateral, and oblique radiographs of the affected finger in isolation (1)[C].

- May require preimaging anesthesia (e.g., digital block)
- Computed tomography (CT) scans are recommended if there is suspicion of joint involvement or for comminuted fractures (4)[A].

TREATMENT

- Fractures at the base (2)[C]:
  - Axial load injury common inciting mechanism
  - Nondisplaced fractures should be splinted for 2 weeks with a dorsal extension block splint and then buddy taped for weeks 2 to 4.
  - Nondisplaced volar fractures, secondary to dorsal extension forces or dislocation, involving <30% of the articular surface are considered stable and may be splinted for 4 to 6 weeks.
  - Fractures affecting the dorsum are frequently associated with central slip attachment and may result in a boutonnière deformity; treatment of these requires 6 weeks in extension splinting.
- Transverse fractures of the shaft (2)[C]:
  - Nondisplaced: may be treated with buddy taping for 2 to 4 weeks
  - Displaced: Attempt reduction under anesthesia (recommend orthopedic referral) with longitudinal traction and manipulation of distal fragment. Tape splint may be necessary for postreduction radiography; generally 15-degree angulation in plane of motion is tolerated; if postreduction films show adequate alignment, splint 4 to 6 weeks.
- Condylar fractures (4)[C]:
  - Nondisplaced: managed with buddy taping for 2 to 4 weeks
  - Displaced: require orthopedic consultation
- Surgical treatment should be considered for comminuted or open fractures, torsional malposition, axis deviation, intra-articular fractures, >15 degrees of angulation, or 6 mm of shortening (2)[C],(6)[C].
  - For those that need surgery, operative intervention should take place within 7 days following the injury or 3 days following a failed conservative approach (6)[C].
  - Open fractures require appropriate antibiotic coverage, washout, sterile dressing, elevation, and splinting until definitive operative treatment is obtained, and tetanus vaccination should be considered.
  - Fractures of the base or shaft of the middle phalanx are often amenable to Kirschner wire (K-wire) fixation (5)[C], although for elite athletes desiring rapid return to play, K-wires are generally less desirable (2)[C].

ONGOING CARE

FOLLOW-UP RECOMMENDATIONS

- Postoperative management of hand fractures aims to balance the following: maintaining stability to allow for fracture healing and encouraging movement to permit restoration of function (6)[C].
- Of note, midshaft phalanx fractures can require longer times to union due to watershed perfusion (5)[C].
- Repeat radiographs at 2 weeks to assess stability and alignment.
- Deformity may result from no treatment, improper reduction, or poor splint compliance.
- Stiffness may result from overtreatment (2)[C].
- Hand or occupational therapy is indicated for loss of function or following surgical intervention (6)[C].
- Return to play is sport and position specific.
- For shaft fractures treated nonoperatively, athletes can return to protected play at 2 weeks and full play at 4 weeks provided the finger is adequately immobilized/protected (1)[C].
- If treated surgically, most athletes can return to play with a cast or semirigid splint (if their sport allows) within 2 weeks yet should wait 6 to 10 weeks to progress to full unprotected play (2)[C].
- A goal of lifelong function should take precedence when making return-to-play decisions.
- Pediatric injuries may require close attention throughout growth and play; iatrogenic physeal arrest may occur in patients with a physeal injury (3)[C].

REFERENCES

1. Wahl EP, Richard MJ. Management of metacarpal and phalangeal fractures in the athlete. *Clin Sports Med.* 2020;39(2):401–422.
2. Gaston RG, Chadderdon C. Phalangeal fractures: displaced/nondisplaced. *Hand Clin.* 2012;28(3):395–401.
3. Abzug JM, Dua K, Bauer AS, et al. Pediatric phalanx fractures. *J Am Acad Orthop Surg.* 2016;24(11):e174–e183.
4. Cavalcanti Kussmaul A, Kuehlein T, Langer MF, et al. The treatment of closed finger and metacarpal fractures. *Dtsch Arztebl Int.* 2023;120(50):855–862.
5. Heifner JJ, Rubio F. Fractures of the phalanges. *J Hand Surg Eur Vol.* 2023;48(2 Suppl):18S–26S.
6. Christodoulou N, Asimakopoulos D, Kapetanos K, et al. Principles of management of hand fractures. *J Perioper Pract.* 2023;33(11):342–349.

ADDITIONAL READING

Zhao W, Wang G, Chen B, et al. The value of ultrasound for detecting hand fractures: a meta-analysis. *Medicine (Baltimore).* 2019;98(44):e17823.

CLINICAL PEARLS

- All fractures require AP, lateral, and oblique radiographs in isolation of the affected digit.
- Splinting and buddy taping remain mainstay of nondisplaced, closed, middle phalangeal fractures, with follow-up 2 to 4 weeks following injury.
- Hand/occupational therapy is only indicated for functional impairment or following surgical intervention.
- Open, unstable, spiral, and comminuted fractures, or those with failure to maintain stability/reduction require orthopedic intervention.
- In pediatric and high-performance athletes, lifelong function should take precedence over return-to-play consideration, requiring close follow-up throughout the healing process.

FRACTURE, NASAL

Suraj A. Achar, MD, FAAFP, CAQSM • Dana Hong, DO, CAQSM

BASICS

EPIDEMIOLOGY

- Most frequently injured and fractured facial structure due to its prominence:
  - Third most commonly fractured structure of the skeleton
- Most fractures occur in the lower half of the nasal bones, where they are thinner and broader.
- Annual incidence in the United States is 53.2/100,000.
- Occurs twice as often in males, most frequently between 15 and 25 years of age and age >60 years

ETIOLOGY AND PATHOPHYSIOLOGY

- The upper third of the nose is a bony tripod formed by a pair of nasal bones that meet in the midline, with the thin perpendicular plate of the ethmoid as a weak center strut.
- A pair of upper and lower lateral cartilages supported by the central quadrangular septal cartilage makes up the lower 2/3.
- Most common cause of injury by age group:
  - <20 years: accident and sports related
  - 21 to 40 years: assault related
  - 41 and older: accident related

COMMONLY ASSOCIATED CONDITIONS

- Fracture of other facial bones
- Septal hematoma
- Septal dislocation
- Cribriform plate injury with leakage of cerebrospinal fluid (CSF)
- Laceration
- Orbital fracture
- Concussion
- Cervical spine injury

DIAGNOSIS

HISTORY

- Force: Low-velocity trauma, such as a blow from an elbow, usually causes a simple fracture pattern. High-velocity trauma from a stick or fast-moving ball/puck more likely causes a complex comminuted fracture as well as associated injuries to the face, head, and cervical spine.
- Direction of blow: Lateral is most common and can cause fracture displacement and dislocation of the septum. Direct blows can lead to nasal obstruction. Inferior blows can disrupt the septal cartilage and nasal tip.

PHYSICAL EXAM

- Nasal deformity
- Epistaxis
- Nasal airway obstruction
- Periorbital swelling and ecchymosis
- Nasal bone reduction: best if done either immediately after the injury or 3 to 5 days later when swelling will not interfere with assessment
- Palpate nasal bones for deformity and crepitus.
- Ring test to rule out CSF leak by collecting fluid from the nose onto filter paper to see if a clear ring of CSF diffuses out beyond the central area of blood.
- Intranasal examination must be performed on each side to evaluate for a bulging septal hematoma or septal dislocation. Use suction and a topical decongestant to control bleeding and then a nasal speculum, otoscope, or rigid nasal endoscope along with a light source for adequate visualization.
- Palpate all bony structures of the face including teeth to assess for associated trauma.
- It is imperative to establish that the airway is not compromised, and there is no other concomitant injury such as a concussion.

DIAGNOSTIC TESTS & INTERPRETATION

- Obtain plain radiographs only if the following criteria are not met:
  - Tenderness and swelling isolated to bony bridge of nose
  - Patient able to breath through each naris
  - No deviation of the septum
  - No septal hematoma present (1)
- If suspicious for fracture of other facial bones, computed tomography (CT) is study of choice.
- Ultrasonography is more accurate than radiography for diagnosis. It also has a higher sensitivity than CT, especially for fractures that involve separation without depression (2)[B].

TREATMENT

GENERAL MEASURES

- Head elevation, lean forward to aid expectoration of blood
- Direct pressure, ice
- Displaced, uncomplicated nasal fractures evaluated within 6 hours of injury should be reduced immediately.
- Isolated nasal fractures >10 days should be referred to an otolaryngologist.
- Topical decongestant
- Cautery of visible bleeding sites in Kiesselbach plexus using silver nitrate sticks
- For refractory epistaxis, may have to pack both sides of the anterior nose with a tampon or antibiotic-soaked petrolatum gauze
- Posterior epistaxis, which is very rare, can require inflation of a Foley bulb or rapid long rhino catheter within the nasal fossa in addition to anterior packing to achieve hemostasis.
- Septal hematomas should be drained as soon as possible due to association with necrosis of the septum; incision, expression of clot, anterior packing for 2 to 3 days, and follow-up with an otolaryngologist (1)

ADMISSION, INPATIENT, AND NURSING CONSIDERATIONS

- Can consider immediate closed reduction before swelling develops if the nose is severely displaced and health care provider is well trained
- In most cases, simply provide analgesics and reexamine in 2 to 5 days.
- Adults with nondisplaced fractures that cause minimal deformity may not require reduction.
- Persistent rhinorrhea that is clear and watery should raise suspicion for potential cribriform damage and CSF leak, in which case the patient needs to be transferred to the hospital for a CT scan and acute consultation with otolaryngologists (3)[C].

ONGOING CARE

- Generally, nasal fractures should be managed within 2 to 3 weeks after injury, and manipulation should occur within 10 days for adults and 7 days for children (4)[B].
- Closed reduction (5)[B]:
  - Ideally performed in first 3 to 6 hours after injury, before significant swelling occurs
  - If delayed, should be done within 10 to 14 days of the injury, before significant bone healing occurs
  - Indications for adult population:
    - Unilateral or bilateral nasal bone fracture
    - Nasal deviation <1/2 of the width of the nasal bridge
  - Provide analgesia with oral medications.
  - Local anesthesia of the nose with cotton pledgets soaked in a topical local anesthetic (e.g., 2% lidocaine) and a vasoconstrictor (e.g., oxymetazoline) packed into the nares; can combine with an infraorbital nerve block
  - A Boies nasal fracture elevator placed intranasally between the septum and nasal bone can be used to reduce depressed segments of nasal bone. Apply steady outward pressure on the posterior aspect of the nasal bone. External pressure may be needed.
  - Walsham or Asch forceps can be inserted to grasp and place the bone back into place, if reduction is unsuccessful.
  - A dorsal splint (adhesive strips with rigid material) should be worn for 7 days.
  - Sinus precautions should be given, including head elevation, avoiding nose blowing and sniffing, and follow-up with a specialist for reevaluation.
  - Contraindications to closed reductions: nasal bone fractures associated with naso-orbital-ethmoid or Le Fort fractures, severely comminuted fractures, open septal fractures, or delayed injury presentation (i.e., >2 weeks) (1)
- Open reduction (5)[B]:
  - Indications for adult population:
    - Extensive or complicated fracture-dislocation of nasal bones and septum
    - Nasal deviation >50% the width of the nasal bridge
    - Open fracture
    - Persistent nasal deformity after closed reduction
    - Involvement of the caudal septum

REFERENCES

1. Mayersak RJ. Initial evaluation and management of facial trauma in adults. Accessed October 2, 2025. https://www.uptodate.com/contents/initial-evaluation-and-management-of-facial-trauma-in-adults
2. Dogan S, Kalafat UM, Yüksel B, et al. Use of radiography and ultrasonography for nasal fracture identification in children under 18 years of age presenting to the ED. *Am J Emerg Med.* 2017;35(3):465–468.
3. Patel Y, Goljan P, Pierce TP, et al. Management of nasal fractures in sports. *Sports Med.* 2017;47(10):1919–1923.
4. Basheeth N, Donnelly M, David S, et al. Acute nasal fracture management: a prospective study and literature review. *Laryngoscope.* 2015;125(12):2677–2684.
5. Mondin V, Rinaldo A, Ferlito A. Management of nasal bone fractures. *Am J Otolaryngol.* 2005;26(3):181–185.

ADDITIONAL READING

- Nigam A, Goni A, Benjamin A, et al. The value of radiographs in the management of the fractured nose. *Arch Emerg Med.* 1993;10(4):293–297.
- Procacci P, Ferrari F, Bettini G, et al. Soccer-related facial fractures: postoperative management with facial protective shields. *J Craniofac Surg.* 2009;20(1):15–20.
- Rubinstein B, Strong EB. Management of nasal fractures. *Arch Fam Med.* 2000;9(8):738–742.

CLINICAL PEARLS

Return to play following a nasal fracture:

- It can take 6 weeks for a nasal fracture to completely heal. An athlete should be advised that returning to competition before complete healing means that even minor contact could disrupt a minimally displaced or previously reduced fracture and require additional intervention. A general guideline is no contact for 1 to 2 weeks followed by return to play while wearing a nasal protective device for another 4 weeks following the initial insult. This is extended to 6 weeks should operative intervention be required.
- If the patient participates in combat sports such as boxing or mixed martial arts, operative intervention is more common, and 10 to 12 weeks is recommended.
- 92% of athletes eventually return to play (3)[C].
- Case reports have been published of return to play within 7 to 10 days with nasal protective device worn for 4-week postreduction with encouraging results.

FRACTURE, OLECRANON

Greg Nakamoto, MD, FACP

BASICS

The issue of fundamental concern when evaluating fractures of the olecranon is determining whether the fracture is displaced or nondisplaced:

- Nondisplaced fractures can be managed with immobilization.
- Displaced fractures should be referred to an orthopedic surgeon for consideration of fixation.

DESCRIPTION

- The olecranon is the curved process extending from the posterior proximal surface of the ulna. It forms a large portion of the articulating surface between the ulna and the trochlea of the humerus. The triceps inserts into the posterior third of the olecranon.
- For a fracture of the olecranon to be considered nondisplaced and stable, the following are required:
  - Displacement <2 mm
  - No change in position with gentle flexion to 90 degrees
  - No change in position with extension against gravity

EPIDEMIOLOGY

- Account for ~10% of fractures of the adult elbow (1),(2),(3),(4)
- Incidence of 12 per 100,000 population (1),(3),(4)
- Olecranon fractures can range from simple nondisplaced fractures to complex fracture-dislocations of the elbow (5).
- Olecranon fractures are uncommon in children because early in life the olecranon process is short, thick, and relatively stronger than the distal humerus. When they do occur, they are often associated with radial head subluxation or dislocation.

RISK FACTORS

- Direct trauma, such as a fall onto the tip of the elbow, may cause a fracture directly:
  - A low-energy mechanism of injury, such as a fall from a standing height, is the most common cause of olecranon fracture in the elderly (especially in older women), and such fractures may best be thought of as fragility fractures (1),(5),(6).
  - A high-energy mechanism of injury, such as a motor vehicle accident, is the most common cause of olecranon fracture in young men (1),(5).
- Indirect trauma, such as a fall onto the hand with the elbow partially flexed, may cause an avulsion owing to eccentric contraction of the triceps (1),(4).
- A combined fracture-dislocation is possible with a high-energy mechanism of injury. The olecranon fragment usually displaces posteriorly.
- Stress fractures of the olecranon are less common, and usually seen in professional throwing athletes (4). The remainder of this chapter is dedicated to the evaluation and management of traumatic olecranon fractures.

COMMONLY ASSOCIATED CONDITIONS

ALERT

The evaluating physician should be aware of the following conditions which can complicate the evaluation and treatment of olecranon fractures:

- **Ipsilateral upper extremity fracture**, the most common being fractures of the radial head and neck
- **Ulnar nerve injury** is reported in 2–5% of cases. It is at risk for injury due to its superficial position at the medial elbow.
- **Discontinuity of the triceps mechanism**
- **Fracture-dislocation** of the elbow
- **Collateral ligament injury** of the elbow
- **Open fracture**
- **Compartment syndrome** of the forearm, although rare, is a surgical emergency.

DIAGNOSIS

HISTORY

Mechanism of injury (1),(4),(5),(6):

- A fall, often from standing height, or blunt trauma to the posterior elbow may cause the fracture directly.
- A fall onto an outstretched hand may cause a fracture indirectly, often through avulsion by the triceps.
- A high-energy mechanism of injury increases the likelihood of fracture-dislocation.

PHYSICAL EXAM

- Pain and swelling over the posterior elbow
- Elbow effusion owing to the intra-articular component of the fracture
- Painful and limited motion at the elbow
- Determine if patient can extend the elbow against gravity. Inability to extend suggests either discontinuity of the triceps mechanism or a mechanical block. Either problem merits surgical consultation.
- Perform distal neurovascular examination. The ulnar nerve may be injured; more common in comminuted fractures
- Excessive soft tissue injury, swelling, or ecchymosis may influence the timing of surgery.

DIFFERENTIAL DIAGNOSIS

- Radial head fracture
- Coronoid process fracture
- Olecranon bursitis

DIAGNOSTIC TESTS & INTERPRETATION

- **Standard radiographs**: Anteroposterior (AP) and lateral views are traditionally considered sufficient for the evaluation of isolated olecranon fractures (3)[C]; some authors also advocate obtaining oblique views.
- A true lateral view is necessary to evaluate for fracture displacement and articular disruption; slightly oblique views are inadequate substitutes for a true lateral.
- Fat pad signs: Collection of intra-articular fluid (e.g., caused by intra-articular fracture) causes displacement and, hence, visualization of the fat pads around the elbow. The anterior fat pad sometimes may be visible in the normal elbow; the posterior fat pad usually is not visible on a normal lateral radiograph and may be the only radiographic evidence of occult fracture.
- Children: often helpful to obtain radiographs of the contralateral elbow for comparison
- **Computed tomography (CT) scan**:
  - Traditional teaching is that good-quality standard radiographs as just listed are essential for accurate diagnosis, classification, and operative planning. In cases of isolated olecranon fracture, they also should be sufficient, and CT scan in such cases rarely provides additional information that alters decision making. CT scan generally is reserved for more complex fracture combinations.
  - However, in one study of surgical plating of olecranon fractures, six of the seven fractures thought to be simple on plain film analysis were found to have occult comminution on CT. The authors concluded that comminution should consequently be considered in all cases of olecranon fractures, even when plain film displays simple patterns, because it may affect choice of surgical fixation (see Wellman et al. in "Additional Reading").
- **Radiographic classification and staging of olecranon fractures can help guide decisions regarding operative versus nonoperative treatment**:
  - There are several systems used for classification of olecranon fractures (including Mayo, AO, Colton, and Schatzker), and no single classification is used universally (3),(4),(5). Studies suggest the Mayo and AO systems have the best interobserver and intraobserver reliability (1),(3)[B].
  - The Mayo classification is useful in determining whether an olecranon fracture should be treated surgically (2),(4)[C].
    - Mayo type I fractures (undisplaced [<2 mm] ± comminution) can be treated nonoperatively.
    - Mayo type II (stable fractures with >3 mm displacement) and type III fractures (unstable, displaced fracture-dislocations) should be treated surgically except as noted below.
    - Mayo type I to III fractures may be further subcategorized into A (non-comminuted) and B (comminuted) fractures (5).
    - Up to 71–90% of all olecranon fractures are Mayo type II (3),(4).
  - The AO classification considers olecranon fractures as a subset of elbow fractures:
    - Type A—extra-articular fractures of the metaphysis of the radius or ulna (thus, olecranon fractures are not included in type A fractures)
    - Type B—intra-articular fractures of the radius or ulna (Olecranon fractures are subclassified as type B1 fractures.)
    - Type C—intra-articular fractures of both the olecranon and radial head
  - As no single classification system is used universally, achieving familiarity with the system most commonly used in your institution may be more practical than trying to learn them all.

TREATMENT

- **Reduction techniques**:
  - Nondisplaced fractures: unnecessary
  - Displaced fractures: surgical reduction and fixation
  - Fracture-dislocation: See "Elbow Dislocation."
- **Nonoperative treatment**:
  - Patients with **nondisplaced fractures** (<2 mm displacement) (Mayo type I) **with intact extensor mechanism** (active extension against gravity) are good candidates for nonoperative management (3),(4)[C].
  - Immobilization of nondisplaced fractures can be done at any degree of flexion. Displacement is generally reduced by keeping the elbow in more extension. However, immobilization at 90 degrees is often more convenient.

- Traditionally, a more **conservative approach** treated all nondisplaced olecranon fractures in a long arm cast with the elbow between 45 to 90 degrees of flexion for 3 to 4 weeks, followed by protected range of motion exercises (3)[C]:
  - Follow-up x-rays are obtained 5 to 7 days after cast application to ensure that displacement has not occurred.
  - No flexion past 90 degrees until complete radiographic bony healing at 6 to 8 weeks
  - To avoid excessive stiffness, elderly patients are allowed to start range of motion before 3 weeks if pain allows.
- Others advocate allowing for **early motion** (3)[C], with immobilization for as little as 7 to 10 days. In such cases, treatment might proceed as follows:
  - Patient is immobilized at 90 degrees in a splint or cast for 7 to 10 days.
  - After 7 to 10 days, the patient starts gentle motion, beginning with pronation and supination.
  - At 2 to 3 weeks, limited flexion and extension exercises can begin.
  - Flexion past 90 degrees can occur when radiographs show complete bone healing.
  - Repeat standard x-rays weekly until evidence of healing to ensure that there is no displacement requiring surgical referral.
  - Lifting can usually be allowed at 6 to 8 weeks.
- **Elderly patients with *nondisplaced* olecranon fractures**: Because of their propensity to develop stiffness at the elbow, elderly patients should spend much less time immobilized. In patients most prone to stiffness, joint immobilization can be achieved with a sling initially and careful range of motion can begin once the patient is comfortable as soon as a few days later.
- **Nonoperative treatment of elderly patients with *displaced* olecranon fractures** (2),(3),(4),(6)[B]:
  - A 2021 meta-analysis of 14 studies of elderly patients (mean age ranged from 70 to 88 years) with stable, displaced olecranon fractures (Mayo type II) found that both nonoperative and operative treatment of these patients achieved excellent and comparable functional outcomes, but the operative group had high reoperation rates for symptomatic hardware or wound problems (6).
  - In one study, nonunion occurred in 85% of patients treated nonoperatively, but did not significantly impact satisfaction scores.
  - On the basis of such data, the nonoperative treatment of displaced olecranon fractures in low-demand elderly patients (approximately ≥75 years old) is consequently increasing in practice and is increasingly seen as an acceptable treatment option for such patients (2),(3),(4),(6)[B].
  - Repeat elbow examination and x-rays are necessary at 2 weeks to ensure there is no evidence of joint instability (that is, a previously unrecognized Mayo type III fracture pattern) that would necessitate surgical intervention.

- **Operative treatment**:
  - Displaced fractures (Mayo type II) in patients <75 years old (3),(4)[B]
  - Any open fracture (Mayo type I–III), for débridement and lavage, with or without fixation (2),(3)[C]
  - All olecranon fracture-dislocation injuries (Mayo type III), regardless of age (2),(3)[C]
  - In the specific case of avulsion fractures that result in impairment of the extensor mechanism of the elbow, treatment is generally operative.

ADDITIONAL THERAPIES

- Splinting: If there is a delay until definitive treatment can be accomplished, then temporary splinting may be done for patient comfort and protection:
  - Nondisplaced fractures should be splinted with the elbow flexed at 90 degrees and hand in neutral position.
  - Displaced fractures should be splinted in a comfortable position with the elbow between 45 and 90 degrees and hand in neutral position; prompt orthopedic consultation should be obtained.
  - In the case of fracture-dislocation, the usual recommendation is that the dislocation should be reduced before splinting is applied.
- Ice and oral analgesics are useful in the prehospital setting. Oral analgesics may be required for several days after casting.
- Nondisplaced fractures: Protected range of motion advanced as described earlier. If the patient still has stiffness, then dynamic splinting and physical therapy referral for elbow range of motion may be of benefit.
- Displaced fractures: range of motion to be initiated as determined by the operating surgeon

SURGERY/OTHER PROCEDURES

Indications for operative treatment include:

- Displaced or unstable fractures
- Avulsion fractures and/or extensor mechanism disruption
- Fracture-dislocations
- Open fractures

ONGOING CARE

FOLLOW-UP RECOMMENDATIONS

- Nondisplaced fractures (Mayo type I): can be released to home in a splint or cast with follow-up x-rays in 1 week. Caution with initial casting because of swelling
- Displaced fractures: disposition determined in consultation with an orthopedic surgeon

COMPLICATIONS

ALERT

- **Loss of motion**: A loss of 10 to 15 degrees of terminal extension in isolated olecranon fractures are common but usually functionally well tolerated. Motion may improve somewhat for up to 2 years after injury.
- **Nonunion** is reported in 1–5% of patients.
- **Heterotopic calcification** occurs in 13–14% of patients.
- For surgical patients, **painful hardware**, sometimes requiring subsequent removal, is one of the most common complications after internal fixation; reported in up to 80% of patients.

REFERENCES

1. Cantore M, Candela V, Sessa P, et al. Epidemiology of isolated olecranon fractures: a detailed survey on a large sample of patients in a suburban area. *JSES Int*. 2022;6(2):309–314.
2. Beaudouin E, Augustin B. Is surgery needed for displaced olecranon fractures in patients aged 75 years or over? *Orthop Traumatol Surg Res*. 2021;107(8):103089.
3. Duckworth AD, Carter TH, Chen MJ, et al. Olecranon fractures: current treatment concepts. *Bone Joint J*. 2023;105-B(2):112–123.
4. Hamoodi Z, Duckworth AD, Watts AC. Olecranon fractures: a critical analysis review. *JBJS Rev*. 2023;11(1).
5. Brüggemann A, Mukka S, Wolf O. Epidemiology, classification and treatment of olecranon fractures in adults: an observational study on 2462 fractures from the Swedish fracture register. *Eur J Trauma Emerg Surg*. 2022;48(3):2255–2263.
6. Chen MJ, Campbell ST, Finlay AK, et al. Surgical and nonoperative management of olecranon fractures in the elderly: a systematic review and meta-analysis. *J Orthop Trauma*. 2021;35(1):10–16.

ADDITIONAL READING

- Marot V, Bayle-Iniguez X, Cavaignac E, et al. Results of non-operative treatment of olecranon fracture in over 75-year-olds. *Orthop Traumatol Surg Res*. 2018;104(1):79–82.
- Veillette CJH, Steinmann SP. Olecranon fractures. *Orthop Clin North Am*. 2008;39(2):229–236.
- Wellman DS, Lazaro LE, Cymerman RM, et al. Treatment of olecranon fractures with 2.4- and 2.7-mm plating techniques. *J Orthop Trauma*. 2015;29(1):36–43.

F

CLINICAL PEARLS

- The goal when evaluating fractures of the olecranon is determining whether the fracture is nondisplaced and stable versus displaced and/or unstable.
- For a fracture of the olecranon to be considered nondisplaced and stable, it must be displaced <2 mm, must not change in position with gentle flexion to 90 degrees, and must not change in position with extension against gravity.
- The assessment of stability and displacement usually can be made with standard radiographs and clinical examination.
- Stable, nondisplaced fractures (Mayo type I) can be treated nonoperatively. Additionally, displaced fractures (Mayo type II) in low-demand elderly patients may also be candidates for nonoperative treatment. All other fractures (Mayo type II in younger patients and all Mayo type III) merit orthopedic consultation for consideration of surgical treatment.
- Physician response to common patient questions:
  - How long do I need to wear this cast/sling?
    - Nondisplaced fractures: In the case of a stable fracture in a reliable patient, immobilization is for comfort and can be discontinued after initial pain and swelling have resolved in 7 to 10 days (even less in the elderly patient prone to stiffness). If the patient is at particular risk for displacing an otherwise stable fracture, immobilization in a long-arm cast for up to 3 weeks may be required.
    - Displaced fractures: depends on the extent of injury and type of repair required

FRACTURE, ORBITAL

Jennifer J. Mitchell, MD, FAAFP, CAQSM, FAMSSM • Kelly T. Mitchell, MD

BASICS

DESCRIPTION

- Fracture of the osseous walls of the orbit due to blunt trauma to the globe, periocular area, or the cheek
- Orbital anatomy:
  - Bony orbit is a conical structure:
    - Base faces anterolaterally
    - Apex originates posteromedially.
    - Seven bones: frontal, maxilla, zygoma, ethmoid, lacrimal, palatine, sphenoid
  - Orbital roof: frontal and sphenoid bones
    - Forms floor of frontal sinus
  - Orbital floor: palatine, maxilla, zygoma bones
    - Forms roof of maxillary sinus
    - Most commonly fractured area of orbit
  - Medial wall: maxilla, lacrimal, ethmoid bones
    - Forms walls of ethmoid sinus, sphenoid sinus, and nasal cavity
    - Second most frequently fractured area of orbit
  - Lateral wall: zygoma, sphenoid bones
    - Not bordered by a sinus
    - Thickest and strongest of the orbital walls (1)
- Types of orbital fractures:
  - Orbital rim: caused by direct blow to bony orbit
  - Orbital wall: caused by blunt trauma to globe:
    - Blowout fracture: most common; fracture fragment is directed away from the bony orbit.
    - Blow-in fracture: trauma typically directed against frontal bone or maxilla; fracture fragment(s) is displaced toward the orbital space, decreasing the orbital volume.
  - Trapdoor orbital fracture:
    - Pure orbital floor fracture, typically in pediatric patient
    - Bony fragment displaces into maxillary sinus
    - Extraocular muscle(s) can become entrapped (inferior oblique or inferior rectus, most commonly).
    - Usually, restriction of upward gaze occurs.
    - Also called white-eyed blowout fracture due to minimal outward signs of trauma
    - Significant oculocardiac reflex can occur (2),(3).

EPIDEMIOLOGY

- 30% of orbital fractures are isolated and 60% combined with other facial fractures.
- Common causes of orbital fractures are assaults, falls, and motor vehicle accidents (MVAs):
  - Sports and assaults more common in the younger and male
  - Falls more common in elderly and female
- 30% of orbital blowout fractures are caused by sports.
- 3–14% of orbital fractures are associated with significant injury to the eye.
- 40% of monocular blindness is due to eye trauma.

ETIOLOGY AND PATHOPHYSIOLOGY

- Blowout fractures:
  - Occur along medial wall and/or orbital floor
  - Orbital rims are intact.
- Two proposed theories:
  - Hydraulic theory:
    - Blunt object of larger than diameter of the orbital entrance strikes the eye.
  - Buckling theory:
    - Fractures occur as a result of direct trauma to the inferior orbital rim (2),(3).

RISK FACTORS

- Most common causes of orbital fracture:
  - Sporting events/falls/assaults/MVAs
- Sports most commonly associated with orbital fracture in the United States:
  - Baseball, basketball, soccer, football, combat sports

GENERAL PREVENTION

- Use of eye protection for any sport where an object or another participant may impact the globe.
- Impact-resistant polycarbonate or Trivex lenses in American Society for Testing and Materials (ASTM) approved frames
- Functionally monocular athletes, best vision 20/40, should wear impact-resistant eye protection at all times, especially for all sports and recreation (1).

COMMONLY ASSOCIATED CONDITIONS

- Ocular injury is associated with blowout fracture 14–40% of the time.
- Potential associated injuries:
  - Mild ocular injuries:
    - Subconjunctival hemorrhage
    - Conjunctival laceration
    - Corneal abrasion
  - Vision-threatening injuries:
    - Hyphema:
      - More likely if decreased acuity and abnormal pupil exam
    - Corneal laceration
    - Globe rupture
    - Traumatic iridocyclitis
    - Acute glaucoma
    - Lens subluxation/dislocation
    - Posttraumatic cataract
    - Vitreous hemorrhage
    - Retinal detachment/tear
    - Commotio retinae, traumatic retinal swelling
    - Foreign body: intraocular or intraorbital
    - Optic nerve injury
    - Orbital emphysema with ocular vascular compromise
    - Retrobulbar hemorrhage
  - Injuries to ocular adnexa:
    - Eyelid contusion ± ecchymosis
    - Eyelid laceration ± margin involvement
    - Canthal injury, laceration, or avulsion
    - Traumatic ptosis
  - Intracranial injuries:
    - Pneumocephalus
    - Cerebral injury
    - Cerebrospinal fluid leak
  - Delayed complications:
    - Enophthalmos
    - Hypoglobus

DIAGNOSIS

HISTORY

- Timing
- Mechanism:
  - Penetrating trauma:
    - Energy/velocity
    - Type of material
    - Size of object
  - Nonpenetrating trauma
- Location
- Protective eyewear in use
- Visual symptoms:
  - Change in vision
  - Diplopia
  - Discharge
  - Flashing lights
  - Floaters
  - Pain
  - Photophobia
- Prior ocular history:
  - Contact lenses use
  - Previous visual impairment/visual correction
  - Prior trauma
  - Surgical history
- Tetanus status

PHYSICAL EXAM

- Signs and symptoms include:
  - Decreased vision
  - Pupil abnormalities
    - Miosis, dilated, afferent pupillary defect (APD)
  - Diplopia
  - Enophthalmos
  - Exophthalmos
  - Hypoesthesia in V2 distribution:
    - Infraorbital, cheek, lateral nose, upper lip
  - Intraorbital emphysema
  - Nosebleed
  - Periorbital ecchymosis
  - Step-off abnormality of bony structures (3)
- Systematic physical examination includes the following:
  - Neurologic survey first
  - If neurologically intact, then initial visual acuity (VA) to evaluate for emergent visual changes; VA before manipulation of eye
  - Vision: near and far (Snellen chart)
  - Patient should use his or her corrective lenses (not contact lenses).
  - Avoid placing pressure on globe; risk of vitreous herniation if globe is ruptured
  - Patient unable to see well enough to read:
    - Display number of fingers
    - Detection of hand motion
    - Light perception
  - Pupil exam:
    - Size, shape, symmetry
    - Reaction to light
  - Swinging flashlight test: APD is present if the pupil of the affected eye dilates when exposed to the light source.
  - Examine head, scalp, face, and periorbital tissues.
  - Lacerations: location, depth, length
  - Lid edema
  - Foreign body
  - Sensory deficit
  - Bony tenderness to palpation around orbital rim
  - Orbital rim fracture
  - Step-offs: blowout fracture
  - Exophthalmos
  - Enophthalmos
  - External eye structures:
    - Conjunctiva:
      - Blood (subconjunctival hemorrhage)
      - Chemosis (swelling)
      - Foreign bodies
    - Cornea:
      - Fluorescein stain/cobalt blue light
      - Irregularities (abrasion, laceration, foreign bodies)
  - Extraocular motility: Generally, decreased motility may be due to edema.
  - Impaired upward gaze: orbital floor fracture
  - Impaired downward gaze: inferior rectus or oblique muscle entrapment
  - Intraocular pressure: Use Tono-Pen.
  - Funduscopic exam:
    - Defer if vision is near normal, and ophthalmology will perform indirect exam less urgently.

- If vision with significant abnormality, defer as ophthalmology evaluation is imminent.
- Red reflex presence or absence
- Decreased intensity can imply vitreous hemorrhage or large retinal detachment.
- Central retinal artery pulsations

– Slit-lamp exam:
- If available: anterior chamber, cornea, iris, lens, or defer to ophthalmology
- If not available, use penlight to look for:
  - Hyphema
  - Obvious laceration
  - Shrunken-appearing globe (3),(4),(5)

DIAGNOSTIC TESTS & INTERPRETATION

- Plain-film radiographs:
  – Rarely used for diagnosis in orbital trauma
  – High false-negative rate: 50%
  – Nondiagnostic rate: 30%
- If plain films ordered:
  – Waters view best displays inferior orbital rims, nasoethmoid bones, and maxillary sinuses.
  – Teardrop sign represents orbital contents herniated into maxillary sinuses.
  – Air–fluid levels/opacifications of sinuses that may indicate fracture
  – Orbital emphysema: medial wall blowout fracture
- Computed tomography (CT) scan, standard imaging modality:
  – Thin-sliced helical CT with coronal reconstructions:
  - Improved image quality
  - Reduced radiation to lens
  – If helical CT scan not available:
  - CT scan with slices of ≤3 mm
  - Axial, coronal, and sagittal planes are useful to assess orbital floor and roof.
  – Sensitivity 79–96%
  – May help distinguish between orbital edema and entrapment of extraocular muscles
  – Findings may predict future enophthalmos or diplopia; may play a role in prompting surgery
- Ultrasound:
  – Contraindicated if high suspicion of globe rupture
- Magnetic resonance imaging (MRI):
  – Limited usefulness in acute stages of ocular trauma
  – Do not perform if metallic intraocular foreign body may be present.
  – Helpful if suspicion of optic nerve injury
  – May identify organic foreign body (4)[C]

TREATMENT

Not emergent unless:

- Visual impairment
- Globe injury
- Immediate referral to ophthalmology if concern for closed globe injury, like hyphema or the more serious open globe injury, symptomatic orbital emphysema, orbital compartment syndrome, retrobulbar hemorrhage, child with trapdoor fracture, optic neuropathy, and to rule out other ophthalmologic injuries (5)[B],(6)[B]
- May need coordinated, immediate care with either ear, nose, and throat (ENT) or facial plastic surgery services as in many centers, they manage the orbital fracture evaluation and treatment, whereas ophthalmology focuses on eyelid and globe injuries
- Prehospital:
  – Airway, breathing, and circulation (ABCs) first priorities
  – Cervical spine immobilization and neurologic evaluation
  – Control active bleeding with direct pressure.
  – No direct pressure to orbit if open globe is possible or suspected
  – Cover with a protective shield and refer to ophthalmologist immediately.

MEDICATION

- Antibiotics may be prudent when fracture communicates with sinus.
- Pain control to include acetaminophen, nonsteroidal anti-inflammatory drugs (NSAIDs), narcotics, and local anesthetics; avoid aspirin.
- Nasal decongestants

ADDITIONAL THERAPIES

- Avoid nose blowing; increased risk of orbital cellulitis
- Avoid Valsalva maneuvers such as coughing.
- Sneeze with mouth open.
- Cold packs for at least 48 hours
- Elevate head of bed.
- Tetanus booster, if not current (3)[A]

SURGERY/OTHER PROCEDURES

- Surgical goal:
  – Remove entrapped orbital tissue/rectus muscle(s).
  – Reconstruct the defect area of the fractured wall if large (4)[C].
- Strong surgical indications:
  Bothersome diplopia that is not improving after all swelling has regressed and not due to a clearly definable restricted muscle
  – Enophthalmos >2 mm
  – Fracture >50% of floor
  – Significant hypoglobus (3)[A]
- Timing of surgery is controversial:
  – Rarely urgent, except when:
  - Oculocardiac reflex present (bradycardia, nausea/vomiting)
  - Ocular motility lesions in children
  - Muscle entrapment in trapdoor fracture:
    - In pediatrics, early surgery (within 24 to 48 hours) appears to be associated with better outcomes (4)[C].
  - Penetrating craniocerebral injuries
  - Concern for optic nerve compression:
    - No clear evidence-based guidance on benefit of optic canal decompression associated with clinical exam findings of optic nerve injury; marked acuity loss and APD
  – Appropriate timing is important for achieving good results:
  - Delay allows for:
    - Orbital swelling resolution
    - Assisting in ensuring accurate diagnosis
    - Strengthening indications for surgery
- No consensus on best material for repair
- If no emergent indications, conservative management, observation with close follow-up, is usually considered because spontaneous improvement is common as most orbital fractures do not require surgery; this may be an emerging paradigm (6)[B].

ONGOING CARE

Return to play:

- Based on significance of ocular injury and associated findings
- Fracture only:
  – Noncontact sport: 2 weeks
  – Contact sport: 4 to 6 weeks
- Surgery for fracture:
  – Return will vary.
  – Depends on specific repair required
- Return to activities with proper eye protection.

PATIENT EDUCATION

Return sooner than planned follow-up for:

- Decline in vision
- Increase in diplopia
- Increased eyelid swelling or bruising
- Concern for enophthalmos or proptosis

REFERENCES

1. Micieli JA, Easterbrook M. Eye and orbital injuries in sports. *Clin Sports Med.* 2017;36(2):299–314.
2. Basnet A, Chug A, Simre S, et al. Comprehensive management of pediatric orbital fractures: a case series and review of literature. *Cureus.* 2024;16(4):e57915.
3. Gart MS, Gosain AK. Evidence-based medicine: orbital floor fractures. *Plast Reconstr Surg.* 2014;134(6):1345–1355.
4. Chung SY, Langer PD. Pediatric orbital blowout fractures. *Curr Opin Ophthalmol.* 2017;28(5):470–476.
5. Zhong E, Chou TY, Chaleff AJ, et al. Orbital fractures and risk factors for ocular injury. *Clin Ophthalmol.* 2022;16:4153–4161.
6. Ray CN, Marsh HD, Gilmore JE, et al. Review of 451 patients presenting with orbital wall fractures: a retrospective analysis. *J Craniofac Surg.* 2023;34(1):126–130.

ADDITIONAL READING

- American Society for Testing and Materials: http://www.astm.org/Standards/F803.htm
- Kontio R, Lindqvist C. Management of orbital fractures. *Oral Maxillofac Surg Clin North Am.* 2009;21(2):209–220.
- Petrigliano FA, Williams RJ III. Orbital fractures in sport: a review. *Sports Med.* 2003;33(4):317–322.
- Uzelac A, Gean AD. Orbital and facial fractures. *Neuroimaging Clin N Am.* 2014;24(3):407–424.
- Young SM, Kim YD, Kim SW, et al. Conservatively treated orbital blowout fractures: spontaneous radiologic improvement. *Ophthalmology.* 2018;125(6):938–944.

CLINICAL PEARLS

- Use of protective masks for infield positions do decrease the risk of orbital/eye injury and may also apply to other ball-related sports not requiring face or head protection.
- Significant changes in VA or pupil changes could indicate a more serious globe injury: hyphema, ruptured globe, or optic nerve injury:
  – Ophthalmic emergency, immediate consultation
  – Significant other exam abnormality: immediate ophthalmology consultation
  – All other abnormalities: ophthalmology consultation within 48 hours
- To diagnose orbital fracture, helical CT scan with coronal reconstructions or CT scan with 3-mm or smaller slices in both axial and coronal planes to assess orbit floor and roof is essential.
- Most orbital fractures will resolve without significant visual sequelae or need for surgical intervention.
- Need 1 week of antibiotics, nasal decongestants, and no forceful sneezing, coughing, or Valsalva

FRACTURE, ORBITAL BLOW OUT

Dana Hong, DO, CAQSM • Ryley Lee, MD

BASICS

DESCRIPTION

Defined as an orbital floor or medial wall fracture without orbital rim involvement owing to blunt trauma to the orbit

EPIDEMIOLOGY

- Sport-related injury accounts for 1/3 of all orbital blowout fractures.
- Frequently associated with other serious injuries (intracranial and intraocular)
- Observed in any sport that puts the athlete at risk for forceful contact to the face
- Most common: soccer, rugby, boxing, martial arts, baseball, wrestling, basketball, action sports
- Object striking the orbital region is usually larger than orbital rim, such as a baseball or fist.
- More common among young adult and adolescent males
- Fractures of orbital floor are relatively rare in children <5 years old as maxillary sinus pneumatization significantly expands from 6 to 12 years old.

ETIOLOGY AND PATHOPHYSIOLOGY

- Force transmitted through the orbital structures to the weakest structural point—most commonly the orbital floor or medial wall—resulting in fracture
- Trapdoor fracture is a linear fracture of the orbital bone that reduces spontaneously to original position, entrapping and strangulating infraocular soft tissue:
  - Usually an intraoperative diagnosis
  - Seen almost exclusively in children
- Orbital floor serves as roof to air-filled maxillary and ethmoid sinuses. Communication between the spaces results in orbital emphysema.
- Orbit contains fat, which holds the globe in place:
  - Orbital floor fracture may result in herniation of the fat on the inferior orbital surface into the maxillary or ethmoid sinuses.
  - Leads to enophthalmos owing to orbital volume loss
  - Sinus congestion and fluid collection occur secondary to edema.
- Infraorbital nerve runs through the bony canal 3 mm below the orbital floor:
  - Injury results in hypoesthesia of the ipsilateral cheek.
  - Distinguished from hypoesthesia owing to swelling by testing for decreased sensation on the ipsilateral gingiva, which is within the infraorbital nerve distribution
- Inferior rectus and inferior oblique muscles run along the orbital floor:
  - Restriction of these extraocular muscles (EOMs) occurs owing to entrapment within the fracture or contusion or cranial nerve dysfunction.
  - Diplopia on upward gaze
  - Inability to elevate the affected eye normally on examination
- Medial rectus muscle is located above the ethmoid sinus:
  - Less commonly entrapped
  - Diplopia on ipsilateral lateral gaze
- Oculocardiac reflex is defined as an increased vagal tone secondary to soft tissue entrapment. Signs and symptoms include nausea, vomiting, bradycardia, and syncope.

GENERAL PREVENTION

Protective eyewear has been shown to decrease eye injuries, although data is insufficient to demonstrate decrease in orbital blowout fractures specifically.

COMMONLY ASSOCIATED CONDITIONS

- Ocular injuries:
  - Ruptured globe (incidence 5–10% of blowout fractures) (1)[B]
  - Subconjunctival hemorrhage
  - Corneal abrasion/laceration
  - Hyphema
  - Iridodialysis
  - Traumatic iridocyclitis (uveitis)
  - Traumatic mydriasis
  - Retinal detachment
  - Vitreous hemorrhage
  - Compressive orbital emphysema
  - Retrobulbar hemorrhage
  - Optic nerve injury
  - Central retinal artery occlusion
  - Acute angle glaucoma
- EOM entrapment:
  - Inferior rectus
  - Inferior oblique
  - Medial rectus (less common)
- Infraorbital nerve injury
- Facial fractures:
  - Nasal bones
  - Zygomatic arch fracture
- Neck injuries
- Intracranial injury

DIAGNOSIS

HISTORY

- Mechanism of injury: significant trauma to the orbit
- Pain
- Swelling
- Bruising
- Double vision with upward gaze

PHYSICAL EXAM

- Periorbital tenderness, swelling, ecchymosis
- Impaired ocular mobility or diplopia:
  - Upward gaze impaired owing to inferior rectus entrapment
  - Ipsilateral lateral gaze impaired with medial rectus entrapment
- Infraorbital hypoesthesia: owing to compression/contusion of infraorbital nerve
- Enophthalmos or hypoophthalmos: owing to herniation of orbital fat through fracture
- Periorbital emphysema
- Normal visual acuity (unless associated ocular injury)
- Epistaxis (indicative of medial wall injury)
- Careful attention not to place pressure on the globe until ruptured globe excluded
- Slit-lamp and funduscopic examination help to identify associated injuries.

DIFFERENTIAL DIAGNOSIS

- Retrobulbar hemorrhage
- Periorbital contusion/ecchymosis
- Cranial nerve palsy
- Ruptured globe
- Orbital hematoma
- Retinal detachment
- Hyphema
- Orbital cellulitis
- Periorbital cellulitis

DIAGNOSTIC TESTS & INTERPRETATION

- Plain radiographs: limited value
- Computed tomography (CT) scan of orbits: study of choice:
  - Defines involved anatomy
  - Location and extent of fractures
  - Presence of intraorbital hemorrhage
  - Globe injury/rupture
  - EOM entrapment
  - Prolapse of orbital fat
  - CT scan findings of orbital floor fracture, EOM displacement, and EOM entrapment may predict diplopia (2)[B].

- Forced duction test:
  - Distinguishes nerve dysfunction from entrapment
  - Topical anesthesia is applied to the conjunctiva, and the globe is pulled away from the expected point of entrapment. If the globe is not mobile, the test is positive for entrapment.
  - Forced duction test in general clinic setting is not standard and is reserved for ophthalmologists for potential of globe manipulation risks.

TREATMENT

GENERAL MEASURES

- Identify life-threatening and/or serious associated injuries.
- Apply cool compresses for the first 24 to 48 hours to decrease swelling in order to minimize or reverse herniation and avoid surgical intervention.
- Avoid Valsalva maneuvers, nose blowing, and sniffing to prevent compressive orbital emphysema.
- Sleep with head of bed elevated.
- Prophylactic antibiotics not routinely required for isolated blowout fractures unless there is evidence of sinus infection or impending surgery to prevent infection
- Nasal decongestants (e.g., phenylephrine nasal spray)
- Analgesics
- Tetanus prophylaxis recommended if there is an open wound or if vaccination is not up to date; not recommended in closed fractures.

MEDICATION

- Phenylephrine nasal spray: BID × 3 to 5 days, caution extended usage for risk of rhinitis medicamentosa
- If evidence of sinus infection or impending surgery:
  - Amoxicillin: 250 to 500 mg PO TID × 10 to 14 days
  - Cephalexin: 250 to 500 mg PO QID × 10 to 14 days
  - Erythromycin: 250 to 500 mg PO QID × 10 to 14 days

ISSUES FOR REFERRAL

- For patients not requiring emergency specialty evaluation, follow-up with a specialist (ophthalmologist or plastic surgeon) should be ensured within 24 hours if patient has muscle entrapment as a result of orbital floor or medial wall fractures; enophthalmos or orbital dystopia; naso-orbital-ethmoid fractures.
- Immediate ophthalmology evaluation if patient has evidence of visual loss, proptosis, extrusion of intraocular contents, conjunctival hemorrhage, tear-shaped pupil (ruptured globe), afferent pupillary defect, signs of orbital compartment syndrome (e.g., "rock hard" eyelids), widened intercanthal distance, limited or painful extraocular motility, orbital dystopic and/or enophthalmos, severe vagal symptoms (nausea, vomiting, bradycardia) associated with EOM

SURGERY/OTHER PROCEDURES

- Most resolve without surgical intervention
- Typically observe for 10 to 14 days until swelling resolves
- Surgery indications:
  - Persistent diplopia
  - Restricted extraocular movements
  - Cosmetically significant enophthalmos or hypoophthalmos
  - Persistent oculocardiac reflex
  - Progressive infraorbital hypesthesia
- Immediate surgical intervention:
  - Orbital "trapdoor" fractures: These fractures, where the bone snaps back and traps tissue, should be surgically repaired within 24 hours to release the entrapped muscle and prevent permanent damage(1)[B].
  - A patient with double vision (diplopia) due to trapped eye muscles who also has a persistent oculocardiac reflex (a dangerous reflex causing a sudden drop in heart rate, nausea, and fainting) requires emergency surgery to relieve the pressure on the muscle and resolve the reflex (3)[A],(4)[C].
- Surgery within 2 weeks:
  - Significant enophthalmos (4)[C]
  - Progressive infraorbital hypesthesia (4)[C]
- There is some debate regarding optimal surgical timing:
  - Early surgery within 14 days is preferred for reducing diplopia and enophthalmos. Surgery after 14 days increases the risk of complications (3)[A],(5)[A].
  - Surgical intervention should be delayed to at least 1 to 2 weeks after injury to allow for resolution of edema but performed before advancement of scarring and fibrosis (4)[C].

ONGOING CARE

COMPLICATIONS

- Sinusitis
- Orbital infection
- Permanent restriction of extraocular movement
- Enophthalmos
- Decreased visual acuity

REFERENCES

1. Chung SY, Langer PD. Pediatric orbital blowout fractures. *Curr Opin Ophthalmol.* 2017;28(5):470–476.
2. Cellina M, Floridi C, Panzeri M, et al. The role of computed tomography (CT) in predicting diplopia in orbital blowout fractures (BOFs). *Emerg Radiol.* 2018;25(1):13–19.
3. Zhang L, Li J, Wells T, et al. Current management strategies in orbital floor fractures. *Otolaryngol Clin North Am.* 2023;56(1):113–127.
4. Pandya RP, Deng W, Hodgson NM. Current guidelines and opinions in the management of orbital floor fractures. *Otolaryngol Clin North Am.* 2023;56(6):1101–1112.
5. Chen A, Patel V, Liu X, et al. Timing of surgical repair in orbital blowout fractures: a systematic review and meta-analysis. *J Oral Maxillofac Surg.* 2022;80(4):716–724.

ADDITIONAL READING

- Aerni GA. Blunt visual trauma. *Clin Sports Med.* 2013;32(2):289–301.
- Lincoln AE, Caswell SV, Almquist JL, et al. Effectiveness of the women's lacrosse protective eyewear mandate in reduction of eye injuries. *Am J Sports Med.* 2012;40(3):611–614.
- Neuman MI, Bachur R. *Orbital Fractures.* UpToDate. Accessed October 2, 2025. https://www.uptodate.com/contents/orbital-fractures
- Shew M, Carlisle MP, Lu GN, et al. Surgical treatment of orbital blowout fractures: complications and postoperative care patterns. *Craniomaxillofac Trauma Reconstr.* 2016;9(4):299–304.

CLINICAL PEARLS

- Pediatric patients >5 years old are more likely to have trapdoor fractures which require immediate surgical intervention.
- CT scan of the orbits is the diagnostic test of choice.
- Most orbital blowout fractures will resolve without intervention; however, significant diplopia, tissue entrapment, and enophthalmos are main indications for surgery.

FRACTURE, PATELLA

Patrick J. Prazak, DO, CAQSM ▪ Haris Vakil, MD

BASICS

Mechanisms of injury:

- Direct trauma: often comminuted; associated with fractures of the tibia, femur, and hip as well as posterior hip dislocation
- Indirect trauma: exertional loading of the extensor mechanism beyond the tensile strength of the patella; often while in knee flexion; frequently transverse with significant displacement and disruption of the extensor retinaculum

ALERT

- Pediatric sleeve fractures: Cartilage of the inferior pole (superior pole less common) of the patella is pulled off, often with a small, avulsed bone fragment. This occurs with a vigorous contraction of the quadriceps muscle group when the knee is in a flexed position.
- Patellar subluxation or dislocation: associated with osteochondral fractures of the medial facet of the patella; avulsion fractures of the medial aspect of the patella can occur at the attachment of the medial retinaculum.

EPIDEMIOLOGY

Incidence

- 1% of all fractures
- Usually 20 to 50 years of age
- Osteochondral fracture of medial patella common in adolescents with patellar dislocation

Pediatric Considerations

- Patellar sleeve fractures are mostly likely to occur from 8 to 16 years of age; osteochondral fractures are also common in the adolescent years.
- Incidence of osteochondral fractures (patellar and femoral) in patients with first-time traumatic patellar dislocations can be as high as 24%.
- Patellar sleeve fractures: male > female (3:1)

DIAGNOSIS

- Transverse: usually displaced, common in the middle or lower third in adults, most patellar fractures sustained during sports participation are of the transverse type. They often result from a strong quadriceps contraction, such as in a fall or jumping sports or can be seen with direct trauma.
- Stellate: usually comminuted and nondisplaced; often secondary to high-impact direct trauma in sport or motor vehicle accidents.
- Longitudinal: due either to trauma (especially of the lateral facet) or to subluxation/dislocation of the patella; adolescents often found to also have osteochondral fragments.

ALERT

- Sleeve fractures: significant articular cartilage and a small bony fragment avulsed from the distal pole; often difficult to see on plain films; may have an ipsilateral patella alta (high-riding patella)
- Stress fractures: Majority have been documented in weightlifters and gymnasts.

HISTORY

- Activity (partial fall, exertional strain, etc.)
- Trauma (object, direction, force)
- Subluxation or dislocation
- Popping or snapping
- Locking or joint instability
- Loss of range of motion (ROM)
- Difficulty weight-bearing
- Speed and extent of swelling
- Characterization of pain
- Constitutional symptoms, especially with delayed presentation or evidence of infection
- Previous knee injuries
- Past medical and surgical history
- Medications and allergies

PHYSICAL EXAM

- Signs and symptoms include:
  - Patellar tenderness to palpation and pain with passive motion of the patella
  - Hemarthrosis or diffuse soft tissue swelling of the knee
  - Limited range in active leg extension due to disruption of soft tissues
- Physical examination includes the following:
  - Pain and tenderness with palpation
  - Pain with passive motion
  - Palpable step-off defect
  - Effusion or soft tissue swelling
  - Full range in active knee extension implies preservation of extensor mechanism.
  - Rule out associated bony or soft tissue injuries (hip, femur, leg and ankle), contamination, and signs of infection.

Pediatric Considerations

Stress testing of ligaments should be delayed until after radiographic evaluation if there are concerns of growth plate injury in children.

ALERT

- Open fractures have a risk of osteomyelitis and septic arthritis.
- Patellar apprehension test is used to help identify acute patellar dislocation.

DIFFERENTIAL DIAGNOSIS

Bipartite patella: usually bilateral with rounded edges at the superior and lateral corners of the patellae and not associated with point tenderness unless fall and fibrous injury

Pediatric Considerations

- Sinding-Larsen-Johansson syndrome: overuse injury of the inferior pole of the patella typically occurring at 10 to 14 years of age
- Acute patellar dislocation: moderate to large hemarthrosis and positive apprehension sign; may or may not have underlying osteochondral defect
- Proximal tibia or distal femur fractures: should be ruled out by x-ray
- Occult physeal injury: may require magnetic resonance imaging (MRI) if not apparent on x-ray
- Anterior cruciate ligament tear: may present with moderate to large hemarthrosis; can have similar mechanism of injury as patellar dislocation

DIAGNOSTIC TESTS & INTERPRETATION

- Anteroposterior (AP) and lateral x-rays: used to evaluate patella, distal femur, proximal tibia, and soft tissues. The AP view can help to determine fracture lines, and the lateral view can help to determine the number of fragments and combination (1)[C].
- Axial (sunrise, merchant) views: help to identify osteochondral medial patellar avulsion and other longitudinal fractures. Comparison views of the contralateral side should be used to help determine fractures from bipartite patellae. Sunrise view (90 degrees of flexion) can be very difficult to obtain with lack of ROM and pain. Merchant view (30 to 60 degrees of flexion) may be easier to obtain acutely.
- Computed tomography (CT) scan: used to detect suspected occult fractures or for surgical planning
- Bone scan: used to evaluate stress reactions, stress fractures and osteomyelitis
- MRI: used to evaluate suspected soft tissue injuries and patellar sleeve and osteochondral fractures. MRI is a critical tool for evaluating the severity of an osteochondral defect and assessing the true extent of injury to the extensor mechanism.

ALERT

All patients with first-time traumatic dislocations should be suspected of having an osteochondral injury until proven otherwise by MRI, CT scan, or continued clinical examination (2)[C].

TREATMENT

- Acute management:
  - Analgesia using nonsteroidal anti-inflammatory drugs (NSAIDs)
  - Ice and elevation to control swelling (avoiding prolonged, direct skin application)
  - Consider aspiration of tense anterior hematomas. Aspiration may be followed by injection of local anesthesia to facilitate assessment of the extensor mechanism. Fatty globules can indicate osteochondral defect or occult patellar fracture.
  - Immobilization: splinting and support in extension to minimize fracture distraction

- Nonoperative treatment:
  - Medically unfit for surgery
  - Closed fracture
  - <2 to 3 mm of articular step-off or <4 mm of fracture widening (1)[C]
  - Full range with active knee extension as compared to the contralateral side
  - Immobilization in a brace or plaster that restricts flexion for 4 to 6 weeks (3)[C]
  - Compressive dressings and aspiration of hemarthrosis (if present) before cast application may help to control edema and discomfort.
  - Repeat radiographs should be obtained periodically to monitor for possible fracture displacement and appropriate healing.
  - Progressive ROM and strengthening are used until the patient can perform a straight leg raise against gravity without extension lag or pain (3)[C].

ADDITIONAL THERAPIES

Special considerations: Open fractures require intravenous (IV) antibiotics and emergent referral for extensive irrigation and débridement, usually followed by internal fixation.

SURGERY/OTHER PROCEDURES

- Open reduction and internal fixation (ORIF): most commonly performed by modified tension-band wiring with either circumferential wire loops or in fragmentary wires or screws (depending on fragment configuration) in conjunction with repair of medial and lateral retinaculum and resection of small fragments not amenable to surgical fixation. Addition of a plate may be necessary to decrease risk of complication or reoperation (4)[A]. Nonmetallic implants are becoming more popular as there is a lower risk of complications and similar outcomes (5)[A].
- Partial patellectomy: indicated with severe patellar comminution or inability to restore a smooth articular surface; involves repair of retinaculum and reinsertion of patellar or quadriceps tendon into remaining patellar fragment near its articular surface
- Total patellectomy: reserved for severe comminution precluding retention of any significant (>25%) patellar fragments; considered a last resort; involves soft tissue repair with shortening of the quadriceps tendon; loss of knee extension strength (up to 40%) is frequently reported.
- Inferior pole avulsion fractures: The normal height of the patella can be maintained by preserving the patellar pole using a combination of a plate with tension-band wiring.
- Osteochondral fractures: difficult to detect on plain films; usually heal if nondisplaced but require arthroscopic removal or screw fixation if displaced; associated patellar instability may be surgically corrected at the same time (2)[C].
- Surgery may be delayed with extensive or contaminated soft tissue injury.

ONGOING CARE

- Immobilization: in a cast or locked brace
- Weight-bearing as tolerated in a cast or locked brace: reduces quadriceps contraction and fragment distraction
- Isometric exercises and straight-leg raises: started within days of cast application or surgical fixation
- ROM exercises: may be started immediately after stable internal fixation with a delay of 4 to 6 weeks for nonoperative treatment or after unstable fracture repair. Exercises should be delayed no more than 6 weeks to reduce pain and stiffness. Active flexion and passive extension are performed until the fracture shows signs of healing on x-ray and are then progressed to resistance exercises (3)[C].
- Resistance exercises: Several months of resistance exercises may be required to achieve full strength and ROM.
- Return to play when bony healing is demonstrated on AP, lateral, and merchant radiographs; complete ROM is achieved; and balance and proprioception are restored (3)[C].

FOLLOW-UP RECOMMENDATIONS

- Check ROM and strength as compared with the contralateral side.
- Repeat plain films (AP, lateral, and merchant) to document signs of healing with callus formation and periosteal reaction.
- Functional testing prior to return to sport
- Orthopedic referral whenever criteria for nonoperative treatment are not met

COMPLICATIONS

- Patellofemoral arthritis is a common complication. Risk factors include incongruence of the articular surface and damage to articular cartilage. Treatment includes physical therapy and can include patellectomy and/or tibial tubercle elevation in severe, refractory cases.
- A slight decrease in flexion is common but not usually clinically significant. Early postoperative motion and physical therapy help to maintain ROM with manipulation under anesthesia and/or arthroscopic lysis of adhesions required if unsuccessful.
- Painful hardware: common complication managed by removal after fracture union (minimum 6 months) or tendon healing (minimum 3 months)
- Infection: local care for superficial infections; osteomyelitis or septic osteoarthritis often requires IV antibiotics with surgical irrigation, débridement, removal of loose hardware and delayed closure.
- Radiographic evidence of avascular necrosis consists of a sclerotic area evident 1 to 2 months after injury, usually of the proximal fragment; mostly asymptomatic and spontaneously resolves within 1 to 3 years.
- Loss of fixation: often owing to unrecognized comminution; requires surgery if fragments are significantly displaced
- Nonunion: uncommon; repeat surgery indicated if symptomatic.
- Periosteal sleeve overgrowth: Patellar sleeve can continue to form new, excess bone which may need to be surgically removed.

REFERENCES

1. Howatt J, Liew AS, Wilkin G. Patellar fractures: anatomy, mechanics, and surgical management. *J Bone Joint Surg Am*. 2021;103(23):2237–2246.
2. Hargett DI, Sanderson BR, Little MTM. Patella fractures: approach to treatment. *J Am Acad Orthop Surg*. 2021;29(6):244–253.
3. Tsotsolis S, Ha J, Fernandes ARC, et al. To plate, or not to plate? A systematic review of functional outcomes and complications of plate fixation in patellar fractures. *Eur J Orthop Surg Traumatol*. 2023;33(8):3287–3297.
4. Edoardo M, Andrea DD, Silvia C, et al. Fixation of patella fractures with metallic implants is associated with a significantly higher risk of complications and re-operations than non-metallic implants: a systematic review and meta-analysis. *Int Orthop*. 2022;46(12):2927–2937.
5. Zhu W, Xu L, Xie K, et al. Design and validation of a smile-necklace plate for treating inferior patellar pole avulsion fractures: a review and hypothesis. *Orthop Surg*. 2022;14(11):2799–2808.

ADDITIONAL READING

- Bauer KL. Osteochondral injuries of the knee in pediatric patients. *J Knee Surg*. 2018;31(5):382–391.
- Safran M, Zachazewski JE, Stone DA, eds. Patellar fracture. In: *Instructions for Sports Medicine Patients*. 2nd ed. Elsevier; 2012:755–760.

CLINICAL PEARLS

- Most athletes with patellar fractures return to play the following season (3 to 6 months) with little residual deficit. Return of function is more limited with comminuted, high-impact mechanisms of injury. Strength of terminal knee extension will be reduced if patellectomy is required.
- If criteria for nonoperative treatment are met, studies have shown a failure rate of <5% for fractures managed nonoperatively.
- MRI is essential for evaluating associated soft tissue injury when there is concern for extensor mechanism disruption, and the results may influence the decision to proceed with surgical intervention.
- Many patients have some residual complaints, but most report good to excellent results after ORIF. Fewer achieve this level of satisfaction after partial patellectomy and even fewer after total patellectomy.

FRACTURE, PELVIC

David Carfagno, DO, CAQSM • Justin Rouintan, DO

BASICS

DESCRIPTION

- Most common mechanisms of injury are motor vehicle accidents, crush injuries, and falls from significant height.
- 3–8% of skeletal injuries, mortality in unstable fractures 8.3% (1); 3 times higher in open fractures
- Typically result from high-energy trauma in young individuals and low energy impact in the elderly (especially those with osteoporosis)
- Stable fractures: tend to be low energy fractures; often only one break in pelvic ring and broken ends line up; include Iliac wing, sacral, superior and inferior pubic ramus fractures
- Unstable fractures: tend to be high-energy fractures; 2+ breaks in the pelvic ring; lateral compression (LC), anterior–posterior compression (APC) and vertical shear (VS) fractures
- The most widely used classification scheme is the Young-Burgess system, considers force, severity, direction, and instability.
- Types of fractures:
  - Iliac wing fractures (Duverney fractures)
  - Sacral fractures
  - Coccygeal fractures
- LC: anterior injury—rami fractures:
  - The most common mechanism of pelvic fractures
  - This usually involves rami fractures anteriorly with a sacral impaction iliac wing fracture. This type of injury is rotationally unstable but usually vertically stable.
  - LC-I: oblique or transverse ramus fracture and ipsilateral anterior sacral compression fracture
  - LC-II: crescent fracture on side of impact (iliac wing fracture)
  - LC-III: type I or II injury on side of impact with contralateral APC fracture
- APC: anterior injury = symphysis diastasis/rami fractures:
  - The first point of failure is the symphysis pubis. As increasing external rotation is applied, the sacrotuberous, sacrospinous, and anterior sacroiliac (SI) ligaments are disrupted.
  - APC-I: minor opening of symphysis <2.5 cm
  - APC-II: opening of symphysis >2.5 cm (open-book fracture), with disruption of sacrospinous and sacrotuberous ligaments and anterior SI; posterior SI ligaments intact
  - APC-III: complete disruption of SI joint and sacrospinous and sacrotuberous ligaments
  - Significant urogenital, vascular, and neurologic injury is accompanied by the APC and VS injuries.
- VS type:
  - Vertical displacement of hemipelvis as a result of axial load to one hemipelvis
  - Symphysis diastasis or rami fractures anteriorly
  - Iliac wing driven up relative to sacrum
  - SI dislocation posteriorly
- Combination (CM type): any combination of above injuries:
  - Multiple breaks in pelvic ring continuity
  - High risk for associated injuries and pelvic hemorrhage
  - Malgaigne fracture
  - Anterior and posterior break in the ring on the same side
  - Straddle fracture:
    - Fractures of all four pubic rami or ipsilateral fracture of two pubic rami with dislocation of symphysis pubis
    - Due to LC or straddle injury (i.e., fall on object)
  - Severe multiple fractures and crush injuries or falls resulting in multiple fractures and gross instability.
- Avulsion fractures:
  - The ischial tuberosity is the most common location for apophyseal avulsion injury in the pelvis and usually results from a forceful contraction of the hamstring muscles.
  - Avulsion of the ischial tuberosity is most often associated with intense athletic activity, such as sprinting, or with excessive passive lengthening of the hamstring muscles, as often occurs during cheerleading or gymnastics.
  - The patient may experience a popping sensation at the time of injury and typically presents with severe posterior thigh or gluteal pain and complains of difficulty walking.

ETIOLOGY AND PATHOPHYSIOLOGY

- The incidence rate of pelvic fractures in the United States is estimated to be 37 out of 100,000 individuals per year, with the highest incidence occurring in those between the ages of 15 and 28 years old (2).
- 60% of pelvic fractures occur from motor vehicle accidents, most commonly pedestrians struck by automobiles.
- In a study on motor vehicle collisions completed by Stein et al. (3), of 1,851 patients studied, 27.6% sustained pelvic fracture injuries.
- 30% are due to falls from heights.
- Represent the third most common cause of death in motor vehicle accidents.
- Mortality rate from pelvic fractures reported is 5–42%.
- Increases to nearly 50% with hemorrhagic shock and open fractures.
- Significant pelvic hemorrhage can occur in unstable pelvic fractures, particularly Type III fractures:
  - Bleeding most commonly arises from the venous plexuses.
  - Significant hemorrhage results in retroperitoneal hematoma formation that may tamponade in the enclosed pelvic space.

RISK FACTORS

Etiologies of pelvic fractures in descending order of frequency:

- Motorcycle crash
- Vehicle-pedestrian collision
- Side-impact motor vehicle collision
- Fall >15 feet
- Motor vehicle crash

DIAGNOSIS

- In awake patients, pain on palpation of the sacrum and SI joints has the highest sensitivity (98%) for posterior pelvic ring fractures (4)[A].
- Multidetector computer tomography (MDCT) is the gold standard for diagnosing pelvic injuries. It has high sensitivity for fractures and can determine additional areas of injury and hemorrhage (5),(6).
- In hospitals without MDCT capabilities or in hemodynamically unstable patients, a single anteroposterior (AP) view of the pelvis should be obtained as early as possible.
  - Most significant unstable pelvic fractures will be seen on the single AP view (2).
  - Once the patient is stable, specialized radiographs (inlet/outlet, Judet) can be obtained.

PHYSICAL EXAM

- Does the patient have pelvic pain?
- Are there neurologic deficits involving sciatic, femoral, or obturator nerves?
- Are there contusions, ecchymoses, or abrasions at or near the bony prominences of the pelvis?
- Are there ecchymoses of the scrotum or perineum?
- Is there blood at the urethral meatus?
- Is there blood in or around the rectum, and is the prostate normal?
- Are there open wounds of the groin, buttock, or perineum?
- Is there a leg length difference, or is the resting position of one leg different from the other?
- Is there pain or abnormal pelvic motion on compression of the anterior iliac spines, LC of the iliac crests, rotation of the lower extremity, or hip flexion-extension?

DIFFERENTIAL DIAGNOSIS

- Normal variants (i.e., os acetabuli epiphyseal line can mimic type I fracture on x-ray)
- Ligamentous injury
- Spinal injury
- Intra-abdominal injury and hemorrhage

DIAGNOSTIC TESTS & INTERPRETATION

- Type and crossmatch
- Hemoglobin/hematocrit, platelet count, and coagulation studies (prothrombin time/partial thromboplastin time)
- Diagnostic studies
  - Prioritization of the studies; computed tomography (CT), angiography, or surgery
- Imaging
  - In the hemodynamically stable patient, the patient can go to CT scan for evaluation of the abdomen, pelvis, and retroperitoneum (7)[C].
  - In the hemodynamically unstable patient, a rapidly performed AP radiograph will reveal 90% of pelvic injuries (2).
  - Patient should also undergo focused assessment with sonography (FAST) in trauma to help assess intraperitoneal bleeding (2).
    - Abdominal US (FAST exam) is highly specific for retroperitoneal bleeding, not very sensitive.
    - Fast exam has largely replaced diagnostic peritoneal aspirate (DPA) or diagnostic peritoneal lavage (DPL) as the initial diagnostic exam of choice in trauma patients. However, DPA is still used in certain circumstances, such as determining if intraperitoneal fluid in the unstable patient is blood or urine.
    - If the FAST is positive, the patient should go for celiotomy with external pelvic fixation and peritoneal packing.
    - If the FAST is negative, DPA should be performed. If DPA is positive for hemorrhage, the patient should go for celiotomy with external pelvic fixation and peritoneal packing.
    - If the FAST and DPA are negative, pelvic stabilization and peritoneal packing should be performed.

- Angiography may be necessary in complicated pelvic fractures where vascular concern is an issue.
  - According to the Pelvic Injury Symposium in 2000 [C], physicians can determine when interventional radiology may be needed based on certain scenarios.
  - Hemodynamic instability, poorly responsive to fluid challenge, no hemoperitoneum, pelvic fracture
  - Hemodynamic stability, little hemoperitoneum, pelvic fracture, >4- to 6-U transfusion over 24 to 48 hours, respectively
  - Large or expanding retroperitoneal hematoma encountered at laparotomy or active bleed on CT scan.
  - Angiography is usually used in these above scenarios within the first 3 hours with a 90% rate of finding extravasation.
- MRI is indicated when there is evidence of neurologic injury.
- Red flags
  - Clinical signs that suggest an increased risk of ongoing pelvic fracture bleeding:
    - Prehospital hypotension
    - Admission base deficit >5
    - Persistent tachycardia in face of normal oxygenation and adequate pain control
    - Recurrent hypotension during resuscitation
    - Requirement for 6-U blood during first 24 hours

TREATMENT

GENERAL MEASURES

- LC-I/APC-I:
  - Protected weight-bearing on the affected side and treated conservatively with bed rest, analgesics, and comfort measures
  - Further surgical treatment may be needed if displacement of the fracture occurs after the patient starts to bear weight.
  - Follow-up x-rays can determine displacement after 2 to 5 days of physical therapy.
- APC-II/LC-I:
  - Marked displacement of the anterior ring without complete ring disruption; consult orthopedic surgery.
- LC-II, LC-III, APC-III, and VS:
  - Complete disruption of the posterior ring, and in general, require stabilization of both the anterior and posterior rings. Consult orthopedic surgery; patient should remain nothing per orem (NPO).
  - May require emergency department pelvic stabilization measures
  - Assess for pelvic hemorrhage (see below).
- Pelvic hemorrhage:
  - Angiography and selective vessel embolization
  - Direct operative control of pelvic bleeding
- Emergency department (ED) course
  - Determine which pelvic fractures are stable and unstable (see "Treatment").
    - *Initial stabilization:*
      - Airway, Breathing, and Circulation (ABCs of trauma care)
      - Avoid using lower extremity intravenous (IV) sites.
      - Aggressive resuscitation with blood or crystalloid, 0-negative or type-specific blood if hemodynamically unstable
      - Immobilize the pelvis to prevent further injury and decrease bleeding.
      - Pneumatic antishock garment (PASG) is an option, particularly when faced with a prolonged transport time or hemodynamically instability.
      - PASG: Use in ED is controversial but allows rapid pelvic immobilization and pelvic compression to slow bleeding.
      - Aggressive fluid resuscitation must occur before deflation of the PASG.
      - External fixator requires more time to place than PASG, but "splints" pelvis in a similar manner; contraindicated in severely comminuted pelvic fracture
      - Placement of a stabilization device should not interfere with further workup and care (DPL, etc.).

MEDICATION

- Crystalloid fluids: normal saline or lactated Ringer, IV bolus 2 L; pediatrics: 20 cc/kg
- Blood products: cross-matched, type-specific, or 0-negative 4 to 6 IU; pediatrics: 10 cc/kg
- Broad-spectrum IV antibiotics should be used in open fractures as prophylaxis against tetanus.

SURGERY/OTHER PROCEDURES

- Several factors play into the initial approach to bony stabilization, including hemodynamic status and response to resuscitation, fracture pattern, associated injury, and inflammatory status.
- Hemodynamic status is of particular concern, as the pelvis may be the primary source of bleeding or be contributing very little to bleeding. In the presence of ongoing thoracic or abdominal hemorrhage, orthopedic management beyond placement of a pelvic binder is delayed. Associated long bone fractures should be immediately splinted with coverage of open wounds.

ADMISSION, INPATIENT, AND NURSING CONSIDERATIONS

- Hospital admission criteria
  - Hemodynamic instability, and pelvic hemorrhage to the ICU
  - "Triad of death" is a term coined to describe patient decompensation in the presence of acute blood loss, resulting in hypothermia, coagulopathy, and acidosis.
  - Type III or IV pelvic fracture
  - Other related injuries (genitourinary, intra-abdominal, neurologic, etc.)
  - Intractable pain
  - Most elderly patients will require hospitalization
- ED discharge criteria
  - Type I or II fractures; hemodynamically stable with no evidence of other injuries.
  - Patient is able to ambulate and pain is adequately controlled.

ONGOING CARE

COMPLICATIONS

- Vascular injury leading to blood loss
- Closed head injuries
- Visceral injury (bladder and urethral, small bowel, diaphragm)
- Neurologic injury
- Chronic Instability; malunion/nonunion
- Infection
- Deep venous thrombosis
- Atelectasis/pneumonia
- Musculoskeletal back pain
- Sexual dysfunction

Pediatric Considerations

- Children can have proportionately greater hemorrhage.
- Nonaccidental trauma is a concern.

REFERENCES

1. Yoshihara H, Yoneoka D. Demographic epidemiology of unstable pelvic fracture in the United States from 2000 to 2009: trends and in-hospital mortality. *J Trauma Acute Care Surg*. 2014;76(2):380–385.
2. Davis DD, Foris LA, Kane SM, et al. *Pelvic Fracture*. StatPearls Publishing; 2022. Accessed February 29, 2024. https://www.ncbi.nlm.nih.gov/books/NBK430734/
3. Stein DM, O'Connor JV, Kufera JA, et al. Risk factors associated with pelvic fractures sustained in motor vehicle collisions involving newer vehicles. *J Trauma*. 2006;61(1):21–31.
4. McCormic JP, Morgan SJ, Smith WR. Clinical effectiveness of the physical examination in diagnosis of posterior pelvic ring injuries. *J Orthop Trauma*. 2003;17(4):257–261.
5. Mohseni S, Talving P, Kobayashi L, et al. The diagnostic accuracy of 64-slice computed tomography in detecting clinically significant arterial bleeding after pelvic fractures. *Am Surg*. 2011;77:1176–1182.
6. Dormagen JB, Tötterman A, Røise O, et al. Efficacy of plain radiography and computer tomography in localizing the site of pelvic arterial bleeding in trauma patients. *Acta Radiol*. 2010;51(1):107–116.
7. Magnone S, Coccolini F, Manfredi R, et al. Management of hemodynamically unstable pelvic trauma: results of the first Italian consensus conference (cooperative guidelines of the Italian Society of Surgery, the Italian Association of Hospital Surgeons, the Multi-specialist Italian Society of Young Surgeons, the Italian Society of Emergency Surgery and Trauma, the Italian Society of Anesthesia, Analgesia, Resuscitation and Intensive Care, the Italian Society of Orthopaedics and Traumatology, the Italian Society of Emergency Medicine, the Italian Society of Medical Radiology -Section of Vascular and Interventional Radiology- and the World Society of Emergency Surgery). *World J Emerg Surg*. 2014;9(1):18.

CLINICAL PEARLS

- Most common mechanism of injury is motor vehicle accidents, therefore assess the pelvis in victims of such accidents.
- Significant vascular injury can accompany pelvic fractures, so rapid diagnosis and intervention is necessary. MDCT is the gold standard, but one AP radiograph should be used in unstable patients.
- Minor fractures can be managed conservatively, fractures with significant displacement will require surgical intervention

FRACTURE, POSTERIOR MALLEOLUS

Kristina Quirolgico, MD, FAAPMR • Zainab Shirazi, MD • Jack Haberl, MD, MBA

BASICS

DESCRIPTION

- Ankle fracture involving the posterior aspect of the distal tibial articular surface
- Also known as malleolus tertius, posterior tibial pilon fracture, or Volkmann fragment

EPIDEMIOLOGY

- Isolated posterior malleolus fractures are uncommon—occurring in about 1–4% of all ankle fractures.
- Posterior malleolus fractures are present in up to 44% of all ankle fractures and 71% of spiral distal tibia fractures.

ETIOLOGY AND PATHOPHYSIOLOGY

Pronation or supination external rotation injury, posterior displacement of the talus, vertical loading during plantar hyperflexion, or a combination of these forces cause fracture of the posterior malleolus.

RISK FACTORS

- Repetitive vertical loading
- Osteoporosis

COMMONLY ASSOCIATED CONDITIONS

- Associated soft tissue and ligamentous ankle injuries (lateral, deltoid, and syndesmosis injuries)
- Bimalleolar or trimalleolar ankle fractures (posterior malleolus in conjunction with lateral malleolus, medial malleolus, or both)
- Fracture patterns can be suggestive of posterior malleolar involvement:
  - Spiral tibial shaft fractures are often associated with occult posterior malleolar involvement.

DIAGNOSIS

Diagnosis of posterior malleolar fractures relies on a high degree of clinical suspicion.

HISTORY

- Very important to obtain exact mechanism of injury:
  - Posterior malleolus fracture has been described in association with supination external rotation and pronation eversion injuries, or high-energy trauma.
  - Can also occur with lower leg fracture caused by rotational force
- History should address chronic versus acute injury.
- Chronic presentation: previously diagnosed ankle "sprain" that persists in being painful but is not unstable.

PHYSICAL EXAM

- Observe for obvious deformity, ecchymosis, and swelling.
- Palpate for pain, starting away from area of maximal tenderness, and compare to uninvolved foot and ankle.
- Check for ligamentous laxity with anterior drawer and talar tilt tests.
- Assess neurovascular status.
- Assess gait and ability to bear weight.
- Consider a fracture if patient is unable to bear weight or has significant swelling or ecchymosis in an acute setting.

DIFFERENTIAL DIAGNOSIS

- Acute setting:
  - High-grade ankle sprain
  - Lateral/medial malleolus fractures
  - Achilles tendon injury
  - Peroneal tendon subluxation and dislocation
- Chronic setting:
  - Posterior ankle impingement (os trigonum syndrome or prominent posterior process of the talus)
  - Retrocalcaneal bursitis
  - Achilles tendinopathy

DIAGNOSTIC TESTS & INTERPRETATION

- Use Ottawa Ankle Rules to decide on getting ankle x-rays to confirm diagnosis (1)[C]:
  - Anteroposterior (AP), lateral, and mortise views should be obtained.
  - Posterior malleolus fractures are often visualized in the lateral view.
- Workup should include x-rays of the knee and lower leg because posterior malleolar fractures often occur with associated injuries, such as Maisonneuve fracture (2)[C].
- Computed tomography (CT) and magnetic resonance imaging (MRI) are used to evaluate complex ankle injuries because they are often associated with occult posterior malleolar involvement (1)[C],(2)[C]:
  - CT is recommended if high clinical suspicion and negative plain radiographs.
  - CT allows for optimal fracture classification (i.e., size of fracture fragment and joint congruency) and management. Addition of 3D reconstruction is preferable for preoperative planning.
  - MRI is advantageous for diagnosing ligamentous injuries and osteochondral lesions.

TREATMENT

Isolated posterior malleolus fractures and nondisplaced posterior malleolus fractures (<25% of distal tibial articular surface) in bimalleolar/trimalleolar ankle fractures are treated nonoperatively (3)[A]:

- Posterior ankle splint with compression wrap
- Ice, elevation
- Non–weight-bearing on crutches for 1 week and then follow-up
- Apply cast for total of 6 weeks if fracture is nondisplaced on plain films.
- If there is fracture displacement (>2 mm or >25% of distal tibial articular surface) or syndesmotic instability, then refer to orthopedic surgeon for evaluation (see "Surgery/Other Procedures").

MEDICATION

Pain management with nonsteroidal anti-inflammatory drugs (NSAIDs) versus opioids (4)[B]:

- NSAIDs are acceptable to use in absolute stability (primary bone healing) and during the first week of healing via callous formation (secondary bone healing).
- Prolonged NSAID use may interfere with successful bone healing, especially in patients using selective COX-2 inhibitors.
- Opioids are associated with negatively impacting fracture healing, but there is no human study that can determine direct causality.

ADDITIONAL THERAPIES

Physical therapy after both operative and nonoperative care (1)[C]:

- Goal is to regain ankle full range of motion, strength, and proprioception.

SURGERY/OTHER PROCEDURES

- If >25% of the articular surface of the distal tibia is involved, or if the fracture is displaced >2 mm, then open reduction and internal fixation (ORIF) is recommended (3)[A],(5)[C],(6)[B].
- When associated with syndesmosis injury, stabilization of the posterior malleolus fracture with posterolateral plating may be preferred over syndesmotic screw (6)[B].
- Postoperative care (1)[C]:
  - Active, compliant patients are treated in boot or walker with partial weight-bearing of 15 to 20 kg for 6 weeks.
  - Older or noncompliant patients are offloaded in a wheelchair and below-knee cast.
  - Those with poor bone quality (osteoporosis, poorly controlled diabetes with neuropathy) are offloaded up to 12 weeks.
  - Gradual increase of weight-bearing and activity once there is radiographic evidence of bony consolidation

ONGOING CARE

FOLLOW-UP RECOMMENDATIONS

Orthopedic referral should be considered for any isolated fractures of the posterior malleolus because they often are complicated by other injuries.

PATIENT EDUCATION

- It is important to discuss that ankle sprains and fractures often are difficult to differentiate.
- If diagnosed with ankle sprain, persistent symptoms (pain, swelling, limp) warrant follow-up and further workup.
- Many different outcomes exist depending on the severity and type of ankle fracture: Compliance is critical.
- Advise patients to avoid smoking and prolonged NSAID use because this can affect fracture healing.

PROGNOSIS

- If diagnosed and treated appropriately, isolated posterior malleolar fractures have good functional outcomes.
- Significant comorbid fractures and/or syndesmotic injuries are much more likely to have long-term issues (see "Complications").

COMPLICATIONS

Variable depending on nonoperative versus operative management and patient comorbidities and compliance:

- Posttraumatic osteoarthritis
- Loss of normal range of motion
- Persistent intra-articular step-off of >2 mm
- Nonunion
- Posttraumatic chronic regional pain syndrome
- Persistent talar subluxation
- Postoperative wound infection
- Postoperative hardware complication

REFERENCES

1. Bartoníček J, Rammelt S, Tuček M. Posterior malleolar fractures: changing concepts and recent developments. *Foot Ankle Clin*. 2017;22(1):125–145.
2. Smeeing DPJ, Houwert RM, Kruyt MC, et al. The isolated posterior malleolar fracture and syndesmotic instability: a case report and review of the literature. *Int J Surg Case Rep*. 2017;41:360–365.
3. Odak S, Ahluwalia R, Unnikrishnan P, et al. Management of posterior malleolar fractures: a systematic review. *J Foot Ankle Surg*. 2016;55(1):140–145.
4. George MD, Baker JF, Leonard CE, et al. Risk of nonunion with nonselective NSAIDs, COX-2 inhibitors, and opioids. *J Bone Joint Surg Am*. 2020;102(14):1230–1238.
5. Rammelt S, Bartoníček J. Posterior malleolar fractures: a critical analysis review. *JBJS Rev*. 2020;8(8):e19.00207.
6. Baumbach SF, Herterich V, Damblemont A, et al. Open reduction and internal fixation of the posterior malleolus fragment frequently restores syndesmotic stability. *Injury*. 2019;50(2):564–570.

ADDITIONAL READING

- Barelds I, Krijnen WP, van de Leur JP, et al. Diagnostic accuracy of clinical decision rules to exclude fractures in acute ankle injuries: systematic review and meta-analysis. *J Emerg Med*. 2017;53(3):353–368.
- Duan X, Kadakia AR. Operative treatment of posterior malleolar fractures. *Open Orthop J*. 2017;11:732–742.
- Prasarn ML, Lorich DG. Posterior malleolus fractures in athletes. *Oper Tech Sports Med*. 2017;25(2):82–86.
- Stringfellow TD, Walters ST, Nash W, et al. Management of posterior malleolus fractures: a multicentre cohort study in the United Kingdom. *Foot Ankle Surg*. 2021;27(6):629–635.
- Tenenbaum S, Shazar N, Bruck N, et al. Posterior malleolus fractures. *Orthop Clin North Am*. 2017;48(1):81–89.
- Veltman ES, Halma JJ, de Gast A. Longterm outcome of 886 posterior malleolar fractures: a systematic review of the literature. *Foot Ankle Surg*. 2016;22(2):73–77.

CLINICAL PEARLS

- Posterior malleolar fractures rarely occur in isolation, so a high index of suspicion is necessary when lateral or medial malleolar fractures and/or syndesmotic injuries are diagnosed.
- An undiagnosed posterior malleolus fracture can be the source of chronic pain in the setting of ongoing pain associated with an ankle "sprain."
- Apply the Ottawa Ankle Rules to catch these on x-ray; posterior malleolar fractures are usually seen on lateral view. CT scan is recommended for fracture classification, future surgical planning, or if there is high clinical suspicion without radiographic findings.
- Treat nonoperatively with splint/cast and non–weight-bearing for at least 6 weeks for isolated, nondisplaced posterior malleolar fractures. Consider orthopedic surgery referral if posterior malleolar fracture involves >25% articular surface or >2 mm displacement.

FRACTURE, PROXIMAL HUMERUS

Julie Chuan, MD, FAAFP, CAQSM

BASICS

- *Caution:* Excessive movement of the arm may produce further neurovascular injury.
- *Controversy:* Prehospital reduction is not recommended because manipulation may lead to neurovascular compromise or further displacement of a fracture.

DESCRIPTION

- Proximal humeral fractures involve fractures of the humeral head, greater and lesser tuberosities, and anatomic and surgical neck (1).
- Mechanisms of injury:
  - Fall onto an outstretched hand
  - High-energy trauma in younger patients
  - Excessive rotation of the arm in the abducted position
  - Low-energy trauma, fall from a standing height, leads to fractures in the elderly.
  - Pathologic fracture from metastatic disease

EPIDEMIOLOGY

Incidence

- Proximal humeral fractures account for 6% of all fractures.
- Predominant gender in adults: female > male, 2 to 3:1
- In children, boys are 3 to 4 times more likely than girls (2).

Prevalence

- Proximal humerus fractures are the second most common upper extremity fractures (1)[C].
- In patients >65 years old, they are the third most common fracture after distal radius and hip fractures.

RISK FACTORS

- Osteoporosis and falls
- Indirect risk factors for falls include depression, epilepsy, diabetes with neuropathy, balance disorders, muscle weakness, and visual and hearing impairment (1)[C].

GENERAL PREVENTION

Increasing moderate physical activity, calcium supplementation to optimize bone density, minimizing psychotropic medications, and fall prevention (nonslip shoes) minimize the risk of proximal humerus fractures (1)[C].

DIAGNOSIS

HISTORY

- History of fall: Simple trip and fall, a low-impact force, is often associated with older (70+ years), osteoporotic women.
- Collision or direct blow: higher impact, occurring more commonly in younger men
- Pain after throwing or pitching
- History of malignancy: Consider metastatic disease for any humerus fracture produced by low-energy mechanism.

Pediatric Considerations

- Proximal humerus physeal fractures are seen in acute trauma and overuse injuries, presenting as "little league shoulder."
- "Unexplained falls" in toddlers or infants are concerning for non-accidental trauma (NAT).
- Check for other bruises and injuries suggesting NAT.
- Examine the elbow in children who are guarding their arm.

PHYSICAL EXAM

- Signs and symptoms include:
  - Pain, swelling, and tenderness about the shoulder, especially around the greater tuberosity
  - Assess for signs of dislocation, neurovascular injuries, open wounds or puncture.
  - Difficulty in initiating active motion
  - Position of the arm is often adducted and held closely against the chest.
  - Crepitus may be present.
  - Shoulder effusion owing to hemarthrosis developing into ecchymoses within 24 to 48 hours at the area of fracture and may spread to chest wall, flank, and distal extremity
  - Diminished peripheral pulses or decreased sensation, especially over the deltoid muscle (axillary nerve)
  - Disruption of the deltoid contour or prominent subacromial sulcus suggests concurrent dislocation, often associated with high impact mechanism of injury (3).
- Neurovascular:
  - Nerve: sensation over the deltoid muscle (axillary nerve) and distal motor and sensory function in the hand and fingers; 45% risk of nerve injury, axillary is the most common with marked displacement of the humeral shaft or anterior fracture-dislocation (4).
  - Vascular: radial and ulnar pulse, capillary refill time
  - Associated injuries: clavicle, scapula, wrist, and elbow for range of motion and tenderness for concomitant injury (1)

DIFFERENTIAL DIAGNOSIS

- Shoulder dislocation
- Acute hemorrhagic bursitis
- Traumatic rotator cuff tear
- Acromioclavicular separation
- Calcific tendinitis
- Pathologic fracture

DIAGNOSTIC TESTS & INTERPRETATION

Initial Tests (lab, imaging)

- AP, lateral, and orthogonal or axillary view to determine glenohumeral joint congruency and fracture pattern
- Computed tomography (CT) scan:
  - Consider for complex fractures
    - Intra-articular fractures to evaluate the glenoid and humeral head
    - Suspected occult fractures
    - Posterolateral compression fractures
    - Evaluate for multipart fractures of humeral head (5).
- Magnetic resonance imaging (MRI):
  - Consideration of rotator cuff integrity is in question.
  - 40% of proximal humerus fractures were in combination with rotator cuff tears, at the time of or within 1 year of injury.
- Classification
  - Neer classification: This system consists of 2- to 4-part fractures, and the locations include the anatomic head, humeral shaft, the greater tuberosity, and the lesser tuberosity.
  - AO/OTA 2018 classification:
    - A: unifocal, extraarticular, 2-part fracture with an intact blood supply
    - B: bifocal, extraarticular, 3-part fracture with possible injury to the blood supply
    - C: articular fracture or 4-part fracture

TREATMENT

GENERAL MEASURES

- Proper immobilization, orthopedic consultation, and pain management
- Operative versus nonoperative treatment is decided in conjunction with orthopedics.
- Nonoperative treatment:
  - About 85% can be managed nonoperatively without significant difference in outcomes.
  - Fragility fractures with weaker osteoporotic bones are harder to stabilize and have a higher surgical failure rate.
  - Younger patients with stronger bone structure and higher functional demands have more benefit from surgical fixation.
  - 2- to 3-part fractures are usually managed conservatively.
  - 4-part fractures in older age group or displaced fracture with high anesthesia risk can be managed conservatively.
- Consult orthopedic surgery urgently if:
  - Any open fractures, fracture-dislocations, vascular or neurologic injuries
  - Closed reduction needs to be performed.

MEDICATION

- Pain medications are indicated for comfort.
- Conscious sedation should be used if attempting a closed reduction.

ADMISSION, INPATIENT, AND NURSING CONSIDERATIONS

- Open fractures for operative management and parenteral antibiotic therapy for open fractures
- Displaced fracture that cannot be treated through closed reduction and therefore require operation
- Significant associated injuries that require admission and observation
- Most do not need hospitalization.

ONGOING CARE

- About 85% are treated nonsurgically.
- Sling, swathe, and axillary pad for 2 to 4 weeks
- Start early passive mobilization as early as second week.
- Weekly radiographs for the first three weeks to monitor for displacement
- Initial immobilization and early motion: succeeds in many cases because most proximal humeral fractures are minimally displaced (5)[B]
- Refer for surgical consideration if:
  - Head splitting fractures
  - Severe varus or valgus displacement of the humeral head
  - Completely off-end fractures
- Surgical interventions (2)[B]:
  - Closed reduction percutaneous pinning
  - Open reduction and internal fixation (ORIF) with locking plates and screws
  - Intramedullary nail
  - Arthroplasty—hemi or reverse shoulder arthroplasty (RSA); RSA for about 50% of fragility fractures are treated surgically.

OUTCOMES

- If axillary artery is disrupted with displaced fractures, higher risk of avascular necrosis of the humeral head
- 1.4% nonunion rate in elderly treated conservatively
- "Nonunion" term is not consistent, varies between 3, 6, and 12 months.
- Nonunions can be treated nonoperatively if pain is minimal with adequate range of motion and function.
- Bone stimulators can be considered for nonoperative treatment of nonunions.
- Nonunions can be surgically reduced with internal fixation if the glenohumeral articular surface is preserved.
- Arthroplasty is preferred for 3- and 4-part fractures if joint surface is compromised (6)[B].
- Risk factors for nonunions include:
  - Displacement of the fracture
  - Inadequate immobilization
  - Aggressive rehabilitation
  - Patient noncompliance
- Comorbidities that can be a risk factor for nonunions include:
  - Disrupted blood supply
  - Osteoporosis
  - Alcoholism
  - Tobacco usage
  - Mental illness
  - Systemic corticosteroids
  - Rheumatologic disease

Pediatric Considerations

Types of fractures:

- Birth fractures
  - Typically clavicle, but can be proximal humerus physeal separations which heal rapidly within 2 to 3 weeks
  - Associated with clavicle and brachial plexus injuries
- Birth trauma with increased risk of fracture include vaginal delivery, breech, prolonged labor, >4.5 kg
- Proximal humerus fracture in <2 years old should raise concern for abuse (5)[B].
- Most proximal humerus fractures in 5 to 11 years old are metaphyseal.
- Boys are 3 to 4 times more likely to sustain proximal humerus fractures.
  - Mechanisms:
    - Direct trauma—fall onto shoulder or a blunt force strike to the posterior shoulder
    - Indirect fall onto out stretch hand with arm abducted and externally rotated
    - Salter-Harris type II are predominantly in >11 years old.
    - Salter-Harris type III and IV are rare and usually with high-energy trauma.

PHYSICAL EXAM

- Symptoms: pain, guarding, arm dysfunction, swelling, ecchymosis, altered contour of the ipsilateral shoulder; refusal to move the shoulder, holding arm internally rotated against the body
  - Neurovascular assessment: Assess function of radial, median, ulnar, axillary (sensation to the lateral aspect of the shoulder), and musculocutaneous nerves (sensation to the extensor aspect of the forearm).
  - Presence of radial, ulnar, and brachial pulses and good capillary refill in all digits
- Shoulder radiographs: AP, scapula Y, and axillary
  - Overuse injuries with repetitive throwing
- "Little league shoulder," proximal humerus growth plate fractures, usually 11 to 14 years old
- Progressive pain over months with throwing
- Weakness secondary to pain with resisted shoulder abduction, internal and external rotation
- Widening of the proximal humerus growth plate on x-ray (4)
- Avulsion fracture of the lesser tuberosity is seen in throwing or fly fishing due to repetitive microtrauma resulting in incomplete traction injury, usually age 12 to 15 years old.
- Neer and Horwitz classification of proximal humerus fractures grades:
  - I is <5 mm displacement.
  - II is <1/3 displacement of the shaft width.
  - III is >1/3 but <2/3 displacement of the shaft width.
  - IV is >2/3 displacement of the shaft width.
  - Grade I and II usually treated nonsurgically unless it is open fracture, vascular injury, or polytrauma.
  - Grade III and IV treatment varies (no consensus) with higher risk of limb shortening and restricted motion.
- Immobilization usually heals in 4 to 6 weeks and then gradual return to activity, ROM, with goal return to all activity by 3 to 4 months with excellent results.

Pediatric Considerations

- In children nearing skeletal maturity, determining the degree of displacement or separation of the proximal humeral epiphysis is essential because exact reduction is important to prevent later growth disturbance.
- Pediatric patients are often less compliant with immobilization and less able to verbalize complaints and may benefit from admission to the hospital for observation and neurovascular checks.

F

REFERENCES

1. Pandey R, Raval P, Manibanakar N, et al. Proximal humerus fractures: a review of current practice. *J Clin Orthop Trauma*. 2023;43:102233.
2. Bhambra T, Souroullas P, Wright A, et al. Evidence-based management of proximal humerus fractures. *Orthop Trauma*. 2023;37:5.
3. Christensen G. Trends in the treatment of proximal humerus fractures in the United States Medicare population. *Seminars Arthroplasty*. 2023:331–336.
4. Misra S, Vaishya R, Trikha V, et al. Practice guidelines for proximal humeral fractures. *J Clin Orthop Trauma*. 2019;10(3):631–633.
5. Popkin C, Levine W, Ahmad C. Evaluation and management of pediatric proximal humerus fractures. *J Am Acad Orthop Surg*. 2015;23(2):77–86.
6. Tapscott DC, Paxton ES. Decision-making and management of proximal humerus nonunions. *Orthop Clin North Am*. 2021;52(4):369–379.

ADDITIONAL READING

AO Foundation. AO/OTA Fracture and Dislocation Classification Introduction to the Classification of Long-Bone Fractures. Accessed date August 24, 2025. https://classification.aoeducation.org/files/download/AOOTA_Classification_2018_Classification_brochure_2107071005.pdf

CLINICAL PEARLS

- Axillary artery is the most common neurovascular injury and can result in avascular necrosis of the humeral head.
- When evaluating shoulder dislocations, consider associated humeral head fractures.
- When the fracture is stable with some callus on radiograph, consider initiating gentle range-of-motion exercises as early as tolerated.

FRACTURE, PROXIMAL PHALANX

Kari J. Rezac, DO • Daniel C. Herman, MD, PhD, FAAPMR, FACSM, FISBS, CAQSM • Brandon Hassid, MD

BASICS

EPIDEMIOLOGY

- The most common fracture of the hand in adults
- Base of proximal phalanx fracture is the most common pediatric hand fracture.
- The 5th ray is most commonly involved, followed by the thumb.
- Males affected 3 times as often as females
- Crush injuries or direct blow to the finger account for >80% of injuries.

ETIOLOGY AND PATHOPHYSIOLOGY

- Intrinsic muscles of the hand (interossei) insert into the extensor expansion on the dorsum of the proximal phalanx.
- Proximal phalangeal fractures usually angulate apex volarly due to the proximal fragment being flexed by interossei and the distal fragment being extended by the central slip's insertion on the base of the middle phalanx.
- Metacarpophalangeal (MCP) joint collateral ligaments are taut in 70 to 90 degrees of flexion and provide stabilization of the MCP joint.

COMMONLY ASSOCIATED CONDITIONS

- Digital nerve injury: contusion, transection
- Digital artery injury: open or closed fracture; usually does not require treatment
- Tendon injury: complete or partial rupture; infrequent with proximal phalangeal fracture
- Thumb avulsion fracture common with ulnar collateral ligament injury (See "MCP [Metacarpophalangeal] Collateral Ligament Sprain.")

DIAGNOSIS

HISTORY

- Mechanism of injury: direct blow, axial load, axial traction, twisting/torque, or "grabbing a jersey"
- History of previous injury, surgery, or deformity

PHYSICAL EXAM

- Pain, swelling, bruising, tenderness, crepitus, instability, loss of motion, and impaired function are typical findings.
- Gross deformity in some cases
- Open (compound) fractures usually are obvious and require emergent care.
- May be mistaken for MCP or proximal interphalangeal (PIP) joint dislocation
- Malrotation is common with spiral and oblique shaft fractures and must be detected and corrected early.
- Inspection/observation: location and degree of deformity, swelling, and ecchymosis
- Rotational malalignment: With MCP and PIP flexed to 90 degrees, all fingers should point toward the scaphoid. When viewed "end on," the plane of all fingernails should be symmetrical.
- Range of motion (ROM): usually decreased; compare with contralateral side.
- Palpation: Feel for crepitus. Determine point of maximal tenderness.
- Provocation: Axial loading or distraction often results in pain at the fracture site (nonspecific).
- Adjacent structures: MCP and PIP joints, tendon function, ligaments (joint stability), and soft tissues
- Neurocirculatory function: sensation, capillary refill, skin color, and temperature

DIFFERENTIAL DIAGNOSIS

- MCP joint dislocation
- PIP joint dislocation
- Soft tissue contusion
- Ligament/capsular sprain
- Flexor/extensor tendon strain or rupture

DIAGNOSTIC TESTS & INTERPRETATION

- Radiographs should be obtained before any manipulative examination.
- Anteroposterior (AP), true lateral, and oblique views of the finger are diagnostic (1)[C].
- Describe rotation of fragments, angulation, and intra-articular versus extra-articular.
- Differences in diameter of fragments suggest rotation.
- Skilled ultrasonographers can detect phalangeal fractures with moderate sensitivity and specificity (2)[B].

TREATMENT

- Prehospital:
  - Apply sterile dressing over any open wounds.
  - Splint in a position of comfort, apply ice if available, and transport for radiographs and definitive treatment.
- Open (compound) fractures: irrigation, sterile wet dressing, ice, elevate, splint, urgently refer to orthopedic surgeon:
  - Prophylactic antibiotics should be administered (3)[A].
  - Empiric antibiotics to cover *Staphylococcus aureus*: cephalosporin, penicillin (methicillin-susceptible *Staphylococcus epidermidis* [MSSE]), or clindamycin, cotrimoxazole (methicillin-resistant *S. aureus* [MRSA])
  - Tetanus toxoid and/or immunoglobulin if indicated
- Reduction of fracture fragments to anatomical positions is desired to speed healing and maximize hand function. Closed reduction is often successful and should usually be attempted (4)[A].
- After reduction, immobilization should be applied, and postreduction imaging should be obtained.
- Fracture management (1),(5),(6)[A]:
  - Stable, nondisplaced without angulation or rotational deformity:
    - Dynamic splinting ("buddy taping") to an adjacent normal digit
    - Use absorbent material between digits for padding and to prevent maceration.
    - Early ROM: Patient should use the hand normally as comfort allows (1)[C].
  - Nondisplaced and impacted fractures:
    - Some degree of intrinsic stability; do not require surgery.
    - Splint with MCP joint flexed 70 to 90 degrees, interphalangeal (IP) joints extended, and buddy taping to adjacent finger to control rotation for 3 weeks. Wrist and distal IP joint (DIP) need not be immobilized (4)[A]. This position of function shifts the extensor aponeurosis distally to cover the majority of the proximal phalanx dorsally, which compresses and stabilizes the fracture.
  - Displaced or angulated transverse midshaft:
    - Apex volar angulation common; generally unstable, with variable response to closed reduction, which should be attempted
    - Technique:
      - Metacarpal or digital block
      - Longitudinal traction and flexion of the MCP joint with manual realignment of fracture fragments
      - If reduction achieved/maintained, apply gutter splint or Burkhalter splint (dorsal slab of stabilizing material placed from the end of a short arm cast to just proximal to the PIP, with MCP joints flexed 70 to 90 degrees).
      - If reduction not achieved after splinting, refer to orthopedics/hand surgeon.

- Oblique fractures:
  - Attempt reduction and splinting (4)[A].
  - If reduction not achieved after splinting, refer to orthopedics/hand surgery.
- Displaced fractures of the base:
  - Significant volar angulation requires reduction.
  - Technique:
    - Metacarpal or digital block
    - Longitudinal traction and flexion of the MCP joint and correct volar angulation with direct pressure
    - If reduction achieved/maintained, apply gutter or Burkhalter splint; if not, refer to orthopedics/hand surgery.
- Unstable: condylar (lateral or medial aspect of base) and displaced intra-articular fractures:
  - Refer to orthopedics/hand surgery for pin fixation or open reduction and internal fixation (ORIF).
- AP, true lateral, oblique x-ray to confirm reduction
- Unacceptable, unstable, or unsure alignment: Early consultation with orthopedic surgeon is advised.
- Persistence of significant displacement, angulation necessitates an orthopedic surgery consultation.
  - >10 to 15 degrees radial or ulnar angulation
  - >15 to 25 degrees apex palmar angulation
  - >0 to 5 degrees rotation (6)[A]

MEDICATION

- Oral analgesics may be used if needed.
- Digital or metacarpal block with local anesthetics may be used if reduction or repair of associated soft tissue injury is required.

ISSUES FOR REFERRAL

The following phalangeal fractures warrant prompt orthopedic consultation because many will require immediate surgery (1),(6)[A]:

- Displaced phalangeal neck or condyle fractures: Failure to treat this injury with pin stabilization can result in a malunion that limits digital flexion.
- Malrotation fractures
- Widely displaced, irreducible proximal phalanx base fractures (due to entrapment of soft tissue)
- Avulsion fractures of the thumb MCP ulnar collateral ligament insertion
  - The pediatric equivalent of skier's thumb typically involves a displaced Salter-Harris type III intra-articular fracture; this also necessitates orthopedic referral.
- PIP joint fracture dislocations involving >30% of the articular surface, as these may be unstable

ONGOING CARE

FOLLOW-UP RECOMMENDATIONS

Any malalignment on follow-up x-rays should prompt an orthopedic surgery consultation.

Patient Monitoring

Monitor specific fractures as follows (6)[A]:

- Stable, nondisplaced without angulation or rotational deformity:
  - Treated with buddy taping
  - Dynamic splinting for 3 weeks; x-ray at 7 to 10 days to check alignment and stability
  - Daily ROM exercises after 1 weeks as comfort allows
  - Continued dynamic splinting for athletic activities for another 4 to 6 weeks
- Nondisplaced and impacted fractures treated with splint or cast:
  - Recheck radiographs in 7 to 10 days to assess healing.
  - After 3 weeks, early protected mobilization with buddy taping
- Displaced or angulated transverse midshaft treated with closed reduction and splint or cast:
  - X-ray at 5 and 10 days to assure reduction is maintained; if not, refer to orthopedics/hand surgery.
  - If reduction maintained, continue splint for 3 to 4 weeks. If reduction fails, refer to orthopedics/hand surgery for ORIF or percutaneous fixation.
- Displaced fractures of the base:
  - X-ray at 5 and 10 days to assure reduction is maintained; if not, refer to orthopedics/hand surgery.

COMPLICATIONS

- Joint stiffness and subsequent functional disability:
  - Adhesions between extensor mechanism and periosteum may result in loss of motion requiring surgical intervention.
  - Adhesions between flexor digitorum superficialis and flexor digitorum profundus may follow prolonged immobilization and require surgical intervention to restore function.
- Arthritis can result from intra-articular fractures.
- Nonunion is rare; however, risk of nonunion is greater when improperly immobilized, patient is noncompliant, or open fractures.

REFERENCES

1. Wahl EP, Richard MJ. Management of metacarpal and phalangeal fractures in the athlete. *Clin Sports Med.* 2020;39(2):401–422.
2. Aksay E, Kilic TY, Yesilaras M, et al. Accuracy of bedside ultrasonography for the diagnosis of finger fractures. *Am J Emerg Med.* 2016;34(5):809–812.
3. Gosselin RA, Roberts I, Gillespie WJ. Antibiotics for preventing infection in open limb fractures. *Cochrane Database Syst Rev.* 2004;2004(1):CD003764.
4. Verver D, Timmermans L, Klaassen RA, et al. Treatment of extra-articular proximal and middle phalangeal fractures of the hand: a systematic review. *Strategies Trauma Limb Reconstr.* 2017;12(2):63–76.
5. Logters TT, Lee HH, Gehrmann S, et al. Proximal phalanx fracture management. *Hand (N Y).* 2018;13(4):376–383.
6. Zhang M, Hirth M, Cole T, et al. A systemic review of conservatively managed isolated extra-articular proximal phalanx finger fractures in adults. *JPRAS Open.* 2024;41:37–51.

ADDITIONAL READING

- Kolovich GP, Heifner JJ. Proximal interphalangeal joint dislocations and fracture-dislocations. *J Hand Surg Eur Vol.* 2023;48(Suppl 2):27S–34S.
- Liao JCY, Chong AKS. Pediatric hand and wrist fractures. *Clin Plast Surg.* 2019;46(3):425–436.
- Meals C, Meals R. Hand fractures: a review of current treatment strategies. *J Hand Surg Am.* 2013;38(5):1021–1031.

CLINICAL PEARLS

- Return-to-play decision based on stability, ROM, current clinical and radiographic healing status, and specific demands of sport
- Most athletes with stable fractures are able to return to sport as early as 2 weeks after the injury with protection such as buddy taping.
- For unstable fractures, early surgical intervention may be desirable for better outcome and earlier return.
- Begin mobilization at 3 weeks to prevent finger stiffness.

FRACTURE, PROXIMAL TIBIAL PLATEAU

Holly J. Benjamin, MD, FAMSSM, FACSM • Stefany J. K. Malanka, MD

BASICS

- Tibial plateau fractures occur as a result of trauma:
  - Shearing force directed either medially (valgus deformity), laterally (varus deformity), axial compression (bicondylar), or combination of forces
- There are six subtypes of fractures (Schatzker classification), which are determined by angulation of the knee and energy applied at time of injury, and bone density (1).
- Associated ligamentous injuries occur due to continued deforming force after the fracture has been sustained.
- 68% of tibial plateau fractures have posterolateral ligamentous corner injury.
- Anterior cruciate ligament (ACL) and posterior cruciate ligament (PCL) tears occur concomitantly in up to 80% and 36% of cases, respectively (2).
- Medial plateau fractures are thought to be a knee dislocation variant.
- Associated with significant functional morbidity due to intra-articular trauma

DESCRIPTION

- Fracture that includes the articular surface of the medial and/or lateral tibial condyles
- Synonym(s): tibial plateau fracture
- First coined a "fender fracture" by Cotton in 1929
- 40–60% of tibial plateau fractures involve an automobile hitting a pedestrian, others are often sports injuries or fall from height.

EPIDEMIOLOGY

- Tibial plateau fractures account for ~1% of all fractures and 8% of fractures in the elderly. Elderly are less likely to have meniscal or ligamentous injury (3).
- Fractures of the lateral plateau account for 55–70%, associated with lower energy mechanisms of injury.
- Medial plateau fractures account for 10–23%, usually from higher energy mechanism of injury.
- Bilateral plateau fractures account for 11–31%.
- In both sexes, the highest frequency was between the ages of 40 and 60 years.

RISK FACTORS

- Osteoporosis
- Perioperative fracture associated with total or unicompartmental knee arthroplasty
- Sports: skiing, football, horseback riding, certain water sports

COMMONLY ASSOCIATED CONDITIONS

- Tibial plateau fractures often accompany a predictable pattern of associated soft tissue knee injury:
  - Medial tibial plateau fracture: lateral collateral ligament and medial meniscus injuries
  - Lateral tibial plateau fracture: medial collateral ligament and lateral meniscus injuries
  - ACL injuries can be seen with either medial or lateral plateau fractures. Also, see intracondylar eminence fractures.
- Owing to brisk hemorrhage and swelling, tibial plateau fractures can be associated with acute compartment syndrome.

DIAGNOSIS

- X-ray: anteroposterior (AP), lateral, oblique; possible tunnel view
- Magnetic resonance imaging (MRI): indicated for assessment of associated ligamentous or cartilaginous injury
- Computed tomography (CT) scan: best to assess bone abnormality
- Schatzker classification system for tibial plateau fractures (4):
  - Type I: lateral split (young patients with strong subchondral bone)
  - Type II: lateral split with depression
  - Type III: pure lateral depression (elderly, osteoporotic patients)
  - Type IV: pure medial depression
  - Type V: bicondylar
  - Type VI: metaphyseal-diaphyseal dissociation
- Other classification systems not as commonly used include AO/Orthopedic Trauma Association and the three-column concept.
- Ancillary studies: Knee aspirate may help to reveal the presence of fat globules (indicating osteochondral injury) and to reduce pain.

HISTORY

- An accurate history will help to determine the direction of the force, velocity (high vs. low), and initial deformity produced.
- Swelling can be immediate or delayed, often indicating osteochondral fracture or internal derangement.

PHYSICAL EXAM

- Signs and symptoms:
  - Painful swollen knee
  - Unable to bear weight
  - May have compartment syndrome signs and symptoms (see below)
- Physical examination:
  - Most accurate way to evaluate the extent of the soft tissue injuries or any open injuries
  - Skin, joint effusion, laxity (stability) testing, compartments, neurovascular exam
  - Check for abrasions or possible open fracture.
  - Visible knee deformity indicates a severe injury.
  - Tenderness to palpation is noted over the medial and/or lateral tibial plateau.
  - Document distal pulses.
  - Check neurologic status with focus on the peroneal nerve and tendon function.
  - Associated ligamentous injuries may show tenderness to palpation and instability of the collateral or cruciate ligaments.
  - Key finding is excursion of endpoint movement.
  - Large hemarthrosis usually is present.
  - If hemarthrosis is not present, it may indicate a torn capsule.
  - Watch for acute compartment syndrome findings.
  - Any signs of compartment syndrome is considered an acute orthopedic emergency, requiring immediate consultation.
    - Pain (severe) out of proportion
    - Pressure or tightness
    - Pallor
    - Paresthesia
    - Paralysis

DIFFERENTIAL DIAGNOSIS

- Intercondylar eminence fracture ± ACL tear: Segond sign on plain film indicates lateral capsule avulsion and ACL tear.
- Collateral ligament avulsion
- Tibial tubercle avulsion
- Proximal fibular fracture
- Patella fracture
- Hemarthrosis from patellar dislocation, ACL tear, or meniscal tear (if in the red or red-white zone)
- Stress fracture
- Physeal injury (pediatric)

DIAGNOSTIC TESTS & INTERPRETATION

- Standard radiographs in AP, lateral, and two oblique views: (sensitivity of 85%)
  - Initial x-rays may miss a small tibial plateau fracture especially in those with osteoporosis.
  - AP views may only show subtle findings as the plateau slope is not well defined in this view.
  - High index of suspicion must be maintained based on mechanism of injury, presence/absence of an effusion, and joint instability.
  - Series provides information allowing for accurate assessment of the fracture pattern:
    - Internal oblique view best assesses the lateral plateau.
    - External oblique view best assesses the medial plateau.
    - Tunnel view is helpful if suspicious for intercondylar eminence fractures.
    - Lateral view demonstrates presence of depressed plateau fracture:
      - Medial side is concave.
      - Lateral side is convex.
  - Posterior collateral ligament injury may show avulsion fracture.
- CT scan:
  - Image of choice if negative films but high index of suspicion for fracture, or for operative planning
  - Assesses articular surface depression, comminution; delineates fracture pattern, fragment size and shape; aids in accurate classification

ALERT

Bicondylar tibial plateau fractures all need CT imaging.

  - If necessary, three-dimensional reconstructions can be provided to enhance the understanding of the fracture pattern.
- MRI: allows for assessment of associated ligamentous injuries; may not show fracture as well as CT
- Arteriography:
  - Should be considered in any tibial plateau fracture where the stability of the joint is in question
  - Also may use ankle brachial index (ABI); if <0.9, indicates arterial insult
  - Medial plateau fractures have a high incidence of vascular insult (owing to greater energy forces).
  - Arteriography/ABI should be performed and documented in almost all cases.
  - Presence of a palpable pulse does not exclude the possibility of intimal tear.
  - A missed vascular injury can result in an intraoperative occlusive thrombosis that could jeopardize the extremity.

TREATMENT

- Successful functional outcomes depend on the restoration of axial and rotational limb alignment coupled with knee joint stability (3).
- Conservative treatment is acceptable if <5 mm (0.5 cm) of depression/displacement and there is no varus/valgus instability through a full arc of motion.
- Key to good outcome is early range of motion (ROM) and non–weight-bearing compliance.
- Important to encourage quadriceps strengthening after bracing discontinued
- Physical therapy: warranted once evidence of fracture healing (4 to 6 weeks); vital if <90 degrees flexion by 4 weeks
- Emergency department (ED) or urgent care treatment:
  - Acute treatment:
    - Non–weight-bearing
    - Long leg splint with knee in full extension, ankle splinted at 90 degrees if instability or dislocation present
    - Hinged knee brace with 0 to 90 degrees of motion preferred for stable fracture
    - Ice, elevation
    - Pain management as needed
    - Monitor compartments closely.
    - Acetaminophen, ice, and elevation are first line with limited use of narcotics and nonsteroidal anti-inflammatory drugs (NSAIDs).

MEDICATION

- Conflicting evidence regarding safety of NSAIDs for pain management; use caution if high risk for nonunion (4),(5).
- Use total range of motion (TROM) brace locked in extension initially if pain control is difficult.

ADDITIONAL THERAPIES

- Patient age, medical condition, history of osteoporosis, and expected level of activity should be taken into consideration on a case-by-case basis in terms of operative versus nonoperative management.
- There are no specific recommendations regarding patient age or comorbid arthritis to dictate operative versus nonoperative management.

ISSUES FOR REFERRAL

- Emergent referral and treatment if there is associated acute compartment syndrome and/or vascular injury
- Referral recommended within 48 hours of fracture depressed or displaced (≥5 mm) or associated with significant ligament/meniscal injuries, or instability

SURGERY/OTHER PROCEDURES

- The goals of treating an intra-articular fracture of the tibia are to preserve pain-free joint mobility, stability, axial alignment, and articular cartilage congruity and diminish risks of posttraumatic osteoarthritis.
- Best accomplished by anatomic reduction of the joint surface and restoration of axial alignment
- Intra-articular fractures, regardless of open or closed treatment, must be mobilized quickly to achieve the best ROM.
- Only percutaneous or open reduction and stable fixation allows early motion without loss of articular cartilage.
- Fractures treated initially by closed reduction often will show persistent displacement of articular cartilage fragments.
- If open reduction cannot be achieved owing to mitigating circumstances, then treatment should consist of skeletal traction and early mobilization.
- Bicondylar tibial plateau fractures are best managed with locked plating in favor of external fixation.
- Absolute surgical indications:
  - Open fractures
  - Acute compartment syndrome
  - Acute vascular injury
- Total knee replacement may be necessary in complex patterns in specific patient populations.
- Timing of surgery: immediate if open fractures, associated compartment syndrome, and fractures with associated vascular injuries
- Careful evaluation of fractures with tomography/CT scan/MRI is recommended.
- Delay of 24 to 48 hours will not compromise the outcome in the absence of emergent surgery indications.
- Patients delayed >48 hours can be placed in skeletal traction.
- Postoperative management:
  - Depends on the degree of stability achieved with fixation and the findings at surgery
  - If stable, early motion by continuous passive motion (CPM) is beneficial.
  - Immobilization in flexion adversely affects postoperative motion.
  - Early non–weight-bearing ambulation is encouraged postoperatively for 8 to 12 weeks.
  - Early motion and non–weight-bearing compliance are critical keys to long-term success.

ONGOING CARE

PROGNOSIS

- High rate of osteoarthritis associated with tibial plateau fractures increases risk of undergoing knee arthroplasty 5-fold (6).
- Prognosis for full return of motion in the presence of osteoarthritis is poor.
- Outcomes are generally better in younger patients.
- Surgical management results in 50–80% return to sport rates in athletes, median time 6 to 7 months.
- However, return to preinjury level of sports is 31–34% average (3).

COMPLICATIONS

- Compartment syndrome (preoperative and postoperative); most common significant short-term complication
- Posttraumatic osteoarthritis
- Infection
- Wound slough
- Loss of ROM
- Loss of normal gait pattern
- Fixation failure
- Loss of articular reduction
- Malunion
- Nonunion (rare)
- Deep vein thrombosis
- Pseudoarthrosis

REFERENCES

1. Schatzker J, Kfuri M. Revisiting the management of tibial plateau fractures. *Injury*. 2022; 53(6): 2207–2218.
2. Cinque ME, Godin JA, Moatshe G, et al. Do tibial plateau fractures worsen outcomes of knee ligament injuries? A matched cohort analysis. *Orthop J Sports Med*. 2017;5(8):2325967117723895.
3. Robertson GAJ, Wong SJ, Wood AM. Return to sport following tibial plateau fractures: a systematic review. *World J Orthop*. 2017;8(7):574–587.
4. Eiff MP, Hatch R. Patellar, tibial, and fibular fractures. In: *Fracture Management for Primary Care*. 4th ed. Elsevier; 2020:263–290.
5. Marquez-Lara A, Hutchinson ID, Nuñez F Jr, et al. Nonsteroidal anti-inflammatory drugs and bone-healing: a systematic review of research quality. *JBJS Rev*. 2016;4(3):e4.
6. Bryson WN, Fischer EJ, Jennings JW, et al. Three-column classification system for tibial plateau fractures: what the orthopedic surgeon wants to know. *Radiographics*. 2021;41(1):144–155.

ADDITIONAL READING

- Elsoe R, Larsen P, Nielsen NPH, et al. Population-based epidemiology of tibial plateau fractures. *Orthopedics*. 2015;38(9):e780–e786.
- Prat-Fabregat S, Camacho-Carrasco P. Treatment strategy for tibial plateau fractures: an update. *EFORT Open Rev*. 2017;1(5):225–232.

CLINICAL PEARLS

- Need to have a high index of suspicion with ligamentous injury, especially in the setting of large swelling shortly after injury
- Although tibial plateau fractures have a low overall incidence, these injury patterns must be thought of in trauma owing to the risk of associated vascular insult (see discussion on arteriography under "Diagnostic Tests & Interpretation").
- Liberal use of advanced imaging is encouraged for full understanding of the extent of the injury.
- Consider compartment syndrome both preoperatively and postoperatively as a potential complication.
- The keys—both for early treatment and for long-term reasonable prognosis—lie in compliance with non–weight-bearing compliance and early ROM.
- Anticipate the development of posttraumatic osteoarthritis and educate these patients accordingly.

FRACTURE, RADIAL HEAD

Ryan C. Fowler, MD, CAQSM • Keith A. Stuessi, MD, CAQSM

BASICS

As classified by modified Mason classification (Johnston adding type IV, Morey adding displacement and percentage affected for type II, and Rineer trying to establish stability for type II):

- Type I: nondisplaced or minimally displaced fracture of head or neck:
  - Intra-articular displacement of the fracture <2 mm and fragment size ≤30% of articular surface
  - Forearm rotation (pronation/supination limited only by acute pain and swelling)
- Type II: displaced fracture of the head or neck:
  - Fracture displaced 2 to 5 mm with fragment size >30% of articular surface
  - Motion may be mechanically limited.
  - Rineer suggests if the fragments have cortical contact, they are more likely to be stable versus if no cortical contact more likely to be unstable.
- Type III: severely comminuted fracture of the radial head and neck
- Type IV (added to Mason classifications by Johnston):
  - Radial head fracture with an associated elbow dislocation (1)

DESCRIPTION

- Fracture of the head of the radius, most often caused by direct axial loading, as with a fall on outstretched hand (FOOSH) injury
- Can also be caused by posterior lateral rotary force, any injury causing posterior dislocation to the elbow that may result in radial head fracture (such as Monteggia fracture or coronoid fracture-dislocation), or rarely, a direct blow

EPIDEMIOLOGY

Radial head fractures are the most common fracture about the elbow, accounting for about 1/3 of all elbow fractures in adults (1); uncommon in children, accounting for only 1% of all fractures

COMMONLY ASSOCIATED CONDITIONS

- 1/3 of patients will have a concomitant injury.
- Essex-Lopresti lesion: disruption of triangular fibrocartilage complex of the wrist and interosseous membrane of the forearm, resulting in instability of the forearm and subluxation of the distal radioulnar joint
- Concomitant capitellar, olecranon, and coronoid fractures (often associated with elbow dislocation)
- Posterior Monteggia fractures: proximal 1/3 ulna fracture with radial head dislocation
- The "terrible triad" includes posterior dislocation of the elbow with radial head fracture and associated coronoid process fracture.
- Medial collateral ligament tear
- Lateral collateral ligament tear
- Presence or absence of mechanical block with rotation; examination achieved after aspiration of hematoma, with or without intra-articular injection of anesthetic; mechanical block associated with displaced fragment of radial head and affects surgical treatment
- Neurologic injuries can occur rarely with isolated radial head fracture but are more commonly associated with dislocation. Ulnar and median nerve are more commonly injured than the radial and posterior interosseous nerve.
- Brachial artery injuries can occur but are rare.

DIAGNOSIS

HISTORY

Determining the mechanism of injury is extremely helpful in differentiating from other elbow fractures. The typical mechanism of injury is a FOOSH in a pronated position, thus creating an axial load to the elbow (2).

PHYSICAL EXAM

- Patient usually holds injured arm gently against the chest with elbow flexed.
- Typically, there is pain and moderate swelling over the lateral side of the elbow.
- Any attempt to flex or extend the elbow or rotate the forearm may accentuate pain.
- Preservation of active elbow range of motion (ROM) was 97% specific for absence of a fracture.
- Focal tenderness over the radial head (located just distal to the lateral epicondyle)
- Palpation of radial head with passive rotation of the forearm typically elicits pain and occasionally, crepitation.
- Forearm and wrist examination required to rule out associated injuries such as acute radioulnar dissociation and/or injury to the interosseous ligament of the forearm
- Palpation of medial ligament necessary for signs of possible disruption
- Neurovascular status checked distally, especially with history of elbow dislocation
- The posterior interosseous nerve is rarely injured but can be tested by having the patient extend or abduct their thumb.

DIFFERENTIAL DIAGNOSIS

- Other fractures of the elbow, including capitellar, olecranon, and coronoid
- Supracondylar fractures (much more prevalent in children)
- Radial head or other bone contusion
- Elbow sprain
- Elbow effusion

DIAGNOSTIC TESTS & INTERPRETATION

Initial Tests (lab, imaging)

- Anteroposterior and lateral radiographs of the elbow are usually sufficient.
- If fat pad sign present (either anterior "sail sign" or "posterior fat pad sign") and fracture not apparent, radiocapitellar views are helpful, taken with forearm in neutral rotation and x-ray beam angled 45 degrees cephalad, also known as the Greenspan view.
- Computed tomography (CT) scan considered for estimating fracture size, degree of fragmentation, and displacement
- If wrist or forearm pain present, x-rays of the forearm and/or wrist in neutral rotation view should be taken.
- Magnetic resonance imaging (MRI) is helpful if there is concern for other soft tissue injury.

Diagnostic Procedures/Other

- Patient may have limited ROM due to pain and effusion.
- Joint aspiration for pain control is performed at the lateral elbow in the soft spot at the center of the dorsal olecranon, radial head, and lateral epicondyle (3)[A].
- If arthrocentesis is avoided, serial exams may be helpful (3)[A].
- Concerns for fracture orientation, severity, or healing should be referred to orthopedics (3)[A].

TREATMENT

GENERAL MEASURES

- Aspiration alone may provide some pain relief versus aspiration with local anesthetic instillation (3)[A].
- Type I:
  - Treated nonoperatively (4)[A]
  - Sling for pain control for 24 to 48 hours and followed by active mobilization. Mobilization should be supported by physical therapy as needed (4)[A].
  - Active ROM can begin as soon as pain permits. Flexion and extension of the elbow and supination and pronation of the forearm should be taken to the point where mild pain begins.
  - If required, hematoma aspiration is safe and effective for pain relief (3)[A].
  - Cast immobilization should be avoided (4)[A], (5)[A].
  - Ice therapy for 2 to 5 days
  - Acetaminophen and oral narcotics as necessary for pain control
- Type II:
  - Orthopedic consultation should be obtained with any type II fracture.
  - Sling or posterior splint for comfort, ice, analgesics can be used for acute treatment until referral to orthopedics.
  - Although there are multiple studies showing similar outcomes in adults with type II fractures treated nonoperatively versus operatively (6)[A], (7)[A],(8)[A], there is still controversy regarding optimal treatment.
  - Associated injuries, especially those causing elbow instability or mechanical block, should be referred for orthopedic consultation and possible open reduction and internal fixation (ORIF).
- Type III:
  - ORIF versus resection and arthroplasty versus resection alone
  - Best treatment strategy for types III and IV is controversial. However, many studies are attempting to address this as new techniques become available (9)[A].
- Type IV:
  - Treated as above, with obvious attention paid to reduction of dislocation and surgical repair of both fractures and associated ligamentous injuries

ADDITIONAL THERAPIES

- Initiate ROM exercises early.
- More aggressive strength and flexibility exercises added progressively as tolerated
- If ROM does not improve on a weekly basis, a mechanical block should be excluded. Once excluded, formal therapy may be needed.
- Only mild restriction of extension and rotation should be expected at 6 weeks.

ONGOING CARE

- Contractures and loss of motion may develop if early active ROM is not initiated.
- Increased sensitivity to cold, which may persist for up to 1 year
- Long-term pain is rarely a complication.
- Nonunion is possible but is frequently asymptomatic.
- Nerve injuries in the form of partial ulnar nerve and posterior interosseous nerve injury have been documented, mainly associated with surgical exploration.

FOLLOW-UP RECOMMENDATIONS

Early orthopedic input is essential in all but type I fractures due to potential need for surgical correction and controversy surrounding treatment.

REFERENCES

1. Kodde IF, Kaas L, Flipsen M, et al. Current concepts in the management of radial head fractures. *World J Orthop*. 2015;6(11):954–960.
2. Jordan RW, Jones AD. Radial head fractures. *Open Orthop J*. 2017;11:1405–1416.
3. Chalidis BE, Papadopoulos PP, Sachinis NC, et al. Aspiration alone versus aspiration and bupivacaine injection in the treatment of undisplaced radial head fractures: a prospective randomized study. *J Shoulder Elbow Surg*. 2009;18(5):676–679.
4. de Muinck Keizer RJO, Walenkamp MMJ, Goslings JC, et al. Mason type I fractures of the radial head. *Orthopedics*. 2015;38(12):e1147–e1154.
5. Unswoth-White J, Koka R, Churchill M, et al. The non-operative management of radial head fractures: a randomized trial of the three treatments. *Injury*. 1994;25(3):165–167.
6. Guzzini M, Vadalà A, Agrò A, et al. Nonsurgical treatment of Mason type II radial head fractures in athletes: a retrospective study. *G Chir*. 2017;37(5):200–205.
7. Yoon A, King GJW, Grewal R. Is ORIF superior to nonoperative treatment in isolated displaced partial articular fractures of the radial head? *Clin Orthop Relat Res*. 2014;472(7):2105–2112.
8. Mulders MAM, Schep NWL, de Muinck Keizer RJO, et al. Operative vs. nonoperative treatment for Mason type 2 radial head fractures: a randomized controlled trial. *J Shoulder Elbow Surg*. 2021;30(7):1670–1678.
9. Miller G, Humadi A, Unni R, et al. Surgical management f Mason Type III radial head fractures. *Indian J Orthop*. 2013;47(4):323–332.

ADDITIONAL READING

- Akesson T, Herbertsson P, Josefsson PO, et al. Primary nonoperative treatment of moderately displaced two-part fractures of the radial head. *J Bone Joint Surg Am*. 2006;88(9):1909–1914.
- Darracq MA, Vinson DR, Panacek EA. Preservation of active range of motion after acute elbow trauma predicts absence of elbow fracture. *Am J Emerg Med*. 2008;26(7):779–782.
- Herbertsson P, Josefsson PO, Hasserius R, et al. Uncomplicated Mason type-II and III fractures of the radial head and neck in adults: a long-term follow-up study. *J Bone Joint Surg Am*. 2004;86-A(3):569–574.
- Kaas L, van Riet RP, Vroemen JP, et al. The incidence of associated fractures of the upper limb in fractures of the radial head. *Strategies Trauma Limb Reconstr*. 2008;3(2):71–74.
- Pike JM, Athwal GS, Faber KJ, et al. Radial head fractures—an update. *J Hand Surg Am*. 2009;34(3):557–565.
- Ring D. Fractures and dislocations of the elbow: radial head fractures. In: Rockwood CA, Green DP, Bucholz RW, eds. *Rockwood and Green's Fractures in Adults*. 6th ed. Lippincott Williams & Wilkins; 2006:1011–1019.
- Rosenblatt Y, Athwal GS, Faber KJ. Current recommendations for the treatment of radial head fractures. *Orthop Clin North Am*. 2008;39(2):173–185.
- Swensen SJ, Tyagi V, Uquillas C, et al. Maximizing outcomes in the treatment of radial head fractures. *J Orthop Traumatol*. 2019;20(1):15.

CLINICAL PEARLS

- In type I fractures, typically, athletes can return to play as early as 6 to 8 weeks, depending on pain, ROM, and strength.
- Protection of the elbow may be needed if returning to contact sports. In types II to IV fractures, return to play is based on extent of associated injuries and surgical correction.

FRACTURE, RIB

Joshua Goldman, MD, MBA ▪ Jeremy Swisher, MD

BASICS

DESCRIPTION

- Rib fractures usually result from acute blunt trauma, particularly in contact sports.
- Nontraumatic mechanisms such as rowing, swinging golf clubs, and throwing can also cause rib fractures.
- Stress fractures can occur because of chronic overuse of the upper body.
- Fractures may be complete, incomplete, or stress related.
- Traumatic rib fractures may often be associated with other fractures, soft tissue injuries, and deep organ trauma. Any trauma-related rib fracture should prompt a thorough evaluation of the deeper organs, such as the heart, lungs, liver, and spleen.

EPIDEMIOLOGY

Isolated fractures of the upper four ribs are rare because they are well protected by the shoulder complex (1),(2)[B].

ALERT

Trauma significant enough to fracture ribs may also fracture other bones in the shoulder and cause injury to deep organs such as the lungs, heart, bronchus, blood vessels, and esophagus (2)[C].

- Blunt trauma to the lower eight ribs commonly results in fractures, most commonly in contact sports, such as football, hockey, and rugby (2),(3)[C].
- Forceful muscle contractions against significant resistance can cause incomplete, complete, or avulsion fractures of the ribs (2),(3)[B].
- Chronic stress of upper body muscles, which attach to the ribs, can result in stress fractures of the ribs; commonly seen in rowing, tennis, golf, gymnastics, and baseball (2),(3)[B].
- First rib fractures can result from falls on an outstretched arm or direct trauma; stress fractures of the first rib, particularly in pitchers, should be considered with high clinical suspicion (1),(2),(4),(5)[B].
- Avulsion fractures of the lower three floating ribs often occur at the attachment of the external oblique muscles; known to occur in baseball pitchers and batters (6)[B].
- Multiple rib fractures occur in high-impact trauma such as automobile, motorcycle, mountain biking, and bicycle racing (2),(6)[B].
- Rib fractures are more common in adults compared to children due to the relative inelasticity of the adult chest wall compared to children (1),(7)[C].

ETIOLOGY AND PATHOPHYSIOLOGY

- There are 12 pairs of ribs. The first seven ribs articulate posteriorly with the spine and anteriorly with the sternum.
- Ribs 8 to 10 attach anteriorly to the costal cartilage.
- The lowest two ribs are "floating" and do not connect anteriorly.
- Immediately below each rib travels its neurovascular bundle, including the intercostal vein, artery, and nerve
- Most acute rib fractures occur because of direct trauma, either blunt or penetrating (i.e., ball, gunshot) (6)[C].
- The ribs relatively long, thin shape makes them susceptible to fractures, with the posterior lateral bend being a common fracture site (8)[C].
- Multiple muscle attachments from the neck and upper extremities to the ribs can lead to stress or fatigue fractures (8)[B]. The first rib is particularly vulnerable due to the insertion of the scalene muscles, which subject it to neck muscle stresses.
- The superior three pairs of ribs, protected by the scapula, clavicle, and soft tissue, are less likely to have isolated fractures. However, the significant force needed to fracture these ribs increases the risk of injury to major vessels and lung parenchyma.
- The inferior "floating" ribs are relatively mobile and more susceptible to injury from blunt trauma.
- The ribs act as a unit during respiration, moving in the anteroposterior and coronal planes. This concerted rib motion, in addition to the actions of the diaphragm and the intercostal muscles, enables inspiration (by increasing intrathoracic volume and decreasing intrathoracic pressure) and expiration (by decreasing intrathoracic volume and increasing intrathoracic pressure). These deep inspirational forces can pull traction on the ribs and result in more pinpoint pain as well as be a clue to further consider a rib fracture.

RISK FACTORS

- Participation in contact and collision sports such as football, hockey, boxing, wrestling, rugby, and soccer, among others (1),(8)[A].
- As with any trauma, injuries can be more severe in athletes unprepared, either from lack of conditioning or contact from the back or blind side.
- Rib stress fractures are more likely to occur in sports with increased upper body demands, such as golf, rowing, gymnastics, baseball, tennis, racquet sports, and weightlifting. Overuse and poor technique can contribute to rib stress fractures (8)[B].
- Other predisposing factors include a history of bone or joint disease, bone tumors, metastatic cancer, poor nutrition, vitamin D deficiency, vitamin C deficiency, and calcium deficiency (1),(2),(6),(7)[C].

COMMONLY ASSOCIATED CONDITIONS

Organ injuries that may occur with acute traumatic rib fractures include:

- Pulmonary contusion
- Pneumothorax
- Tension pneumothorax
- Hemothorax
- Liver laceration, especially with lower rib fractures
- Spleen laceration, especially with lower rib fractures
- Esophageal rupture
- Great vessel injury, aorta, and superior vena cava with upper and middle rib fractures (1),(2)[C]

DIAGNOSIS

HISTORY

- Acute rib fracture usually presents after chest trauma; can also result from a fall on an outstretched arm
- Often, the pain may be localized to one or two ribs (3)[C].
- Patients can frequently reproduce or exacerbate the pain by taking a deep breath.
- Athletes may experience the sensation of having "the wind knocked out of them."
- Athlete may recall feeling a "pop" when the trauma occurred.
- Abdominal pain may be present if the lower (11th and 12th) ribs are involved.
- Stress fractures usually occur in elite athletes who train intensely. These fractures tend to be more insidious in onset and are more common in unilateral arm sports (7),(8)[C].
- Rib stress fractures present with a gradual onset of activity-related chest wall pain, similar to stress fractures of other bones. Often, the pain first occurs only with the inciting activity (e.g., rowing, swinging a golf club, throwing) and then progresses to pain with deep breathing or simple movements, such as rolling over in bed or reaching overhead (7),(8)[B].

PHYSICAL EXAM

- Localized pain, swelling, or ecchymosis may be present over the involved rib(s).
- A palpable deformity may be noted in cases of complete displaced fractures.
- Pain is generally exacerbated by deep inspiration, leading to shallow, rapid breathing.
- An auscultated click caused by movement of the rib fracture and can be heard with a stethoscope placed over the fracture site.
- Pain can be aggravated by coughing and sneezing.
- Other symptoms, such as increasing shortness of breath, increasing pain, cyanosis, and subcutaneous emphysema, may indicate serious life-threatening conditions requiring emergent attention.
- Vital sign changes such as hypoxia, tachypnea, or respiratory distress should raise suspicion of more serious pathology.
- With significant chest trauma, a thorough cardiopulmonary examination must be performed to evaluate for complications or associated injuries (1),(2)[B].
- For upper chest trauma, special attention should be given to the neck, shoulders, and major vessels (2),(3)[B].
- For lower chest trauma, a thorough abdominal examination should be performed to rule out injury to the liver, spleen, gastrointestinal (GI) tract, and kidneys (1),(2)[C].
- Diminished breath sounds may reflect splinting from the pain of a simple chest wall contusion or the presence of significant injury (e.g., pneumothorax, hemothorax, or pulmonary contusion).

DIFFERENTIAL DIAGNOSIS

- Rib/chest wall contusion
- Muscle strain
- Rupture of pectoralis major
- Costochondral separation/sprain
- Sternal fracture (anterior)
- Intervertebral joint/disc injury
- Apophyseal joint sprain
- Costovertebral joint sprain
- Scheuermann disease (posterior)
- Other causes of chest pain, such as cardiac causes, peptic ulcer disease, gastroesophageal reflux disorder, pneumothorax, pulmonary embolism, asthma, pleurisy, herpes zoster

DIAGNOSTIC TESTS & INTERPRETATION

- Standard posteroanterior and lateral chest radiographs are adequate to identify some rib fractures, but overall sensitivity is poor (1),(2),(7)[C].
- A dedicated rib series, which includes oblique views of the chest wall not typically included in standard chest series, can be more informative.
- Clinicians can base their diagnosis and management on plain radiographs and clinical findings, and a rib series is unnecessary (1),(2)[C].
- In the case of pathologic fractures, other blood work, such as complete blood count, comprehensive metabolic panel, and isoenzymes of alkaline phosphatase, may be directed by history and physical exam (1),(2),(3)[B].

- Routine repeat films are generally not necessary unless there are complications, continued pain, or poor healing.
- A bone scan of the chest wall can be used to diagnose rib stress fractures early in the pathologic process and can be seen as early as 7 hours after injury (8)[C].
- Due to the oblique nature of the bones, CT is less sensitive than other modalities. An angulated thin-section helical CT can be more helpful.
- MRI remains the gold standard for bone stress injuries because it evaluates bone edema and fracture. Ordering an MRI chest wall (3T) early can be useful in the diagnostic process (6),(7),(8)[C].
- With upper thoracic rib fractures, arteriography is indicated if there is evidence of vascular insufficiency, hemorrhage, or concomitant brachial plexus injury; marked displacement of the rib fragments; fractures of the scapula, vertebrae, or sternum; widening of the mediastinum; left apical cupping; or downward displacement of the left main stem bronchus (1),(2),(3)[B].
- Point-of-care ultrasonography can detect rib fractures and complications such as pneumothorax with higher sensitivity than radiographs, but it is operator dependent (5),(8)[C].

TREATMENT

GENERAL MEASURES

- Treatment is generally supportive.
- Pain control is the cornerstone of treatment and may be required for up to 3 to 6 weeks after injury.
- Ice and nonsteroidal anti-inflammatory drugs (NSAIDs) can help control symptoms, although stronger oral pain medications may be needed in rare cases.
- Local intercostal nerve blocks remain an option if other pain control techniques fail (1),(2)[B].
- Epidural anesthesia is also an option for pain control (1),(2)[C].

ALERT

Strapping or a chest binder has been advocated to help with pain. Caution should be exercised because immobilization techniques may result in inhibition of deep breathing, leading to atelectasis and possibly pneumonia (1),(6)[C].

- If immobilization is deemed necessary for comfort, its use should be minimized.
- Rib stress fractures are treated similarly to other low-risk stress fractures: with restriction of the inciting activity for 4 to 6 weeks, followed by a gradual return to the activity as tolerated.
- Rehabilitation should include proper mechanics and eliminating training errors to avoid recurrence of rib stress fractures (7),(8)[C].

MEDICATION

- For isolated injuries, generally begin treatment with NSAIDs without opioids for up to 14 days (1),(2)[B].
- For more severe injuries, and if ventilation is compromised, admission and invasive treatments such as intercostal nerve blocks may be indicated (1),(2),(3)[C]. Cadaveric studies show that ultrasound guidance dramatically improves the accuracy of intercostal nerve block injections compared to landmark-based (unguided) techniques (9)[C]. Real-time visualization of the needle and pleura helps minimize the risk of complications like pneumothorax, which has been reported in up to 6% of unguided intercostal blocks (10)[C].

ADDITIONAL THERAPIES

- For stress fractures, biomechanics of their upper thoracic and shoulder areas based on sport should be evaluated and corrected if necessary (2)[C].
- Use of incentive spirometry can prevent atelectasis and its complications.
- Rib belts or binders are not recommended because they compromise respiratory function.

SURGERY/OTHER PROCEDURES

- The need for surgery is rare in cases of isolated rib fractures (1)[C].
- An exception is in the case of flail chest, where open reduction and internal fixation may be necessary (1),(2),(3)[C].
- Surgical fixation may be of benefit with chest wall deformity, flail chest, or symptomatic nonunion.
- Suspected internal injuries associated with rib fractures should be referred for possible surgical repair.
- Chronic pain due to recurrent stress fracture, nonunion, or recurrent dislocation or subluxation may improve with surgical excision of the involved rib (7),(8)[B].

ONGOING CARE

FOLLOW-UP RECOMMENDATIONS

- Pain from rib fractures can be severe for several days following the injury.
- The athlete should be encouraged to continue activities as tolerated, except for contact sports (7)[C].
- Contact should be limited for the first 3 weeks following injury. Consider rib protection in contact sports after return (8)[C].
- Most rib fractures heal within 6 to 8 weeks. Rib stress fractures may take up to 12 weeks for full return to play (7),(8)[C].
- Monitor regularly for signs of delayed complications (8)[B].
- Delayed injuries from isolated rib fractures sustained during blunt trauma are rare.
- A follow-up examination 6 to 8 weeks after the injury is advisable to assess the patient's progress, especially if they are unable to return to sports or work by that time.

PROGNOSIS

- Intensive training for athletes with stress fractures is not recommended for at least the first 3 weeks.
- Athletes with isolated rib fractures can gradually increase activity as pain permits.
- Full healing usually takes 6 to 8 weeks; however, athletes may return to participation in noncontact sports when pain free.
- Early return to contact sports may be possible prior to 6 weeks if pain is controlled, and the area can be protected adequately until full healing occurs (7),(8)[C].

COMPLICATIONS

- Nonunion of the ribs is rare in general. Symptomatic nonunion can occur and would be an indication for surgery (4),(8)[B].
- Pseudoarthrosis of the 1st rib is described in the literature and has been a cause for discontinued participation (4),(8)[B].
- Early and adequate pain relief is essential to prevent complications such as splinting and atelectasis, which can potentially lead to pneumonia.
- Significant complications may include pneumothorax, pulmonary contusion, pneumonia, and intercostal hemorrhage.

REFERENCES

1. Sirmali M, Türüt H, Topçu S, et al. A comprehensive analysis of traumatic rib fractures: morbidity, mortality and management. *Eur J Cardiothorac Surg*. 2003;24(1):133–138.
2. Brasel KJ, Moore EE, Albrecht RA, et al. Western Trauma Association critical decisions in trauma: management of rib fractures. *J Trauma Acute Care Surg*. 2017;82(1):200–203.
3. Chien CY, Chen YH, Han ST, et al. The number of displaced rib fractures is more predictive for complications in chest trauma patients. *Scand J Trauma Resusc Emerg Med*. 2017;25(1):19.
4. Murphy CE IV, Raja AS, Baumann BM, et al. Rib fracture diagnosis in the Panscan era. *Ann Emerg Med*. 2017;70(6):904–909.
5. Watson TS. The benefits and limitations of ultrasound in the diagnosis of rib fractures from the emergency department to the sports field: a narrative review. *Brit Columbia Med J*. 2021;63(2):75–82.
6. Chapman BC, Overbey DM, Tesfalidet F, et al. Clinical utility of chest computed tomography in patients with rib fractures CT chest and rib fractures. *Arch Trauma Res*. 2016;5(4):e37070.
7. Marcussen B, Negaard M, Hosey RG, et al. A case series and literature review: isolated traumatic first rib fracture in athletes. *Clin J Sport Med*. 2020;30(3):257–266.
8. Schowalter S, Le B, Creps J, et al. Rib fractures in professional baseball pitchers: mechanics, epidemiology, and management. *Open Access J Sports Med*. 2022;13:89–105.
9. Bhatia A, Gofeld M, Ganapathy S, et al. Comparison of anatomic landmarks and ultrasound guidance for intercostal nerve injections in cadavers. *Reg Anesth Pain Med*. 2013;38(6):503–507.
10. Shanti CM, Carlin AM, Tyburski JG. Incidence of pneumothorax from intercostal nerve block for analgesia in rib fractures. *J Trauma*. 2001;51(3):536–539.

CLINICAL PEARLS

- In most cases of isolated rib fractures, simple chest films are sufficient. A dedicated rib series may be considered based on clinical findings.
- Patients should continue to be as active as they can tolerate, limiting contact, and may use NSAIDs or acetaminophen for pain for isolated fractures.
- Multiple rib fractures correlate more closely with serious intrathoracic and intra-abdominal injuries. Fractures of superior ribs (numbers 1 to 3) reflect trauma involving significant force and the potential for injury to major blood vessels and lung parenchyma.
- Displaced fractures increase the risk of internal injury and delayed bleeding and generally warrant admission.
- Rib stress fractures are treated with restriction of the inciting activity for 4 to 6 weeks, followed by a gradual return to the activity as tolerated.
- Most rib fractures heal well with conservative management, and routine follow-up chest radiographs are unnecessary unless clinically indicated by symptoms.

FRACTURE, SACRAL

Craig Pille, MD • Brendan Dempsey, MD

BASICS

- Sacral injuries are rare, but most authors believe that sacral fractures are generally underrecognized.
- A high degree of suspicion is required to make the diagnosis:
  - Only 10–30% of sacral fractures are seen on standard radiographs.
  - 10.5% sensitivity of pelvic radiographs reported (1)
  - Advanced imaging is often required to appreciate sacral injury.

DESCRIPTION

- Traumatic fractures of the sacrum are most commonly described using the Denis system of fracture orientation:
  - Zone 1:
    - Most common fracture type, usually stable
    - Fracture line usually vertically through the sacral ala
    - Entirely lateral to foramina
    - Typically, strength of sacroiliac (SI) ligaments spares SI joint from injury, but fractures that enter SI joint are at greater risk for instability.
    - Neural elements typically spared; <10% with neurologic involvement
  - Zone 2:
    - Fracture line through one or more neural foramina but sparing the central spinal canal
    - 20–30% with neurologic injury
    - Usually structurally stable
  - Zone 3:
    - Fracture line medial to neural foramina; typically includes transverse fractures and involving the spinal canal
    - >50% with neurologic injury
    - Often unstable
- Atraumatic injuries result from a mismatch between bone stress and bone strength:
  - Stress fractures in athletes
  - Insufficiency fractures in elderly:
    - Typically, bilateral in those with normal gait and unilateral in those with altered gait mechanics

EPIDEMIOLOGY

Sacral fractures need to be considered in several clinical scenarios:

- Multitrauma patients with other pelvic or thoracolumbar injury:
  - Sacral fractures rarely occur as isolated injury (<5%).
- Osteoporotic patients with low back or gluteal pain:
  - Atraumatic or trivial injury
- Athletes with activity-related pain of low back/SI region:
  - 1.6% of sports-related low back pain (2)
  - Usually in running-based sports:
    - Often after increases in training intensity
  - May produce thigh pain as well

ETIOLOGY AND PATHOPHYSIOLOGY

Sacral fractures may occur by the following mechanisms:

- Posttraumatic injuries:
  - Producing large forces and fracture across healthy bone:
    - Typically, motor vehicle accidents or falls from a height
- Atraumatic injuries:
  - Normal stresses (or trivial injury) producing fractures across relatively weakened bone:
    - Insufficiency fractures in the elderly/ill
    - Fractures often bilateral
  - Increased stress or overuse, producing fracture across relatively normal bone:
    - Stress fractures in the younger, athletic population
    - Fractures often unilateral

RISK FACTORS

- Insufficiency fractures are most common in elderly osteoporotic females:
  - May occur in others at risk for poor bone density, including the following:
    - Chronic corticosteroid use
    - History of pelvic irradiation
- Stress fractures occur most commonly in running athletes:
  - As with other stress fractures, risk increases with the following:
    - Training errors (inadequate recovery, increasing training, etc.)
    - Biomechanical factors (leg length discrepancy, poor core, and pelvic stabilization)
    - Increased impact forces (footwear, training surface)
    - Nutritional/hormonal impacts on bone density (relative energy deficiency in sport [RED-S], inadequate calcium [Ca++]/vitamin D)

COMMONLY ASSOCIATED CONDITIONS

Acute sacral fractures may be seen in conjunction with:

- Other bony injury:
  - Other pelvic ring disruptions
  - Other spinal fractures:
    - May be noncontiguous
  - Fracture-dislocations of lower facet joints or disruption of lumbosacral junction
- Neurologic injury:
  - Should be described according to the Gibbons grading system:
    - Grade 1: no neurologic deficit
    - Grade 2: paresthesias/sensory changes only
    - Grade 3: motor deficit but gastrointestinal (GI)/genitourinary (GU) function normal
    - Grade 4: loss of GI/GU function
- Injury to other pelvic contents:
  - Rectal perforation most common
- Atraumatic sacral fractures
- Osteoporosis
- RED-S

DIAGNOSIS

Prehospital:

- Traumatic sacral fractures typically occur in the multitrauma patient.
- Initial assessment and treatment should proceed as per Advanced Trauma Life Support for patients with suspected spine injury:
  - Airway, breathing, and circulation (ABCs)/resuscitation
  - Spine precautions/backboard
  - Transport

HISTORY

- Injury to sacrum is suggested by pain in lower back/pelvis and can radiate to the leg, groin, buttocks, or thigh (3).
- Pain is often worse with weight-bearing activity; improved with rest
- Important to inquire about possible nerve root involvement:
  - Incontinence of bowel or bladder, sexual dysfunction
  - Sciatica
  - Paresthesias, especially of saddle region
- Patients without history of trauma should be asked about:
  - Change in activity or footwear, especially in running-based sports
  - Risk factors for poor bone density:
    - Osteopenia/osteoporosis in patient or family members
    - Past or present disordered eating pattern
    - Oligomenorrhea or amenorrhea in females

PHYSICAL EXAM

- Trauma patient:
  - Inspect for ecchymosis/bruising over sacral prominence.
  - Palpate entire spinal column and bony pelvis in addition to the sacrum.
  - Test for pelvic ring instability with external and internal rotation of iliac wings.
  - Neurologic testing of L5–S5 nerve root function should be completely assessed initially and then periodically reevaluated:
    - Pinprick sensation, rectal sphincter contraction and tone, as well as cremasteric, bulbocavernosus, perianal wink reflexes
    - L5 injuries most common with zone 2 injuries
    - Sacral roots have bilateral input, and unilateral injuries to S2–S5 are difficult to detect.
  - Digital rectal and vaginal evaluation to exclude open fractures; need chaperones for all genital exams
  - Morel-Lavallée lesion may be present.
- Atraumatic patient with possible insufficiency or stress fracture:
  - No pathognomonic findings
  - Typically with tenderness over sacrum, paraspinal, and/or over region of SI joint
  - Flexion, abduction, external rotation (FABER) test (with hip in FABER) often positive
  - Tenderness with lateral compression
  - Squish test—patient supine, palpate anterior superior iliac spine (ASIS) bilaterally
  - Distal neurovascular assessment typically normal
  - Gait may be antalgic; pain with hop test may be present.

DIFFERENTIAL DIAGNOSIS

- Differential diagnosis for acute fractures:
  - Contusion
  - Other pelvic or lumbar fractures
  - Nerve root injuries
- Differential diagnosis for atraumatic/stress fractures:
  - Lumbar disc disease
  - Mechanical low back pain
  - SI dysfunction
  - Spondylolysis/spondylolisthesis

DIAGNOSTIC TESTS & INTERPRETATION

- Trauma patients should have stool assessed for occult blood.
- Consider secondary osteoporosis such as hyperthyroidism, hyperparathyroidism, and osteomalacia (thyroid-stimulating hormone [TSH], parathyroid hormone [PTH], Ca++, phosphate [Phos], albumin, 25-hydroxy vitamin D, urinary Ca++, complete blood count [CBC], liver function test [LFT], C-reactive protein [CRP], erythrocyte sedimentation rate [ESR]).
- Traumatic injury:
  - Although radiographs typically only reveal about 30% of sacral fractures, they may be useful for initial assessment of suspected sacral injury:
    - Anteroposterior (AP) views of the pelvis are standard in multitrauma patients.
    - Visualization of suspected sacral injuries may be enhanced with the addition of pelvic inlet view: 35- to 40-degree caudal tilt of radiograph tube; pelvic outlet view: 45-degree cranial tilt of radiograph tube; lateral view of sacrum
    - Look for transverse L5 fractures, which can be seen in up to half of pelvic and sacral fractures.
    - Stepladder sign: results from the overriding displacement of transverse fracture fragments, seen on AP view
  - Computed tomography (CT) scanning is now standard for definitive assessment of suspected acute sacral fracture:
    - Routine CT scans often not satisfactory
    - Close consultation with radiologist on gantry alignment recommended.
    - Useful to help plan surgical intervention
    - Thin section (1.0- to 1.5-mm cuts) with coronal and sagittal reconstructions; relatively high radiation exposure: 10 to 20 mSv
  - Magnetic resonance imaging (MRI) may help delineate neural compression or injury:
    - Multiplanar nature may show better assessment of fracture alignment.
- Atraumatic injury:
  - Initial lumbar spine series as well as AP views of the pelvis are often obtained:
    - Usually unremarkable
  - MRI of sacrum appropriate for diagnosis:
    - Gold standard for sacral stress fracture
    - Most bony stress injuries will have high signal on T2-weighted images, low signal on T1-weighted images.
    - Fracture line may or may not be present.
  - CT is an alternative to MRI:
    - Increased radiation
    - Can see sclerotic healing or fresh fracture line
  - Bone scan most sensitive but not specific for bony stress injury:
    - Stress fractures in athletes; typically, with unilateral uptake sacral ala
    - Insufficiency fractures; often with multiple sites of injury; classic "H" sign seen in about 40% of patients; bilateral vertical fractures with horizontal component
    - Uptake can be obscured by residual in bladder; outlet views in addition to standard anterior and posterior projections are suggested.

TREATMENT

- Presence of instability, displacement, neurologic injury, and additional injuries determine treatment.
- Acute fracture:
  - See below for surgical indications.
  - Stable injuries without neurologic involvement treated with initial activity modification with gradual ambulation and advancement as tolerated (1)[A]:
    - Fractures through S3 and distally often require protection with sitting until pain free.
- Stress fracture: average ±6 weeks for return to sport (but some may take up to 3 months):
  - Protected weight-bearing if limp or pain with ambulation:
    - Advance weight-bearing as tolerated
  - Discontinue painful activity/relative rest.
  - Maintain cardiovascular conditioning with pain-free activity:
    - May need to begin with non–weight-bearing activity (typically swimming or cycling)
  - Begin progressive rehabilitation typically after 3- to 5-day pain-free interval:
    - Core/pelvic stabilization; address underlying biomechanical deficiencies.
    - Cardiovascular cross-training progression through following sequence when activity is pain free: non–weight-bearing (i.e., pool running, bicycling), weight-bearing/nonimpact (i.e., elliptical-type trainer), impact (i.e., running), sports-specific functional progression
- Insufficiency fractures in elderly may have prolonged symptoms (up to 9 months):
  - Initial treatment is usually nonoperative, even for patients with neurologic deficit:
    - Many authors recommend initial period bed rest followed by progressive ambulation.
    - Neurologic symptoms appear to improve as pain resolves.
  - Consider surgery if severe pain after 3-month trial conservative treatment.

MEDICATION

- Analgesics should be titrated for symptom relief:
  - Should not be used to allow for progression of activity or sport participation
  - Scheduled doses for first several days may allow for pain-free rest:
    - Over-the-counter analgesics often sufficient for stress fractures: acetaminophen up to 1,000 mg q4h PRN; pediatric dosage 10 to 15 mg/kg up to q4h; nonsteroidal drugs often beneficial, although theoretically may impair bony healing
- Supplemental vitamin D and Ca++ for stress or insufficiency fractures:
  - 1 g Ca daily
  - 800 to 1,000 IU vitamin D daily

SURGERY/OTHER PROCEDURES

- Surgical consideration for traumatic sacral fractures:
  - Neurologic impairment
  - Unstable injuries
  - Severe disruption of sagittal or coronal alignment:
    - In AP plane displacement, >1 cm generally recognized as unstable
  - Injuries with persistent pain after about 6 months
- Insufficiency fractures considered for surgery if with persistent, severe pain after 3 months conservative treatment—sacroplasty technique has a growing body of literature to support (4),(5)[B].

ADMISSION, INPATIENT, AND NURSING CONSIDERATIONS

- Acute traumatic sacral fractures often require hospitalization for additional injury:
  - Isolated and stable zone 1 or 2 fractures with no neurologic deficit and adequate pain control may be considered for outpatient treatment.
- Stress fractures and insufficiency fractures are generally managed in outpatient setting.

ONGOING CARE

Sacral stress or insufficiency fractures may be a bellwether for underlying metabolic bone disease:

- Bone density testing or other laboratory evaluation should be considered.

DIET

Patients with insufficiency or stress fractures should be counseled on appropriate intake of Ca++ and vitamin D.

PATIENT EDUCATION

Education should focus on biomechanical issues and training errors predisposing to injury:

- Importance of maintaining adequate strength and flexibility of core and pelvic musculature.
- Advance training volume by ~10% per week to minimize risk of additional overuse injury.
- Especially in the running athlete, the importance of appropriate footwear selection:
  - Effective life span of most running shoes is 300 to 400 miles.

PROGNOSIS

- Presence of a neurologic defect is the most important factor.
- Healthy athletes with sacral stress injury:
  - Usually able to return to normal activity 4 to 6 weeks
  - Usually able to return to sport 6 to 10 weeks
- Elderly patients with insufficiency fractures may have pain for many months.
- Fractures requiring surgery often with instrumentation:
  - Up to 1/3 may have hardware failure.

COMPLICATIONS

- Deformity or bony callus formation after acute injury may lead to nerve root entrapment.
- Prolonged pain common in elderly with insufficiency fractures

REFERENCES

1. Barber LA, Katsuura Y, Qureshi S. Sacral fractures: a review. *HSS J.* 2023;19(2):234–246.
2. Kaneko H, Murakami M, Nishizawa K. Prevalence and clinical features of sports-related lumbosacral stress injuries in the young. *Arch Orthop Trauma Surg.* 2017;137(5):685–691.
3. Longhino V, Bonora C, Sansone V. The management of sacral stress fractures: current concepts. *Clin Cases Miner Bone Metab.* 2011;8(3):19–23.
4. Gutierrez-Gomez S, Wahl L, Blecher R, et al. Sacral fractures: an updated and comprehensive review. *Injury.* 2021;52(3):366–375.
5. Gibbs WN, Doshi A. Sacral fractures and sacroplasty. *Neuroimaging Clin N Am.* 2019;29(4):515–527.

ADDITIONAL READING

Ner EB, Rabau O, Dosani S, et al. Sacral stress fractures in athletes. *Eur Spine J.* 2022;31(1):1–9.

CLINICAL PEARLS

- Consider sacral injury in any acute injury resulting in other pelvic or spinal injury.
- Consider sacral injury in chronic cases of low back, thigh, or buttock pain.
- Sacral fractures are typically occult on plain radiographs and often require advanced imaging for definitive diagnosis.

F

FRACTURE, SCAPHOID

Jason A. Krystofiak, MD, CAQSM

BASICS

DESCRIPTION

- Most commonly fractured carpal bone
- Fractures occur in three anatomic sections: proximal, waist, and distal.
- Mechanism of injury is normally a fall onto an outstretched hand (FOOSH).
- Proximal pole fractures have an increased risk of nonunion.

EPIDEMIOLOGY

- The scaphoid is the most commonly fractured carpal bone, accounting for over 85% of sport-related carpal bone fractures (1).
- Increased rate in males aged 20 to 24 years and less common in children and older adults (In children, distal radial physeal injuries occur more often than scaphoid [Salter-Harris fracture types 1 and 2]; in older adults, distal radius metaphyseal fractures occur before scaphoid fractures)

Incidence

- Varying incidence but overall greater in men compared to women
- Higher risk in sports such as football and rugby

ETIOLOGY AND PATHOPHYSIOLOGY

- Classic injury: Mechanism is an axial load of a hyperextended, radially deviated wrist.
- Normally associated with falls, athletic injuries, or motor vehicle trauma
- Increased risk of nonunion in proximal pole fractures due to a retrograde blood supply

DIAGNOSIS

HISTORY

- Patients report falling on an outstretched hand or a forced wrist extension.
- Pain and swelling at the radial wrist near the 1st metacarpal base
- Characterized as a deep and dull pain made worse with gripping or squeezing

PHYSICAL EXAM

- Tenderness at the anatomic snuffbox:
  - Bordered by the extensor pollicis longus tendon medially and extensor pollicis brevis and abductor pollicis longus tendons laterally
  - Sensitivity 86%, specificity 30% (2)
  - False positives may occur by compression of the radial nerve sensory branch as it passes through the snuffbox.
- Tenderness of scaphoid tubercle:
  - Extend patient's wrist and apply pressure to the tuberosity at the proximal wrist crease.
  - Sensitivity 95%, specificity 74% (2)
- Scaphoid compression test:
  - Axially/longitudinally compressing patient's thumb along the 1st metacarpal
  - Poor specificity 30% (2)
- Pronated wrist to a supinated position against resistance causing pain:
  - Appears to be the most accurate predictor of an occult scaphoid fracture (3)
  - Sensitivity 100%, specificity 98% (3)

DIFFERENTIAL DIAGNOSIS

- Scapholunate dissociation
- Distal radius fracture (Colles and Smith)
- Extensor carpi radialis sprain
- 1st metacarpal fracture
- Flexor carpi radialis sprain
- Carpometacarpal or radiocarpal arthritis

DIAGNOSTIC TESTS & INTERPRETATION

- Plain radiographs of the wrist:
  - Obtain posteroanterior (PA), true lateral, and oblique views. Also, include a scaphoid specific view: PA of the wrist in full pronation and ulnar deviation.
  - May request additional views: PA wrist with clenched fist in radial and ulnar deviation
  - Plain radiographs may be normal immediately after injury, with a false-negative rate near 20% (occult distal radius fracture) (2).
  - Fracture may become apparent 10 to 14 days after injury (immobilization allows demineralization of the fracture line).
  - Examine radiographs for evidence of scapholunate widening (Terry Thomas sign) evidenced by >3 mm between the scaphoid and the lunate:
    - Indicates injury to the scapholunate ligament
- Magnetic resonance imaging (MRI):
  - Consider when initial radiographs are negative and/or ligamentous injury is suspected.
  - Sensitivity 94%, specificity 98% (2)
  - MRI shows diminished signal in T1-weighted and increased signal in T2-weighted images.
  - Cost-effective when compared to immobilization followed by repeat radiographs (2)
- Computed tomography (CT) scan: can be used to help diagnose, but best for characterizing displacement and assessing for fracture union/healing
  - Sensitivity 82%, specificity 96% (2)
- Bone scan:
  - Consider in patients with persistent tenderness but negative plain radiographs.
  - Sensitivity (93%), but specificity (91%) is less than MRI and computed tomography (CT) (2)
  - Positive scan shows focal increased uptake at the scaphoid 72 hours after the injury.
- Ultrasound:
  - Accessible and cost-effective, but operator dependent
  - Findings include disruption of the scaphoid cortex and scapho-trapezium-trapezoid effusion.
  - Sensitivity 82%, specificity 77% (2)

TREATMENT

GENERAL MEASURES

Scaphoid fractures or suspected fractures with negative radiographs (4)[C]:

- Immobilize in a thumb spica.
- Sling for comfort
- Ice and elevation

MEDICATION

Tylenol or nonsteroidal anti-inflammatory drugs (NSAIDs) as needed (The use of NSAIDs for >3 days at higher doses during the postoperative or acute phase of fracture healing may lead to increased rates of nonunion, delayed union, and pseudarthrosis in adults.)

ADDITIONAL THERAPIES

- Classification systems exist (Herbert, Russe, etc.); however, classifications are not reliably prognostic (5).
- <1 mm separation of the fracture is considered nondisplaced (4).
- Most nondisplaced fractures (distal pole, incomplete waist) can be treated successfully with short arm spica cast immobilization (4)[C],(6)[B].
- Time to fracture union with cast immobilization varies by location:
  - Distal pole (6 to 8 weeks) < waist (8 to 12 weeks) < proximal pole (3 to 6 months) (4),(7)
- Thumb immobilization does not appear to affect the rate of nonunion (7)[C].
- Long-arm cast (vs. short-arm cast) does not improve nonunion rates (4)[C],(6)[B],(7)[C].
- Displaced fractures and proximal pole fractures (prone to nonunion and avascular necrosis) should be referred for surgical fixation (4)[C],(7)[C].
- Postoperative or postcasting hand therapy (occupational therapy [OT])

SURGERY/OTHER PROCEDURES

- Operative fixation is recommended for displaced fractures (>1 mm) and proximal pole fractures (4)[C],(6)[B].
- Surgical management can improve return times to sport as well as return rates (1)[A].
- Consider surgery for nondisplaced fractures in high-demand athletes/patients where the necessary length of casting would interfere significantly with competition, training, or work (4)[C].
- Multiple surgical techniques can be used (dorsal open reduction internal fixation [ORIF], volar ORIF, percutaneous, arthroscopic assisted):
  - Each has advantages and disadvantages.
  - Surgeon preference and experience is often the deciding factor in operative technique.

ONGOING CARE

FOLLOW-UP RECOMMENDATIONS

- Nondisplaced waist or distal pole fractures can be managed closely by a primary care physician.
- Refer patients with displaced fractures, complete waist, and proximal pole fractures.
- Patients with a delayed presentation, carpal ligament instability, and evidence of nonunion should also be referred.
- Refer high-demand athletes/patients with nondisplaced fractures.

COMPLICATIONS

- Avascular necrosis of the proximal fracture fragment, leading to wrist dysfunction and early osteoarthritis
- High incidence of fibrous nonunion (15%) (1)
- Frequent malunion
- Chronic scapholunate advanced collapse (SLAC)
- Posttraumatic arthritis

REFERENCES

1. Goffin JS, Liao Q, Robertson GA. Return to sport following scaphoid fractures: a systematic review and meta-analysis. *World J Orthop*. 2019;10(2):101–114.
2. Bäcker HC, Wu CH, Strauch RJ. Systematic review of diagnosis of clinically suspected scaphoid fractures. *J Wrist Surg*. 2020;9(1):81–89.
3. Coventry L, Oldrini I, Dean B, et al. Which clinical features best predict occult scaphoid fractures? A systematic review of diagnostic test accuracy studies. *Emerg Med J*. 2023;40(8):576–582.
4. Winston MJ, Weiland AJ. Scaphoid fractures in the athlete. *Curr Rev Musculoskelet Med*. 2017;10(1):38–44.
5. Ten Berg PW, Drijkoningen T, Strackee SD, et al. Classifications of acute scaphoid fractures: a systematic literature review. *J Wrist Surg*. 2016;5(2):152–159.
6. Grewal R, King GJ. An evidence-based approach to the management of acute scaphoid fractures. *J Hand Surg Am*. 2009;34(4):732–734.
7. Fowler JR, Hughes TB. Scaphoid fractures. *Clin Sports Med*. 2015;34(1):37–50.

ADDITIONAL READING

- Ram AN, Chung KC. Evidence-based management of acute nondisplaced scaphoid waist fractures. *J Hand Surg Am*. 2009;34(4):735–738.
- Shehab R, Mirabelli MH. Evaluation and diagnosis of wrist pain: a case-based approach. *Am Fam Physician*. 2013;87(8):568–573.
- Wheatley BM, Nappo KE, Christensen DL, et al. Effect of NSAIDs on bone healing rates: a meta-analysis. *J Am Acad Orthop Surg*. 2019;27(7):e330–e336.

CLINICAL PEARLS

- A scaphoid fracture is unlikely in the absence of tenderness in the anatomic snuffbox and at the scaphoid tubercle.
- High-demand athletes may do better with early surgical fixation of even nondisplaced fractures because this allows earlier return to activity.

FRACTURE, SPINOUS AND TRANSVERSE PROCESSES

Priya Sharma, DO • Suraj A. Achar, MD, FAAFP, CAQSM

BASICS

DESCRIPTION

- Transverse and spinous process fractures are considered minor spine injuries and usually are stable and benign. Both types can be markers of considerable trauma and should encourage the physician to look for additional injury.
- Transverse process fractures most commonly occur within the lumbar spine. Fractures of the spinous process typically occur at C7 or any of the lower cervical or upper thoracic vertebrae. They are commonly avulsion-type injuries resulting from contraction of the surrounding musculature.
- Spinous process fractures of the lower cervical or upper thoracic vertebrae are traditionally referred to as "clay shoveler injuries" but now are found mostly after sudden deceleration in motor vehicle accidents (MVAs) or forced flexion of the neck, often in football players and weightlifters.
- Synonym(s): minor spinal fracture

EPIDEMIOLOGY

- Transverse process fractures are commonly identified with high-energy trauma (such as MVAs or falls).
- Spinous process fractures may also be seen in sports with direct blow, fall, or collision or in relation to osteoporosis.
- Overuse injuries with deadlifts or rows, repetitive golf swings and twisting and turning movements in wrestling can be associated.
- "Sentinel spinous process fractures" are associated with fractures of lamina and facets, which can lead to instability.

ALERT

Nonspinal injuries as high as 68.9% are common with transverse process fractures due to a typically high-energy trauma mechanism, so detection of a transverse process fracture should raise suspicion for other injury (1),(2).

- Liver lacerations, splenic injury, rib fractures, ureteral injuries
- L2 is the most frequently fractured level followed by L3 in high-energy trauma (2).
- Transverse process fractures resulting from low-energy trauma (e.g., playing football) do not generally have associated spinal, nerve root, or visceral injuries.

RISK FACTORS

- High-energy trauma (falls, MVAs, etc.)
- Growth spurts, training errors, improper technique, and repetitive trauma predispose the athlete to spine fractures.

DIAGNOSIS

HISTORY

Forceful hyperflexion of the neck (e.g., spearing in football) is associated with lower cervical spinous process fractures. Lumbar transverse process fractures usually result from direct trauma.

PHYSICAL EXAM

- Localized pain over injured area without radiation
- Pain increased with neck flexion (lower cervical spinous process fracture) or hip flexion (iliopsoas attachment to lumbar transverse process fracture) as well as extension or rotation of the spine
- Careful neurologic examination for weakness, reflex changes, or sensory changes in a dermatomal distribution; because neurologic injuries are not commonly associated with minor fractures, abnormal results should raise suspicion of additional spinal injury.
- Benign abdominal examination does not exclude coexistent intra-abdominal injury.

DIFFERENTIAL DIAGNOSIS

- Spinal "burst" fracture
- Paraspinal muscle strain
- Ligamentous spinal injury
- Disc herniation
- Spondylolysis and/or spondylolisthesis

DIAGNOSTIC TESTS & INTERPRETATION

- CT scan: gold standard for identification of spinal fractures; superior to plain films to evaluate extent of spinal fractures and evaluate for serious spine injury but has limited field of view and high radiation dose
- Urgent MRI: necessary if neurologic symptoms are present to evaluate extrinsic spinal cord compression or intrinsic cord injury
- Radiographic appearance often lags behind clinical healing and should not be used as the primary criterion for return to play.
- Cervical lateral radiograph:
  - Very important to visualize C7 spinous process, which often is obscured by the shoulders
  - Obtain "swimmer's view" if necessary to visualize C7–T1 junction.
  - Anteroposterior (AP) radiograph may show double shadow of spinous process due to avulsion.
  - Flexion-extension films to rule out ligamentous instability and lamina or facet injury
- Thoracolumbar AP radiograph:
  - Relatively insensitive at identifying transverse process fractures
  - May show double shadow of spinous process due to avulsion
  - Hematoma may obscure evidence of transverse process fracture. Loss of normal psoas shadow may be most prominent finding indicating retroperitoneal pathology.

TREATMENT

GENERAL MEASURES

- Short-term rest is often the most effective treatment for isolated injury.
- Cryotherapy repeated frequently within initial 36 to 48 hours may help prevent muscle spasm.
- Nonopioid medication (e.g., nonsteroidal anti-inflammatory drugs [NSAIDs] or short-term muscle relaxants) and gentle range of motion exercises may be helpful in lumbar transverse process fractures.
- Use of orthoses is debated but can be provided for comfort and is typically not needed for stabilization of fractures (1),(3).
- In all cases of suspected spine injury, immobilization with a backboard and rigid cervical collar is mandatory until the patient can be cleared radiographically.

ADDITIONAL THERAPIES

- If transverse process fractures result from high-energy trauma, there should be a high index of suspicion for associated visceral and orthopedic injuries.
- Cervical transverse process fractures warrant additional imaging to assess for vascular injury given proximity of the vertebral artery (1).

- Thoracic and L1 fractures found to be associated with thoracic injury, so additional evaluation for rib fractures, pulmonary contusions, vascular injury, and urinary tract injury is warranted (1)[B],(2).
- Urinalysis should be performed; if >8 red blood cells (RBCs) per high-power field are seen, perform cystogram and intravenous (IV) pyelogram to evaluate for possible urinary tract injury (1)[B].
- Recent research has found an association with lower lumbar transverse process fracture with pelvic injury, notably L4 transverse process fracture with acetabular fractures and L5 transverse process fracture with pelvic ring injuries (1),(2)[B].

ALERT
If transverse process fractures are identified on plain radiographs, abdominal CT should be performed due to possible associated visceral, abdominal, and orthopedic injuries (1)[B],(2)[B].

ALERT
With cervical injury, protection against flexion with an orthosis should be provided for 4 to 6 weeks:

- Obtain flexion/extension radiographs at end of immobilization period.
- Return to play once fracture is healed and patient has full, painless range of motion and no neurologic deficits (4)[B].
- There is controversy whether bracing is beneficial in thoracolumbar fractures without associated spinal injury. Some authors have suggested the use of bracing for symptomatic relief. Others have shown that it is not effective in immobilization and can result in complications such as skin breakdown. At the time of publication, there is no evidence for the effectiveness of bracing in patients with thoracolumbar fractures (1),(3)[B],(5)[C].
- If there is associated spinal injury, a rigid orthosis is needed. The patient should be limited to isometric exercises, with restricted upper extremity exercises, until full range of motion and no tenderness to palpation are present.
- Isolated fractures of the transverse process usually cause disability for a few weeks and carry a very low likelihood of long-term sequelae. Early mobilization and physical therapy are important in rehabilitation:
  - Healing of the transverse process often does not occur because of distraction of the fracture fragment from muscle pull. Healing is often determined by radiographs and palpation at site of injury.
  - Return to play once range of motion is painless and the trunk has been strengthened.
  - Likely, no equipment changes will be needed in noncontact sports, but padded equipment modification may be helpful in reducing the risk for reinjury in contact sports.
- Contiguous transverse process fractures should be observed carefully for development of pseudoarthrosis or myositis ossificans.

Pediatric Considerations
There is an association between transverse process fractures and spinous process fractures, with chest injury being common with higher thoracic injuries and abdominal injuries with lower thoracic or lumbar fractures. Pediatric patients benefit from conservative management and aggressive treatment of their comorbidities (6).

SURGERY/OTHER PROCEDURES
Nonunion of fractured fragments is common in both injuries, but most authors advocate avoiding excision of fragments unless pain persists beyond the period of immobilization (3).

ONGOING CARE

FOLLOW-UP RECOMMENDATIONS
Patients with isolated fractures without concomitant neurologic injury do not need orthopedic or neurosurgical referral.

REFERENCES

1. Arena JD, Kvint S, Ghenbot Y, et al. Thoracolumbar transverse process fractures are more frequently associated with nonspinal injury than clinically significant spine fracture. *World Neurosurg*. 2021;146:e1236–e1241.
2. Acree JS, Schlechter J. Level-specific thoracic and lumbar transverse process fractures and concomitant orthopedic injuries: is there an association? *Curr Orthop Pract*. 2015;26(4):411–413.
3. Awad K, Spencer D, Ramakrishnan D, et al. Adult trauma patients with isolated thoracolumbar spinous and transverse process fractures may be managed conservatively to improve emergency department throughput. *J Trauma Inj*. 2021;34(1):31–38.
4. Boden BP, Jarvis CG. Spinal injuries in sports. *Neurol Clin*. 2008;26(1):63–78.
5. Peterson A, Behrens J, Salari P, et al. Isolated thoracic and lumbar transverse process fractures: do they need spine surgeon evaluation? A high-volume level I trauma center experience with cost analysis. *N Am Spine Soc J*. 2023;15:100242.
6. Akinpelu BJ, Zuckerman SL, Gannon SR, et al. Pediatric isolated thoracic and/or lumbar transverse and spinous process fractures. *J Neurosurg Pediatr*. 2016;17(6):639–644.

ADDITIONAL READING

- Homnick A, Lavery R, Nicastro O, et al. Isolated thoracolumbar transverse process fractures: call physical therapy, not spine. *J Trauma*. 2007;63(6):1292–1295.
- Krueger MA, Green DA, Hoyt D, et al. Overlooked spine injuries associated with lumbar transverse process fractures. *Clin Orthop Relat Res*. 1996;(327):191–195.
- Nicholas J, Hershman E. *The Lower Extremity and Spine in Sports Medicine*. Mosby; 1995.
- Sturm JT, Perry JF Jr. Injuries associated with fractures of the transverse processes of the thoracic and lumbar vertebrae. *J Trauma*. 1984;24(7):597–599.
- Tewes DP, Fischer DA, Quick DC, et al. Lumbar transverse process fractures in professional football players. *Am J Sports Med*. 1995;23(4):507–509.

CLINICAL PEARLS

- Transverse process fractures, especially those with high injury mechanism, should raise suspicion for nonspinal injury and thorough evaluation for concomitant injury should be performed (1),(2)
- Isolated transverse process fractures can be treated conservatively without concern for long-term outcome sequelae such as pain, neurologic deficits, or ambulatory difficulties (4),(5).
- Athletes involved in contact sports may feel more comfortable in a flak jacket, although there is no evidence that they prevent reinjury or accelerate return to competition.

FRACTURE, STERNUM

Steven Cuff, MD, FAAP, CAQSM • Justin Leasure, MD

BASICS

DESCRIPTION

- Direct:
  - Results from direct force applied to the sternum, most often from a blow to the body of the sternum in the lower part
  - Fracture typically occurs near manubrium.
- Indirect:
  - Results from an indirect flexion-compression injury of the cervicothoracic spine, usually a forced flexion of the cervical spine that causes the upper two ribs to pull the manubrium posteriorly (downward and posterior force on the manubrium and upper two ribs)
  - May be exacerbated by chin striking the manubrium
  - Always involves the upper two segments of the sternum
- Stress fracture:
  - Results from repetitive motion of chest wall muscles, ribs, and clavicles with associated stress transmitted to sternum
- Muscular:
  - Results from violent muscular action that causes fracture through opposing muscle groups (i.e., tetanus)
  - Extremely rare

EPIDEMIOLOGY

- Sternal fractures are not common, especially in children and adolescents, due to elasticity of sternum and costal cartilage.
- Incidence and prevalence of sternal fractures have not been well defined in the general population.
- Accounts for about 3–8% of all blunt trauma, <0.5% of traumatic fractures (1)
- More common in men (60–80%) (2)

ETIOLOGY AND PATHOPHYSIOLOGY

- In adults, most commonly related to automobile accidents (68–84%) (1),(2), typically from a direct mechanism
- Striking the steering wheel or dashboard
- Flexion of the sternum across the diagonal part of the seat belt, which acts as a fulcrum
- Although seatbelts decrease the risk of serious injury, they do not seem to decrease the risk of sternal fractures during motor vehicle accidents (MVAs); however, they do decrease the risk of internal injury, likely because of the fracture mechanism.
- Other causes from direct trauma include auto versus pedestrian, cardiopulmonary resuscitation (CPR), direct impact sports, falls, and assaults (3).
- In children, more likely to be caused by low-energy trauma such as a fall off a bicycle (direct) or trampoline injury (indirect) (4)
- Indirect forces more likely to result in pathologic or insufficiency fractures (3)

RISK FACTORS

- Insufficiency fractures caused by decreased bone density or weakened bone can occur spontaneously in patients with underlying bone density problems (especially women), those on long-term steroids, and those with severe thoracic kyphosis (3).
- Repetitive upper body exercise transmitting force to the sternum, such as in golf, wrestling, and weight lifting, can lead to stress fracture (3).

COMMONLY ASSOCIATED CONDITIONS

ALERT

The overall mortality from isolated sternal fractures is low (0.8%); however, because of the high energy associated with these injuries, 2/3 of sternal fractures will have secondary injuries that have a mortality of up to 7.9% (5).

- Trauma to heart, mediastinum, great vessels, tracheobronchial tree, lung parenchyma, or liver: mediastinal injury much less common with an indirect mechanism. Always consider cardiac contusion, especially with double or comminuted fracture and in fracture involving the sternal angle.
- Pulmonary contusion
- Myocardial laceration
- Bone marrow embolization
- Pneumothorax
- Hemothorax
- Pericardial tamponade
- Retrosternal hematoma
- Sternoclavicular dislocation
- Clavicular fracture
- Rib fractures: can cause flail chest
- Vertebral fracture: most commonly thoracic vertebrae but also may occur in lower cervical or upper lumbar vertebrae
- Head/brain injury
- Limb fracture

DIAGNOSIS

HISTORY

- Mechanism of injury: direct blow to chest wall
- Forced flexion of cervical spine (heavy blow to back of head or fall onto head or upper back)
- Pain with inspiration
- Crepitus with respiratory excursion
- Dyspnea, usually transient; if persistent, consider more severe underlying injury like cardiopulmonary contusions.
- Symptoms in patients with spontaneous insufficiency or stress fracture may create a greater diagnostic challenge because the symptoms may resemble other serious conditions.

PHYSICAL EXAM

- Pain
- Localized tenderness over the fracture site that is readily reproducible
- Bruising
- Swelling
- Deformity
- Possible dyspnea
- Palpable or visible step-off (deformity present only with displaced fracture)
- Palpable crepitus with respirations (more rare)
- Edema, ecchymosis
- Screen for associated rib fracture, clinical evidence of pulmonary contusion, vascular injury, pneumothorax, and pericardial friction rub.

DIFFERENTIAL DIAGNOSIS

- Costochondral dislocation
- Sternoclavicular dislocation
- Sternal contusion
- Costochondritis/Tietze syndrome
- Rib fracture/dislocation
- Cardiac causes: contusion, laceration, ischemia, myocarditis
- Aortic dissection
- Pleurisy
- Sickle cell crisis
- Osteomyelitis

DIAGNOSTIC TESTS & INTERPRETATION

- Chest posteroanterior (PA) and lateral radiographs gold standard (3)[C] (fracture missed in >80% of anteroposterior views); possible pneumothorax or mediastinal injury. Widened mediastinum could indicate hematoma due to underlying vascular injury until ruled out. Sternal fracture displacement and sternal dislocation occur in the sagittal plane.
- One should not confuse nonossified intrasternal cartilage in young patients with fractures.
- Ultrasound has higher sensitivity but lower specificity (6)[A].
- Chest computed tomography (CT) scanning is less sensitive than plain radiographs because the fracture line can occur between image cuts.

- Bone scintigraphy may be more sensitive than plan radiographs, especially early on following trauma; however, its use is limited (3)[C].

ALERT

Electrocardiogram (ECG): may see ECG changes in >50%, especially if from a direct mechanism. No single test is consistently reliable for diagnosis of myocardial contusion. If initial ECG is normal, consider repeat in 24 hours; may see ST- or T-wave abnormalities or bundle branch block; may see major arrhythmia in first 24 hours (rare)

- Cervical, thoracic, lumbar spine radiographs: especially if from an indirect mechanism
- Consider other studies (echocardiogram, CT, aortography, serial troponins) if underlying injury is suspected.

TREATMENT

GENERAL MEASURES

- Evaluate and treat any associated life-threatening injuries.
- Most nondisplaced fractures are treated conservatively with rest, ice, and analgesia until symptoms subside.
- Consider hematoma block using ultrasound if reduction is necessary.
- Some displaced fractures can be reduced by having the patient lay supine and hyperextending the thoracic spine by placing a sandbag transversely under the shoulders, slightly below the level of the spines of the scapulae. Extension can be maintained by bracing or bed rest.
- For simple displaced fractures, some authors recommend having the patient lay supine and simultaneously lifting the head and the extended lower extremities, thus separating the upper and lower parts of the sternum. Use thumb to place pressure on the anteriorly displaced fragment (should infiltrate with local anesthetic first, or can use intravenous [IV] procedural sedation).
- Immobilization typically is not necessary with nondisplaced fractures.

ADDITIONAL THERAPIES

- Consider cardiac monitoring while performing reduction if available.
- Avoid aggravating activities and contact sports.
- May start general conditioning within the limits of discomfort

SURGERY/OTHER PROCEDURES

- Open reduction internal fixation: Primary indication is cardiopulmonary function compromise or pain with respiration that limits respiratory excursion; also flail chest; if not stabilized, can have pseudoarthrosis that can be source of ongoing pain or instability
- Surgical treatment for displaced fractures as above
- Consider surgical repair if nonunion (rare).
- Short-term immobilization may be necessary after surgical repair.

ADMISSION, INPATIENT, AND NURSING CONSIDERATIONS

Consider 24-hour inpatient observation and monitoring due to the relatively high likelihood of associated underlying injuries.

ONGOING CARE

FOLLOW-UP RECOMMENDATIONS

- Usually heals without any sequelae
- Consider early orthopedic referral if displaced fracture, open fracture, or flail chest.
- Early consultation as appropriate if there are associated underlying thoracic injuries (pneumothorax, cardiac contusion, etc.)
- Patients should know that sternal pain will last for 8 to 12 weeks for all age groups.
- *Precautions*:
  - Brace the chest when coughing, sneezing, or turning. You may need a pillow or to cross your arms over your chest (splinting). This may help to prevent pneumonia.
  - Do not lift, push, or pull anything >10 lb (4.5 kg).
  - Avoid any maneuvers that cause you pain such as repetitive overhead reaching.
  - Do not reach back with both arms at the same time.
  - Do not push or pull with your arms when moving or getting out of bed. Use your legs to change position in bed; lower yourself to the side and bring your feet onto the bed.

COMPLICATIONS

- Malunion or nonunion
- Infection
- Chronic pain (5)

REFERENCES

1. Alent J, Narducci DM, Moran B, et al. Sternal injuries in sport: a review of the literature. *Sports Med*. 2018;48(12):2715–2724.
2. Yeh DD, Hwabejire JO, DeMoya MA, et al. Sternal fracture—an analysis of the National Trauma Data Bank. *J Surg Res*. 2014;186(1):39–43.
3. Khoriati A, Rajakulasingam R, Shah R. Sternal fractures and their management. *J Emerg Trauma Shock*. 2013;6(2):113–116.
4. Moënne Bühlmann K, Araneda Castiglioni D, Ortega Flores X, et al. Clinical and radiological study of sternal fractures in pediatrics. *Radiologia (Engl Ed)*. 2019;61(3):234–238.
5. Doyle JE, Diaz-Gutierrez I. Traumatic sternal fractures: a narrative review. *Mediastinum*. 2021;5:34.
6. Yousefifard M, Baikpour M, Ghelichkhani P, et al. Comparison of ultrasonography and radiography in detection of thoracic bone fractures; a systematic review and meta-analysis. *Emerg (Tehran)*. 2016;4(2):55–64.

ADDITIONAL READING

- Athanassiadi K, Gerazounis M, Moustardas M, et al. Sternal fractures: retrospective analysis of 100 cases. *World J Surg*. 2002;26(10):1243–1246.
- Baker JC, Demertzis JL. Manubrial stress fractures diagnosed on MRI: report of two cases and review of the literature. *Skeletal Radiol*. 2016;45(6):833–837.
- Celik B, Sahin E, Nadir A, et al. Sternum fractures and effects of associated injuries. *Thorac Cardiovasc Surg*. 2009;57(8):468–471.
- Dixit S, Chang C. Sternal fracture. In: Madden C, Putukian M, McCarty E, et al, eds. *Netter's Sports Medicine*. 2nd ed. Elsevier; 2018:403.
- Ferguson LP, Wilkinson AG, Beattie TF. Fracture of the sternum in children. *Emerg Med J*. 2003;20(6):518–520.
- Lahham S, Patane J, Lane N. Ultrasound of sternal fracture. *West J Emerg Med*. 2015;16(7):1057–1058.
- Miller AC, Rosati SF, Suffredini AF, et al. A systematic review and pooled analysis of CPR-associated cardiovascular and thoracic injuries. *Resuscitation*. 2014;85(6):724–731.
- Recinos G, Inaba K, Dubose J, et al. Epidemiology of sternal fractures. *Am Surg*. 2009;75(5):401–404.

CLINICAL PEARLS

- ECG: may see ECG changes in >50%, especially if from a direct mechanism
- Contact sports should be avoided until symptoms subside, typically 6 to 12 weeks.
- General conditioning or training program permitted within the limits of discomfort posed by the injury
- When returning to play, should consider chest protector if likelihood of reinjury

F

FRACTURE, STRESS: METATARSAL, NAVICULAR

Christopher Jordan, MD, ATC, CAQSM ▪ Jacob Walker, MD

BASICS

DESCRIPTION
- Overload, repetitive stress injury to bone
- Manifest as fatigue fractures to otherwise normal bone

EPIDEMIOLOGY
- Stress fractures account for up to 15% of overuse injuries in sports (1). Stress fractures of the 2nd and 3rd metatarsals are most common in running and dancing (2),(3).
- Tarsal navicular stress fractures are rare in the general population but relatively common in sprinting and jumping athletes.
- Tarsal navicular stress fractures have been reported in athletes as young as 13 years old.
- High-risk stress fractures include the proximal 5th metatarsal and tarsal navicular due to high-tensile load and diminished blood flow (4).
- 5th metatarsal is the most frequently fractured metatarsal bone.

RISK FACTORS
- Training errors: number, frequency, intensity, and duration of strain cycles
- Impact attenuation: muscle fatigue, training surfaces, footwear
- Gait mechanics: foot type, lower extremity alignment, altered gait
- Bone health: nutrition, genetics, hormones, bone disease
- Foot kinematics: short 1st ray, long 2nd metatarsal (5),(6)

DIAGNOSIS

HISTORY
- Pain onset usually insidious
- Pain location typically at site of fracture; forefoot for metatarsal stress fractures and dorsomedial midfoot for tarsal navicular stress fractures; some patients may report ankle pain related to the tarsal navicular stress fractures.
- Usually minimal or no swelling with stress fractures. Tendinitis pain often improves as the injured tissue warms up, but stress fracture pain persists or worsens during the activity.

PHYSICAL EXAM
- Metatarsals: forefoot pain that progressively worsens with activity
- Tarsal navicular: vague, dorsal midfoot pain sometimes radiating along the medial arch or into the ankle
- Minimal or no forefoot swelling
- Tenderness at the base, head, or midshaft of the metatarsal
- Axial load applied to head of the metatarsal causes pain at the fracture site (shaft), even though the examiners pressure is applied distal on the metatarsal.
- Examine callous patterns, which may clue the examiner to excessive loads to individual metatarsals.
- Tender over the dorsum of the navicular at the "N" spot in the space between the anterior tibial tendon and the extensor hallucis longus tendon
- Biomechanical examination, joint range of motion, strength, and flexibility to assess predisposing conditions

DIFFERENTIAL DIAGNOSIS
- Tendinitis
- Tendon rupture, partial or complete
- Metatarsalgia
- Symptomatic accessory ossicle
- 5th metatarsal apophyseal injury
- Mueller-Weiss syndrome (5)

DIAGNOSTIC TESTS & INTERPRETATION
- Radiographs:
  - Metatarsals: Anteroposterior and lateral radiographs are often initially normal; 2 to 3 weeks following symptom onset, periosteal thickening and sometimes a radiolucent line can be appreciated; initial imaging modality due to low cost and wide availability (6)[C]
  - Tarsal navicular: Plain radiographs often are normal throughout the course of a navicular stress fracture (5)[C].
- Bone scan:
  - Metatarsals: very sensitive, but necessary only if a diagnosis is needed quickly, as with a competitive athlete; not specific and must be correlated with clinical history and examination (1)
  - Navicular: no longer preferred due to poor specificity (5)[C]
- Computed tomography (CT) scan:
  - Metatarsals: not helpful
  - Navicular: Thin-sliced cuts in the plane of the talonavicular joint reveal the curvilinear fracture extending from the dorsal cortex surrounded by exuberant bony sclerosis. CT scan is helpful to determine an incomplete fracture versus a complete dorsoplantar transection of the navicular. CT scan can also help differentiate between navicular stress fracture and a stress reaction (5)[C].
  - Helpful for bone healing assessment and surgical planning when necessary (6)[C]
- Magnetic resonance imaging (MRI):
  - Although generally not necessary, metatarsals will demonstrate intramedullary edema.
  - Edema seen on short TI inversion recovery (STIR) or T2-weighted MRI images may help distinguish an active tarsal navicular stress fracture from a persistent, chronic mature fracture as sometimes seen on CT scan (1)[C].
- Pathologic findings:
  - Navicular fracture types (5)
    - Type 0.5: stress reaction; signal change on MRI but no fracture on CT scan
    - Type I fractures involve only the dorsal cortex.
    - Type II fractures are fractures that extend into the navicular body.
    - Type III fractures traverse the entire navicular and extend into the plantar cortex.
  - 5th metatarsal high-risk fracture zones (1):
    - Zone 1—metatarsal tuberosity; avulsion fracture
    - Zone 2—metaphyseal/diaphyseal junction; Jones fracture (high-risk area)
    - Zone 3—proximal diaphyseal junction (high-risk area)

TREATMENT

GENERAL MEASURES
- Metatarsals:
  - Cease sporting activities.
  - Non–weight-bearing only needed for pain control
  - Rest period, average 6 weeks

- Navicular:
  - Type 0.5: non–weight-bearing in CAM boot (5)[C]
  - Non–weight-bearing on crutches with below-the-knee cast or removable brace for 6 to 8 weeks; high failure rate with weight-bearing rest (2),(6)[C]
  - Studies continue to show poorer outcomes with early weight-bearing (2)[B].
  - Follow-up clinical assessment for tenderness at the "N" spot. Radiographic assessment is not helpful. Continued tenderness should extend non–weight-bearing for another 2 to 3 weeks.

SURGERY/OTHER PROCEDURES

- Surgery is rarely required for metatarsal stress fractures.
- 90% of navicular stress fractures can be managed with non–weight-bearing cast. However, type III fractures should be referred for surgical management.
- Surgical fixation with internal screw, bone grafting, or both is necessary for fractures not clinically healed by nonoperative means.
- Recent studies show comparative long-term outcomes between conservative non–weight-bearing and surgery.
- 5th metatarsal stress fracture: surgery recommended for athletes to return early to sport

ONGOING CARE

- Metatarsals:
  - Modify activity level and training activities to provide relative rest (4)[C].
  - Address abnormal biomechanics.
  - Consider calcium and vitamin D supplementation.
  - Return to progressive gradual training only after pain-free walking and no local tenderness at the fracture site.
  - Orthotics may be used, although there is only anecdotal evidence of benefit.
  - Proximal 5th metatarsal: Surgical fixation may result in quicker return to sport.
- Navicular (4),(6)[C]:
  - Time to full recovery may take >4 months (6)[C].
  - May benefit from formal physical therapy
  - Reexamine patient every 2 to 3 weeks to ensure adequate recovery.
  - First 2 weeks following cast removal: activities of daily living, swimming, water running
  - Second 2 weeks: Assess "N" spot; if nontender, then 5-minute jogging on grass every other day; gradually increase to 10 minutes per session.
  - Third 2 weeks: Assess "N" spot; if nontender, then faster running for short distances; that is, 50 m on alternate days; gradual speed increase
  - Fourth 2 weeks: Assess "N" spot; if nontender, then gradual return to full training over several weeks. Average time to return to sport is 5 to 6 months from diagnosis.
  - Attention throughout the rehabilitation time to soft-tissue massage and joint mobilization to the talocrural, subtalar, and midtarsal joints
  - Strength training to reverse the atrophy acquired during immobilization

FOLLOW-UP RECOMMENDATIONS

- Metatarsal stress fractures not healing in a reasonably expected period should be referred to orthopedic surgery or podiatry. Consider referring for biomechanical evaluation for recurrent stress fractures.
- Navicular: Refer the persistently symptomatic navicular stress fracture that does not heal by the above outlined protocol.
- Consider early referral to orthopedic surgeon or podiatrist for zone 2 or 3 fractures of the 5th metatarsal.

REFERENCES

1. Khan M, Madden K, Burrus MT, et al. Epidemiology and impact on performance of lower extremity stress injuries in professional basketball players. *Sports Health*. 2018;10(2):169–174.
2. McInnis KC, Ramey LN. High-risk stress fractures: diagnosis and management. *PM R*. 2016;8(Suppl 3):S113–S124.
3. Ellison MA, Akrami M, Fulford J, et al. Three dimensional finite element modelling of metatarsal stresses during running. *J Med Eng Technol*. 2020;44(7):368–377.
4. Hoenig T, Eissele J, Strahl A, et al. Return to sport following low-risk and high-risk bone stress injuries: a systematic review and meta-analysis. *Br J Sports Med*. 2023;57(7):427–432.
5. Patel KA, Christopher ZK, Drakos MC, et al. Navicular stress fractures. *J Am Acad Orthop Surg*. 2021;29(4):148–157.
6. Constantinou D, Saragas NP, Ferrao PN. Bilateral navicular stress fractures with nonunion in an adolescent middle-distance athlete: a case report. *Curr Sports Med Rep*. 2021;20(5):236–241.

ADDITIONAL READING

- Attia AK, Mahmoud K, Bariteau J, et al. Return to sport following navicular stress fracture: a systematic review and meta-analysis of three hundred and fifteen fractures. *Int Orthop*. 2021;45(10):2699–2710.
- Cheung CN, Lui TH. Proximal fifth metatarsal fractures: anatomy, classification, treatment and complications. *Arch Trauma Res*. 2016;5(4):e33298.
- Morimoto S, Iseki T, Morooka T, et al. The effectiveness of intramedullary screw fixation using the Herbert screw for fifth metatarsal stress fractures in high-level athletes. *Am J Sports Med*. 2021;49(14):4001–4007.
- Saxena A, Behan SA, Valerio DL, et al. Navicular stress fracture outcomes in athletes: analysis of 62 injuries. *J Foot Ankle Surg*. 2017;56(5):943–948.
- Thompson P, Patel V, Fallat LM, et al. Surgical management of fifth metatarsal diaphyseal fractures: a retrospective outcomes study. *J Foot Ankle Surg*. 2017;56(3):463–467.
- Toren AJ, Hahn DB, Brown WC, et al. Vascularized scapular free bone graft after nonunion of a tarsal navicular stress fracture: a case report. *J Foot Ankle Surg*. 2013;52(2):221–226.
- Torg JS, Moyer J, Gaughan JP, et al. Management of tarsal navicular stress fractures: conservative versus surgical treatment: a meta-analysis. *Am J Sports Med*. 2010;38(5):1048–1053.

CLINICAL PEARLS

- Risk factors for stress fractures include overuse or training errors, biomechanical factors, choice and/or age of shoe, nutrition, and menstrual issues for women.
- Careful attention to the risk factors, particularly training errors, will minimize the risk of reinjury.
- Surgery is rarely indicated for metatarsal and tarsal navicular stress fractures.
- High-risk stress fractures of the foot include the tarsal navicular and proximal 5th metatarsal.

FRACTURE, TALUS

Brian Atkinson, MD, CAQSM, DipABLM • Karl B. Fields, MD, CAQSM, FAMSSM

BASICS

DESCRIPTION

- Relatively uncommon fracture usually involving the talar neck, lateral process, or osteochondral fracture of talar dome
- Excluding smaller osteochondral fractures, talar neck fractures account for 50% of talar fractures, talar body fractures 40%, and talar head fractures 5–10%.
- Osteochondral fractures (a subset of talar body fractures) can occur in up to 6.5% of acute ankle sprains.
- Shepherd fracture (posterior tubercle fracture) represents the largest single group of talar body fractures.
- "Snowboarder's ankle," a lateral process fracture, is the second most common type of talar body fracture.
- Stress fractures of the talus have been reported but are rare (1).

EPIDEMIOLOGY

- Talar fractures constitute 3–6% of all foot fractures and are estimated at 1% of all fractures in the entire human body.
- "Snowboarder's ankle" (lateral process fracture) appears to be increasing in frequency.

ETIOLOGY AND PATHOPHYSIOLOGY

- 60–70% of the talar surface consists of cartilage, accommodating seven different articulations.
- The talus has no muscular insertions or origins and is held in place by its osseous neighbors and constraining ligamentous attachments.
- The talar neck is the only section of the talus that is primarily extra-articular.
- The tibiotalar articulation is responsible for hindfoot motion in the plantar/dorsiflexion plane; the subtalar joint provides hindfoot inversion/eversion motion.
- The tibiotalar joint has more loads per unit area than any other joint in the body (2).
- Only 40% of the talus can be perfused by blood vessels. The other 60% is covered by articular cartilage. As a result, talus fractures are at a high risk of avascular necrosis.

RISK FACTORS

- In general, fractures of the talar head and neck are the result of high-energy trauma.
- Snowboarding is associated with acute dorsiflexion/inversion injuries to the ankle, which can cause lateral process fractures.

DIAGNOSIS

HISTORY

- Fractures of the talar head and neck usually are found after high-velocity trauma (e.g., motorcycle accidents).
- Fractures of the talar neck occur as a result of hyperdorsiflexion and axial loading of the foot against a stationary tibia.
- Anterolateral osteochondral fractures are associated with an inversion-dorsiflexion injury of the ankle.
- Posterolateral osteochondral fractures are associated with plantar flexion, inversion, and external rotation of the ankle.
- Chronic osteochondral fractures present with pain following an adequate healing time for ligamentous injury, complaints of ankle "giving out," catching, or locking up.
- Historically, lateral process fractures involved dorsiflexion and inversion with an axial load, but more recent cadaveric studies have suggested that eversion can also be involved (3).

PHYSICAL EXAM

- Talar head fractures cause swelling and tenderness at the talonavicular joint.
- Talar neck fractures present with swelling and tenderness of the proximal dorsal foot. With displaced fractures, the normal ankle contours will be changed.
- Acute inversion injuries of the ankle that remain painful after conservative treatment should make the clinician suspicious for osteochondral lesion of the talus or a lateral process fracture.
- Acute osteochondral fractures present with edema, ecchymosis, range of motion limited by guarding, and pain to palpation.
- Displaced talar neck fractures can lead to skin necrosis due to significant stretching of the soft tissues (4).

ALERT

Thoracolumbar compression spinal fractures have been found in association with fractures of the talar neck and talar body, particularly after a jump or fall from a height (4).

ALERT

Lateral talar process fractures have the same symptoms as an acute sprain of the anterior talofibular ligament. Findings may include tenderness inferior and anterior to the tip of the lateral malleolus associated with pain on active and passive range of motion of the ankle and subtalar joints.

DIFFERENTIAL DIAGNOSIS

Conditions that can mimic osteochondral fractures of the talar dome include osteochondritis dissecans, degenerative joint disease, and/or loose bodies.

DIAGNOSTIC TESTS & INTERPRETATION

- Initial radiographic workup of most talar fractures should include ankle mortise views with routine anteroposterior (AP) and lateral views.
- The Canale view (foot internally rotated 15 degrees with x-ray angled at 75 degrees from the plane of the table) gives a direct AP view of the talus and is very useful in evaluating talar neck fractures.
- To best view lateral osteochondral lesions with plain x-rays, films should be obtained with 10 to 35 degrees of internal rotation and maximal plantar flexion.
- Lateral osteochondral fractures have a thin, wafer-like appearance; medial osteochondral lesions have a deep, cup-shaped appearance.
- If plain x-rays show abnormalities of the talar dome, computed tomography (CT) scan should be performed to determine size and nature of lesion, essential in preoperative planning.

ALERT

If an injury to the talar dome or lateral talar process is suspected but plain radiographs are unremarkable, further imaging, ideally with a magnetic resonance imaging (MRI) or CT, is indicated.

- Fractures of the posterolateral process can be potentially mistaken as an os trigonum (5).
- Ultrasound can be used as a screen in minor injuries and recurrent ankle pain. Studies correlate excellent ability to determine articular cartilage thickness at the talar dome.

TREATMENT

- Displaced talar fractures require anatomical reduction to prevent arthrosis and avascular necrosis and usually require surgical fixation.
- Reduction of a displaced talar neck fracture can be attempted by plantar flexion of the foot, bringing the head and body into line. This is an orthopedic emergency if there are signs of skin necrosis.
- Clinical signs and symptoms correlated with repeated radiographic examination are important during conservative treatment to assure proper healing.
- Although nondisplaced talar fractures may be treated in a short, non–weight-bearing leg cast for 6 to 12 weeks, it is recommended only for non-ambulatory patients or those medically unable to tolerate surgery (1)[C].
- Surgical indications for lateral process talar fractures remain unclear. Up to 67% of displaced fractures fail nonoperative management. Given this, it is recommended that all displaced fractures be referred for surgical intervention.
- Stress fractures are treated with 3 to 6 weeks of non–weight-bearing immobilization with a controlled ankle motion (CAM) walker, followed by progressive mobilization, rehabilitation, and return to activity based on case reports.

ADDITIONAL THERAPIES

- 50% of talar neck fractures go on to avascular necrosis, as do 25–50% of talar body fractures.
- Treatment of osteonecrosis is primarily conservative, and patient can begin weight-bearing once there is evidence of stable changes on x-ray. Failure of conservative measures to allow weight-bearing may require surgery (4).
- Talar head fracture complications include midtarsal instability, talonavicular arthritis, and avascular necrosis of the talar head.
- Standard range of motion, strengthening, and proprioceptive rehabilitation are appropriate after the fracture has healed.

SURGERY/OTHER PROCEDURES

ALERT

Any talar fracture that is displaced, even minimally, requires surgical treatment, given the risks of avascular necrosis and future arthritis.

- Nondisplaced osteochondral fractures can be managed conservatively for up to 12 months without compromising subsequent surgical outcomes.
- Any loose body associated with a fracture may require arthroscopic removal.

REFERENCES

1. Vallier HA. Fractures of the talus: state of the art. *J Orthop Trauma*. 2015;29(9):385–392.
2. Boon AJ, Smith J, Zobitz ME, et al. Snowboarder's talus fracture. Mechanism of injury. *Am J Sports Med*. 2001;29(3):333–338.
3. Grear BJ. Review of talus fractures and surgical timing. *Orthop Clin North Am*. 2016;47(3):625–637.
4. Fortin PT, Balazsy JE. Talus fractures: evaluation and treatment. *J Am Acad Orthop Surg*. 2001;9(2):114–127.
5. Majeed H, McBride DJ. Talar process fractures: an overview and update of the literature. *EFORT Open Rev*. 2018;3(3):85–92.

ADDITIONAL READING

- Mandracchia VJ, Buddecke DE Jr, Giesking JL. Osteochondral lesions of the talar dome. A comprehensive review with retrospective study. *Clin Podiatr Med Surg*. 1999;16(4):725–742.
- Mayer D. Isolated talus fractures: description of a new clinical sign. *Am J Emerg Med*. 1997;15(4):412–414.
- Ross H, Marchand L, Cardon J, et al. Patient-reported outcomes after lateral process talus fracture. *J Orthop Trauma*. 2021;35(12):e470–e474.
- Schachter AK, Chen AL, Reddy PD, et al. Osteochondral lesions of the talus. *J Am Acad Orthop Surg*. 2005;13(3):152–158.
- Sormaala MJ, Niva MH, Kiuru MJ, et al. Outcomes of stress fractures of the talus. *Am J Sports Med*. 2006;34(11):1809–1814.

CLINICAL PEARLS

- "Snowboarder's fracture" is becoming more common with the increasing popularity of the sport.
- If ankle pain persists after adequate time for a simple ankle sprain to heal, be suspicious of a possible osteochondral fracture or other injury to the talus.
- Most talar fractures need referral to orthopedic surgery for consultation. Even nondisplaced fractures may require open reduction and internal fixation (ORIF).

FRACTURE, TIBIAL PLATEAU

Larry Balle II, MD, MPH, CAQSM • Ramon Ylanan, MD, CAQSM

BASICS

DESCRIPTION

- Fracture and/or depression of the proximal tibial articulating surface (1)
- Largest and most kinematically complex joint (2)
- Also referred to as *tibial condylar fractures*
- Impact force, patient age, and degree of knee flexion at the time of injury will impact type of fracture (3).
- Most commonly used classification: Schatzker (1),(3),(4)
  - Type I—pure cleavage, lateral femoral condyle driven into articular surface of tibial plateau, wedge-shaped split-off fracture of the lateral tibial plateau displaced outward and down (1): best prognosis
  - Type II—cleavage combined with depression, lateral wedge is split with varying portions of remaining lateral plateau and articular surface area comminuted and depressed downwards into metaphysis (1): commonly occurs in patients with osteopenia (2)
  - Type III—pure central depression, articular surface of the lateral plateau is depressed and driven into lateral tibial condyle, no lateral wedge split-off and lateral cortex is intact (1)
  - Type IV—medial condyle fracture (1), most commonly posteromedial aspect (2):
    - A—split-off wedge fragment of medial plateau (1)
    - B—medial fragment depressed or comminuted
    - Either may be combined with fracture of tibial spine
- Type V—bicondylar fracture, both plateaus fractured, appearance of inverted Y, may be associated with fracture of intercondylar eminence, metaphysis, and diaphysis intact (1)
- Type VI—tibial plateau fracture with dissociation of tibial metaphyseal-diaphyseal junction via oblique or transverse fracture, with varying degrees of comminution of one or both tibial condyles and articular surface (1)

ALERT

- With high-energy mechanisms, associated major life-threatening injuries take precedence.
- Immobilize early to prevent further neurologic or vascular injury.

EPIDEMIOLOGY

Incidence

- ~1.2% of all fractures (2), 8% of elderly fractures (3)
- Highest frequency in both sexes between ages 40 and 60 years old (2)
- Recent trends indicate greater incidence in elderly women (3),(5).
- 55–70% are lateral tibial plateau in isolation.
- 10–25% are medial tibial plateau in isolation.
- ~15% are bicondylar.
- In as many as 90%, some degree of soft tissue injury occurs with 1–3% presenting as open fractures.

COMMONLY ASSOCIATED CONDITIONS

- Meniscus injuries occur in 10–47% of cases (3).
- Nerve injuries—posterior tibial nerve and common peroneal nerve
- Ligament injuries occur in 20–30% of cases.
- *Lateral* plateau fractures commonly associated with medial collateral ligament.
- *Medial* plateau fractures (types IV, V, VI) are less common overall but more common in younger patients with high-energy injuries and associated soft tissue injuries (2),(3):
  - Associated injuries include posterior lateral corner injuries, lateral collateral ligament, posterior cruciate ligament, medial meniscus, and neurovascular injury to peroneal nerve (1% incidence) and popliteal vessels.

ALERT

Isolated medial plateau fractures (type IV) may be associated with knee dislocation-relocation injury with neurovascular injury in posterior knee.

- Compartment syndrome is most common in Schatzker types IV to VI (up to 18% in Schatzker VI injuries and 53% in medial plateau fractures) (2).

DIAGNOSIS

HISTORY

- Mechanism of injury important in diagnosis
- Valgus/varus load with or without an axial load
- Lateral plateau is most common (3),(5) due to direct blow to lateral knee mechanism.
- Medial requires higher force/energy mechanism.
- *High-energy injuries*:
  - Pedestrian struck in the lower leg by an automobile
  - Passenger in motor vehicle collision
  - Fall from a height
  - Violent twisting force (e.g., skiing or dancing)

Pediatric Considerations

- Occurs in patients with higher demand and good bone stock, the tibial plateau resists depression (2)
- Tibia plateau fractures have a very high incidence of soft tissue injury (ligament followed by meniscus).
- Careful assessment of the physis is crucial to monitor for long-term complications such as growth arrest or deformity.

Geriatric Considerations

Elderly patients and osteoporotic patients present more often with low-energy lateral tibial plateau fractures without insult to soft tissue often radiographically occult (2).

PHYSICAL EXAM

- Painful, swollen knee
- Significant pain with ambulation or the inability to bear weight on the injured leg
- Knee effusion (hemarthrosis)
- Decreased (both active and passive) range of motion (ROM) of the knee
- Tenderness along the proximal tibia (either medial or lateral tibial plateau)
- Possible varus or valgus deformity of the knee
- Possible joint instability associated with ligamentous injury
- Neurovascular examination (2)[A]:
  - Evaluate for neurovascular damage and compartment syndrome.
  - Check popliteal, posterior tibial, and dorsalis pedis arterial pulse (consider ankle brachial index if knee dislocation in the differential normal >0.9).
  - Check the integrity of peroneal nerve: ankle and toe dorsiflexion, and sensation in the web space between the great and 2nd toes.

DIFFERENTIAL DIAGNOSIS

- Knee dislocation
- Cruciate ligament tears/avulsion
- Collateral ligament tears/avulsion
- Meniscal tears
- Quadriceps tendon rupture
- Patellar fracture
- Patellar dislocation

DIAGNOSTIC TESTS & INTERPRETATION

Initial Tests (lab, imaging)

- Plain radiography—initial investigation of choice (2)[A]
- Anteroposterior (AP) and lateral views of the knee and proximal tibia—79% sensitivity for predominantly lateral plateau fractures (2),(5)
- Tibial plateau view—AP view with the knee in 10 to 15 degrees of flexion helps to visualize depressions.
- Oblique views increase sensitivity to approximately 85% (2).
- Caudal tilt plateau view—determines the degree of articular step off
- Subtle fractures—if lipohemarthrosis (fat-fluid level) seen on lateral view and no obvious fracture seen on x-ray, a computed tomography (CT) should be performed to avoid missing covert fracture (2).
- Cross-sectional imaging: CT and magnetic resonance imaging (MRI):
  - More detailed image of fracture (1),(6)
  - Helpful in preoperative planning and identification of associated injuries (2),(4),(5),(6)
  - CT coupled with angiography quantifies magnitude of fracture or depression and evaluates vascular involvement (2).
  - CT/MRI is indicated if (4):
    - High-energy mechanism
    - Schatzker type IV, V, or VI fracture

ALERT

Consider angiography if:

- Alteration in distal pulses
- Expanding hematoma
- Bruit on exam
- Injury to anatomically related nerves

- MRI can be used to better identify soft tissue (ligamentous, chondral, meniscus, and neurovascular) injuries (2),(4) and classify fracture using the Schatzker system, especially in the pediatric population.

Diagnostic Procedures/Other

- Compartment pressures if compartment syndrome clinically suspected:
  - Pain not over fracture site
  - Pain on passive stretch
  - Paresthesia
  - Abnormality of pulses
  - Pressures >30 mm Hg—indication for fasciotomy
- Arthrocentesis to look for fat globules if effusion present and mechanism strongly suggests that fracture present without x-ray findings (2)

TREATMENT

GENERAL MEASURES

- Airway, breathing, and circulation (ABCs)/advanced trauma life support (ATLS) protocol in multiple trauma victim
- Long-leg splint/immobilizer initially
- Ice
- Elevation
- Emergency department (ED)/clinic management:
  - Nonoperative management:
    - Schatzker type I—nondisplaced fractures in low-demand patients (2)
  - Coronal plane stabilizing brace (2),(6)
  - Clinic setting—may consider a long leg cast (once swelling has improved) but will limit early ROM (6)
  - Restricted weight-bearing
  - Permit full ROM.
  - Rest, ice, compression, and elevation

ALERT
Non–weight-bearing and early ROM are critical.

- Average time to heal is 12 to 20 weeks.
- Consider aspiration of hemarthrosis and injection of local anesthetic.
- Timetables
  - Non–weight-bearing for 4 to 6 weeks or until radiographic evidence of healing is noted and then may proceed with partial weight-bearing with brace and crutch assistance.
  - Initial 10 to 14 days in hinged brace locked in full extension
  - Consider unlocking the brace as tolerated at the 2-week follow-up to allow for early ROM.
  - Begin gradual ROM, with goal of 90 degrees of flexion by 4 weeks.
  - Follow up with repeat x-rays every 2 to 3 weeks.
- Pain control
- Early orthopedic follow-up if knee is ligamentously unstable

ISSUES FOR REFERRAL

- Indications for orthopedic consultation for closed fractures (2)[A],(6):
  - Lateral plateau fracture with:
    - Articular step off >3 mm (2) to >4 mm (6)
    - Condylar widening >5 mm (2)
    - Coronal plane instability
  - Displaced medial plateau fracture (60% of weight-bearing through medial plateau)
  - Bicondylar fractures
- Fracture dislocations, vascular injuries, and compartment syndrome (2)[A]:
  - Emergent orthopedic consultation
- Open fractures:
  - Emergent orthopedic consultation
  - Remove contaminants.
  - Apply moist sterile dressing.
  - Assess tetanus immunity.
  - Consider empiric antibiotics.

SURGERY/OTHER PROCEDURES

- Depending on severity of injury, may require staged management due to compromise of soft tissue and physiology (2)
- Operative options:
  - Open reduction and internal fixation (ORIF)/ standard plating (5)
  - Arthroscopic techniques, types I–III
  - Percutaneous techniques
  - Definitive external fixation
  - Primary arthroplasty (6)

ALERT
Complicated fractures may be referred for total knee arthroplasty (6).

ADMISSION, INPATIENT, AND NURSING CONSIDERATIONS

Admission criteria:

- Open fractures for débridement, irrigation, and intravenous (IV) antibiotics
- Comminuted bicondylar fractures for traction
- High-energy mechanism for observation of neurovascular status
- Suspected compartment syndrome
- Pain control

ONGOING CARE

FOLLOW-UP RECOMMENDATIONS

Patient Monitoring

- Nonoperative treatment: biweekly follow-up initially with x-rays to evaluate fracture
- If knee is unstable, early follow-up with orthopedics to evaluate ligamentous injury

PATIENT EDUCATION

Formal physical therapy early for ROM can help to restore function.

COMPLICATIONS

- Joint stiffness, decreased lower limb mobility (3)
- Posttraumatic osteoarthritis common sequelae (2),(3)
- Surgical site infection following ORIF (3)

REFERENCES

1. Millar SC, Arnold JB, Thewlis D, et al. A systematic literature review of tibial plateau fractures: what classifications are used and how reliable and useful are they? *Injury*. 2018;49(3):473–490.
2. Mthethwa J, Chikate A. A review of the management of tibial plateau fractures. *Musculoskelet Surg*. 2018;102(2):119–127.
3. Aguilar JR, Rios X, Edery EG, et al. Epidemiological characterization of tibial plateau fractures. *J Orthop Surg Res*. 2022;17(1):106.
4. Schatzker J, Kfuri M. Revisiting the management of tibial plateau fractures. *Injury*. 2022;53(6):2207–2218.
5. Le Baron M, Cermolacce M, Flecher X, et al. Tibial plateau fracture management: ARIF versus ORIF—clinical and radiological comparison. *Orthop Traumatol Surg Res*. 2019;105(1):101–106.
6. Vaartjes TP, Assink N, Nijveldt RJ, et al. Functional outcome after nonoperative management of tibial plateau fractures in skeletally mature patients: what sizes of gaps and stepoffs can be accepted? *Clin Orthop Relat Res*. 2022;480(12):2288–2295.

ADDITIONAL READING

- Eiff MP, Hatch RL, et al. *Fracture Management for Primary Care*. 3rd ed. Saunders; 2011.
- Markhardt BK, Gross JM, Monu JUV. Schatzker classification of tibial plateau fractures: use of CT and MR imaging improves assessment. *Radiographics*. 2009;29(2):585–597.
- Porrino J, Richardson ML, Hovis K, et al. Association of tibial plateau fracture morphology with ligament disruption in the context of multiligament knee injury. *Curr Probl Diagn Radiol*. 2018;47(6):410–416.
- Sanders E, Policicchio AL, Phillips L. High incidence of soft tissue injury in pediatric proximal tibia fractures: a systematic review. *Arthrosc Sports Med Rehabil*. 2023;5(5):100771.
- Schatzker J, Mcbroom R, Bruce D. The tibial plateau fracture. The Toronto experience 1968–1975. *Clin Orthop Relat Res*. 1979;(138):94–104.
- Simon RR, Sherman SC, Koenigsknecht SJ, eds. Proximal tibia fractures. In: *Emergency Orthopedics: The Extremities*. 5th ed. Appleton & Lange; 2007:396–403.

CLINICAL PEARLS

- Mechanism of injury important in diagnosis: high-energy axial force with coronal force component
- Lateral tibial plateau more commonly injured
- Pediatric tibial plateau fractures with high incidence of ligament and meniscal pathology
- X-rays—AP, lateral, and obliques
- Schatzker type I may be treated nonoperatively.
- Schatzker type IV associated with dislocation-relocation injury (check ankle/brachial index)
- In Schatzker types IV to VI, neurovascular compromise is high-risk, emergent orthopedic consultation.

FRACTURE, TIBIAL SPINE AVULSION

Chris Koutures, MD, FAAP • Alana Ryan, DO, CAQSM

BASICS

DESCRIPTION

- Tibial spine avulsion fractures occur when the anterior cruciate ligament (ACL)–tibial spine bone interface is ruptured by undue stress.
- In children, the weaker incompletely ossified bone will fail before the ligament is injured resulting in fracture.
- Thus, an injury that typically would result in a midsubstance ACL tear in an adult instead would cause a fracture through the anterior tibial spine via pull of the ACL.
- Fracture through the posterior tibial spine (where the posterior cruciate ligament attaches) is rare and generally occurs in skeletally mature patients.
- Mechanism of injury:
  - Hyperextension ± valgus stress or rotation about the knee
  - Fracture also can occur with a direct blow to the distal end of the femur with the knee flexed.
- Synonym(s): tibial eminence fracture; intercondylar eminence fracture

EPIDEMIOLOGY

- Avulsion fractures of the ACL attachment to the tibial spine are relatively rare, accounting for three fractures per 100,000 children annually and approximately 2% of all knee injuries in children (1)[C].
- Most prevalent in children 8 to 14 years of age but are also seen in adults >35 years of age who have low bone density.
- ACL avulsion from the femoral attachment is less common, as is posterior cruciate ligament avulsion from the posterior tibial eminence.
- Tibial spine fractures classically have been associated with a fall from a bicycle or motorcycle on an outstretched leg (1)[C].
- The injury is now also commonly seen in sporting activities (1)[C].

RISK FACTORS

- Children <16 years of age
- Adults >35 years of age who are osteopenic or undergo high-energy trauma (1)[C]

COMMONLY ASSOCIATED CONDITIONS

- In adolescents and adults, tibial spine avulsion fractures are commonly associated with concomitant knee injury.
- These most commonly include meniscal entrapment or tear, chondral injury, bone contusion, intrinsic ACL injury, and collateral ligament pathology (1)[C],(2)[B].

DIAGNOSIS

HISTORY

- In children aged 8 to 11 years, often due to hyperextension injury
- Above this age, owing to either hyperextension injury or single-leg landing from a jump, both associated with a rotational or twisting stress to the knee
- Audible "pop" at the time of injury
- Immediate (within 1 to 2 hours) prominent swelling of the knee (acute hemarthrosis)
- Frequently unable to bear weight after injury

PHYSICAL EXAM

- Signs and symptoms:
  - Presence of a large, tense knee effusion (especially in a child <16 years of age) should raise concern for a potential ACL avulsion fracture.
  - Examination findings of an ACL tear should raise suspicion.
- Physical examination:
  - Large, tense effusion noted with loss of range of motion (ROM)
  - ACL stress tests (Lachman, anterior drawer, and pivot shift) show more forward translation of the tibia compared with the noninjured side.
  - A positive posterior drawer sign or if the tibia is displaced posteriorly relative to the femur when compared with the noninjured knee may suggest posterior cruciate ligament avulsion from the tibial spine.
  - Evaluate other ligamentous and meniscal structures, particularly the menisci and collateral ligaments, for concomitant pathology.

DIFFERENTIAL DIAGNOSIS

- Midsubstance ACL tear
- Congenital absence or deficiency of the ACL
- Midsubstance tear of the posterior cruciate ligament
- Tibial plateau fracture
- Patellar dislocation or subluxation
- Osteochondral fracture of the femoral condyle

DIAGNOSTIC TESTS & INTERPRETATION

- Plain radiographs should include anteroposterior (AP), lateral, and tunnel views. The latter outlines the femoral notch and tibial eminence.
- The lateral view is most helpful to assess fracture position and degree of displacement.
- Radiographs should be obtained on an urgent basis at the first evaluation.
- Types of anterior tibial spine avulsion fractures are based on degree of displacement. The Meyers and McKeever classification scheme is the most widely accepted:
  - Type I: minimal displacement of the anterior eminence
  - Type II: elevation of the anterior third to half of the eminence with hinging on posterior eminence
  - Type IIIA: complete displacement and separation of fragment without rotational malalignment
  - Type IIIB: complete displacement and separation of fragment with rotational malalignment
- Types II and III are of equal incidence, are more common than type I, and more likely to be associated with concomitant knee injury (2),(3)[B].
- Consideration for computed tomography (CT) or magnetic resonance imaging (MRI) to evaluate degree of displacement and surrounding injury may be important in clinical decision making (1)[C].
- With negative plain radiographs, nondisplaced fracture or ligament injury still must be suspected in patients with acute hemarthrosis. MRI should be obtained in these instances to further evaluate extent of injury.

TREATMENT

- Acute treatment
- Analgesia:
  - Nonsteroidal anti-inflammatory drugs (NSAIDs) are used initially for pain control.
  - Frequent application of ice for 20-minute periods as tolerated by patient.
- Aspiration of the joint may enhance comfort and allow further knee extension. Lack of full knee extension may imply a mechanical block (i.e., fracture fragment or meniscal entrapment).
- Immobilization:
  - Initial care can include complete knee immobilization with minimal knee flexion for 2 to 3 days until effusion begins to resolve.
  - Crutch ambulation is recommended in this initial stage.

ISSUES FOR REFERRAL

- All suspected ACL avulsion fractures should promptly be referred to an orthopedic surgeon.
- Tibial spine avulsions in patients with open growth plates would benefit from urgent consultation with a pediatric orthopedic specialist.

ADDITIONAL THERAPIES

- Type I fracture: After effusion resolves, type I fractures are best managed by long leg cast immobilization with knee flexed at ~0 to 20 degrees (degree that supports confirmed fragment reduction) for 6 weeks (1)[C].
- Type II and III fractures:
  - Controversy exists regarding optimal treatment for fractures with greater degrees of displacement.
  - Type II tibial spine fractures can be managed by either closed reduction with the knee immobilized as in type I fractures or surgically with arthroscopy or open reduction and internal fixation (1)[C].
- Type III fractures generally require open or arthroscopic reduction with fragment fixation with either suture or metal fixation (1)[C].
- Special considerations:
  - The knee should be immobilized while awaiting surgical consultation.
- After completion of cast immobilization, focus should be on recovering knee ROM followed by strengthening of knee extensors.
- Aggressive rehabilitation and early achievement of ROM is predictive of successful functional outcomes (1)[C].
- Proprioception is another key part of the rehabilitation process.

SURGERY/OTHER PROCEDURES

- Arthroscopic or open reduction with internal fixation should be performed for displaced type II fractures if closed methods fail to obtain or maintain reduction of fracture fragment.
- Many authors prefer arthroscopic reduction owing to less surgical trauma and prompt initiation of the postoperative rehabilitation course.

ONGOING CARE

FOLLOW-UP RECOMMENDATIONS

- In the immediate postinjury or postoperative period, follow-up radiographs are necessary to evaluate for loss of fracture reduction.
- Radiographic demonstration of proper fracture union should be obtained before discontinuing knee immobilization and allowing knee mobilization.

PROGNOSIS

- Tibial spine fractures generally have an excellent prognosis, even when the fracture fragment is completely displaced.
- Despite true anatomic reduction, about 50% of pediatric patients may have mild objective, measurable ACL laxity owing to interstitial ligament damage that occurs before the avulsion. However, it generally does not result in functional instability.
- Fewer data on treatment outcome are available for skeletally mature patients, with one study reported symptomatic knee instability as the main complication of nonoperative treatment of tibial spine fractures (4)[C].

COMPLICATIONS

Although overall prognosis is remarkably good, some complications may include:

- Patients >18 years old are more likely to experience loss of motion and joint stiffness due to arthrofibrosis than those <18 years old.
- Meniscal entrapment may represent significant blocks to anatomic reduction resulting in nonunion (2).
- Some cases of residual ACL laxity require ACL reconstruction.
- Physeal arrest is a rare complication of surgical reduction (1)[C].

REFERENCES

1. Shin YW, Uppstrom TJ, Haskel JD, et al. The tibial eminence fracture in skeletally immature patients. *Curr Opin Pediatr*. 2015;27(1):50–57.
2. Rhodes JT, Cannamela PC, Cruz AI, et al. Incidence of meniscal entrapment and associated knee injuries in tibial spine avulsions. *J Pediatr Orthop*. 2018;38(2):e38–e42.
3. Mayo MH, Mitchell JJ, Axibal DP, et al. Anterior cruciate ligament injury at the time of anterior tibial spine fracture in young patients: an observational cohort study. *J Pediatr Orthop*. 2019;39(9):e668–e673.
4. Aderinto J, Walmsley P, Keating JF. Fractures of the tibial spine: epidemiology and outcome. *Knee*. 2008;15(3):164–167.

ADDITIONAL READING

Accousti WK, Willis RB. Tibial eminence fractures. *Orthop Clin North Am*. 2003;34(3):365–375.

CLINICAL PEARLS

- History of either hyperextension or rotational stress to the knee (e.g., landing single legged from a jump)
- Similar mechanism of injury for a midsubstance ACL injury
- Thus, in any case of a suspected ACL injury, obtain urgent radiographs at the first evaluation to look for a potential tibial spine avulsion fracture. Images should include AP, tunnel, and lateral (most helpful to assess fracture position and degree of displacement) views.
- Initial care can include complete knee immobilization with minimal knee flexion for 2 to 3 days until effusion begins to resolve.
- All suspected ACL avulsion fractures should be urgently referred to an orthopedic surgeon.
- Tibial spine fractures generally have an excellent prognosis, even when the fracture fragment is completely displaced.

FRACTURE, VOLKMANN (POSTEROLATERAL MALLEOLUS)

Holly J. Benjamin, MD, FAMSSM, FACSM • Shaheen Jadidi, DO

BASICS

Pediatric Considerations

- Volkmann fracture is a rare injury in children <14 years of age, given the relative weak physis of the tibia.
- Salter-Harris fractures occur during external rotation and abduction injuries, which only occasionally involve the posterior tubercle. The fracture fragment usually is contiguous with the medial malleolar fragment.

DESCRIPTION

- Ankle fracture involving avulsion of the posterior lip of the tibia at its articular surface (Volkmann tubercle or posterior malleolus)
- The name is confusing because there is also a Volkmann contracture, which is a flexion contracture of the upper extremity.
- Fracture occurs via a force through the posterior inferior tibiofibular ligament (PITFL) at its tibial attachment.
- The Lauge-Hansen (L-H), Danis-Weber, Bartoníček/Rammelt, and Orthopaedic Trauma Association/Arbeitsgemeinschaft für Osteosynthesefragen systems have been used to describe ankle injury patterns. The L-H system can aid in closed reduction maneuvers.
- **Supination external rotation (SER):** the ankle rolled outward. Before the Volkmann fracture, the front-lower ankle ligament tears and the fibula (lower leg bone) breaks spirally.
- **Pronation external rotation (PER):** the foot twisted outward while pronated. Before the Volkmann fracture, the inner ankle ligament (deltoid) tears, the inner ankle bone (medial malleolus) breaks, the front-lower ankle ligament tears, and the fibula breaks spirally.
- **Pronation abduction (PA):** the foot rotated outward while pronated. The inner ankle ligament tears or the inner ankle bone breaks first.

EPIDEMIOLOGY

- The prevalence of isolated posterior malleolar fracture (PMF) is low, accounting for 1–4% of all ankle fractures.
- Volkmann fracture more commonly occurs concurrently with other malleolar fractures, spiral fibular fractures, and deltoid ligament and syndesmotic membrane injuries.
- Posterior malleolus fractures occur in up to 44% of all ankle fractures (1)[C].
- Fracture usually involved a significant portion of the articular surface or fibular displacement.

ETIOLOGY AND PATHOPHYSIOLOGY

- Volkmann tubercle or triangle is part of the posterior aspect of the distal tibia and is commonly referred to as the posterior malleolus.
- The posterior malleolus extends from the fibular notch of the tibia to the medial malleolus.
- The PITFL's attachment to the posterior malleolus resists posterior translation of the talus.
- The PITFL is also referred to as the posterior tibiofibular ligament and is one of four syndesmotic ligaments that maintain integrity between the tibia and fibula.
- The PITFL provides >40% of ankle syndesmotic stability (1)[B].
- Given that the PITFL is markedly stronger than the anterior inferior tibiofibular ligament (AITFL), the torsional/rotational forces rupture the AITFL but avulse the posterior tibial tubercle through an intact PITFL.

DIAGNOSIS

HISTORY

- Ankle injury involving a Volkmann fracture is rarely subtle, given typical concomitant fractures and ligament tears.
- A mechanism of injury involving a significant external rotation or abduction force and the presence of associated injuries should evoke suspicion.
- Any floor or field sport, particularly contact sports, can result in a PMF.
- Patients should be questioned for specific injury mechanism, associated sounds such as "pops" or "cracks," and weight-bearing ability.

PHYSICAL EXAM

- Emergent examination:
  - Should focus on neurovascular compromise secondary to joint dislocation or leg compartment syndrome and skin integrity
  - Doppler ultrasound (US) should be used if pulses are nonpalpable, and a detailed sensorimotor examination of the foot should be done.
  - Concern for early compartment syndrome should prompt measurement of leg compartment pressures.
- Nonemergent examination:
  - Systematic ankle, foot, leg, and knee examination should be performed, including soft tissues and neurovascular assessment.
  - Observation, palpation, and careful range of motion should be done, followed by stability testing.
  - Acute examination will reveal a painful, tender, and swollen ankle with limited or inability to bear weight consistent with a moderate or severe injury.
  - Possible findings include an increased posterior drawer test, increased internal rotation, and, with associated syndesmotic instability, a positive squeeze and external rotation tests.

DIAGNOSTIC TESTS & INTERPRETATION

- Radiographs: anteroposterior, lateral, and mortise views are standard (1)[C]. Weight-bearing films unless otherwise contraindicated or too painful; typically, that may help to show any tibiofibular diastasis if there is syndesmotic disruption
- Lateral films generally show the PMF but do not reliably estimate the size of the avulsion or the articular surface involvement (2)[B].
- The use of radiographs for size estimation of PMF has been found to be limited, leading to an increasing reliance on computed tomography (CT) for diagnosing trimalleolar ankle fractures. There has been a shift in focus from size to fracture morphology as crucial for improving outcomes (3)[A].
- Standard views will help diagnose associated injuries that are almost always present.
- Stress radiographs are controversial and not routinely indicated.
- If Volkmann fracture is seen on plain film evaluation, CT is recommended to elucidate the extent of articular involvement, size of the fragment, and integrity of the anterior tibiofibular joint and syndesmosis, which are often used in determining treatment (1)[C].

- Several new CT-based classifications have emerged in the literature as a result of a recent shift toward CT imaging to characterize fracture morphology including Haraguchi, Mason, and Bartoníček/Rammelt which has emerged as preferred since 2015 due to its ascending severity and therapy recommendations (3)[A].
- Magnetic resonance imaging (MRI) is used for evaluation of soft tissues, including the syndesmosis, but is generally not indicated unless CT films are inadequate for detailing the injury characteristics. Both CT and MRI can help with surgical decisions.

TREATMENT

GENERAL MEASURES

- Closed reduction is generally not indicated prior to definitive treatment, unless the neurovascular structures or skin are compromised.
- If compromised, reduction of dislocation or deformity should be accomplished immediately by closed reduction using the L-H classification to reverse the order of injury or, if on the field, carefully attempt to restore anatomic alignment.
- Isolated, nondisplaced fractures can be considered for conservative treatment in a short-leg walking cast (1)[C],(4)[A].
- Use of a modified Jones compression dressing and posterior splint is important to reduce swelling. Severe or untreated swelling is associated with a poor surgical outcome.
- Compression dressing with frequent icing and elevation can allow for operative intervention in the first 2 to 3 days.

SURGERY/OTHER PROCEDURES

- Indications for surgical fixation are debated and varied.
- Most prominent indications are >25% of articular surface involvement, fragment displacement >2 mm, or joint instability (5)[C].
- If factors such as displacement of malleoli, talar subluxation, plafond articular incongruity, or syndesmotic instability exist, internal fixation is recommended.
- Surgical fixation of the posterior malleolus can restore up to 70% of syndesmotic stability compared to 40% from syndesmotic screw fixation without fracture fragment reduction (1)[B].
- Operative approaches, methods of fixation, and recovery times are similarly varied based on fracture characteristics and associated injuries.

ONGOING CARE

PROGNOSIS

- Posterior tubercle fractures adversely affect the prognosis of ankle fractures compared to single or bimalleolar fractures (1)[C],(4)[A],(6)[B].
- Although often used as an indication for surgery, the size of the posterior malleolar fragment is not strongly correlated to outcomes (4)[A].
- Factors such as fracture displacement, congruency of the articular surface, and residual tibiotalar subluxation are related to outcomes (4)[A].
- Overall incidence of posttraumatic osteoarthritis, including surgical and nonoperative management, is 33% (4)[A].

REFERENCES

1. Irwin TA, Lien J, Kadakia AR. Posterior malleolus fracture. *J Am Acad Orthop Surg*. 2013;21(1):32–40.
2. Haraguchi N, Haruyama H, Toga H, et al. Pathoanatomy of posterior malleolar fractures of the ankle. *J Bone Joint Surg Am*. 2006;88(5):1085–1092.
3. Terstegen J, Weel H, Frosch KH, et al. Classifications of posterior malleolar fractures: a systematic literature review. *Arch Orthop Trauma Surg*. 2023;143(7):4181–4220.
4. Odak S, Ahluwalia R, Unnikrishnan P, et al. Management of posterior malleolar fractures: a systematic review. *J Foot Ankle Surg*. 2016;55(1):140–145.
5. Bartoníček J, Rammelt S, Tuček M, et al. Posterior malleolar fractures of the ankle. *Eur J Trauma Emerg Surg*. 2015;41(6):587–600.
6. Kang C, Hwang DS, Lee JK, et al. Screw fixation of the posterior malleolus fragment in ankle fracture. *Foot Ankle Int*. 2019;40(11):1288–1294.

ADDITIONAL READING

- Clare MP. A rational approach to ankle fractures. *Foot Ankle Clin*. 2008;13(4):593–610.
- Stanitski CL. Pediatric and adolescent sports injuries. *Clin Sports Med*. 1997;16(4):613–633.
- van den Bekerom MPJ, Haverkamp D, Kloen P. Biomechanical and clinical evaluation of posterior malleolar fractures. A systematic review of the literature. *J Trauma*. 2009;66(1):279–284.
- Vander Griend RA, Savoie FH, Hughes JL. Fractures of the ankle. In: Rockwood CA Jr, Green DP, Bucholz RW, eds. *Rockwood and Green's Fractures in Adults*. Vol 2. 3rd ed. JB Lippincott; 1991:1983–2039.

CLINICAL PEARLS

- Volkmann fractures are avulsion fractures of the posterior lip of the tibia at its articular surface via a significant external rotation or abduction force through the PITFL.
- Lateral ankle radiographs generally show the PMF best and when found should prompt CT evaluation to assess the extent of articular involvement, size of the fragment, and integrity of the anterior tibiofibular joint.
- Indications for surgical fixation are debated, but most prominent indications are >25% of articular surface involvement, fragment displacement >2 mm, or joint instability.
- Because the PITFL accounts for 40% of syndesmotic stability, significant (>2 mm) displacement of the Volkmann fragment causes some syndesmotic instability and should prompt surgical evaluation and fixation. This is also why only isolated, nondisplaced posterior malleolus fractures should be considered for nonoperative management.

FRACTURE, ZYGOMA (ZF)

Jina Libby, DO, FAAPMR • Lawrence Chang, DO, MPH

BASICS

- Zygoma: major support between the maxilla and the skull (1)[B]
- Comprises of the lateral wall and floor of the orbit, the zygomatic arch, and malar eminence (1)[B]
- Zygoma fracture (ZF) results from any blunt trauma to the side *of the face.*

EPIDEMIOLOGY

- Second most common fracture of the face after nasal bone fractures (2)[B]
- Males > females (2)[B]
- 20 to 40 years old range (3)[B]
- Accidental falls more in older patients (3)[B]
- Professionals > amateurs
- Associated with substance abuse (3)[B]

ETIOLOGY AND PATHOPHYSIOLOGY

- Known as "cheek bone" or "malar bone"
- Found on anterior-lateral aspect of the face
- Posteriorly is the "zygomatic arch"—part of the temporal bone.
- Zygomatic bone and arch contain:
  - Zygomaticofacial and zygomaticotemporal arteries
  - Second division of the trigeminal nerve provides sensation to check and anterior temple.
  - Infraorbital nerve
  - Muscle attachments: the masseter, the zygomaticus major, and temporalis fascia
  - The Whitnall tubercle: maintains the eyelid contour
- The *direction* and *magnitude* of force are important factors (4)[B]:
  - A side blow directed posteriorly and medially causes a zygomatic body (tripod) fracture.
  - A lateral blow often results in an isolated zygomatic arch fracture.
- Any blow to the cheek potentially causes a ZF.
- Most common causes are:
  - Motor vehicle collisions (4)[B]
  - Falls (4)[B]
  - Physical assault (4)[B]
  - Sport injuries (4)[B]:
    - Combat sports (boxing, taekwondo, kickboxing, and Muay Thai) (5)[B]
    - Kickboxing causes the most maxillofacial injuries (5)[B].
    - Skiing, soccer, biking, and rugby has also shown to have high traumatic injury rates, including facial fractures (5)[B].
    - Blunt-force trauma from athletic equipment, including ball(s) or disc(s)

Pediatric Considerations

- Facial trauma is rarely seen in the pediatric population (6)[B].
- Children have a relatively larger cranium to facial skeleton, thus higher incidence of head trauma.
- Ages 12 to 18 years account for the majority of facial trauma in children (6)[B].
- Most common cause: motor vehicle accidents, sports, and bike riding(6)[B]

GENERAL PREVENTION

- Appropriate use of athletic helmet/face shield
- Safety apparel and protective guards during combat sports if facial injury is to be prevented (4)[B].
- Seatbelts and airbags use, although not prevalent in all countries (2)[B],(4)[B]
- Public/athletes education
- Workplace safety regulations (4)[B]

DIAGNOSIS

HISTORY

- Trauma: accident, physical assault, fall, sports injury
- Direct ocular injury or intraorbital hemorrhage
- Abnormal vision, diplopia
- Paresthesia of face in equivalent dermatome
- Periorbital edema
- Trismus—difficulty with mastication
- Abnormal bite (6)[B]
- Flattening of the cheek (4)[B]
- Epistaxis from ruptured maxillary sinus mucosa (6)[B]

PHYSICAL EXAM

- Evaluation for associated injuries (cervical spine, head, intracranial, globe, other maxillofacial bones, etc.) (4)[B]
- Mental status assessment (4)[B]
- Pain with palpation of zygoma/cheekbone (4)[B]
- Edema over the zygoma (4)[B]
- Maxillary vestibular edema (4)[B]
- Maxillary vestibular ecchymosis (4)[B]
- Ophthalmic evaluation:
  - Extraocular muscle movement abnormalities (4)[B]
  - Proptosis (4)[B]
  - Periorbital edema (4)[B]
  - Orbital dystopia (4)[B]
  - Subconjunctival hemorrhage (4)[B]
  - Enophthalmos—sunken eyes (4)[B]
  - Diplopia (4)[B]
  - Infraorbital nerve paresthesia (4)[B]
  - Maxillary branch of the trigeminal nerve injury causing upper lip numbness (6)[B]
- Crepitus from subcutaneous emphysema
- Proptosis and visual loss may occur with forceful nose blowing due to emphysema.
- Associated skull base fractures: Watch out for rhinorrhea (Halo test) (4)[B].
- Paranasal sinus fractures
- Trismus
- Flattening of the cheekbone: depression of malar eminence (4)[B]
- "Step off" palpable defect along the infraorbital rim (4)[B]
- Evaluate for other globe injuries.

Pediatric Considerations

- Sedation may be required to properly examine some children.
- If a head injury is suspected, sedation is not recommended.

DIFFERENTIAL DIAGNOSIS

- Other maxillary facial bone fractures and injuries
- Enophthalmos
- Floor orbital fracture
- Globe retraction
- Medial wall orbital fracture
- Facial contusions
- "Le Fort" fractures: transfacial fracture of the midface

DIAGNOSTIC TESTS & INTERPRETATION

- X-ray: first line (3)[B]
- Computed tomography (CT) scan of the face: gold standard (3)[B],(4)[B]
  - Consider brain and C-spine CT scan if concerned about associated injury (4)[B].
- Ultrasonography: useful as a screening
- Classification:
  - Type 1: isolated zygomatic arch fracture
  - Type 2: zygomaticomaxillary complex fracture (mechanical force applied in one direction)
  - Type 3: zygomaticomaxillary complex fracture (application of force in two directions)
  - Type 4: comminuted zygomatic arch fractures (6)[B]

TREATMENT

- Airway, breathing, circulation (ABCs) (4)[B]
- If there is bleeding, apply gentle pressure and elevate the head (4)[B].
- Avoid shifting or worsening the fracture position (4)[B].
- Closed ZF, displaced or nondisplaced, is stable for outpatient reduction in 1 to 3 days (4)[B].
- Isolated, nondisplaced zygomatic arch fractures may be treated nonoperatively (6)[B].
- Displaced zygomatic arch fractures typically require surgical treatment (6)[B].
- Surgical repair is recommended within 2 weeks of displaced fracture to avoid functional and aesthetic complications (6)[B].
- Avoidance of nose blowing is *mandatory* because air can be forced between the disrupted orbital walls into the retrobulbar space causing pain and permanent visual loss.
- Consider starting soft diet.
- Goal is restoration of:
  - Normal facial contour
  - Normal sensory nerve function
  - Normal globe position
  - Normal masticatory function
- Indications for surgical repair include:
  - Displacement or instability of the fracture
  - Mechanical restriction of mandibular movement (chewing)
  - Alteration in facial contour
  - Globe dystopia
  - Enophthalmos
  - Diplopia
  - Sensory nerve deficit

Pediatric Considerations

- Multiple injuries are often seen: head trauma, skull fracture, and orthopedic injuries.
- Definitive repair of facial fractures should not be delayed beyond 3 or 4 days.
- Facial bones heal rapidly in children.
- Delays >3 to 4 days can lead to malunion and cosmetic defect.

MEDICATION

- The treatment of zygomatic complex fractures is primarily surgical.
- Supportive treatment may include analgesics and nasal decongestants.
- The routine use of systemic antibiotics is not recommended.
- The efficacy and safety of perioperative intravenous corticosteroids are inconclusive.

ISSUES FOR REFERRAL

- Patients with altered mental status or intracranial involvement need emergent neurosurgical evaluation (4)[B]
- Patients with frontal bone fractures need to follow-up with a facial reconstructive surgeon (4)[B].

ONGOING CARE

PATIENT EDUCATION

- Avoid nose blowing for fear of orbital emphysema and potential blindness.
- Warn about signs and symptoms of orbital/retrobulbar hemorrhage.
- Advise patients to call the surgeon at any time if orbital bleeding is suspected.

PROGNOSIS

Favorable outcome includes:

- Early intervention especially in children
- Bony union
- Absence of skeletal or soft tissue deformity
- Normal range of mandibular movement

COMPLICATIONS

- Associated ophthalmic or intracranial trauma
- Ectropion
- Epiphora
- Cosmetic deformities such as cheek flatness (6)[B]
- Decreased mandibular movement (6)[B]
- Hypoesthesia of face
- Postoperative orbital hemorrhage: rare but may lead to permanent blindness
- Malunion from inadequately or unreduced zygomatic fracture

REFERENCES

1. Ali AAA. Epidemiological study of zygomatic fractures: a five-year retrospective analysis in a single hospital experience. *Egypt J Plast Reconstr Surg*. 2020;44(4):527–533.
2. Hanif S, Riaz N, Ehsan-Ul Haq M, et al. Frequency, etiology and presenting complaints associated with zygomatic complex fractures. *Pakistan J Ment Health Sci*. 2022;16(1):53–55.
3. Homer A, Homer B, Sullivan SR, et al. The natural history of treated and untreated zygomatic arch fractures. *J Craniofac Surg*. 2019;30(7):e631–e633.
4. Chukwulebe S, Hogrefe C. The diagnosis and management of facial bone fractures. *Emerg Med Clin North Am*. 2019;37(1):137–151.
5. Shirani G, Kalantar Motamedi MH, Ashuri A, et al. Prevalence and patterns of combat sport related maxillofacial injuries. *J Emerg Trauma Shock*. 2010;3(4):314–317.
6. Bukhsh A, Majrashi F, Almutairi A, et al. Epidemiology, classification and management of zygomatic fractures among children. *J Health Care Sci*. 2022;02(06):124–129.

CLINICAL PEARLS

- Suspect a ZF if blow to the side of the face.
- Consider coexisting ocular, head, and cervical spine injury.
- X-ray is used first but CT scan is the modality of choice.
- Tell the patient not to blow their nose for 10 days.
- Consult surgery if unstable ZF, worsening symptoms or simply if in doubt.

FREIBERG DISEASE

Christopher McGrew, MD, FACSM, CAQSM

BASICS

DESCRIPTION

- Osteonecrosis of the superior portion of the metatarsal head of unknown etiology
- Freiberg first described this entity in 1914, in six patients as an infraction (incomplete fracture without displacement of the fragments).
- Fourth most common osteochondrosis
- Affects women more commonly than men
- Synonym(s): Freiberg infraction; eggshell fracture; Koehler second disease; metatarsal flat-head; metatarsal epiphysitis; osteochondritis deformans metatarsojuvenilis

EPIDEMIOLOGY

- Incidence unknown
- Male:female ratio is 1:5.
- Peak onset around 11 to 17 years, but reported age range of 10 to 77 years
- Has been hypothesized that the condition is progressive, beginning in adolescence and remaining asymptomatic until later in life when symptoms occurs secondary to joint arthrosis
- Most common involvement is the 2nd metatarsal head, approximately 2/3 of cases.
- Second most common involvement is the 3rd metatarsal head, involved in 27% of cases.
- 4th and 5th metatarsal heads rarely involved
- Bilateral involvement is seen in <10% of cases.
- Usually affects the longest metatarsal
- Occasionally seen in sports requiring sprinting and jumping

ETIOLOGY AND PATHOPHYSIOLOGY

- No single clear etiologic factor exists.
- Several theories have been postulated:
  - Traumatic factors include metatarsal stress during normal activity and/or abnormal biomechanics of the forefoot intrinsically or as a result of footwear, causing repetitive microtrauma on the dorsal aspect of the distal metatarsal head.
  - Vascular factors include abnormal metatarsal head vascular variations as well as trauma-induced vessel damage, spasm, and eventual ischemia.
  - Mechanical factors include immobility of the 2nd metatarsal due to its "keystone" position at its articulation with the midfoot, a longer 2nd metatarsal, a short 1st metatarsal, a hypermobile 1st metatarsal, hallux abducto valgus (bunion), use of high-heeled shoes, and rapid weight gain.
  - Systemic factors are thought to be possible contributors including infection, endocrine disturbance, hormonal changes, osteopenia, steroid use, inflammatory diseases such as systemic lupus erythematous, and hypercoagulable states.

RISK FACTORS

- No known risk factors
- May be related to repetitive microtrauma versus vascular deficiency or both

DIAGNOSIS

HISTORY

- Slow development of significant, dull, aching pain over affected metatarsal head
- Patient may notice loss of range of motion.
- Pain increases with activity and motion.
- Pain worsens with weight-bearing, especially barefoot or in high-heeled footwear.
- Pain often relieved by rest, but pain may awaken patient from sleep.

PHYSICAL EXAM

- Surrounding soft tissue swelling
- Tenderness over affected metatarsal head
- May be painful with motion
- May be limited motion of metatarsophalangeal (MTP) joint
- Palpable bony prominences and crepitus possible in advanced disease
- Other foot deformities may be present such as hallux valgus.

DIFFERENTIAL DIAGNOSIS

- Fracture: acute or stress
- Tendonitis
- Capsulitis
- Septic joint
- Neuroma
- Gout
- Metatarsalgia

DIAGNOSTIC TESTS & INTERPRETATION

ALERT

Radiography normal in early stages:

- Asymmetric joint space widening may be seen 3 to 6 weeks following symptom onset, differentiating it from other arthritides whose characteristic finding involves joint space narrowing.
- As the disease progresses, osteonecrotic changes are seen on the superior/central head.
- Eventually, the superior/central head collapses and flattens.
- Medial and lateral dorsal osteophytes develop.
- Osteophytes may break free, becoming loose bodies, best seen on lateral oblique radiographs.
- Cystic changes may be seen in the head.
- The inferior portion of the metatarsal head is usually not involved.
- Radiographic staging of disease, based on correlation with Smillie classification:
  - Stage I: MTP joint space widening, with increased subchondral bone density
  - Stage II: metatarsal head flattening (anteroposterior view)
  - Stage III: collapse of the central portion of the dorsal part of the distal metatarsal head

- Stage IV: medial and lateral fractures of the projections of the remaining metatarsal head (multiple loose bodies in the joint)
- Stage V: complete loss of joint anatomy and integrity

- Three-phase bone scan in the early stages will reveal a photopenic area surrounded by a focal uptake. Later stages show generalized increased uptake of the entire affected metatarsal head (1)[C].
- Magnetic resonance imaging (MRI) has been purported to be the gold standard in early diagnosis of Freiberg as radiographs are often normal in the early stages.
- Early stages of Freiberg will have a hypointense signal on T1-weighted images and heterogeneous increased on T2-weighted images.
- In addition to MRI, 3D computed tomography (CT) scans have also been used to determine the exact Smillie stage and aid in preoperative planning.

TREATMENT

GENERAL MEASURES

Nonoperative management should be the first line of treatment regardless of stage at time of presentation.

ALERT

Goal is to restrict weight-bearing for a sufficient time to allow healing to take place.

- Immediate cessation of sports and high-impact activities
- Use of crutches to restrict weight-bearing may be indicated in early stages when most painful.
- As symptoms subside, may progressively bear weight with use of metatarsal pads, bars, and/or a custom orthosis
- Occasionally may need a walking boot or short-leg walking cast with a toe plate
- By restricting weight-bearing, the lesion may heal over a period of 6 to 12 weeks.
- Return to sports when asymptomatic with custom foot orthosis
- Operative treatment indicated if nonoperative treatment fails or if disease is advanced
- Smillie stages I to III have a good chance of success with nonoperative, conservative management.
- Smillie stages IV to V are more likely to require operative management.
- There is a wide range of surgical procedures described in the literature for management of Freiberg.
- Joint-preserving procedures are typically performed in the early stages of disease, whereas joint-destructive procedures are reserved for advanced stages (2)[A].

MEDICATION

Symptomatic treatment with acetaminophen or short-term nonsteroidal anti-inflammatory drugs (NSAIDs) as indicated (3)[C]

ISSUES FOR REFERRAL

Orthopedic surgery or podiatry referral indicated if nonoperative treatment fails or if disease is advanced

SURGERY/OTHER PROCEDURES

- Surgery is reserved for those patients who fail conservative therapies or those with late stage and demonstrated degenerative joint progression.
- Examples of joint-sparing procedures include core decompression, bone grafting, metatarsal osteotomies, joint débridement, and microfracture surgery.
- Examples of joint-destructive procedures include arthroplasty, implant arthroplasty, interpositional arthroplasty, metatarsal head resection, and osteochondral distal metatarsal allograft replacement.

ONGOING CARE

FOLLOW-UP RECOMMENDATIONS

No standard return to participation protocol has been established. Protocol should be individualized and based on radiographic confirmation of healing as well as symptom resolution.

PATIENT EDUCATION

Patient education should focus on the need for activity modification and a functional symptom-based rehabilitation program.

PROGNOSIS

- For most nondegenerative lesions, conservative therapy is likely to lead to healing and resolution of symptoms.
- Current surgical procedures are demonstrating satisfactory results but continue to be an investigative topic.

COMPLICATIONS

Joint degeneration or destruction with resultant chronic pain and/or loss of function

REFERENCES

1. Talusan PG, Diaz-Collado PJ, Reach JS Jr. Freiberg's infraction: diagnosis and treatment. *Foot Ankle Spec.* 2014;7(1):52–56.
2. Alhadhoud MA, Alsiri NF, Daniels TR, et al. Surgical interventions of Freiberg's disease: a systematic review. *Foot Ankle Surg.* 2021;27(6):606–614.
3. Seybold JD, Zide JR. Treatment of Freiberg disease. *Foot Ankle Clin.* 2018;23(1):157–169.

ADDITIONAL READING

- Ishimatsu T, Yoshimura I, Kanazawa K, et al. Return to sporting activity after osteochondral autograft transplantation for Freiberg disease in young athletes. *Arch Orthop Trauma Surg.* 2017;137(7):959–965.
- Pereira BS, Frada T, Freitas D, et al. Long-term follow-up of dorsal wedge osteotomy for pediatric Freiberg disease. *Foot Ankle Int.* 2016;37(1):90–95.
- Wax A, Leland R. Friberg disease and avascular necrosis of the metatarsal heads. *Foot Ankle Clin.* 2019;24(1):69–82.

CLINICAL PEARLS

Typical presentation is an adolescent female in a growth spurt who presents with forefoot pain with walking or activity.

GANGLION CYST

Michael Jake Peterson, MD • Daniel C. Herman, MD, PhD, FAAPMR, FACSM, FISBS, CAQSM • Alexandra E. Warrick, MD, CAQSM

BASICS

DESCRIPTION

- Benign fluid-filled cysts overlying a joint or tendon sheath that contains a mucinous, gelatinous fluid
- Synovial tissue has been seen under electron microscopy at the base of ganglions (1).
- Most commonly arise in the wrist and hand but can occur less commonly at other joints such as the knee and foot or arise from tendon sheaths (1)
- Sites:
  - 60–70% are found on dorsum of the wrist.
  - 13–20% are found on volar aspect of the wrist.
  - 10% are found arising from the tendon sheath of the hand.
  - 10% are found elsewhere.
- Another term for ganglion cysts at the distal interphalangeal (DIP) joints of the fingers is mucous cysts. These are associated with Heberden nodules, which are signs of osteoarthritis, and are most commonly found in women 40 to 70 years old.

EPIDEMIOLOGY

- Most common soft tissue mass found within the hand or wrist (accounts for 60–70% total)
- Usually arises between 2nd and 5th decades of life
- Female > male predominance with reported ratio ranging from 2:1 to 3:1. This is also true in the pediatric population (1).

ETIOLOGY AND PATHOPHYSIOLOGY

- The etiology is currently unknown, but several theories exist.
- The most modern theory is that chronic and repetitive microtrauma results in mucinous degeneration of fibrous tissue. The proposed pathophysiology behind this is that the repetitive microtrauma stimulates fibroblasts to produce hyaluronic acid which accumulates and forms the mucin of the cyst (1).
- Another theory is that the herniation of capsular synovium forms the ganglion cysts (1).

RISK FACTORS

Sports such as gymnastics with repetitive microtrauma and strain of the hands and wrists

DIAGNOSIS

HISTORY

- Typically presents with a painless cyst over a joint or tendon sheath.
- If compression of local structures such as nerves or arteries is occurring, they can present with pain, numbness, decreased range of motion, or, rarely, weakness.
- If pain is present, most patients rate it as mild and report that it is bothersome rather than debilitating.
- Patients may report concern about the cosmetic appearance or concern that it is a malignant tumor, when it is a benign growth.
- Ganglion cysts can enlarge over time or remain stable in size.

PHYSICAL EXAM

- Firm, smooth, mobile, well-circumscribed mass usually 1 to 3 cm in size
- Typically fixed to deeper structures as opposed to the skin
- Ganglion cysts associated with joints can be made more prominent with flexion of the joint away from the cyst.
- Readily transilluminates
- No warmth or erythema

DIFFERENTIAL DIAGNOSIS

- Epidermal inclusion cyst
- Lipoma
- Rheumatoid nodule
- Tophus
- Infectious tenosynovitis
- Tenosynovial giant cell tumor
- Synovial sarcoma
- Aneurysmal bone cyst
- Simple bone cyst
- Chondroblastoma
- Chondromyxoid fibroma
- Enchondroma
- Nonossifying fibroma
- Osteoid osteoma
- Osteoblastoma

DIAGNOSTIC TESTS & INTERPRETATION

- Diagnosis is clinical and imaging is not typically necessary.
- Imaging is typically used in patients with atypical presentations of symptoms or with entrapment at unusual sites (2)[A].
- Radiographs are generally unremarkable but can be used to rule out any underlying related osseous abnormality.
- On magnetic resonance imaging (MRI), intraneural ganglion cysts have a hypointense appearance on T1 sequences and a hyperintense appearance on T2-weighted sequences (2)[A].
- Of note, there are several signs on MRI that can be helpful in further characterizing ganglion cysts and include the signet ring sign, transverse limb sign, and tail sign (2)[A].
- Ultrasound imaging shows an anechoic, cystic fluid collection that is nonvascular; ultrasound can help to visualize adjacent neurovasculature, particularly on the volar aspect of the wrist (2)[A].
- Postoperative imaging is rarely performed and its clinical utility is unknown (2)[A].

TREATMENT

GENERAL MEASURES

- Explain that spontaneous resolution of untreated ganglion cysts ranges from 40% to 58% and that will often correlate with the volume of activity (resolve with decreased repetitive activity) (3)[A].
- Invasive measures such as injections and surgery may be unnecessary.
- Reassure on the benign nature of the cyst.

MEDICATION

No medications have shown any efficacy in treating ganglion cysts.

SURGERY/OTHER PROCEDURES

- Aspiration:
  - Aspiration of ganglion cysts provides short term improvement; however recurrence rates are high ranging from 35% to 69% (4)[A].
  - Aspiration is performed with a larger bore needle as the mucinous contents are thick and may not easily be aspirated through a small gauge needle.
  - Local anesthetic infiltration is used at designated aspiration sites prior to large gauge needle insertion.
  - Multiple punctures of ganglion cysts during aspiration has not been shown to reduce recurrence rate (4)[A].
  - Complications other than recurrence from aspiration include infection and damage to nearby structures (most commonly median nerve and radial artery injury for volar wrist ganglion cysts).
  - A high degree of caution is exercised before aspirating volar wrist cysts adjacent to the radial artery even with ultrasound guidance and not advisable if there are safety risks to the neurovasculature.
  - Ultrasound-guided aspiration can be used to reduce but not eliminate the risk of damaging nearby structures.
- Injection:
  - Many studies have investigated the effectiveness of aspiration and injection of ganglion cysts with different substances such as alcohol, antibiotics, hypertonic saline, anesthetic agents, phenol, corticosteroids, hyaluronidase, sodium tetradecyl sulfate, but none showed improved outcomes, and many had higher risks of complications (5)[C].
- Thread technique:
  - Threading of a ganglion cyst with sutures at right angles whose ends are tied together then subsequently massaging the area at different intervals has been tried as an alternative treatment method in the past, but has a high risk of infection and high recurrence rates and has fallen out of favor.
- Surgery:
  - Surgical removal of ganglion cysts has the lowest rate of recurrence but has a slightly higher complication risk than aspiration.
  - Intraoperative findings of ganglion cysts with joint connections is more likely if preoperative imaging is done (2)[A].
  - A technique developed by Angelides and Wallace is considered to be the most effective surgical technique: It removes the entire cyst, stalk, and pedicle, as well as any attachments to nearby structures or joints as well as a small segment of an associated joint capsule (3)[A].
  - Recurrence rates using the Angelides and Wallace technique range from 1% to 31% (3)[A].
  - Arthroscopic approach is preferred over open excision as studies have demonstrated a statistically significant lower rate of recurrence (9.4% compared to 11.2%) and complications (0–8.5% vs. 0–28%).
  - Complications from surgery include wound infection, neuroma formation, scar, keloid, and damage to nearby structures such as median nerve or radial artery for volar ganglion cysts.
  - Complication rates for volar wrist ganglion cysts are higher than dorsal wrist ganglion cysts because of the proximity of the median nerve and radial artery.

Pediatric Considerations

- Overall, the literature supports observation as initial management and advancing to further medical treatment when there is significant pain and/or decreased range of motion. There is no treatment algorithm consensus.
- Observation results in spontaneous resolution in 64–83% of cases over 4 months to 5 years with most self-resolving within 2 years.
- Volar wrist ganglions are more likely to self-resolve than dorsal wrist ganglions.
- Aspiration has limited data as children have more difficulty tolerating the procedure. One small case series reported an 86% success with aspiration followed by triamcinolone acetonide injection, but one quarter of the patients had a persistent sclerotic lump for 6 months.
- Surgical excision is indicated for pain or decreased range of motion. Recurrence rates vary between 3% and 28.5% over 4 months to 11 years. Lower rates were achieved with excision of volar wrist ganglions compared to dorsal and/or when the ganglion and stalk were excised in their entirety. Complications are similar in adults but have lower reported rates ranging from 5.5% to 8.7%.
- Arthroscopic resection is not routinely done. There is one published study that consisted of eight patients with an average age of 15 years where only one patient (11%) had recurrence after 3 years.

REFERENCES

1. Zhou J, Al-Ani S, Jester A, et al. Wrist ganglion cysts in children: an update and review of the literature. *Hand (N Y)*. 2022;17(6):1024–1030.
2. Lenartowicz KA, Wolf AS, Desy NM, et al. Preoperative imaging of intraneural ganglion cysts: a critical systematic analysis of the world literature. *World Neurosurg*. 2022;166:e968–e979.
3. Clark DM, Nelson SY, O'Hara M, et al. Surgical and patient-centered outcomes of open versus arthroscopic ganglion cyst excision: a systematic review. *J Wrist Surg*. 2022;12(1):32–39.
4. Suen M, Fung B, Lung CP. Treatment of ganglion cysts. *ISRN Orthop*. 2013;2013:940615.
5. Kuliński S, Gutkowaska O, Gosk J. Chemical substances used in the treatment of ganglions located in the hand and wrist. *Polim Med*. 2016;46(1):95–100.

G

CLINICAL PEARLS

- Ganglion cysts are benign fluid-filled cysts overlying a joint or tendon sheath, most commonly the wrist or hand that contain a mucinous, gelatinous fluid.
- Diagnosis is clinical and imaging is typically only needed to rule out other potentially concerning diagnoses or plan for surgery if needed.
- Spontaneous resolution of untreated ganglion cysts ranges from 40% to 58%.
- Aspiration of ganglion cysts will decrease the size of a cyst in the short term; however, recurrence rate is high ranging from 35% to 69%.
- Surgical removal of ganglion cysts has the lowest rate of recurrence but has slightly higher complication risk than aspiration. In adults, arthroscopic resection has lower rates of recurrence and complications compared to open excision.

GLENOHUMERAL DISLOCATION, ANTERIOR

Argin Haritounian, DO ▪ Bernadette Pendergraph, MD

BASICS

DESCRIPTION

- Humeral head is displaced anteriorly beyond the glenoid fossa due to external rotation while arm is in abduction (1).
- Direct contact to the posterior shoulder less common mechanism (2)

EPIDEMIOLOGY

- Most dislocated major joint; 50% of all dislocations are of the shoulder with an incidence rate of 23.9 per 100,000 person-years (1).
- Bimodal incidence with peaks in the 2nd and 6th decades of life (1)
- 96% of glenohumeral dislocations are anterior (2).
- Most common complication related to dislocation is recurrent glenohumeral instability, ranging from 14% to 100%, depending on age of first dislocation and continued risky behavior (3).

RISK FACTORS

- History of previous dislocation (1)
- Generalized ligamentous laxity (3)
- Sports such as wrestling, football, rugby, skiing, and skateboarding

COMMONLY ASSOCIATED CONDITIONS

- Bankart lesions: detachment of inferior glenohumeral ligament-labral complex from anterior glenoid rim; very common in younger patients; strongly associated with dislocation recurrence (1),(3)
- Rotator cuff tears: Between 14% and 63% of anterior dislocations are associated with rotator cuff tears, often subscapularis, with increasing frequency in older individuals (1),(3).
- Fractures: Humeral head and neck (significant displacement may be a contraindication to closed reduction), glenoid rim (bony Bankart), and greater tuberosity avulsions; seen especially with traumatic etiology (3),(4)
- Hill-Sachs lesion: depression fracture of posterolateral humeral head. In patients <40 years old, >50% of anterior dislocations are associated with this type of lesion (1),(2),(4).
- Neurologic injury: common complication with 10% suffering injury to the axillary nerve. Less frequently injured are the brachial plexus or musculocutaneous nerve (2). Most often, these injuries recover spontaneously.
- Vascular injury: infrequent complication (1–2%), axillary artery most frequently injured in anterior dislocation, higher incidence in older individuals given the loss of arterial elasticity secondary to atherosclerosis (2)

DIAGNOSIS

HISTORY

- Often occurs after a fall on the outstretched arm or with reaching (making a tackle) and having arm forcibly abducted (1)
- First time event versus recurrence (may affect ease of reduction and long-term treatment plan) (1)
- Amount of trauma involved (traumatic vs. atraumatic) can give clues as to whether there is a component of ligamentous instability (2).
- Duration shoulder has been dislocated (helps in decision concerning analgesia) (2).

PHYSICAL EXAM

- Anterior fullness of the shoulder (1),(2)
- Forearm of affected arm often cradled with shoulder in an internally rotated, partially adducted position (3).
- Perform distal neurovascular exam, both before and after reduction to check for previously mentioned neurovascular injuries (3).
- Check deltoid muscle strength and lateral shoulder sensation to assess axillary nerve function (former not always practical prior to reduction of dislocated shoulder) (2).
- Check proximal and distal muscle function and (if no obvious deformity is present) range of motion (active and passive) before and after relocation (1),(2).
- No crepitus should be felt or heard during relocation. Some special exam maneuvers such as a sulcus sign, load and shift, and apprehension test may not be appropriate to perform in the acute setting.

DIFFERENTIAL DIAGNOSIS

- Acute glenohumeral subluxation
- Acromioclavicular joint separation
- Fractures of humeral head, coracoid, acromion, proximal humerus, clavicle, rib
- Rotator cuff injury
- Posterior dislocation

DIAGNOSTIC TESTS & INTERPRETATION

- Acute traumatic shoulder dislocations are evaluated with a trauma series that includes an axillary view, a trans-scapular (Y) lateral view, and a true shoulder anterior-posterior view (1)[A],(2)[C].
- Standard anteroposterior: head of humerus displaced medially on glenoid; difficult to distinguish anterior from posterior dislocations (2)[C]
- True lateral (trans-scapular [Y]) view: humeral head displaced toward coracoid process
- Axillary view: allows easier visualization of associated injuries but requires movement of an already uncomfortable patient. A Velpeau view is an alternative if axillary view cannot be accomplished.
- West Point view (reverse axillary lateral) helps in showing bony Bankart lesions (1)[A].
- Stryker notch view (anteroposterior internal rotation of humerus) good to demonstrate Hill-Sachs deformity
- Computed tomography (CT) scan is used for fracture/dislocation to quantify loss of glenoid bone. Bone loss >7 mm in width or >20–30% of total glenoid surface area is associated with recurrent glenohumeral instability (4)[C].
- Magnetic resonance imaging (MRI) can evaluate for soft tissue injuries but may miss bony abnormalities. MRI arthrogram may further evaluate the surrounding ligaments (labrum ligamentous complex).
- Point-of-care ultrasound (POCUS) can identify glenohumeral joint dislocation and reduction with 100% sensitivity and specificity (5)[A].

TREATMENT

- Analgesia often not needed if reduction is performed immediately after dislocation (1)[A],(2)[A].
- Verbal coaching to help relax the patient is helpful.
- Analgesic and benzodiazepine medications may be required, if reductions are not performed early, to relax spasm and ease relocation (1)[A],(4)[C].
- Some sources recommend local glenohumeral joint anesthesia using 10 to 20 mL of 1% lidocaine (4)[C].

ALERT

Intra-articular lidocaine has been shown to have similar relocation success rates versus intravenous (IV) analgesia and sedation, and a significant decrease in cost and length of stay in the emergency department, although patient satisfaction tends to be higher with the use of IV agents (2)[A].

- Reduction techniques:
  - Traction methods: Stimson (prone traction with weight applied to arm hanging down). Success rate: not reported; supine traction/countertraction (gentle traction at 45 degrees of abduction while countertraction applied with folded sheet under axilla); success rate: not reported
  - Leverage methods: Kocher (with patient supine, flex elbow to 90 degrees, adduction, externally rotate arm, and forward flexion of the shoulder); success rate: 81–100%
  - Axillary pressure by assistant's hand may help guide the humeral head over the glenoid.
  - Combination methods: Milch: Stabilize the humeral head, fully abduct the arm, apply traction, and push humeral head over glenoid rim. Success rate: 70–100%; scapular manipulation: patient prone or seated with arm at 90 degrees of flexion with mild traction applied (10 to 15 lb), apply medially directed force to inferolateral border of scapula; may also do when patient is supine to assist with other techniques; success rate: 79–96%

- Self-reduction techniques are also available and are highly successful if used early and for recurrent dislocations. Manual assist can also help. The best technique described is to have the patient lock hands in front of ipsilateral knee and relax backward allowing gentle traction with the relaxation of shoulder muscles.
- Experience, familiarity, and available resources (time and help) are important considerations when deciding which technique to use (1)[A].
- Postreduction:
  - Recheck neurovascular exam and rotator cuff; postreduction radiographs (2)[A]
  - Controversy exists as to best approach to post dislocation management, but many authors at this time would recommend immobilization in a sling for comfort about 1 week, followed by range-of-motion exercises and then progression to strengthening exercises, with an emphasis placed on periscapular muscle strengthening. Shorter immobilization period decreases the risk of adhesive capsulitis in the older patient (aged >30 years) (1)[A].
  - Although still controversial, immobilization in external rotation may decrease recurrence of primary shoulder dislocation by 44% compared to immobilization in internal rotation for individuals 20 to 40 years of age (6)[A].
  - Immobilization theoretically allows time for "scarring" of injured anterior structures and healing of pathologic lesions (2)[A].
  - Contraindications to closed reduction:
    - Humeral head and neck fractures
    - Significantly displaced (<1 cm) greater tuberosity fractures
    - Severe scapula fractures
    - Intrathoracic humeral head fractures

ADDITIONAL THERAPIES

- Early range of motion in older patients (aged >30 years) to prevent adhesive capsulitis (3)[C]
- Strengthening of rotator cuff muscles and scapular stabilizers help in maintaining dynamic stability (1)[A].
- Most helpful in nontraumatic dislocations in patients who have multidirectional instability or generalized ligamentous laxity (traumatic unilateral Bankart lesions, surgery [TUBS] vs. atraumatic, multidirectional, bilateral shoulders, rehabilitation, inferior capsular shift [AMBRI]).
- Glenohumeral joint stability braces aid in return to play and prevention of recurrence (1)[A],(3)[C].

SURGERY/OTHER PROCEDURES

- Surgical stabilization recommended for many athletic first-time dislocators, especially if "throwing shoulder, younger athletes, or participation in high-risk sports" (1)[A],(2)[A].
- Surgery recommended for those with recurrent dislocations, especially if the episodes appear to require less "trauma" than prior episodes (1)[A],(2)[A]
- Surgery likely needed for large Hill-Sachs deformity involving 20–40% of the anterior articular surface (3)[C]
- Most athletes return to sport 4 to 6 months following surgical stabilization (2)[A].

ONGOING CARE

- No clear data to guide safe to return to sport, but most experts recommend when pain free, functional range of motion, symmetrical rotator cuff strength, and bilateral scapular strength (2)[A].
- Recurrence:
  - Risk factors for recurrent instability: male, age ≤40 years and hyperlaxity (1)[A]
  - Ongoing instability can result in glenohumeral bone loss and articular damage leading to osteoarthritis and chronic instability (3)[C].

ALERT
Athletes returning to play with history of instability are at risk for recurrence, with one study showing 37% incidence of repeat dislocation during the ongoing season (2)[A].

- There is 39% chance of recurrent instability after sustaining a traumatic shoulder dislocation, but recurrence rate varies inversely with age.
- Up to 95% recurrence in athletic patients with initial dislocation at <20 years old without surgical intervention (1)[A],(2)[A]
- Presence of a Hills-Sachs lesion associated with recurrent dislocation (1)[A]

FOLLOW-UP RECOMMENDATIONS

- Growing consensus for early arthroscopic stabilization after primary anterior shoulder dislocation in young athletic patients (15 to 25 years old) unwilling to modify their risk factors because numerous studies have shown a high rate of recurrence in nonoperative treated subjects in this group; often procedure delayed until post season.
- When surgically stabilized, athletes show significant decreased rates of dislocation recurrence and higher return to sports (2)[A].
- Recurrent instability patients likely to benefit from orthopedic referral for arthroscopic or open surgical repair as warranted
- Patients with multidirectional instability should be treated with traditional methods, although surgical repair may be necessary with recurrences.
- Early sports medicine referral indicated for all except uncomplicated, recurrent anterior dislocations (Recurrent anterior dislocation patients should be referred to orthopedic surgery.)
- Orthopedic referral indicated for humeral head or neck fractures and irreducible dislocations

REFERENCES

1. Alkaduhimi H, van der Linde JA, Flipsen M, et al. A systematic and technical guide on how to reduce a shoulder dislocation. *Turk J Emerg Med*. 2016;16(4):155–168.
2. Cutteridge J, Dixon J, Garrido P, et al. A systematic review and meta-analysis of operative versus non-operative management for first time traumatic anterior shoulder dislocation in young adults. *Shoulder Elbow*. 2025;17(2):130–139.
3. Baker HP, Krishnan P, Meghani O, et al. Protective sport bracing for athletes with mid-season shoulder instability. *Sports Health*. 2023;15(1):105–110.
4. Bao MH, DeAngelis JP, Wu JS. Imaging of traumatic shoulder injuries—understanding the surgeon's perspective. *Eur J Radiol Open*. 2022;9:100411.
5. Gottlieb M, Patel D, Marks A, et al. Ultrasound for the diagnosis of shoulder dislocation and reduction: a systematic review and meta-analysis. *Acad Emerg Med*. 2022;29(8):999–1007.
6. Shinagawa K, Sugawara Y, Hatta T, et al. Immobilization in external rotation reduces the risk of recurrence after primary anterior shoulder dislocation: a meta-analysis. *Orthop J Sports Med*. 2020;8(6):2325967120925694.

ADDITIONAL READING

- Eljabu W, Klinger HM, von Knoch M. The natural course of shoulder instability and treatment trends: a systematic review. *J Orthop Traumatol*. 2017;18(1):1–8.
- Hasebroock AW, Brinkman J, Foster L, et al. Management of primary anterior shoulder dislocations: a narrative review. *Sports Med Open*. 2019;5(1):31.
- Watson S, Allen B, Grant JA. A clinical review of return-to-play considerations after anterior shoulder dislocation. *Sports Health*. 2016;8(4):336–341.

CLINICAL PEARLS

- Understand patient subtypes: Patient history helps classify the instability and guide treatment. The two classic types are:
  - **TUBS**: These patients typically have a history of a specific traumatic dislocation, and their instability is in one direction. They often have a Bankart lesion and usually respond best to surgical repair.
  - **AMBR**: These patients often have looser joints without a specific major injury, and their shoulders are unstable in multiple directions. The primary treatment is an intensive rehabilitation program.
- High-risk population: Young male athletes (<20 years of age) who suffer a traumatic dislocation have an extremely high recurrence rate (up to 95%) without surgical stabilization.
- **Prereduction checklist**: Always perform a thorough neurovascular exam (especially checking the axillary nerve) before and after reduction. Do not attempt a closed reduction if a significant fracture is suspected.
- **Reduction technique**: No single reduction method is universally superior. The best technique is the one with which the clinician is most familiar and comfortable.
- **Immobilization**: For patients aged 20 to 40 years who are managed nonsurgically, consider immobilizing the shoulder in external rotation, as this may reduce the risk of recurrence compared to a traditional sling.

GLENOHUMERAL DISLOCATION, POSTERIOR

Vincent Marshall, DO ▪ Benjamin L. Boswell, DO

BASICS

DESCRIPTION

- A posterior glenohumeral dislocation (PGHD) occurs when the humeral head disarticulates from the glenoid and rests posteriorly to its normally seated position on the glenoid.
- Glenohumeral (GH) instability is classified by:
  - Mechanism (traumatic or atraumatic)
  - Direction (anterior, posterior, superior, inferior, or multidirectional)
  - Circumstance (acute, chronic, or recurrent)
  - Degree (subluxation or dislocation)
- Other names:
  - Posterior shoulder dislocation

EPIDEMIOLOGY

- Glenohumeral dislocation (GHD) is frequent, but PGHD is rare, with an incidence of 1–4% of all GHD (1). Approximately 15% of these cases involve bilateral shoulders.
- The highest incidence is in males aged 35 to 55 years.
- Diagnosis can be a challenge: Sometimes, it can be omitted due to incorrect diagnosis, absence of consideration in differential diagnosis, suboptimal radiographic evaluation, and absence of characteristic signs and symptoms; missed diagnosis reaches 60–79%, and the diagnosis can delay from 24 hours to a year (1).
- Extremely rare in pediatrics because force necessary to cause a dislocation will instead cause a proximal humerus fracture

ETIOLOGY AND PATHOPHYSIOLOGY

- In the absence of trauma, posterior dislocations occur most often because of a seizure (contraction of the internal rotators) or electrocution.
- Traumatic dislocation can occur when an axial load is applied to the upper extremity in the "at-risk" position: forward flexion, adduction, and internal rotation.
- Injury can occur in athletes with a fall on a flexed elbow and adducted arm or by a direct axial load to the humerus.

RISK FACTORS

- The "Es" of posterior shoulder dislocation: epilepsy, electrocution, or extreme trauma
- History of posterior shoulder dislocation or instability
- Disorders such as Charcot shoulder and Ehlers-Danlos syndrome have been well documented.
- Congenital anomalies, such as scapular aplasia, increase the risk of dislocation.
- Glenoid hypoplasia and excessive glenoid retroversion increase risk.
- At-risk sports/positions for posterior instability and/or dislocation include offensive linemen in American football with arms in blocking position, backhand stroke in racquet sports, pull-through phase of swimming, and follow-through phase in golf or throwing motion (2)[C].
- The group aged 15 to 19 years was at the highest risk for recurrent dislocations and instability (3)[C].
- Gender was not a significant predictor of instability (3)[C].

GENERAL PREVENTION

- Rotator-cuff strength and control
- General muscle strength
- Overall core stability

COMMONLY ASSOCIATED CONDITIONS

- Multiple trauma
- Epilepsy
- Connective tissue disorders
- Scapular dysplasia
- Scapular dyskinesia

DIAGNOSIS

HISTORY

- Traumatic mechanism of injury is generally direct trauma to anterior aspect of shoulder.
- Epileptic or electrocution event with complaint of shoulder pain and inability to range GH joint
- Direction of applied force and position of the arm (the "at-risk" position)
- Can be acute or chronic
- History of previous injury or pain in affected shoulder
- Previous or present description of pain, including location, intensity, and duration
- Previous or present history of tingling, weakness, catching, and locking
- Any aggravating or alleviating factors

PHYSICAL EXAM

- Severe shoulder pain that increases with movement
- An arm held in internal rotation and adduction
- Key feature: External rotation is blocked, a critical feature of the examination that should raise suspicion.
- Prominence in the posterior aspect of the shoulder with flattening of the normal anterior contour of the deltoid
- There may be prominence of the coracoid process and squaring off the anterolateral acromion.
- The humeral head may be visible or palpable posteriorly.
- Routine observation, gentle palpation, range of motion, and strength of the affected extremity should be performed.
- Limitation with passive external rotation and abduction may be noted.

ALERT

It is of utmost importance to monitor the neurovascular status of the affected arm. Injury to the axillary vessels is rare but potentially catastrophic.

- Although neurovascular compromise is less common than with anterior shoulder dislocation, the axillary nerve is most commonly injured and results in shoulder badge weakness and numbness. This usually resolves without intervention.
- Evaluate for atrophy of posterior rotator cuff muscles as an indication of chronic posterior instability.
- Assess for generalized ligamentous laxity.
- Scapulothoracic mechanics and rhythm should be observed if position not "fixed."

DIFFERENTIAL DIAGNOSIS

- Acute subluxation
- Anterior shoulder dislocation
- Fractures (clavicle, scapula, and humerus)
- Rotator cuff pathology (strain, partial or complete tear)
- Adhesive capsulitis/frozen shoulder
- Acromioclavicular joint pathology
- Intra-articular pathology (labral, glenoid, or ligamentous)
- Scapular winging/instability

DIAGNOSTIC TESTS & INTERPRETATION

Initial Tests (lab, imaging)

Plain radiographs for a suspected posterior shoulder dislocation should include an anteroposterior (AP) view, a transscapular lateral view (Y view), and a modified axillary view.

ALERT

Evidence of posterior dislocation on a standard AP view is subtle and may be undiagnosed in 50% of cases.

- The normal lateral projection of the greater tuberosity in the AP view is lost in a posterior shoulder dislocation.
- The anterior aspect of the humeral head becomes impacted against the posterior rim of the glenoid, causing a compression fracture on the anterior aspect of the humeral head. This causes a reverse Hill-Sachs lesion that gives the appearance of a "trough sign" on the radiographic AP view.
- With disarticulation of the humeral head posteriorly, the anterior rim of the glenoid is void of the humeral head, which is displaced medial to the glenoid convexity. This is visualized best with the radiographic axillary view.
- Axillary view is helpful for evaluating glenoid rim fracture and morphology (hypoplasia, retroversion).
- Bedside ultrasound has a very high sensitivity and specificity, approaching 100% in some studies (4)[B].
- US reduces time to diagnosis and time to reduction and is valuable in confirming reduction immediately, especially when procedural sedation is used (4).

Follow-Up Tests & Special Considerations

Advanced imaging (computed tomography [CT], magnetic resonance imaging [MRI], or arthrography) should be reserved for evaluating the extent of associated humeral head fractures/impression defect, glenoid fractures, rotator cuff tears, labral pathologies, morphology of the glenoid, and articular surface integrity. However, if surgery is warranted, CT scan for preoperative planning is acceptable (2)[B].

TREATMENT

GENERAL MEASURES

- Expedited reduction is key. Delay in reduction leads to worsening muscle spasm and tightness, making reduction attempts more difficult.
- Early attempts at reduction should be performed in all cases, except if associated fractures of the anatomic or surgical neck of the humerus.
- On-field or sideline reduction attempts are associated with risk because there may be an associated fracture.
- Closed reduction attempts should only be attempted if posterior dislocation has been present for 3 weeks or less.
- At times, reduction may be delayed due to multiple traumatic injuries, hemodynamic instability, or other comorbidities.
- Multiple factors influence the choice of anesthesia. For example, a patient with multiple dislocations and shoulder instability may only require pain management with opioids, whereas a first-time dislocation with delayed time to reduction attempt may require procedural sedation.

- Intra-articular lidocaine for anesthesia has been used in anterior dislocation reduction and has shown similar effectiveness to procedural sedation. This method could be used in posterior dislocation reductions when sedation is not feasible or presents too many risks (5).
- Procedural sedation or general anesthesia may be necessary if a gentle and atraumatic reduction cannot be obtained.
- With the patient supine, gentle longitudinal traction is applied to the affected arm while the elbow is flexed at 90 degrees. Countertraction used with a sheet wrapped around patient's chest by an assistant is often necessary. While traction is applied, gentle internal rotation of the arm often unlocks the humeral head from the rim of the glenoid. It may also be necessary to use direct anterolateral pressure on the humeral head to unlock it from the glenoid rim.
- An alternative technique is to apply gentle internal rotation and lateral traction to disimpact the humeral head.
- If dislocation is seen hours or even days after occurring, it may be impossible to reduce nonsurgically.
- If an atraumatic reduction cannot be achieved, reduction in the operating room under general anesthesia should be considered.
- Open reduction should also be considered for persistent dislocation (>6 weeks), chronic dislocations, and humeral head compression fracture with involvement >25%.
- Associated fractures also may require operative intervention, and open reduction may be necessary.
- Confirm intact neurovascular status after any reduction attempt.
- Obtain postreduction radiographs to confirm reduction and to evaluate humeral or glenoid fractures.
- Consider repeating physical exam, taking care not to cause repeat dislocation.

ALERT
Immobilization should not include the use of a sling and swathe because internal rotation should be avoided.

- Immobilize in neutral to external rotation, allowing for healing of the posterior capsulolabral complex.
- A shoulder spica cast or commercial brace for posterior shoulder dislocation; arm held in 20 degrees of external rotation and 0 to 20 degrees of abduction.
- Duration of immobilization depends on age, chronicity, associated fractures, and operative intervention.
- For first-time, uncomplicated dislocations: 7 to 14 days of immobilization for patients >45 years of age to avoid shoulder stiffness.

Pediatric Considerations
Younger patients are immobilized 4 to 6 weeks to allow capsular scarring to occur.

MEDICATION
Postreduction pain management can be at provider's discretion, but some avoid nonsteroidal anti-inflammatory drugs (NSAIDs) due to theoretical increased malunion rate if a fracture is present.

ISSUES FOR REFERRAL
If unable to perform closed reduction, patient should be referred to orthopedic surgery urgently for operative management.

ADDITIONAL THERAPIES
- Independent of the duration of immobilization, aggressive physical therapy should be completed.
- Isometric external rotation strengthening can occur during the immobilization stage in the brace.
- Progressive range of motion with strengthening of the internal and external rotators
- Advanced rehabilitation program for athletes concentrating on sport-specific activities and proprioception
- Return to athletics for first-time nonoperative dislocators is not fully understood due to limited data. It should be individually based on GH functionality and strength.
- Repeat nonoperative dislocators may return to activity once pain free and full strength has been recovered. These patients are likely to have recurrent dislocations.

SURGERY/OTHER PROCEDURES
- A conservative nonoperative trial of physical therapy may allow an individual with an uncomplicated dislocation to resume pain-free daily activities.
- Patients with a defect size <25% of the articular surface are treated conservatively with a favorable outcome (6)[B].

ALERT
Athletes (specifically overhead athletes) may continue to have disability that is not amenable to an extended conservative trial of rehabilitation (3 to 6 months). In these patients, operative intervention should be considered following the initial dislocation.

- Surgical intervention is indicated with associated injuries, such as fractures, rotator cuff tears, and suspected labral pathology.
- Although the posterior capsulolabral complex often heals with nonoperative management, recurrent instability may necessitate the need for surgical repair and additional soft tissue repair for improved posterior stability.
- Operative interventions often include examination under anesthesia, diagnostic arthroscopy, and arthroscopic or open stabilization procedures.
- Arthroscopic stabilization procedures for posterior shoulder instability have undergone significant evolution since earlier reports. Current literature, including long-term studies with follow-up often exceeding 10 years, indicates that although many patients achieve good to excellent functional outcomes and durable stability, reported recurrence rates can vary, generally ranging from approximately 5% to over >20%. These outcomes are influenced by patient-specific factors, the chronicity of instability, associated injuries, and evolving surgical techniques (7)[B].

ADMISSION, INPATIENT, AND NURSING CONSIDERATIONS
Consider admission for patients who have failed initial closed reduction attempts.

ONGOING CARE

FOLLOW-UP RECOMMENDATIONS
Orthopedic referral should be considered for all PGHD. Potentially associated injuries of fractures, rotator cuff tears, and labral pathology require evaluation and long-term management.

PROGNOSIS
Prognosis is favorable when managed properly. There is limited data on recurrence rate specifically for PGHD, although general recurrence rates for all GHDs are higher in the population ages 15 to 19 years with no difference between genders (3)[C].

COMPLICATIONS

ALERT
Although neurovascular injury is less common in PGHD, it can occur. Axillary nerve injury is most common, causing shoulder badge weakness and numbness. This often resolves without intervention. Always evaluate neurovascular bundle with any shoulder dislocation.

- Reverse Hill-Sachs lesion, compression fracture of the anterior humeral head, leading to joint instability
- Reverse Bankart lesion, detachment of the posteroinferior capsular periosteum, leading to laxity of the posterior band of the inferior GH ligament and a labral tear, resulting in joint instability

REFERENCES

1. Rosas-Medina JA. Undetected traumatic posterior glenohumeral dislocation. Article in Spanish. *Acta Ortop Mex*. 2017;31(4):196–201.
2. Bradley JP, Forsythe B, Mascarenhas R. Arthroscopic management of posterior shoulder instability: diagnosis, indications, and technique. *Clin Sports Med*. 2008;27(4):649–670.
3. Shields DW, Jefferies JG, Brooksbank AJ, et al. Epidemiology of glenohumeral dislocation and subsequent instability in an urban population. *J Shoulder Elbow Surg*. 2018;27(2):189–195.
4. Gottlieb M, Patel D, Marks A, et al. Ultrasound for the diagnosis of shoulder dislocation and reduction: a systematic review and meta-analysis. *Acad Emerg Med*. 2022;29(8):999–1007.
5. Sithamparapillai A, Grewal K, Thompson C, et al. Intra-articular lidocaine versus intravenous sedation for closed reduction of acute anterior shoulder dislocation in the emergency department: a systematic review and meta-analysis. *CJEM*. 2022;24(8):809–819.
6. Guehring M, Lambert S, Stoeckle U, et al. Posterior shoulder dislocation with associated reverse Hill-Sachs lesion: treatment options and functional outcome after a 5-year follow up. *BMC Musculoskelet Disord*. 2017;18(1):442.
7. Savoie FH III, Holt MS, Field LD, et al. Arthroscopic management of posterior instability: evolution of technique and results. *Arthroscopy*. 2008;24(4):389–396.

ADDITIONAL READING

- Andrews JR, Wilk KE. *The Athlete's Shoulder*. Churchill Livingstone; 1994.
- Canale TS. *Campbell's Operative Orthopaedics: Fractures and Dislocations*. Mosby; 1998.
- Dee R, Mango E, Hurst LC. *Principles of Orthopaedic Practice*. McGraw-Hill; 1989.
- Miller MD, Thompson SR. *DeLee and Drez's Orthopaedic Sports Medicine Principles and Practice*. Vol 1. 4th ed. Saunders; 2014.

CLINICAL PEARLS
- Due to the high rate of missed posterior shoulder dislocations, one must include an axillary view to the standard series of shoulder radiographs. Have a low threshold to check advanced imaging such as CT or MRI if the diagnosis is suspected and initial radiographs are negative. US shows promise in diagnosis of shoulder dislocation and can be used as a dynamic imaging tool.
- Early reduction attempts increase rate of successful closed reduction.
- All PGHDs should be referred to orthopedics for long-term follow-up.

GLENOID LABRAL TEARS/SLAP LESIONS

Brian Lowell, MD, CAQSM

BASICS

DESCRIPTION

- The anatomy of the glenohumeral (GH) joint is complex, and stability is provided from combination of the capsule, tendons, muscles, bones, and the labrum:
  - Labrum acts by increasing surface area for humeral head contact by deepening the glenoid socket cavity.
  - Provides attachment site for GH ligament and the tendon of the long head of the biceps
  - Composed of fibrocartilage and dense fibrous collagenous tissue
  - The superior aspect is more mobile than the inferior portion that is tightly attached to the glenoid rim.
  - Multiple anatomic variations exist: congenitally absent portions of the labrum, different anchor sites for the GH ligament, different biceps tendon origins, and superior labral recesses (1).
- There are currently 10 described superior labrum anterior-to-posterior (SLAP) lesions, of which the four originally described by Snyder are the most common:
  - Type I is degenerative fraying of the labrum.
  - Type II is a detached labral/biceps complex from superior glenoid rim.
  - Type III is a bucket-handle tear of superior labrum, but bicep tendon remains intact.
  - Type IV is a bucket-handle tear with extension into the biceps tendon (2).
- SLAP lesions occur as acute injuries or with chronic degradation.

EPIDEMIOLOGY

- Incidence of SLAP lesion occurs in approximately 6–26% of all arthroscopic shoulder cases from 1985 to 2000 (3).
- Reported to occur in up to 25% of patient with symptomatic shoulder instability
- More common in men than women
- Most commonly seen in individuals in their mid-20s

ETIOLOGY AND PATHOPHYSIOLOGY

- SLAP lesion development consists of an internal rotation deficit, tightening of the posterior capsule, posterior superior GH shift, maximization of external rotation forces at the biceps anchor and superior labral attachment, and "peel back" of the labrum. Alterations in scapular movements (dyskinesis) and grinding forces with internal rotation exacerbate this mechanism (1).
- Mechanisms of injury to the glenoid labrum occur via acute trauma or repetitive microtrauma from overhead motions:
  - Acute mechanism of injury:
    - Compression due to a fall on an outstretched arm or onto an adducted shoulder.
    - Traction injury from a swift pull
    - Humeral head shearing such as during vehicle accidents from seat belt restraint, or shoulder dislocation.
  - Chronic mechanism of injury:
    - Secondary to repetitive motions that result in micro trauma accumulation
    - Chronic instability

RISK FACTORS

- Repetitive overhead motions (sports or occupational):
  - Baseball (commonly pitchers)
  - Football (quarterbacks)
  - Weightlifters (military press)
  - Swimmers
  - Tennis (serving)
  - Volleyball (serving)
- Shoulder instability/trauma
- Anatomic variation or underlying generalized laxity/instability

GENERAL PREVENTION

- There are no definitive guidelines for prevention of SLAP lesions. Generally, physical therapy (PT) practices are followed:
  - Rotator cuff strengthening
  - Scapular stabilizer strengthening
  - Posterior capsule stretching
  - Limiting internal rotation deficits
  - Ensuring proper overhead mechanics
- Additionally, monitoring pitch counts in the youth has been implemented as a preventative technique.

COMMONLY ASSOCIATED CONDITIONS

Labral tears are commonly associated with other underlying shoulder problems, as forces that cause labral injuries can cause other pathology. Thus, a high index of suspicion is required when evaluating for SLAP lesion, as other shoulder pathology coexist in approximately 85% of cases (Bankart lesions, GH instability, rotator cuff, and bicipital tendon pathology). This can significantly confound the diagnosis.

DIAGNOSIS

Labral tear diagnosis is made by history, physical, and appropriate imaging. The gold standard for diagnosis of a SLAP lesion is direct visualization via arthroscopy.

HISTORY

- Most individuals complain of nonspecific shoulder pain. Pain is commonly located anterior and superior. Patient's experience is extremely variable.
- Other pertinent positives in the history may include:
  - Acute injury or repetitive overhead motion (sport, hobby, occupational)
  - Mechanical symptoms: catching, painful clicking, or popping deep within the shoulder with overhead movements
  - Decrease in athletic performance (strength, velocity, accuracy, precision)
  - Weakness in the upper extremity
  - Sense of instability

PHYSICAL EXAM

- Examination maneuvers are generally inaccurate due to frequent concurrent shoulder pathology; there is **no gold standard clinical test**.
- Combinations of clinical tests provide higher accuracy. Combining two tests from a group with relatively high sensitivity (compression rotation test, anterior apprehension test, or O'Brien test) with one test from a group with relatively high specificity (Yergason test, biceps load test, or Speed test) results in sensitivity and specificity of nearly 75% and 90%, respectively (4).
- Relatively high-sensitivity tests:
  - **Compression rotation test:** With patient supine, the patient's arm is abducted to 90 degrees and the elbow is flexed to 90 degrees while the examiner applies axial force to the humerus; positive if pain or clicking is noted
  - **Anterior apprehension test:** With patient supine, examiner passively abducts and externally rotates the humerus; positive if pain or sensation of instability is noted
  - **O'Brien test:** With patient standing, the arm is forward flexed to 90 degrees with the elbow in full extension. With an adducted arm to 10 degrees and an internally rotated humerus, the examiner applies downward force to the arm as the patient resists. Patient then fully supinates the arm and repeats resistance; positive if pain is elicited with internal rotation and reduced with external rotation (supination)
- Relatively high-specificity tests:
  - **Yergason test:** With patient standing with elbow at 90 degrees of flexion, patient supinates forearm against examiner's resistance while examiner palpates long head of biceps tendon; positive if pain at biceps tendon; lower sensitivity except with distal biceps injury
  - **Biceps load II test:** With patient supine, examiner grasps patient's wrist and elbow. The arm is abducted 120 degrees and fully externally rotated (apprehension position), with elbow held in 90 degrees of flexion and forearm supinated. Examiner then resists elbow flexion by patient; positive if pain is noted (test with most utility for patients with a SLAP-only lesion) (5)[C]
  - **Speed test:** With patient seated, elbow extended and forearm in full supination, the clinician resists active forward flexion from 0 to 60 degrees; positive if pain is increased in the shoulder and the patient localizes the pain to the bicipital groove (4)[C]

DIFFERENTIAL DIAGNOSIS

- GH arthritis
- Rotator cuff impingement, tendinopathy, or tear
- Biceps tendinopathy, tear, or subluxation
- Shoulder instability
- Adhesive capsulitis
- Acromioclavicular (AC) joint disorder
- Cervical radiculopathy or other referred pain
- Paralabral ganglion cyst
- Pain syndromes (complex regional pain or Parsonage-Turner syndrome)

DIAGNOSTIC TESTS & INTERPRETATION

Initial Tests (lab, imaging)

- Plain radiographs are useful in identifying bony pathology such as fracture, GH arthritis, AC joint arthritis, and calcific deposits.
- Ultrasound is useful in evaluating for coexistent injuries (biceps tendon, rotator cuff tendons, joint capsule, and AC joint) but is insensitive for labral pathology. Joint effusion, bicipital sheath effusion, and paralabral cysts are secondary findings that suggest intra-articular pathology, which may include SLAP lesion.
- Magnetic resonance imaging (MRI) and magnetic resonance arthrography (MRA) are the mainstays in imaging for SLAP lesions.

- Arthrography with contrast medium improves imaging by outlining the intra-articular and synovial surfaces through slight distension of the capsule:
  - Direct (intra-articular) MRA is superior to plain MRI and vascular contrast-enhanced MRI for detecting SLAP lesions with respect to both sensitivity and specificity.

Diagnostic Procedures/Other

GH arthroscopy:

- Gold standard
- Most sensitive and specific test for labral pathology
- Evaluation of the biceps labral complex should be done with a probe because it may appear normal with just visualization.

TREATMENT

GENERAL MEASURES

- Ideal treatment of SLAP injuries remains unclear. Current recommendations support an initial nonsurgical approach prior to surgical intervention.
- Initial therapy (nonoperative):
  - Relative rest from aggravating activities
  - PT with a focus on endurance and strengthening of the rotator cuff and scapular stabilizers and posterior capsule stretching to assist with limitations on internal rotation (1)
  - A history of trauma or participation in overhead activities is strongly associated with failure of nonoperative treatment.

MEDICATION

- Short course ~8 to 10 days nonsteroidal anti-inflammatory drugs (NSAIDs) or acetaminophen.
- With minimal pain relief from oral pharmacologic intervention and failure of one round of PT, subacromial or intra-articular corticosteroid injection can be considered.

ISSUES FOR REFERRAL

- Referral to a surgical specialist should be made if a patient is experiencing persistent symptoms despite 3 to 6 months of adequate PT.
- Consider early referral in elite and overhead athletes for possible faster return to sport.

SURGERY/OTHER PROCEDURES

- Evaluation with diagnostic arthroscopy and treatment is indicated if initial treatment interventions do not appropriately manage symptoms.
- Although there is no uniform approach to SLAP lesion surgical repair, several options are available (débridement, SLAP repair/fixation, subacromial decompression, tenotomy of the long head of the biceps tendon, and tenodesis of the long head of the biceps) (2)[C].
- Due to discouraging surgical results (poor outcomes with respect to return to previous level of play and surgical complications) with SLAP repair, biceps tenodesis is becoming a more favorable option with better rates of return to sports and lower reoperation rates (2)[C].
- Other surgical intervention may be required depending on associated conditions such as rotator cuff tears or instability.

ONGOING CARE

- Postoperative care varies among individuals and depends on overall surgical intervention. Therapy is largely patient directed.
- Example of postoperative therapy are as follows:
  - Sling immobilization to protect shoulder for first 4 weeks
  - Shoulder, elbow, and hand range of motion (ROM) for first 4 weeks; full ROM typically achieved by 10 weeks
  - Restore strength/balance and begin isotonic rotator cuff strengthening 8 to 12 weeks postoperatively.
  - Plyometric training at approximately 20 weeks
  - Throwing exercises between 24 and 28 weeks
  - Return to activity 6 to 9 months

FOLLOW-UP RECOMMENDATIONS

Rigorous follow-up is recommended with nonsurgical and surgical management of SLAP lesions.

PROGNOSIS

- Contact athletes typically return to sport quicker than overhead athletes and had a greater percentage of athletes return to their prior level of play. The evidence is rather unfavorable for overhead athletes returning to prior level of play status post SLAP repair (40–70%).
- Return to play and return to previous level was limited in pitchers compared to other positional players in baseball (3).
- Individuals with isolated SLAP lesions (rare) return to activity much quicker than individuals with concomitant shoulder pathology, specifically rotator cuff injuries which is a negative prognostic indicator for returning to play (6).
- Bicep tenodesis had a higher return to sports rate (84.5%) compared to SLAP repairs (79.5%) (5)[C].
- Age appears to affect outcomes because younger athletes appear to do better overall.

COMPLICATIONS

Complications of untreated SLAP tears include chronic pain, loss of function, and decreased physical performance. Complications associated with surgical intervention include infection, hemarthrosis, failed surgical intervention, instability, adhesive capsulitis, and chondral injury.

REFERENCES

1. Abrams GD, Safran MR. Diagnosis and management of superior labrum anterior posterior lesions in overhead athletes. *Br J Sports Med.* 2010;44(5):311–318.
2. Popp D, Schöffl V. Superior labral anterior posterior lesions of the shoulder: current diagnostic and therapeutic standards. *World J Orthop.* 2015;6(9):660–671.
3. de Sa D, Arakgi ME, Lian J, et al. Labral repair versus biceps tenodesis for primary surgical management of type ii superior labrum anterior to posterior tears: a systematic review. *Arthroscopy.* 2019;35(6):1927–1938.
4. Oh JH, Kim JY, Kim WS, et al. The evaluation of various physical examinations for the diagnosis of type II superior labrum anterior to posterior lesion. *Am J Sports Med.* 2008;36(2):353–359.
5. Abdul-Rassoul H, Defazio M, Curry EJ, et al. Return to sport after the surgical treatment of superior labrum anterior to posterior tears: a systematic review. *Orthop J Sports Med.* 2019;7(5):2325967119841892.
6. LeVasseur MR, Mancini MR, Hawthorne BC, et al. Slap tears and return to sport and work: current concepts. *J ISAKOS.* 2021;6(4):204–211.

CLINICAL PEARLS

- Glenoid labral tears are relatively uncommon shoulder injuries but are more commonly seen in overhead athletes and those who participate in contact sports.
- Labral injuries typically cause vague pain, decreased performance, and mechanical symptoms. Physical exam, although helpful, is unreliable for definitive diagnosis, so have a low threshold for imaging in appropriate cases.
- Generally, nonsurgical treatment is indicated prior to surgical intervention.
- Evaluation with diagnostic arthroscopy and treatment is appropriate if nonsurgical therapy does not manage symptoms.
- Consider early referral in elite and overhead athletes for possible faster return to sport.
- The evidence is rather unfavorable for overhead athletes returning to prior level of play status post SLAP surgical repair. If no labral pathology is identified, broaden differential to include cervical or brachial plexus pathology.

GOUT

Kenneth S. Taylor, MD, FAAFP, CAQSM ▪ Suraj A. Achar, MD, FAAFP, CAQSM

BASICS

- Gout is an acute disease that can progress to a chronic state.
- The most common inflammatory arthropathy, affecting >8 million Americans (1)
- Consists of painful inflammatory deposition of monosodium urate crystals into joints and may also form at the joint space and soft tissues (tophaceous gout)
- Pseudogout is a similar but distinct entity in which the inflammatory process is instigated by calcium pyrophosphate dihydrate (calcium pyrophosphate deposition disease [CPPD]) crystal deposition instead of monosodium urate.

DESCRIPTION

- Gout has three stages:
  - Acute phase: inflammatory monarthritic; resolves within several days to just over a week
  - Interval phase: The patient is asymptomatic.
  - Chronic phase: intermittent repeated flairs of monarticular or polyarticular gout and soft tissue deposition of tophi
- Common joints affected by gout: 1st metatarsophalangeal (MTP) joint (most common site of initial presentation; also known as *podagra*), olecranon, ankle, wrist, knee, tarsal joints, and interphalangeal joints of the hand
- Much less commonly affected joints include shoulder, sternoclavicular joint, spine, and sacroiliac joints.
- Tophaceous gout can extend to periarticular structures (tendons, skin, and soft tissue) and rarely can affect visceral organs.
- Up to 20% of gout patients may present with polyarticular or tophaceous gout at initial presentation.

EPIDEMIOLOGY

Incidence

- Commonly presents in middle-aged men (30 to 50 years old)
- Also commonly seen in elderly men and postmenopausal women, typically in those with multiple medical comorbidities
- Predominant gender: male > female (2 to 4:1)

Prevalence

- Prevalence of gout in United States is ~3–6% in men, 1–3% in women, and increases with increasing age (2),(3).
- Others have found a prevalence of 8.4 per 1,000 (4).

ETIOLOGY AND PATHOPHYSIOLOGY

- Precipitation of monosodium urate crystals in a joint space or soft tissue
- This triggers immune activation with the release of cytokines and neutrophil recruitment.
- This inflammatory process results in localized pain, swelling, and erythema of the affected joint.
- This disease process closely resembles infection.

RISK FACTORS

- Male
- Pacific islander
- Excessive alcohol intake (especially beer and liquor)
- Hypertension and cardiovascular disease
- Chronic diuretic use (thiazide and loop)
- Organ transplant recipients treated with calcineurin inhibitors
- Recent surgery
- Hyperuricemic state (from either overproduction or underexcretion of uric acid)
- Rapid changes in uric acid level
- Diets high in purine-containing products
- Diets low in dairy or high in meat or fish (hazard ratio up to 1.41 in high-quantity meat eaters and 1.51 in high-quantity fish eaters) (5); total protein intake is not correlated with risk for gout.
- Risk factors for the presence of tophaceous gout at initial diagnosis:
  - Postmenopausal women
  - Coexisting chronic renal disease
  - Diuretic therapy
- Dehydration (a very important risk factor)

GENERAL PREVENTION

- Factors that can reduce risk of gout:
  - High-quantity dairy product intake (hazard ratio of 0.56) (5)
  - Minimizing diuretic use and dose (particularly thiazides)
  - Minimizing alcohol intake
- The Dietary Approaches to Stop Hypertension (DASH) diet demonstrated significantly decreased serum urate levels, particularly in younger adults (6).
- Urate-lowering agents are used for the prevention of chronic gout. See "Medication."

COMMONLY ASSOCIATED CONDITIONS

- Hypertension
- Chronic diuretic therapy
- Obesity
- Hyperlipidemia
- Chronic renal disease
- Cardiovascular disease
- Hyperuricemic syndromes such as myeloproliferative or lymphoproliferative disorders, psoriasis, cyclosporine A use (in organ transplant patients), and inherited defects in purine metabolism
- Patients with gout are at increased risk for uric acid nephrolithiasis.

DIAGNOSIS

HISTORY

- Initially a severely painful, erythematous, and swollen joint (noninfectious monarthritis)
- There is no significant trauma of the joint preceding the attack.
- Rarely, there may be polyarticular involvement at first onset.
- Maximal pain reaches peak at 24 to 48 hours (1),(7).

PHYSICAL EXAM

- Gout:
  - Swelling, erythema, warmth, and tenderness of affected joint
  - 80% of flares involve a single joint (1st MTP, knee, ankle, and other joints).
  - Sometimes overlying skin can be erythematous and desquamated, resembling cellulitis.
- Tophi:
  - Subcutaneous nodules (resembling rheumatoid arthritis) or a bulky mass overlying a joint
  - ± Tenderness or erythema of tophi
  - Aspirated tophi contents appear as white pasty or chalky material.

DIFFERENTIAL DIAGNOSIS

- Pseudogout
- Rheumatoid arthritis
- Psoriatic arthritis
- Septic arthritis
- Osteoarthritis
- Reactive arthritis
- Osteomyelitis
- Malignancy
- Joint trauma

DIAGNOSTIC TESTS & INTERPRETATION

Initial Tests (lab, imaging)

- Distinction from an infectious process may be difficult.
- Complete blood count (CBC): Leukocytosis may be extremely high.
- C-reactive protein (CRP) and erythrocyte sedimentation rate (ESR) are often elevated as well.
- Chemistry panel to assess renal function: Not only is renal impairment associated with gout, but chronic hyperuricemia can lead to urate nephropathy.
- Uric acid level often will be high during an acute gout attack but may be normal:
  - Incidence of gout in patients with uric acid levels >9 mg/dL is 6 times greater than in patients at 7.0 to 8.9 mg/dL (7).
  - In a group of 339 patients with acute gout, 14% had uric acid levels ≤6 mg/dL and 32% were ≤8 mg/dL (8).
  - Thus, uric acid level on its own cannot be used to diagnose or rule out gout, but a high uric acid level in the appropriate clinical context can be suggestive of gout (8)[B].
- Although sometimes helpful, imaging is not necessary to make a diagnosis of gout (9)[A].
- Can be used to evaluate for an alternate diagnosis such as rheumatoid arthritis
- Chronic gout is often characterized by subcortical cysts, bony erosions, overhanging edges, and diffuse soft tissue calcifications on x-ray or magnetic resonance imaging (MRI) (9).
- Large tophi can be identified on MRI but often will need to be aspirated to confirm the diagnosis (9)[A].
- Pseudogout, on the other hand, does not typically have bony abnormalities but instead consists of chondrocalcinosis (calcification of fibrocartilage).

Diagnostic Procedures/Other

- The "gold standard" diagnosis of gout is made by aspiration (arthrocentesis) of the affected joint's synovial fluid (10)[A].
- Characteristic needle-shaped, negatively birefringent monosodium urate crystals are seen under polarized light microscopy.
- In contrast, pseudogout consists of rhomboid-shaped crystals with weakly positive birefringence.
- Aspirate: Check cell count, Gram stain, and bacterial culture to evaluate for infection (with a negative Gram stain and negative culture).
- Aspirate white blood cell (WBC) count: 2,000 to 50,000 seen in gout (also pseudogout or rheumatoid arthritis); >50,000 is suspicious for septic arthritis.
- It is important to look for septic arthritis, which can mimic gout (and rarely may coexist with gout).
- Ultrasound-guided aspiration can improve accuracy.
- Baseline diagnostic ultrasound scores based on urate deposits including aggregates, double contour sign, and tophi were significantly lined with occurrence of flares (11)

TREATMENT

GENERAL MEASURES

- See "Risk Factors" for what to avoid.
- Therapy for gout includes diet modification (see "Risk Factors"), using medications that reduce overall uric acid levels (such as losartan, calcium channel blockers, and fenofibrate), and minimizing medications that are known to increase gout flairs (such as diuretics and aspirin) when appropriate.

MEDICATION

- Acute treatment:
  - Nonsteroidal anti-inflammatory drugs (NSAIDs) are first-line therapy; typically naproxen (500 mg BID) or indomethacin (50 mg TID) is used (12)[A]; should be given within 24 to 48 hours of symptom onset for best results (7)[B]
  - Cyclooxygenase-2 (COX-2) inhibitors are equally effective according to recent studies (13)[B].
  - Duration of treatment varies, often ranging from 3 to 10 days until the attack subsides.
  - Within several days of treatment, the dosing can be decreased if clinical improvement (1)[B].
  - Corticosteroids oral, or intra-articular are an effective alternative first-line agent if NSAIDs are contraindicated (2),(14)[A]:
    - Begin oral prednisone at 30 to 40 mg/d or prednisolone 30 mg/d × 2 to 3 days, then taper over total of 5 to 10 days (7),(10)[C].
    - Intra-articular injections; can use:
      - Betamethasone 3 to 6 mg
      - Dexamethasone 5 to 10 mg
      - Methylprednisolone 20 to 40 mg
      - Triamcinolone 20 to 40 mg
  - Septic arthritis is an absolute contraindication to intra-articular corticosteroid treatment.
  - Colchicine is very effective for treatment of acute gout (15)[A].
  - Use oral colchicine 0.6 mg 2 to 3 times per day or 1 to 2 times per day in patients with renal impairment or elderly patients:
    - For best results, colchicine should be given within 24 to 48 hours of symptom onset (15)[B].

– IV colchicines should not be used and are no longer approved by the U.S. Food and Drug Administration (FDA) owing to the high level of toxicity (15)[A].
– A pegylated recombinant form of urate-oxidase enzyme (Krystexxa) that converts uric acid to an inactive water-soluble form has been FDA approved for use in refractory gout (3).

- Preventive treatment:
  - Dietary modifications:
    - Reduce or eliminate:
      - Beer and liquor (no increased risk with wine)
      - High-fructose products/sweetened beverages
      - Meat/seafood (5)
    - Increase/beneficial:
      - Dairy/skim milk
      - Coffee (Tea does not reduce risk.)
      - Vitamin C 500 mg/d
      - Cherry/cherry extract had shown promise (5) but had no impact on gout flares over a 28-day period, based on data from 50 adult patients (16).
- Indications for chronic preventative therapy include (17)[B]:
  - Recurrent or disabling gout attacks (specifically >2 gout attacks per year)
  - Persistent tophi
  - Joint damage noted on imaging
  - Uric acid nephropathy or nephrolithiasis
- The symptom-free period required prior to starting prophylactic therapy once the acute attack has resolved is unclear:
  - Some advocate using concomitant colchicine or NSAID treatment the first 3 to 6 months of urate-lowering treatment (18)[C].
  - Some suggest waiting about 2 to 6 weeks after the acute attack before starting prophylactic medication, although recent evidence shows it is safe in conjunction with NSAIDs (1),(7)[C].
- If a gout attack occurs while on urate-lowering treatment, the urate-lowering medication should *not* be stopped (1),(7)[B].
- Uric acid level should be monitored for a goal of <6 mg/dL (355 μmol/L) because this is associated with a significantly lower incidence of gout (7)[B].
- Allopurinol is a xanthine oxidase inhibitor that decreases uric acid production:
  - Most commonly used
  - Therapeutic dose is 100 to 300 mg/d: Start at a lower dose (50 or 100 mg/d), and titrate up slowly over several weeks (e.g., by 100 mg every 2 to 4 weeks) to target uric acid goal of <6 mg/dL (10)[C].
  - Patients with renal insufficiency require lower doses.
  - Periodic laboratory testing (liver enzymes and CBC) should be considered.
  - Chinese, Thai, or Korean descent has a higher risk of hypersensitivity skin reactions—genetic testing is available (1).
  - Drug rash with eosinophilia and systemic symptoms (DRESS) syndrome: A rare but serious drug reaction with symptoms like:
    - Extensive skin rash
    - Involvement of internal organs (liver, kidney, lungs)
    - Swollen lymph nodes (lymphadenopathy)
    - Increased eosinophils (a type of WBC) in the blood (eosinophilia)
    - Abnormal lymphocytes (a type of WBC) in the blood (atypical lymphocytosis)
  - Although DRESS syndrome can be caused by various medications, allopurinol is a well-known culprit. The risk of DRESS with allopurinol typically occurs within 2 to 8 weeks of starting the medication (19).
- Febuxostat is a newer medication:
  - Cleared through the liver and therefore an appropriate alternative in renal disease
- Probenecid is a uricosuric agent that increases uric acid secretion:
  - Second-line medication for prophylaxis (12)
  - Ineffective in patients with impaired creatinine clearance
  - Avoid in patients with nephrolithiasis.
  - Caution for multiple medication interactions
- NSAIDs (naproxen 250 mg 2 times per day) or colchicine (≤0.6 mg 1 to 2 times per day) can be used as chronic suppression therapy in the place of or in addition to urate-lowering agents (7)[B].
- Low-dose prednisone (≤10 mg) also can be considered, but it has long-term side effects (7)[B].
- Recently approved drug lesinurad is being studied as an adjunct to allopurinol to improve efficacy. Lesinurad: Uric acid reabsorption inhibitor combined with allopurinol in 200 mg or 300 mg increments is superior to allopurinol alone in lowering uric acid levels.

ISSUES FOR REFERRAL

- Rheumatology if refractory condition, multiple comorbidities, or unusual presentation
- Orthopedics if suspected septic arthritis

ADMISSION, INPATIENT, AND NURSING CONSIDERATIONS

- Consider for severe cases of gout, especially if needed for pain control or for diagnostic confirmation.
- Suspected septic arthritis requires IV antibiotics and orthopedic referral.

ONGOING CARE

PROGNOSIS

Prior to advent of preventative therapy up to 2/3 patients undergoing a gout attack will have another one within 12 months.

COMPLICATIONS

- It takes on average, about 10 years for chronic tophaceous gout to develop after the initial attack (7).
- Chronic gout can lead to joint damage and destruction.
- Frequent attacks can be very painful and disabling and have a negative impact on quality of life.
- Chronic urate nephropathy

REFERENCES

1. Hainer BL, Matheson E, Wilkes RT. Diagnosis, treatment, and prevention of gout. *Am Fam Physician*. 2014;90(12):831–836.
2. Rainer TH, Cheng CH, Janssens HJ, et al. Oral prednisolone in the treatment of acute gout: a pragmatic, multicenter, double-blind, randomized trial. *Ann Intern Med*. 2016;164(7):464–471.
3. Clebak KT, Morrison A, Croad JR. Gout: rapid evidence review. *Am Fam Physician*. 2020;102(9):533–538.
4. Lawrence RC, Felson DT, Helmick CG, et al. Estimates of the prevalence of arthritis and other rheumatic conditions in the United States. Part II. *Arthritis Rheum*. 2008;58(1):26–35.
5. Beyl RN Jr, Hughes L, Morgan S. Update on importance of diet in gout. *Am J Med*. 2016;129(11):1153–1158.
6. Castilla-Ojo N, Turkson-Ocran RA, Conlin PR, et al. Effects of the DASH diet and losartan on serum urate among adults with hypertension: results of a randomized trial. *J Clin Hypertens (Greenwich)*. 2023;25(10):915–922.
7. Keith MP, Gilliland WR. Updates in the management of gout. *Am J Med*. 2007;120(3):221–224.
8. Schlesinger N, Norquist JM, Watson DJ. Serum urate during acute gout. *J Rheumatol*. 2009;36(6):1287–1289.
9. Schumacher HR Jr, Becker MA, Edwards NL, et al. Magnetic resonance imaging in the quantitative assessment of gouty tophi. *Int J Clin Pract*. 2006;60(4):408–414.
10. Terkeltaub RA. Clinical practice. Gout. *N Engl J Med*. 2003;349(17):1647–1655.
11. Cao L, Zhao T, Xie C, et al. Performance of ultrasound in the clinical evaluation of gout and hyperuricemia. *J Immunol Res*. 2021;2021:5550626.
12. Zhang W, Doherty M, Bardin T, et al. EULAR evidence based recommendations for gout. Part II: management. Report of a task force of the EULAR Standing Committee for International Clinical Studies Including Therapeutics (ESCISIT). *Ann Rheum Dis*. 2006;65(10):1312–1324.
13. Wortmann RL. Recent advances in the management of gout and hyperuricemia. *Curr Opin Rheumatol*. 2005;17(3):319–324.
14. Janssens HJ, Janssen M, van de Lisdonk EH, et al. Use of oral prednisolone or naproxen for the treatment of gout arthritis: a double-blind, randomised equivalence trial. *Lancet*. 2008;371(9627):1854–1860.
15. Terkeltaub RA. Colchicine update: 2008. *Semin Arthritis Rheum*. 2009;38(6):411–419.
16. Stamp LK, Chapman P, Frampton C, et al. Lack of effect of tart cherry concentrate dose on serum urate in people with gout. *Rheumatology*. 2020;59(9):2374–2380.
17. Shoji A, Yamanaka H, Kamatani N. A retrospective study of the relationship between serum urate level and recurrent attacks of gouty arthritis: evidence for reduction of recurrent gouty arthritis with antihyperuricemic therapy. *Arthritis Rheum*. 2004;51(3):321–325.
18. Borstad GC, Bryant LR, Abel MP, et al. Colchicine for prophylaxis of acute flares when initiating allopurinol for chronic gouty arthritis. *J Rheumatol*. 2004;31(12):2429–2432.
19. Aatif T, Fatihi J, El Annaz H, et al. Allopurinol-induced drug reactions with eosinophilia and systemic symptoms syndrome with interstitial nephritis. *Indian J Nephrol*. 2018;28(6):477–481.

CLINICAL PEARLS

- Gout is an acute inflammatory arthritis of rapid onset that can mimic infection.
- A painful, warm, erythematous, swollen joint should be aspirated to evaluate for septic arthritis versus gout.
- Tophaceous gout is the chronic form of gout that, in rare cases, can present acutely.
- Prophylactic treatment should be considered in recurrent patients because it has been shown to reduce chronic flairs and joint damage.
- Dietary modifications and losing weight can greatly reduce the risks of gout.
- Pseudogout is a disease that is distinct from gout but has various similarities, is generally less debilitating, and less common.

GREATER TROCHANTERIC PAIN SYNDROME (TROCHANTERIC BURSITIS)

Whitney Liehr, DO • Daniel C. Herman, MD, PhD, FAAPMR, FACSM, FISBS, CAQSM

BASICS

DESCRIPTION

Historically, the condition of pain and tenderness in the area of the greater trochanter had been referred to as *trochanteric bursitis*. Recent literature has referred to this condition as *greater trochanteric pain syndrome*. This change has come about owing to the recognition that the etiology of this pain can be from multiple sources, including the bursa and gluteal tendons, snapping hip or the iliotibial band. This includes tendinosis and tendon tears of the gluteus medius and gluteus minimus that insert on the greater trochanter (1).

EPIDEMIOLOGY

- Incidence peaks between the 4th and 6th decades of life.
- Predominant gender: female > male (4:1)
- Most common lower extremity tendinopathy in adults
- Common in runners

ETIOLOGY AND PATHOPHYSIOLOGY

- Etiology of bursitis:
  - Inflammation of the bursae can come from repetitive friction between the bony structures of the trochanter and the muscle, tendon, or fascial tissue that overlies the bursae.
  - Inflammation of the bursae also can come about owing to direct trauma to the lateral hip.
- Etiology of tendinopathy:
  - Tendon changes can develop from acute or chronic overuse of a muscle tendon unit.
  - Weakness or tightness of the muscle tendon unit contributes to this condition.

Genetics

No genetic predisposition is known.

RISK FACTORS

- Ipsilateral or contralateral hip arthritis
- Degenerative changes of the lumbar spine
- Degenerative changes of the knees
- Leg-length discrepancy
- Total hip arthroplasty
- Obesity
- Fibromyalgia
- Iliotibial band syndrome
- Weakness of hip abductors and/or external rotators of the hip
- Pes planus
- Greater trochanteric width
- Excessive or rapidly increased activity
- Training on hard or banked surfaces
- Poorly cushioned shoes
- Limitation of internal rotation of the hip
- Local trauma

GENERAL PREVENTION

- Strengthening of hip external rotators and hip abductors
- Stretching of muscles around the hip
- Avoid sudden increase in activity (including intensity, duration, or pace).
- Avoid exercise on banked surfaces.
- Proper shoe wear
- Avoid direct trauma (use protection when appropriate).
- Weight loss (if appropriate)

COMMONLY ASSOCIATED CONDITIONS

See "Risk Factors."

DIAGNOSIS

HISTORY

- Pain localized to the area of the lateral hip is the key historical finding. This pain may radiate down the lateral thigh or into the groin.
- Pain is often aggravated by:
  - Prolonged walking
  - Rising after sitting
  - Lying on affected side
  - Squatting
  - Climbing
- Patient also may report other related conditions as seen in "Risk Factors."

PHYSICAL EXAM

- Tenderness over the greater trochanter is the key diagnostic finding.
- Pain reported within 30 seconds of standing on the affected limb (LR = 12) (2).
- Other exam tests may be positive but are less specific and/or lack sensitivity:
  - Pain with end range combined flexion, abduction, and external rotation (FABER), particularly when adding resistance to internal rotation (2)
  - Pain with end range adduction, particularly when adding resisted hip abduction (2)
- Other testing to evaluate for associated conditions:
  - Positive Patrick or FABER testing for sacroiliac joint dysfunction or hip joint pathology
  - Ober test for iliotibial band flexibility
  - Hip range of motion for hip joint pathology
  - Leg-length measurement for leg-length discrepancy
  - Foot inspection for pes planus or overpronation
  - Lower extremity neurologic assessment for lumbar radiculopathy or neuromuscular disorders

DIFFERENTIAL DIAGNOSIS

A wide variety of conditions should be considered:

- Lumbosacral disc disease
- Spinal stenosis
- Radiculopathy
- Degenerative disease of the hip
- Osteonecrosis of the hip
- Stress fracture of the hip
- Slipped capital femoral epiphysis
- Fracture
- Contusion
- Soft tissue infection

DIAGNOSTIC TESTS & INTERPRETATION

Initial Tests (lab, imaging)

- Blood tests are not altered by this condition.
- Imaging is not essential for the diagnosis.
- If radiography is done, it should include anteroposterior view and frog-leg lateral view of the affected hip.

- Radiographs typically are normal but can show irregular bone formation or bony spurring at the greater trochanter owing to chronic bursitis or chronic tendinopathy.
- Radiographs also may show associated degenerative disease of the hip joint or the lumbar spine.

Diagnostic Procedures/Other

- Advanced imaging is rarely necessary.
- Detection of abnormalities on magnetic resonance imaging (MRI) is a poor predictor of clinical syndrome
- MRI may be used in refractory cases.
- Ultrasound can be used to aid in diagnosis and management of gluteal tendon tears and may be more accurate than MRI (3)[A].
- Ultrasound guided diagnostic injections may aid in diagnosis.

TREATMENT

GENERAL MEASURES

- Multimodal conservative approach including (4)[A]:
  - Ice
  - Analgesics
  - Nonsteroidal anti-inflammatory drugs (NSAIDs)
  - Minimize aggravating activities such as running or prolonged standing or walking.
  - Avoid lying on affected side and consider placing a pillow between knees while sleeping.
- Physical therapy or home exercises program focusing on (4)[A]:
  - Strengthening (including hip abductors and external rotators of the hip)
  - Stretching (including the piriformis and iliotibial band)
  - Address flexibility of hip and low back.
- Platelet-rich plasma (PRP) injections may provide longer lasting effects compared to corticosteroid injections (CSI) (5)[C].
- Corticosteroid injection (4),(5)[A]:
  - Ultrasound-guided of injections may be helpful, particularly for patients with large body habitus.
- Extracorporeal shock wave therapy (6)
- Deep friction massage of greater trochanteric, gluteal, and iliotibial band areas
- Weight loss (if applicable)
- Address leg-length discrepancy (if applicable).
- Address pes planus or overpronation (if applicable).

MEDICATION

- Analgesics:
  - Acetaminophen 1,000 mg PO TID
- NSAIDs:
  - Ibuprofen 800 mg PO TID
  - Naproxen 500 mg PO TID
  - Others
- Injectable corticosteroids:
  - 1 mL of dexamethasone 4 mg/mL
  - 1 mL of triamcinolone 40 mg/mL
- Anesthetics:
  - Injection of anesthetic alone can be diagnostic.
  - Can be used along with corticosteroids during injection
  - 5 mL of 1% lidocaine, 5 mL of 0.5% bupivacaine, or a combination of both can be used.

ISSUES FOR REFERRAL

- Recalcitrant pain and failure of nonsurgical treatments
- Septic bursitis

SURGERY/OTHER PROCEDURES

- Surgery is rarely needed and should be reserved for recalcitrant cases that have failed nonsurgical measures.
- Various surgical procedures have been described. They include:
  - Open surgery with fenestration or release of the iliotibial band and excision of the subgluteal bursae
  - Arthroscopic bursectomy
  - Gluteal tendon repair

ONGOING CARE

COMPLICATIONS

- Bursal thickening and fibrosis
- Tendon thickening, fibrosis, or tearing

REFERENCES

1. Redmond JM, Chen AW, Domb BG. Greater trochanteric pain syndrome. *J Am Acad Orthop Surg.* 2016;24(4):231–240.
2. Grimaldi A, Mellor R, Nicolson P, et al. Utility of clinical tests to diagnose MRI-confirmed gluteal tendinopathy in patients presenting with lateral hip pain. *Br J Sports Med.* 2017;51(6):519–524.
3. Grimaldi A, Mellor R, Hodges P, et al. Gluteal tendinopathy: a review of mechanisms, assessment, and management. *Sports Med.* 2015;45(8):1107–1119.
4. Gazendam A, Ekhtiari S, Axelrod D, et al. Comparative efficacy of nonoperative treatments for greater trochanteric pain syndrome: a systematic review and network meta-analysis of randomized controlled trials. *Clin J Sport Med.* 2022;32(4):427–432.
5. Migliorini F, Kader N, Eschweiler J, et al. Platelet -rich plasma versus steroids injections for greater trochanter pain syndrome: a systematic review and meta-analysis. *British Med Bull.* 2021;139(1):86–99.
6. Korakakis V, Whiteley R, Tzavara A, et al. The effectiveness of extracorporeal shockwave therapy in common lower limb conditions: a systematic review including quantification of patient-rated pain reduction. *Br J Sports Med.* 2018;52(6):387–407.

ADDITIONAL READING

- Paluska SA. An overview of hip injuries in running. *Sports Med.* 2005;35(11):991–1014.
- Williams BS, Cohen SP. Greater trochanteric pain syndrome: a review of anatomy, diagnosis and treatment. *Anesth Analg.* 2009;108(5):1662–1670.

CLINICAL PEARLS

- Greater trochanteric pain syndrome, previously referred to as trochanteric bursitis, is best diagnosed with tenderness of the lateral hip and reproduced pain with single leg stance.
- Treatment modalities including ice, analgesics, anti-inflammatories, physical therapy, and steroid injections are reasonable first-line interventions for pain and improved function.
- Ultrasound is an emerging diagnostic tool and can be used to assist in guidance for injections.

GREENSTICK FRACTURE

Thomas Munro, MD • Greg Canty, MD

BASICS

DESCRIPTION

Greenstick fractures are incomplete fractures that occur when a bone is exposed to angulation and rotational bending forces. The bending forces are strong enough that the bone begins to fracture on the tension side, but the force is not sufficient enough to result in a complete fracture with the compression side maintaining its integrity:

- The fracture appears on the tension (convex) side of the bone as a break in the periosteum and the cortex.
- The compression side of the bone, or the concave surface, remains intact and appears as a hinge.
- This fracture pattern is most commonly described in forearm fractures of growing children.
- Greenstick fractures may be isolated or may coexist with other complete fractures in forearm injuries.

EPIDEMIOLOGY

- Studies suggest up to 5% of childhood and adolescent fractures are of the greenstick variety (1).
- Some studies suggest an even greater percentage of childhood fractures may be of the greenstick variety.
- Although extremely rare, there have been a few case reports of greenstick fractures in the young adult population.
- Forearm (radius or ulna) = most common
- Proximal humerus
- Tibia

ETIOLOGY AND PATHOPHYSIOLOGY

Greenstick fractures occur in children and adolescents because the bone is more:

- Porous
- Compliant
- Resilient
- Soft

COMMONLY ASSOCIATED CONDITIONS

- Complete fracture of an accompanying bone (common)
- Fracture/dislocation like a Monteggia variant (proximal 3rd ulna fracture with anterior disruption of radial head) (rare)

DIAGNOSIS

Prehospital:

- Suspect with any forearm injury having a mild angular deformity, swelling, and pain.

HISTORY

- Establish mechanism of injury, which is often a fall on an outstretched hand with rotational force.
- Inquire about any numbness, tingling, or pain out of proportion to exam findings.

PHYSICAL EXAM

- Pain and localized tenderness to palpation
- Unwillingness to use or mobilize the affected extremity
- Mild to moderate angular deformity
- Swelling
- Ecchymosis
- Palpation of bony deformities
- Crepitus
- Assess the distal portion of the affected extremity for:
  - Circulation (capillary refill and pulses)
  - Motor function
  - Sensation
- Assess proximal and distal joints/bones for related injuries.

DIFFERENTIAL DIAGNOSIS

- Complete fracture
- Compound fracture
- Plastic deformation/bowing deformity
- Torus (buckle) fracture
- Contusion
- Sprain

DIAGNOSTIC TESTS & INTERPRETATION

- Anteroposterior and lateral radiographs required for diagnosis
- Look for tearing of the periosteum and the cortex on the convex side of the affected bone with an intact periosteum on the concave surface.
- Plastic deformation of bone may also be apparent.
- Oblique views may occasionally be helpful.
- Radius crossover sign may be helpful in determining rotational malalignment after reduction (2)[B]. The typical radiographs, where the radius crossover sign is present, demonstrate a pronated appearance of the proximal forearm with a neutral position of the distal forearm.
- Repeat radiographs after reduction.

TREATMENT

GENERAL MEASURES

- Prehospital:
  - Ice to affected region for control of pain and swelling
  - Splint in comfortable position using:
    - Air splint or board
    - Tape
    - Rolled towels
- Emergency department (ED) treatment:
  - Pain control (see "Medication")
  - Fracture reduction (3)[C]:
    - Most greenstick fractures of the forearm are reduced by rotating the palm toward the apex of the fracture.
    - Distal greenstick fractures have a higher reduction success rate than proximal greenstick fractures (4)[A].
    - Greenstick fractures are incomplete fractures and may require completing the fracture in order to obtain adequate reduction.
  - Immobilize the injury with either a cast or splint:
    - Immobilize in reduced position.
    - Long-arm cast/splint with elbow at 90 degrees if fracture of proximal or middle third of forearm
    - May consider below-the-elbow cast or removable splint if fracture is in distal third of forearm (5)[B]
    - Ensure proper three-point molding to maintain any reduction.
    - Postreduction films after casting/splinting (Look for radius crossover sign discussed in imaging.)
  - Ensure reduction is maintained with immobilization and good perfusion persists prior to discharge from ED.

MEDICATION

First Line

- Ibuprofen PO: 10 mg/kg every 6 to 8 hours (maximum of 800 mg/dose)
- Oxycodone PO (available as an elixir containing 1 mg/1 mL)]: 0.1 to 0.2 mg/kg every 4 to 6 hours (maximum 5 to 10 mg/dose)

Second Line

- Fentanyl IV 0.5 to 1.0 μg/kg every 1 to 2 hours (maximum dose 50 μg); may also consider intranasal 1.5 to 2.0 μg/kg (maximum 100 μg)
- Morphine PO 0.15 to 0.30 mg/kg every 3 to 4 hours (maximum 20 mg)

ISSUES FOR REFERRAL

- Refer if unable to maintain reduction.
- Refer for any signs of median nerve or tendon entrapment.
- Refer for any progressive deformity.

SURGERY/OTHER PROCEDURES

Rarely indicated unless nerve/tendon entrapment or inability to maintain reduction

ADMISSION, INPATIENT, AND NURSING CONSIDERATIONS

- Admission criteria:
  - Any suspicion of a nonaccidental injury (NAI):
    - History is the best predictor of NAI.
    - Best predictor of NAI is whether history is consistent with injury pattern/severity.
- Discharge criteria:
  - Pain is well controlled.
  - Orthopedic referral available within 1 week
  - Splint/cast care/pain management instructions:
    - Ice/cold pack application
    - Elevation of the injured limb
    - Analgesic plans for mild, moderate, and severe pain
    - Return precautions

ONGOING CARE

FOLLOW-UP RECOMMENDATIONS

Patient Monitoring

- With greenstick fractures of the forearm, clinical follow-up and radiographs obtained at 2 to 6 weeks postinjury reduce overall care costs and radiation exposure without compromising clinical results.
- Greenstick fractures of the tibia are at risk for valgus deformity and may be followed for 1 to 2 years.
- Loss of reduction or progression of any deformity warrants surgical consideration, although younger patients have excellent capability of remodeling and rarely require surgery.

PROGNOSIS

- Greenstick fractures are expected to heal completely.
- Complications are rare.
- Remodeling capabilities are tremendous in young patients.
- Excellent prognosis

COMPLICATIONS

- 10–15% of greenstick fractures may lose reduction after immobilization.
- Nerve or tendon sheath entrapment
- Unrecognized accompanying injuries
- Increased refracture risk after a healed greenstick fracture (6)

REFERENCES

1. Cheng JC, Shen WY. Limb fracture pattern in different pediatric age groups: a study of 3,350 children. *J Orthop Trauma*. 1993;7(1):15–22.
2. Wright PB, Crepeau AE, Herrera-Soto JA, et al. Radius crossover sign: an indication of malreduced radius shaft greenstick fractures. *J Pediatr Orthop*. 2012;32(4):e15–e19.
3. Noonan KJ, Price CT. Forearm and distal radius fractures in children. *J Am Acad Orthop Surg*. 1998;6(3):146–156.
4. Rimbaldo KM, Fauteux-Lamarre E, Babl FE, et al. Deformed pediatric forearm fractures: predictors of successful reduction by emergency providers. *Am J Emerg Med*. 2021;50:59–65.
5. Boutis K, Howard A, Constantine E, et al. Evidence into practice: pediatric orthopaedic surgeon use of removable splints for common pediatric fractures. *J Pediatr Orthop*. 2015;35(1):18–23.
6. Bhanushali A, Axelby E, Patel P, et al. Re-fractures of the paediatric radius and/or ulna: a systematic review. *ANZ J Surg*. 2022;92(4):666–673.

ADDITIONAL READING

- Casey PJ, Moed BR. Greenstick fractures of the radius in adults: a report of two cases. *J Orthop Trauma*. 1996;10(3):209–212.
- Drendel AL, Gorelick MH, Weisman SJ, et al. A randomized clinical trial of ibuprofen versus acetaminophen with codeine for acute pediatric arm fracture pain. *Ann Emerg Med*. 2009;54(4):553–560.
- Koller DM, Myers AB, Lorenz D, et al. Effectiveness of oxycodone, ibuprofen, or the combination in the initial management of orthopedic injury-related pain in children. *Pediatr Emerg Care*. 2007;23(9):627–633.
- Mencio GA, Frick SL, eds. *Green's Skeletal Trauma in Children*. 6th ed. Saunders; 2019.
- Ting BL, Kalish LA, Waters PM, et al. Reducing cost and radiation exposure during the treatment of pediatric greenstick fractures of the forearm. *J Pediatr Orthop*. 2016;36(8):816–820.
- Waters PM, Skaggs DL, Flynn JM, eds. *Rockwood and Wilkins' Fractures in Children*. 9th ed. Lippincott Williams & Wilkins; 2020.
- Wenger DR, Pring ME, Pennock AT, et al, eds. *Rang's Children's Fractures*. 4th ed. Lippincott Williams & Wilkins; 2018.

CLINICAL PEARLS

- Examine surrounding bones/joints closely for accompanying injuries such as a both-bone forearm fracture or a Monteggia-variant fracture/dislocation.
- Incomplete fractures, like the greenstick, may require completing the fracture for adequate reduction.
- Reduce radial greenstick fractures by rotating the forearm so that the palm is pointing toward the apex of the fracture.
- Forearm fractures have tremendous potential for remodeling, but greenstick fractures require monitoring after reduction to ensure reduction is maintained.
- Beware of the long-term risk for a valgus deformity following greenstick fractures of the tibia.

GYMNAST'S WRIST/DISTAL RADIAL EPIPHYSITIS

Jeremy Swisher, MD ▪ Neil L. Sparks, DO, MS, FAAFP ▪ Kimberly Burbank, MD

BASICS

DESCRIPTION

- Distal radial epiphysitis, commonly known as gymnast's wrist, is an overuse injury that affects the growth plate at the distal radius.
- Patients will typically complain of chronic wrist pain on the radial side that is worsened with wrist loading movements. X-ray (XR) may show widening of the distal radial epiphyseal plate.

EPIDEMIOLOGY

- Distal radial epiphysitis is prevalent among adolescent athletes who participate in sports requiring repetitive wrist loading, such as gymnastics, weightlifting, softball, and baseball.
- Average age: 8 to 15 years old
- Peak age: 11 years old
- Predominant sex: female

Pediatric Considerations

- The distal radial epiphyseal plate closes at ~17 years of age. Female growth plates typically close before males.
- Distal radial epiphysitis occurring before the growth plate closes places the pediatric population at risk for uneven or restricted growth of the radius.

ETIOLOGY AND PATHOPHYSIOLOGY

- Distal radial epiphysitis is primarily caused by repetitive and forceful wrist extension activities, leading to increased stress on the distal radial epiphyseal plate.
- Microtrauma and cumulative stress can contribute to inflammation, pain, and potential disruption of the normal growth process in this epiphyseal plate.

RISK FACTORS

- Accelerated growth spurt
- High body mass index (BMI)
- History of previous injury
- High training volume
- Poor flexibility

GENERAL PREVENTION

- Avoiding early sports specialization by taking a minimum of 3 to 4 months out of the year off from each sport
- Using a wrist brace to limit wrist hyperextension
- Working on mobility to improve strength and flexibility of the smaller muscles of the wrist and hand

DIAGNOSIS

HISTORY

- Gymnast's wrist typically presents as a gradual onset of distal radius pain, and athletes may complain of swelling, tenderness, or limited range of motion of the wrist.
- They are typically involved in weight-bearing activities of the wrist, such as handstands or weightlifting.
- The pain is exacerbated with wrist-loading movements but may also be present at rest.

PHYSICAL EXAM

- On exam, patients will have tenderness to palpation over the distal radial epiphyseal plate.
- There can also be reduced grip strength as well as pain that is worsened with axial wrist loading or wrist hyperextension.

DIFFERENTIAL DIAGNOSIS

- Scaphoid stress reaction
- Distal radial fracture
- Dorsal impingement syndrome
- Triangular fibrocartilage complex (TFCC) injury

DIAGNOSTIC TESTS & INTERPRETATION

Gymnast's wrist can be diagnosed clinically. However, if there is clinical uncertainty, radiography and magnetic resonance imaging (MRI) can assist in making a diagnosis or ruling out more concerning pathology.

Initial Tests (lab, imaging)

- Initial imaging of choice is plain radiography (anteroposterior [AP] and lateral) of the wrist to examine for widening of the distal radial epiphyseal plate. XR may also show spurring of the metaphysis and sclerotic changes. A contralateral view is helpful for comparison (1)[C].
- MRI can also be used to look for irregular widening of the epiphyseal plate or paraphyseal edema, but it is typically unnecessary.

Follow-Up Tests & Special Considerations

- Follow-up imaging is not required if patients are making good clinical improvements.
- Consider repeat imaging or more advanced imaging if there is worsening pain or you have concerns about premature closure of the physis.
- Positive ulnar variance (when the distal ulnar articular surface projects more distal than the radius) can be seen on XR and can increase the risk of developing other wrist pathologies (1)[C],(2)[C].

TREATMENT

GENERAL MEASURES

- It is important to take 4 to 6 weeks of rest from activities that load the wrist (1)[C],(3)[C].
- Gradual return to activity after this period of rest and immobilization can begin if pain-free.
- Ice, nonsteroidal anti-inflammatory drugs (NSAIDs), and acetaminophen are appropriate in the short term.
- Wrist bracing can decrease stress through the growth plate, due to limiting wrist dorsiflexion (1)[C],(4)[C].

MEDICATION
Medications are not required for the treatment of gymnast's wrist. However, the following NSAIDs can be considered in the short term to assist with decreasing pain and inflammation in the pediatric patient:
- diclofenac (25 mg 4 times daily)
- naproxen (5 to 7 mg/kg/dose every 8 to 12 hours)
- or ibuprofen (400 mg every 4 to 6 hours)

First Line
- Rest and immobilization are the mainstays of treatment. Physical therapy can play an important role in strengthening the surrounding muscles and connective tissue after immobilization to prevent further injury (1)[C],(3)[C].
- An initial rest period of 4 to 6 weeks is recommended to decrease the loading and shearing forces through the physis. Further rest and immobilization can then be considered based on their clinical recovery.

ISSUES FOR REFERRAL
Follow-up is important in the first 2 months at regular intervals. If pain persists or becomes more severe despite conservative measures, an orthopedic surgery referral is appropriate.

SURGERY/OTHER PROCEDURES
- Although surgery is rarely required, it is indicated in cases of severe growth arrest.
- Operative management should focus on achieving neutral ulnar variance (joint leveling).
- The level of skeletal maturity guides surgical intervention. For children >12, epiphysiodesis of the longer bone is recommended. For those <12, physis stapling is recommended. After skeletal maturity, surgical intervention to lengthen the radius or shorten the ulna can be performed through various surgical approaches (5)[B].

COMPLEMENTARY & ALTERNATIVE MEDICINE
Physical therapy and occupational therapy play a vital role in the rehabilitation of these patients. Improving the strength and flexibility of the smaller stabilizing muscles of the wrist is helpful for recovery and preventing future injury.

ONGOING CARE

FOLLOW-UP RECOMMENDATIONS
- Patients should have follow-up in clinic every 2 weeks in the first 2 months to evaluate their clinical response. Clinic appointments can then be spaced as appropriate if they have recovered and are beginning a return to activity.
- Rate of recurrence: ~12% (6)[C]

PATIENT EDUCATION
- Early sports specialization can place an athlete at increased risk of overuse injuries.
- 3 to 4 months out of the year, one should be encouraged to take a break from their primary sport and allow other muscle groups and joints to be active.
- Do not train through the pain. Premature closure of the growth plate is a real complication if distal radial epiphysitis is not treated appropriately.
- The average duration of symptoms before a diagnosis: ~3 months (6)[C].
- Tell your coach or physician early if you are experiencing symptoms.

PROGNOSIS
- With appropriate management, there is typically a great prognosis for those diagnosed with distal radial epiphysitis.
- Initial improvements are typically observed in the first 4 to 6 weeks of treatment.
- Full recovery can occur within 2 to 3 months when following the recommended rest and rehabilitation plan.
- A delay in diagnosis or presentation to a healthcare provider can lead to a worse prognosis.

COMPLICATIONS
- Some complications to be aware of include disruption of the growth plate, premature closure of the growth plate, chronic wrist pain, reduced range of motion, and potential bone stress injury.
- Important preventative measures for these complications include adherence to rest and immobilization to allow the body to heal. Having close follow-up with patients can be helpful to stress the importance of this and to look for complications.
- Madelung-type deformity: premature closure of the ulnar aspect of the distal radial physis; this can lead to increased volar tilt with the ulna dorsally displaced.

REFERENCES

1. Lintner LJ, Swisher JR, Sitton ZE. Childhood and adolescent sports-related overuse injuries. *Am Fam Physician.* 2023;108(6):544–553.
2. Tomori Y, Nanno M, Takai S. Premature closure of the distal radial physis without evident history of trauma: a case report. *Medicine (Baltimore).* 2020;99(31):e21515.
3. Arnold A, Thigpen CA, Beattie PF, et al. Overuse physeal injuries in youth athletes: risk factors, prevention, and treatment strategies. *Sports Health.* 2017;9(2):139–147.
4. Hart E, Whited A, Bae DS, et al. Wrist guards/supports in gymnastics: are they helping or hurting you? *Am J Sports Med.* 2023;51(13):3426–3433.
5. Mauck B, Kelly D, Sheffer B, et al. Gymnast's wrist (distal radial physeal stress syndrome). *Orthop Clin North Am.* 2020;51(4):493–497.
6. Heyworth BE, Sullivan N, Hart E, et al. Gymnast's wrist: a retrospective analysis of descriptive epidemiology, clinical & radiologic features, treatment & outcomes. *Orthop J Sports Med.* 2019;7(Suppl 3):2325967119S00064.

ADDITIONAL READING

- Saxena TA, Mckie J. *Madelung Deformity.* StatPearls Publishing; 2025. https://www.ncbi.nlm.nih.gov/books/NBK580535/
- Sports Medicine Review. Gymnast's wrist (radial epiphysitis). https://www.sportsmedreview.com/blog/gymnasts-wrist-radial-epiphysitis/

G

CLINICAL PEARLS
- Characterized by insidious onset of radial sided wrist pain along the growth plate
- 4 to 6 weeks of rest from wrist-loading activities is recommended as initial treatment.
- Short-arm wrist splints can decrease stress through the joint by limiting wrist dorsiflexion.
- A delay in diagnosis or treatment can have serious complications, including premature closure of the growth plate.
- There are relatively high rates of recurrence for this condition, so it is important to have close follow-up and stress adherence to the prescribed regimen.

HAGLUND DEFORMITY (PUMP BUMP)

Shaun P. Garff, DO • Rohan M. Sebastian, MD, MBA

BASICS

DESCRIPTION

- Haglund deformity is an abnormal prominence of the posterosuperior surface of the calcaneus. It can give rise to Haglund disease, which consists of retrocalcaneal bursitis, insertional Achilles tendinitis, and pre-Achilles (superficial) bursitis. These occur due to compression of the distal Achilles tendon and the surrounding soft tissues.
- Named after the Swedish orthopedic surgeon Patrick Haglund in 1928 (1)
- Often chronic process but can present with acute exacerbation of pain
- Synonyms(s): Haglund disease; Haglund syndrome; pump bump; Mulholland deformity

EPIDEMIOLOGY

Haglund deformity affects females more than males and is seen in all active age groups.

- Seen in individuals/athletes wearing shoes with rigid heel counters (e.g., pumps, ice skates, work boots, high heels) or experience an increase in training (e.g., increase in miles, running on hard surfaces)
- Incidence increases with age and significantly higher in patients with diabetes mellitus (DM) and hypothyroidism (2).

RISK FACTORS

- Heel varus
- Pes cavus
- Rigid plantarly flexed 1st ray
- Rigid or poorly shaped heel counters
- Tight Achilles tendon

GENERAL PREVENTION

- Appropriate shoe wear (avoiding high heels and shoes with rigid heel counters)
- Heel lift/pad
- Stretching Achilles tendon
- Avoiding running on hard surfaces or uphill

DIAGNOSIS

HISTORY

- Posterior heel pain with palpable bump
- Increase in training program, specifically number of miles run or changing running surface
- Change in shoe wear (shoes with rigid heel counters can irritate the subcutaneous tissues and can inflame the underlying bursae)
- May be an incidental finding on imaging without any symptoms

PHYSICAL EXAM

- Dull, achy, exertional posterior heel pain
- Tenderness and thickening of the overlying skin at the Achilles tendon attachment
- Palpable swelling anterior or posterior to the Achilles tendon
- Pain intensified with active or passive dorsiflexion of the ankle
- Prominent-appearing posterosuperior portion of the calcaneus
- Careful, discrete palpation may differentiate between swelling in the Achilles tendon and swelling in the retrocalcaneal bursa.
- Assessment for gastrocnemius/soleus tightness is imperative.

DIFFERENTIAL DIAGNOSIS

- Retro-Achilles bursitis
- Achilles tendinitis/tendinosis
- Retrocalcaneal bursitis
- Calcaneal stress fracture
- Ankle impingement
- Tibiotalar degenerative joint disease

DIAGNOSTIC TESTS & INTERPRETATION

- Weight-bearing radiographs of both feet and/or ankles can assist in determining enthesopathic spurring and thus concern for state of the Achilles tendon degradation (1).
- Lateral radiographs may show a 2- to 3-mm bony extrusion on the posterosuperior angle of the calcaneus.
- Calcaneal body index assesses the shape of the calcaneus, and the calcaneal inclination angle assesses the orientation of the calcaneus; good predictors of posterior heel pain
- Calcaneal pitch lines and Fowler lines have been used in the past for diagnosis but in recent studies have been found to have no statistically significant relationship to posterior heel pain (3).
- Consider ordering magnetic resonance imaging (MRI) or musculoskeletal ultrasound (US) to evaluate the integrity of the Achilles tendon and the retrocalcaneal bursa.

TREATMENT

GENERAL MEASURES

- Shoe modification
- Ensure the shoe's heel counter (trim line) sits below or well above the bony protrusion to avoid direct pressure.

- Use a heel lift (0.25 to 0.5 inch) to slightly elevate the heel, reducing tension on the Achilles and shifting pressure from the prominence.
- Apply a tongue pad or an Achilles heel pad to the shoe to reduce friction over the bump (4)[C].
- Achilles stretching program
- Decrease in mileage and hill running
- Minimization of hard-surface running
- Nonsteroidal anti-inflammatory drugs (NSAIDs) (topical and/or short-term oral)
- Immobilization with a short leg cast or walking boot
- Soft tissue modalities (i.e., ice, US, iontophoresis, ASTYM, Graston Technique)

ALERT
Corticosteroid injections are generally avoided to prevent injury or damage to Achilles tendon (5)[C].

ADDITIONAL THERAPIES
Although evidence is limited, dry needling of the gastrocnemius/soleus for insertional tendinopathy that can coexist with Haglund deformity can be helpful.

SURGERY/OTHER PROCEDURES
- Partial (posterosuperior) calcaneal osteotomy (open or endoscopic) with excision of Haglund prominence; may include complete resection of the bursal projection or Achilles tendon débridement
- Endoscopic surgery has the advantage of shorter operative times, lower complication rates, and better cosmesis (6)[A].
- Postoperative course: immobilization in short leg cast or walking boot for 2 to 6 weeks, followed by 2 weeks partial weight-bearing, then full weight-bearing over succeeding 6 weeks; course shortened with endoscopic procedure
- Results of open surgery have generally shown good results, although failure rates have occurred in up to 25–30% (1).
- Rehabilitation program consisting of conditioning exercises and functional retraining

ONGOING CARE

FOLLOW-UP RECOMMENDATIONS
Return to clinic in 4 to 6 weeks for reevaluation and discussion of management options after initial conservative interventions.

COMPLICATIONS
- Achilles tendon rupture
- Postoperatively: infection, hematoma, recurrent exostosis, persistent pain, hypoesthesia (1)
- Chronic heel pain
- Sural nerve injury

REFERENCES

1. Syed TA, Perera A. A proposed staging classification for minimally invasive management of Haglund's syndrome with percutaneous and endoscopic surgery. *Foot Ankle Clin*. 2016;21(3):641–664.
2. Via AG, Oliva F, Padulo J, et al. Insertional calcific tendinopathy of the Achilles tendon and dysmetabolic diseases: an epidemiological survey. *Clin J Sport Med*. 2022;32(1):e68–e73.
3. Bulstra GH, van Rheenen TA, Scholtes VAB. Can we measure the heel bump? Radiographic evaluation of Haglund's deformity. *J Foot Ankle Surg*. 2015;54(3):338–340.
4. Choo YJ, Park CH, Chang MC. Rearfoot disorders and conservative treatment: a narrative review. *Ann Palliat Med*. 2020;9(5):3546–3552.
5. Thomas JL, Christensen JC, Kravitz SR, et al. The diagnosis and treatment of heel pain: a clinical practice guideline—revision 2010. *J Foot Ankle Surg*. 2010;49(3 Suppl):S1–S19.
6. Yuen WLP, Tan PT, Kon KKC. Surgical treatment of Haglund's deformity: a systematic review and meta-analysis. *Cureus*. 2022;14(7):e27500.

ADDITIONAL READING

Almaawi A, Boszczyk AM, Daniels TR. Exostosis (osteochondrosis, apophysites, and Haglund's deformity). In: Valderrabano V, Easley M, eds. *Foot and Ankle Sports Orthopaedics*. Springer; 2017:209–218.

CLINICAL PEARLS
- Posterior heel pain consistent with Haglund deformity needs foot/ankle x-rays.
- Not all radiographic evidence of a Haglund deformity produce symptoms.
- Initial treatment with conservative measures can be very successful.
- Return to play is dependent on the severity and number of associated conditions involved. Return to play after conservative treatment ranges from 2 to 8 weeks, whereas surgery and postoperative course limit and prevent strenuous activity for 4 to 6 months. Athletes may return to strenuous activity when local symptoms have resolved.

HALLUX VALGUS (BUNIONS)

Alan Shahtaji, DO, CAQSM • Jonathan Mason, DO, CAQSM, RMSK

BASICS

DESCRIPTION

- Hallux valgus (HV) refers to a subluxation of the 1st metatarsophalangeal (MTP) joint with lateral or valgus deviation of the great toe and medial (varus) deviation of the 1st metatarsal, leading to a bony prominence at the medial aspect of the joint (medial eminence or bunion).
- Synonym(s): bunion; hallux abducto valgus (HAV); metatarsus primus varus

EPIDEMIOLOGY

- More common in females; female:male = 10:1
- It occurs in approximately 23% of adults aged 18 to 65 years and up to 36% of adults >65 years but can occur in adolescents F > M 10 to 15 years of age.
- Familial tendency
- Almost exclusively seen in shoe-wearing societies
- Prevalence is highest in women in their 4th through 6th decades of life; potential worsening with aging
- Subset of juvenile/adolescent onset

ETIOLOGY AND PATHOPHYSIOLOGY

- The dorsal, plantar, medial, and lateral structures attach to proximal phalanx and maintain alignment of MTP articulation. There are no attachments on the distal metatarsal, so deviation of proximal phalanx dictates deformity.
- As HV deformity develops, the abductor hallucis tendon is displaced in a plantar direction and the joint loses most of its medial support.
- The adductor hallucis then pulls the proximal 1st phalanx laterally and exerts a rotational force, resulting in pronation of the 1st phalanx.
- With worsening of the HV deformity, the extensor hallucis longus shifts into the 1st metatarsal interspace and becomes a lateral force on the great toe.
- The plantar sesamoid complex may shift laterally if the 1st metatarsal continues to deviate medially.
- Pes planus and forefoot pronation likely accelerate the progression when HV is present. These conditions increase pressure on the medial aspect of the great toe and attenuation of the medial capsular structures at the 1st MTP joint.

RISK FACTORS

- Hereditary influences
- Constrictive footwear, mostly with narrow toe box; conflicting literature regarding high-heeled shoes; neuromuscular disorders and collagen-deficient disorders
- A rounded MTP articulation and longer 1st metatarsal
- Metatarsus primus varus and an increased 1st and 2nd intermetatarsal angle (IMA) are often implicated in juvenile or adolescent HV.
- Possible associations:
  - Tight gastrocnemius-soleus complex and Achilles tendon
  - Hypermobility of the 1st tarsometatarsal joint
  - Pes planus/planovalgus and forefoot pronation

GENERAL PREVENTION

Avoid tight-fitting shoes with narrow toe box.

COMMONLY ASSOCIATED CONDITIONS

- Lesser toe abnormalities, including hammertoes, crossover toes, and claw toes; ingrown toenails in the great toe or the 2nd toe
- Metatarsalgia (lateral)
- Plantar keratosis beneath the 2nd metatarsal head
- Bursitis with pressure erythema over deformed areas

DIAGNOSIS

HISTORY

- Pain over the medial MTP eminence aggravated by tight or rigid footwear is the most common complaint.
- Pain under the 2nd metatarsal head with a plantar keratosis is also common.
- Blisters, swelling, callus formation, or bursitis over the medial eminence may occur with athletic activities.
- Patients may describe forefoot widening or difficulty wearing shoes comfortably. Concern about foot appearance and footwear exists (1)[B]. Numbness or tingling of the medial aspect of the great toe may occur from compression of medial cutaneous nerve.
- May have weight shift and gait compensation to lateral foot resulting in metatarsalgia

ALERT

Lateral metatarsalgia may be presenting complaint (2)[B].

PHYSICAL EXAM

- Note the severity of HV and rotational deformity of the great toe in both the standing and non–weight-bearing positions.
- Assess for alignment of arch and hindfoot.
- Check active and passive range of motion (ROM) at the 1st MTP joint (normal extension is ~70 degrees) and tarsometatarsal joint.
- Evaluate sensation of the great toe.
- Assess for pain and location of great toe sesamoids.
- Evaluate for tightness of the gastrocnemius-soleus complex.

DIFFERENTIAL DIAGNOSIS

- Hallux rigidus (degenerative arthritis of the great toe MTP joint with dorsal bunion)
- Trauma with torn medial capsule
- HV interphalangeus (valgus at the interphalangeal joint, not the MTP joint)
- Gout and other inflammatory conditions
- Osteoarthritis of the 1st MTP joint

DIAGNOSTIC TESTS & INTERPRETATION

Weight-bearing anteroposterior (AP), oblique, and lateral foot radiographs along with sesamoid views may be helpful.

ALERT

- Using the AP radiographs, the HV angle (HVA) can be measured. HVA is calculated using the bisection of the longitudinal axes from the proximal phalanx and the 1st metatarsal. Normal HVA is <15 degrees.
- The 1st to 2nd IMA is formed by the intersection of the longitudinal axis of the 1st and 2nd metatarsals; normal IMA <9 degrees
- Radiographs can assess MTP joint congruity and presence of arthritis. Subluxation of the MTP, position of the sesamoids, and shape of the metatarsal head are also evaluated (3)[B].

TREATMENT

GENERAL MEASURES

- Initial treatment consists of footwear modification and patient education.
- Nonsurgical interventions may improve pain outcomes in the short-to-intermediate term (1)[A].
- Nonsurgical interventions are unlikely to improve HVA (1)[A].
- Treatment of an athlete with HV should be nonoperative until pain and symptoms are significantly affecting athletic performance.
- Wider toe box footwear will help decrease pressure and friction on the medial eminence.
- Shoes with flexible and nonconstricting stitching over the medial eminence are recommended (shoes can be professionally stretched to provide additional room).
- Medial longitudinal arch support may decrease pressure on the 1st metatarsal, especially in patients with pes planus. Custom-fabricated orthotics improve foot pain (4)[A] but do not change radiographic progression (5).
- Activity modification in joggers and runners (substituting bicycling or other nonimpact activities) may significantly decrease symptoms and stress on the forefoot.
- Bunion splints, spacers, and slings/guards may help alleviate symptoms but do not slow progression nor permanently "fix" HV.

MEDICATION

Topical and occasional use of short term oral nonsteroidal anti-inflammatory drugs (NSAIDs) may be beneficial in decreasing pain and inflammation.

ADDITIONAL THERAPIES

- Felt pads to protect the medial eminence
- Metatarsal pads to help unload the joint

Pediatric Considerations

- Similar to adults in that it is predominantly a female preponderance
- More common bilaterally with unilateral symptomology
- Necessitating further work-up
- Nonoperative treatments are similar to adults including mostly shoe modifications
- Surgery recommended for unrelenting pain as there are high recurrence rates in the juvenile patient
- Consideration should be given to wait until physis are closed.

SURGERY/OTHER PROCEDURES

- Surgery should be considered after nonsurgical treatment has failed and is not solely indicated for cosmesis.
- Numerous surgical procedures have been developed to correct HV.
- Operative procedures include various osteotomies and soft tissue releases. MTP fusions are considered in severe HV, arthritic, inflammatory, and/or neuromuscular conditions.
- A distal chevron osteotomy may be beneficial in alleviating pain in mild and moderate HV (4)[A], whereas proximal crescentic osteotomy and distal soft-tissue repair has been used with moderate to severe cases (2)[A].
- With the minimally invasive chevron osteotomy, radiologic and clinical outcome is comparable to the open technique (1)[B].

ONGOING CARE

FOLLOW-UP RECOMMENDATIONS

Patients should be referred for surgical consideration when nonoperative treatments, including footwear and activity modification, have not adequately relieved symptoms.

COMPLICATIONS

- Increased risk of falls secondary to pain and postoperative footwear, especially in the elderly
- Lesser toe deformities and local skin breakdown and ulceration
- Considerations: Stiffness, decreased ROM, and reduced function of the MTP joint are potential risks of surgery and may hamper athletic performance (especially in sprinters and dancers who require MTP motion for strength in toe push-off).
- It is important that patients understand that the bunion may still be present and not all patients will be able to wear desired shoes.

REFERENCES

1. Nix SE, Vicenzino BT, Collins NJ, et al. Characteristics of foot structure and footwear associated with hallux valgus: a systematic review. *Osteoarthritis Cartilage*. 2012;20(10):1059–1074.
2. Coughlin MJ, Jones CP. Hallux valgus and first ray mobility: a prospective study. *J Bone Joint Surg Am*. 2007;89(9):1887–1898.
3. Nix SE, Vicenzino BT, Smith MD. Foot pain and functional limitation in healthy adults with hallux valgus: a cross-sectional study. *BMC Musculoskelet Disord*. 2012;13:197.
4. Kuhn J, Alvi F. *Hallux Valgus*. StatPearls Publishing; 2023. Updated September 29, 2022. Accessed August 8, 2025. https://www.ncbi.nlm.nih.gov/books/NBK553092/
5. Redfern D. Minimally invasive chevron akin (MICA) for correction of hallux valgus. *Tech Foot Ankle Surg*. 2020;19(3):132–141.

ADDITIONAL READING

- Coughlin MJ, Jones CP. Hallux valgus: demographics, etiology, and radiographic assessment. *Foot Ankle Int*. 2007;28(7):759–777.
- Hawke F, Burns J, Radford JA, et al. Custom-made foot orthoses for the treatment of foot pain. *Cochrane Database Syst Rev*. 2008;(3):CD006801.
- Hurn SE, Matthews BG, Munteanu SE, et al. Effectiveness of nonsurgical interventions for hallux valgus: a systematic review and meta-analysis. *Arthritis Care Res (Hoboken)*. 2022;74(10):1676–1688.
- Kaufmann G, Dammerer D, Heyenbrock F, et al. Minimally invasive versus open chevron osteotomy for hallux valgus correction: a randomized controlled trial. *Int Orthop*. 2019;43(2):343–350.
- Reina M, Lafuente G, Munuera P. Effect of custom-made foot orthoses in female hallux valgus after one-year follow up. *Prosthet Orthot Int*. 2013;37(2):113–119.

CLINICAL PEARLS

- HV deformities mostly occur in females > males with a hereditary predisposition in shoe wearing cultures.
- Activity modification, proper footwear, and selective use of orthotic arch supports may be used to control symptoms.
- Refractory symptoms are a surgical indication, but the bunion may remain, and loss of ROM postoperatively is significant for some athletes.
- Do not confuse with traumatic entity of medial capsule injury.

HAMMER/CLAW/MALLET TOE

Antonio Howard, MBBS, MSc, FAAPMR, CAQSM ▪ Robert D. Martin, MD

BASICS

DESCRIPTION

- Toe joint deformities result from an imbalance between flexor and extensor forces about the interphalangeal (IP) and metatarsophalangeal (MTP) joints. Pain often results from abnormal distribution of pressure and increased friction against other toes or footwear:
  - Mallet toe is a flexion deformity at the distal interphalangeal (DIP) joint.
  - Hammer toe is a flexion deformity affecting the proximal interphalangeal (PIP) joint. Concomitant extension at the MTP joint may be present.
  - Claw toe is a flexion deformity affecting the PIP and DIP joints. Concomitant extension at the MTP joint is always present.
- Acute deformities are usually flexible/reducible. Chronic deformities may become rigid/fixed.

EPIDEMIOLOGY

- Incidence increases with age.
- Female preponderance, especially after age 70 years
- Claw toe deformity may be present in up to 46% of patients within the first year after a severe stroke.
- Hammer toe deformity is the most common lesser toe deformity. The 2nd toe is most commonly affected.

ETIOLOGY AND PATHOPHYSIOLOGY

Imbalance between flexor and extensor forces about the IP and MTP joints, secondary to:

- Toe crowding in ill-fitting footwear leading to chronic shortening of the flexor tendons and eventual flexion contracture
- Traumatic injury to the:
  - Terminal extensor tendon of the extensor expansion resulting in reduction of extensor forces and predominance of flexor tone at the DIP joint, or
  - Metatarsal/plantar plate resulting in dorsal subluxation of the MTP joint and predominant flexor tone at the IP joints
- Chronic synovitis leading to injury of the terminal extensor tendon, sagittal bands, and/or metatarsal/plantar plate
- Neurologic disease, such as:
  - Peripheral neuropathy and associated intrinsic foot muscle weakness. The foot intrinsic muscles are responsible for flexion at the MTP joint and extension at the IP joints. Weakness of the foot intrinsic muscles with preservation of the long flexor tone leads to the predominance of MTP extension and IP flexion forces that result in claw toe.
  - Spasticity leading to increased tone in the extrinsic muscles of the foot—the long flexors/extensors which overpower the small intrinsic muscles of the foot and have the combined effect of extension at the MTP joint and flexion at the IP joints
- Long flexor tendon contracture as a complication of posterior leg compartment syndrome

RISK FACTORS

- Constricting footwear—high heels, narrow and shallow toe box
- Abnormally long metatarsal and/or toe, relative to adjacent ray
- Neuromuscular disorders (more commonly associated with claw toe deformity), such as:
  - Peripheral neuropathy (e.g., secondary to diabetes mellitus and Charcot-Marie-Tooth disease)
  - Muscular dystrophies
  - Equinovarus associated with spasticity and/or dystonia (e.g., with stroke, cerebral palsy)
- Inflammatory joint disease
- Older age
- High body mass index
- Acute trauma

GENERAL PREVENTION

Avoidance of constrictive footwear

DIAGNOSIS

HISTORY

- Trauma
- Personal or family history of neuromuscular disorder
- Risk factors for peripheral neuropathy: diabetes mellitus, alcohol abuse, renal failure

PHYSICAL EXAM

- Inspect for:
  - Toe deformity and position of the MTP, PIP, and DIP joints. Observations should be made in the weight-bearing and non–weight-bearing position.
  - Signs of abnormal pressure: callous formation (usually dorsal IP joints, at the tip of the toe or at the metatarsal heads on the plantar surface), skin ulcers, injury to nails.
  - Other associated foot/toe deformities: equinovarus, pes planus/cavus, hallux valgus, under-riding or over-riding toes
  - Gait evaluation: Observe for antalgic gait. Often times, spasticity is more pronounced during ambulation.
  - Palpate to assess for:
    - The point of maximal tenderness to guide the need for pressure relief
    - The presence or absence of synovitis
    - Joint range of motion
    - Laxity of the MTP joint plantar plate
    - Flexible versus fixed deformity; this may be assessed by passively ranging the MTP and/or IP joints or by moving the ankle into plantar flexion and observing for resolution of hammer or claw toe deformities. Alternatively, dorsally directed pressure on the plantar surface of the involved metatarsal may reduce a flexible hammer toe deformity (push up test).
    - Heel cord tightness using the Silfverskiold test (It measures the dorsiflexion [DF] of the foot at the ankle joint [AJ] with knee extended and flexed to 90 degrees. The test is considered positive when DF at the AJ is greater with knee flexed than extended.)
    - Neurovascular integrity and muscular tone.
- Examination considerations:
  - Patients should be examined in weight-bearing and non–weight-bearing positions because MTP extension may be more manifest during weight-bearing.
  - Similarly, hammer and claw toe deformities may be less apparent with certain ankle positions. Ankle equinus should be manually corrected and the toes reexamined for deformity in this position.
  - It is important to distinguish between flexible versus fixed deformity. If a deformity is correctable with manipulation, it is typically considered a "flexible" deformity. Flexible deformities are more likely to respond to nonoperative measures. Fixed deformities are more likely to require surgery.

DIAGNOSTIC TESTS & INTERPRETATION

Initial Tests (lab, imaging)

- Imaging is typically not necessary to make a diagnosis. When obtained, weight-bearing x-rays of the feet—anteroposterior (AP), lateral, and oblique—should:
  - Confirm the presence of IP joint deformity
  - Identify other associated foot abnormalities (e.g., MTP joint subluxation)

- Consider rheumatologic workup as guided by the clinical index of suspicion: erythrocyte sedimentation rate (ESR), C-reactive protein (CRP), complete blood count (CBC), rheumatoid factor (RF), and antinuclear antibody (ANA).
- Advanced imaging—bone scan or magnetic resonance imaging (MRI)—may be indicated in cases of ulceration with suspected underlying osteomyelitis.

Diagnostic Procedures/Other
- Nerve conduction study and electromyography (NCS/EMG) may be useful in the workup for neuromuscular causes.
- Motor nerve blocks with local anesthetic may be helpful in distinguishing between spasticity and contracture.

TREATMENT

GENERAL MEASURES
- Patient education about shoe selection/modification—flat/low heel, wider, and taller toe-box and adequate length (1)[C]. A good rule of thumb is, there should be a circumference of 1 cm around the foot and at the distal tip of the toes when standing on the insole.
- Orthotics/measures to reduce flexible deformities (e.g., Budin splint, figure of 8 taping) (1),(2)[C]
- Other pressure relief measures:
  - Toe sleeves, typically with foam padding to relieve pressure over the dorsal toe
  - Toe crests relieve pressure at the tip of the toes.
  - Metatarsal pads relieve pressure under the metatarsal heads.
  - Rocker bottom sole can help reduce forefoot pressure during gait (3)[C].
- Attention to nail care and callous trimming, as necessary

MEDICATION
- Oral analgesics for pain—acetaminophen, nonsteroidal anti-inflammatory drugs (NSAIDs)
- Chemodenervation/neurolysis:
  - Alcohol or phenol neurolysis (e.g., tibial nerve motor branch block to treat equinus)
  - Botulinum toxin injection at muscle motor points in the flexor digitorum longus (FDL) and flexor hallucis longus and brevis (FHL and FHB) muscles (4)[B]
- Medication considerations:
  - Exercise the usual precautions in cases of known liver, renal, gastrointestinal, pulmonary, or cardiac disease.

ISSUES FOR REFERRAL
- Surgery *may* be indicated when nonoperative treatment is unsuccessful in relieving symptoms.
- Surgery may also be indicated to promote ulcer healing or to reduce the risk of ulcer progression and/or recurrence in patients at high risk for morbidity e.g. diabetics (5)[B].
- The acute onset of toe deformity or pain, particularly in the athlete or in the presence of associated trauma, should lead to more prompt and urgent evaluation by a surgeon.

ADDITIONAL THERAPIES
Consider prescribing exercises for heel cord stretching (in subtalar neutral) and foot core strengthening as clinically indicated.

SURGERY/OTHER PROCEDURES
- Differentiation between flexible and rigid deformity must be incorporated into surgical planning:
  - Flexible hammer/claw toes may be repaired with flexor and extensor percutaneous tenotomies (1)[C].
  - Flexible mallet toes may be treated with percutaneous release of the FDL tendon (1)[C].
  - Transfer of the FDL tendon to the extensor mechanism is an option in some flexible deformities (1),(6)[C].
  - Rigid deformities often require a capsulotomy or treatment with arthroplasty (joint resection) or arthrodesis (joint fusion) (6)[C].
- Involvement of the MTP joint may require additional soft tissue (i.e., capsulotomy, collateral ligament release, plantar plate repair) and/or bony (i.e., shortening osteotomy) procedures.

ONGOING CARE

FOLLOW-UP RECOMMENDATIONS
In the absence of any pressing surgical indication (e.g., acute trauma, competitive athlete, ulcer/infection), nonsurgical treatment may be a long-term option provided that the patient's expectations are being met, and symptoms do not create significant interruption in activities of daily living (ADLs).

PROGNOSIS
- Surgery may be unnecessary if nonsurgical treatment is started early.
- Postoperative recovery time varies depending on the complexity and invasiveness of the procedure.
- Most patients are allowed to bear weight through the heel immediately following surgical intervention.
- Return to activity is highly dependent on the type of procedure performed. For example, after plantar plate repair, return to play may be delayed for 3 months following surgery.

COMPLICATIONS
- Fixed toe deformity
- Toenail injury
- Callous formation
- Ulceration with the potential for osteomyelitis
- If surgery is performed:
  - Excessive shortening of the toe may lead to poor motor control of the affected digit.
  - Excessive shortening of the metatarsal may lead to a floating toe in addition to causing transfer metatarsalgia (adjacent metatarsal pain).
  - Persistent numbness of the toe and surrounding areas may occur as a result of nerve injury.
  - FDL tendon transfer results in the inability to actively flex the affected toe at the distal interphalangeal joint.

REFERENCES

1. Frey-Ollivier S, Catena F, Hélix-Giordanino M, et al. Treatment of flexible lesser toe deformities. *Foot Ankle Clin*. 2018;23(1):69–90.
2. Federer AE, Tainter DM, Adams SB, et al. Conservative management of metatarsalgia and lesser toe deformities. *Foot Ankle Clin*. 2018;23(1):9–20.
3. Malhotra K, Davda K, Singh D. The pathology and management of lesser toe deformities. *EFORT Open Rev*. 2017;1(11):409–419.
4. Takekawa T, Takagi S, Kitajima T, et al. Claw toe: anatomic guide for injection of botulinum toxin into foot muscles. *Can J Neurol Sci*. 2022;49(1):102–108.
5. Andersen AH, Rasmussen A, Frimodt-Møller M, et al. The effect of needle tenotomy on hammer, mallet and claw toe deformities in patients with diabetes, a retrospective study. *J Clin Transl Endocrinol*. 2019;12(18):100208.
6. Manz WJ, Bariteau JT. Complications of lesser toe surgery: how to avoid them before surgery and how to assess and treat them when they have occurred. *Foot Ankle Clin*. 2022;27(2):233–251.

ADDITIONAL READING

- Hagedorn TJ, Dufour AB, Riskowski JL, et al. Foot disorders, foot posture, and foot function: the Framingham foot study. *PLoS One*. 2013;8(9):e74364.
- Hannan MT, Menz HB, Jordan JM, et al. High heritability of hallux valgus and lesser toe deformities in adult men and women. *Arthritis Care Res (Hoboken)*. 2013;65(9):1515–1521.
- Laurent G, Valentini F, Loiseau K, et al. Claw toes in hemiplegic patients after stroke. *Ann Phys Rehabil Med*. 2010;53(2):77–85.
- Lim EC, Ong BK, Seet RC. Botulinum toxin-A injections for spastic toe clawing. *Parkinsonism Relat Disord*. 2006;12(1):43–47.
- Mens MA, van Netten JJ, Busch-Westbroek TE, et al. Biomechanical and musculoskeletal changes after flexor tenotomy to reduce the risk of diabetic neuropathic toe ulcer recurrence. *Diabet Med*. 2022;39(4):e14761.
- Shirzad K, Kiesau CD, DeOrio JK, et al. Lesser toe deformities. *J Am Acad Orthop Surg*. 2011;19(8):505–514.

CLINICAL PEARLS
- Remember: The joint will deform or pull to the strong (intact) side.
- Injecting botulinum toxin to both the long and the short flexors of the toes is well tolerated and efficacious in the treatment of toe clawing from spasticity, allowing for lower dosages to be used than injecting the long flexors alone.
- Surgery for cosmesis alone should be strongly discouraged.

H

HAMSTRING STRAIN

Alan Shahtaji, DO, CAQSM • Alec Gabriel Contag, MD

BASICS

DESCRIPTION

- Hamstring injuries are among the most common reported muscle injuries in sports medicine.
- The musculotendinous unit (biceps femoris [BF], semitendinosus [ST], and semimembranosus [SM]) can be injured at multiple sites, including the proximal bony attachment, the proximal free tendon, the musculotendinous junction, the intramuscular tendon, the central muscle belly, and the distal tendon.
- The injury often occurs due to an excessive load during an eccentric contraction, such as with running or jumping.
- Time lost to this injury is significant, and rate of recurrence is high among athletes.
- Proximal hamstring tendinopathy is often a chronic process seen in runners.

EPIDEMIOLOGY

The BF is the most commonly injured muscle, with the myotendinous junction being most often affected.

Incidence

Hamstring injury incidence is 0.81 per 1,000 hours of activity, or about 10% of new injuries in field sports. Strains specifically occur at a rate of 0.67 per 1,000 hours (1)[A].

Prevalence

- Research has focused on male athletes, but no gender, body mass, or height predisposition exists.
- Injury prevalence across field sports was 13% over a 9-month course (1)[A].
- Prevalence varies but has been reported up to 29% in athletes (2)[A].
- Reinjury is common and is reported at rates of 12–31%.

ETIOLOGY AND PATHOPHYSIOLOGY

- Strains are classified by severity of muscle fiber injury:
  - Stretch type injury with few muscle fibers injured, causing only minor swelling/pain and minimal loss of strength/motion
  - Partial tear with strength loss and functional limitations due to more extensive muscle injury
  - Extensive or complete tear across whole muscle with disabling loss of muscle function
  - Magnetic resonance imaging (MRI) classifications vary and are either based on extent of edema and signal change versus location of injury.
  - The healing process in muscle injury includes initial muscle fiber insult with immediate hemorrhage followed by inflammatory cell introduction to the damaged tissue, production of connective scar tissue, and regeneration of damaged muscle fibers.
- The hamstring musculotendinous unit (BF, ST, and SM) is susceptible to injury for many reasons:
  - The hamstrings cross two joints, which can be moving in opposing directions.
  - The short head of the BF has a long, inconstant origin along the femur.
  - The hamstrings (specifically the biceps) have dual innervation, which causes forceful, uncoordinated contractions (the hamstrings, including the long head of the biceps, are innervated by the tibial branch of the sciatic nerve, with the exception being the short head of the biceps, which alone is innervated by the peroneal branch of the sciatic nerve).
- The usual mechanism of injury occurs in the later part of the swing phase as the hamstrings rapidly change from eccentrically working to decelerate knee extension to concentrically becoming an extensor of the hip.

RISK FACTORS

Individual factors include, strength imbalances, flexibility, core strength, lumbopelvic position, age, previous injury, and fatigue. Risk of strain specifically is similar at all ages, despite increasing injury risk overall in older athletes. Population factors include higher risk on grass fields over turf, and a 9.4 times higher risk during competition than training (1)[A].

ALERT

Previous history of hamstring injury increases risk of reinjury by 2 to 6 times. A proposed multifactorial model for hamstring injury includes poor flexibility, strength imbalances, inadequate warm-up, and muscle fatigue, with hamstring weakness and inflexibility being the largest contributors to injury (2)[A].

GENERAL PREVENTION

Primary prevention of acute hamstring injuries has been proven highly effective with a 50% reduction in injury using eccentric strengthening like Nordic hamstring exercises. Muscle soreness of these regimens limit adherence and compliance (2)[A].

COMMONLY ASSOCIATED CONDITIONS

Pediatric Considerations

Apophyseal injury, like traction apophysitis must be considered with the emergence of ischial apophyses at ages 13 to 15 years until ages 20 to 25 years when they fuse with the pelvis:

- Proximal avulsion injuries at the ischial tuberosity can occur with eccentric contraction during knee extension with hip flexion (i.e., hurdling in track with lead leg).
- This contrasts with adults, who tend to suffer complete tendon rupture proximally at the ischium.

DIAGNOSIS

Most hamstring strain injuries occur in an acute setting with sudden onset of posterior thigh pain that often limits participation. The diagnosis can be made with history and physical exam.

HISTORY

- Hamstring strain is most seen in kicking or speed athletes.
- In cases of avulsion injury, other activities are often reported, such as water skiing, dance, weightlifting, and ice skating.
- Acute or chronic:
  - Some hamstring strain injuries are more chronic in nature with recurring "tightness" or muscle "pull" complaints.
- Severity: Discontinuation of activity, inability to ambulate following the injury, and/or describing an audible pop at the time of injury can point toward a more severe strain or an avulsion injury.
- Location of pain (distal, mid, or proximal posterior thigh)

PHYSICAL EXAM

- A "stiff-legged" gait may occur as patient tries to avoid hip flexion with knee extension.
- Position patient prone and inspect for swelling and/or ecchymosis.
- Palpate the entire length of each hamstring muscle going from common origin on ischial tuberosity moving distally until insertion on fibular head (BF), medial femur (SM), and medial tibia (ST).
- Note location of pain and presence of defect. Test active range of motion, strength, flexibility, and neurovascular testing of bilateral lower extremities.
- Note severity of injury using maximal tolerance of passive straight leg raise/knee extension.

DIFFERENTIAL DIAGNOSIS

In addition to the associated injuries listed above, consider these in the differential diagnosis:

- Lumbar radiculopathy
- Direct hamstring injury, including muscle laceration or contusion (common direct mechanism for injury as opposed to indirect strain mechanism)
- Posterior lateral corner knee injury, meniscal injury, or popliteal cyst formation or rupture
- Pelvic or proximal femoral stress fracture
- Gluteus medius injury or adductor strain
- Hip injury

DIAGNOSTIC TESTS & INTERPRETATION

- History and physical exam alone are sufficient for diagnosis, but radiographs, MRI, and sonography may be useful in guiding selection of treatment.
- Radiographs: Anteroposterior pelvis can be helpful acutely if an avulsion is suspected.

- Ultrasound (US) and MRI can help determine more accurate location and extent of injury:
  - US is as useful as MRI for acute hamstring injury and has added benefit of low cost.
  - US images of complete tendon bundle avulsion from ischial tuberosity appear as an absence of tissue over the tuberosity with hypoechoic signs of hemorrhage, although partial tears show hypoechoic clefts without full tendon retraction.
  - MRI images of an acute injury appear as high signal in or around the muscle on T2-weighted images.
  - There is no significant change in MRI appearance over the first 7 days after acute hamstring injury.
  - MRI findings do not reliably predict time for return to play (RTP) (3)[A],(4)[C].
  - There is debate in the literature regarding the significance of injury to intramuscular tendon.

TREATMENT

- The treatment protocol is different for acute versus chronic injury as well as for initial versus recurrent injury. Location and type of injury also dictate treatment considerations (3)[A].
- 86% of injuries tend to be myofascial and can benefit from nonoperative treatment alone (4)[C].
- Acute:
  - Goals: control pain, swelling, hemorrhage, and muscle fiber adhesion; restore normal gait (5)[C]
  - Treatment:
    - Protection, rest, ice, compression, and elevation (PRICE):
      - Avoid nonsteroidal anti-inflammatory drugs (NSAIDs) because no proven benefit and may disrupt natural healing process; also, risk of side effects (5)[C]
      - Platelet-rich plasma (PRP) research has been divided regarding its effectiveness in acute hamstring injuries. Presently the literature does not show PRP to be effective in reducing time to RTP (3)[A].
- Subacute/rehab and functional (days to weeks/months):
  - Goals: advance activity as tolerated and work toward regaining strength, flexibility, and psychological readiness (5)[C]
  - Treatment:
    - Several different protocols exist, and hamstring rehabilitation could be an entire chapter unto itself. Criteria-based programs are being employed at most sports medicine institutions.
    - There is variability but attention to core strength, neuromuscular influences, and lumbar stability (3)[A].
      - Eccentric or lengthening programs tend to have better outcomes when compared to concentric-based rehab (3)[A].
- RTP:
  - Goals: Safe and timely RTP with best possible functionality and least risk of repeat injury
  - The absence of any structural injury on MRI is associated with accelerated RTP (3)[A].
  - Factors associated w/ RTP readiness: pain-free sports-specific activity, triple hopping, and muscular strength within 10% of uninjured side (4)[C]
  - Factors associated with delayed RTP include greater passive knee extension in uninjured leg, BF injury, bruising, pain severity at time of injury, and "popping" sound (3)[A].
  - Treatment:
    - May RTP when able to perform pain-free sport-specific activity along with a normal physical examination and psychological readiness (5)[C]
    - Use sports medicine RTP models that incorporate biopsychosocial influences.

SURGERY/OTHER PROCEDURES

- Surgical referral is indicated in proximal injuries with bony avulsions that are >2 cm displaced, two tendons that are retracted ≥2 cm, or three tendon avulsions (6)[A].
- More research is required regarding certain populations who may benefit from acute surgical intervention regardless of retraction length.
- No established guidelines exist defining what length of time counts as an acute versus chronic injury (6)[A].
- Distal tendon avulsions are less common but deserve special attention and may need primary surgical intervention, especially in high-level athletes.
- Surgical research suggests improved patient reported outcomes after surgery; however, no significant comparative studies exist between operative and nonoperative treatments in regard to RTP (6)[A].

ONGOING CARE

FOLLOW-UP RECOMMENDATIONS

- Recovery time after hamstring strain injury can be as short as 2 weeks and as long as several months, depending on the severity and chronicity of the injury.
- Although reinjury is common, proper functional rehab and appropriate RTP can minimize the risk.
- Maintenance and prevention protocols should focus on eccentric-based exercises and modifiable risk factors.

REFERENCES

1. Maniar N, Carmichael DS, Hickey JT, et al. Incidence and prevalence of hamstring injuries in field-based team sports: a systematic review and meta-analysis of 5952 injuries from over 7 million exposure hours. *Br J Sports Med*. 2023;57(2):109–116.
2. Rudisill SS, Varady NH, Kucharik MP, et al. Evidence-based hamstring injury prevention and risk factor management: a systematic review and meta-analysis of randomized controlled trials. *Am J Sports Med*. 2023;51(7):1927–1942.
3. Rudisill SS, Kucharik MP, Varady NH. Evidence-based management and factors associated with return to play after acute hamstring injury in athletes: a systematic review. *Orthop J Sports Med*. 2021;9(11):23259671211053833.
4. Chang JS, Kayani B, Plastow R, et al. Management of hamstring injuries: current concepts review. *Bone Joint J*. 2020;102-B(10):1281–1288.
5. Valle X, Tol JL, Hamilton B, et al. Hamstring muscle injuries, a rehabilitation protocol purpose. *Asian J Sports Med*. 2015;6(4):e25411.
6. Jokela A, Stenroos A, Kosola J, et al. A systematic review of surgical intervention in the treatment of hamstring tendon ruptures: current evidence on the impact on patient outcomes. *Ann Med*. 2022;54(1):978–988.

ADDITIONAL READING

- Askling CM, Tengvar M, Thorstensson A. Acute hamstring injuries in Swedish elite football: a prospective randomized controlled clinical trial comparing two rehabilitation protocols. *Br J Sports Med*. 2013;47(15):953–959.
- Bengtzen RR, Ma OJ, Herzka A. Point-of-care ultrasound diagnosis of proximal hamstring rupture. *J Emerg Med*. 2018;54(2):225–228.
- Brukner P, Connell D. 'Serious thigh muscle strains': beware the intramuscular tendon which plays an important role in difficult hamstring and quadriceps muscle strains. *Br J Sports Med*. 2016;50(4):205–208.
- Hamilton B, Tol JL, Almusa E, et al. Platelet-rich plasma does not enhance return to play in hamstring injuries: a randomised controlled trial. *Br J Sports Med*. 2015;49(14):943–950.
- Reurink G. Managing acute hamstring injuries in athletes. *Br J Sports Med*. 2017;51(7):614–615.
- Reurink G, Goudswaard GJ, Moen MH, et al. Platelet-rich plasma injections in acute muscle injury. *N Engl J Med*. 2014;370(26):2546–2547.
- van der Horst N, Backx F, Goedhart EA, et al. Return to play after hamstring injuries in football (soccer): a worldwide Delphi procedure regarding definition, medical criteria, and decision-making. *Br J Sports Med*. 2017;51(22):1583–1591.
- van der Made AD, Almusa E, Whiteley R, et al. Intramuscular tendon involvement on MRI has limited value for predicting time to return to play following acute hamstring injury. *Br J Sports Med*. 2018;52(2):83–88.
- Wangensteen A, Bahr R, Van Linschoten R, et al. MRI appearance does not change in the first 7 days after acute hamstring injury—a prospective study. *Br J Sports Med*. 2017;51(14):1087–1092.

CLINICAL PEARLS

- Previous history of hamstring injury is a significant risk factor for hamstring strain injury.
- Compliance with eccentric protocols like the Nordic hamstring protocols is essential for prevention of hamstring injuries.
- Functional rehab with criteria-based progression and incorporation of eccentric strengthening is effective for acute hamstring injuries.
- Evidence is inconclusive regarding PRP for RTP.
- Severe proximal and distal injuries may require surgery.

HEEL PAIN: HEEL FAT PAD SYNDROME, LATERAL PLANTAR NERVE ENTRAPMENT

Reno Ravindran, MD, FAAFP, CAQSM • Richard E. Rodenberg Jr., MD, FAAP, CAQSM

BASICS

DESCRIPTION

- Heel fat pad syndrome (HFPS):
  - The heel pad is composed of columns of adipose tissue (globules) separated by fibrous septae extending from the skin to the calcaneal periosteum.
  - The fibroelastic septae are arranged in a honeycombed structure, which runs vertically, diagonally, and transversely.
  - The encapsulated fat acts in a hydraulic fashion to absorb shock by resisting compressive loads.
  - The heel pad is located directly below the calcaneus and acts as a shock-absorbing layer allowing the heel to tolerate repetitive high load bearing, allowing for pain-free ambulation (1).
- Lateral plantar nerve (LPN) entrapment:
  - LPN and the first branch of the LPN (FBLPN), also known as Baxter nerve, are branches of the tibial nerve, which supplies autonomic, sensory, and motor fibers to the plantar foot. The LPN is the most common cause of plantar heel pain of neural origin (2).
- Synonym(s): calcaneodynia; heel pain syndrome; heel pad atrophy; calcaneal neuritis; policeman's heel; runner's heel; tennis heel; stone bruise; tuber calcanei pain; subcalcaneal bursitis

EPIDEMIOLOGY

- 1 in 10 people develop heel pain in their lifetime.
- Peak age 40 to 60 years (3)
- More common with increasing age, obesity, and diabetes
- LPN: relationship with long-distance running, ballerinas and gymnasts (4)
- More common with prolonged standing or walking on hard surfaces (3)

ETIOLOGY AND PATHOPHYSIOLOGY

- HFPS:
  - With aging, the heel pad becomes less elastic, making the patient more prone to atrophy of the pad which results in less shock absorption.
  - Trauma and inflammation may also lead to degeneration of the heel pad or rupture of the fibrous tissue septa, leading to decreased compressibility and heel pad atrophy.
  - The cause is often multifactorial leading to heel pad atrophy and pain (1),(3).
- LPN entrapment can occur at different sites:
  - Where the nerve passes at the sharp edge of the deep fascia of the abductor hallucis
  - Distal to the medial edge of the calcaneus
  - Between the abductor hallucis and the medial head of quadratus plantae muscle (2),(3)
  - Predisposing factors include abductor hallucis, muscle hypertrophy, local trauma, local venous engorgement, or calcaneal enthesophytes.

RISK FACTORS

- Elderly, advancing age
- Obesity
- Prolonged standing, walking, and running on hard surfaces
- Overuse in recreational and athletic activities
- Poorly constructed shoes
- Repetitive steroid injection due to potential for heel pad atrophy (3),(5)
- Possible associated altered biomechanics, including hyperpronation, decreased ankle dorsiflexion, decreased metatarsophalangeal joint extension, pes cavus, and pes planus
- Presence and absence of heel spurs do not correlate with heel pain.

DIAGNOSIS

HISTORY

- Gradual onset of plantar heel pain, which may be unilateral or bilateral
- May have a history of local trauma
- Pain may radiate into the arch or proximally to the medial heel area.
- If pain is severe enough, a patient may walk on the ball or lateral aspect of the foot.
- HFPS
  - Pain primarily with weight-bearing and relieved with rest
  - Symptoms can be exacerbated by walking barefoot or on hard surfaces; progressively worse with standing/walking (5)
  - Pain is described as deep and nonradiating involving the central weight-bearing portion of the calcaneal tuberosity and commonly misdiagnosed as plantar fasciitis. Plantar fasciitis pain is typically on medial calcaneal tuberosity.
  - Pain does not tend to radiate or increase with dorsiflexion (1),(3)[C].
- LPN entrapment:
  - Burning, sharp, shooting, shock-like pain; localized to the medial inferior aspect of the heel and proximally into the medial ankle region; pain may radiate across the plantar aspect of the heel to the lateral aspect of the foot.
  - Pain worse during or after weight-bearing activities and improves with rest
  - Pain at night may be due to nerve compression as a result of venostasis and venous engorgement.
  - Poststatic dyskinesia: plantar heel pain when patient first stands after periods of rest; can be typical in patients with heel pain of neural origin, but this can also occur in plantar fasciitis
  - Sensory deficit may not be common but occasionally, can cause tingling and/or numbness in the heel or foot (2)[C].

PHYSICAL EXAM

- HFPS:
  - Thorough examination of the lower extremity, including neurovascular exam, is recommended.
  - Exam is facilitated by having the patient lie prone.
  - Observe for any signs of fat pad atrophy.
  - Observe gait for signs of pes planus, pes cavus, hindfoot deformity, hyperpronation, as well as look for indications of posterior tibial tendon dysfunction.
  - Observe ankle range of motion (ROM) and pain is not reproducible with passive motion of the ankles or toes which may be more indicative of plantar fasciitis.
  - Tenderness directly over the central weight-bearing portion of the calcaneal tuberosity rather than on the distal tuberosity
  - Typically, negative calcaneal squeeze test
  - In prolonged cases, the underlying bone can be felt underneath the skin due to significant fat pad atrophy (1),(3).
- LPN entrapment:
  - FBLPN diagnosis is mainly clinical but a thorough physical exam is important to help rule out other etiologies of heel pain.
  - Palpation over the FBLPN deep to the abductor hallucis muscle or medial calcaneal tuberosity with reproduction of pain/symptoms proximally and distally; should have minimal tenderness over the plantar fascia origin
  - Dorsiflexion with eversion of the ankle can reproduce symptoms; although not specific, can help with diagnosis
  - Plantar flexion-inversion may reproduce symptoms, although not specific (5)[C].
  - Positive Tinel test (4)[C]
  - Medial heel or foot sensory disturbances are suggestive of an alternative nerve disorder because the FBLPN is purely motor (2).

DIFFERENTIAL DIAGNOSIS

- Calcaneal fracture or stress fracture
- Plantar fasciitis/fasciopathy
- Plantar aponeurosis rupture
- Local inflammatory conditions (subcalcaneal bursitis, osteomyelitis, tendonitis/tenosynovitis)
- Systemic inflammatory conditions (enthesitis, ankylosing spondylitis, Reiter syndrome, psoriatic arthritis, rheumatoid arthritis, inflammatory bowel–induced inflammation, gout, and pseudogout)
- Entrapment neuropathy (tarsal tunnel syndrome, medial calcaneal nerve, LPN/Baxter nerve)
- Infectious (osteomyelitis, tuberculosis)
- Benign neoplasm (glomus tumor of heel pad, osteoid osteoma, intraosseous lipoma, giant cell tumor)
- Malignant neoplasm (osteogenic sarcoma, chondrosarcoma, Ewing sarcoma, metastatic tumor)
- Neuropathy (diabetes mellitus, alcoholism, reflex sympathetic dystrophy)

- Metabolic (osteomalacia, Paget disease)
- Calcaneal apophysitis
- Referred pain from the low back (S1 radiculopathy) (3)

DIAGNOSTIC TESTS & INTERPRETATION

Initial Tests (lab, imaging)

- Radiographic studies are typically not needed to diagnose HFPS or LPN but can be used to rule in or out other diagnoses in the differential (3)[C].
- Anteroposterior, lateral, and oblique plain radiographs; radiographs may reveal calcaneal spurs or calcifications, fractures, tumors, arthrosis, or other unusual causes of heel pain.
- High-resolution ultrasound (US) or magnetic resonance imaging (MRI) to look for benign tumors or neuromas entrapping a nerve
- US quantified fat pad thickness <9 mm may be predictive of HFPS (5).
- MRI may reveal edema in abductor hallucis or quadratus plantae muscle or surrounding fascia along with fibrosis, edema and septal defects. (5)[C].
- Lumbar spine radiographs and MRI to rule out causes of lumbar radiculopathy
- Consider bone scan or MRI to rule out suspected stress fracture.

Diagnostic Procedures/Other

LPN:

- Electromyography and nerve conduction studies can reveal abnormalities in LPN (6)[C].
- Quantitative sensory testing, also known as the pressure-specified sensory device, determines pain mechanisms by assessing function of large and small sensory nerve fibers.
- If nerve entrapment is suggested by history and exam, a diagnostic injection with local anesthetic providing complete pain relief can be diagnostic (4)[C].

TREATMENT

- The earlier treatment is started generally often leads to improvement in most patients.
- Nonsteroidal anti-inflammatory drug (NSAID) of choice
- Physical therapy to focus on Achilles tendon and plantar fascia flexibility and strengthening exercises of foot intrinsics and posterior tibial tendon (2)
- Rest, modified weight-bearing activities
- Injections of local anesthetics/steroids at site of nerve entrapment for LPN; caution should be exercised with repeated injections of steroid or improper technique due to the risk of irreversible damage to the heel pad by mechanical disruption of the heel septae and by steroid-induced fat necrosis (4)[C].
- Immobilization rarely necessary, symptom directed
- Orthotics, heel cups
- Treatment of other associated conditions (e.g., night splints in plantar fasciitis)

ADDITIONAL THERAPIES

Various methods for altering the biomechanical forces on the heel have been advocated but little evidence-based proof is available:

- Low-quality evidence for shock wave therapy (6)[A]
- Low-quality evidence that orthoses were effective in the reduction of heel pain. A well-fitted heel cup cushions the heel and prevents the heel pad from splaying, thereby improving the intrinsic cushioning of the calcaneus. There is no consensus as to which type of orthosis is best. Regardless of whether over-the-counter heel cups/orthoses versus custom orthoses are used; consistent features should be support of the arch, presence of adequate cushioning material, recess for area of pain beneath the heel, and slight medial elevation (6)[A].
- Moderate quality evidence that low-level laser therapy, dry-needling of lower leg and foot muscle trigger points, and calcaneal taping were effective in the reduction of persistent heel pain. Taping of the heel in fat pad syndrome can provide support and limit movement of the heel's fat pad (6)[A].
- High-quality evidence that US-guided pulsed radiofrequency (USGPRF) achieved heel pain reduction (6)[A].
- Weight control
- Shoes with softer midsoles, which provide more cushioning of the fat pad
- Raising the heel may thereby transfer the weight-bearing anteriorly with heel strike and in midstance.
- Medial heel wedge to relieve the pressure on the medial tuberosity, causing more lateral pressure
- Platelet-rich plasma injections are a non-evidence-based treatment.

SURGERY/OTHER PROCEDURES

- HFPS:
  - Surgery is reserved for patients when conservative treatment fails to provide adequate pain relief and should be considered a last resort. There are no proven techniques that can recreate or replace the normal anatomy of the heel pad (1)[C].
  - Surgical options are directed toward the cause of heel pain and include spur resection, wide release of plantar fascia, drilling decompression, and neurolysis.
- LPN entrapment:
  - Considered after failure of conservative treatment for 6 to 12 months (5)[C]
  - Surgical nerve decompression of the first branch of LPN or fascial release provides good to excellent results in >85% of surgically treated patients (4)[C].

ONGOING CARE

FOLLOW-UP RECOMMENDATIONS

- HFPS responds very well to conservative treatment and is usually self-limited.
- LPN: Approximately 90% of patients improve with nonoperative management.
- 52% of patients required at least 6 months to reach maximum improvement (5)[C].

REFERENCES

1. Balius R, Bossy M, Pedret C, et al. Heel fat pad syndrome beyond acute plantar fasciitis. *Foot (Edinb)*. 2021;48:101829.
2. Meadows JR, Finnoff JT. Lower extremity nerve entrapment in athletes. *Curr Sports Med Rep*. 2014;13(5):299–306.
3. Ferkel E, Davis WH, Ellington JK. Entrapment neuropathies of the foot and ankle. *Clin Sports Med*. 2015;34(4):791–801.
4. Chang AH, Rasmussen SZ, Jensen AE, et al. What do we actually know about a common cause of plantar heel pain? A scoping review of heel fat pad syndrome. *J Foot Ankle Res*. 2022;15(1):60.
5. Delee J, Drez D. Peripheral nerve entrapment around the foot and ankle. In: *DeLee, Drez, & Miller's Orthopaedic Sports Medicine*. 5th ed. Elsevier; 2020.
6. Salvioli S, Guidi M, Marcotulli G. The effectiveness of conservative, non-pharmacological treatment, of plantar heel pain: a systematic review with meta-analysis. *Foot (Edinb)*. 2017;33:57–67.

ADDITIONAL READING

- Aldridge T. Diagnosing heel pain in adults. *Am Fam Physician*. 2004;70(2):332–338.
- Alvarez-Nemegyei J, Canoso JJ. Heel pain: diagnosis and treatment, step by step. *Cleve Clin J Med*. 2006;73(5):465–471.
- Bateman JE. *Disorders of the Foot and Ankle, Medical and Surgical Management*. WB Saunders; 1991.
- Franson J, Baravarian B. Tarsal tunnel syndrome: a compression neuropathy involving four distinct tunnels. *Clin Podiatr Med Surg*. 2006;23(3):597–609.
- Toomey EP. Plantar heel pain. *Foot Ankle Clin*. 2009;14(2):229–245.

CLINICAL PEARLS

- Both soft heel cups and more rigid ones have been used with some success. The hard cups are intended to encompass the heel pad beneath the calcaneus, helping to restore some of its compressibility. The softer cups are designed primarily to cushion the fat pad. Athletes who run a lot in their sport often prefer softer heel cups or orthotics.
- To prevent HFPS, training errors should be identified and corrected. The athlete should wear proper shoes with an energy-absorbing heel cushion, avoiding excessive wear of the shoes. Mileage should be increased gradually, and running on steep hills should be avoided. Training on safe and shock-absorbing surfaces is essential (e.g., running on an all-weather track or on a surface softer than concrete or asphalt).

H

HEMATOMAS, EPIDURAL AND SUBDURAL

Greg Nakamoto, MD, FACP

BASICS

DESCRIPTION

Both epidural hematoma (EDH) and subdural hematoma (SDH) are structural brain injuries that can result from traumatic brain injury (TBI). However, they can follow different courses and have different prognoses.

- In EDH, blood is confined to the space between the inner table of the calvaria (inner surface of the skull and the dura mater).
- In SDH, localized bleeding occurs below the dura mater, directly adjacent to brain parenchyma.
- SDH can be acute or chronic (this topic focuses on acute SDH, commonly defined as an SDH diagnosed within 72 hours of TBI).
- Successful treatment of EDH and acute SDH involves treatment principles of TBI as well as considerations specific to EDH and SDH.
- Synonyms:
  - EDH: epidural hemorrhage, extradural hematoma, extradural hemorrhage
  - SDH: subdural hemorrhage
  - EDH and SDH: intracranial hematoma, intracranial hemorrhage, extra-axial hematoma, extra-axial hemorrhage

ALERT

EDH and acute SDH are neurosurgical emergencies. With prompt appropriate treatment, a patient with an EDH can often achieve complete neurologic recovery, whereas a missed diagnosis may result in death within hours. Mortality for patients with acute SDH is much higher (36–79%) due to greater associated underlying injury to the brain tissue itself.

EPIDEMIOLOGY

- EDH: Incidence is reported between 2.7% and 4% of TBI admissions (1):
  - Peak incidence is in the 2nd decade.
  - More frequently located in temporoparietal and temporal regions; bilateral in 2–5% of patients
  - Typically attributed to bleeding from the middle meningeal artery due to a temporal skull fracture; other sources of EDH blood include the middle meningeal vein, the diploic veins, or the venous sinuses.
- Acute SDH: Incidence is reported between 12% and 29% of TBI admissions (2):
  - Mean age reported to be between 31 and 47 years, with the vast majority being male.
  - Most SDH are caused by motor vehicle accidents (MVAs), falls, and assaults; predominant mechanism varies by age.
  - Acute SDH occurs either secondary to a parenchymal laceration (which implies a severe underlying brain tissue injury) or due to disruption of a surface or bridging vessel (in which case underlying brain injury may be less severe).
  - SDH is the most common athletic injury resulting in death.

RISK FACTORS

- EDH and SDH: high-energy head trauma
- SDH:
  - Low-energy head trauma (e.g., fall from a standing height) can cause SDH in susceptible persons (i.e., elderly, or any person with cortical atrophy).
  - Bridging veins can be torn during acceleration-deceleration injuries without actual head impact.
  - Intentional head injury is also a source of SDH in infants and children ("shaken baby syndrome").

COMMONLY ASSOCIATED CONDITIONS

- EDH: associated temporal or other skull fracture
- SDH: underlying brain parenchymal injury
- EDH and SDH:
  - Sequelae of increased intracranial pressure (ICP), including obtundation, Cushing reflex (bradycardia, hypertension, and irregular respiration), respiratory distress, and death
  - Due to high-energy mechanisms of injury, cervical spine and other orthopedic trauma are often seen.

DIAGNOSIS

Prehospital:

- EDH: <50% of the patients have the classically described "lucid interval" that is commonly associated with EDH (2):
  - Patient suffers TBI, which is often followed by an initial period of altered consciousness.
  - The patient subsequently improves, exhibiting for a period of the appearance of recovery.
  - The period of improvement, however, ends with secondary deterioration of the patient's mental status, ending the so-called "lucid interval."
- SDH: Lucid interval has been described in between 12% and 38% of patients with SDH (2):
  - Between 37% and 80% of patients with acute SDH present with initial Glasgow Coma Scale (GCS) scores of 8 or less, thus meeting criteria for severe head injury (2).

HISTORY

- Mechanism: High-energy trauma resulting in skull fracture is a risk factor for EDH. Acute SDH due to high-energy trauma implies more underlying brain tissue damage. Mechanism of injury can also guide the search for associated traumas in the poorly responsive patient.
- Lucid interval: more common with EDH
- Deterioration in mental status: Regardless of mechanism or level of recovery after initial injury, any patient with a deterioration of mental status after TBI should be evaluated for a possible neurosurgical emergency.

PHYSICAL EXAM

- Trauma assessment as necessitated by search for coexisting injuries
- Complete neurologic exam initially, followed by serial exams to assess for herniation (ipsilateral pupillary dilatation, contralateral hemiparesis) and signs of increased ICP (obtundation, Cushing reflex)
- Calculation of GCS, which helps guide treatment (mild TBI: GCS ≥13; moderate TBI: GCS 9 to 12; severe TBI: GCS ≤8)
- EDH: skull exam to look for fracture

DIFFERENTIAL DIAGNOSIS

- Concussion
- Uncomplicated skull fracture
- Intracerebral hemorrhage/cerebrovascular accident
- Subarachnoid hemorrhage
- Second impact syndrome

DIAGNOSTIC TESTS & INTERPRETATION

- Perform appropriate laboratories for any associated trauma and coagulation studies for neurosurgical planning.
- Computed tomography (CT) is the study of choice in EDH and SDH (1),(2)[A]:
  - EDH: Lesion is hyperdense (acute blood), biconvex, sharply demarcated, and adjacent to the skull; mass effect is common.
  - SDH: Lesion can be slightly less dense than in EDH (from mixing with cerebrospinal fluid [CSF]), concave, and conforming to the underlying brain; accompanying parenchymal injury and edema may be seen; may become isodense with brain parenchyma as early as 4 days

TREATMENT

In addition to the primary structural injury caused by TBI, neurotrauma also results in an inflammatory response that causes secondary brain injury. The goal of presurgical neuroresuscitation is minimization of secondary injury by maintaining adequate cerebral perfusion and minimizing elevated ICP (3),(4),(5)[C].

GENERAL MEASURES

- Prehospital:
  - Athletes with neurologic findings on exam and a concerning mechanism of injury should be transported to a trauma center for evaluation via emergency medical services (EMS).
  - As would be expected for any trauma patient:
    - Stabilize vital signs, achieve airway control, support blood pressure (BP), and address acute life-threatening injuries.
    - Establish intravenous (IV) access.
    - Cervical spine precautions as indicated
- Emergency room (ER) treatment:
  - Complete prehospital care steps not already addressed as per *Advanced Trauma Life Support* guidelines.
  - If intubation is indicated, consider esmolol at 1.5 mg/kg IV to blunt the hemodynamic response to intubation (use only if hypotension not a concern) (3)[C]. Preferred induction agents include ketamine and etomidate (for their hemodynamic sparing properties) or propofol (for neuroprotective effects, although can lead to hypotension) (3)[C].

- Once spine is cleared, elevate the head of the bed to 30 degrees to reduce ICP and increase venous drainage (3),(4)[C].
- Maintain systolic BP >100 mm Hg (>110 mm Hg if 15 to 49 or >70 years of age) (3),(4),(6)[B].
- Maintain goal temperature between 35°C and 37°C (i.e., normothermia) (4),(5)[C].
- Consider 7-day course of prophylactic phenytoin in all patients with severe TBI to reduce early posttraumatic (within 7 days of injury) seizures (3),(4),(6)[C].
- Once the patient is stabilized and any suspected ICP elevation is controlled, head CT is the preferred imaging modality in TBI (1),(2)[A].
- If clinical signs of increased ICP despite the above, then consider osmotic agents (mannitol or hypertonic saline); followed by propofol or pentobarbital coma and hyperventilation
- Reversal of coagulopathy and discontinuation of platelet inhibition medications
- ICP monitoring:
  - Patients with a GCS ≤8 should undergo placement of an ICP monitor if (i) any acute abnormality is seen on CT (hematomas, contusions, swelling, herniation, or compressed basal cisterns) or (ii) normal CT but 2 or more of the following on admission: age >40 years, unilateral or bilateral motor posturing, or a systolic BP <90 mm Hg (3),(4),(6)[B].
  - Treatment of ICP >22 mm Hg is recommended as values above this level are associated with increased mortality in patients with TBI (4),(6)[B].
- Rapid neurosurgical consultation for any symptomatic EDH or SDH or for any asymptomatic EDH or SDH meeting the CT criteria listed under "Surgery/Other Procedures"
- Medical interventions to control elevated ICP should not delay definitive neurosurgical treatment.

ALERT

Corticosteroids have been shown to increase mortality when used acutely in patients with head injury (6)[A].

ADDITIONAL THERAPIES

- If there is a high index of suspicion of EDH or SDH but a negative CT scan, such patients should be admitted for observation because EDH and SDH can evolve slowly. If headache or other symptoms persist, or the patient otherwise simply fails to improve, repeat CT in 6 to 12 hours before considering discharge:
  - Delayed EDH (hematoma not present on initial CT but found on follow-up scan) comprises up to 10% of cases in most series.
- Drilling burr holes (trephination):
  - Reserved for patients with raised and deteriorating ICP refractory to medical management when neurosurgical intervention is not available (3)[C].
  - Contraindications to drilling burr holes include GCS >8, no imaging obtained, and neurosurgical intervention is available (3)[C].

SURGERY/OTHER PROCEDURES

Acute neurosurgical referral is merited for any patient who is found to have either an EDH or acute SDH:

- Indications for surgical management of EDH include any of the following (1),(3)[A]:
  - GCS <9 with anisocoria
  - Hematoma size >30 cm^3 on CT
  - Hematoma growth causing elevated ICP or neurologic deterioration
    - Because enlargement of an EDH is common, in patients initially being treated nonoperatively, the first follow-up CT scan should be obtained within 6 to 8 hours after TBI (1)[C].
- Indications for surgical management of SDH include any of the following (2),(3)[A]:
  - GCS decline by >2
  - Hematoma thickness >10 mm or midline shift (MLS) >5 mm on CT (regardless GCS)
  - Fixed and dilated or asymmetric pupils
  - ICP >20 mm Hg
  - Patients who present with coma (GCS <9) but with an SDH with a thickness <10 mm and an MLS <5 mm can be treated nonoperatively, provided they undergo ICP monitoring, are neurologically stable because the injury have no pupillary abnormalities, and have no intracranial hypertension (no ICP >20 mm Hg) (2)[B].
- Any patient with known EDH or SDH who is initially stable but later develops new symptoms suggestive of mass effect, herniation, or increased ICP is a candidate for emergent neurosurgical intervention.

ONGOING CARE

FOLLOW-UP RECOMMENDATIONS

- EDH: In the case of nonsurgical EDH, the consulting neurosurgeon may consider discharge if the patient is neurologically stable after some period of observation. For patients treated both surgically and nonsurgically, follow-up CT scan in 1 to 2 weeks is commonly pursued in even asymptomatic patients to monitor for signs of progression or recurrence (6)[C], although the preferred timing of follow-up CT scans is not established in the literature and largely institution dependent.
- SDH: Due to its association with underlying brain injury (2), period of observation required before determination of clinical stability in SDH may be longer than for EDH. Furthermore, patients with an underlying brain injury may be more likely to need rehabilitation or temporary/permanent skilled nursing care.

PROGNOSIS

- EDH: Mortality is about 10% (range 7–12%) for EDH, as low as 5% if treated optimally within a few hours. The mortality rate is twice as high if there was no lucid interval, presumably because of associated brain parenchyma injury (1).
- SDH: Mortality in SDH is more varied but generally worse than for EDH; ranges from 40% to 60% in those requiring surgery and up to 68% in surgical cases presenting to the hospital in coma (2).

COMPLICATIONS

- Complications seen in patients with TBI include:
  - Neurologic deficits associated with parenchymal brain injury, which is more commonly seen in acute SDH than EDH.
  - Neurologic deficits associated with increased ICP and subsequent herniation
  - Posttraumatic seizures, which can occur early or late after TBI
- Postoperative complications include:
  - Recurrent or residual hematoma, which may require repeat operations
  - Wound infection, meningitis, or cerebral abscess after craniotomy
  - CSF leak

REFERENCES

1. Bullock MR, Chesnut R, Ghajar J, et al. Surgical management of acute epidural hematomas. *Neurosurgery*. 2006;58(Suppl 3):S7–S15.
2. Bullock MR, Chesnut R, Ghajar J, et al. Surgical management of acute subdural hematomas. *Neurosurgery*. 2006;58(Suppl 3):S16–S24.
3. Long B, Koyfman A. Secondary gains: advances in neurotrauma management. *Emerg Med Clin North Am*. 2018;36(1):107–133.
4. Robinson CP. Moderate and severe traumatic brain injury. *Continuum (Minneap Minn)*. 2021;27(5):1278–1300.
5. Bernard F. Neurotrauma and intracranial pressure management. *Crit Care Clin*. 2023;39(1):103–121.
6. Carney N, Totten AM, O'Reilly C, et al. Guidelines for the management of severe traumatic brain injury, fourth edition. *Neurosurgery*. 2017;80(1):6–15.

ADDITIONAL READING

- Al-Mufti F, Mayer SA. Neurocritical care of acute subdural hemorrhage. *Neurosurg Clin N Am*. 2017;28(2):267–278.
- Davanzo JR, Sieg EP, Timmons SD. Management of traumatic brain injury. *Surg Clin North Am*. 2017;97(6):1237–1253.

CLINICAL PEARLS

- EDH and acute SDH are neurosurgical emergencies that merit rapid neurosurgical evaluation.
- Athletes with neurologic findings on exam and a concerning mechanism of injury should be transported to a trauma center for evaluation via EMS.
- CT is the study of choice in evaluating intracranial lesions in a patient with head injury (1),(2)[A].
- Nonsurgical interventions are aimed at minimizing secondary injury by maintaining adequate cerebral perfusion and minimizing elevated ICP.
- In patients who need operative treatment, delay in time to surgery is associated with poorer outcomes.

HEMATURIA IN SPORTS

Charles W. Webb, DO, FAMSSM, FAAFP, CAQSM • Shelby Rider, MD, MS

BASICS

Exercise-induced hematuria (EIH):

- Occurs with or without trauma in males and females; resolves with rest in 2 to 3 days (1)
- Although a benign condition, it is a diagnosis of exclusion.
- Directly correlated with exercise intensity, duration, core temperature, acidosis, oxidative stress (1)
- EIH is found in 95–100% of cases after exercise in both trained athletes and the general population (1).
- Traumatic mechanisms:
  - Direct urologic trauma (1)
  - Foot strike and bladder trauma (2)
- Atraumatic mechanisms:
  - Physiologic decreased renal blood flow during exercise causing hypoxic damage to the nephron and leading to increased permeability for red blood cells (RBCs) and proteins
  - Increased glomerular filtration pressure favoring excretion of RBCs and protein
  - Hydration and a partially full bladder during exercise may help to prevent or minimize this condition (2).
- Persistent recurrent, symptomatic, or traumatic hematuria warrants further evaluation (1),(2),(3),(4).

DESCRIPTION

- Microscopic hematuria: $\geq$3 RBCs per high-powered field (HPF) in two of three properly collected urine samples (5):
  - $\geq$3 RBCs per HPF is abnormal in children, $\geq$5 RBCs per HPF is abnormal in adults (3).
  - A urine dipstick of 1+ blood corresponds to ~1 to 5 RBCs/HPF and can detect as little as 150 ug/L of hemoglobin (3).
  - Can also be caused by free hemoglobin, myoglobin, or other substances (see "Diagnosis")
  - Urine dipstick is *not* diagnostic of hematuria (5).
  - Prompt microscopic analysis is important for detection.
- Gross hematuria: red-brown urine with numerous RBCs seen on microscopy:
  - *Note*: 1 mL of blood per liter of urine can produce a visible color change (3).
  - Lower urinary tract causes of hematuria generally have isomorphic RBCs (3),(5).
  - Glomerular causes of hematuria generally have dysmorphic RBCs (3),(5).
- EIH: transient, usually microscopic hematuria following physical exertion
- Symptomatic hematuria: gross or microscopic hematuria in the presence of any lower or upper urinary tract symptoms (e.g., flank pain, renal colic, dysuria, urgency)
- Asymptomatic hematuria: either gross or microscopic hematuria in the absence of any urinary tract symptoms

EPIDEMIOLOGY

- EIH: idiopathic
- All other causes:
  - Age $<$40 years: usually infection
  - Age $>$40 years: increasing incidence of tumor
  - Males age $>$60 years: usually prostatic obstruction, calculi, or tumor
  - Females age $>$60 years: usually malignancy (4),(5),(6)

Prevalence

- Prevalence of hematuria in the general population ranges from 2.5% to 20% (1),(5).
- Prevalence increases to 18–80% following athletic competition and usually resolves in 48 hours (1),(2).

RISK FACTORS

- Previous or chronic urinary tract infection (UTI)
- Anticoagulation
- Strenuous exercise
- History of calculi, prostatitis, trauma, malignancy, coagulopathy, or sexually transmitted illness
- Travel to Africa, India, or the Middle East (5)

GENERAL PREVENTION

Routine screening of adults for microscopic hematuria with urinalysis (UA) is not indicated.

DIAGNOSIS

- Hematuria is rarely a medical emergency but may be a sign of underlying pathology.
- History and exam will help to guide which patients need further workup.
- Benign asymptomatic microscopic hematuria can be achieved with urine microscopy on $\geq$2 separate urine samples (6).
- $>$50 RBCs/HPF is generally considered significant hematuria and may warrant *immediate* further investigation.
- Symptomatic or gross hematuria warrants further workup regardless of age.
- Causes:
  - Unexplained/idiopathic: 87% of all cases of microhematuria
  - Spurious:
    - Menstruation
    - Sexual intercourse
  - Pseudohematuria (or dipstick hematuria)
  - Rhabdomyolysis
  - Foods (beets, rhubarb, blackberries)
  - Drugs (doxorubicin, chloroquine, rifampin)
  - UTI: acute cystitis or pyelonephritis
    - If UTI is suspected, obtain urine culture, treat infection, and repeat test in 6 weeks before further workup.
  - Prostatitis or urethritis
  - Urinary tract calculi
  - Exercise induced: Clinically significant hematuria is common after exercise (3).
  - Trauma to flank or abdomen (renal fracture)
  - Genitourinary mucosal injury by instrumentation
  - Cancer: renal, bladder, prostate, ureter
    - Present in 19–25% of gross hematuria but increases dramatically in older population in those over 60 years old the majority are related to cancer
    - Less common $<$40 years old (4),(6)
    - Low-risk populations: young, female, nonsmoker, without irritative voiding symptoms (6)
  - Transient/intermittent hematuria is common.
  - Benign prostatic hyperplasia (BPH)
  - Glomerular disease
  - Sickle cell disease
- Rare causes: Polycystic kidney disease (PCKD), *Schistosoma haematobium,* radiation cystitis, urethral strictures, tuberculosis, medullary sponge kidney, cyclophosphamide-induced cystitis, arteriovenous malformation, renal artery thrombosis, papillary necrosis of any cause, loin pain hematuria syndrome
- EIH (1),(2):
  - Not fully understood; thought to be multifactorial, etiology unclear
  - Diagnosis of exclusion
  - Can make the diagnosis without further workup in athletes $<$40 years old who have hematuria within 12 hours of vigorous activity that resolves completely within 48 to 72 hours
  - More likely to present with microscopic hematuria
  - More common with increased intensity of exercise
  - Contact sports more likely to case direct urinary tract injury
  - Noncontact sports more likely to cause physiologic changes that indirectly lead to hematuria
  - Bladder trauma in runners; can be alleviated by voiding before running
  - Cyclist can experience direct trauma to the prostate and urethra.
  - Hemoglobinuria can be caused by RBC lysis for a number of reasons.
  - Dehydration and increased blood viscosity
  - Increased body temperature
  - Exercise-induced catecholamines shunt blood away from kidneys and into muscles, resulting in hypoxic damage to nephrons, increased glomerular permeability, and subsequent hematuria
  - March, or foot-strike, hematuria is thought to occur from trauma to the foot capillaries after prolonged weight-bearing.
- Traumatic hematuria:
  - More likely to present as gross hematuria
  - Children are more likely to have renal injury following trauma owing to lack of perinephric fat and less protection by the ribs.
  - There is a lower threshold for imaging of children.
  - In children, additional criteria for imaging include $>$50 RBCs/HPF and abdominal/flank pain or ecchymosis.
  - Serious renal injury is much more likely to occur after a fall, bike, or motor vehicle accident (high-velocity accidents and/or collisions) than with athletic participation.
  - Football was the most common sport causing traumatic renal injury.

HISTORY

- Recent physical activity: type, intensity, and duration; EIH can occur up to 12 hours after activity (1).
- Trauma (5)
- Urinary tract symptoms: Flank pain, renal colic, dysuria, weak stream are not related to EIH (5).
- Medication use, including herbals and over-the-counter drugs: Anticoagulants do not increase the risk of hematuria and should not influence the workup.
- Family history of sickle cell disease/trait or hematuria
- Red flags for malignancy or tuberculosis such as fevers, night sweats, and weight loss or gross hematuria
- Assess risk factors for significant urologic disease:
  - Abuse of analgesic drugs (nonsteroidal anti-inflammatory drugs [NSAIDs])
  - Age $>$40 years and male sex increases likelihood of cancer (4),(5).
  - Exposure to pelvic radiation
  - Irritative voiding symptoms
  - Occupation exposure to chemicals or dyes
  - Smoking
  - Recent sore throat could suggest poststreptococcal glomerulonephritis or immunoglobulin A (IgA) nephropathy.
  - Travel to developing nations
  - Unilateral flank pain suggests calculi or pyelonephritis.

PHYSICAL EXAM

- Many patients will not have any signs or symptoms. Nearly all patients with EIH will be asymptomatic. The symptoms listed below suggest something *other than* benign EIH: fever, urethral discharge, flank pain or ecchymosis, painless red or brown urine, dysuria, frequency, hesitancy, suprapubic pain

- Physical examination: vitals, abdominal and flank exam, Genitourinary exam
- Stepwise approach to the patient (4),(5):
  - Step 1: history and physical as above:
    - If patient <40 years of age, observe and repeat UA after 48 to 72 hours.
    - If UA is normal, no further studies are warranted. Observe the patient for recurrence.
    - If hematuria persists or exam suggests cause other than EIH, proceed to step 2.
  - Step 2: Obtain the following laboratory tests:
    - Urine culture and serum creatinine, blood urea nitrogen (BUN), complete blood count (CBC), prothrombin time (PT), partial thromboplastin time (PTT), sickle-cell preparation
    - Consider serum creatine kinase.
    - If serum creatinine is normal, obtain intravenous pyelogram (IVP) to evaluate for obstruction, mass, and kidney function.
    - If results of these tests are normal, proceed to step 3.
  - Step 3: cystoscopy; if normal or patient is at moderate risk, proceed to step 4.
  - Step 4: ultrasound (US) or computed tomography (CT) scan (3),(4):
    - Include bladder, especially if patient >40 years of age.
    - If normal, proceed to step 5.
  - Step 5: Consider renal arteriogram:
    - Evaluate for vasculitis, arteriovenous (AV) malformation, and renal infarction/thrombosis.
    - If normal, proceed to step 6.
  - Step 6: Consider renal biopsy:
    - If at any time concurrent proteinuria, dysmorphic RBCs, or casts are present, obtain 24-hour urine for protein, creatinine, calcium, citrate, and uric acid.
    - Consider antistreptolysin O (ASO) titer, venereal disease research laboratory (VDRL), antineutrophil cytoplasmic antibodies (ANCA), compliment levels, antiglomerular basement membrane antibody levels, and hepatitis serology.

DIFFERENTIAL DIAGNOSIS

- Painless:
  - EIH
  - Malignancies
  - Glomerulonephropathy, especially in children
  - PCKD
  - Sickle cell trait or disease
  - Coagulation defect (clotting factor deficiency, thrombocytopenia, polycythemia)
  - Vasculitis (lupus, goodpasture syndrome)
  - Infection (endocarditis, tuberculosis, syphilis)
  - Iatrogenic: anticoagulation, catheterization, NSAIDs
  - Early calculi formation: hypercalciuria, hyperuricosuria, hypocitraturia (Citrate helps to prevent stone formation.)
  - Myoglobinuria—rhabdomyolysis (no RBCs on microscopy)
  - Hemolysis—"march hematuria" (no RBCs on microscopy)
  - Medications: phenothiazine, phenolphthalein laxatives, rifampin, phenazopyridine, phenytoin, quinine
  - Porphyria
  - Vegetable dyes (beets, rhubarb)
  - Vaginal blood contamination
- Painful: pyelonephritis, prostatitis, cystitis, urethritis, calculi, trauma, bladder or renal tumor, renal artery aneurysm, renal vein thrombosis

DIAGNOSTIC TESTS & INTERPRETATION

Initial tests (lab, imaging)

- UA with microscopy; further testing indicated if UA not clear in 48 to 72 hours (1):
  - Must include cell count
  - RBCs alone suggest prostatic disease, pelvic or ureteral calculi, trauma, heavy exercise, or malignancy.
  - Dysmorphic RBCs can be seen in EIH as well as intrinsic renal disease.
  - White blood cells (WBCs) + RBCs suggests infection.
  - RBCs + protein/casts/dysmorphic RBCs or absence of clots suggests glomerular disease.
  - RBC casts are virtually diagnostic of glomerulonephritis or vasculitis.
  - RBC clots usually indicate extraglomerular bleeding.
  - Proteinuria suggests renal disease.
- Urine culture
- 24-hour urine protein, creatinine, calcium, uric acid, and citrate
- Spot urine protein: creatine ratio usually sufficient
- CBC, PT, and PTT
- Serum creatinine/BUN/electrolytes
- Urine cytology is rarely helpful.
- Imaging is needed only if microhematuria does not clear on UA after 48 to 72 hours of rest (1),(4).
- Imaging is rarely needed, unless there is a traumatic incident or suspected nephrolithiasis or tumor.
- Non–contrast-enhanced CT scan is the preferred modality for evaluating calculi with a sensitivity of 98–100% and a specificity of 92–100%. Many institutions have a renal stone CT scan protocol to minimize radiation exposure.
- CT urography is preferred test to evaluate urologic malignancy or obstruction.
- The combination of CT urography and cystoscopy generally is considered sufficient to evaluate for serious urinary tract pathology.
- US can be used safely in children and pregnant women but low sensitivity for calculi or tumors <3 cm.
- Retrograde pyelography also can be used to visualize the bladder and collecting system.
- Voiding cystourethrogram (VCUG) is used to detect vesicoureteral reflux.
- Magnetic resonance (MR) urography can be used in place of CT scan.
- Arteriography detects renovascular hypertension, polyarteritis nodosa, thromboemboli, mass, and aneurysm (3).

TREATMENT

- General:
  - Treatment targeted to the underlying condition
  - Antibiotics for infection
  - Pain control, if applicable; avoid NSAIDs until renal injury and nephritis are ruled out.
  - Pyridium can be given for cystitis.
- EIH:
  - Rest and reassurance
  - Emphasize hydration during exercise and avoidance of urination within 15 to 20 minutes of onset of exercise to minimize bladder trauma.
- Traumatic hematuria:
  - Assess life-threatening and coexisting injuries.
  - Immediate surgical consultation for signs of shock or severe trauma
  - Evaluate need for imaging.
- Management of asymptomatic microscopic hematuria:
  - Confirm in 2/3 properly collected specimens (5)
  - No further workup needed if present in only one sample or no RBCs seen on microscopic analysis
  - Further workup if >50 RBCs/HPF in single sample
  - Rule out transient or spurious causes; treat if present.
  - If age ≥40 years, refer for urologic evaluation with imaging and cystoscopy.
  - If age <40 years, assess for:
    - Glomerular filtration rate (GFR) <60 mL/min
    - Proteinuria (albumin:creatinine ratio ≥30 or protein:creatine ratio ≥50).
    - Hypertension (BP ≥140/90 mm Hg).
  - If any of the above are abnormal, refer to nephrology.
  - If no diagnosis is found, monitor GFR, proteinuria, and hypertension yearly.
- Management of symptomatic microscopic hematuria:
  - Evaluate for transient and spurious causes.
  - Consider immediate referral to urology.
  - May follow the same algorithm as for anti-müllerian hormone (AMH)
- Management of gross hematuria:
  - Consider referral to urology.
  - Evaluate and treat transient causes.
  - Assess renal function and consider imaging before referral (1),(5).

ONGOING CARE

Referral to urology or nephrology useful when other etiologies cannot be found and the hematuria persists

PROGNOSIS

- Based on underlying diagnosis, if known
- Unexplained hematuria is relatively common in the general population and carries a favorable prognosis as long as an appropriate diagnostic workup has been done (1),(4),(5).

REFERENCES

1. Akiboye RD, Sharma DM. Haematuria in sport: a review. *Eur Urol Focus*. 2019;5(5):912–916.
2. Urakami S, Ogawa K, Oka S, et al. Macroscopic hematuria caused by running-induced traumatic bladder mucosal contusions. *IJU Case Rep*. 2018;2(1):27–29.
3. Imam AA, Saadeh SA. Evaluation of proteinuria and hematuria in ambulatory setting. *Pediatr Clin North Am*. 2022;69(6):1037–1049.
4. Woldu SL, Ng CK, Loo RK, et al. Evaluation of the New American Urological Association guidelines risk classification for hematuria. *J Urol*. 2021;205(5):1387–1393.
5. Ingelfinger JR. Hematuria in adults. *N Engl J Med*. 2021;385(2):153–163.
6. Samson P, Waingankar N, Shah P, et al. Predictors of genitourinary malignancy in patients with asymptomatic microscopic hematuria. *Urol Oncol*. 2018;36(1):10.e1–10.e6.

CLINICAL PEARLS

- Return to play is acceptable if hematuria resolves after 48 to 72 hours of rest; otherwise, counsel patients on an individual basis depending on the diagnosis.
- Transient hematuria is usually benign but should be worked up further in people ≥40 years of age.
- Persistent hematuria always should be evaluated further.
- Painless gross hematuria should be considered bladder cancer until proven otherwise.

HEMOGLOBINOPATHIES IN SPORT: THALASSEMIA, SICKLE CELL TRAIT

Bernadette Pendergraph, MD • Neel Kotrappa, MD • Claudia Alvarez, DO

BASICS

DESCRIPTION

Thalassemia and sickle cell trait are genetic disorders of hemoglobin production. Thalassemias are a mixed collection of quantitative abnormal production, leading to either absent or decreased production of normal α or β subunits. Sickle cell trait is inheritance of a normal hemoglobin gene and an abnormal *β-globin sickle gene*.

EPIDEMIOLOGY

Incidence

- Thalassemia: 1 in 1,000 people has thalassemia in the United States.
- Sickle cell trait: United States (screened newborns)—73 cases per 1,000 African Americans; 7 per 1,000 Hispanics; 3 per 1,000 whites; 1 in 3 persons in West Africa; 1 in 5 persons in the eastern province of Saudi Arabia (1).

Prevalence

- Thalassemia is the most common single genetic disorder known. In the thalassemia belt (Mediterranean, Turkey, Iran, India, Thailand, Cambodia, and southern China), the prevalence is 2.5–15%.
- Sickle cell trait affects 2.5 million people in the United States and 300 million people worldwide (2).

ETIOLOGY AND PATHOPHYSIOLOGY

- Thalassemia occurs when there is an abnormal gene on chromosome 16 or 11 that impairs the production of α or β subunits of hemoglobin, respectively. Abnormalities include point mutations, total deletions, or the rearrangement of gene loci. Thalassemia minor occurs when a single abnormal gene is inherited, resulting in normal or low-normal hemoglobin measurement with significant microcytosis. More severe forms of β thalassemia impair erythropoietin production, cause hemolytic anemia, and reduce oxygen capacity (2).
- Sickle cell trait occurs from the inheritance of one normal hemoglobin gene (HbA) and one abnormal B1 globin gene (HbS). In this carrier state, hemoglobin A1 and hemoglobin S are produced in a 60:40 ratio. The B1 gene is found on the short arm of chromosome 11. Red blood cells (RBCs) will sickle and polymerize under certain conditions, such as severe tissue hypoxia, acidosis, dehydration, increased viscosity, and hypothermia (1).

Genetics

Both conditions are caused by the inheritance of an autosomal-recessive gene.

GENERAL PREVENTION

Genetic screening and preconception counseling

COMMONLY ASSOCIATED CONDITIONS

- Sickle cell trait: increased incidence of hyposthenuria, microhematuria, renal papillary necrosis, exertional rhabdomyolysis, exercise-related sudden death, and renal medullary carcinoma; 2-fold increase in venous thrombosis; 4-fold increased risk for pulmonary embolism; splenic infarcts reported at high altitude (>7,500 feet) (1)
- Thalassemia minor is usually asymptomatic. Other forms of thalassemia are associated with erythroid hyperplasia (extramedullary erythropoietic tissue development in face, chest, abdomen, and pelvis), resulting in frontal bossing, coarse facies, and splenomegaly. Heart failure occurs secondary to hemolytic anemia. Bone abnormalities include shortened upper extremities, pathologic fractures of long bones and vertebral bodies, notching, and osteolytic lesions of the ribs because of marrow masses. Growth retardation, delayed pubertal development, insulin resistance, hypothyroidism, and hypoparathyroidism are also possible complications.

DIAGNOSIS

Prehospital:

- Thalassemia minor: usually asymptomatic
- Sickle cell trait: usually asymptomatic; may present with cramping or collapse, usually within the first 30 minutes of intense exercise and initial conditioning with normal core temperature (3).

HISTORY

- Thalassemia: symptoms of anemia—dizziness, fatigue, light-headedness, weakness
- Sickle cell trait: usually asymptomatic; may present with gradual deterioration over minutes with symptoms of muscle cramping/pain, dyspnea, severe weakness, fatigue provoked by multiple bursts of vigorous exertion often combined with ambient temperatures ≥80°C or high altitude (4)

PHYSICAL EXAM

- Thalassemia: no findings or signs of anemia—pallor, elevated heart rate, low blood pressure, cool extremities, brittle nails
- Sickle cell trait: Muscles are soft and nontender to palpation; no visible contractions

DIFFERENTIAL DIAGNOSIS

- α-Thalassemia minima (5):
  - One-gene deletion
  - Asymptomatic; normal hematologically
- α-Thalassemia minor (5):
  - Two-gene deletion
  - Microcytosis and mild anemia, not reversed with iron
- β-Thalassemia trait (5):
  - One normal gene and one abnormal
  - Microcytosis and mild anemia not reversed with iron
  - Asymptomatic
- Sickle disease: sickle cell trait combined with β-thalassemia minor, α-thalassemia, hemoglobin C, or traditional double sickle cell hemoglobin:
  - Symptomatic
- Iron deficiency anemia:
  - Microcytosis, decreased iron stores; improves with iron repletion
- Dilutional pseudoanemia:
  - Increased volume expansion related to exercise; normal RBC indices and iron stores

DIAGNOSTIC TESTS & INTERPRETATION

- Sickle solubility test: initial screening test that detects HbS. It cannot differentiate between sickle cell disease or trait; needs confirmation by hemoglobin electrophoresis, high-performance liquid chromatography (HPLC), or isoelectric focusing (IEF). HPLC and IEF identify α-thalassemias (1)[C].
- Hemoglobin electrophoresis: Sickle cell trait shows hemoglobin AS (hemoglobin A1, 55–60%, and hemoglobin S, 40–45%) (2)[C].
- Complete blood count (CBC): Both sickle cell trait and thalassemia lead to microcytosis and hypochromia.
- Reticulocyte count: normal in sickle cell trait but increased when combined with α- or β-thalassemia
- Indirect bilirubin: normal in sickle cell trait but increased when combined with α- or β-thalassemia
- DNA analysis and HPLC: Identify α-thalassemias (5)[C].

TREATMENT

- No treatment for asymptomatic sickle cell trait; focus is on prevention of exertional rhabdomyolysis and exertional collapse.
- Collapse in sickle cell athlete (3)[C]:
  - Occurs from sickling of RBCs in exerting limbs, with resultant rhabdomyolysis from continued exertion in the face of ischemia
  - Severe lactic acidosis from anaerobic metabolism of ischemic muscles can develop, leading to eventual shock.
  - Rapid diagnosis and treatment are necessary to prevent acute renal failure from the rhabdomyolysis, subsequent hyperkalemia, eventual ventricular fibrillation, and death.
- Prehospital:
  - Thalassemia: fluid resuscitation if abnormal vital signs
  - Sickle cell trait: If with cramping or collapse, check vital signs, administer high-flow oxygen, cool athlete if necessary, and activate emergency medical services (if patient is obtunded or vital signs are unstable).
- Emergency department (ED) treatment:
  - Continued support: oxygen, intravenous (IV) fluids
  - Evaluation for rhabdomyolysis: CBC, comprehensive metabolic panel, coagulation panel, lactate dehydrogenase (LDH), creatinine kinase
  - Correction of hyperkalemia
- Return to duty/play (3)[C]:
  - Can return if asymptomatic at rest and with normal end-organ function
  - Exercise and environmental reacclimatization
  - Risk factors for recurrence: hyposthenuria, early chronic kidney disease, associated hemoglobinopathy, pyruvate kinase deficiency

ISSUES FOR REFERRAL

Hematology referral: patients with symptomatic sickle cell trait, concern for misdiagnosis and need for more advanced testing, thalassemias requiring transfusions

ADDITIONAL THERAPIES

- Thalassemia: in severe cases, transfusions to keep the hemoglobin 9.0 to 10.5 g/L; chelation therapy in those receiving transfusions with deferasirox, deferoxamine, or deferiprone (2)[C]:
  - Deferasirox: 20 to 30 mg/kg/d orally; associated with nausea, abdominal pain, diarrhea, rash, or liver/kidney dysfunction
  - Deferoxamine: 20 to 40 mg/kg/d subcutaneous (SC) infusion; minimal side effects
  - Deferiprone: 25 to 33 mg/kg TID orally; associated with neutropenia and agranulocytosis
- Stem cell transplant: curative (2)[C]
- Sickle cell trait:
  - Education of the athlete on importance of conditioning and identification of cramping as a sign of sickling
  - All athletes with the sickle cell trait should be counseled on preseason strength and conditioning programs, gradual progression during session training, and stopping activity if cramping, difficulty catching breath, weakness, or pain (3)[C].
  - When performing repetitive sprints/interval training, longer periods should be allowed for athlete to recover in between exertional activities.
  - Exertion should be limited when conditions exist that may precipitate sickling: illness, high ambient temperature, dehydration, asthma, and altitude (3)[C].

ONGOING CARE

PATIENT EDUCATION

- Centers for Disease Control and Prevention (CDC) Keeping Workers Hydrated and Cool Despite the Heat: https://blogs.cdc.gov/niosh-science-blog/2011/08/12/heat-2/
- Consortium for Health and Military Performance (CHAMP) Sickle Cell Trait Awareness: https://www.hprc-online.org/resources-partners/whec/educational-tools/sickle-cell-trait-awareness-videos
- National Collegiate Athletic Association (NCAA) Student Athlete Fact Sheet—Sickle Cell Trait: http://fs.ncaa.org/Docs/health_safety/SickleCellTraitforSA.pdf
- Sickle Cell Disease Association of America: http://www.sicklecelldisease.org/about/sickle-cell-101/
- Thalassemia International Federation: http://www.thalassemia.org.cy/education/

PROGNOSIS

Excellent, if prevention measures are instituted

REFERENCES

1. Pecker LH, Lanzkron S. Sickle Cell Disease. *Ann Intern Med*. 2021;174(1):ITC1–ITC16.
2. Sanchez-Villalobos M, Blanquer M, Moraleda JM, et al. New insights into pathophysiology of β-thalassemia. *Front Med (Lausanne)*. 2022;9:880752.
3. O'Connor FG, Franzos MA, Nye NS, et al. Summit on exercise collapse associated with sickle cell trait: finding the "way ahead." *Curr Sports Med Rep*. 2021;20(1):47–56.
4. Maron BJ, Harris KM, Thompson PD, et al. Eligibility and disqualification recommendations for competitive athletes with cardiovascular abnormalities: task force 14: sickle cell trait: a scientific statement from the American Heart Association and American College of Cardiology. *J Am Coll Cardiol*. 2015;66(21):2444–2446.
5. Baird DC, Batten SH, Sparks SK. Alpha- and beta-thalassemia: rapid evidence review. *Am Fam Physician*. 2022;105(3):272–280.

ADDITIONAL READING

- Munkongdee T, Chen P, Winichagoon P, et al. Update in laboratory diagnosis of thalassemia. *Front Mol Biosci*. 2020;7:74.
- Quattrone RD, Eichner ER, Beutler A, et al. Exercise collapse associated with sickle cell trait (ECAST): case report and literature review. *Curr Sports Med Rep*. 2015;14(2):110–116.

CLINICAL PEARLS

- Universal precautions that include liberal hydration, gradual conditioning, and acclimatization can minimize the risk for an exertional injury such as rhabdomyolysis and exercise collapse associated with sickle cell trait (ECAST).
- Although all states are required to perform newborn screening for genetic disorders, many individuals still do not know their sickle cell trait status making mandated testing an important aspect of the prevention program.
- Recognize thalassemia as a cause of microcytic anemia and avoid iron supplementation unless athlete is truly iron deficient.
- Additional testing beyond hemoglobin electrophoresis is necessary to identify different types of thalassemias.

HEREDITARY MULTIPLE OSTEOCHONDROMAS

Scott L. Paradise, MD, CAQSM, FAAFP • Janelle Marra, DO, FAAFP, CAQSM

BASICS

DESCRIPTION

- Inherited condition characterized by the development of multiple osteochondromas
- Osteochondromas vary in number and size, involved bones, and subsequent physical deformity.
- Also known as *diaphyseal aclasis*, multiple hereditary exostoses, Bessel-Hagen disease, and familial exostoses

EPIDEMIOLOGY

- Prevalence varies (1):
  - 1:1,000 in the indigenous people of Guam and the Mariana Islands
  - 1:50,000 to 1:100,000 in Western populations
- Patients without osteochondroma development by age 12 years are highly unlikely to develop later in life (1).

ETIOLOGY AND PATHOPHYSIOLOGY

- Autosomal dominant, approximately 10% of cases are *de novo* (1)
- Most with loss of function or missense mutations in *EXT1* (56–78%) or *EXT2* (21–44%) responsible for heparan sulfate synthesis, which is involved in the regulation of chondrocyte proliferation and differentiation (1)
- Animal studies implicate a two-hit model of loss of heterozygosity in the pathogenesis of hereditary multiple osteochondromas (HMO) which may contribute to varying degrees of severity and age of onset (1).
- Caused by epiphyseal chondrocyte proliferation and subsequent bony overgrowth in the first decade of life

RISK FACTORS

- There is a higher penetrance in males.
- *EXT1* mutations are associated with more severe phenotype (1).

GENERAL PREVENTION

Knowledge of the pathogenic variant can allow preimplantation genetic testing and prenatal counseling.

DIAGNOSIS

PHYSICAL EXAM

- Osteochondromas commonly involve the appendicular skeleton: femur (30%), radius and ulna (13%), tibia (20%), and fibula (13%) (1).
- Osteochondromas of the axial skeleton may be difficult to observe or palpate on physical exam.
- HMO is associated with shortened stature, scoliosis, and hip dysplasia.
- Appendicular deformities include limb-length discrepancy, angular deformities of the forearm or leg, and hand deformity from shortened metacarpals (1),(2).
- May present with pathologic fracture or pain or symptoms from local mass effect on neurovascular structures

DIFFERENTIAL DIAGNOSIS

- Solitary osteochondroma
- Subungual exostosis
- Metachondromatosis
- Ollier disease (enchondromatosis)
- Maffucci syndrome
- Trevor disease (*dysplasia epiphysealis hemimelica*)
- Langer-Giedion syndrome (trichorhinophalangeal syndrome type 2)
- Potocki-Shaffer syndrome (11p11 deletion syndrome)

DIAGNOSTIC TESTS & INTERPRETATION

- Often identified by the presence of multiple osteochondromas on plain radiographs:
  - Cartilage-capped bony outgrowths from the epiphyseal plate
  - Continuity of cortical and medullary bone with underlying parent bone is highly characteristic (3).
  - Pedunculated or sessile
  - Sessile lesions or osteochondromas of flat bones with complex anatomy may require advanced imaging.
- Computed tomography (CT) is best for demonstrating cortical and marrow continuity but may poorly evaluate cartilage cap (3).
- Magnetic resonance imaging (MRI) is ideal for evaluating cartilage cap thickness (3)[C],(4)[B]:
  - No radiation exposure
  - May require sedation in younger patients
  - Best for evaluating adjacent soft tissue (e.g., dural compression from intracanal spinal osteochondromas)
- Ultrasound has been used to evaluate cartilage cap thickness and differentiate from overlying bursitis (3).
- Technetium bone scans may show increased radiotracer uptake in lesions that have undergone malignant transformation (1).

TREATMENT

ISSUES FOR REFERRAL

- May be optimally managed at specialty centers with experience in managing HMO.
- Consultation with a geneticist may be considered for genotype testing and prenatal counseling.
- Orthopedics or neurosurgery referral is recommended for management of intracanal spinal osteochondromas.
- Patients with malignant transformation should be managed by multidisciplinary care team.

SURGERY/OTHER PROCEDURES

- Excision may be performed due to locally irritating lesions or to relieve compressive symptoms (1)[C].
  - Intracanal spinal osteochondromas require specialist consultation.
- Growth deformities may be treated by corrective osteotomy, limb-lengthening procedures, or epiphysiodesis of the contralateral limb in children.

ONGOING CARE

FOLLOW-UP RECOMMENDATIONS

- Patients should be educated on the possibility of development of intracanal spinal osteochondromas, which may cause emergent spinal cord compression.
  - Patients should be made aware of concerning symptoms including weakness, numbness, paresthesia, incontinence, unsteady gait, and neck or back pain and advised to urgently seek medical advice if any of these symptoms occur.
- Osteochondromas that grow or become symptomatic after puberty should raise concern for malignant transformation (1)[C].

PROGNOSIS

Most patients will lead healthy lives. However, some may experience chronic pain, labor dystocia, problems at school, bullying, and lower rates of participation in competitive sports (5).

COMPLICATIONS

- Most symptoms arise from local mass effect causing neurovascular compression or traction or causing bursa formation.
- Fractures may occur at the base of pedunculated osteochondromas.
- Spinal osteochondromas occur in 3–68% of patients with HMO (6).
  - Males more likely to have spinal involvement
  - Cervical spine lesions may be more common than thoracic and lumbar spine lesions (6).
- 2–5% of patients experience malignant transformation into chondrosarcoma (1).
  - Rates of transformation may be higher in males and patients with the *EXT1* genotype (2).
  - Cartilage caps thicker than 20 to 30 mm are associated with increased risk of chondrosarcoma (1).
- Rarely, osteomyelitis, infarction of cartilage cap, or hemarthrosis may occur (3).

SCREENING FOR COMPLICATIONS

- No universal screening protocols for detection of intracanal spinal osteochondromas.
  - Recommendations vary from one-time spinal imaging during developmental years (e.g., when able to cooperate without general anesthesia) to spinal imaging only at the onset of myelopathic symptoms (1)[C],(6)[B].
  - Some authors advocate spinal imaging in the presence of harbinger lesions (pelvic or rib osteochondromas, which may indicate more severe phenotype and higher likelihood of spinal involvement) (6)[B].
- There are no universal screening methods or optimal intervals to screen for malignant transformation (1)[C],(2)[C].
  - Clinical monitoring of osteochondroma size may alert clinicians to malignant degeneration (1)[C],(2)[C].
  - Consider imaging of pelvic or scapular osteochondromas every 2 to 3 years (1)[C].
    - Some experts recommend annual screening from ages 20 to 40 years; however, it is not clear if the benefits outweigh the risks of this approach and it has not been prospectively validated (4)[B].
  - Consider total body noncontrast MRI to screen asymptomatic individuals with HMO (1)[C].

REFERENCES

1. Wuyts W, Schmale GA, Chansky HA, et al. Hereditary multiple osteochondromas. In: Adam MP, Feldman J, Mirzaa GM, et al, eds. *GeneReviews®*. University of Washington, Seattle; 1993–2023. Updated August 6, 2020. Accessed August 8, 2025. https://www.ncbi.nlm.nih.gov/books/NBK1235/
2. Porter DE, Lonie L, Fraser M, et al. Severity of disease and risk of malignant change in hereditary multiple exostoses. A genotype-phenotype study. *J Bone Joint Surg Br*. 2004;86(7):1041–1046.
3. Murphey MD, Choi JJ, Kransdorf MJ, et al. Imaging of osteochondroma: variants and complications with radiologic-pathologic correlation. *Radiographics*. 2000;20(5):1407–1434.
4. Fei L, Ngoh C, Porter DE. Chondrosarcoma transformation in hereditary multiple exostoses: a systematic review and clinical and cost-effectiveness of a proposed screening model. *J Bone Oncol*. 2018;13:114–122.
5. Goud AL, de Lange J, Scholtes VA, et al. Pain, physical and social functioning, and quality of life in individuals with multiple hereditary exostoses in The Netherlands: a national cohort study. *J Bone Joint Surg Am*. 2012;94(11):1013–1020.
6. Jackson TJ, Shah AS, Arkader A. Is routine spine MRI necessary in skeletally immature patients with MHE? Identifying patients at risk for spinal osteochondromas. *J Pediatr Orthop*. 2019;39(2):e147–e152.

ADDITIONAL READING

National Organization for Rare Disorders. Hereditary multiple osteochondromas. Published 1993. Updated September 19, 2012. Accessed November 30, 2023. https://rarediseases.org/rare-diseases/hereditary-multiple-osteochondromas/

CLINICAL PEARLS

- Most patients will lead healthy lives with increased likelihood of chronic pain and decreased participation in competitive sports.
- There are no universal screening protocols for identifying intracanal osteochondromas, and estimates of prevalence vary widely; all patients should be aware of myelopathic symptoms and should seek immediate medical care if they occur.
- Rate of malignant transformation is estimated at 2–5%; there are no universally accepted surveillance protocols.
- Lesions that grow or begin to cause symptoms after skeletal maturity should be evaluated for malignancy.

HERPES GLADIATORUM

Stephen Shaheen, MD, CAQSM, FACEP

BASICS

DESCRIPTION

Variant of cutaneous herpes disease caused by herpes simplex virus type 1 (HSV-1) or type 2 (HSV-2) occurring among athletes of contact sports, especially wrestlers; it is transmitted almost exclusively by direct skin-to-skin contact—especially after prolonged periods of time. It is also known as "mat herpes."

EPIDEMIOLOGY

Affects 2.6% of high school wrestlers and 7.6% of collegiate wrestlers. Current estimates from the National Collegiate Athletic Association (NCAA) indicate possible increased yearly incidence rates of 20–40% in collegiate wrestlers (1). With wrestlers, 94–97% of infections are caused by infection by HSV-1 (2).

RISK FACTORS

- Abrasions or physical traumas increase the likelihood of acquiring infection.
- Physical and mental stressors (i.e., weight loss, sleep deprivation, competition, school responsibilities) may increase likelihood of recurrence.

GENERAL PREVENTION

- Isolate infected wrestler to prevent skin contact with other wrestlers (control outbreaks among previously infected wrestlers).
  - Almost a third of athletes in select study groups carried the virus but awareness was low; only 3% knew of their infection (2).
- Regular wrestling mat cleaning and general hygiene (e.g., avoid sharing towels, soap, razors)
  - Several studies have shown that mats and other fomites likely play an insignificant role in infection spread (2).
- Consider using prophylactic antiviral medications during the season or before competition (3).
- Acyclovir 200 mg BID
- Valacyclovir 500 mg or 1 g daily
- Famciclovir 250 mg BID
- Teach skin hygiene (e.g., showering after activity) and protect other skin abrasions from secondary contact.
- Educate athletes on how to identify lesions/recurrence, seek early treatment, and have a high index of suspicion.
  - In one smaller study, the correct HSV diagnosis was made at initial presentation in only 10% of cases (2).

DIAGNOSIS

HISTORY

- Initial versus recurrent eruption
- Similar location as previous infection
- Previous treatment and length of infection
- History of recent stressors (e.g., school, sleep, weight loss, emotional, sun exposure, trauma) (4)

PHYSICAL EXAM

- Incubation period for primary infection is 2 to 14 days.
  - >90% of infections occur within the first 8 days of initial virus exposure (2).
  - Sore throat (40%), intermittent fever and chills (25% and 27%), headache (22%) typically occur only with initial infection (4).
- Prodrome of burning, stinging pain, or itching at the infected site, followed by clusters of vesicles on an erythematous base
- Common locations include head, neck, and upper body.
  - In wrestling, >70% of outbreaks involve the face or neck (2).
- Erythema and grouped vesicles, ulcers, or crusts on head, face, neck, or upper extremities most common but may occur anywhere on the body
- Symptoms of fever, localized lymphadenopathy, malaise, myalgia, or pharyngitis may accompany infection, especially with initial episode.
- Repeated outbreaks usually are less severe and involve a smaller area.
- Infections around the eye increase the risk of corneal or retinal involvement, such as keratoconjunctivitis or retinal necrosis.
- Consider herpes if infection fails to improve after 3 to 4 days of oral antibiotic therapy and if lesions cross the midline and involve the face and scalp.

DIFFERENTIAL DIAGNOSIS

- Impetigo
- Herpes zoster
- Folliculitis
- Allergic or contact dermatitis
- Tinea gladiatorum
- Cellulitis

- Diagnosis can be made by viral culture or Tzanck smear of vesicle fluid, although neither is as sensitive as polymerase chain reaction (PCR).
- PCR testing is a sensitive but costly method to determine viral presence and is considered the gold standard for detecting HSV-1 or HSV-2 in individuals with a rash suggestive of a herpes infection.

TREATMENT

- Initial infection:
  - Started early in the clinical course, during vesicle formation, oral antiviral medications can arrest viral replication and shorten the duration of infection (3)
  - Acyclovir 200 mg 5 times a day or 400 mg TID for 10 days
  - Valacyclovir 1 g BID for 10 days
  - Topical application of the two above drugs is of limited benefit. One agent, cetrimide/diphenhydramine/moroxydine has moderate effect if used when paresthesias begin (4).
  - During the ulcer stage, benzoyl peroxide and use of a hair dryer can help dry crusts more rapidly and minimize secondary bacterial infections.
- Recurrent infection:
  - Antiviral medications begun during the prodromal phase can effectively shorten the duration of recurrent infections (3).
  - According to a recent study, treatment with 1 g valacyclovir daily reduced herpes gladiatorum (HG) outbreaks by 92% in individuals with a <2-year history of recurrent HG, and treatment with 300-mg valacyclovir daily reduced HG outbreaks in 88% of those with a <2-year history of recurrent infection (3).
  - Valacyclovir 1 g PO daily or 500 mg BID for 3 to 7 days
  - Valacyclovir 2 g × 1 dose; repeat in 12 hours.
  - Acyclovir 800 mg BID for 5 days or 400 mg TID for 5 days
  - Famciclovir 125 mg BID for 5 days or 1 g PO BID for 1 day

- Treatments and levels of evidence:
  - Level 1 (strong, good quality, patient-oriented evidence): treatment with systemic oral antivirals in initial and recurrent infections (1),(3),(5)
  - Level 2 (limited-quality, patient-oriented evidence): prevention of outbreak via season-long antiviral prophylaxis for players with history of HG outbreak (1)
  - Level 3 (limited, case-oriented, disease-oriented evidence): isolating players with weeping lesions, educating players on importance of not returning to play with active lesions, covered or not (5)

REFERENCES

1. Wilson EK, Deweber K, Berry JW, et al. Cutaneous infections in wrestlers. *Sports Health.* 2013;5(5):423–437.
2. Peterson AR, Nash E, Anderson BJ. Infectious disease in contact sports. *Sports Health.* 2019;11(1):47–58.
3. Anderson BJ, McGuire DP, Reed M, et al. Prophylactic valacyclovir to prevent outbreaks of primary herpes gladiatorum at a 28-day wrestling camp: a 10-year review. *Clin J Sport Med.* 2016;26(4):272–278.
4. Nassani LM. "Herpes gladiatorum in sports: an appraisal for health care worker and team dentists." *J Oral Maxillofac Surg Med Pathol.* 2023;35(5):468–472.
5. Shah N, Cain G, Naji O, et al. Skin infections in athletes: treating the patient, protecting the team. *J Fam Pract.* 2013;62(6):284–291.

ADDITIONAL READING

- Anderson BJ. Managing herpes gladiatorum outbreaks in competitive wrestling: the 2007 Minnesota experience. *Curr Sports Med Rep.* 2008;7(6):323–327.
- Anderson BJ. The effectiveness of valacyclovir in preventing reactivation of herpes gladiatorum in wrestlers. *Clin J Sport Med.* 1999;9(2):86–90.
- Anderson BJ. The epidemiology and clinical analysis of several outbreaks of herpes gladiatorum. *Med Sci Sports Exerc.* 2003;35(11):1809–1814.
- Anderson BJ. Valacyclovir to expedite the clearance of recurrent herpes gladiatorum. *Clin J Sport Med.* 2005;15(5):364–366.
- Annunziato PW, Gershon A. Herpes simplex virus infections. *Pediatr Rev.* 1996;17(12):415–423.
- Johnson R. Herpes gladiatorum and other skin diseases. *Clin Sports Med.* 2004;23(3):473–484.
- Stacey A, Atkins B. Infectious diseases in rugby players: incidence, treatment, and prevention. *Sports Med.* 2000;29(3):211–220.

CLINICAL PEARLS

- Return to play: National Federation of State High School Associations Sports Medicine Advisory Committee guidelines:
  - Herpetic lesions (simplex, fever blisters/cold sores, zoster, gladiatorum): To be considered "noncontagious," all lesions must be scabbed over with no oozing or discharge, and no new lesions should have occurred in the preceding 48 hours, with no lymph node swelling near affected area. For primary (first episode of HG), wrestlers should be treated and not allowed to compete for a minimum of 10 days. If general body signs and symptoms like fever and swollen lymph nodes are present, that minimum period of treatment should be extended to 14 days. Recurrent outbreaks require a minimum of 120 hours or 5 full days of oral antiviral treatment, again so long as no new lesions have developed and all lesions are scabbed over. Herpesvirus may spread prior to vesicle formation; therefore, anyone in contact with the infected individual during the 3 days prior to the outbreak must be isolated from any contact activity for 8 days and be examined daily for suspicious skin lesions.
- NCAA guidelines on herpes simplex:
  - Primary infection: (i) Wrestler must be free of systemic symptoms of viral infection (fever, malaise, etc.). (ii) Wrestler must have developed no new blisters for 72 hours before the examination. (iii) Wrestler must have no moist lesions; all lesions must be dried and surmounted by a *firm adherent crust* with no evidence of secondary bacterial infection. (iv) Wrestler must have been on appropriate dosage of systemic antiviral therapy for at least 120 hours before and at the time of the meet or tournament. (v) Active herpetic infections shall not be covered to allow participation. See above criteria when making decisions for participation status.
  - Recurrent infection: (i) Blisters must be completely dry and covered by a *firm adherent crust* at time of competition, or wrestler shall not participate. (ii) Wrestler must have been on appropriate dosage of systemic antiviral therapy for at least 120 hours before and at the time of the meet or tournament. (iii) Active herpetic infections shall not be covered to allow participation. See above criteria when making decisions for participation status.
  - Questionable cases:
    - Tzanck preparation and/or HSV antigen assay (if available)
    - Wrestler's status deferred until Tzanck preparation and/or HSV assay results complete
    - Wrestlers with a history of recurrent herpes labialis or HG could be considered for season-long prophylaxis. This decision should be made after consultation with the team physician.

H

HIGH ANKLE SPRAIN

Chelsea Rubis, DO ▪ Delmas J. Bolin, MD, PhD, FACSM

BASICS

- A syndesmosis is a fibrous joint in which two adjacent bones (in this case, tibia and fibula) are linked by a strong membrane or ligaments. It provides stability to the mortise of the talocrural joint.
- Symptoms result from disruption of ligaments supporting the integrity of the ankle mortise joint.
- Associated with prolonged symptoms of pain and dysfunction
- Relevant injured structures can include anterior tibiofibular, posterior tibiofibular, and transverse tibiofibular ligaments; interosseous membrane; and interosseous ligament; which serve to prevent lateral displacement of distal fibula during weight-bearing.
- Synonym(s): syndesmodial injury of the lower leg

DESCRIPTION

- Mechanism of injury involves passive forceful external rotation of the ankle or rapid pivoting in internal rotation off an externally rotated planted foot, valgus load to the lateral aspect of the leg with a planted foot, or hyperdorsiflexion (less common) (1).
- The talus is pressed against the fibula, opening the distal tibiofibular articulation and rupturing the tibiofibular syndesmosis and tibiofibular ligaments.

EPIDEMIOLOGY

- 1–10% of all ankle sprains (Underdiagnosis may be common.)
- Higher percentage (as high as 35%) involves the syndesmosis when occurring in collision sports such as football, rugby, and lacrosse.

RISK FACTORS

- Collision sports are at higher risk:
  - Football
  - Rugby
  - Lacrosse
- Sports that immobilize the foot in a high ankle shoe or boot:
  - Hockey
  - Slalom skiing; catching inner ski on gate
  - Wrestling
- Sports played on turf (e.g., soccer)

COMMONLY ASSOCIATED CONDITIONS

- Deep deltoid ligament tear
- Fibular or medial malleolar fracture
- Pronation-external rotation (PER) and supination-external rotational (SER) fractures
- Proximal fibular fractures (Maisonneuve injuries)
- Heterotopic ossification or synchondrosis of the syndesmosis in 25–100% of cases
- Tibiofibular synostosis resulting in prolonged pain and chronic disability
- Longer healing time and more missed practices
- Occult talar dome fracture

DIAGNOSIS

HISTORY

- Patient is often unable to adequately or completely describe mechanism; patients commonly report an inversion mechanism.
- The clinician should delineate any prior ankle injuries.
- Focus history on mechanism of injury and direct location of pain; raise index of suspicion with history of forceful external rotation, hyperdorsiflexion, or hyperplantarflexion.
- Examples of common mechanisms include soccer (player tackling ball), football (player prone, has foot stepped on, leading to forceful external rotation), and skiing (slalom skiers, catch ski on gate).
- Pain is usually between anterior distal tibia and fibula and also posteromedially at ankle joint.
- Pain can be persistent on weight-bearing or an unusually long period of recovery after the initial injury.
- Pain is also worse with pushing off or with external rotation.

PHYSICAL EXAM

- Palpation of the syndesmosis is the most sensitive:
  - Can present with pain along the distal anterolateral ankle radiating above the leg with/without edema/ to the distal tibiofibular region accompanied
- Squeeze test: Compression above midcalf produces distal pain in the anterior ankle joint (syndesmosis).
- External rotation stress test: Distal lower leg is stabilized with ankle in neutral position while mediolateral force/external rotation of the foot is performed; positive test noted by pain and/or increased rotation relative to unaffected side
- Push-off test: Push off/heel raise on affected side may be weak or absent.
- Fibular translation (drawer) test: pain or increased translation of fibula from anterior to posterior or loss of firm end point relative to uninjured side
- Stabilization test: Distal syndesmosis is stabilized with athletic tape and assess if symptoms are decreased with running and jumping.
- Cotton test: increased translation or pain with translation of talus from medial to lateral (may indicate deltoid ligament tear)
- Crossed-leg test: pain at syndesmosis with gentle pressure exerted on the medial side of the knee while resting the midtibia of affected leg on uninjured knee
- Dorsiflexion lunge test: decreased pain or increased range of motion after compression is applied on the ankle syndesmosis during a lunge on the injured side
- Evaluate distal neurovascular status with any lower leg injury to rule out acute compartment syndrome (2)[B].

DIFFERENTIAL DIAGNOSIS

- PER ankle fracture (Weber C)
- SER ankle fracture (Weber B)
- Fracture of the proximal fibula (Maisonneuve)
- Ossification of the syndesmosis
- Calcification of the syndesmosis
- Deltoid ligament tear
- Talar dome fracture
- Tibiofibular synostosis resulting in prolonged pain and chronic disability

DIAGNOSTIC TESTS & INTERPRETATION

ALERT

- X-rays: Initial studies are static films. 50% of syndesmotic injuries have avulsion fractures associated:
  - Weight-bearing anteroposterior view:
    - Tibiofibular clear space is among most sensitive indicators of syndesmotic injuries; measured 1 cm proximal to ankle joint; widening demonstrated by >6 mm between medial border of fibula and medial cortical density of tibia
    - Tibiofibular overlap; measured 1 cm proximal to joint; normal is >6 mm overlap between medial border of fibula and lateral border of tibia.
    - Medial clear space should be <4 mm; >4 mm termed *diastasis*

- Standing mortise view to evaluate talocrural angle; the angle of a line drawn across tips of malleoli intersecting with a line perpendicular to a line drawn across the superior aspect of tibial plafond. Variation from contralateral side of >5 degrees is significant.
- Lateral
- Dynamic radiographs:
  - Varus and valgus ankle stress views can be helpful to assess instability.
  - External rotation stress views not considered reliable indicators of syndesmotic injury
- Magnetic resonance imaging (MRI) can clarify diagnosis and extent of soft tissue injury:
  - Although sensitive and specific for syndesmotic injuries, MRI is not predictive for instability because it is a static test.
- Computed tomography (CT) helpful for bony detail of suspected talar dome injuries (3)[B]
- Ultrasound (US) imaging can be used to diagnose ligament ruptures of the lower leg (4)[B].

TREATMENT

- High ankle sprains/syndesmosis injuries without fracture (2)[B]: Consensus is three- to four-phase rehabilitation protocol. If no frank diastasis, most injuries result in inability to bear weight without symptoms:
  - Phase I is to limit inflammatory response and protect the joint, usually with short-term (10 days to 2 weeks) non–weight-bearing protection in a cast, boot, or brace with crutches. Include protection, rest, ice, compression, and elevation and modalities to minimize edema. Orthoses that prevent external rotation and dorsiflexion are recommended (5)[B].
  - Phase II is typically restoration of strength, range of motion, and normalization of gait pattern. In this phase, high ankle braces (DonJoy Velocity and others) may facilitate rehabilitation.
  - Phase III progression once patient can ambulate and hop without dysfunction. Progress to agility drills, plyometrics, sports-specific tasks, and strengthening.
  - Return to play is challenging and is typically based on a functional testing evaluation and physical examination; usually 6 to 8 weeks
  - Patient may return to play with demonstration of tasks such as backward pedaling, vertical hopping, or running in figure-8 pattern.
- Syndesmosis injuries with fracture or diastasis noted on radiographs:
  - Referral to orthopedic surgeon indicated if frank diastasis is noted on radiographs or if fracture is present
- Screw fixation followed by non–weight-bearing cast immobilization for 6 weeks, followed by appropriate rehabilitation (2)[B]
- Suture-button fixation followed by non–weight-bearing cast immobilization for 6 to 8 weeks, followed by appropriate rehabilitation
- Platelet-rich plasma injections under US guidance have been used in elite athletes for faster return to play (4).

REFERENCES

1. Fermín TM, Symenidis PD. Physical examination of ankle sprain and ankle instability: can we really divide it into low and high ankle sprains? *Foot Ankle Clin N Am.* 2023;28:217–229.
2. Fort NM, Aiyer AA, Kaplan JR, et al. Management of acute injuries of the tibiofibular syndesmosis. *Eur J Orthop Surg Traumatol.* 2017;27(4):449–459.
3. Herscovici D Jr, Anglen JO, Archdeacon M, et al. Avoiding complications in the treatment of pronation-external rotation ankle fractures, syndesmotic injuries, and talar neck fractures. *J Bone Joint Surg Am.* 2008;90(4):898–908.
4. Laver L, Carmont MR, McConkey MO, et al. Plasma rich in growth factors (PRGF) as a treatment for high ankle sprain in elite athletes: a randomized control trial. *Knee Surg Sports Traumatol Arthrosc.* 2015;23(11):3383–3392.
5. Williams GN, Allen EJ. Rehabilitation of syndesmotic (high) ankle sprains. *Sports Health.* 2010;2(6):460–470.

ADDITIONAL READING

- Amendola A, Williams G, Foster D. Evidence-based approach to treatment of acute traumatic syndesmosis (high ankle) sprains. *Sports Med Arthrosc Rev.* 2006;14(4):232–236.
- Hopkinson WJ, St Pierre P, Ryan JB, et al. Syndesmosis sprains of the ankle. *Foot Ankle.* 1990;10(6):325–330.
- Kellett JJ. The clinical features of ankle syndesmosis injuries: a general review. *Clin J Sport Med.* 2011;21(6):524–529.
- Sman AD, Hiller CE, Rae K, et al. Prognosis of ankle syndesmosis injury. *Med Sci Sports Exerc.* 2014;46(4):671–677.
- Switaj P, Mendoza M, Kadakia A, et al. Acute and chronic injuries to the syndesmosis. *Clin Sports Med.* 2015;34(4):643–677.
- Vopat ML, Vopat BG, Lubbarts B, et al. Current trends in the diagnosis and management of syndesmotic injury. *Curr Rev Musculoskelet Med.* 2017;10(1):94–103.

CLINICAL PEARLS

- A high ankle sprain involves ligaments that stabilize the ankle mortise joint. It is not a "routine ankle sprain" and must be treated differently.
- High ankle sprains should be immobilized as soon as the diagnosis is made for a variable period ranging from a few days in elite professional and collegiate athletes to 2 weeks for high school athletes. Suspect a high ankle sprain in a "regular ankle sprain" that is not improving as you expect.
- Although anecdotal, some find high ankle stirrup braces helpful in the subacute setting for stabilizing the mortise joint, limiting rotational stress at the ankle, and permitting a more vigorous rehabilitation.

HIGH-ALTITUDE ILLNESS

Edgar M. VanHorne, MD • Keenan Wheeler, DO

BASICS

- Altitude sickness was described and documented by missionaries to South America in the late 16th century.
- High-altitude illness (HAI) is primarily caused by hypobaric hypoxemia. Rapid ascent to elevation in excess of 2,000 m, without adequate physiologic acclimatization, can result in a spectrum of HAI, ranging from a mild acute mountain sickness (AMS) to more severe and potentially fatal forms of high-altitude pulmonary edema (HAPE) and high-altitude cerebral edema (HACE).
- High-altitude environment:
  - Intermediate: 1,520 to 2,440 m (5k to 8k feet).
  - High: 2,440 to 4,270 m (8k to 14k feet).
  - Very high: 4,270 to 5,500 m (14k to 18k feet).
  - Extreme altitude: above 5,500 m (>18k feet).
- Optimal prevention of HAI involves slow, graded ascent to altitude. Certain medications and portable oxygen or hypobaric chamber may mitigate and alleviate symptoms.

ALERT
Once symptoms are recognized, the definitive solution to HAI is descent to lower altitude.

DESCRIPTION

- The atmospheric percentage of oxygen is a constant 21%. However, the partial pressure of oxygen decreases with increasing altitude resulting in less inspired oxygen per respiratory cycle. Hypobaric hypoxia forms the physiologic basis for the HAIs, AMS, HAPE, and HACE.
- Initial AMS symptoms are typically mild and self-limited, progressing to more severe HACE if not adequately recognized and treated.
- HAPE or HACE can present independently and progress rapidly, with or without initial warning of AMS symptoms.
- Untreated, HAPE or HACE can be fatal.

EPIDEMIOLOGY

- Incidence and severity of HAI increase with higher altitude, speed of ascent, and physical exertion.
- At high altitude, AMS may affect 25% of unacclimated individuals, increasing to 50–85% afflicted at very high altitude (>4,000 m, e.g., Mt. Everest base camp, and Mt. Kilimanjaro).
- HAPE and HACE are rarely seen <4,000 m, accounting for an estimated 0.1–0.4% of all cases.
- Children are as susceptible as adults with a slight decrease in incidence in those >50 years of age.

GENERAL PREVENTION

ALERT

- Graded ascent is the best means of acclimatization and HAI prevention.
- Avoid same-day travel from sea level to a sleeping elevation above 2,750 m.
- Never ascend to a higher sleeping altitude with HAI symptoms.
- Avoid alcohol use within the first 48 hours at altitude.
- If travel is planned from sea level to above 2,500 m, spend one night at an intermediate elevation.
- Above 2,500 m, do not ascend >500 m sleeping altitude per day.
- Spend an extra night of acclimatization for every 1,000 m altitude gained.
- It is recommended that any person with underlying cardiopulmonary or hematologic conditions consult with a physician familiar with high-altitude medicine prior to travel.
- Pharmaceutical agents: Acetazolamide and dexamethasone may be used for prevention of AMS/HACE and sustained-release; nifedipine for individuals prone to HAPE

ETIOLOGY AND PATHOPHYSIOLOGY

- Hypobaric hypoxia:
  - With ascent to high altitude comes decreased partial pressure of oxygen. Decreased atmospheric PaO_2 affects absorption into the circulation at the alveolar level. Hypoxemia at the cellular level causes a myriad of physiologic stress responses.
  - Decreased partial pressure of oxygen triggers the carotid body to signal the respiratory centers in the medulla to increase ventilation. The extent of compensatory hypoxic ventilatory response (HVR) is thought to be determined at the genetic level. Increased ventilatory rate causes hypocapnia and respiratory alkalosis, which results in an increase in renal excretion of bicarbonate.
- **AMS:**
  - Hypoxic stress induces the trigeminovascular system (TVS), leading to increased cerebral blood flow and resultant nausea, headache, and malaise.
  - The central respiratory center responds to HVR-induced respiratory alkalosis with periods of apnea causing disturbed sleep.
- **HACE:**
  - Vasogenic cerebral edema, caused by a myriad of responses to hypobaric hypoxia, including TVS induction, endothelial activation, and sympathetic activity.
- **HAPE:**
  - Acute pulmonary edema induced by hypoxic pulmonary hypertension increases capillary hydrostatic pressure causing extravasation of fluid across the vascular endothelium and into the alveolar space.
  - Impaired reabsorption of alveolar fluid and amplified inflammatory mediator response then accelerate and exacerbate the process.

RISK FACTORS

- Rapid ascent
- Sleeping at altitude >2,000 m; exceeding >500 m/d sleeping altitude above 2,500 m
- Lack of acclimatization
- Young age
- Strenuous exertion at high altitude
- Previous history and/or individual susceptibility to altitude illness
- Obesity
- Chronic obstructive pulmonary disease (moderate), OSA (severe), uncompensated congestive heart failure, pulmonary hypertension (mild), obesity Class 3, sickle cell trait well-controlled hypertension and asthma are not considered risk factors.
- Physical fitness does not predict or prevent altitude illness.

ALERT
Ascent contraindicated (per Centers for Disease Control and Prevention [CDC] guidelines):

- Angina (unstable)
- Asthma (unstable, poorly controlled)
- Cerebral space-occupying lesions
- Cerebral vascular aneurysms or arteriovenous malformations (untreated, high risk)
- Chronic obstructive pulmonary disease (severe/very severe)
- Cystic fibrosis (forced expiratory volume in the first second of expiration [FEV_1] <30% predicted)
- Heart failure (decompensated)
- Myocardial infarction or stroke (<90 days before ascent)
- Pregnancy (high risk)
- Pulmonary hypertension (pulmonary artery systolic pressure >60 mm Hg)
- Sickle cell anemia

DIAGNOSIS

- AMS:
  - Nausea
  - Light-headedness
  - Headache
  - Insomnia
  - Anorexia
  - Malaise
  - Fatigue
  - Weakness
  - Impaired memory
  - Inability to focus or concentrate
- HAPE: Symptoms of AMS may present initially and then progress 2 to 5 days after ascent to dyspnea on exertion and/or dyspnea at rest:
  - Persistent cough, progressing to pink, foamy sputum
  - Chest tightness
  - Fatigue
  - Muscle weakness
- HACE: Ataxia and confusion are hallmark symptoms heralding progression from AMS to HACE:
  - Headache
  - Vomiting
  - Incoordination
  - Disorientation
  - Irrational behavior
  - Auditory or visual hallucination
  - Lethargy
  - Altered level of consciousness
  - Unconsciousness or coma within 24 hours after the onset of ataxia

HISTORY

- Rapid ascent to high altitude
- AMS:
  - Onset of symptoms typically 12 to 24 hours and self-limited (as early as 2 hours after arrival but rarely after 36 hours)
- HAPE:
  - Symptoms usually begin 2 to 5 days after arrival to high altitude and classically the second night sleeping at high altitude.
  - May have a sudden onset (e.g., gondola or helicopter ascent), especially in sedentary individuals at altitude
  - Decreased exercise performance and increased recovery time, cough, dyspnea on exertion, and progressive worsening of symptoms, especially at night; pink, frothy sputum is usually a late finding.
- HACE:
  - AMS symptomatology with progressive worsening of neurologic symptoms, including ataxia, extreme lassitude, mental status changes, and coma
  - Commonly associated with HAPE
  - AMS progression to HACE at altitude may be within 12 hours but more commonly 1 to 3 days.
  - HACE generally occurs above 3,000 m but has been described at altitude as low as 2,100 m.

PHYSICAL EXAM

- AMS:
  - Specific physical findings are uncommon in mild AMS.
  - Tachycardia or bradycardia
  - Normotensive
- HAPE:
  - Breathlessness at rest
  - Cyanosis
  - Crackles in right middle lobe are typical but can be anywhere in the lung field.
  - Tachycardia
  - Tachypnea
  - Low-grade fever
  - Orthopnea
- HACE:
  - Inability to perform activities such as dressing or eating
  - Truncal ataxia demonstrated by poor heel-toe walking
  - Mental status changes
  - Occasionally focal neurologic deficits
  - Funduscopic examination can demonstrate papilledema and retinal hemorrhages (not diagnostic).

DIFFERENTIAL DIAGNOSIS

- AMS:
  - Dehydration
  - Exhaustion
  - Viral syndrome
  - Gastroenteritis
  - Hangover
  - Hypothermia
  - Carbon monoxide exposure
  - Hyponatremia
  - Seizures or focal neurologic deficits are uncommon.
- HAPE:
  - Pneumonia
  - Asthma
  - Pulmonary embolism
  - Congestive heart failure
  - Myocardial infarction
  - Fever >101°F, chills, or mucopurulent sputum are typically absent.
- HACE:
  - In addition to AMS differential:
    - Cerebrovascular accident
    - Alcohol intoxication
    - Brain tumor
    - Central nervous system (CNS) infection (e.g., meningitis)
    - Acute psychosis/delirium

DIAGNOSTIC TESTS & INTERPRETATION

Initial Tests (lab, imaging)

- HAPE:
  - Chest x-rays demonstrate normal heart size with patchy infiltrates.
- HACE:
  - Brain magnetic resonance imaging (MRI) T2-weighted images show increased signal in the white matter, particularly the splenium of the corpus callosum, consistent with vasogenic edema and microhemorrhage.

TREATMENT

ALERT

- Descent to a lower altitude is the mainstay of treatment for any HAI.
- Low-intensity descent of at least 500 m is recommended.
- Avoid further ascent until symptoms resolve.
- Supplemental oxygen 2 to 4 L/min if available
- Preventative/treatment options

MEDICATION

- Oral acetaminophen 650 to 1,000 mg or ibuprofen 600 mg for pain or headache; ondansetron orally disintegrating tablet (ODT) 4 mg PO q4–6h for nausea and vomiting
- Acetazolamide 125 to 250 mg PO BID, starting 8 to 24 hours prior to ascent (1)[A]/pediatric dosing 1.25 mg/kg (max 125 mg q12h)
- Ibuprofen 600 mg PO TID for AMS prevention and symptomatic relief of headache (2)[B]
- Dexamethasone 2 mg PO q6h or 4 mg PO q12h, can be used as alternative for AMS prevention if sulfa/acetazolamide allergic. Start the day of ascent, continuing for first 2 days at altitude, or for rapid increase in altitude (1)[A],(3)[A].
- For treatment of HAPE, dexamethasone 4 mg PO/intramuscular (IM)/intravenous (IV) q6h
- For treatment of HACE, dexamethasone 8 mg loading dose, followed by 4 mg PO/IM/IV q6h

ALERT

Rebound symptoms of AMS have been described after discontinuation of dexamethasone and continued ascent should be avoided.

- Budesonide 200 μg inhaled BID starting 3 days prior to ascent has been shown effective in preventing AMS (4)[B].
- Nifedipine 30 mg extended-release PO BID to treat HAPE if oxygen unavailable and rapid descent is delayed (5)[C].
- Tadalafil 10 mg PO BID, as an alternative to nifedipine (due to potential hypotension with concomitant use), has been described for treatment of HAPE in case reports (2)[C].
- When extreme weather or additional factors preclude rapid descent, medical treatment has been shown to be a viable option up to 4,240 m (6)[B].
- If available, a portable hypobaric chamber, or Gamow bag, manually inflated to 2 psi, may be effectively used to simulate a descent of 1,000 to 3,000 m.
- On return to low altitude, transition to inpatient hospital care as soon as possible

COMPLEMENTARY & ALTERNATIVE MEDICINE

Limited research on Ginkgo biloba for AMS prophylaxis has produced conflicting results but may be a viable alternative for those seeking natural sources. Coca preparations have shown potential for increasing blood oxygenation and decreasing AMS symptoms in some studies (7)[B].

ONGOING CARE

- General measures:
  - Minimize heavy exertion for 2 to 3 days on arrival to high altitude.
  - Maintain adequate hydration.
  - Eat frequent, small, high-carbohydrate meals.
  - Avoid alcohol or other sedative/hypnotic medications which could suppress respiratory drive.
  - Smoking worsens hypoxia and should be avoided.
- In critically ill patients:
  - Monitor vital signs periodically because hypotension may lead to cerebral hypoperfusion.
  - Intravenous fluid (IVF) is not contraindicated in HAPE. Administer if available to treat dehydration and maintain cardiac perfusion.
  - Gradually decompress portable hypobaric chambers to minimize potential barotrauma to the middle ear.
  - HACE progressing to coma warrants advanced airway management and bladder decompression if possible. Hyperventilation may lead to further cerebral ischemia and should be avoided.

REFERENCES

1. Kitsteiner JM, Whitworth JD, Nashelsky J. FPIN's clinical inquiries. Preventing acute mountain sickness. *Am Fam Physician*. 2011;84(4):398–400.
2. Lipman GS, Kanaan NC, Holck PS, et al. Ibuprofen prevents altitude illness: a randomized controlled trial for prevention of altitude illness with nonsteroidal anti-inflammatories. *Ann Emerg Med*. 2012;59(6):484–490.
3. Eide RP III, Asplund CA. Altitude illness: update on prevention and treatment. *Curr Sports Med Rep*. 2012;11(3):124–130.
4. Chen GZ, Zheng CR, Qin J, et al. Inhaled budesonide prevents acute mountain sickness in young Chinese men. *J Emerg Med*. 2015;48(2):197–206.
5. Davis C, Hackett P. Advances in the prevention and treatment of high altitude illness. *Emerg Med Clin North Am*. 2017;35(2):241–260.
6. Fagenholz PJ, Gutman JA, Murray AF, et al. Treatment of high altitude pulmonary edema at 4240 m in Nepal. *High Alt Med Biol*. 2007;8(2):139–146.
7. Biondich AS, Joslin JD. Coca: high altitude remedy of the ancient Incas. *Wilderness Environ Med*. 2015;26(4):567–571.

ADDITIONAL READING

- Centers for Disease Control and Prevention. High-altitude travel and altitude illness. https://wwwnc.cdc.gov/travel/yellowbook/2024/environmental-hazards-risks/high-elevation-travel-and-altitude-illness
- Flaherty G, O'Connor R, Johnston N. Altitude training for elite endurance athletes: a review for the travel medicine practitioner. *Travel Med Infect Dis*. 2016;14(3):200–211.
- Hackett P, Shlim D. High elevation travel and altitude illness. Updated April 23, 2025. Accessed August 18, 2025. https://www.cdc.gov/yellow-book/hcp/environmental-hazards-risks/high-altitude-travel-and-altitude-illness.html
- Luks AM, Beidleman BA, Freer L, et al. Wilderness Medical Society clinical practice guidelines for the prevention, diagnosis, and treatment of acute altitude illness: 2024 update. *Wilderness Environ Med*. 2024;35(Suppl 1):2S–19S.
- Smedley T, Grocott MP. Acute high-altitude illness: a clinically orientated review. *Br J Pain*. 2013;7(2):85–94.

CLINICAL PEARLS

- Proper acclimatization (i.e., graded ascent) is the best method for preventing HAI.
- Never ascend to a higher sleeping altitude if symptoms of HAI are present.
- Acetazolamide 125 to 250 mg PO BID remains a safe and effective means to prevent and treat AMS in both adults and children (max 125 mg per dose).
- Dexamethasone is effective for treating significant AMS as well as HACE.
- Early recognition and treatment of HAPE/HACE are critical.
- Once the symptoms of HAI are recognized, supplemental oxygen (if available), and/or controlled descent to a lower altitude are the mainstay of treatment.

HIP APOPHYSITIS

Anthony J. Saglimbeni, MD, CAQSM ▪ Anthony Kwon, MD

BASICS

DESCRIPTION

- Hip apophysitis is a chronic inflammatory injury seen only in child, adolescent, and skeletally immature athletes.
- Repetitive overload of hip muscles applies excessive forces to pelvic apophyses resulting in hip pain and inflammation.

EPIDEMIOLOGY

Incidence

- Hip apophysitis is common among young athletes.
- Hip apophyses appear and fuse later than growth plates in long bones, placing adolescents at increased risks for apophysitis, especially during periods of growth spurts (boys 13 to 14 years old, girls 11 to 12 years old).
- Apophysitis of the hip occurs more commonly in male athletes compared to females.

ETIOLOGY AND PATHOPHYSIOLOGY

- In the immature skeleton, the apophysis refers to a secondary ossification center that often forms an insertion point for a tendon or ligament.
- Given the differential strength of the physeal cartilage compared with attaching tendons and ligaments, the apophysis can be subject to injury from compounded stress from repetitive microtrauma.
- Overuse and repetitive exercise of the larger pelvic muscles exerts excessive force on hip apophyses causing inflammation and pain.

RISK FACTORS

- Skeletal immaturity
- Limited flexibility
- Rapid bone growth
- Early sport specialization
- Excessive sport participation
- Running, kicking sports, dancing

GENERAL PREVENTION

- Strength and flexibility program to improve hip range of motion and symmetrical balance between hip muscles
- Caution should be taken to avoid repetition and overuse.
- Engagement in a variety of sports or cross-training activities may be beneficial.

COMMONLY ASSOCIATED CONDITIONS

Increased stress on an injured apophysis or rapid eccentric loading of the attached muscle can cause a hip avulsion fracture.

DIAGNOSIS

HISTORY

- Increase in physical activity duration, frequency, and intensity
- Recent growth spurt
- Gradually increasing pain, exacerbated by physical activity (i.e., running or jumping) (1)[A]
- Limited range of motion (1)[A]
- Biomechanical and gait changes (2)[A]

PHYSICAL EXAM

- Localized tenderness and swelling near the affected apophysis (Commonly affected apophyses include anterior superior iliac spine [ASIS], anterior inferior iliac spine [AIIS], and ischial tuberosity.) (2),(3)[A]
- Pain near the tendon-bone junction that worsens with resisted activation of the associated muscle tendon complex (2),(3)[A].
- Diminished range of motion (1)[A]

DIFFERENTIAL DIAGNOSIS

Avulsion fracture, femoral or pubic bone stress fractures, slipped capital femoral epiphysis (SCFE), femoral head epiphysis, (Legg-Calvé Perthes disease), femoral acetabular and ischiofemoral impingement, malignancy (3),(4),(5)[A]

DIAGNOSTIC TESTS & INTERPRETATION

Initial Tests (lab, imaging)

- Anteroposterior radiographs of the hip and pelvis may show open apophysis (1)[A].
- Affected apophysis may or may not show minimal widening on radiography (1)[A].
- Ultrasound findings may include regional hypoechogenicity, widening or fragmentation of the hypoechoic physis, or hyperemia (1),(3)[A].
- Ultrasound is more sensitive than radiography and can also confirm the absence of a muscle and tendon injury (3)[A].
- Magnetic resonance imaging may show increased edema within the apophysis on fluid-sensitive sequences and slight widening of the apophysis (4)[A].

TREATMENT

GENERAL MEASURES

- Dependent on degree of pain and instability
- Relative rest while maintaining activities as tolerated (3)[A]
- Ice and limited use of oral or topical nonsteroidal anti-inflammatory drugs (3)[A]
- Alternative activities (i.e., biking, swimming) (1),(3)[A]
- Protected weight-bearing
- Physical therapy (1)[A]
- Gentle stretching; avoid vigorous stretching (2)[A].

ISSUES FOR REFERRAL

Physical therapy referral is indicated for hip and abdominal strengthening and flexibility. Consider sports medicine or orthopedic referral for pain persisting after fusion of the apophyseal sites or cases refractory to conservative management (3)[A].

ADDITIONAL THERAPIES

Neoprene shorts for warmth and compression (2)[A]

SURGERY/OTHER PROCEDURES

Surgery consult may be necessary in cases of severe avulsion fracture (1),(2)[A]. Adolescent pelvic avulsion fractures rely on the amount of displacement to guide treatment. Conservative management recommendations include rest and avoiding use of the muscle(s) attached to the avulsed fragment. Operative treatment is typically reserved for widely displaced fractures or symptomatic nonunions (6)[A].

ONGOING CARE

FOLLOW-UP RECOMMENDATIONS

Follow up weekly or as needed intervals on a case-by-case basis. Once athlete achieves full range of motion without pain, gradual return to sport may begin ideally under the supervision of an athletic trainer or physical therapist.

PROGNOSIS

- Dependent on severity of pain and disability
- Most patients respond well to conservative therapy, with gradual return to pain free activity, often within several weeks to months.
- Only a small minority requiring surgical intervention

REFERENCES

1. Belair JA, Hegazi TM, Roedl JB, et al. Core injuries remote from the pubic symphysis. *Radiol Clin North Am*. 2016;54(5):893–911.
2. Weiss JE, Stinson JN. Pediatric pain syndromes and noninflammatory musculoskeletal pain. *Pediatr Clin North Am*. 2018;65(4):801–826.
3. Achar S, Yamanaka J. Apophysitis and osteochondrosis: common causes of pain in growing bones. *Am Fam Physician*. 2019;99(10):610–618.
4. Baal JD, Cecil KL, Patel R, et al. Imaging of overuse injuries of the hip. *Radiol Clin North Am*. 2023;61(2):191–201.
5. Samet JD. Pediatric sports injuries. *Clin Sports Med*. 2021;40(4):781–799.
6. Yeager KC, Silva SR, Richter DL. Pelvic avulsion injuries in the adolescent athlete. *Clin Sports Med*. 2021;40(2):375–384.

ADDITIONAL READING

- Arnaiz J, Piedra T, de Lucas EM, et al. Imaging findings of lower limb apophysitis. *AJR Am J Roentgenol*. 2011;196(3):W316–W325.
- Houghton KM. Review for the generalist: evaluation of pediatric hip pain. *Pediatr Rheumatol Online J*. 2009;7:10.

CLINICAL PEARLS

- Hip strength and flexibility are key to reducing the risk of hip apophysitis.
- Ensure that athletes recover to full pain-free range of motion before returning to sport.
- Hip apophysitis can recur in the growing athlete; be cautious to avoid overtraining.

HIP POINTER

Keifer P. Walsh, DO, MS

BASICS

DESCRIPTION

A hip pointer or "bruised hip" is a contusion of the iliac crest and surrounding soft tissues. It is a common injury in contact or collision sports that is primarily managed with conservative modalities.

EPIDEMIOLOGY

- Hip/groin injuries account for 10–14% of all sport injuries with hip pointers representing a small subset (1),(2),(3).
- One study demonstrated an incidence of 0.3% with an average of 5.6 days training loss in professional American football (1).

ETIOLOGY AND PATHOPHYSIOLOGY

- Most common in contact/collision sports (football, hockey, rugby, soccer, lacrosse, wrestling, martial arts)
- Traumatic contusion results in subperiosteal edema of bony surface and possible hematoma of surrounding soft tissue (3),(4).

RISK FACTORS

- Collision sports
- Inadequate iliac crest protection
- Youth athletes with iliac crest apophysis that is not fused

DIAGNOSIS

HISTORY

- Typical presentation with pain and/or bruising over hip from recent collision or fall
- Patient may also present with inability to perform sport if trauma is uncertain.

PHYSICAL EXAM

- Posture often flexed to side of injury
- Swelling and/or deformity
- Tenderness with palpation along the iliac crest
- Palpable or visible hematoma
- Weakness and pain with active hip flexion and abduction, abdominal contraction, trunk rotation and side-bending
- Absence of abdominal wall bruising or tenderness

DIFFERENTIAL DIAGNOSIS

- Hip apophyseal injuries (5)
- Hip avulsion fractures
- Ischial pubic or femoral neck stress injuries
- Intra-abdominal injury
- Intra-articular hip etiologies (labral pathology, avascular necrosis/osteonecrosis, slipped capital femoral epiphysis, Legg-Calvé-Perthes disease) (6)
- Hip flexor or external rotator tendinopathy
- Cutaneous nerve injury (lateral femoral cutaneous, iliohypogastric ilioinguinal, superior cluneal nerves)

DIAGNOSTIC TESTS & INTERPRETATION

- Plain radiographs to rule out fracture (anteroposterior and lateral views)
- Bilateral imaging for contralateral comparison if concerned about growth plate injury (closure expected around 14 to 16 years of age)
- Musculoskeletal ultrasound can be used to rule out avulsion injury, evaluate for hematoma, and aid in return-to-sport decisions.

TREATMENT

GENERAL MEASURES

- Analgesia:
  - Minimize swelling with immediate ice and compression.
  - Nonsteroidal anti-inflammatory drugs (NSAIDs) are indicated at onset until resolution.
  - Injection with local anesthetic and/or aspiration of hematoma may provide pain relief outside of the acute period, although minimal data supports this (4).
- Physical therapy:
  - Gentle abdominal and hip stretching when tolerated, followed by gradual progression to abdominal and hip strengthening
- Hip spica wrap or neoprene strap may be helpful for compression and comfort.

- Return to sport/activity:
  - Once pain and swelling resolve with minimal tenderness at contusion site and patient returns to normal function
  - Protection with sport-specific padding

ADDITIONAL THERAPIES

- If intra-abdominal trauma is suspected, consider emergent transport for imaging and surgical evaluation.
- Crutches for partial or non–weight-bearing may be necessary for first few days of treatment (3).
- Advanced imaging should be considered for pain or functional limitations not improving with conservative measures.
- Injection with corticosteroid should be used with caution given potential for soft tissue injury with return to sport.

SURGERY/OTHER PROCEDURES

Not indicated for hip pointer injuries

ONGOING CARE

PROGNOSIS

Most patients gradually return to previous level of activity within 2 to 3 weeks.

COMPLICATIONS

- Recurrent or recalcitrant injury or worsening hematoma for return earlier than indicated
- Myositis ossificans or dystrophic soft tissue calcification (seen on radiograph or advanced imaging)

REFERENCES

1. Feeley BT, Powell JW, Muller MS, et al. Hip injuries and labral tears in the National Football League. *Am J Sports Med*. 2008;36(11):2187–2195.
2. Werner J, Hägglund M, Ekstrand J, et al. Hip and groin time-loss injuries decreased slightly but injury burden remained constant in men's professional football: the 15-year prospective UEFA Elite Club Injury Study. *Br J Sports Med*. 2019;53(9):539–546.
3. Knapik DM, Salata MJ. Hip injuries in the contact athlete. *Oper Techn Sport Med*. 2019;27(3):145–151.
4. Hall M, Anderson J. Hip pointers. *Clin Sports Med*. 2013;32(2):325–330.
5. Herring SA, Kibler WB, Putukian M, et al. Initial assessment and management of select musculoskeletal injuries: a team physician consensus statement. *Med Sci Sports Exerc*. 2024;56(3):385–401.
6. Chamberlain R. Hip pain in adults: evaluation and differential diagnosis. *Am Fam Physician*. 2021;103(2):81–89.

ADDITIONAL READING

Varacallo M, Bordoni B. *Hip Pointer Injuries*. StatPearls Publishing; 2023. Updated August 4, 2023. Accessed August 19, 2025. https://www.ncbi.nlm.nih.gov/books/NBK538258

CLINICAL PEARLS

- Hip pointer refers to an iliac or femoral contusion primarily seen in contact sports that is typically managed conservatively with return to sport/activity within 2 to 3 weeks.
- Alternate etiologies including hip avulsion fractures (loss of passive range of motion) and intra-abdominal trauma (bruising patterns and/or tenderness concerning for spleen, liver, or kidney injury) must be ruled out.
- Adequate sport-specific hip padding may decrease the incidence of injury or reinjury and allow for sooner return to activity.

HOFFA FAT PAD SYNDROME

Donald Kasitinon, MD, CAQSM, RMSK

BASICS

DESCRIPTION

- First reported by Albert Hoffa in 1904
- Also known as infrapatellar fat pad (IFP) syndrome
- Burning or aching infrapatellar anterior knee pain that can be reproduced with knee extension (1)
- Occurs when the IFP becomes inflamed, leading to impingement of the tibiofemoral joint or lateral aspect of the patellofemoral joint (2)

EPIDEMIOLOGY

- Largely unknown
- In one study over a 10-year period, only 1% of patients undergoing arthroscopy had confirmed findings of the syndrome (3).
- Low documented incidence likely due to:
  - Difficulty in diagnosing condition
  - Success in treatment with conservative management (2)
- Predominantly seen in young women and in those participating in jumping sports or with ligamentous laxity (4)
- Can also be seen in runners, cyclists, and soldiers (2)

ETIOLOGY AND PATHOPHYSIOLOGY

- Usually results from a single traumatic event or repetitive microtrauma
- The IFP is an intracapsular, extrasynovial structure that fills the anterior knee compartments and is richly vascularized and innervated by nociceptive type IVa free nerve endings (1).
- Substance P targets these nerve endings and causes vasodilation; promotes immune cell recruitment contributing to edema in tissue; can cause thickening and fibrosis of the IFP
- Scar tissue gradually accumulates and causes impingement at the intercondylar notch and trochlea with full extension of knee (2).

Genetics

No evidence of genetic predisposition

RISK FACTORS

- Jumping sports
- Repetitive sports such as cycling
- Ligament laxity
- History of prior patellar dislocation or other ligamentous knee injury (2)
- Patella alta
- Increased tibial tubercle-tibial groove distance
- Increased trochlear angle (5)

GENERAL PREVENTION

Focus on closed-chain quadriceps exercises that promote appropriate patellar tracking and increased awareness of the condition (2).

COMMONLY ASSOCIATED CONDITIONS

- Patellofemoral pain syndrome
- Patellar tendinosis
- Chondromalacia patella

DIAGNOSIS

HISTORY

- Burning or aching to the anterior knee deep to or on either of side of the patellar tendon just distal to inferior pole of patella
- Usually occurs with knee at full extension, dynamic extension (such as with stair ascent), or prolonged flexion
- Pain usually occurs over a prolonged period of time and may be associated with a previous knee injury (2).

PHYSICAL EXAM

- Tender around patellar tendon, typically close to inferior pole of patella
- At least some degree of range of motion restriction and pain at end range extension
- Hoffa test: Apply firm pressure with the thumb inferior to the patella just outside the margin of the patellar tendon with knee in 30 degrees of flexion. Knee is fully extended with steady pressure, and increased pain is a positive test. This is then repeated on medial or lateral side of tendon (2).
- Can be difficult to differentiate from patellar tendinosis, but patellar tendon pathology typically worsens with loaded knee flexion (particularly eccentric quadriceps contraction) (1)

DIFFERENTIAL DIAGNOSIS

- Keep in mind that Hoffa fat pad syndrome is a diagnosis of exclusion.
- Bursitis (prepatellar, superficial infrapatellar, deep infrapatellar, and pes anserine)
- Patellar tendinosis
- Osteoarthritis
- Plica syndrome
- Meniscal tears
- Articular cartilage injuries or osteochondral lesions
- "Cyclops lesion" following anterior cruciate ligament (ACL) reconstruction (2)

DIAGNOSTIC TESTS & INTERPRETATION

- Radiographs are not necessary but may help rule out fractures or degenerative joint disease that may also cause range-of-motion restriction (see Figs. 82 and 83 in Appendix A).
- Sagittal magnetic resonance imaging (MRI) is the gold standard for assessing IFP pathology (2)[A].
  - Edema of the superior/posterior fat pad and inflamed infrapatellar bursa (6)
  - Also excludes other potential pathologies (2)
- Ultrasound may also be helpful:
  - Static images: can show inflammation of the IFP and fluid in the deep infrapatellar bursa
  - Dynamic exam: can show IFP herniating during knee flexion and extension
  - Power Doppler: can visualize inflammation within the IFP

TREATMENT

- Mainstay of treatment is physical therapy with the following goals (1),(2)[A]:
  - Restore the biomechanics of patellar tracking via vastus medialis oblique strengthening.
  - Taping to off-load the patellar tendon and fat pad (using the "V" formation across the proximal half of the patella to tilt the inferior patella anterior and decrease impingement)
  - Stretching
  - Gluteal strengthening to improve pelvic control
- Topical and oral nonsteroid anti-inflammatory drugs (NSAIDs) can be helpful for pain control (4),(6)[B].
- May also consider injections:
  - Ultrasound-guided steroid injections into the fat pad may assist by providing anti-inflammatory effects and secondarily fat pad atrophy. This may require 1 to 3 injections at intervals of 4 to 6 weeks (1),(2),(4),(5)[A].
  - Ultrasound-guided Hoffa fat pad hydrodissection (with anesthetic, normal saline, and potentially corticosteroid) can assist in releasing adhesions, mobilizing the fat pad, and removing any neovascularization that may be contributing to symptoms.
- If conservative treatment has been exhausted, arthroscopic resection of the IFP is the primary surgical treatment (1),(2),(3),(4),(5)[A].
- Patients with no other concurrent disease may anticipate long-term improvement in their symptoms and function following arthroscopic excision.

REFERENCES

1. Dragoo JL, Johnson C, McConnell J. Evaluation and treatment of disorders of the infrapatellar fat pad. *Sports Med.* 2012;42(1):51–67.
2. DuBose M, Taqi M. *Hoffa Pad Impingement Syndrome.* StatPearls Publishing. Updated February 22, 2023. Accessed October 10, 2025. https://www.ncbi.nlm.nih.gov/books/NBK58963/
3. Ogilvie-Harris DJ, Giddens J. Hoffa's disease: arthroscopic resection of the infrapatellar fat pad. *Arthroscopy.* 1994;10(2):184–187.
4. Larbi A, Cyteval C, Hamoui M, et al. Hoffa's disease: a report on 5 cases. *Diagn Interv Imaging.* 2014;95(11):1079–1084.
5. Abelleyra Lastoria DA, Benny CK, Hing CB. Predisposing factors for Hoffa's fat pad syndrome: a systematic review. *Knee Surg Relat Res.* 2023;35(1):17.
6. Munday CE, Patel SU, Jain N, et al. A rare cause of Hoffa's fat pad impingement: the crossed-doubled patellar tendon. *BJR Case Rep.* 2023;9(6):20220049.

ADDITIONAL READING

- Kumar D, Alvand A, Beacon JP. Impingement of infrapatellar fat pad (Hoffa's disease): results of high-portal arthroscopic resection. *Arthroscopy.* 2007;23(11):1180–1186.
- Mace J, Bhatti W, Anand S. Infrapatellar fat pad syndrome: a review of anatomy, function, treatment, and dynamics. *Acta Orthop Belg.* 2016;82(1):94–101.

CLINICAL PEARLS

- Hoffa fat pad syndrome is a rare, but likely underdiagnosed, cause of anterior knee pain.
- Typically presents as burning or aching to the anterior knee deep to the proximal patellar tendon.
- Sagittal MRI is the gold standard for assessing IFP pathology.
- Mainstay of treatment is physical therapy focusing on the biomechanics of patellar tracking and taping to offload the IFP. This can be supplemented with injections.
- If conservative treatment fails, arthroscopic resection of the IFP is the primary surgical treatment and yields good results in those without other concurrent pathologies.

HYPERMOBILITY SUBTYPE OF EHLERS-DANLOS SYNDROME

Adrian Tabares, MD, CAQSM, RMSK

BASICS

DESCRIPTION

- Joint hypermobility syndrome is a term previously used and was once viewed as a distinct clinical entity comprising of joint laxity and skin fragility. It currently falls under the classification for Ehlers-Danlos syndrome hypermobility subtype (hEDS) (1),(2).
- It is a diagnosis of exclusion that requires the absence of other features of Ehlers-Danlos syndrome (EDS), of which there are currently 13 recognized subtypes, in addition to other connective tissue disorders. Although there is still ongoing debate on how the clinical diagnosis is made, it is currently based on a combination of clinical history and physical exam findings (1),(2),(3).
- There is no confirmatory genetic test, and the phenotype is variable.
- Manifestations in individuals can range from asymptomatic to chronic widespread pain (3).
- Many affected individuals pursue athletics that require a large degree of flexibility, such as yoga, dance, and gymnastics.

EPIDEMIOLOGY

Incidence

Actual incidence is unknown.

Prevalence

The prevalence of joint hypermobility syndrome may be up to 1 in 500 based on a 2019 national survey in Wales. It was previously estimated to be between 1:5,000 and 1:15,000 (1),(4).

ETIOLOGY AND PATHOPHYSIOLOGY

- The pathophysiology of the hEDS is poorly understood because there are no observable structural abnormalities on examination of collagen fibers or other associated molecules or the genes encoding for them in the majority of patients.
- This is in contrast to other disorders such as classical EDS and Marfan syndrome, which can be distinguished, based on genetic markers (1).

Genetics

- No genetic marker identified to date
- Believed to be inherited through an autosomal dominant pattern
- Incomplete penetrance and variable phenotype (1),(2)

RISK FACTORS

More commonly seen in childhood, adolescence, female gender, and people of Asian and West African descent (1),(3)

GENERAL PREVENTION

Unknown

COMMONLY ASSOCIATED CONDITIONS

- Recurrent joint subluxation and dislocation
- Pes planus
- Chronic pain
- Anxiety and depression
- Gastroesophageal reflux disease (GERD)
- Irritable bowel syndrome (IBS)
- Syncope
- Orthostatic hypotension
- Piezogenic papules
- Recurrent or multiple abdominal hernias
- Mild skin hyperextensibility (1),(2),(3)

DIAGNOSIS

HISTORY

- The diagnosis of the hEDS relies on appropriate history taking and the exclusion of other types of connective tissue disorders, joint arthritides, and myopathy. A family history should be elicited to determine if genetic testing for other conditions is warranted (1),(2),(3)[B].
- The 2017 International Classification of EDS recommends the following diagnostic criteria in order to establish the diagnosis including the presence of criterion 1, 2, and 3 (2).

1. Generalized joint hypermobility (GJH) as determined by Beighton score >6 in prepubertal children, >5 in pubertal men and women up to age 50 years, and >4 in those over the age of 50 years. If the Beighton score is 1 point below the cut-off and the 5-point questionnaire referenced below is positive, GJH can be diagnosed (2).
2. Two or more of the following features (A to C): Feature A: systemic manifestations of a more generalized connective tissue disorder (total of 5 must be present) unusually soft or velvety skin; mild skin hyperextensibility; unexplained striae such as striae distensae or rubrae of the back, groin, thighs, breasts or abdomen in adolescents, men, or prepubertal women without a history of significant gain or loss of bodyfat or weight; bilateral piezogenic papules of the heel; recurrent or multiple abdominal hernias (umbilical, inguinal, crural); atrophic scarring of at least two sites and without formation of truly papyraceous or hemosideric scars as seen in classical EDS, pelvic floor, rectal, and/or uterine prolapse in children, men, or nulliparous women without a history of morbid obesity or other known predisposing medical condition; dental crowding and high or narrow palate; arachnodactyly as defined in one or more of the following: positive wrist (Steinberg) sign bilaterally, positive thumb (Walker) sign bilaterally, arm span:height ratio >1.05, mitral valve prolapse (MVP) mild or greater based on strict echocardiographic criteria, aortic root dilation with Z-score >+2 (2). Feature B: positive family history, with one or more first-degree relatives independently meeting the current diagnostic criteria for hEDS. Feature C: musculoskeletal complications (must have at least one): (i) musculoskeletal pain in two or more limbs, recurring daily for at least 3 months; (ii) chronic widespread pain for ≥3 months; (iii) recurrent joint dislocations or frank joint instability, in the absence of trauma (i or ii): (i) three or more atraumatic joint dislocations in the same joint or two or more atraumatic dislocations in two different joints occurring at different times; (ii) medical confirmation of joint instability at two or more sites not related to trauma (2).
3. All of the following prerequisites must be met: (i) absence of unusual skin fragility, which should prompt consideration of other types of EDS; (ii) exclusion of other heritable and acquired connective tissue disorders, including autoimmune rheumatologic conditions. In patients with an acquired connective tissue disorder such as lupus or rheumatoid arthritis, additional diagnosis of hEDS requires meeting both features A and B of criterion (ii) feature C of criterion 2 cannot be counted toward the diagnosis in this situation; (iii) exclusion of alternative diagnoses that may also include joint hypermobility by means of hypotonia and/or connective tissue laxity. Alternative diagnoses and diagnostic categories include, but are not limited to, neuromuscular disorders such as myopathic EDS, Bethlem myopathy, or other heritable connective tissue disorders (HCTD) such as other types of EDS, Loeys-Dietz syndrome, Marfan syndrome, and skeletal dysplasias. Exclusion of these considerations may be based on history, physical exam, and/or molecular genetic testing, as indicated (2).

PHYSICAL EXAM

- The Beighton score has been developed to assess joint hypermobility and consists of a 9-point scoring system. One point is given for each positive test: (i) if the patient is able to demonstrate apposition of the thumb to the forearm, (ii) extension of the 5th finger beyond 90 degrees, (iii) extension of the elbow beyond 10 degrees, (iv) extension of the knee beyond 10 degrees, and (v) being able to place both palms flat on the floor with forward flexion of the trunk while keeping the legs straight (1),(2),(3).
- The sum of all positive tests is then calculated with a maximum score of 9/9.
- Major criteria include a score of 4/9 or greater or arthralgia for >3 months among four or more joints.
- Minor criteria include the following:
  - A Beighton score of 1 to 3/9 (0 to 3 if age 50 years or older)
  - Arthralgia >3 months in one to three joints, or back pain for >3 months
  - Dislocation/subluxation in more than one joint or on more than one occasion
  - Soft tissue rheumatism with more than three lesions
  - Marfanoid habitus (tall, thin, wingspan to height ratio >1.03, upper-to-lower body ratio <0.89, arachnodactyly [positive Steinberg wrist sign])
  - Abnormal skin: striae, hyperextensibility, thin skin, papyraceous scars
  - Drooping eyelids, myopia, or "antimongoloid slant"
  - Varicose veins, hernia, or rectal/uterine prolapse
- Previously, the diagnosis of joint hypermobility was made if any of the following were met: (i) two major criteria, (ii) one major and two minor criteria, (iii) four minor criteria, or (iv) two minor criteria and an affected first-degree relative (1),(2),(3)[B].
- If joint hypermobility is suspected but the individual does not meet Beighton score criteria, a 5-point questionnaire may be used to assess for historical joint hypermobility. This consists of the following questions:
  - Could you ever place your hands flat on the floor without bending your knees?
  - Could you ever bend your thumb to touch your forearm?
  - As a child, did you amuse your friends by contorting your body into strange shapes *or* could you do the splits?

- As a child or teenager, did your shoulder or kneecap dislocate on more than one occasion?
- As a child or teenager, did you consider yourself "double-jointed?"

- A positive answer to two or more questions is consistent with GJH (1),(2)[B].

DIFFERENTIAL DIAGNOSIS

- EDS classic and other types
- Marfan syndrome
- Loeys-Dietz syndrome
- Ankylosing spondylitis
- Rheumatoid arthritis
- Fibromyalgia
- Multiple sclerosis
- Amyotrophic lateral sclerosis
- Autonomic polyneuropathies
- Myopathy
- Chronic fatigue syndrome
- Osteogenesis imperfecta
- Arterial tortuosity syndrome
- Lateral meningocele syndrome

DIAGNOSTIC TESTS & INTERPRETATION

Initial Tests (lab, imaging)

There are no diagnostic labs or imaging to confirm hEDS, and the diagnosis relies on history and physical exam findings (1),(2).

Follow-Up Tests & Special Considerations

Additional testing may be performed to rule out other conditions or to evaluate for other pathology and may include:

- X-ray, diagnostic ultrasound, computed tomography (CT), or magnetic resonance imaging (MRI) of involved joints.
- Inflammatory markers, uric acid levels, autoimmune markers, evaluation for endocrine or hematologic conditions, muscle biopsy
- Echocardiography if EDS or Marfan syndromes are suspected
- Bone mineral density testing for osteogenesis imperfecta (1)[C]

Pediatric Considerations

In pediatric patients, a second evaluation in adult age is recommended or laboratory testing to exclude other disorders before the diagnosis is made (1)[C].

Diagnostic Procedures/Other

Arthrocentesis may be considered if joint infection or other arthritides such as gout or pseudogout are suspected.

Test Interpretation

Tissue pathology does not play a role in diagnosis.

TREATMENT

GENERAL MEASURES

- Although there are no treatment options that lead to the resolution of the hEDS, treatment should be individualized and focus on symptom management (3),(5).
- Physical and occupational therapy: There is limited evidence to suggest therapy can be effective in pain reduction, improved proprioception, strength, balance, and improvement of quality of life. However, joint-specific exercise has not been found to be more effective than exercise in general (5)[A].
- Splints and orthotics may provide additional support but high-quality evidence is lacking (5)[C].
- Pain management using a team approach, including behavioral therapy and pharmacologic and nonpharmacologic methods can provide an adjunct to overall symptom control (3)[C].

MEDICATION

Medication has not been found to be effective for the long-term treatment of the hEDS. However, analgesics, such as acetaminophen; nonsteroidal anti-inflammatories; muscle relaxants; antidepressants, such as selective serotonin reuptake inhibitors (SSRIs) and tricyclics; and antiseizure medications, such as gabapentin, may prove helpful in reducing acute and chronic pain (3)[C].

ISSUES FOR REFERRAL

- A referral to a rheumatologist or clinical geneticist may be considered for additional testing if the diagnosis remains uncertain.
- Cardiology, endocrinology, gastroenterology, neurology, ophthalmology, orthopedic surgery, and podiatry referrals may be considered for additional evaluation.
- Psychiatry, clinical psychology, and pain management referrals may be indicated for assistance in management (1)[C].

SURGERY/OTHER PROCEDURES

Surgery may be recommended for recurrent joint dislocations and instability on an individualized basis.

COMPLEMENTARY & ALTERNATIVE MEDICINE

- A number of supplements have been proposed to treat joint hypermobility syndrome including calcium, carnitine, coenzyme Q10, glucosamine, magnesium, methylsulfonylmethane, Pycnogenol, silica, vitamin C, and vitamin K.
- However, large-scale, randomized controlled trials demonstrating efficacy are lacking (6)[C].

ONGOING CARE

FOLLOW-UP RECOMMENDATIONS

Patient Monitoring

Follow-up is recommended at the clinicians discretion based on the specific needs of the individual.

PATIENT EDUCATION

- The goal of education is to help individuals understand the nature of the condition and recommended treatment options.
- Education may help reduce rates of joint dislocations and other associated injuries.
- Self-help groups such as the Hypermobility Syndromes Association (HMSA) located in the United Kingdom may provide further support (3).

PROGNOSIS

- The hEDS is a lifelong condition that in many individuals may manifest as recurrent episodes of joint pain and instability.
- Some individuals experience reduction in symptoms along with reduced flexibility that occurs with age.
- Longitudinal studies examining the progression of the condition are currently unavailable (1),(3).

COMPLICATIONS

- Although recurrent joint subluxation, dislocation, and pes planus are commonly associated conditions, exact rates of these complications remain unknown (2),(3).
- Physical therapy including a strengthening protocol is thought to reduce the rates of these complications, but high-quality studies that provide measurement of these outcomes are lacking (3),(4).

REFERENCES

1. Colombi M, Dordoni C, Chiarelli N, et al. Differential diagnosis and diagnostic flow chart of joint hypermobility syndrome/Ehlers-Danlos syndrome hypermobility type compared to other heritable connective tissue disorders. *Am J Med Genet C Semin Med Genet*. 2015;169C(1):6–22.
2. Malfait F, Francomano C, Byers P, et al. The 2017 international classification of the Ehlers-Danlos syndromes. *Am J Med Genet C Semin Med Genet*. 2017;175(1):8–26.
3. Pacey V, Tofts L, Wesley A, et al. Joint hypermobility syndrome: a review for clinicians. *J Paediatr Child Health*. 2015;51(4):373–380.
4. Demmler JC, Atkinson MD, Reinhold EJ, et al. Diagnosed prevalence of Ehlers-Danlos syndrome and hypermobility spectrum disorder in Wales, UK: a national electronic cohort study and case-control comparison. *BMJ Open*. 2019;9(11):e031365.
5. Palmer S, Bailey S, Barker L, et al. The effectiveness of therapeutic exercise for joint hypermobility syndrome: a systematic review. *Physiotherapy*. 2014;100(3):220–227.
6. Mantle D, Wilkins RM, Preedy V. A novel therapeutic strategy for Ehlers-Danlos syndrome based on nutritional supplements. *Med Hypotheses*. 2005;64(2):279–283.

ADDITIONAL READING

- Grahame R, Bird HA, Child A. The revised (Brighton 1998) criteria for the diagnosis of benign joint hypermobility syndrome (BJHS). *J Rheumatol*. 2000;27(7):1777–1779.
- Hakim AJ, Grahame R. A simple questionnaire to detect hypermobility: an adjunct to the assessment of patients with diffuse musculoskeletal pain. *Int J Clin Pract*. 2003;57(3):163–166.

SEE ALSO

Connective Tissue Disorders; Benign Hypermobility Syndrome, Joint Hypermobility Syndrome

CLINICAL PEARLS

- The hEDS is a chronic condition and a diagnosis of exclusion that includes joint laxity and skin fragility.
- The diagnosis is based on history and physical exam and relies on the exclusion of other connective tissue disorders such as Marfan syndrome and EDS.
- The 2017 International Classification of EDS diagnosis guidelines provide criteria to aid the clinician in making the diagnosis but make establishing the diagnosis more time-consuming.
- Treatment should be tailored to address symptoms and include physical therapy to improve strength, balance, proprioception, and quality of life.

HYPERTHERMIA: HEAT STROKE, EXHAUSTION, AND CRAMPS

Christopher C. Trigger, MD, FACEP, CAQSM

BASICS

DESCRIPTION

- Heat illness is the result of increased heat production and impaired heat dissipation.
- May also be caused by endotoxin release leading to a systemic inflammatory response
- Exertional heat illness is possibly a continuum, based on signs and symptoms, and can be divided into the following groups:
  - Heat cramps
  - Heat exhaustion
  - Heat stroke
  - Heat injury

EPIDEMIOLOGY

Incidence

- Roughly 3 deaths per year in sports since 1995 are attributed to exertional heat stroke, mainly in high school football (1).
- Exertional heat stroke is the third leading cause of death in athletes (2).

Prevalence

- Exact numbers of heat illness across all sports are unknown.
- American football, running, cycling, and adventure races have been identified as the sports with the greatest number of heat-related illnesses.

ETIOLOGY AND PATHOPHYSIOLOGY

- Heat dissipation occurs via four processes (1),(3):
  - Radiation is the direct release of heat from the body to the environment.
  - Conduction occurs with direct transfer of heat during contact with a cooler object.
  - Convection is when cooler air passes over the warmer exposed skin, lifting the heat away.
  - Evaporation through perspiration is the body's most effective way of eliminating heat, although limited when humidity is high.
- Leaky gut hypothesis and endotoxemia (1),(3)
  - Increased intestinal permeability leading to endotoxin release into the circulation leading to systemic inflammatory response syndrome (SIRS)

RISK FACTORS

- Hot, humid weather
- Dehydration
- Sickle trait
- Age (<15 years or >65 years)
- Poorly trained and/or overweight athletes
- Cumulative heat load from previous days exposures
- Improper attire (plastic suits)
- Equipment (football pads/helmet)
- Poor acclimatization
- Medications:
  - Dietary supplements (i.e., ephedra, diet pills)
  - Antihypertensives (i.e., diuretics, β-blockers, calcium channel blockers)
  - Tricyclic antidepressants
  - Monoamine oxidase inhibitors
  - Antihistamines
  - Amphetamines
  - Illicit drugs (i.e., cocaine, heroin, phencyclidine)
- Concurrent illness (viral illness, skin disorders, cardiac disease)

GENERAL PREVENTION

- Prehydration/posthydration
- Modify time; intensity; and exposure in hot, humid weather:
  - Exercise in the early morning or evening.
  - Limit sun exposure if possible.
  - Remove unnecessary equipment and/or clothing.
- Heat acclimatization is the primary strategy in reducing the risk of heat illness (usually takes 1 to 2 weeks) (1)[A].
- Increase electrolyte intake, mainly sodium (Na), using sports drinks.
- Wet bulb globe temperature (WBGT) monitoring and categorization California rules
  - Schools must use WBGT devices to precisely measure heat stress levels.
  - Areas are categorized (e.g., California category 1, 2, 3 based on climate), with category 3 having the highest WBGT thresholds for outdoor activity due to hotter conditions.
- Heat acclimatization
  - A 5-day acclimatization period is mandatory for fall sports. This involves gradually increasing practice duration and intensity to help athletes adapt to heat.
- Practice modifications based on WBGT levels
  - Below are the specific thresholds and required adjustments to practice schedules, rest breaks, and equipment:
    - <27.8°C (<82°F)
      - Normal activities permitted
      - Ensure at least three rest breaks per hour.
    - 27.8–30.5°C (82.0–86.9°F)
      - Implement more frequent and longer rest breaks.
      - Football players should be restricted to helmets, shoulder pads, and shorts.
    - 30.6–32.2°C (87.0–90.0°F)
      - Reduce practice time to a maximum of 2 hours.
      - Provide more frequent and longer rest breaks.
      - Full pads may be allowed if the WBGT rises during practice, but caution is advised.
    - 32.3–33.3°C (90.1–92.0°F)
      - Limit practice time to a maximum of 1 hour.
      - No conditioning activities allowed
      - Ensure 20 minutes of rest per hour.
    - 33.4°C (92.1°F) and above
      - No outdoor workouts or contests are permitted.
- Emergency preparedness
  - Schools are required to have comprehensive emergency action plans in place to effectively address any heat-related illnesses that may occur.
- These guidelines are designed to minimize the risk of heat-related illness by proactively adjusting activities based on environmental conditions. Staying vigilant and adhering to these thresholds is key to athlete safety.

DIAGNOSIS

HISTORY

- Heat cramps:
  - Painful involuntary contractions of muscles, most commonly the calf, quadriceps, and abdomen
  - Heat cramps are more commonly thought of as an electrolyte problem than a heat issue.
- Heat exhaustion:
  - Fatigue
  - Shortness of breath
  - Dizziness or syncope
  - Nausea and vomiting
  - Normal mental status
- Heat stroke:
  - Central nervous system (CNS) symptoms with the correct environmental conditions (hot and humid)
  - May be combative
  - Previous history of heat exhaustion
- Heat injury:
  - End-organ damage without evidence of CNS depression
  - Laboratory testing required for diagnosis
  - May be a consequence of delayed recognition and/or inadequate cooling

PHYSICAL EXAM

- Heat cramps:
  - Normal temperature and vital signs
  - Tense, tender, involuntary contraction of the muscle belly
- Heat exhaustion:
  - Normal or elevated core temperature but <40°C (104°F)
  - Vital signs usually normal but can be variable depending on severity
  - Normal mental status
  - Flushed skin
  - Profuse sweating
  - Cold, clammy skin
- Heat stroke:
  - Core (rectal) temperature >40°C (104°F) (1),(2)
  - CNS disturbances (confusion, ataxia, irritability, coma)
  - Tachycardic, tachypneic, and hypotensive
  - Hot skin with or without sweating
  - End-organ damage/failure

- Heat injury:
  - Elevated core temperature
  - End-organ damage (usually dark urine, severe muscle pain, and abnormal blood chemistry levels)
  - Organ dysfunction may persist for several weeks.

DIFFERENTIAL DIAGNOSIS

- Dehydration
- Electrolyte abnormality
- Cardiovascular disease
- Exercise-associated collapse
- CNS lesion
- Thyroid dysfunction
- Infection

DIAGNOSTIC TESTS & INTERPRETATION

Initial Tests (lab, imaging)

Routine lab work typically unnecessary for minor heat illness, but depending on the clinical picture, you may need to check the following:

- Complete blood count (CBC)
- Basic metabolic panel
- Urinalysis to detect myoglobin
- Serum creatine kinase to evaluate for rhabdomyolysis
- Toxicology screen
- Cardiac enzymes
- Liver function tests
- Coagulation studies to evaluate disseminated intravascular coagulation

Diagnostic Procedures/Other

Electrocardiography (ECG): Consider in heat stroke to look for cardiac damage/dysfunction.

TREATMENT

- Acute treatment:
  - Use basic or advanced cardiac life support for all unstable patients and transfer them to the nearest medical facility.
  - The goal in treating all heat illnesses is to lower the core temp to an acceptable (38–39°C) level within 30 minutes of recognition.
  - Consider heat illness as a code and get athletes out of the sun and cool quickly and before transport.
- Heat cramps (2):
  - Rest
  - Oral replacement of fluids and electrolytes (Na) using sports drinks (2)
  - Intravenous (IV) fluids if unable to tolerate by mouth
  - Passive stretching and/or ice massage of the affected muscles
- Heat exhaustion (1),(2):
  - More aggressive cooling techniques:
    - Move to cool environment.
    - Rest and remove excess clothing.
    - Apply ice bags to neck, axilla, and/or groin (2)[C].
  - Place in supine position and elevate legs.
  - Replacement of fluids and electrolytes
  - IV fluids if unable to tolerate oral rehydration
- Heat stroke (1),(2),(4):
  - Support airway, breathing, and circulation (ABCs).
  - Rapid cooling of the patient is first line:
    - Ice water immersion most rapid form of cooling (1)[A]
    - Cooling rates >0.15°C/min are best for survival without medical complications (1)[A].
    - If immersion unavailable, place wet towels/sheets and ice bags to neck, axilla, and groin (1),(2)[C].
  - Oral fluids preferred if able to tolerate PO, and IV fluids can complicate especially if hyponatremia but if needed for resuscitation proceed.
  - If a physician is onsite and cooling occurs immediately and patient is asymptomatic 1 hour after cooling, transport to emergency department (ED) may be unnecessary (2)[B].
- Heat injury:
  - Similar to above focusing on rapid cooling while supporting the ABCs
  - IV fluids
  - Serial testing needed to determine severity of end-organ damage/injury
- ED treatment:
  - The patient should be immediately cooled on field/site and prior to transporting to the ED.
  - Once in the ED, the patient should continue similar cooling techniques as noted above.
  - Prepare and start treatment of possible end-organ injury as soon as possible.

ONGOING CARE

FOLLOW-UP RECOMMENDATIONS

Return to activity/play recommendations should be individualized (1),(2),(4):

- Heat cramps (2)[C]:
  - May return immediately after symptoms resolve with rest and fluid replacement
  - Depending on severity, may require 24 hours of relative rest
- Heat exhaustion (1),(2)[C]:
  - Immediate return not recommended
  - Generally, can return to activity within 24 to 48 hours
  - Gradually increase intensity and volume of training.
- Heat stroke and heat injury (1),(2)[B]:
  - Consider at least 7 days of rest or until asymptomatic and lab values have normalized.
  - Consider follow-up no later than 1 week after event or even sooner based on severity of symptoms and lab abnormalities.
  - Start with 1 to 2 weeks of everyday activities followed by training in a cool environment and then increase intensity while acclimating to heat over a 4- to 6-week period.
  - Clear the athlete for full competition if heat tolerance exists after roughly 6 weeks of training.
  - If an athlete does not tolerate return-to-play progression or has recurrent heat illnesses, consider laboratory exercise-heat tolerance test.

PATIENT EDUCATION

- Avoid risks listed above.
- Acclimate and hydrate preexercise and postexercise to reduce risk.
- "Salty sweaters" may be at higher risk for heat cramps due to loss of Na; encourage increased salt intake with meals and hydration with electrolytes.

COMPLICATIONS

- Death
- End-organ failure
- Seizures
- Cardiovascular collapse
- Acute respiratory distress syndrome
- Liver failure
- Acute renal failure
- Rhabdomyolysis
- Disseminated intravascular coagulation

REFERENCES

1. Roberts WO, Armstrong LE, Sawka MN, et al. ACSM expert consensus statement on exertional heat illness: recognition, management, and return to activity. *Curr Sports Med Rep*. 2021;20(9):470–484.
2. Casa DJ, DeMartini JK, Bergeron MF, et al. National Athletic Trainers' Association position statement: exertional heat illnesses. *J Athl Train*. 2015;50(9):986–1000.
3. Garcia CK, Renteria LI, Leite-Santos G, et al. Exertional heat stroke: pathophysiology and risk factors. *BMJ Med*. 2022;1(1):e000239.
4. Pryor RR, Bennett BL, O'Connor FG, et al. Medical evaluation for exposure extremes: heat. *Clin J Sport Med*. 2015;25(5):437–442.

CLINICAL PEARLS

- Remember the principle "cool first, transport second."
- General Heat Stress Index (3),(4)
- Consider prevention protocols (e.g., acclimatization, monitoring, hydration).
- Include serious heat illness protocols in your emergency action plan.

HYPERTROPHIC CARDIOMYOPATHY

Anne M. Garrison, DO, CAQSM • Lisa Falotico, DO, CAQSM

BASICS

DESCRIPTION

- Genetic disorder of cardiac myocytes characterized by cardiac hypertrophy
- Asymmetric nondilated left ventricular hypertrophy (LVH), with or without outflow obstruction
- Mostly inherited autosomal dominant disease, but many cases are sporadic
- Hypertrophic cardiomyopathy (HCM) accounts for approximately 8–12% of sudden cardiac death (SCD)
- Death results from ventricular tachycardia either due to, or in the absence of, left ventricle (LV) outflow obstruction (some patients have arrhythmogenic foci).

EPIDEMIOLOGY

- Incidence of SCD in athletes <35 years old, mostly due to HCM, is 1:250,000.
- General population prevalence of 1:200 to 1:500 inferring that about 750,000 Americans are affected by HCM, but only 10–20% identified clinically.
- Many patients remain undiagnosed.
- Timely accurate diagnosis is a priority is treatable and consistent with normal longevity.
- More than a dozen gene mutations are known to cause HCM; however, in about 40% of patients, no causal genes have been identified.
- Underlying cause for about 1/3 of nontrauma-related sudden deaths in young asymptomatic patients

RISK FACTORS

- Family history of unexplained or early (<40 years old) cardiac death
- Age from 12 to 30 years
- Prior history of syncope
- Male > female
- Previously, an abnormal blood pressure (BP) response to exercise was seen as an independent marker of sudden death risk. This is now unfounded by emergence of new risk markers.

DIAGNOSIS

HISTORY

- History is negative for most patients.
- Family history of HCM or SCD
- Direct and specific questions are important, and parents should be questioned as well: chest pain, palpitations, dyspnea with exertion, syncope, exercise intolerance, orthopnea.
- Providers should also inquire about prescription medications and drugs of abuse.

PHYSICAL EXAM

- Most common initial presentation is syncope or SCD with exertion
- Most patients with HCM have a completely normal physical examination.
- Murmur: In rare cases where murmur is detected, it is usually midsystolic and heard at the midleft sternal border:
  - Murmur is ominous if it increases with maneuvers to decrease LV end-diastolic (LVED) filling. These maneuvers cause dynamic obstruction in the LV outflow tract.
  - Maneuvers include rising from squatting to standing, moving from supine to vertical position, and performing the Valsalva maneuver.
  - Murmur decreases when LVED filling increases while moving from standing to squatting (LV free wall moves away from the septum with increased filling)
  - Benign murmurs usually become louder while squatting and decrease on rising.
  - Benign murmurs are common with improved fitness from training, as described with the athletic heart syndrome (AHS).
  - Athletes with significant outflow obstruction eventually may have pansystolic blowing murmur of mitral regurgitation radiating to the axilla.
- Any diastolic murmur indicates other cardiac pathology requiring workup.
- Screening electrocardiogram (ECG) as part of the preparticipation exam can help detect cardiac disorders with the potential to cause SCD (such as HCM), but are best interpreted by clinicians proficient in interpreting athlete ECGs.

DIFFERENTIAL DIAGNOSIS

- Athlete's heart syndrome
- Myocarditis/pericarditis
- Coronary artery anomalies
- Aortic stenosis
- Prolonged QT syndrome
- Marfan syndrome
- Wolff-Parkinson-White syndrome
- Arrhythmogenic right ventricular dysplasia
- Exercise-induced asthma
- Costochondritis
- Gastroesophageal reflux

DIAGNOSTIC TESTS & INTERPRETATION

Initial Tests (lab, imaging)

- ECG recommended as initial evaluation and periodic follow-up every 1 to 2 years (1)[B]
  - ECG is abnormal in 75–95% of patients with phenotypic HCM.
  - Typical abnormalities: deep T-wave inversions, especially in inferolateral leads, ST-segment depression or elevation, pathologic Q waves, and intraventricular conduction delay
  - However, evidence of LVH and repolarization changes do not correlate with the severity or pattern of hypertrophy (1).
  - Abnormal ECG findings should prompt additional investigation/imaging (2).
- Recommended as component of screening first-degree relatives for HCM (1)[B]
- Holter monitoring:
  - 48 hours—30 days of monitoring recommended as initial evaluation and periodic monitoring to identify patients at risk of SCD and manage arrhythmias (1)[B]
- Echocardiogram
  - Comprehensive 2D echocardiography (ECHO) helps establish diagnosis of HCM, determine pattern of hypertrophy, presence of LV apical aneurysms, LV systolic and diastolic function, mitral valve function as well as the presence and severity of left ventricular outflow tract obstruction (LVOTO).
  - Transthoracic echocardiogram (TTE) recommended for initial evaluation (1)[B]
  - Adult patient's maximal end-diastolic wall thickness of 15 mm, or greater, anywhere in the LV (which is approximately 6 standard deviations above the mean) (1)
  - For pediatric patients, the diagnostic threshold is different. A diagnosis has traditionally been made when the heart's wall thickness measures two or more standard deviations above the average, which is represented by a Z-score of +2.0 or greater. This Z-score is essential because it adjusts the measurement to account for the child's specific gender, body size, and stage of growth.
  - Approximately 2% white athletes and 18% of black athletes have increased LV wall thickness, the "gray zone" below the diagnostic threshold for HCM but above usual measurements (13 to 14 mm in men and 12 to 13 mm in women) (2).
- Cardiac magnetic resonance imaging (CMR)
  - CMR can identify areas of LVH not well visualized on ECHO.
  - CMR provides high spatial resolution and fully tomographic images of the heart.
  - If HCM suspected but ECHO is inconclusive, CMR is recommended (1)[B].
  - If suspicion of alternate diagnoses, including infiltrative/storage diseases or athlete's heart, CMR is recommended (1)[B].

- CMR can also evaluate myocardial fibrosis after injection of late gadolinium enhancement (LGE) contrast. The sharp contrast images provide highly accurate measurements of the LV thickness, LV chamber, right ventricle (RV) chamber, LV mass, and systolic function as well as assess LV apical aneurysm and ejection fraction—all of which are beneficial if considering an implantable cardiac defibrillator (ICD).
- However, CMR is not always an option for testing due to availability, cost, contraindications (pacemakers, ICDs, renal function, and patient factors (claustrophobia, body habitus, pediatric age, etc.).

- Computed tomography (CT)
  - Not commonly used but can provide good spatial resolution defining LV structure and function
  - Can be used for adult patients with suspected HCM if ECHO is not diagnostic and CMR is not available (1)[C]
- Genetic testing
  - Has an important role in diagnosis and management of HCM for patients and their families
  - Most cases are autosomal dominantly inherited, with a 50% change of offspring inheriting the same disease-causing genetic variant.
  - Getting at least a three-generation family history of HCM and SCD events is important.
  - The potential social, legal, ethical, psychological, and professional implications of having a genetic disease should be discussed.
  - Appropriate counseling should be performed by trained cardiac genetic counselor or similar genetics expert (1)[B].
  - However, the usefulness of genetic testing to assess the risk of SCD in HCM is uncertain (1)[B].
  - First-degree relatives of patients with HCM with pathogenic variant identified/suspected should be offered clinical screening including ECG and 2D echocardiogram and cascade genetic testing. (1)[B].

Diagnostic Procedures/Other

- Exercise stress testing is reasonable to determine functional capacity and provide initial prognostic information in patients with HCM (1)[B].
- LVOTO is present at rest and intensifies with exercise in about 1/3 of patients, and LVOTO can be provoked in another 1/3 of patients with HCM, making exercise stress testing useful (3).
- Not useful for younger children who are unable to cooperate with exercise testing (1)
- Recommended to detect and quantify dynamic LVOTO in symptomatic HCM patients without resting or provocable outflow tract obstruction ≥50 mm Hg on TTE (1)[B]

TREATMENT

- Acute treatment/emergency action plan:
  - Cardiopulmonary resuscitation (CPR) for syncope or arrest and defibrillation with automated external defibrillator (AED) as soon as possible if indicated
- Long-term treatment (for symptomatic patients):
  - Treatment is individualized based on degree/location of LV thickening, symptoms, and concomitant cardiac pathology. Considerations include:
    - ICD for primary or secondary prevention of SCD (3)[B]
    - Lifestyle—Avoid dehydrating situations: hot tubs, hot showers, saunas, as well as exercising during concomitant illness (2).
    - Medication (typically β-blockers) (3)[B]
    - Nondihydropyridine calcium channel antagonists
    - Myomectomy or ablation (3)[B]
    - Activity restrictions (3)[C]

ONGOING CARE

- 2020 American Heart Association/American College of Cardiology recommendations:
  - Genotype (+) phenotype (−): Participation in competitive sports of any intensity is reasonable (2)[C].
  - Phenotype (+): High-intensity recreational/moderate- to high-intensity competition may be considered after comprehensive evaluation and shared discussion repeated annually with an expert provider who conveys that the risk of sudden death and ICD shocks may be increased and with the understanding that eligibility decisions for competitive sports often involve third parties (2)[C].
  - Mild- to moderate-intensity recreation is beneficial for most patients with HCM—to improve cardiopulmonary fitness, physical functioning, and quality of life (1)[B].
  - Most patients with HCM: Low-intensity competition is reasonable (2)[C].
- HCM patients in high-intensity recreational activities or moderate- to high-intensity competitive sports activities may be considered after comprehensive evaluation and shared discussion with experts who convey the risk of SCD and ICD shocks may increase, and with the understanding that eligibility decisions for competitive sports often involve other parties (team medical staff, institutional leadership) acting on behalf of the team or school (1)[C].

Pregnancy Considerations

It is reasonably safe for women with clinically stable HCM to become pregnant—but should involve discussion of maternal and fetal risks as well as genetic counseling.

REFERENCES

1. Ommen SR, Mital S, Burke MA, et al. 2020 AHA/ACC guidelines for the diagnosis and treatment of patients with hypertrophic cardiomyopathy: a report of the American College of Cardiology/American Heart Association Joint Committee on Clinical Practice Guidelines. *Circulation*. 2020;142(25):e558–e631.
2. Lander BS, Phelan DM, Martinez MW, et al. Hypertrophic cardiomyopathy: updates through the lens of sports cardiology. *Curr Treat Options Cardiovasc Med*. 2021;23(8):53.
3. Maron BJ, Desai MY, Nishimura RA, et al. Diagnosis and evaluation of hypertrophic cardiomyopathy. *J Am Coll Cardiol*. 2022;79(4) 372–389.

ADDITIONAL READING

Marian AJ, Braunwald E. Hypertrophic cardiomyopathy: genetics, pathogenesis, clinical manifestations, diagnosis, and therapy. *Circ Res*. 2017;121(7):749–770.

CLINICAL PEARLS

- Individuals with suspected HCM should avoid moderate to intense physical exertion while awaiting definitive diagnosis. This is critical to prevent exacerbation of a potentially life-threatening condition, such as sudden cardiac arrest. In settings where a timely evaluation may be challenging, it is recognized that mild exertion (e.g., activities of daily living that do not significantly increase heart rate or breathlessness) may be permissible, but a thorough risk assessment should guide such decisions.
- Genotype positive/phenotype negative patients may spontaneously convert to LV hypertrophy, often without cardiac symptoms, at any age, but appears to occur most often between the ages of 12 and 20 years.
- HCM is a relatively benign disease with about 2/3 HCM patients experiencing a normal life without significant morbidity—particularly in patients without significant LVOTO. However, prognosis is guarded in patients deemed at risk of SCD.
- ICD should not be placed for the sole purpose of participation in competitive athletics (1)[B].

HYPHEMA

Jennifer J. Mitchell, MD, FAAFP, CAQSM, FAMSSM • Kelly T. Mitchell, MD

BASICS

DESCRIPTION

- Blood in the anterior chamber of the eye
- Traumatic hyphema grading:
  - Microhyphema:
    - Circulating red blood cells (RBCs) usually seen by slit lamp exam only
  - Grade I:
    - <1/3 anterior chamber with layered blood
  - Grade II:
    - 1/3 to 1/2 of anterior chamber filled with blood
  - Grade III:
    - >1/2 anterior chamber filled with blood
  - Grade IV:
    - 100% anterior chamber filling (total or 8-ball hyphema) (1)

EPIDEMIOLOGY

Incidence

- Annual incidence of traumatic hyphema:
  - 17/100,000 <18 years old (2)
  - 20.7/100,000 <20 years old (1)
  - 0.52/100,000 emergency department (ED) visits in United States; 66% male (3)
- Pediatrics: males:females 3:1 (2)

ETIOLOGY AND PATHOPHYSIOLOGY

- Trauma:
  - Blunt trauma 2/3
  - Lacerating injury 1/3 (2)
- Spontaneous: association with certain medical conditions
- Postocular procedure: laser, surgery

RISK FACTORS

- Traumatic hyphema:
  - High-risk sports causing blunt injury to eye with projectile or body part:
    - Soccer is the most common.
    - Badminton and pickleball increasing in frequency as popularity grows
    - Basketball, baseball, Australian rules football
    - Paintball and air dart
    - Any combat sport
    - Hockey, lacrosse, racquetball decreasing due to enforced eye protection rules
  - Work injuries: grinding, weed trimming
- Spontaneous hyphema:
  - Neovascularization; diabetes mellitus, uveitis
  - Blood dyscrasias/hemoglobinopathies
  - Ocular tumors: xanthogranuloma

GENERAL PREVENTION

- Protective eyewear during sports involving contact or use of a ball (4),(5)
- Impact-resistant polycarbonate or Trlvex lenses in American Society for Testing and Materials (ASTM)-approved frames (4)
- Functionally monocular athletes, best vision 20/100, should wear impact-resistant eye protection at all times, especially for all sports and recreation.

COMMONLY ASSOCIATED CONDITIONS

- Eyelid swelling and bruising
- Orbital fracture
- Subconjunctival hemorrhage or hemorrhagic chemosis
- Corneal abrasion or corneal scleral laceration
- Ruptured globe
- Foreign body: eyelid, ocular surface, intraocular
- Iridodialysis

DIAGNOSIS

HISTORY

- Acute vision loss, eye pain, photophobia, and visible blood in anterior chamber
- Mechanism of injury to determine whether associated injuries such as open globe or orbital fracture may be present (2)
- Presence of sickle cell disease or blood dyscrasias, which changes prognosis and management (2); sickle-shaped RBCs clog trabecular meshwork and cause more severe type of glaucoma.
- Predisposing medical conditions and medications related to increased risk of spontaneous hyphema
- Higher suspicion in context of blunt force trauma with ball or body part and decline in vision
- If mechanism does not match degree of injury, evaluate for child abuse or intimate partner violence (IPV), diabetes mellitus, clotting disorder, or tumors (1),(2).

PHYSICAL EXAM

Acute systematic exam (4):

- Sports-related ocular trauma evaluated on site
- Mechanism of injury, if not personally witnessed
- Best corrected visual acuity, pocket Snellen chart or smart phone app
- External exam looking for conjunctival, corneal, or orbital injury
- Pupil exam with penlight, including evaluation for afferent pupillary defect
- Penlight exam of the anterior chamber looking for haziness with red tinge (microhyphema) or boat-shaped layering of blood inferiorly
- Ocular motility
- Topical anesthetic may be used to facilitate exam.
- Intraocular pressure evaluation should be deferred to ophthalmology.
- If concern for ruptured globe, place protection (shield or sturdy sunglasses) over affected eye, advise nothing by mouth (NPO); refer emergently; defer further ocular exam or manipulation to ophthalmologist.

DIFFERENTIAL DIAGNOSIS

- Iris tear, traumatic mydriasis
- Orbital fracture
- Retrobulbar hematoma
- Ruptured globe:
  - Anterior corneal scleral rupture
  - Occult posterior scleral rupture
- Traumatic cataract
- Traumatic subconjunctival hemorrhage or hemorrhagic chemosis
- Vitreous hemorrhage

DIAGNOSTIC TESTS & INTERPRETATION

Initial Tests (lab, imaging)

- Sickle cell rapid preparation in high-risk populations (African American, Afro-Caribbean, Hispanic); if positive, hemoglobin electrophoresis (2)[B]
- Spontaneous hyphema: complete blood count (CBC), prothrombin time, partial thromboplastin time, international normalized ratio, liver function to screen for bleeding dyscrasias
- Orbital computed tomography (CT) scan if concern for globe rupture, intraocular foreign body, orbital fracture
- CT: thin-sliced helical CT with coronal reconstructions; if helical CT not available, CT scan with ≤3 mm cuts in axial/coronal/sagittal view
- Plain film x-ray for ocular or orbital injury has a high false-negative rate and is not useful to plan therapeutic intervention.
- Magnetic resonance imaging (MRI) is contraindicated in cases of possible metallic foreign body.
- Use of ultrasound in this setting should be deferred to the consulting ophthalmologist as it has questionable diagnostic yield in this clinical context and carries risk of further injury from inadvertent compression of the injured eye.

Diagnostic Procedures/Other

- A gonioscopy exam, to assess for glaucoma, puts pressure on the eye and is contraindicated with an acute hyphema; can also precipitate rebleeding if done too early, before hyphema resolution
- Performed by ophthalmologist due to requirement for a specialized lens and advanced training
- Once the blood is completely resolved, no earlier than 4 weeks, the managing ophthalmologist will perform gonioscopy to check for angle recession (trauma to the angle) to determine whether there is increased risk for hyphema-related glaucoma.

TREATMENT

GENERAL MEASURES

- Prehospital:
  - Cannot return to contest or activity
  - Place rigid eye shield to protect the eye.
  - Minimize mobility of the patient.
  - Head of transport bed elevated 30 to 45 degrees so blood will settle inferiorly.
  - Do not give any nonsteroidal anti-inflammatory drugs (NSAIDs) or aspirin due to platelet inhibition.
  - Keep NPO in case surgery is required.
- ED treatment:
  - Assess and treat life-threatening injuries.
  - To facilitate further exam, provide additional pain control with topical anesthetic: proparacaine or tetracaine ophthalmic drops
  - Fluorescein dye can be used to assess for corneal abrasion.
  - Examine carefully for ocular perforation (open globe).
  - Treat emesis and pain to prevent sudden intraocular hypertension and extrusion of ocular contents.
  - Evaluate for underlying hemoglobinopathy or bleeding dyscrasias, if indicated. When not being examined, keep eye protected with shield and head of bed elevated to 30 to 45 degrees.
  - Arrange for urgent ophthalmology assessment.
  - Strict limitation of activity is required until the clot resolves as rebleeding worsens long-term visual prognosis. Therefore, at home, near bedrest for 5 to 7 days.
  - Return-to-play or strenuous activity is only allowed after hyphema is completely resolved, likely 7 to 14 days.
  - Frequency of follow-up will depend on initial ophthalmology evaluation of severity of ocular injury, level of hyphema, and intraocular pressure. It could be daily or every other day for the first 5 to 10 days.

MEDICATION

- Medication management should be directed by ophthalmology.
- Anticoagulant medications risk: hyphema persistence or rebleed, so risk of continuation versus benefit for underlying medical conditions are made on a case-by-case basis (1)[A]
- Mydriatics and cycloplegics permit visualization of the posterior pole, provide comfort from iritis, facilitate clot resolution, and decrease the risk of posterior synechiae related to scarring of the iris to the lens:
  - Cyclopentolate ophthalmic drops 1 gtt BID
  - Atropine ophthalmic drops 1 gtt QD to BID (1)[A]
- Ophthalmic topical steroids help decrease intraocular inflammation, minimize long-term iris scarring, and may facilitate clot stabilization to minimize rebleeding, which is a priority early in the course of hyphema (1)[A].
- Oral steroids may have a role to decrease inflammation and minimize rebleeding risk.
- Antifibrinolytic agents lower the rate of rebleeding but may delay clot resorption. Their use is controversial for a variety of reasons. They do not offer any major advantage in preventing most complications related to hyphema (1)[A]:
  - Aminocaproic acid:
    - 50 mg/kg PO q4h for 5 days, adult dosing
    - 30% gel q6h for 5 days, adult dosing
    - Side effects: nausea, vomiting, hypotension; more likely with oral versus topical
    - Contraindicated in pregnancy, renal disease, hemophilia, thromboembolic disease
  - Tranexamic acid:
    - 75 mg/kg divided TID for 5 days, adult dosing
    - 5% solution 1 gtt q6h for 5 days, adult dosing
    - *Not U.S. Food and Drug Administration (FDA) approved*

ISSUES FOR REFERRAL

Any hyphema warrants early (same or next day) ophthalmologic referral to categorize the severity of the ocular injury and hyphema which is critical in management decisions.

ADDITIONAL THERAPIES

- Eye protection with hard plastic eye shield at all times, including sleep, until hyphema is resolved.
- Strict bed rest for severe hyphema, sickle cell trait/disease, children, bleeding predisposition and noncompliant patients; this may require hospitalization.
- Bed rest with quiet activity at home otherwise
- Consulting ophthalmologist will guide the care regarding continued use of medications and management of intraocular pressure.
- Traumatic hyphema and intraocular hypertension require medication to decrease intraocular pressure:
  - Topical medications used: β-adrenergic blocker eye drops (timolol), α-agonist eye drops (brimonidine—avoid in children <3 years old due to risk of apnea), prostaglandin analogs (latanoprost), and topical carbonic anhydrase inhibitors (CAIs), if sickle cell hemoglobinopathy has been ruled out
  - In sickle cell, CAIs may cause increased sickling in anterior chamber due to decreasing the pH.
- After complete resolution of the hyphema, and usually at the 2- to 4-week follow-up appointment, the ophthalmologist will perform a complete exam with gonioscopy to check for posttraumatic glaucoma and a dilated retinal exam for occult breaks or tears.
- If vision is still blurrier than expected, an optical coherence tomography (OCT) or fluorescein angiography may be performed to assess for occult, posttraumatic injury to the macula or retinal vessels.

SURGERY/OTHER PROCEDURES

- 5–7% requires surgery (1)[A].
- Indications for surgical intervention after hyphema:
  - Corneal blood staining
  - Intraocular pressure >24 mm Hg for >24 hours in patient with sickle cell disease
  - Intraocular pressure >60 mm Hg for >2 days
  - Intraocular pressure ≥50 mm Hg for 5 days
  - 50% or greater hyphema unresolved for 7 days (1)[A],(2)[A]
- Other surgeries considered by ophthalmologist to optimize vision:
  - Trabeculectomy glaucoma surgery to treat persistently elevated intraocular pressure even after clot evacuation
  - Corneal transplant if blood staining has occurred, impacting visual axis; can cause amblyopia in children
  - Cataract surgery for associated posttraumatic cataract

ADMISSION, INPATIENT, AND NURSING CONSIDERATIONS

Inpatient management is recommended for:

- Other ocular or facial injuries requiring hospital care
- Bleeding dyscrasias or sickle hemoglobinopathy
- Active young children or unstable home
- Large hyphemas (grade III or IV) with early signs of elevated intraocular pressure
- Suspected child abuse
- Evidence of secondary rebleeding on follow-up examination

ONGOING CARE

PATIENT EDUCATION

- Patient must understand need for strict compliance with all activity restrictions, medication dosing, and follow-up appointments.
- Review symptoms of rebleeding or elevated intraocular pressure (sudden decreased vision and pain).
- Provide medications and medication schedule prior to discharge to improve adherence.

PROGNOSIS

- Final visual acuity depends on size of hyphema and related complications.
- Secondary hemorrhages usually result in hyphemas that are larger than the initial injury. When this complication occurs, the patients usually have a poorer outcome due to the higher occurrence of severe glaucoma and blood staining of the cornea.
- A final vision of 20/50 or worse is seen in 10% of patients with grade I and in 50–75% with grade III or IV. The poorer visual outcome is usually due to more severe optic atrophy secondary to the initial trauma or secondary glaucoma or visually significant blood staining.
- 14% of hyphema patients have poor visual outcomes because of associated sequelae (vitreous hemorrhage, retinal detachment, ocular rupture).
- Blunt eye injury and hyphema increase risk of late-developing traumatic glaucoma.
- Anticipate return to normal activities within a week, but no athletic participation for up to a month (6).

COMPLICATIONS

- Potential for permanent significant vision loss
- Rebleeding
- Glaucoma: early or late developing
- Corneal blood staining
- Traumatic cataract: early or late developing

REFERENCES

1. Bansal S, Gunasekeran DV, Ang B, et al. Controversies in the pathophysiology and management of hyphema. *Surv Ophthalmol*. 2016;61(3):297–308.
2. Trief D, Adebona OT, Turalba AV, et al. The pediatric traumatic hyphema. *Int Ophthalmol Clin*. 2013;53(4):43–57.
3. Zafar S, Canner JK, Mir T, et al. Epidemiology of hyphema-related emergency department visits in the United States between 2006 and 2015. *Ophthalmic Epidemiol*. 2019;26(3):208–215.
4. Micieli JA, Easterbrook M. Eye and orbital injuries in sports. *Clin Sports Med*. 2017;36(2):299–314.
5. Dockery DM, Harrington MA, Gardiner MF, et al. A 5-year retrospective assessment of clinical presentation associated with sports injury in young people presenting to a tertiary eye center. *J Pediatr Ophthalmol Strabismus*. 2021;58(6):377–384.
6. Iftikhar M, Mir T, Seidel N, et al. Epidemiology and outcomes of hyphema: a single tertiary centre experience of 180 cases. *Acta Ophthalmol*. 2021;99(3):e394–e401.

ADDITIONAL READING

- American Academy of Ophthalmology. *Protective Eyewear for Young Athletes*. Accessed October 4, 2025. https://www.aao.org/clinical-statement/protective-eyewear-young-athletes
- Ashraf G, Arslan J, Crock C, et al. Sports related ocular injuries at a tertiary eye hospital in Australia: a 5-year retrospective descriptive study. *Emerg Med Australas*. 2022;34(5):794–800.
- Black AM, Eliason PH, Patton DA, et al. Epidemiology of facial injuries in sport. *Clin Sports Med*. 2017;36(2):237–255.
- Cass SP. Ocular injuries in sports. *Curr Sport Med Rep*. 2012;11(1):11–15.
- Gharaibeh A, Savage HI, Scherer RW, et al. Medical interventions for traumatic hyphema. *Cochrane Database Syst Rev*. 2013;12(12):CD005431.
- Hong S, Choi KE, Kim J, et al. Analysis of patients with blowout fracture caused by baseball trauma. *J Craniofac Surg*. 2022;33(4):1190–1192.
- Romaniuk VM. Ocular trauma and other catastrophes. *Emerg Med Clin North Am*. 2013;31(2):399–411.
- Walton W, Von Hagen S, Grigorian R, et al. Management of traumatic hyphema. *Surv Ophthalmol*. 2002;47(4):297–334.

CLINICAL PEARLS

- Significant and permanent vision loss can occur related to the initial hyphema or rebleed or associated ocular injuries.
- Appropriate protective eyewear is needed for all athletic events involving a ball, projectile, or physical contact: Soccer, basketball, baseball, and badminton are common causes.
  - The ASTM has established performance standards for selected eyewear that are most appropriate for sports with a risk of ocular injury.
  - The American Academy of Ophthalmology has helpful guidelines online.
- Concern for hyphema requires urgent/emergent evaluation and referral to an ophthalmologist.
- Detailed education of the patient for adherence to activity restrictions is essential.
- Return to athletic competition may be prolonged.

H

HYPOTHENAR HAMMER SYNDROME

Holly J. Benjamin, MD, FAMSSM, FACSM ▪ Alvin Au-Yeung, DO, MPH

BASICS

DESCRIPTION

Digital ischemia of the superficial palmar arch of the ulnar artery in the hand caused by repetitive compression, blunt trauma, or a single severe trauma over the hook of the hamate-hypothenar eminence, usually as a result of occupational or sporting activities (1),(2),(3),(4)[A].

EPIDEMIOLOGY

- Traditionally regarded as a rare condition (<1 per 100,000), in the general population, although may be underdiagnosed
- Incidence in patients with secondary Raynaud phenomenon (RP) is approximately 1.1–1.3%.
- No known prevalence
- Male:female ratio is 9:1.
- Age bracket is 40s to 50s.

ETIOLOGY AND PATHOPHYSIOLOGY

- Etiology (1),(2):
  - *Trauma*: frequent use of the hand as a "hammer"
  - *Vascular pathology*: thrombosis, abnormal anatomy, prothrombotic factors, or aneurysm of the ulnar artery; unilateral symptoms with hypothenar hammer syndrome (HHS) are suspected to occur when persons with preexisting palmar ulnar artery fibrodysplasia experience repetitive palmar trauma. This revised theory for the etiology of HHS explains why HHS does not develop in most patients with repetitive palmar trauma (1),(4).
  - *Work related*: auto mechanics, metal workers, lathe operators, miners, machinists, butchers, bakers, carpenters, and brick layers
  - *Sport related*: golf, baseball catchers, heavy weightlifting, martial arts, mountain biking
- Pathophysiology:
  - Hypothenar relates to the muscles of the 5th finger.
  - Unilateral, dominant ring finger +/− small finger
  - Less commonly, index and middle fingers
  - Raynaud episodes noted, thumb is spared.
  - Triphasic color change often absent
  - "AFO" mnemonic:
    - A—abductor digiti minimi
    - F—flexor digiti minimi
    - O—opponens digiti minimi
  - The hand obtains its arterial supply from the ulnar and radial arteries. The ulnar artery and nerve pass through Guyon canal next to the hamate bone before dividing into the superficial and deep palmar branches. Just distal to the canal, a short segment (about 2 cm) of the superficial branch that forms the origin of the superficial palmar arch is unprotected between the skin and the bone in the hypothenar area. Here the artery is directly anterior to the hook of the hamate, covered only by the palmaris brevis, subcutaneous tissue, and skin, and therefore vulnerable to injury. Chronic trauma to this area can lead to pathology of the ulnar artery.
  - Types of HHS (2),(3)
    - *Type 1*: stenosis of superficial palmar arch around the hook of the hamate
    - *Type 2a*: occlusion of the superficial palmar arch around the hook of the hamate
    - *Type 2b*: occlusion of superficial and deep palmar arches around the hook of the hamate
    - *Type 3a*: occlusion of the ulnar artery at the proximal part of the wrist
    - *Type 3b*: occlusion of the ulnar artery near the wrist

DIAGNOSIS

Early diagnosis allows more effective therapeutic strategies and is important in preventing long-term negative medical sequelae.

HISTORY

Symptoms (2):

- Paresthesia in fingers; pins and needles sensation
- Pain in fingers caused by cold temperatures or repetitive movements.
- Raynaud-like phenomenon that spares the thumb

PHYSICAL EXAM

- A hypothenar mass or callus
- Pulsatile mass if aneurysm is present
- Tenderness over the hypothenar eminence
- RP–like symptoms in the fingers and on the ulnar side of the hand (5),(6)
- Positive Allen test (see below)
- Dependent rubor
- Fingertip ulceration, blanching, mottling, cyanosis, pallor, gangrene (rare)
- *Allen test*: assesses for which part of the hand is perfused by the radial artery
- The technique is as follows:
  - Patient elevates the hand and makes a fist for 20 seconds.
  - Firm pressure is held against both the radial and ulnar arteries.
  - The patient opens the hand, and it should blanche (changes color to white).
  - The examiner releases compression of the ulnar artery, but not the radial artery.
  - A normal hand flushes within 5 to 7 seconds.
  - If the hand remains white, then there is an abnormal circulation—positive Allen test.

DIFFERENTIAL DIAGNOSIS
- Hand–arm vibration syndrome (5)
- RP (2)[A]: Primary RP involves the thumb, whereas HHS does not. HHS is a cause of secondary RP.

DIAGNOSTIC TESTS & INTERPRETATION
- Complete blood count (CBC) and international normalization ratio (INR) if thrombosis is suspected
- Doppler ultrasound (US)—first line; measure digital brachial index: <0.7 necessitates reconstruction (2)[B].
- Arteriography (gold standard)
- Magnetic resonance (MR) angiography
- Computed tomography (CT) angiography
- *Findings*: tortuous "corkscrew" ulnar artery, occlusion or aneurysm at the hook of hamate

TREATMENT

Optimal therapy for HHS has not been determined.
- Nonsurgical:
  - Lifestyle modifications: Avoid further trauma, smoking cessation, alteration of sporting activity.
  - Urokinase has been used to clear obstruction, as has prostaglandin E1 with heparin. Because the etiology of acute hand ischemia is not always obvious at the time of presentation, a trial of Urokinase infusion is warranted because it is relatively safe, and its use may obviate the need for complex microsurgical reconstruction.
  - Calcium channel blockers, vasodilators, and platelet inhibitors have also been used (2)[B].
  - Treat underlying atherosclerosis and prothrombotic factors (e.g., smoking, diabetes, and hyperlipidemia).
- Surgical:
  - Surgical reconstruction (end-to-end anastomosis of the ulnar artery): This requires microsurgical techniques. Arteries may be transplanted from other sites, or a venous graft may be used (3)[B].
  - Sympathectomy appears to give poor results.

ONGOING CARE

- *Complications*: gangrene of the fingers in severe cases, which may require surgery
- *Prognosis*: Many patients improve with nonsurgical treatments as mentioned above (about 80% success). Results of reconstructive surgery are variable, and recurrence is common (2)[B].
- *Prevention*: education focusing on improving work practices, sports modification, hand protection, and avoiding palmar hand use as a hammer to pound, push, or twist objects (2)[A]

REFERENCES

1. Ferris BL, Taylor LM Jr, Oyama K, et al. Hypothenar hammer syndrome: proposed etiology. *J Vasc Surg*. 2000;31(1 pt 1):104–113.
2. Yuen JC, Wright E, Johnson LA, et al. Hypothenar hammer syndrome: an update with algorithms for diagnosis and treatment. *Ann Plast Surg*. 2011;67(4):429–438.
3. Estíbaliz AT, Eztizen LS, Osman-Alberto SA, et al. Bilateral Hypothenar hammer syndrome case presentation and literature review. *Case Rep Vasc Med*. 2022;2022:2078772.
4. Trommeter RA, Freeman CL, Shah KS, et al. Hypothenar hammer syndrome. *J Emerg Med*. 2019;56(1):105–106.
5. Brodmann M, Stark G, Aschauer M, et al. Hypothenar hammer syndrome caused by post-traumatic aneurysm of the ulnar artery. *Wien Klin Wochenschr*. 2001;113(17–18):698–700.
6. Piessat C, De Almeida YK, Athlani L. Hypothenar hammer syndrome: outcomes after ulnar artery reconstruction with autologous vein graft. *Hand Surg Rehabil*. 2023;42(3):203–207.

ADDITIONAL READING

- Schröttle A, Czihal M, Lottspeich C, et al. Hypothenar hammer syndrome. *Vasa*. 2015;44(3):179–185.
- Swofford BP, Swofford DP. Management of hypothenar hammer syndrome a case report. *Am J Case Rep*. 2018;19:150–152.

CLINICAL PEARLS

- Avoid using the hand as a hammer.
- Rare condition but needs high suspicion in certain groups
- Doppler US—first line
- CT angiography is the gold standard.
- Prevention is the best management modality.
- Conservative treatment if no ischemia
- Surgical treatment for ischemia and to prevent further complications from thrombus or aneurysms

H

HYPOTHERMIA AND FROSTBITE

Kurtis Lawton, DO • Craig C. Young, MD

BASICS

DESCRIPTION

- Frostbite:
  - Severe, local cold-related injury, resulting in freezing of soft tissue:
    - Superficial: partial or complete freeze of skin
    - Deep: involvement of skin and underlying tissue (may include muscles, vessels, nerves, fat, and bone)
- Hypothermia:
  - Systemic cold injury, classified as:
    - Mild: core body temperature 32–35°C (90–95°F)
    - Moderate: 30–32°C (86–90°F)
    - Severe: <30°C (86°F)

EPIDEMIOLOGY

Incidence

- True incidence of hypothermia and frostbite is unknown in athletes:
  - Mild cases of both are likely common in cold environments.
  - Accidental hypothermia estimated at 5.6 per 1,000,000 people in the United States
- Annual incidence of hypothermia-related deaths <1 per 100,000:
  - More common in men especially in rural areas
  - Incidence and mortality data very limited in accidental/cold exposure–related hypothermia and in individuals in lower socioeconomic groups.

ETIOLOGY AND PATHOPHYSIOLOGY

- Frostbite:
  - Fluids in body tissues and cellular spaces freeze and crystallize.
  - Cyclic vasodilation and vasoconstriction contribute to hypoxia/ischemia of affected tissue.
  - Severe or prolonged exposure can lead to irreversible tissue damage.
- Hypothermia:
  - Body heat is lost to the environment at a rate that overwhelms normal temperature homeostasis, resulting in decreased core body temperature.
  - With decreasing temperature, heart rate, cardiac output, and cerebral blood flow decrease:
    - May lead to cardiac rhythm disturbance and death

RISK FACTORS

- Hypothermia:
  - Environmental factors: cold temperature, wind chill, prolonged exposure, high altitude
  - Wet clothing (increases heat loss 2 to 5 times) or immersion (increases heat loss 10 to 25 times)
  - Fatigue
  - Low body fat (decreased tissue insulation), malnutrition
  - Alcohol use (inhibits shivering, enhances heat loss through peripheral vasodilation, and may lead to false sense of warmth)
  - Extremes of age (very young or old)
  - Infants have high body-surface-area-to-mass ratio, dependent on others to seek shelter.
  - Older persons have lowered ability to vasoconstrict and generate metabolic heat.
  - Underlying medical disease (e.g., sickle cell anemia, peripheral vascular disease, diabetes, seizure disorder, hypothyroidism)
  - Use of neuroleptic drugs
  - Psychiatric disorders
  - Low socioeconomic status
- Frostbite:
  - Environmental factors:
    - Cold temperature, wind chill, prolonged exposure, high altitude:
      - Risk of frostbite is <5% with temperatures >5°F (−15°C), but significant risk of frostbite increases with wind chill temperature ≤−18°F (−27°C).
  - Wet clothing (increases heat loss 2 to 5 times) or immersion (increases heat loss 10 to 25 times)
  - Prior cold injury
  - Constrictive clothing or shoes
  - Smoking
  - Vasospastic disorders (i.e., Raynaud syndrome)

GENERAL PREVENTION

Best treatment for hypothermia and frostbite is prevention:

- Event planning based on the potential temperature ranges
- Proper clothing, including hats, mittens, and multiple layers, as necessary
- Avoid alcohol and other mood-altering drugs.
- Recognize the signs and symptoms of hypothermia that indicate a need to seek shelter (shivering, slurred speech, somnolence).

DIAGNOSIS

- Frostbite:
  - Skin may appear erythematous and swollen, or waxy, white, yellow, or blue-purple.
  - Vesicles/blisters may be present.
  - Patients with superficial frostbite complain of numbness and pain in affected area, but in severe/deep frostbite, pain may be absent.
  - Technetium 99 triple-phase bone scan is currently the standard imaging modality for establishing disease severity, but microangiography may better predict prognosis (1)[B].
- Hypothermia:
  - Mild: Patient displays shivering and mild mental status changes, including confusion, amnesia, dysarthria, and ataxia.
  - Moderate: As core temperature declines, patient may develop severely impaired judgment or stupor, loss of deep tendon reflexes, loss of shivering with muscle rigidity, and cardiac arrhythmias.
  - Severe: Patient may have dilated pupils and appear comatose, with nearly undetectable blood pressure (BP) and respiration.

HISTORY

- Duration and severity of cold exposure (Prolonged exposure to very cold temperatures increases risk of severe frostbite or hypothermia.)
- Recent alcohol or drug use (impairs judgment and increases susceptibility to cold injury)
- History of cold-water immersion (Wet clothing and skin significantly increase continued heat loss.)
- Underlying medical conditions (increases risk of severe frostbite or hypothermia)
- Pain in affected area suggests superficial versus deep frostbite.

PHYSICAL EXAM

- Measure core body temperature with a thermometer capable of measuring hypothermic temperatures:
  - To avoid further cold exposure, rectal temperature is not advisable until the patient is in a warm environment (2)[C].
  - Oral temperature is inadequate for diagnosis but can rule out hypothermia (2)[C].
  - Esophageal temperature has greatest accuracy but should be used only when patient's airway is secured (2)[C].
  - Epitympanic thermometer (not to be confused with the widely available much less accurate infrared tympanic thermometer) may be used if airway is not secured (2)[C].
- Assess pulse and cardiac rhythm:
  - Tachycardia may be seen with mild hypothermia.
  - May progress to bradycardia, atrial fibrillation, or ventricular fibrillation with more severe hypothermia
  - In severe hypothermia, may be difficult to manually palpate pulse
- Assess mental status:
  - Degree of mental status alteration correlates with severity of hypothermia.
- Perform complete neurologic examination:
  - Intact sensation to pinprick indicates a better prognosis for patients with frostbite.
  - Decreased muscle coordination, delayed deep tendon reflexes, and slowed pupillary reflexes suggest more severe hypothermia.
  - Focal neurologic deficit suggests etiology of mental status changes other than hypothermia.
- Inspect appearance of skin:
  - Cold, yellow-white, or purple skin suggests frostbite.
  - Tissue pliability suggests superficial frostbite; hard tissue without pliability suggests deep frostbite.
- Electrocardiogram (ECG): may see tachycardia; bradycardia; atrial fibrillation; ventricular fibrillation; prolonged PR, QRS, and QT intervals; and J waves (positive deflection occurring at junction of QRS complex and ST segment)
- Electrolytes and basic chemistries: Hypothermic patients are at high risk for acid–base disturbances.

DIFFERENTIAL DIAGNOSIS

- Frostbite:
  - Frostnip: freezing injury to superficial skin layers
  - Trench foot: swelling, cyanosis, and erythema of extremity without freezing of tissue
  - Chilblains: local cold-related erythematous skin lesions
  - Raynaud phenomenon: cold-induced vasospasm resulting in sequential pallor, cyanosis, and erythema of digits
- Hypothermia:
  - Altered mental status from metabolic abnormalities, alcohol/toxic ingestion, or closed head injury

TREATMENT

- Prehospital:
  - Frostbite:
    - Avoid thawing until no further risk of refreezing.
    - Immerse affected part in 37–39°C (98.6–102.2°F) (2)[C].
    - Remove wet clothing and protect from further cold injury.
    - Ensure adequate hydration with warmed oral or intravenous (IV) fluids.

    - Avoid rubbing or massaging skin, which may compound tissue damage (3)[C].
    - Monitor and treat for concurrent hypothermia. Moderate and severe hypothermia should be treated before treating frostbite injury (4)[C].
    - Arrange transport to medical facility for moderate or severe frostbite.
  - Hypothermia:
    - Mild:
      - Passive external rewarming: Prevent further heat loss with blankets, dry clothing, shared body heat, and moving patient to shelter (2)[C].
      - Active external rewarming: direct application of heat sources (heating pad, hot water bottle, warm water immersion, electric blanket) applied to trunk and used cautiously. Application of heat sources to extremities can result in rapid reversal of cold-induced peripheral vasoconstriction, leading to hypotension (rewarming shock) and further decreases in core temperature ("afterdrop").
      - Hot drinks for patients who are coherent with normal gag reflex
    - Moderate/severe: in addition to the above measures:
      - Active emergency medical system. Perform a primary survey and institute cardiopulmonary resuscitation (CPR) if needed.
      - Attempts at field rewarming should not delay transport to emergency facility for patients with moderate or severe hypothermia.
      - Avoid agitation or jarring due to high risk of arrhythmias.
- Emergency department (ED) treatment:
  - Frostbite:
    - After rewarming, débride white blisters and apply topical aloe vera. For hemorrhagic blisters, apply aloe vera without débridement (4)[C].
  - Hypothermia (moderate or severe):
    - Continuous cardiac monitoring
    - Active external rewarming with forced-air rewarming blanket
    - Active internal rewarming with heated (40–42°C) [104–108°F]) IV fluid or heated humidified air or oxygen (42°C) (2)[C]:
      - Peritoneal, gastric, pleural, or bladder lavage with heated (40°C [104°F]) fluids may be used.
      - For severe cases, cardiopulmonary bypass may improve survival in young, otherwise healthy individuals.
    - Monitor electrolytes; rewarming usually corrects electrolyte and acid–base disturbances.
    - Conventional wisdom has held that hypothermia with cardiac arrest requires a modified Advanced Cardiac Life Support (ACLS) protocol; however, evidence to support this is insufficient, and the recommendation of administering or withholding medications is not clear:
      - In the case of hypothermia with cardiac arrest, establish airway and start CPR. It may be reasonable to consider administration of a vasopressor according to the standard ACLS algorithm concurrent with rewarming strategies.

MEDICATION

- Frostbite:
  - Administer tetanus prophylaxis if indicated according to standard tetanus guidelines (3)[C].
  - Administer analgesics/nonsteroidal anti-inflammatory medications unless contraindicated.
  - Administration of penicillin G (500,000 IU every 6 hours for 48 to 72 hours) prophylactically is controversial and not shown to reduce amputation rate (5)[C].
  - Administration of intra-arterial or IV tissue plasminogen activator within 24 hours of rewarming may decrease amputation rate (4)[C].
  - Consider IV prostaglandin (iloprost) (2)[C] or thrombolytic treatment (6)[B] which appears to reduce the risk of digital amputations from frostbite. Strongly recommended for first-line therapy for grades 3 and 4 frostbite <48 hours after thawing and possibly up to 72 hours. (iloprost U.S. Food and Drug Administration [FDA] approval February 2024, available from specialty pharmacy).
- Hypothermia:
  - No evidence to support routine use of antibiotics, steroids, or barbiturates

ADDITIONAL THERAPIES

Range-of-motion and strengthening exercises may benefit frostbite-affected limbs.

SURGERY/OTHER PROCEDURES

Surgical débridement or amputation may be indicated for late treatment of necrotic or gangrenous tissue due to frostbite.

ONGOING CARE

PROGNOSIS

- Mild to moderate cases of both hypothermia and frostbite generally recover fully without complication.
- Severe cases may lead to significant disability and death
- Frostbite prognosis:
  - Poor: cool skin after rewarming, numbness, no pain with rewarming, dusky/blue digits, hemorrhagic bullae
  - Good: warm skin after rewarming, intact sensation, pain with rewarming, pink digits, clear bullae

COMPLICATIONS

- Frostbite:
  - Limb and digit loss
  - Premature closure of the epiphysis (younger athletes)
  - Autonomic dysfunction of affected extremity
  - Permanent cold sensitivity and susceptibility to cold injury
- Hypothermia:
  - Cardiac arrhythmias
  - Electrolyte and acid–base disorders
  - Inefficient clotting leading to disseminated intravascular coagulation

REFERENCES

1. Lacey AM, Fey RM, Gayken JR, et al. Microangiography: an alternative tool for assessing severe frostbite injury. *J Burn Care Res*. 2019;40(5):566–569.
2. Dow J, Giesbrecht GG, Danzl DF, et al. Wilderness Medical Society clinical practice guidelines for the out-of-hospital evaluation and treatment of accidental hypothermia: 2019 update. *Wilderness Environ Med*. 2019;30(4S):S47–S69.
3. Zaramo TZ, Green JK, Janis JE. Practical review of the current management of frostbite injuries. *Plast Reconstr Surg Glob Open*. 2022;10(10):e4618.
4. McIntosh SE, Freer L, Grissom CK, et al. Wilderness Medical Society clinical practice guidelines for the prevention and treatment of frostbite: 2019 update. *Wilderness Environ Med*. 2019;30(4S):S19–S32.
5. Crooks S, Shaw BH, Andruchow JE, et al. Effectiveness of intravenous prostaglandin to reduce digital amputations from frostbite: an observational study. *CJEM*. 2022;24(6):622–629.
6. Rogers C, Lacey AM, Endorf FW, et al. The effects of rapid rewarming on tissue salvage in severe frostbite injury. *J Burn Care Res*. 2022;43(4):906–911.

ADDITIONAL READING

- Castellani JW, Eglin CM, Ikaheimo TM, et al. ACSM expert consensus statement: injury prevention and exercise performance during cold-weather exercise. *Curr Sports Med Rep*. 2021;20(11):594–607.
- Falat C. Environmental hypothermia. *Emerg Med Clin North Am*. 2024;42(3):493–511.
- Gauthier J, Morris-Janzen D, Poole A. Iloprost for the treatment of frostbite: a scoping review. *Int J Circumpolar Health*. 2023;82(1):2189552.
- Hickey S, Whitson A, Jones L, et al. Guidelines for thrombolytic therapy for frostbite. *J Burn Care Res*. 2020;41(1):176–183.
- Lipatov K, Komarova E, Asatryan A, et al. Frostbite of the upper extremities: hot issues in diagnosis and surgical treatment (review). *Burns*. 2022;48(6):1279–1286.
- Lowe J, Warner M. Can iloprost be used for treatment of cold weather injury at the point of wounding in a forward operating environment? A literature review. *Int J Circumpolar Health*. 2023;82(1):2210340.
- McDaniel L. Hypothermia and cold injury in children. *Pediatr Rev*. 2022;43(1):58–60.
- Persitz J, Essa A, Ner EB, et al. Frostbite of the extremities—recognition, evaluation and treatment. *Injury*. 2022;53(10):3088–3093.
- Schimelpfenig SS, Jacobsen B. Pediatric environmental cold injuries. *Pediatr Rev*. 2022;43(8):449–457.
- Sheridan RL, Goverman JM, Walker TG. Diagnosis and treatment of frostbite. *N Engl J Med*. 2022;386(23):2213–2220.
- Sidhar K, Elliott K, Ibrahem M. Heat, cold, and environmental emergencies in athletes. *Clin Sports Med*. 2023;42(3):441–461.
- Soar J, Becker LB, Berg KM, et al. Cardiopulmonary resuscitation in special circumstances. *Lancet*. 2021;398(10307):1257–1268.
- Vogel K, Hulsopple C. Cold weather injuries: initial evaluation and management. *Curr Sports Med Rep*. 2022;21(4):117–122.
- Zafren K, Hollis S, Weiss EA, et al. Prevention and treatment of nonfreezing cold injuries and warm water immersion tissue injuries: a supplement to Wilderness Medical Society clinical practice guidelines. *Wilderness Environ Med*. 2023;34(2):172–181.

CLINICAL PEARLS

- Hypothermia can occur even at moderate temperatures (50–65°F [10–18°C]) if wind, rain, sweat, or wet clothing lead to heat loss that is greater than metabolic heat production.
- Prolonged exposure to cold temperatures, wet clothing, drug or alcohol use, and underlying medical conditions increase risk of hypothermia and frostbite.
- Avoid freeze-thaw-freeze cycles which worsen tissue damage.
- Prevention is the best treatment for hypothermia and frostbite.
- Delayed surgical intervention is associated with increased tissue salvage.

ILIOPSOAS INJURY

Margaret E. Gibson, MD, FAMSSM • Andrew Hurvitz, MD, FAAOS

BASICS

- The iliopsoas is the most powerful hip flexor with a major role in posture, walking, and running.
- Pathology can include iliopsoas tendonitis, bursitis, impingement, and snapping hip (coxa saltans).
- The iliopsoas tendon is often considered the "innocent bystander" of the hip and tendonitis symptoms are caused by underlying pathology.
- Patients usually present with aching groin pain.
- Most commonly, the onset of pain is insidious, exacerbated by running, climbing stairs, getting in/out of bed, or rising from a seated position.
- Occasionally, it presents acutely with sharp pain; more common with tendon tears (usually after eccentric contraction) or direct trauma
- Iliopsoas bursitis is often associated with inflammatory and degenerative arthritis (1).
- After total hip arthroplasty, impingement of the iliopsoas tendon can be a cause of persistent groin pain.

DESCRIPTION

- Iliopsoas pathology usually causes anterior groin pain, but it can also be referred down the medial thigh or the ipsilateral lower back.
- It is one of four defined clinical entities of groin pain in athletes.
- Tendonitis is acute inflammation that can chronically lead to tendinosis.
- Bursitis is inflammation and pain in a bursa.
- The iliopsoas bursa (iliopectineal bursa) is the largest synovial bursa in the body and is present in >95% of adults. It averages 3 cm (width) × 6 cm (length) in size. There is often communication with the hip joint capsule (~15% of adults).
- Iliopsoas impingement is often used interchangeably with internal snapping hip, and the patient will have groin pain due to a tight iliopsoas that impinges with hip extension.
- Snapping may or may not produce pain. Extra-articular snapping hip is caused by the iliopsoas tendon rubbing over a bony prominence (anterior inferior iliac spine, iliopectineal eminence, lesser trochanter) is termed *internal* or *medial*. Extra-articular snapping from the iliotibial band and greater trochanter is termed *external* or *lateral*.
- Avulsion fractures/apophyseal separations of the lesser trochanter can occur in skeletally immature patients and are rare.

EPIDEMIOLOGY

- Reported in patients of all ages, but average age is 25 years (12 to 56 years)
- Iliopsoas disorders have been reported in one review to be the primary cause of chronic groin pain in 12–36% of athletes and in 25–30% of athletes with acute groin injury (2).
- A recent scoping review highlights the following (3):
  - 207 athletes who presented with 2 months of groin pain, iliopsoas related pain was the primary pathologic entity in 35% and a secondary pathology in 20% of athletes.
  - 110 patients with acute pain, iliopsoas pathology was the leading cause of pain, caused by kicking in soccer players and change of direction in other athletes.
  - Snapping hip syndrome often asymptomatic is more common in females than males and reported in >90% of elite ballet dancers.

ETIOLOGY AND PATHOPHYSIOLOGY

- The psoas muscle originates from the transverse processes of T12–L5 and the iliacus muscle originates from the internal aspect of the iliac fossa. They converge to form the iliopsoas muscle-tendon complex and insert distally on the lesser trochanter.
- The function is hip flexion, external rotation of the femur, and trunk stabilization.
- The muscle-tendon complex crosses over the anterior pelvic brim, hip capsule, and anterior labrum. The iliopsoas bursa lies between the tendon and the bony pelvic brim.
- Frictional compression of the bursa between these structures leads to an inflammatory reaction.

RISK FACTORS

- Rheumatoid arthritis, osteoarthritis (OA), acute trauma, overuse, mechanical factors (tightened hip flexors), total hip arthroplasty
- Sports with a high volume of running, change of direction and kicking
- Common sports associated: soccer, hockey, competitive track and field, strength training, rowing, uphill running, dancing, aerobics

COMMONLY ASSOCIATED CONDITIONS

- OA
- Rheumatoid arthritis
- Pigmented villonodular synovitis
- Synovial chondromatosis
- Infection
- Trauma
- Status post total hip arthroplasty
- Avascular necrosis of the femoral head
- Leg-length discrepancy
- Hip dysplasia
- Hip instability
- Femoroacetabular impingement (FAI)

DIAGNOSIS

- Groin pain ± snapping
- If pain is the predominant feature, it will be in the groin or anterior thigh.
- Irritation of the femoral nerve can be a cause of anterior thigh pain.
- If there is remarkable bursal swelling, a pelvic or inguinal mass may be palpated.

HISTORY

- Pain is typically achy but may be sharp and located in the groin or anterior thigh.
- Hip flexion and extension may cause pain.
- Actions with increased hip flexion angles such as squatting, putting on socks and shoes, rising after prolonged sitting, walking up stairs and inclines, running, kicking, dancing, and cycling may increase pain (3).
- The patient may complain of popping or snapping, which may or may not be painful.

PHYSICAL EXAM

- Examine the hip, low back, and sacroiliac joints.
- There is no pathognomonic sign for iliopsoas tendinopathy and none of the listed tests are specific.
- The hip may be passively held in flexion, and the stride length on the affected side may be shortened to avoid hip extension.
- Local tenderness to palpation beneath the midpoint of the inguinal ligament
- Test hip flexion strength in a seated position.
- Iliopsoas test: Pain or weakness of the iliopsoas on flexion and external rotation of the hip against resistance was 94% sensitive in dancers (4).
- Positive Thomas test (tight iliopsoas)
- Active iliopsoas snapping test: Palpate the groin while extending a flexed, abducted, external rotated hip (2).
- Hip microinstability may cause the iliopsoas to be overused. Microinstability testing is pain with hip abduction-hypertension-external rotation, prone instability, or hyperextension and external rotation (3).

DIFFERENTIAL DIAGNOSIS

- Inguinal mass present: lymphadenopathy, malignant tumor, hernia, vascular malformation, hematoma
- Pain or paresthesia present: L1 disk disease, meralgia paresthetica, hip arthritis, stress fracture of the hip, FAI, hip dysplasia, labral tear, proximal rectus femoris avulsion fracture at the anterior inferior iliac spine in an adolescent
- Acute trauma leading to muscle/tendon tear or avulsion fracture of the lesser trochanter

DIAGNOSTIC TESTS & INTERPRETATION

Initial Tests (lab, imaging)

- X-rays: weight-bearing anteroposterior (AP) views of the pelvis, cross-table lateral views of each hip; radiographs evaluate bony pathology including (FAI, developmental hip dysplasia, and OA).
- Ultrasound (US): Musculoskeletal US (MSKUS) is a noninvasive, cost-effective diagnostic modality that can demonstrate the fluid nature of an enlarged bursa (1)[A]. Dynamic US can demonstrate abnormal snapping or movement of the tendon over the anterior pelvic brim.
- Flexion, abduction, and external rotation (FABER) position increases the sonographic tendon exposure.
- MSKUS also can be used to guide aspiration/injection of the bursa (5)[A].
- Computed tomography (CT) scan: can demonstrate abnormal bony pathology causing friction at the pelvic brim or a malpositioned lesser trochanter (not often used)

- Magnetic resonance imaging (MRI) is a more sensitive and specific means of identifying lesions other than the bursa as the source of hip pain.
- MR arthrography may be required to increase the sensitivity of detecting an acetabular labral tear.

TREATMENT

- In mild cases of tendonitis/bursitis, relative rest, nonsteroidal anti-inflammatory drugs (NSAIDs), and heat or other physical therapy modalities (3)[C].
- US-guided aspiration and injection of a steroid preparation can help decrease pain.

GENERAL MEASURES

- Two basic premises: reduce pain and inflammation and rehabilitation and prevention of reinjury
- Treatment depends on the severity and nature of the underlying cause.
- Acute tendon injuries and avulsions should undergo conservative treatment unless the avulsion fragment is separated >2 cm (6)[C].

ADDITIONAL THERAPIES

- Different studies have examined physical therapy and manual treatments.
- Stretching of the hip flexors, including iliopsoas and quadriceps
- Strengthening of the same and of hip rotators (internal and external)
- Eccentric hip and core loading protocols (7)[C]
- Myofascial release of the psoas and proprioceptive neuromuscular facilitation exercises may help.
- Modification of any underlying mechanical abnormality (i.e., correcting leg length discrepancy)

SURGERY/OTHER PROCEDURES

- Injections of local anesthetic with or without corticosteroid can help manage iliopsoas related pain.
- A systematic review, in which 5/6 studies targeted the iliopsoas bursa, showed injections significantly decreased pain and improved the Harris Hip Score, with only 28.9% progressing to surgery (5)[A].
- US injections for patients with iliopsoas tendinopathy after total hip arthroplasty are also successful, with a recent study showing 79% resolution of groin pain. However, 5 of 20 (25%) patients with malposition of the acetabular component ultimately required revision surgery (8)[B].
- Surgery should only be considered for refractory cases unresponsive to 3 to 6+ months of conservative treatment.
- Iliopsoas tendinopathy is often secondary to other underlying hip pathology (i.e., FAI, hip dysplasia/microinstability, increased femoral version) and these conditions should be specifically evaluated in patients with psoas symptoms (3)[C].
- In the absence of other contributing hip pathology, partial release/fractional lengthening can be considered (after an appropriate trial of nonoperative management), but outcomes from the procedure are varied and may have consequences such as residual atrophy (25% volume loss) and weakness (19% reduction in seated hip flexion strength) (9)[B].
- Complete tenotomy is no longer favored in the literature, with the exception of patients with psoas impingement associated with the acetabular component of a total hip arthroplasty (10)[A].

ONGOING CARE

PATIENT EDUCATION

- A home-based exercise program led to pain improvement in 77% of individuals (11)[B].
- The program included:
  - Daily stretching targeting the hip flexor, quadriceps, and lateral hip/piriformis and hamstrings
  - Hip internal and external exercises performed in a seated position with an elastic resistance strap
  - Progression included decreasing hip flexion and then adding side-lying abduction and external rotation with the hip at 45 degrees of flexion.
  - One-legged mini squat on the affected side was the final step.

PROGNOSIS

Good prognosis with reduction of inflammation, appropriate rehabilitation, and proper attention to alteration of mechanical issues

REFERENCES

1. Jonczy ML, Büchler L, Mahenthiran Y, et al. Epidemiology, clinical manifestation, diagnosis, and treatment of bursitis iliopectineal: a systematic review. *SAGE Open Med.* 2025;13:20503121251317899.
2. Anderson CN. Iliopsoas: pathology, diagnosis, and treatment. *Clin Sports Med.* 2016;35(3):419–433.
3. Tramer JS, Holmich P, Safran MR. The iliopsoas: anatomy, clinical evaluation, and its role in hip pain in the athlete: a scoping review. *J Am Acad Orthop Surg.* 2024;32(13):e620–e630.
4. Andronic O, Nakano N, Daivajna S, et al. Non-arthroplasty iliopsoas impingement in athletes: a narrative literature review. *Hip Int.* 2019;29(5):460–467.
5. Katz L, Feinberg G, Kent V, et al. Iliopsoas injections: a systematic review of patient outcomes and progression to surgery. *JBJS Rev.* 2025;13(1).
6. Homma Y, Baba T, Ishii S, et al. Avulsion fracture of the lesser trochanter in a skeletally immature freestyle footballer. *J Pediatr Orthop B.* 2015;24(4):304–307.
7. Rauseo C. The rehabilitation of a runner with iliopsoas tendinopathy using an eccentric-biased exercise—a case report. *Int J Sports Phys Ther.* 2017;12(7):1150–1162.
8. Weintraub MT, Barrack TN, Burnett RA III, et al. Ultrasound-guided iliopsoas bursal injections for management of iliopsoas bursitis after total hip arthroplasty. *J Arthroplasty.* 2023;38(7 Suppl 2):S426–S430.
9. Brandenburg JB, Kapron AL, Wylie JD, et al. The functional and structural outcomes of arthroscopic iliopsoas release. *Am J Sports Med.* 2016;44(5):1286–1291.
10. Giai Via R, Giachino M, Elzeiny A, et al. Arthroscopic and endoscopic techniques for iliopsoas release in THA are safe and effective: a systematic review of the literature. *Eur J Orthop Surg Traumatol.* 2024;34(6):2845–2857.
11. Johnston CA, Lindsay DM, Wiley JP. Treatment of iliopsoas syndrome with a hip rotation strengthening program: a retrospective case series. *J Orthop Sports Phys Ther.* 1999;29(4):218–224.

ADDITIONAL READING

- Chopra A, Robinson P. Imaging athletic groin pain. *Radiol Clin North Am.* 2016;54(5):865–873.
- Smith J, Brennan P, Klug K, et al. Clinical efficacy of ultrasound-guided iliopsoas corticosteroid injection for hip pain. *Kans J Med.* 2024;17(6):146–149
- Weir A, Brukner P, Delahunt E, et al. Doha agreement meeting on terminology and definitions in groin pain in athletes. *Br J Sports Med.* 2015;49(12):768–774.
- Zimmerer A, Hauschild M, Nietschke R, et al. Results after arthroscopic treatment of iliopsoas impingement after total hip arthroplasty. *Arch Orthop Trauma Surg.* 2022;142(2):189–195.

CLINICAL PEARLS

- The iliopsoas is the most powerful hip flexor.
- The iliopsoas bursa is the largest synovial bursa in the body and is present in >95% of adults and in 15% of people, it communicates with the hip joint.
- Pain involving the iliopsoas can come from tendon overuse or injury, or inflammation of the bursa from activity or intra-articular pathology.
- Diagnostic US or MRI are the best means of imaging.
- Aspiration and/or injection of inflamed bursa can be successfully performed with US guidance.
- Rehabilitation focuses on improving flexibility and strengthening.
- Surgery should only be considered in refractory cases.

ILIOTIBIAL BAND FRICTION SYNDROME

Peter Clements, MD ▪ Alexandra Tee, MD, CAQSM

BASICS

DESCRIPTION

- Iliotibial band friction syndrome (ITBS or ITBFS) is an overuse tendinopathy that occurs from compression of the iliotibial band (ITB) against the lateral femoral epicondyle.
- Pain is especially sharp after foot strike in the gait cycle, usually at ~30 degrees of knee flexion
- Synonym(s): ITB tendinopathy

EPIDEMIOLOGY

- Incidence as high as 12% of all running-related overuse injuries
- Second to patellofemoral syndrome as the most common running injury
- Also a common overuse injury in cyclists

ETIOLOGY AND PATHOPHYSIOLOGY

- The ITB is composed of dense fibrous connective tissue that originates off the iliac crest. Its course runs inferiorly, passing over the lateral femoral epicondyle prior to insertion distally on the tibia at Gerdy tubercle.
- The ITB is compressed against the lateral femoral epicondyle with knee flexion, with the greatest compression at 30 degrees of knee flexion.
- Etiology is unclear, but it appears that the repetitive compression leads to inflammation of the band as well as inflammation of the connective tissue and fat pad between the band and the epicondyle (1).

RISK FACTORS

- Training factors: higher weekly mileage, downhill running, rapid increase in mileage, disproportionate running on a track in the same direction
- Increased peak hip adduction (possibly owing to significant weakness of the hip abductors of one limb as compared with the other), genu varum, and increased knee internal rotation during stance phase, with running (2),(3)

DIAGNOSIS

HISTORY

- Lateral knee sharp pain or burning
- Pain is not present when the patient starts exercising but begins at a predictable time or distance within the workout.
- Symptoms that subside shortly after the workout but return with the next workout
- Pain worse with downhill running, stride lengthening, or sitting for long periods of time with a flexed knee
- Involvement in distance running or sport that requires continuous running (i.e., soccer) or repeated knee flexion/extension (i.e., cycling, Nordic skiing)

PHYSICAL EXAM

- Lateral knee pain made worse with running (4)[C]
- Pain with ascending and descending stairs
- Stiff-legged walking in advanced cases
- Extensive musculoskeletal exam with particular attention to the lower extremities: With a patient with ITBS, the clinician may notice local tenderness and swelling as well as crepitation, snapping, or pitting edema over the distal ITB where it passes over the lateral femoral epicondyle, and there may be pain or paresthesia along the length of the band (4)[C].
- Perform Ober test: Position the patient on the unaffected side with the involved knee in 90 degrees of flexion. The leg is abducted at the hip, and the examiner then grasps the ankle and extends leg, allowing the knee to return to an adducted position. A person with ITB tightness will remain abducted (5).
- Perform Noble compression test: With the patient on his or her side with the affected knee up and flexed at 90 degrees, apply pressure on the ITB at the lateral femoral epicondyle and extend the knee. A positive test occurs when pain occurs as the knee approaches 30 degrees of flexion (5).
- Evaluate for excessive ankle pronation and causes of it, including evaluation for tight gastrocnemius or soleus muscles, pes planus, or femoral or tibial torsion. Excessive ankle pronation increases knee flexion.
- Evaluate for muscle imbalances, especially hip and core musculature.
- Exclude lumbar spine and intra-articular hip pathology.
- Feet and footwear should be evaluated closely. Footwear can give clues to the pronation pattern.
- Evaluate iliac crests and leg length. Discrepancies of leg length can cause tightening of the ITB.

DIFFERENTIAL DIAGNOSIS

- Patellofemoral syndrome
- Degenerative joint disease
- Lateral meniscal damage or pathology
- Lateral collateral ligament sprain
- Lateral synovial plica syndrome
- Distal femoral bone stress injury
- Superior tibiofibular joint sprain
- Popliteal or biceps femoris tendinopathy
- Peroneal nerve injury
- Gout and other metabolic arthropathy
- Referred pain

DIAGNOSTIC TESTS & INTERPRETATION

- Generally not needed except to rule out other disease processes
- Consider a standing anteroposterior (AP) view of pelvis (in adult) to assess leg length discrepancy if clinically indicated.
- Ultrasound is typically reserved for recurrent or refractory cases. In ITBFS, it may show soft-tissue edema and discrete fluid collection between the ITB and the lateral femoral epicondyle. Cortical irregularity of the adjacent femoral epicondyle can also be observed (3).

TREATMENT

GENERAL MEASURES

- Initially, patient should rest and avoid offending activities, such as running and cycling (4),(6)[C].
- Control inflammation and pain with ice and nonsteroidal anti-inflammatory drugs (NSAIDs) (4),(5)[C].
- Physical therapy should focus on hip and core strengthening, progressive loading, and stretching. Foam rolling is a controversial treatment strategy but may be beneficial (6).
- Gait training should focus on increasing gait width, reducing hip adduction changing from heel strike to forefoot landing, and avoiding excess pronation (5),(6).
- Relative rest is important, but no forms of immobilization are used.
- It is important to acknowledge that there remains a lack of consensus in the scientific literature in terms of best treatment strategies for ITBFS.

ADDITIONAL THERAPIES

- Corticosteroid injections have been shown to be more effective than placebo in controlling pain related to ITBS. They may be performed under ultrasound guidance for improved target accuracy (3),(5)[B]. However, cases of ITB rupture after steroid injection have been documented.
- There is currently no conclusive data regarding the effectiveness of platelet-rich plasma (PRP), prolotherapy, or stem cell therapy in treating this condition.

SURGERY/OTHER PROCEDURES

- Only after exhaustive nonoperative therapy
- Techniques include ITB release, open partial excision, or lengthening. Bursectomy and synovial recess excision have also been reported (5).

ONGOING CARE

FOLLOW-UP RECOMMENDATIONS

If no improvement is seen after extensive therapy and training modification, then referral to an orthopedic surgeon is warranted.

REFERENCES

1. Díaz FJ, Gitto S, Sconfienza LM, et al. Ultrasound of iliotibial band syndrome. *J Ultrasound*. 2020;23(3):379–385.
2. Barton CJ, Bonanno DR, Carr J, et al. Running retraining to treat lower limb injuries: a mixed-methods study of current evidence synthesized with expert opinion. *Br J Sports Med*. 2016;50(9):513–526.
3. Fredericson M, Wolf C. Iliotibial band syndrome in runners: innovations in treatment. *Sports Med*. 2005;35(5):451–459.
4. Strauss EJ, Kim S, Calcei JG, et al. Iliotibial band syndrome: evaluation and management. *J Am Acad Orthop Surg*. 2011;19(12):728–736.
5. Fairclough J, Hayashi K, Toumi H, et al. The functional anatomy of the iliotibial band during flexion and extension of the knee: implications for understanding iliotibial band syndrome. *J Anat*. 2006;208(3):309–316.
6. Noehren B, Davis I, Hamill J. ASB clinical biomechanics award winner 2006 prospective study of the biomechanical factors associated with iliotibial band syndrome. *Clin Biomech (Bristol)*. 2007;22(9):951–956.

CLINICAL PEARLS

- An attempt to return too early with pain can result in significant delay. Activity can be resumed when symptoms have improved nearly 100% or have resolved.
- Earlier return can be accomplished using non–weight-bearing activities such as swimming or running in the deep end of a pool. Return should be gradual with gentle buildup on level ground progressing in distance/resistance and elevation.
- Most patients recover in about 6 weeks and are able to resume full activity at that time.
- To prevent ITBFS, avoid rapid increases in training volume and maintain flexibility with adequate warm-up periods and stretching before and after exercise.

I

IMPETIGO

Arturo J. Aguilar, MD, FAAFP, CAQSM

BASICS

DESCRIPTION

- Superficial skin infection of the epidermis with *Staphylococcus aureus*, group A β-hemolytic *Streptococcus* (GAS), a combination of *Staphylococcus* and *Streptococcus*, or methicillin-resistant *S. aureus* (MRSA). Impetigo is classically characterized as well-defined erythematous papules and pustules with honey-colored crust located on the face, neck, and hands (1),(2).
- Divided into bullous and nonbullous types (1)
  - Bullous (1),(3):
    - Caused by exfoliative toxins from *S. aureus*
    - Favors intertriginous areas
    - Starts as a vesicular eruption that develops into bullae and then may rupture to form honey crusts
  - Nonbullous (70% of cases) (1),(3):
    - Caused by *S. aureus* and GAS
    - Starts as macules or pustules and progresses to vesicular eruption, which rupture to form erosions with honey crusts.
- Divided into primary and secondary infection (3)
  - Primary infection is direct bacterial invasion of intact skin (3).
  - Secondary infection is an infection of an area of compromised skin barrier such as an abrasion, insect bites, scabies, or eczema (3).
- Impetiginous (or common) impetigo is a nonbullous subtype that is a complication of systemic diseases such as diabetes mellitus or HIV. It may also develop as a secondary infection of a cut, scrape, or insect bite (4),(5).
- May be transmitted person to person or person to athletic equipment by direct contact (4),(5)
- Can also be spread by autoinoculation from skin excoriations in contact with other parts of the body (4),(5)
- Synonym: scrum strep (4)

EPIDEMIOLOGY

- Most common bacterial skin infection in children (3)
- Most common in areas of skin-to-skin contact between athletes (4),(5)
- Most common on face, neck, and hands (1)
- Incidence is greatest in the summer months (4).

ETIOLOGY AND PATHOPHYSIOLOGY

- Bullous (1),(3):
  - Epidermolytic toxin from *S. aureus*
- Nonbullous (1),(3):
  - *S. aureus* and/or GAS

RISK FACTORS

- Abrasions or open cuts allow passage of bacteria through the epidermis (3),(4).
- Sweat-soaked and water-soaked clothes allow easy passage of bacteria through the first protective layer of the epidermis (stratum corneum) (4).
- Poor hygiene (4)

GENERAL PREVENTION

Techniques (4),(5):

- Avoid sharing equipment, towels, tape, and ointments.
- Avoid dispensing ointments from common containers.
- Clean equipment and clothes daily.
- Shower immediately after sports activity with antibacterial soap.
- Avoid communal hot tubs.
- Wear moisture-wicking, synthetic clothing.
- Discourage body shaving in contact sports.
- Frequent skin checks by athletic trainers and athletes in contact sports
- Frequent handwashing by athletic trainers and affected athletes
- Cover any injured skin immediately.

DIAGNOSIS

HISTORY

- Mild itching and soreness (4)
- May be an infection of a minor previous skin injury or occur on unimpaired skin (3),(4)
- Bullous (1),(3),(6):
  - Starts with superficial vesicles, which progress to flaccid bullae without surrounding erythema
  - When the bullae rupture, they ooze and create honey-colored crusts.
  - Self-limited and may spontaneously resolve in 7 days if left untreated
- Nonbullous (more contagious) (1),(3),(6):
  - Starts as a single macule or papule that develops into a vesicle
  - Vesicle may rupture and form an erosion and the contents become honey-colored crusts that are often pruritic.
  - May spontaneously resolve without scarring if left untreated for 7 days

PHYSICAL EXAM

Findings (1),(2),(3):

- Clear vesicles in the early stages
- Some may progress to pustules and/or bullae.
- When vesicles or pustules/bullae break, they will have a honey-colored crust with erythematous papules or erosions.
- Lesions may range from millimeters up to several centimeters in diameter.
- Mainly located on face and upper extremities
- Regional lymphadenopathy
- Diagnosis is based on history and clinical appearance (1).
- Cultures can be done if history or epidemic of MRSA.

DIFFERENTIAL DIAGNOSIS
- Acne vulgaris
- Folliculitis
- Poison ivy
- Atopic dermatitis (2)
- Herpes gladiatorum
- Tinea corporis gladiatorum

DIAGNOSTIC TESTS & INTERPRETATION
Wound culture to confirm or rule out MRSA if recent epidemic on the athletic team (4)

TREATMENT
Methods (4)[C]:
- Crusts should be gently washed away with soap and water to remove honey-colored crusts and improve antibiotic penetration.

MEDICATION
First Line
- Mild (2),(3),(4)[A]:
  - Topical 2% mupirocin 2 times a day for 5 days
  - Topical 1% ozenoxacin cream 2 times a day for 5 days
  - Topical fusidic acid (not available in the United States)
  - Topical 1% retapamulin 2 times a day for 5 days
- Moderate or widespread (adult dosing) (3),(4)[A]:
  - Topical therapy in combination with oral antibiotic coverage or oral antibiotics, alone
  - Cephalexin 250 to 500 mg 3 to 4 times a day for 7 days
  - Dicloxacillin 250 to 500 mg 3 to 4 times a day for 7 days
- Penicillin-allergic oral therapy (3),(5)[B]:
  - Clindamycin
  - MRSA-suspected lesions or areas of high prevalence of MRSA should be treated with doxycycline or clindamycin orally for at least 7 days (4)[B].
  - Topical 1% ozenoxacin cream for 7 days (1)[A]

ADDITIONAL THERAPIES
- Clean clothes in bleach and water at a temperature of at least 71°C (4)[C].
- Clean equipment with diluted bleach solution (4)[B].

ONGOING CARE
Return-to-play guidelines (5)[C]:
- College:
  - National Collegiate Athletic Association wrestling rules for competition:
    - Oral antibiotics for at least 72 hours prior to competition
    - No new lesions for 48 hours before a meet or tournament
    - No moist, exudative, or purulent lesions at the meet or tournament time
    - Active purulent lesions shall not be covered to allow participation.
    - Noninfectious lesions may be covered with a nonpermeable dressing that will not dislodge.
- High school:
  - Each state's high school association has varying guidelines for competition.

PATIENT EDUCATION
Educate athletes and athletic staff regarding the importance of good hygiene (5).

PROGNOSIS
Up to 74% of cases may heal in 7 days, if left untreated (6).

COMPLICATIONS
Secondary (1),(4):
- Poststreptococcal glomerulonephritis up to 3 weeks after skin infection:
  - Occurs in 20% of nonbullous-type impetigo
  - Risk not decreased with antibiotic treatment
- Hyperpigmented area after healed lesions mostly in dark-skinned athletes
- Cellulitis
- Lymphangitis
- Guttate psoriasis
- Toxic shock syndrome
- Staphylococcal scalded skin syndrome
- Sepsis
- Osteomyelitis
- Pneumonia

REFERENCES

1. Abrha S, Tesfaye W, Thomas J. Intolerable burden of impetigo in endemic settings: a review of the current state of play and future directions for alternative treatments. *Antibiotics (Basel)*. 2020;9(12):909.
2. Rosen T, Albareda N, Rosenberg N, et al. Efficacy and safety of ozenoxacin cream for treatment of adult and pediatric patients with impetigo: a randomized clinical trial. *JAMA Dermatol*. 2018;154(7):806–813.
3. Gahlawat G, Tesfaye W, Bushell M, et al. Emerging treatment strategies for impetigo in endemic and nonendemic settings: a systematic review. *Clin Ther*. 2021;43(6):986–1006.
4. Adams BB, ed. Bacterial skin infections. In: *Sports Dermatology*. New York, NY: Springer; 2006:3–8.
5. National Collegiate Athletic Association. *Sports Medicine Handbook*. National Collegiate Athletic Association; 2025. Accessed October 3, 2025. https://ncaaorg.s3.amazonaws.com/ssi/publications/SSI_SMHB.pdf
6. Hoffmann TC, Peiris R, Glasziou P, et al. Natural history of non-bullous impetigo: a systematic review of time to resolution or improvement without antibiotic treatment. *Br J Gen Pract*. 2021;71(704):e237–e242.

CLINICAL PEARLS
- Impetigo is a superficial skin infection caused by *Staphylococcus* or *Streptococcus*.
- Signs include vesicles, with or without bullae, erythematous papules, and honey-colored crusts.
- Treat mild or localized infection with 1% ozenoxacin cream, mupirocin 2% cream, retapamulin 1% cream, or fusidic acid.
- Treat moderate or widespread infection with topical treatment plus oral antibiotics such as dicloxacillin or cephalexin.
- Treat MRSA-positive infection with oral doxycycline, oral clindamycin, or topical ozenoxacin.
  - NCAA wrestling guidelines require 72 hours of oral treatment and no new lesions for 48 hours before competition.

IMPINGEMENT, SUBACROMIAL BURSITIS AND ROTATOR CUFF TENDINOSIS

Jeswin Jacob, DO ▪ Mark E. Lavallee, MD, CSCS, FACSM, FAMSSM

BASICS

DESCRIPTION

- Pathologic mechanism is a spectrum of clinical findings; structural narrowing in the subacromial space and irritation of the tendons of the rotator cuff muscles
- Repetitive shoulder activity causes breakdown in the rotator cuff muscles from tensile overload and failed healing response which results in tendinopathy.
- Weakness in the rotator cuff muscles (supraspinatus, infraspinatus, teres minor, or subscapularis) results in loss of effective dynamic glenohumeral movement.
- This causes impingement of the cuff muscles under the acromion, enhancing the pain and inflammation.
- Synonym(s): subacromial bursitis; shoulder impingement syndrome

EPIDEMIOLOGY

- One of the most common causes of shoulder pain
- Very common in athletes, especially in those with repetitive motion of the arms (i.e., throwing, racquet sports, swimming, weight lifting)
- In individuals <25 years of age, impingement is usually related to laxity caused by instability.
- In those 25 to 40 years of age, impingement is usually due to overuse of the rotator cuff.
- In those >40 years of age, impingement is caused by use of the cuff muscles over threshold. This may result in partial- or full-thickness tears in addition to impingement.

RISK FACTORS

- Repetitive shoulder activity at or above the shoulders
- Weight lifting (Olympic style) and high intensity interval training (HIIT)
- Throwing sports, racquet sports, swimming, volleyball
- "Industrial" athletics (repetitive, overhead motion)
- Shoulder instability or scapular dyskinesis
- Previous shoulder surgery or trauma (to ipsilateral or contralateral shoulder)
- Individuals with more "hooked" acromial morphology (type III > type II > type I)
- Smoking
- Diabetes

COMMONLY ASSOCIATED CONDITIONS

- Rotator cuff tear (partial or full)
- Adhesive capsulitis
- Thoracic outlet syndrome
- Brachial plexus injury
- Axillary nerve entrapment
- Pancoast tumor
- Suprascapular nerve palsy

DIAGNOSIS

HISTORY

- Rule out cervical spine disease, neck pain.
- Symptoms: weakness, crepitation, numbness, "slipped out," night pain, dead arm
- Exacerbation: Pain presents more at rest or with activity.
- Duration: chronic (overuse) versus acute (traumatic)
- Activation: right or left handed, type of job, sports, hobby
- History of previous trauma or surgery

PHYSICAL EXAM

- Shoulder pain with overhead activity
- Weakness in the shoulder musculature
- Crepitus
- Numbness/paresthesias (usually between the lateral neck to the elbow)
- Night pain
- Pain at rest (usually in more severe cases)
- Medial upper scapular border or medial upper trapezius pain
- Observation:
  - How the athlete carries arm/shoulder (e.g., recent dislocation, guarding, obvious asymmetry)
  - Deltoid atrophy (i.e., C5 plexus injury)
  - Scapular winging (i.e., long thoracic nerve palsy, cranial nerve XI palsy)
  - Infraspinatus fossa scalloping (inferior branch of the suprascapular nerve)
- Palpation:
  - Cervical spinous process: Rule out cervical neck pathology as cause of shoulder pain.
  - Subacromial bursa: distal to acromion
  - Biceps tendon (long head)/bicipital groove
  - Insertion of the deltoid on the humerus: pain at site but no pain with palpation; axillary nerve pain referral site
  - Coracoid process: pain referral site for impingement
- Range of motion (ROM):
  - Abduction (0 to 180 degrees)
  - Adduction (0 to 50 degrees)
  - Flexion: forward (0 to 180 degrees) and horizontal (0 to 130 degrees)
  - Extension (0 to 90 degrees)
  - Internal rotation (0 to 100 degrees) (adduction and internal rotation: "bra strap")
  - External rotation (0 to 60 degrees) (abduction and external rotation: "shampoo hair")
- Manual muscle testing:
  - Deltoid: full abduction, resist at 90 degrees
  - Supraspinatus: abduction to 90 degrees forward flexion to 30 degrees, resist downward pressure (empty can/Jobe test)
  - Infraspinatus and teres minor: arm at side, 90 degrees at elbow, resist external rotation (i.e., "opening the door")
  - Subscapularis: hand on lower back, push against resistance; Gerber lift-off test or hand on belly and out against resistance; belly-press test
- Special tests:
  - Hawkins test: 90 degrees of forward flexion at the shoulder and elbow, support elbow, pain with internal rotation of arm
  - Arc test: Shoulder abduction gets "stuck" or painful at 60 to 120 degrees.
  - Infraspinatus test: 90 degrees of flexion at the elbow; elbow held against body while patient attempts to externally rotate arm against examiner's resistance, pain in shoulder with external rotation
  - Neer test: arm straight, thumb down, passive forward flexion (pain at 60 to 120 degrees)
  - Impingement test: Inject subacromial bursa with lidocaine; helps to differentiate between impingement and cuff tear or joint pathology; after injection, pain, ROM, and strength should improve if impingement and not a tear or joint pathology.
  - Drop arm test: Patient cannot hold arm at 90 degrees of abduction; indicates cuff tear
  - Speed test: arm straight, forward flexion to 90 degrees, palm up, resisted downward pressure; palpate the bicipital tendon at groove; pain indicates bicipital tendonitis.

DIFFERENTIAL DIAGNOSIS

- Rotator cuff tear (partial or full thickness)
- Adhesive capsulitis
- Acromioclavicular sprain/injury
- Labral tear
- Bicipital tendonitis
- Thoracic outlet syndrome
- Brachial plexus injury
- Fracture: clavicle, humerus, scapula
- Subluxation of the glenohumeral joint
- Axillary nerve entrapment
- Pancoast tumor
- Bankart lesion (avulsion fracture of glenoid labrum)
- Hill-Sachs lesion (impact fracture of humeral head)
- Septic arthritis
- Glenohumeral arthritis
- Thrombosis of subclavian or brachial artery

DIAGNOSTIC TESTS & INTERPRETATION

- Imaging is often not needed in light of a good history, physical exam, and a straightforward case.
- Radiography (1),(2):
  - Anteroposterior (AP) view and axillary (transscapular) views bare minimum to order; radiographs helpful for acute injuries to rule out fractures, dislocations; with impingement, may be helpful to get additional views
  - Internal and external AP rotational views help to visualize humerus (i.e., Hill-Sachs lesions).
  - Stryker notch view helps to visualize posterolateral humeral head deformity (i.e., Hill-Sachs lesions).
  - West Point (modified axillary) view allows visualization of the anterior/inferior glenoid (i.e., Bankart lesions).
  - Outlet or Alexander view allows for visualization of subacromial space; helpful in elderly patients with severe impingement
  - Calcification on the tendon is associated with bicipital tendonitis or severe impingement.
- Ultrasound (US):
  - Dependent on skill and comfort of practitioner, can be cost-effective in-office imaging choice for static and dynamic view of soft tissue structures of the shoulder (i.e., rotator cuff muscles, biceps tendons, subacromial bursa, calcification in tendons)
  - Also, can be used to guide injections into biceps tendon sheath, subacromial bursa, or glenohumeral joint
- Magnetic resonance imaging (MRI):
  - In severe or confusing cases, MRI is helpful in the diagnosis of rotator cuff tears, labrum tears, biceps tendon rupture as well as assessing volume and capsule thickening in adhesive capsulitis (1).
  - An MRI arthrogram is often useful to further evaluate for a torn labrum, thus improving visualization of the anatomy.
- Electromyography/nerve conduction study: helpful if there is weakness in addition to an altered neurologic exam (sensation, reflexes); has the highest sensitivity when symptoms have persisted >3 weeks

TREATMENT

MEDICATION

- Oral analgesia: nonsteroidal anti-inflammatory drugs (NSAIDs), acetaminophen, tramadol; in severe cases, short-term pain relief with narcotics
- Dermal: topical cream or transdermal patches (NSAID or lidocaine based)
- Injectable: subacromial bursa injection (5 to 10 mL 2:2:1 mixture of lidocaine/bupivacaine, corticosteroid; use a 22- to 25-gauge, 1.5-inch long needle)
  - US-guided injection of corticosteroids shown to be superior versus anatomic landmark-guided injection in improving the clinical symptoms of subacromial impingement syndrome (3)

ADDITIONAL THERAPIES

- Management of acute phase (4):
  - Relative rest: Decrease the use of the affected shoulder with overhead activities.
  - Home exercise program (HEP): exercise done daily, three sets per exercise
  - ROM: dangling arm circles, finger wall-walking, broom-handle exercises
  - Strengthening: sword-from-sheath exercises, posterior dumbbell raises, proprioceptive neuromuscular facilitation (PNF), augmented soft tissue mobilization (ASTM), scapular stabilizing exercises using light weights or flexible elastic cords
- Rehabilitation for long-term treatment:
  - Formal physical therapy: pain relief via contrast baths, hydrocollator, ice, mobilization/manipulation, modalities (e.g., electrostimulation, US therapy)
  - ROM strengthening: deltoid, rotator cuff musculature, scapular stabilizers, biceps
  - ROM flexibility: biceps, triceps, glenohumeral joint
  - Transmembrane corticosteroid (i.e., phonophoresis, iontophoresis)
  - Return to normal function.
  - Sports-specific retraining
- In the younger athlete, impingement is often due to another underlying problem (i.e., instability, scapular dyskinesis, muscular imbalance).
- Certain athletes (i.e., mentally challenged, unmotivated, etc.) may need assistance with formal physical therapy without a trial of HEP.

SURGERY/OTHER PROCEDURES

- Anterior acromioplasty (shoulder decompression): The acromion is "shaved" to allow more space for the rotator cuff. It is used only if conservative measures fail. There is a less favorable outcome in younger (50% success rate) than older athletes.
- Surgical débridement/repair of rotator cuff: often accompanies an anterior acromioplasty
- Surgical débridement/repair of labrum

COMPLEMENTARY & ALTERNATIVE MEDICINE

- Mentioned in literature for recalcitrant cases: prolotherapy, platelet-rich plasma (PRP) injections, acupuncture, dry needling, autologous stem cell therapy, and topical nitrates
- Tenex (percutaneous ultrasonic tenotomy) or TenJet (hydrostatic tenotomy) are minimally invasive options that can treat tendinopathic rotator cuff and are now becoming popular in failed conservative cases (5).

ONGOING CARE

FOLLOW-UP RECOMMENDATIONS

- Presence of a fever and a tense joint capsule (i.e., a potentially septic joint, orthopedic surgical emergency)
- Severe disease that is refractory to physical therapy, modalities, and steroid injections
- Rotator cuff tear, full or partial thickness, unresponsive to conservative care
- Cervical rib, causing shoulder symptoms
- Superior labrum anterior and posterior (SLAP)
- Gross instability of shoulder not improved with physical therapy

REFERENCES

1. Pesquer L, Borghol S, Meyer P, et al. Multimodality imaging of subacromial impingement syndrome. *Skeletal Radiol.* 2018;47(7):923–937.
2. Spicer PJ, Fain AD, Soliman SB. Ultrasound in sports medicine. *Radiol Clin North Am.* 2019;57(3):649–656.
3. Deng X, Zhu S, Li D, et al. Effectiveness of ultrasound-guided versus anatomic landmark-guided corticosteroid injection on pain, physical function, and safety in patients with subacromial impingement syndrome: a systematic review and meta-analysis. *Am J Phys Med Rehabil.* 2022;101(12):1087–1098.
4. Steuri R, Sattelmayer M, Elsig S, et al. Effectiveness of conservative interventions including exercise, manual therapy, and medical management in adults with shoulder impingement: a systematic review and meta-analysis of RCTs. *Br J Sports Med.* 2017;51(18):1340–1347.
5. Vajapey S, Ghenbot S, Baria MR, et al. Utility of percutaneous ultrasonic tenotomy for tendinopathies: a systematic review. *Sports Health.* 2021;13(3):258–264.

ADDITIONAL READING

- Bolia IK, Collon K, Bogdanov J, et al. Management options for shoulder impingement syndrome in athletes: insights and future directions. *Open Access J Sports Med.* 2021;12:43–53.
- Monica J, Vredenburgh Z, Korsh J, et al. Acute shoulder injuries in adults. *Am Fam Physician.* 2016;94(2):119–127.

I

CLINICAL PEARLS

- If caught early with no other shoulder pathology and treated with aggressive conservative therapy, many athletes are able to return to their prior level of competition.
- With subacromial injections, often pain relief is immediate, due to the analgesia (i.e., lidocaine/bupivacaine). This will wear off. Corticosteroid injections may have a delay in onset.
- If no other shoulder pathology is present, and the injury is treated with aggressive conservative therapy, most athletes respond well and are able to avoid surgery.

INGROWN TOENAIL

Nicole L. Leonard, MD ▪ Daniel C. Herman, MD, PhD, FAAPMR, FACSM, FISBS, CAQSM ▪ Kevin J. Burnham, MD, CAQSM

BASICS

DESCRIPTION

- Onychocryptosis is commonly called ingrown toenail and most commonly affects the great toe.
- Occurs when nail plate grows into the periungual skin of the lateral nail fold, resulting in inflammation and possible infection (1)[C]
- Three stages (2)[C]:
  - Stage 1 (mild): erythema, slight edema, and pain when pressure is applied to the lateral nail groove
  - Stage 2 (moderate): increased stage 1 symptoms coupled with infection
  - Stage 3 (severe): worsening stage 1 symptoms, chronic inflammation with granulation tissue formation and nail fold hypertrophy
- Can be chronic and cyclical; recurrence is not uncommon.
- Synonym(s): *unguis incarnatus*; in-fleshed toenail; embedded toenail

EPIDEMIOLOGY

- Prevalence ranging from 2.5% to 5% (2)[C]
- Bimodal peak; adolescents and young adults and then in the elderly (2)[C],(3)[B]
- Gender predominance is uncertain, possibly women > men (3)[B].
- Most commonly affects the great toe at the distal-lateral margin (2)[C]

ETIOLOGY AND PATHOPHYSIOLOGY

- Most often multifactorial (2)[C]
- Improper nail trimming performance is a recognized risk factor, leading to nail spicules to anchor into periungual tissue and penetrate as the nail grows (2)[C].
- Inflammatory reaction can lead to granuloma and permanent hypertrophy of the nail fold.

RISK FACTORS

- Shoes with tight-fitting toe box
- Improper nail-trimming techniques (including tearing of nails)
- Nail plate shape abnormalities
- Onychomycosis
- Diabetes
- Hyperhidrosis
- Obesity
- Subungual neoplasms
- Peripheral edema
- Repetitive minor trauma
- Family history of incurvated nails
- Congenital or acquired foot deformities
- Medications (indinavir, ritonavir, retinoids, docetaxel, cyclosporine, oral antifungals, gefitinib, cetuximab)

GENERAL PREVENTION

- Proper foot hygiene
- Avoidance of shoes with a tight-fitting toe box
- Properly trimming nails (cutting the nail straight across)
- Avoidance of repetitive trauma

COMMONLY ASSOCIATED CONDITIONS

- Paronychia
- Cellulitis
- Osteomyelitis

DIAGNOSIS

HISTORY

- Initial presentation mostly characterized by signs of inflammation and/or acute infection, including erythema, edema, pain, drainage
- Ask about chronology, risk factors (i.e., tight-fitting shoes, prior trauma, activities).
- Assess pain at rest, standing, and ambulating.
- Ask about recurrence and previous treatment: may affect treatment choice.
- History of immune deficiency or abnormal wound healing: increased chance for severe infection and possibly requires the use of antibiotics

PHYSICAL EXAM

- Signs and symptoms:
  - Pain, swelling, and limitation of activities
  - Cardinal signs of inflammation (redness, warmth, and drainage)
  - Incurvated nail margin
- Physical examination:
  - Tenderness, erythema, edema, drainage
  - Inspect for foreign bodies.
  - Cardinal signs of ascending infection (redness traveling up the foot); this is more common in individuals with poor circulation or diabetes.
  - Presence of excess medial or lateral nail fold

DIFFERENTIAL DIAGNOSIS

- Osteomyelitis
- Cellulitis
- Paronychia
- Felon
- Foreign body
- Pyogenic granuloma
- Herpetic whitlow
- Subungual exostosis
- Tumor

DIAGNOSTIC TESTS & INTERPRETATION

- Labs and imaging usually not necessary (4)[C]
- Consider tissue cultures, complete blood count (CBC), erythrocyte sedimentation rate (ESR), C-reactive protein (CRP) ± blood cultures if there is concern for a more severe infection (e.g., osteomyelitis).
- Radiographs, magnetic resonance imaging (MRI) with contrast, and/or bone scan may be required for a severely infected toe if osteomyelitis or subungual exostosis are suspected.

TREATMENT

- Indications for treatment: significant pain or infection, nail deformity, chronic or recurrent paronychia (1)[C]
- General measures should also include management of underlying factors.
- Conservative measures versus surgical intervention depends mainly on the stage.

CONSERVATIVE THERAPY

Recommended in mild to moderate lesions or stage 1 and stage 2 (1)[C],(2)[C],(4)[C],(5)[A]

- Soak affected toe in warm, soapy water followed by high-potency topical corticosteroid ointment for 2 weeks.
- Cotton-wick insertion: cotton wisp placed under the ingrown nail edge (also may be done with dental floss)
- Gutter splint: plastic tubing (e.g., intravenous [IV] infusion tubing) with a vertical slit and placing this over the ingrown nail edge
- Taping procedure: one end of tape placed under against the side of ingrown toenail, with the rest twisted around the toe; pulls the side of nail fold away from the nail to decrease pressure
- If infection is suspected, it is important to remove the source of infection. When using antibiotics, they should be directed against gram-positive bacteria (e.g., *Staphylococcus aureus* and *Streptococcus* spp.).

SURGERY/OTHER PROCEDURES

- Surgery may be recommended for severe or recurrent lesions and in cases where initial efforts of noninvasive managements are ineffective (1)[C],(2)[C],(4)[C],(5)[A].
- Surgical interventions more effectively prevent recurrence than nonsurgical treatments (6)[A].
- Ablation of the nail matrix with phenol may reduce the risk of recurrence (5)[A],(6)[A].
- Oral or topical antibiotics are not recommended unless significant cellulitis is present (1)[C].
- Various techniques; performed under local anesthesia (1)[C],(2)[C],(4)[C],(5)[A],(6)[A]
  - Partial nail avulsion with chemical matrixectomy: mechanical avulsion or excision of lateral nail edge followed by application of phenol to prevent further growth
  - Winograd technique or wedge resection: removal of the wedge up to germinal matrix and hypertrophied bone tissue; remaining soft tissue is sutured to the nail.
  - Vandenbos procedure: incision made at nail base while the lateral nail fold is removed with a lateral elliptical sweep
  - Zadik procedure: total nail avulsion
- Contraindications include disorders causing digital ischemia (e.g., diabetes, peripheral vascular disease, and collagen diseases).
- An incomplete matrixectomy can result in regrowth of a nail spicule which can result in an inflammatory reaction or recurrence, necessitating another procedure.

ONGOING CARE

FOLLOW-UP RECOMMENDATIONS

- After nail plate excision: Rest and elevate the toe first 12 to 24 hours; change dressing after 24 to 48 hours and resume normal ambulation; expect sterile exudate from the nail bed for 2 to 3 weeks.
- Immunocompromised individuals with a severe infection may require hospitalization for administration of IV antibiotics.

PATIENT EDUCATION

- Properly fitting footwear
- Proper nail trimming (and foot hygiene)
- Online patient handouts:
  - https://familydoctor.org/condition/ingrown-toenails/
  - https://www.aafp.org/pubs/afp/issues/2019/0801/p158.html

COMPLICATIONS

- Recurrence
- Scarring of nail fold
- Narrowing or loss of nail (when matrix ablation performed)
- Secondary infection of the nail fold
- Osteomyelitis
- Pyogenic granuloma

REFERENCES

1. Mayeaux EJ Jr, Carter C, Murphy TE. Ingrown toenail management. *Am Fam Physician.* 2019;100(3):158–164.
2. Geizhals S, Lipner SR. Review of onychocryptosis: epidemiology, pathogenesis, risk factors, diagnosis and treatment. *Dermatol Online J.* 2019;25(9):13030.
3. Cho SY, Kim YC, Choi JW. Epidemiology and bone-related comorbidities of ingrown nail: a nationwide population-based study. *J Dermatol.* 2018;45(12):1418–1424.
4. Hassan RE, Khan L, Shah SH, et al. Surgical strategies for ingrown toenails: a comprehensive review of techniques, outcomes, and advancements. *Cureus.* 2024;16(1):e52501.
5. Eekhof JAH, Van Wijk B, Knuistingh Neven A, et al. Interventions for ingrowing toenails. *Cochrane Database Syst Rev.* 2012;(4):CD001541.
6. Exley V, Jones K, O'Carroll G, et al. A systematic review and meta-analysis of randomised controlled trials on surgical treatments for ingrown toenails part I: recurrence and relief of symptoms. *J Foot Ankle Res.* 2023;16(1):35.

CLINICAL PEARLS

- Reoccurrence is common and therefore preventative measures are essential.
- Treatment should include addressing the ingrown toenail as well as the underlying etiology.
- Antibiotics have not been shown to change the healing from ingrown toenails when using surgical treatment options.
- Impact activities should be avoided until the patient is pain free and clear of infection.

INNER EAR INJURIES (TYMPANIC MEMBRANE PERFORATION)

Connie Hsu, MD • Holly J. Benjamin, MD, FAMSSM, FACSM

BASICS

DESCRIPTION

Disruption of the tympanic membrane, leading to a connection between the middle ear and the external auditory canal

EPIDEMIOLOGY

Incidence

The incidence of tympanic membrane perforation in the general population has not been studied. Overall, tympanic membrane perforation is more common in men than women (1).

ETIOLOGY AND PATHOPHYSIOLOGY

- Blunt trauma (slap to the ear)
- Penetrating trauma (Q-tip)
- Rapid pressure change (diving, flying)
- Extreme noise (blast)
- Lightning
- Spontaneous perforation associated with acute otitis media
- Spontaneous perforation from otitis externa secondary to *Aspergillus niger*
- Acute necrotic myringitis

DIAGNOSIS

HISTORY

- Sudden onset of pain followed by relief
- Otorrhea (purulent or bloody)
- Ear pain (mild)
- Decreased hearing (partial)
- Tinnitus
- Vertigo
- Severe pain or complete hearing loss in the affected ear may suggest additional injuries.

PHYSICAL EXAM

- Often a clinical diagnosis
- Direct visualization of tympanic membrane with otoscope
- Otoscope fogging may be present.
- Test hearing in both ears:
  - Weber test (tuning fork on midline bone):
    - Sound should be equal or louder in the injured ear, consistent with decreased conduction.
    - Sound localizing to the opposite side of injury indicates possible otic nerve injury.
  - Rinne test: usually normal (air conduction detected after bone conduction fades) or shows a small conductive loss
  - Audiogram may also be used.
- Note any nystagmus with changes of position or pressure on the tragus occluding the canal (fistula sign).
- Insufflation via pneumatic otoscope:
  - The perforated tympanic membrane will not move normally.
  - Holding pressure for 15 seconds (the fistula test) may cause nystagmus or vertigo if the pressure is transmitted through the middle ear and into a labyrinthine fistula.

DIFFERENTIAL DIAGNOSIS

- Temporal bone fracture
- Serous otitis media
- Suppurative otitis media
- Otitis externa
- Cerumen impaction
- Barotrauma
- Acoustic trauma
- Foreign body
- Child abuse

DIAGNOSTIC TESTS & INTERPRETATION

- Radiography and magnetic resonance imaging (MRI) are of no value unless the clinical picture suggests ossicular destruction and/or cholesteatoma.
- Asymptomatic perforations, especially if hearing is near normal, require no imaging studies.
- Definitive diagnosis requires otomicroscopy or middle ear impedance studies, performed outpatient.

TREATMENT

GENERAL MEASURES

- Treatment is primarily supportive.
- Medical treatment for perforations is directed at controlling otorrhea and keeping the ear dry (2).
- Clean debris from the ear canal.
- Acute otitis media with tympanic membrane perforation should be treated with an oral antibiotic (2)[A].
- Oral antibiotic choices (administered for 7 to 10 days):
  - Amoxicillin
  - Trimethoprim-sulfamethoxazole
  - Amoxicillin/clavulanic acid (Augmentin)
- Topical quinolone antibiotics are useful for chronic suppurative otitis media and tympanostomy tube otorrhea in the absence of systemic disease.
- Ofloxacin otic drops may improve rate and time to closure of perforation for traumatic perforations but do not affect hearing loss or infection rate complications (3)[A].
- Penetrating traumatic perforations in the posterosuperior quadrant should be referred to otolaryngology for consideration for surgery.
- Analgesics if needed for pain

ALERT

Do not prescribe topical ototoxic eardrops such as gentamicin, neomycin sulfate, or tobramycin.

MEDICATION

- Amoxicillin: 250 to 500 mg (children: 20 to 40 mg/kg/24 h) PO TID
- Trimethoprim-sulfamethoxazole (Bactrim DS): 1 tablet (children: 6 to 12 mg/kg/24 h) PO BID
- Amoxicillin/clavulanic acid (Augmentin): 250 to 500 mg (children: 20 to 40 mg/kg/24 h) PO TID
- Ofloxacin otic topical 0.3%: 10 drops in affected ear BID × 7 days
- Ciprofloxacin 0.3% and dexamethasone (Ciprodex) 0.1% otic suspension: 4 drops in affected ear BID × 7 days (2)

ISSUES FOR REFERRAL

Arrange ear, nose, throat (ENT) specialist follow-up:

- After detailed examination and formal audiometric tests, most otolaryngologists follow the perforation with monthly examinations.
- Operative repair is reserved for the 10–20% that do not heal spontaneously.

SURGERY/OTHER PROCEDURES

- Office procedures such as paper patch myringoplasty method (85.3–91.4%) (4)[A]
- Surgical tympanoplasty under local or general anesthesia (82.8–90.2% success) (4)[A]
- Regenerative treatment using gelatin sponge, basic fibroblast growth factor, and fibrin glue is safe and effective for tympanic membrane perforation repair (5)[A].

ADMISSION, INPATIENT, AND NURSING CONSIDERATIONS

Admission criteria:

- Associated injuries requiring admission
- Severe vertigo impairing ambulation

ONGOING CARE

PATIENT EDUCATION

- Provide detailed discharge instructions.
- Occlude the ear canal with cotton coated in petroleum jelly or antibiotic ointment when showering to prevent entry of water into the middle ear, which can be painful.
- Swim only with fitted earplugs.
- Avoid forceful blowing of the nose.
- Avoid Q-tips.
- Patients may return to play when all clinical symptoms are improved, including inner ear symptoms and hearing, and the tympanic membrane is intact.

PROGNOSIS

ALERT

Most perforations heal spontaneously over a few months (76% within 1 month, 97% within 3 months) (6).

- Size of perforation and secondary infection are leading causes for delayed or nonclosure.
- Delayed closure and chronic perforations are indications for surgery.
- Morbidity associated to tympanic membrane perforations is primarily related to hearing loss, which would benefit from repair.
- Overall, mortality and morbidity are low.

ALERT

Chronic otitis media leading to hearing loss is a complication of perforated tympanic membrane. These patients should be referred for prompt evaluation by an otolaryngologist.

COMPLICATIONS

- Infection
- Dislocation of ossicles
- Perilymph leak
- Cholesteatoma

REFERENCES

1. Carniol ET, Bresler A, Shaigany K, et al. Traumatic tympanic membrane perforations diagnosed in emergency departments. *JAMA Otolaryngol Head Neck Surg*. 2018;144(2):136–139.
2. Wright D, Safranek S. Treatment of otitis media with perforated tympanic membrane. *Am Fam Physician*. 2009;79(8):650–654.
3. Kutbi AH, Malas M, Al-Talhi AA, et al. The effect of using ofloxacin ear drops in traumatic tympanic membrane healing: a systematic review and meta-analysis. *Ear Nose Throat J*. 2024:1455613241264479.
4. Jungbauer WN Jr, Jeong S, Nguyen SA, et al. Comparing myringoplasty to type I tympanoplasty in tympanic membrane repair: a systematic review and meta-analysis. *Otolaryngol Head Neck Surg*. 2023;168(5):922–934.
5. Kanemaru SI, Kanai R, Omori K, et al. Multicenter phase III trial of regenerative treatment for chronic tympanic membrane perforation. *Auris Nasus Larynx*. 2021;48(6):1054–1060.
6. Tachibana T, Kariya S, Orita Y, et al. Spontaneous closure of traumatic tympanic membrane perforation following long-term observation. *Acta Otolaryngol*. 2019;139(6):487–491.

ADDITIONAL READING

Huang J, Teh BM, Shen Y. Butterfly cartilage tympanoplasty as an alternative to conventional surgery for tympanic membrane perforations: a systematic review and meta-analysis. *Ear Nose Throat J*. 2023;102(7):NP369–NP378.

CLINICAL PEARLS

- Infections are responsible from more tympanic membrane perforations than sports-related trauma.
- No imaging is needed for uncomplicated tympanic membrane perforations.
- Avoid ototoxic eardrops/solutions in the setting of tympanic membrane perforations.
- Most tympanic membrane perforations heal spontaneously.

INTERMETATARSAL (MORTON) NEUROMA

Steven Reece, MD, CAQSM ▪ Elizabeth Walker, DO ▪ Annemarie Beran, DO

BASICS

DESCRIPTION

- Fibrosis, demyelination, and inflammation of an interdigital nerve of the foot; not a true neuroma
- Occurs at the common planter nerve bifurcation into the interdigital nerve (1)
- Most commonly occurs at the 3rd intermetatarsal space—between the heads of the 3rd and 4th metatarsals; but can also involve the 2nd or 4th intermetatarsal spaces
- Most often, symptoms are unilateral; if bilateral, typically requires further workup and investigation for etiologies such as neuropathy
- Diagnosed clinically through history and examination, without need for routine imaging (2)

EPIDEMIOLOGY

- The second most compressive neuropathy behind carpal tunnel syndrome (3)
- Most common in women in the 4th or 5th decade of life
- Athletes most at risk include combat sports (barefoot), ballet or pointe dancers, and runners.
- Nonathletic risk seen with narrow toe box shoes, high heels, or barefoot walking

ETIOLOGY AND PATHOPHYSIOLOGY

- Epineural and perineural fibrosis causing subsequent demyelination and inflammatory thickening of the interdigital nerve (3)
- No single causative factor demonstrated in literature, but common suggestions include compression of the nerve due to intermetatarsal bursa swelling, vascular degeneration, trauma, and/or compression at intermetatarsal ligament (2).
- Trauma and neuropathic degeneration causes reactive inflammation and swelling of the interdigital nerve leading to typical neuropathic entrapment symptoms of numbness, tingling, burning, pins, and needles (1),(2).

GENERAL PREVENTION

- Correct footwear—avoid narrow toe box and high heels.
- Longitudinal arch support

DIAGNOSIS

HISTORY

- Intermittent plantar foot pain usually between the 3rd and 4th metatarsals with accompanying neuropathic descriptors such as numbness, tingling, burning, pins and needles
- Localized metatarsalgia at the ball of foot with radiation of pain dorsally into the webspace or accompanying toes and interdigital space
- Subjective clicking reported by patient is highly specific for Morton neuroma (MN) (4)[A].
- Common descriptors include "walking on a pebble" and "burning pain" of the web space (4)[A].
- Aggravating activities—wearing shoes with narrow toe box, barefoot walking, prolonged weight-bearing

PHYSICAL EXAM

- Tenderness to palpation on the plantar surface of the foot at the affected intermetatarsal space (2)[B]
- Neuropathic symptoms present on either plantar or dorsal aspect of the foot, with radiation into the toes
- Sensory deficits, but typically no strength deficits or weakness
- Mulder click: palpable click and pain with compression of the metatarsal heads (4)[A]
- Thumb-index finger squeeze test: pain or reproducible neurologic symptoms distally with compression of affected webspace (4)[A],(5)[B]; ensure anatomically correct palpation to avoid metatarsal shafts; can consider utilization of Q-tip or pen to ensure accurate testing of webspace
- Positive Tinel sign at the plantar aspect of the foot with repetitive nerve stimulation

DIFFERENTIAL DIAGNOSIS

- Nonspecific metatarsalgia
- Ganglion cyst
- Neuropathy—diabetic or nutritional deficiency, particularly if symptoms are bilateral
- Metatarsal stress fracture
- Avascular necrosis of metatarsal bones
- Plantar plate injury or tear (5)

DIAGNOSTIC TESTS & INTERPRETATION

- A clinical diagnosis where imaging is usually not required (2)[A]
- If symptoms are persistent or atypical, x-ray imaging can evaluate for bony abnormalities.
- Electromyography not warranted; can be helpful for evaluation of other neuropathies but not diagnostic for MN
- Ultrasound (US) examination can reveal hypoechoic lesion within normal tissue of the intermetatarsal space (6)[C].
- US can offer real-time correlation between symptoms and imaging findings.
- MRI may show increased signal and edema surrounding the interdigital nerve.
- US and MRI have similar diagnostic sensitivity; however, US is typically more convenient and cost-effective (5)[B].

TREATMENT

GENERAL MEASURES

- Conservative treatment with lifestyle modification and anti-inflammatory medications are first line.
- Redistribute, offload, and decrease pressure on metatarsal heads to decompress impacted nerve with proper shoe wear—avoid narrow toe box, high heels, barefoot walking.
- Metatarsal pad placement proximal to the affected interspace (1)[C]; improper pad placement may alter responses to conservative treatment.
- If conservative measures fail to alleviate symptoms, can pursue corticosteroid injection of the intermetatarsal bursa (5)[B]
- Injection technique: dorsal approach, 45-degree entry into intermetatarsal space
- No consensus on recommended steroid, provider preference—usually 0.5- to 1.0-mL steroid and 0.5-mL anesthetic (6)[C]
- Common steroid doses include but are not limited to 20-mg triamcinolone, 20-mg methylprednisolone, or 3-mg betamethasone; avoid epinephrine to prevent necrosis.
- Recommended maximum of two corticosteroid injections of bursa/MN due to concerns of fat atrophy and joint capsule degeneration (3)[C]

SURGERY/OTHER PROCEDURES

- Literature is sparse, but MN can also be treated with chemical neurolysis and/or radiofrequency thermal neurolysis (6)[B].
- Surgical consultation and/or evaluation warranted if symptoms fail to respond to conservative treatment

REFERENCES

1. McKean KA. Neurologic running injuries. *Neurol Clin*. 2008;26(1):281–296.
2. Pastides P, El-Sallakh S, Charalambides C. Morton's neuroma: a clinical versus radiological diagnosis. *Foot Ankle Surg*. 2012;18(1):22–24.
3. Cooper MT. Common painful foot and ankle conditions: a review. *JAMA*. 2023;330(23):2285–2294.
4. Pitcher M, Moulson A, Pitcher D, et al. Diagnostic accuracy of subjective features and physical examination tests for Morton neuroma: a systematic review. *Foot Ankle Orthop*. 2024;9(4):24730114241291055.
5. Shapiro BE, Preston DC. Entrapment and compressive neuropathies. *Med Clin North Am*. 2009;93(2):285–315.
6. Klontzas ME, Koltsakis E, Kakkos GA, et al. Ultrasound-guided treatment of Morton's neuroma. *J Ultrason*. 2021;21(85):e134–e138.

ADDITIONAL READING

Bignotti B, Signori A, Sormani MP, et al. Ultrasound versus magnetic resonance imaging for Morton neuroma: systematic review and meta-analysis. *Eur Radiol*. 2015;25(8):2254–2262.

CLINICAL PEARLS

- Pain, numbness, paresthesia in the intermetatarsal space, typically the 3rd
- Typically diagnosed clinically through history and physical exam without need for routine imaging
- Treatment first with conservative measures
- Shoe wear with wide toe box and/or metatarsal pads can offload pressure on metatarsal heads to alleviate neuropathic symptoms.
- Diagnosis of MN should not limit or restrict an athlete or patient activity levels so long as symptoms do not cause a limp or other alteration in gait; condition may be painful but is not dangerous.
- If imaging is pursued, MRI and US have similar sensitivities with no statistical significance—US examination often preferred over MRI for dynamic nature of testing and cost efficiency.

INTERPHALANGEAL COLLATERAL LIGAMENT SPRAIN

Lindsay A. Lafferty, MD ▪ Shawn Phillips, MD, MSPT ▪ Matthew L. Silvis, MD, FAMSSM

BASICS

DESCRIPTION

- Injury to a collateral ligament at the interphalangeal (IP) joint of the finger, usually the proximal IP (PIP) joint:
  - 1st degree: pain but no laxity
  - 2nd degree: pain and laxity but firm end point when ligament is stressed
  - 3rd degree: pain and loss of firm end point when ligament is stressed
- Mechanisms: axial loading with radial or ulnar stress applied to the finger, usually while extended
- Synonym(s): jammed finger

EPIDEMIOLOGY

Incidence

- PIP joints represent the most common sites of ligament injuries in the fingers.
- 1st- and 2nd-degree sprain more common than 3rd-degree sprain
- Index finger most often affected
- Combined injury to both collateral ligaments is more common than isolated radial collateral ligament (RCL) or ulnar collateral ligament (UCL) injury.

RISK FACTORS

- Ball handling, collision, and contact sports: football, basketball, volleyball, wrestling
- Prior injury or dislocation of the PIP joint

DIAGNOSIS

HISTORY

- Finger struck by player or ball during play
- Axial trauma causing forced ulnar or radial deviation
- Usually presents acutely but may become chronic

PHYSICAL EXAM

- Pain and swelling over radial or ulnar aspects of PIP joint
- Decreased range of motion (ROM) secondary to pain and edema
- Confirm neurovascular integrity, especially with on-field assessment.
- Ensure that maximum tenderness is over lateral aspects and not dorsal or volar.
- Dorsal pain may suggest central slip injury.
- Collateral ligament stability is best evaluated with the metacarpophalangeal (MCP) joint in 90 degrees of flexion and the IP joint stressed in extension and in 30 degrees of flexion (1)[C].
- Hyperextension is concerning for a volar plate injury.
- Compare with uninjured fingers.
- Instability with lateral stress (opening beyond 10 degrees or lack of firm end point) suggests loss of integrity (1)[C].
- Assess function of flexor and extensor tendons by isolating MCP, PIP, and distal IP (DIP) joints separately to rule out tendon injury.
- Loss of active ROM may be due to either pain or volar plate/central slip injury, so digital block may be necessary to test ROM (2)[C].

DIFFERENTIAL DIAGNOSIS

- Phalangeal fracture
- IP dislocation
- Central slip injury
- Volar plate injury
- Often associated with one or more of above

DIAGNOSTIC TESTS & INTERPRETATION

- Plain radiographs are generally not required for 1st-degree injuries but may be considered for 2nd- or 3rd-degree injuries or to rule out associated fracture.
- Posteroanterior, true lateral, and oblique radiographs of involved fingers (1),(3)[C]
- Avulsion fracture may be seen at ligamentous insertion.
- Look for dorsal subluxation to suggest instability.
- Ultrasound (US) is a cost saving modality that may be used to evaluate dynamic finger ligament integrity and comparative examination of the contralateral side (1),(4)[C].

TREATMENT

GENERAL MEASURES

- Immobilization:
  - Guided by level of activity, degree of pain, and disability
  - Mild injures may be "buddy taped," and patient may consider immediate return to play depending on function and sport requirements (1)[C].
  - 1st and 2nd degree: protected motion with "buddy tape" continuously for up to 3 weeks (5)[B]; consider taping during physical activity for an additional 2 to 4 weeks (2)[C].
  - 3rd degree: Treat as severe 2nd degree. Surgery may be warranted if "unstressed instability," tissue interposition limiting joint motion, or lack of joint congruity is observed on radiographs (1)[C].

- In general, "buddy tape" to adjacent finger; for example, long finger to index and ring to small finger to prevent additional trauma to the index or small finger (5)[B]
- Continuous immobilization for >3 weeks may lead to permanent stiffness.
- Rehabilitation: Depending on severity, begin passive ROM exercises in 1st week and active ROM after 1 to 2 weeks, later for more severe injuries (2)[C].

ADDITIONAL THERAPIES

- Displaced intra-articular and large avulsion fractures with displacement may require open reduction and internal fixation (ORIF) (1)[C].
- Hyperextension and/or dorsal dislocation injuries and central tenderness over the volar aspect should raise concern for volar plate injuries requiring different treatment.
- Central tenderness over the dorsal PIP joint suggests central slip injury, which can lead to a chronic boutonnière deformity and requires a different management approach.

Pediatric Considerations

Collateral ligament injury in children should raise concern for growth plate involvement, and there should be a low threshold for referral to a hand specialist (6)[C].

SURGERY/OTHER PROCEDURES

- Generally necessary if instability with active ROM, tissue interposition limiting joint motion, or lack of joint congruity is observed on radiographs (1)[C].
- Most complete tears heal well with conservative treatment, and operative trauma may limit joint motion.
- Although surgical repair for complete tears are described as a viable treatment option, there is insufficient high quality evidence to inform current practice. Based on current literature no evidence-based conclusions can be made regarding the superiority of acute surgical repair over conservative management (1)[C],(4)[A].

ONGOING CARE

FOLLOW-UP RECOMMENDATIONS

- Follow up in 1 to 2 weeks for reevaluation of laxity.
- Refer significant fractures for possible ORIF.
- If uncertain of possible central slip/volar plate injury, refer to surgeon or follow up in 7 to 10 days for reevaluation (6)[C].
- Chronic symptoms may respond to extended splinting and "buddy taping" with protected ROM exercises for several weeks to months (6)[C].
- Surgical repair may be indicated if disability and instability persist after a sufficient trial of conservative treatment (6)[C].

PATIENT EDUCATION

Advise patients that some persistent deformity may be noted after injury has healed.

REFERENCES

1. Carruthers KH, Skie M, Jain M. Jam injuries of the finger: diagnosis and management of injuries to the interphalangeal joints across multiple sports and levels of experience. *Sports Health*. 2016;8(5):469–478.
2. Freiberg A, Pollard BA, Macdonald MR, et al. Management of proximal interphalangeal joint injuries. *Hand Clin*. 2006;22(3):235–242.
3. Draghi F, Gitto S, Bianchi S. Injuries to the collateral ligaments of the metacarpophalangeal and interphalangeal joints: sonographic appearance. *J Ultrasound Med*. 2018;37(9):2117–2133.
4. Bui D, Jenkins M, Schick B, et al. Outcomes of acute operative repair of complete digital proximal interphalangeal joint collateral ligament ruptures: a systematic review. *J Hand Surg Asian Pac Vol*. 2021;26(4):644–653.
5. Roh YH, Koh YD, Go JY, et al. Factors influencing functional outcome of proximal interphalangeal joint collateral ligament injury when treated with buddy strapping and exercise. *J Hand Ther*. 2018;31(3):295–300.
6. Leggit JC, Meko CJ. Acute finger injuries: part I. Tendons and ligaments. *Am Fam Physician*. 2006;73(5):810–816.

ADDITIONAL READING

- Alexy C, De Carlo M. Rehabilitation and use of protective devices in hand and wrist injuries. *Clin Sports Med*. 1998;17(3):635–655.
- Khouri JS, Bloom JMP, Hammert WC. Current trends in the management of proximal interphalangeal joint injuries of the hand. *Plast Reconstr Surg*. 2013;132(5):1192–1204.
- Palmer RE. Joint injuries of the hand in athletes. *Clin Sports Med*. 1998;17(3):513–531.

CLINICAL PEARLS

- Ensure active ROM in all affected and surrounding joints to rule out more significant ligamentous injuries.
- Return to play depends on severity and demands of sport, but frequently, immediate return to play can be accomplished with "buddy taping."
- Most injuries can be managed with protected motion through "buddy taping" for up to 3 weeks and early ROM to prevent stiffness.
- Some residual soreness can be expected for months and sometimes up to a year.
- The joint affected may appear permanently enlarged owing to scarring during the healing process.

INTERSECTION SYNDROME

Eric Yuan, MD, FAAFP, CAQSM

BASICS

DESCRIPTION

- Intersection syndrome is a painful condition located in the distal radial forearm caused by friction where the tendons of the 1st extensor compartment cross-over the tendons of the 2nd compartment.
- Patient usually presents with pain, crepitus, and squeaky sensation in the dorsal distal forearm; may have localized swelling
- Pain usually occurs about 4 cm (range of 4 to 8 cm) proximal to the radial styloid.
- Synonym(s): Oarsman wrist; crossover syndrome; squeaker wrist

EPIDEMIOLOGY

- Most common in rowing, weightlifting, and racket sports
- Skiers, other athletes, or workers who do repetitive forceful wrist flexion and extension activities are also at risk.

ETIOLOGY AND PATHOPHYSIOLOGY

- The abductor pollicis longus (APL) and extensor pollicis brevis (EPB) tendons comprise the 1st dorsal wrist compartment.
- The extensor carpi radialis longus (ECRL) and extensor carpi radialis brevis (ECRB) tendons comprise the 2nd compartment.
- Friction occurs at the intersection where the APL and EPB of the 1st compartment crossover the tendon sheath of the ECRL and ECRB in the 2nd compartment (1), leading to tenosynovitis.

RISK FACTORS

Sports with increased risk include:

- Rowing
- Weightlifting
- Skiing
- Racquetball
- Tennis
- Any activity with repetitive forceful flexion and extension of the wrist

GENERAL PREVENTION

Avoid or modify activity involving repetitive forceful flexion and extension of the wrist.

DIAGNOSIS

HISTORY

- Commonly misdiagnosed as de Quervain tenosynovitis
- Symptoms typically have insidious onset over weeks to months.
- History of increase in activity that requires repetitive wrist flexion/extension
- Athletes will report pain in the distal forearm or radial side of wrist, typically 4 cm (range of 4 to 8 cm) proximal to the radial styloid; may complain of localized swelling and a squeaking sensation

PHYSICAL EXAM

- Localized swelling 4 to 8 cm proximal to the radial styloid may be present.
- Crepitus on palpation is classic for intersection syndrome.
- Pain exacerbated by ulnar deviation of the hand
- Movement of wrist typically causes more pain than movement of thumb, as seen in de Quervain.
- Bony palpation is typically nontender, and neurovascular status should be intact.
- Redness, warmth, and a "squeaking" sound at the tendon intersection site may be present.

DIFFERENTIAL DIAGNOSIS

- De Quervain tenosynovitis
- Extensor pollicis longus tendinitis (drummer boy palsy)
- Triangular fibrocartilage complex (TFCC) injury
- Wartenberg syndrome (neuritis of superficial radial nerve)
- Degenerative joint disease of carpometacarpal joint
- Radial styloid fracture
- Scaphoid fracture
- Forearm stress fracture

DIAGNOSTIC TESTS & INTERPRETATION

Initial Tests (lab, imaging)

- Radiographs should be taken to evaluate for any underlying abnormalities. Anteroposterior, lateral, and oblique views of the wrist and distal forearm are the images of choice.
- If diagnostic ultrasound (US) is available, this can be helpful for differentiating intersection syndrome from other disorders. US features include peritendinous edema (hyperechoic area) and synovial fluid within the compartments' tendon sheaths. The portability of US offers a distinct advantage compared with magnetic resonance imaging (MRI), which may require an extended field of view (2)[C].
- MRI would not be indicated in the initial evaluation of this syndrome. If diagnosis is not clear or pain is persistent, MRI could be considered to evaluate for soft tissue masses or bony abnormalities. The MRI should include the forearm in addition to the wrist (3)[B].

Follow-Up Tests & Special Considerations

If symptoms persist and diagnosis is not clear, electromyography (EMG)/nerve conduction testing (NCT) may be helpful to evaluate for nerve entrapment.

TREATMENT

GENERAL MEASURES

Initial treatment (for 2 to 3 weeks) (4)[C]:

- Rest and/or activity modification
- Ice
- Nonsteroidal anti-inflammatory drugs (NSAIDs)
- Thumb spica splint in 15 degrees of extension

ADDITIONAL THERAPIES

- All treatment requires subsequent activity modification to prevent recurrence.
- Occupational therapy may be helpful for stretching program, local swelling reduction, and to help with activity modification. Manual therapy may be used in chronic cases to reduce scar tissue or tendinopathy.
- Injection is usually reserved after no improvement with 2 to 3 weeks of splinting and activity modification.
- A 1:1 mixture of a local anesthetic and steroid combination (1 to 2 mL total) may be injected into the area of maximal swelling or guided into intersection of 1st and 2nd compartment under US guidance.
- Saline hydro dissection or prolotherapy under US guidance is an additional treatment option (5)[C].

SURGERY/OTHER PROCEDURES

- Surgery is reserved for recalcitrant cases.
- Surgery for intersection syndrome aims to decompress the tendons at their crossover point. This may involve a combination of tenosynovectomy (removing the inflamed tendon sheath), fasciotomy (releasing the overlying connective tissue), and débridement of the bursa (6)[C].

ONGOING CARE

FOLLOW-UP RECOMMENDATIONS

- If no improvement after adequate course of conservative therapy, surgical referral is warranted.
- Surgery may be needed if fibrosis of the tendon sheath has occurred.

PROGNOSIS

- Recovery is achieved in majority of patients after initial treatment of activity modification, splinting, and NSAIDs for 2 to 3 weeks.
- If surgery is necessary, postoperative rehabilitation typically lasts 4 to 6 weeks.
- Return to play may occur once symptoms have resolved.

REFERENCES

1. Adams JE, Habbu R. Tendinopathies of the hand and wrist. *J Am Acad Orthop Surg*. 2015;23(12):741–750.
2. Flores DV, Murray T, Jacobson JA. Diagnostic and interventional US of the wrist and hand: quadrant-based approach. *Radiographics*. 2023;43(8):e230046.
3. Lee RP, Hatem SF, Recht MP. Extended MRI findings of intersection syndrome. *Skeletal Radiol*. 2009;38(2):157–163.
4. Schmidt E, Kobayashi Y, Gottschalk AW. It's not de Quervain tenosynovitis—a diagnosis to consider in persistent wrist pain. *Ochsner J*. 2021;21(2):120–122.
5. Beutel BG, Taylor K, Michols NJ, et al. *Intersection Syndrome*. StatPearls Publishing. Updated May 23, 2025. Accessed October 3, 2025. https://www.ncbi.nlm.nih.gov/books/NBK430899
6. Balakatounis K, Angoules AG, Angoules NA, et al. Synthesis of evidence for the treatment of intersection syndrome. *World J Orthop*. 2017;8(8):619–623.

ADDITIONAL READING

- Patrick NC, Hammert WC. Hand and wrist tendinopathies. *Clin Sports Med*. 2020;39(2):247–258.
- Skinner TM. Intersection syndrome: the subtle squeak of an overused wrist. *J Am Board Fam Med*. 2017;30(4):547–551.

CLINICAL PEARLS

- Intersection syndrome is an overuse syndrome.
- Pain is located 4 to 8 cm proximal to radial styloid.
- Athletes will often report a squeaking sensation in their wrist.
- Be able to consider both intersection syndrome and de Quervain tenosynovitis in the differential of distal forearm pain.
- The mainstay of treatment is conservative, using activity modification and a short course of NSAIDs and possibly thumb spica splinting.

I

ISCHIOFEMORAL IMPINGEMENT

Navdeep Rai, MD, MS ▪ Priya Sharma, DO ▪ Kenneth S. Taylor, MD, FAAFP, CAQSM

BASICS

DESCRIPTION

- Ischiofemoral impingement (IFI) syndrome is a lesser known cause of hip pain that occurs due to narrowing of the space between the ischium and femur.
- The impingement occurs between the lateral aspect of the os ischium and the lesser trochanter of the femur, leading to compression of the quadratus femoris muscle and sometimes adjacent neurovascular structures.
- It is usually correlated with trauma or prior hip surgery (1),(2),(3).

EPIDEMIOLOGY

Most cases in the literature are female, likely due to gender-specific differences in pelvic anatomy that may be associated with reduced ischiofemoral distance (4),(5).

ETIOLOGY AND PATHOPHYSIOLOGY

Causes of IFI may be acquired, congenital, or functional in nature.

- Acquired: traumatic deformities (such as intertrochanteric fractures or malunion of pelvic or proximal femoral fractures), total hip arthroplasty, valgus producing intertrochanteric osteotomy, osteoarthritis (leading to superomedial migration of femur), space-occupying lesions, sequelae of Perthes disease, pathologies of bordering soft tissues such as hamstring enthesopathy or rupture (1),(4)
- Congenital: coxa valga as well as developmental dysplasia of the hip (DDH)
- Functional: dynamic or positional factors that alter hip kinematics, such as increased femoral anteversion, hip or pelvic instability, muscular imbalances, or leg length discrepancy (3),(5)

RISK FACTORS

- Female sex
- Congenital disorders (coxa valga, DDH, etc.)
- Trauma
- Prior hip surgery
- Idiopathic

COMMONLY ASSOCIATED CONDITIONS

- Quadratus femoris edema, tear, atrophy (1),(4),(6)
- Psoas and hamstring tendon pathology
- Neobursa formation in vicinity of impinging structures (6)
- Concomitant sciatic nerve entrapment (3)

DIAGNOSIS

HISTORY

- Pain in the hip, lower/deep buttock, medial groin, or thigh; +/− radiation to the knee (1),(2)
- Worsened with walking or weight-bearing (4)
- A snapping, clunking, or locking sensation of the hip joint is often described during long-stride walking (caused by the lesser trochanter forcefully bypassing the os ischium) (1),(4),(5).

PHYSICAL EXAM

- Test of choice: IFI
  - Patient in lateral decubitus with symptomatic side up. Hip is passively extended, adducted, and externally rotated while maintaining knee at 90 degrees (3),(5).
  - Test is positive if symptoms are reproduced.
  - Hip extension and abduction relieve pain (5).
  - Sensitivity of 82% and specificity of 85% (3),(5)
- Long stride walking test: pain evoked by the patient taking exaggerated large steps, which increases hip extension and external rotation
  - Sensitivity of 94% and specificity of 85% (5)
- Additional exam findings may include functional leg length discrepancy due to compensatory abduction of the leg to increase the distance between the lesser trochanter and ischium (5).

DIFFERENTIAL DIAGNOSIS

- Femoroacetabular impingement
- Piriformis syndrome
- Hamstring injury
- Lumbosacral radiculopathy
- Sciatica
- Sacroiliac (SI) joint dysfunction
- Spinal stenosis
- Quadriceps femoris tear
- Adductor tendonitis

DIAGNOSTIC TESTS & INTERPRETATION

- Test of choice is hip magnetic resonance imaging (MRI) and typically demonstrates a decreased distance (<15 mm) between the ischial tuberosity and lesser trochanter, edema, or injury of the quadratus femoris muscle, and sometimes tendon or nerve involvement (1),(3),(6).
- Plain radiographs recommended to assess for bony abnormalities, prior trauma, or other contributing pathologies
- Ultrasound measurements of IFI have been shown to be similar to MRI, but interrater reliability can vary and sonographer experience may limit assessment (3).
- Injection of quadratus femoris/ischiofemoral space with local anesthetic or corticosteroid that relieves symptoms can be diagnostic (1),(2).

TREATMENT

- Activity modification
- Medication: short-term nonsteroidal anti-inflammatory drugs (NSAIDs), acetaminophen (Tylenol), +/− gabapentin
- Structured rehabilitation program focusing on hip and core strength, flexibility, and stabilizers, and addressing biomechanical contributors
- Consider for symptomatic relief: heat, ultrasound therapy, electrical stimulation, shockwave therapy.
- Image-guided steroid and/or local anesthetic injection may provide therapeutic benefit, although duration of response may vary (1),(2),(3).
- Surgery (for refractory cases): Resection of lesser trochanter may consider correction of leg length discrepancy.

REFERENCES

1. Torriani M, Souto SCL, Thomas BJ, et al. Ischiofemoral impingement syndrome: an entity with hip pain and abnormalities of the quadratus femoris muscle. *AJR Am J Roentgenol*. 2009;193(1):186–190.
2. Wilson MD, Keene JS. Treatment of ischiofemoral impingement: results of diagnostic injections and arthroscopic resection of the lesser trochanter. *J Hip Preserv Surg*. 2016;3(2):146–153.
3. Wu WT, Chang KV, Mezian K, et al. Ischiofemoral impingement syndrome: clinical and imaging/guidance issues with special focus on ultrasonography. *Diagnostics (Basel)*. 2022;13(1):139.
4. Ali AM, Teh J, Whitwell D, et al. Ischiofemoral impingement: a retrospective analysis of cases in a specialist orthopaedic centre over a four-year period. *Hip Int*. 2013;23(3):263–268.
5. Gomez-Hoyos J, Martin RL, Schroder R, et al. Accuracy of 2 clinical tests for ischiofemoral impingement in patients with posterior hip pain and endoscopically confirmed diagnosis. *Arthroscopy*. 2016;32(7):1279–1284.
6. Akca A, Safak KY, Ilis ED, et al. Ischiofemoral impingement: assessment of MRI findings and their reliability. *Acta Ortop Bras*. 2016;24(6):318–321.

ADDITIONAL READING

- Ali AM, Whitwell D, Ostlere SJ. Case report: imaging and surgical treatment of a snapping hip due to ischiofemoral impingement. *Skeletal Radiol*. 2011;40(5):653–656.
- Ganz R, Slongo T, Turchetto L, et al. The lesser trochanter as a cause of hip impingement: pathophysiology and treatment options. *Hip Int*. 2013;23(Suppl 9):S35–S41.
- Gollwitzer H, Banke IJ, Schauwecker J, et al. How to address ischiofemoral impingement? Treatment algorithm and review of the literature. *J Hip Preserv Surg*. 2017;4(4):289–298.
- Johnson KA. Impingement of the lesser trochanter on the ischial ramus after total hip arthroplasty. Report of three cases. *J Bone Joint Surg Am*. 1977;59(2):268–269.
- Lee S, Kim I, Lee SM, et al. Ischiofemoral impingement syndrome. *Ann Rehabil Med*. 2013;37(1):143–146.
- López-Sánchez MC, Armesto Pérez V, Montero Furelos LÁ, et al. Pinzamiento isquiofemoral: dolor de cadera de causa poco frecuente. *Reumatol Clin*. 2013;9(3):186–187.
- Ozdemir ZM, Aydingoz U, Gormeli CA, et al. Ischiofemoral space on MRI in an asymptomatic population: normative width measurements and soft tissue signal variations. *Eur Radiol*. 2015;25(8):2246–2253.
- Patti JW, Ouellette H, Bredella MA, et al. Impingement of lesser trochanter on ischium as a potential cause for hip pain. *Skeletal Radiol*. 2008;37(10):939–941.
- Safran M, Ryu J. Ischiofemoral impingement of the hip: a novel approach to treatment. *Knee Surg Sports Traumatol Arthrosc*. 2014;22(4):781–785.
- Singer AD, Subhawong TK, Jose J, et al. Ischiofemoral impingement syndrome: a meta-analysis. *Skeletal Radiol*. 2015;44(6):831–837.
- Tosun O, Cay N, Bozkurt M, et al. Ischiofemoral impingement in an 11-year-old girl. *Diagn Interv Radiol*. 2012;18(6):571–573.

CLINICAL PEARLS

- IFI should be considered as a cause of refractory groin/hip pain, particularly in females.
- Usually involves anatomic narrowing of the space between the ischium and femur
- Pain is worse with walking or weight-bearing and can involve clunking or clicking sensation.
- Diagnosed by exam (+IFI or long stride tests) and confirmed with MRI
- Treated conservatively with surgery as last resort

I

KLIPPEL-FEIL SYNDROME: FUSION OF CERVICAL VERTEBRAE

Erika Pruss, MD • Allison Cotter, MD

BASICS

- A malformation sequence
- Clinical triad of short neck, low hairline, and fusion of multiple cervical vertebrae resulting in decreased range of motion (ROM)

DESCRIPTION

- First described independently by Maurice Klippel and Andre Feil in 1912. They described patients who had the triad of short, webbed neck; decreased ROM in the cervical spine; and a low hairline.
- Original classification by Gunderson et al. (1):
  - Type I: massive fusion of cervical spine
  - Type II: fusion of one or two cervical interspaces
  - Type III: thoracic or lumbar vertebrae involved
- The primary modern classification system was created by Samartzis and is as follows (2),(3):
  - Type I: single-level fusion
  - Type II: multiple noncontiguous fused segments
  - Type III: multiple contiguous fused segments

EPIDEMIOLOGY

- Occurrence is sporadic.
- However, cases with autosomal dominant and autosomal recessive inheritance with variable expression have been reported.
- Most commonly involves C2–C3 and C5–C6 levels (4)

Incidence

- The true incidence of Klippel-Feil syndrome is unknown.
- Estimated as 1:40,000 to 42,000; recent computed tomography (CT) study of asymptomatic patients demonstrated a prevalence of 1 in 172 (3) and a similar study on patients who presented to ED after trauma found a prevalence of 1 in 83 (5).

ETIOLOGY AND PATHOPHYSIOLOGY

- Etiology of Klippel-Feil syndrome and its associated conditions are unknown.
- The sequence may be a part of a serious neural tube development caused by a failure in the normal segmentation or division of the cervical vertebrae during the early weeks (3rd and 8th weeks) of fetal development.
- Other possible etiologies include vascular disruption and global fetal insult.
- Recent molecular studies have suggested genetic mutations (MEOX1 gene, GDF6, GDF3, PAX1, RIPPLY2) may be involved in the pathogenesis (4).

GENERAL PREVENTION

- Prevention of complications can be done by initial broad evaluation of systems commonly affected by Klippel-Feil syndrome and regular evaluation of associated features. It is important to keep in mind that patients are often asymptomatic until an injury occurs.
- Motion at each intervertebral space should be evaluated annually by lateral flexion–extension radiographs of the cervical spine.

COMMONLY ASSOCIATED CONDITIONS

- Klippel-Feil triad is associated with congenital abnormalities of the genitourinary (GU) tract, musculoskeletal system, spinal cord/neurologic system, cardiovascular system, and auditory system.
- GU tract:
  - GU tract structure abnormalities occur in 30–40% of patients with Klippel-Feil syndrome; double collecting systems, renal aplasia, horseshoe kidney, and recurrent pyelonephritis are common; however, absence of a kidney is the most common finding.
  - The extent of cervical abnormality does not correlate with severity of GU abnormalities; thus, thorough GU evaluation is indicated in all patients.
- Musculoskeletal:
  - Concomitant spinal abnormalities occurred in ~19% of Klippel-Feil syndrome patients (6).
  - Short stature
  - Atlantoaxial instability
- Scoliosis is present in ~50–60% of patients with Klippel-Feil syndrome. Scoliosis may be due to fusion in the thoracic or lumbar spine, or a developmental compensation for the cervical/cervicothoracic scoliosis.
  - Cervical spinal stenosis can also occur in association with Klippel-Feil syndrome; although uncommon, when present, cervical stenosis can increase risk of neurologic involvement.
  - Sprengel anomaly (congenital elevation of the scapula) occurs in 20–30% of those with Klippel-Feil syndrome. A higher-than-expected incidence of scoliosis occurs in those with Sprengel anomaly.
  - Upper extremity abnormalities, including syndactyly, hypoplastic thumb, supernumerary digits, and hypoplasia of the upper extremity
- Cardiovascular:
  - Septal defect, primarily ventricular septal defect (VSD)
  - Situs inversus
  - Coarctation of the aorta
- Pulmonary:
  - Lobar agenesis
- Neurologic:
  - Chiari I malformation
  - Syringomyelia
  - Diastematomyelia
  - Sleep-disordered breathing
  - Dermoid cyst in the posterior fossa
  - Hereditary neuropathies
- Auditory system:
  - Hearing impairment: occurs in >1/3 of Klippel-Feil syndrome patients
- Other:
  - Ptosis of the eye
  - Duane eye contracture
  - Lateral rectus palsy
  - Facial nerve palsy
  - Cleft palate
  - Synkinesia or mirror movement
  - Facial asymmetry
  - Craniosynostosis

DIAGNOSIS

- Clinical presentation is variable due to the presence/absence of different associated anomalies.
- Often, Klippel-Feil syndrome is discovered incidentally on physical examination.
- The complete triad is present in <50% of cases.

HISTORY

- Often asymptomatic
- Neck/back pain +/− neurologic symptoms, including numbness, tingling, weakness
- Decreased hearing

PHYSICAL EXAM

- Low hairline
- Short neck
- Decreased cervical ROM; rotational loss is usually more pronounced than loss of flexion and extension.
- Torticollis
- Facial asymmetry
- Heart examination to evaluate for heart position and murmurs
- Chest examination to evaluate for rib fusion and other chest wall anomalies
- Back examination for Sprengel deformity and scoliosis

DIFFERENTIAL DIAGNOSIS

- Congenital muscular torticollis
- Acquired spinal fusion (postinfection, spine inflammatory disorders)
- Wildervanck (cervico-oculo-acoustic) syndrome
- Mayer-Rokitansky-Küster syndrome
- Cervical spina bifida
- Congenital scoliosis
- Brachial plexus injury
- Central nervous system (CNS) lesion (brain tumor)
- Iniencephaly
- Dyssegmental dysplasia

DIAGNOSTIC TESTS & INTERPRETATION

Initial Tests (lab, imaging)

- Plain radiography (anteroposterior/later land open-mouth odontoid views of the cervical spine) is the basis for the diagnosis of Klippel-Feil syndrome.
- Flexion–extension radiographs are indicated if instability is suspected at the craniocervical junction or if two fused segments are separated by an open segment.
- Plain radiographs of the entire spine must be obtained to detect other spinal anomalies.
- Rib series radiography to evaluate for possible rib anomalies, such as multiple rib fusions, also is necessary.
- CT scanning may be done in patients being evaluated for surgery but is not required for diagnosis.

- Magnetic resonance imaging (MRI) is indicated in patients with neurologic deficits to assess subluxation most accurately, cord compression, spinal stenosis, and additional CNS anomalies.
- Ultrasound (US) of the kidneys: Indicated to screen for renal anomalies. Intravenous (IV) pyelography should be performed if further definition of a kidney abnormality is required.
- Echocardiogram may be indicated if concern for concomitant cardiac abnormalities on exam.

Diagnostic Procedures/Other

Full age–appropriate hearing screening: due to the high incidence of hearing loss

TREATMENT

GENERAL MEASURES

- No known treatment for underlying etiology
- Treatment is symptomatic, which includes modification of activities, bracing, and for subluxation, traction. Response to traction may also predict the success of surgery.
- Surgical interventions should be delayed as long as possible. Indications for surgery include progressive symptomatic segmental instability and neurologic compromise.
- Physical therapy may help to maximize ROM and minimize functional limitations.
- General activity limitations, even without presence of symptoms or instability:
  - Avoid contact sports.
  - Avoid occupations and recreational activities with risk of head and neck trauma.
- Sports participation limitations: **Risk stratification involves individualized assessment and should include detailed history, neurologic examination, and appropriate imaging annually. Regular surveillance for any progression of symptoms or comorbidities is important.**
  - All types: Generally, avoid contact sports and activities with risk of head and neck trauma; absolute contraindication in patients with any evidence of instability, stenosis, cord compression, or with upper cervical/occipitocervical fusion
  - Type I: may participate in noncontact sports with caution; avoid contact/collision sports if any instability, hypermobility, neurologic symptoms, or high-risk features are present; individualized risk assessment with detailed history, exam, and imaging is required.
  - Type II/III:
    - Fusion of one or two interspaces at C2 or above with limited cervical ROM, occipitocervical anomalies, involvement of C2, instability, disk disease, or degenerative changes—absolute contraindication
    - Fusion of one or two interspaces at C3 or below with full cervical ROM and no occipitocervical anomalies, no involvement of C2, no instability, no disk disease, and no degenerative changes—no additional contraindications; may participate in contact sports provided no neurologic symptoms or other high-risk features are present

SURGERY/OTHER PROCEDURES

- Referral to otolaryngology for airway issues and evaluation for hearing loss (7)
- Surgical interventions should be delayed as long as possible.
- Indications for surgery include progressive symptomatic segmental instability, neurologic compromise, and/or severe scoliosis.
- Surgical techniques involve occipitocervical arthrodesis, halo immobilization, and atlantoaxial arthrodesis.
- A recent study separated patients who received surgery into four groups: subaxial cervical spine fusions, axial cervical spine abnormalities including subluxation, Chiari malformation, and thoracic anomalies (6).

ONGOING CARE

FOLLOW-UP RECOMMENDATIONS

Patient Monitoring

- Annual evaluation with cervical spine imaging to evaluate for instability or progression of symptoms
- Additional follow-up studies based on individual system involvement

PATIENT EDUCATION

- If hypermobility is noted in the upper cervical segment, there is increased risk of developing neurologic impairment and patients should not be cleared for activities that increase risk of neck injury (i.e., gymnastics, cheerleading, contact sports).
- If hypermobility is noted in the lower cervical segment, there is increased risk of degenerative disk disease, and patients should be treated symptomatically and held from sports based on symptoms and clinical evaluation.

PROGNOSIS

Prognosis is good if features of the disorder are treated early and appropriately.

REFERENCES

1. Gunderson CH, Greenspan RH, Glaser GH, et al. The Klippel-Feil syndrome: genetic and clinical reevaluation of cervical fusion. *Medicine (Baltimore)*. 1967;46(6):491–512.
2. Samartzis D, Herman J, Lubicky JP, et al. Sprengel's deformity in Klippel-Feil syndrome. *Spine (Phila Pa 1976)*. 2007;32(18):E512–E516.
3. Gruber J, Saleh A, Bakhsh W, et al. The prevalence of Klippel-Feil syndrome: a computed tomography—based analysis of 2,917 patients. *Spine Deform*. 2018;6(4):448–453.
4. Litrenta J, Bi AS, Dryer JW. Klippel-Feil syndrome: pathogenesis, diagnosis, and management. *J Am Acad Orthop Surg*. 2021;29(22):951–960.
5. Moses JT, Williams DM, Rubery PT, et al. The prevalence of Klippel-Feil syndrome in pediatric patients: analysis of 831 CT scans. *J Spine Surg*. 2019;5(1):66–71.
6. Hachem LD, Mathieu F, Lamberti-Pasculli M, et al. Klippel-Feil syndrome: clinical phenotypes associated with surgical treatment. *Spine (Phila Pa 1976)*. 2020;45(11):718–726.
7. Kenna MA, Irace AL, Strychowsky JE, et al. Otolaryngologic manifestations of Klippel-Feil syndrome in children. *JAMA Otolaryngol Head Neck Surg*. 2018;144(3):238–243.

ADDITIONAL READING

- Brown MW, Templeton AW, Hodges FJ III. The incidence of acquired and congenital fusions in the cervical spine. *Am J Roentgenol Radium Ther Nucl Med*. 1964;92:1255–1259.
- Driscoll DJ, Rigamonti D, Gailloud P. Klippel-Feil syndrome. In: *NORD Guide to Rare Disorders*. Lippincott Williams and Wilkins; 2003:720.
- Gjorup PA, Gjorup L. Klippel-Feil's syndrome. *Dan Med Bull*. 1964;11:50–53.
- Hensinger RN, Lang JE, MacEwen GD. Klippel-Feil syndrome: a constellation of associated anomalies. *J Bone Joint Surg Am*. 1974;56(6):1246–1253.
- Klippel-Feil syndrome. In: Behrman RE, Kliegman RM, Jenson HB. *Nelson Textbook of Pediatrics*. 16th ed. W.B. Saunders Company; 2000:2090.
- Klippel-Feil sequence. In: Jones KL, Jones MC, del Campo M. *Smith's Recognizable Patterns of Human Malformation*. 7th ed. Elsevier Saunders; 2013:810–811.
- McGaughran JM, Kuna P, Das V. Audiological abnormalities in the Klippel-Feil syndrome. *Arch Dis Child*. 1998;79(4):352–355.
- Samartzis DD, Herman J, Lubicky JP, et al. Classification of congenitally fused cervical patterns in Klippel-Feil patients: epidemiology and role in the development of cervical spine-related symptoms. *Spine (Phila Pa 1976)*. 2006;31(21):E798–E804.
- Samartzis D, Kalluri P, Herman J, et al. Cervical scoliosis in the Klippel-Feil patient. *Spine (Phila Pa 1976)*. 2011;36(23):E1501–E1508.
- Thomsen MN, Schneider U, Weber M, et al. Scoliosis and congenital anomalies associated with Klippel-Feil syndrome types I–III. *Spine (Phila Pa 1976)*. 1997;22(4):396–401.
- Tracy MR, Dormans JP, Kusumi K. Klippel-Feil syndrome: clinical features and current understanding of etiology. *Clin Orthop Relat Res*. 2004;(424):183–190.
- Wheeless CR. Klippel-Feil syndrome. In: *Wheeless' Textbook of Orthopaedics*. Data Trace Internet Publishing; 1995–2009.
- Zhou PL, Poorman GW, Wang C, et al. Klippel-Feil: a constellation of diagnoses, a contemporary presentation, and recent national trends. *J Craniovertebr Junction Spine*. 2019;10(3):133–138.

CLINICAL PEARLS

- When examining the back, always look at the scapula for Sprengel deformity.
- If Sprengel deformity is observed, consider cervical spine x-rays to rule out fusion associated with Klippel-Feil syndrome.
- Remember that many patients are asymptomatic so be sure to thoroughly assess neck ROM in all patients.

KNEE DISLOCATION

Tricia Prince, DO, MS, AOCPMR • Timothy Tiu, MD, FAAPMR, CAQSM

BASICS

- Traumatic knee dislocation is defined as complete disruption of the integrity of the tibiofemoral articulation (1),(2),(3).
- A multiligamentous knee injury is defined as a grossly unstable knee with disruption of at least two of the four major ligamentous structures (2),(4),(5).
- Knee dislocation is a rare but potentially devastating injury. It may lead to amputation or inability to return to full function.
- The true incidence of knee dislocations is unknown, as up to 80% spontaneously reduce. Neurovascular evaluation is a critical aspect as delays in diagnosis can lead to catastrophic results, particularly missed popliteal artery injury (1),(2).
- High-velocity injuries involving a sudden violent force, such as a motor vehicle accident (MVA), falls from skiing, and injuries from gymnastics and extreme sports, are usually associated with an increased risk for neurovascular damage, owing to more extensive disruption to the joint capsule.
- Low-velocity injuries are usually due to sports, such as football or rugby, and usually have less soft tissue damage with better prognosis.
- Ultra low–velocity injuries are attributed to increasing rates of obesity (2).
- There are six structures within the knee that are at risk of injury with knee dislocation: anterior cruciate ligament (ACL), posterior cruciate ligament (PCL), medial cruciate ligament (MCL), lateral cruciate ligament (LCL), medial meniscus, and lateral meniscus. *Cautions*:
  - Documentation of pulses and motor response (ankle dorsiflexion) is essential.
  - Splint in slight flexion to prevent traction or compression of the popliteal artery (6)[C].

DESCRIPTION

- Categorized by the position of the tibia in relationship to the distal femur
- Anterior dislocation (40%):
  - Hyperextension of the knee of at least 30 degrees
  - Rupture of the posterior capsule followed by the PCL
- Posterior dislocation (33%):
  - Direct blow to the anterior tibia with the knee flexed at 90 degrees ("dashboard" injury or falling onto flexed knee)
  - ACL is usually spared.
- Medial dislocation (4%):
  - Varus stress causing tear to ACL, PCL, and LCL; highest risk of posterolateral corner (PLC) damage and thus the highest risk of irreducible dislocation
  - Associated with tibial plateau fracture
- Lateral dislocation (18%):
  - Valgus stress causing tear to ACL, PCL, and MCL
  - Associated with tibial plateau fracture
- Rotatory dislocation:
  - Twisting mechanism (planted foot and body twisting in opposite direction) that can be further divided into anteromedial, anterolateral, posterolateral
  - Posterolateral dislocations are nearly impossible to be reduced by closed method.
- Popliteal artery injury:
  - Reported in as high as 64% of dislocations. Recent large-scale study reports frequency of 3.3% (1).
  - Artery is fixed proximally at the fibrous insertion of the adductor magnus onto the medial femoral epicondyle and distally tethered by the tendinous arch of the soleus (1),(5),(7).
  - The popliteal artery (PA) sits within the popliteal fossa with branches to the collateral artery supply. The geniculate collateral arteries cannot compensate for a ruptured PA.
  - If vascular injury is not reversed within 6 to 8 hours, amputation rate approaches 90% (2).
  - Anterior dislocations place traction on the PA and cause contusion or intimal injury, which may result in delayed thrombosis.
  - Posterior dislocations (most common) cause direct intimal fracture or transection of the artery with immediate thrombosis.
- Fibular nerve injury:
  - The fibular nerve wraps around the fibular head.
  - May occur in up to 25–40% of dislocations
  - Characterized by hypesthesia of anterolateral leg and dorsum of foot, weakness of ankle dorsiflexion
  - Poor prognosis for recovery
  - Medial dislocations cause injury by traction to the nerve.
  - Rotatory injuries have a high incidence of traction and transection.

EPIDEMIOLOGY

- Incidence is estimated to be 0.18% of all trauma admissions (1).
- The most common mechanism of injury is an MVA.
- Most commonly anterior (40%), followed by posterior (33%); most common types associated with PA damage (5),(7),(8)
- PA injury rate previously reported up to 64%; newer data reports 3.3% (1).
- Full recovery of the fibular nerve is unlikely.

Prevalence

- MVAs (50–60%)
- Sports (30–50%)
- Falls (1–17%)

ETIOLOGY AND PATHOPHYSIOLOGY

- High-energy injuries such as MVAs, auto versus pedestrian accidents, and athletic injuries
- Football is the most common source of athletic injuries.
- Ground-level falls in obese patients

RISK FACTORS

- Morbid obesity is a potential risk factor for posterior dislocations.
- Contact or high-velocity sports

DIAGNOSIS

HISTORY

- Patient will usually hear a pop at time of injury.
- Have patient describe mechanism of injury, if possible.

PHYSICAL EXAM

- The initial physical exam may be difficult, owing to excessive swelling and pain.
- Subjective pain, instability, and swelling
- Grossly deformed knee/asymmetry
- Grossly unstable knee in anterior/posterior plane or on varus/valgus stress:
  - ACL and PCL, collateral ligament injuries
  - Suspect a relocated knee dislocation if the patient had a high-impact injury with multiple ligamentous laxity.
- Lateral/posterolateral (irreducible) dislocation:
  - Grossly deformed
  - Dimple sign: dimple of the medial skin and soft tissues
  - Pucker sign: Puckering of skin results from its attachment to the invaginated capsule (6).
- Evaluate vasculature:
  - By palpation, Doppler, ankle-brachial pressure indexes, and distal perfusion (5),(7)[C]
  - Dorsalis pedis, posterior tibialis, popliteal
  - Popliteal thrill or expanding pulsatile hematoma
  - Signs of distal ischemia: pallor, paresthesia, pain, paralysis, unequal temperature
  - If peripheral pulses are normal initially, it is essential to do serial, frequent exams with documentation of pulses (5),(7)[C].
  - Estimated 5–15% of knee dislocations may have a strong distal pulse initially with delayed expansion of intimal tear (2)[B].
- Neurologic examination:
  - Sensory: anterolateral lag, dorsum of foot, 1 web space
  - Motor: ankle dorsiflexion, eversion

DIFFERENTIAL DIAGNOSIS

- Tibial plateau fracture
- Supracondylar femoral fracture
- Isolated fibular nerve injury
- ACL injury/rupture

DIAGNOSTIC TESTS & INTERPRETATION

Initial Tests (lab, imaging)

- Complete blood count (CBC)
- Basic metabolic protein with blood urea nitrogen/creatinine (BUN/Cr)
- International normalized ratio (INR)/coagulation studies

- Knee x-rays: fractures common (periarticular, avulsion fracture, tibial plateau). Stress radiography enables assessment of ligamentous integrity (2).
- Ankle brachial index (ABI): systolic blood pressure (BP) from all four extremities with Doppler probe and BP cuff; ABI: highest pressure from dorsal pedal pulse or posterior tibial pulse/highest brachial BP (5),(6),(7):
  - Prospective study: ABI >0.90 had 100% negative predictive value for arterial injury requiring surgical repair (1),(2),(5),(8).
  - Patients with asymmetric pulses, normal reperfusion, and ABI <0.90 should undergo arteriography (2)[C].
- Angiography remains the "gold standard," but because of risks, there is evidence to support the use of selective angiography or computed tomography (CT) angiography (1),(2),(5),(7).
- Duplex Doppler
- Magnetic resonance imaging (MRI) may identify ligamentous injuries.

TREATMENT

- Prehospital:
  - If covering a game or event with potential high-impact injuries, initially assess for life-threatening injuries.
  - Basic life support: circulation, airway, breathing (CAB), assess for head and neck injury.
  - If knee dislocation is suspected, immediate neurovascular assessment becomes the focus of evaluation. If safe, remove shoes and socks for better neurovascular exam.
  - Splint knee in 20 degrees flexion in order to prevent spontaneous posterior tibia translation and preserve safety of the popliteal neurovascular structures (6)[C].
  - Plan for reduction in emergency room (ER).
- ER treatment:
  - Reduction to reduce pressure on both the neurovascular structures and the skin; successful under conscious sedation in most cases; intraoperative closed and, rarely, open reduction may be necessary (5)
  - If a "pucker sign" or "dimple sign" is evident, suspicion of an irreducible posterolateral knee dislocation should be raised and an emergency open reduction in the operating room is to be undertaken (6).
  - Intravenous (IV) analgesia for patient comfort
  - Vascular and orthopedic surgical consultation for open injury, evidence of PA injury, or unable to reduce dislocation

SURGERY/OTHER PROCEDURES

- All vascular injuries will need a vascular surgeon consult ASAP.
- Orthopedic consult
- Patients with hard signs of vascular injury should undergo immediate surgical exploration with or without intraoperative arteriography (6)[C],(7).
- Ligamentous repair/reconstruction versus conservative treatment with splinting alone depends on activity level of patient.
- Goal of repair is to provide a functional, stable joint:
  - Nonoperative care is reserved only for sedentary patients or if unable to undergo surgery (8)[C].
- Physical therapy will be essential for conservative and postoperative treatment.
- Rehabilitation depends on specific ligaments torn.
- Goal of 90 degrees knee flexion 6 weeks postoperatively and 120 degrees at 12 weeks (3).
- No return to full activity or sports before 9 months (5),(6)[C]

ADMISSION, INPATIENT, AND NURSING CONSIDERATIONS

- All patients with knee dislocation require admission for either arterial injury repair or observation of limb perfusion.
- Patients with normal pulses and ABI >0.90 should undergo 24 to 48 hours of serial examinations (1),(2),(5),(6)[C],(8).

ONGOING CARE

PROGNOSIS

- Prognosis depends on neurovascular damage, which depends on velocity of injury.
- Fibular nerve damage portends a worse prognosis. Full recovery is unlikely, but younger patients may have better nerve recovery (9).
- Complications include joint stiffness, joint contractures, ongoing knee instability, joint pain, and swelling (5).
- Recovery to good function of the knee for daily activities of living is likely, but return to demanding sports is not predictable (5).

COMPLICATIONS

- Amputation
- Compartment syndrome
- Neurovascular deficit
- Chronic pain
- Stiffness
- Instability
- Posttraumatic arthritis

REFERENCES

1. Chowdhry M, Burchette D, Whelan D, et al. Knee dislocation and associated injuries: an analysis of the American College of Surgeons National Trauma Data Bank. *Knee Surg Sports Traumatol Arthrosc*. 2020;28(2):568–575.
2. Ockuly AC, Imada AO, Richter DL, et al. Initial evaluation and classification of knee dislocations. *Sports Med Arthrosc Rev*. 2020;28(3):87–93.
3. Mühlenfeld N, Berthold DP, Münch LN, et al. Epidemiology of complete knee dislocations: an updated classification system. *Arch Orthop Trauma Surg*. 2022;142(10):2711–2718.
4. Wascher DC, Schenck RC Jr, Treme GP, et al. The knee dislocation classification system is simple, reproducible, and allows communication among surgeons. *J Knee Surg*. 2022;35(09):1044–1045.
5. Henrichs A. A review of knee dislocations. *J Athl Train*. 2004;39(4):365–369.
6. Gottlieb M, Koyfman A, Long B. Evaluation and management of knee dislocation in the emergency department. *J Emerg Med*. 2020;58(1):34–42.
7. Mohseni M, Simon LV. *Knee Dislocation*. StatPearls Publishing; 2025. Updated February 27, 2024. Accessed August 8, 2025. https://www.ncbi.nlm.nih.gov/books/NBK470595/
8. Ng JWG, Myint Y, Ali FM. Management of multiligament knee injuries. *EFORT Open Rev*. 2020;5(3):145–155.
9. Tan L, Wang J, Liu X, et al. Risk factors for common peroneal nerve injury in knee dislocation: a retrospective study. *Research Square*. Preprint posted online March 4, 2020. doi:10.21203/rs.3.rs-15922/v1

ADDITIONAL READING

Piedade SR, Hutchinson MR, Parker D, et al. *Sideline Management in Sports*. Springer Nature; 2024:135–150.

CLINICAL PEARLS

- Knee dislocations often reduce spontaneously. If it is a high-impact injury with knee deformity or multiple ligamentous laxity, suspect a knee dislocation (1),(2),(3),(4).
- All knee dislocations need a vascular surgery consult ASAP.
- Normal pulse does not necessarily indicate normal PA. Angiography remains the "gold standard," but there is evidence to support the use of selective angiography or CT angiography (1),(2),(5),(8)[C].
- Neurologic deficit indicates worse injury and prognosis.
- Splint knee in 20 degrees flexion to protect neurovascular structures (6)[C].
- PA damage that is not surgically repaired within 8 hours is likely to result in above-knee amputation (2),(5),(6),(8).
- Ultra low–velocity injuries are more common in obese individuals and due to falls (1).

KNEE FABELLA SYNDROME

Keifer P. Walsh, DO, MS

BASICS

DESCRIPTION

Knee fabella syndrome is an overuse disorder of the fabella, a sesamoid bone in the posterolateral knee. Similar to the patella for the extensor mechanism, the fabella redirects forces of knee flexion. It is uncommon and therefore should be considered a diagnosis of exclusion when treatment modalities for related conditions are unsuccessful.

EPIDEMIOLOGY

- Prevalence of the fabella (regardless of symptoms) across most European countries ranges from 10% to 30%, although has been reported in up to 87% in specific Asian populations (1)
- Bilateral in nearly 50% if present
- Incidence of those which become symptomatic is unclear

ETIOLOGY AND PATHOPHYSIOLOGY

Anatomy:

- Sesamoid within the posterolateral capsule of the knee joint
- Embedded in the muscle fibers of the lateral gastrocnemius muscle and articulates with the lateral femoral condyle
- Fabellofibular ligament (ligament of Vallois) inserts at the fibular head superficial to the popliteus muscle
- Considered a static stabilizer of the posterolateral corner (PLC)
- Presence of fabella has been associated with decreased width and thickness of the common fibular nerve adjacent to the bone compared to proximal portions of the nerve in cadaver studies (2).
- Histologically can either be bony (compact bone surrounded by trabecular bone, surfaced with fibrocartilage and collagen fibers) or less commonly cartilaginous (hyaline cartilage with flattened chondrocytes) (3)

RISK FACTORS

- Anatomic variations including size of fabella or proximity to other bony or soft tissue structures
- Biomechanical factors such as changes in gait or knee alignment including genu recurvatum
- Direct trauma to posterior knee
- Overuse including repetitive knee flexion causing mechanical irritation of local structures or tightness of the lateral gastrocnemius muscle
- Postoperative status from total knee arthroplasty or high tibial osteotomy has been well-demonstrated in the literature (4).

DIAGNOSIS

HISTORY

- Posterior knee pain that is worse in full or prolonged knee extension
- Catching/clicking sensation with deep knee flexion
- Occupational or recreational requirement for repetitive knee flexion
- Foot drop or radicular symptoms in the lateral leg or foot (sparing the heel)

PHYSICAL EXAM

- Tenderness with palpation over posterolateral knee
- Recreation of clicking/catching with passive flexion from 90 degrees into full extension or active deep squat

DIFFERENTIAL DIAGNOSIS

- Baker cyst
- Biceps femoris tendinopathy (insertional)
- Iliotibial (IT) band pain/syndrome
- Lateral gastrocnemius tendinopathy
- Lateral meniscus injury
- Osteoarthritis
- Osteochondritis dissecans (femoral condyle)
- Popliteal tendinopathy
- PLC injury (lateral collateral ligament [LCL], popliteus tendon, popliteofibular ligament or dynamic stabilizers)
- Tibiofibular joint instability

DIAGNOSTIC TESTS & INTERPRETATION

Considered a clinical diagnosis, imaging studies should be used to both rule out other etiologies and confirm the presence of a fabella at the site of typical symptoms.

Initial Tests (lab, imaging)

- X-ray or ultrasound to identify fabella
- Magnetic resonance imaging (MRI) may demonstrate fabella irritation, inflammation, thickening of lateral gastrocnemius tendon, or damage to articular surface of posterolateral femoral condyle.

TREATMENT

GENERAL MEASURES

- Conservative management includes activity modification to minimize or alter excess knee flexion or twisting.
- Physical therapy to strengthen muscles of the knee extensor mechanism, improve knee flexibility, and provide manual therapy.
- Nonsteroidal anti-inflammatory drugs (NSAIDs) may be beneficial for acute symptoms taken either orally or topically.
- There is no consensus that bracing reduces symptoms or prevents complications from knee fabella syndrome, although may help reinforce proper biomechanics/alignment or aid in patient confidence during activity or sport.

ADDITIONAL THERAPIES

- Injection with corticosteroid may provide pain relief for inflammation of adjacent tissues.
- Nerve hydrodissection for secondary common fibular entrapment neuropathy can be considered.
- Radial extracorporeal shockwave therapy has shown benefit for pain (5)[B].

SURGERY/OTHER PROCEDURES

Surgical excision (fabellectomy) is definitive and can often be done arthroscopically (6)[B].

ONGOING CARE

PROGNOSIS

Most individuals recover with conservative measures and therefore have a good prognosis, although those with predisposing anatomic factors are more likely to require surgical intervention.

COMPLICATIONS

- Common fibular neuropathy
- Fabella fracture or stress fracture
- Popliteal artery entrapment syndrome

REFERENCES

1. Driessen A, Balke M, Offerhaus C, et al. The fabella syndrome—a rare cause of posterolateral knee pain: a review of the literature and two case reports. *BMC Musculoskelet Disord*. 2014;15:100.
2. Dalip D, Iwanaga J, Oskouian RJ, et al. A comprehensive review of the fabella bone. *Cureus*. 2018;10(6):e2736.
3. Kawashima T, Takeishi H, Yoshitomi S, et al. Anatomical study of the fabella, fabellar complex, and its clinical implications. *Surg Radiol Anat*. 2007;29(8):611–616.
4. Okano E, Yoshioka T, Yanai T, et al. Fabella syndrome as an uncommon cause of posterolateral knee pain after total knee arthroplasty: a case report and review of the literature. *Case Rep Orthop*. 2016;2016:4328462.
5. Seol PH, Ha KW, Kim YH, et al. Effect of radial extracorporeal shock wave therapy in patients in fabella syndrome. *Ann Rehabil Med*. 2016;40(6):1124–1128.
6. Weng SP, Wu TM, Chien CS, et al. Treatment of fabella syndrome with arthroscopic fabellectomy: a case series and literature review. *BMC Musculoskelet Disord*. 2021;22(1):748.

ADDITIONAL READING

- Provencher MT, Sanchez G, Ferrari MB, et al. Arthroscopy-assisted fabella excision: surgical technique. *Arthrosc Tech*. 2017;6(2):e369–e374.
- Zipple JT, Hammer RL, Loubert PV. Treatment of fabella syndrome with manual therapy: a case report. *J Orthop Sports Phys Ther*. 2003;33(1):33–39.

CLINICAL PEARLS

- Knee fabella syndrome is very uncommon, and therefore, other disorders of the posterolateral knee should be considered first.
- At-risk populations include those with repetitive knee flexion activities or those who have had injuries or surgical procedures involving posterolateral structures.
- Most cases of knee fabella syndrome can be managed conservatively with activity modification and physical therapy, although surgical excision is effective.

KÖHLER DISEASE (ASEPTIC NECROSIS OF THE TARSAL NAVICULAR)

Peter Clements, MD

BASICS

DESCRIPTION

- Pediatric osteochondrosis of the tarsal navicular, first described by Alban Köhler in 1908 (1)
- Osteochondrosis is a disease process that causes necrosis of the ossification center of a developing bone and is followed by regeneration.

EPIDEMIOLOGY

- Predominant age: occurs in children 2 to 7 years of age (average age 5 years) (2)
- Predominant gender: males > females (4 to 6:1)
- Usually occurs unilaterally; bilateral in only ~15–20% of cases
- Appears to be no relation between body weight and incidence
- Consideration:
  - Adult-onset navicular osteonecrosis is known as Mueller-Weiss disease (also known as Brailsford disease).

ETIOLOGY AND PATHOPHYSIOLOGY

- Navicular development:
  - The navicular becomes evident on radiographs between 18 and 24 months in girls and between 30 and 36 months in boys.
  - A denser and more irregularly shaped navicular is often present in children whose navicular ossifies later.
  - These findings are similar in appearance to those in Köhler disease.
  - The navicular ossifies from a single center in 2/3 of children and from multiple centers in the remainder. Those ossifying later than normal tend to be from multiple centers.
  - A dense perichondral network of blood vessels has been described on the nonarticular surfaces with numerous penetrating arteries.
- Theories of etiology:
  - Questionably a normal variant but does not explain why some individuals are asymptomatic
  - Some believe that it is avascular necrosis secondary to compression prior to ossification (3); however, this does not explain acute onset of pain, lack of correlation with radiographic changes in a short amount of time, and that regardless of treatment, a normal navicular is the end result (true necrosis should cause deformity).
  - Most likely a syndrome or continuum of disease because radiographic changes can be seen in asymptomatic individuals. Perhaps those who are symptomatic have experienced a stress injury to the ossifying bone. This may explain radiographic changes, with remodeling to a normal-appearing bone.

RISK FACTORS

- May be caused by repetitive microtrauma to the maturing navicular ossification center (the last tarsal bone to ossify) (4)
- Compression of the bony nucleus at a critical phase of growth may occlude the penetrating blood vessels and produce ischemia and aseptic necrosis of the bone.
- Delayed ossification leading to irregular ossification centers may predispose to disease.
- Occurrence has not shown to be related to acute macrotrauma, age at first walking, foot type, or family history.

DIAGNOSIS

Although variations in morphology of the navicular have been described, the diagnosis of Köhler disease is made on the basis of both clinical and radiographic findings.

HISTORY

- It is often difficult for young children to localize pain, but it should be over the midfoot area.
- Repetitive microtrauma (running, sports) may be a risk factor.
- A history of macrotrauma should lead the practitioner to consider other causes of foot pain.

PHYSICAL EXAM

- Signs and symptoms:
  - Insidious onset of foot pain and limp aggravated by activity
  - Time to presentation varies from days to months after onset of pain.
- Physical examination:
  - Look for localized edema and warmth in the area of the tarsal navicular.
  - Palpate the entire foot and ankle; tenderness should be localized to the medial midfoot.
  - Check the range of motion of the ankle and subtalar joints, which should be normal.
  - Examine the knee and hip, which can be the source of referred pain and limp.

DIFFERENTIAL DIAGNOSIS

- Normal variants: Variations of size and shape of the navicular ossification center may be indistinguishable from Köhler disease except for the absence of symptoms.
- Osteochondritis dissecans
- Occult fracture of the midfoot

DIAGNOSTIC TESTS & INTERPRETATION

Radiographs:

- Standard anteroposterior, lateral, and oblique radiographs of the foot should be obtained.
- Findings (5):
  - Varying degrees of navicular sclerosis
  - Diminished size or flattening of the navicular ("Alka-Seltzer-on-end" appearance)
  - Occasional loss of trabecular pattern and fragmentation

- A person with an asymptomatic foot with abnormal radiographic features found incidentally does not have Köhler disease.
- Bone scintigraphy (5)[C]:
  - If diagnosis is not clear based on x-rays, a bone scan may show decreased uptake in the navicular, indicating decreased or interrupted blood supply.
  - In the later phases, may show increased uptake indicating revascularization
- Pathologic findings:
  - Patchy areas of bone destruction and dead trabeculae with interference of normal ossification

TREATMENT

GENERAL MEASURES

- Acute treatment:
  - Ice for inflammation/pain reduction
  - Nonsteroidal anti-inflammatory drugs (NSAIDs) or acetaminophen for analgesia
- Despite not altering the long-term outcome, immobilization has been shown to decrease the duration of symptoms (5)[C].
- Immobilization:
  - Patients with cast immobilization are typically pain free at 3 months, whereas those treated without casting were symptomatic until 15 months on average.
  - Those casted for a minimum of 2 months were asymptomatic in the shortest time.
  - Weight-bearing status does not appear to affect outcome.

ADDITIONAL THERAPIES

- Orthoses have not been found to be effective.
- Rehabilitation: usually not indicated

SURGERY/OTHER PROCEDURES

Rarely required

ONGOING CARE

FOLLOW-UP RECOMMENDATIONS

Orthopedic referral is indicated if symptoms do not resolve with conservative management.

Patient Monitoring

- In a study of 12 cases, complete restoration of normal bone structure occurred in 8 months (minimum of 6 months and maximum of 13 months) (6)[C].
- At 30-year follow-up, zero patients showed degenerative changes at the talonavicular joint, and no radiographic differences were seen compared to the unaffected foot (6)[C].

PROGNOSIS

- Complete resolution of symptoms with reconstitution of the navicular can be expected in all patients.
- No evidence of cartilage degeneration in long-term follow-up studies.

REFERENCES

1. Köhler A. A frequent disease of individual bones in children. *Munch Med Wochenschr*. 1908;55:1923–1925.
2. Chan JY, Young JL. Köhler disease: avascular necrosis in the child. *Foot Ankle Clin*. 2019;24(1):83–88.
3. Trammell AP, Davis DD, Scott A. *Kohler Disease*. StatPearls Publishing; 2023. Updated August 7, 2023. Accessed September 20, 2025. https://www.ncbi.nlm.nih.gov/books/NBK507831/
4. Santos L, Estanqueiro P, Matos G, et al. Köhler disease: an infrequent or underdiagnosed cause of a child's limping? *Acta Reumatol Port*. 2015;40(3):304–305.
5. Alhamdani M, Kelly C. Köhler's disease presenting as acute foot injury. *Am J Emerg Med*. 2017;35(11):1787.e5–1787.e6.
6. Khoury J, Jerushalmi J, Loberant N, et al. Köhler disease: diagnoses and assessment by bone scintigraphy. *Clin Nucl Med*. 2007;32(3):179–181.

ADDITIONAL READING

- Borges JL, Guille JT, Bowen JR. Köhler's bone disease of the tarsal navicular. *J Pediatr Orthop*. 1995;15(5):596–598.
- Gips S, Ruchman RB, Groshar D. Bone imaging in Köhler's disease. *Clin Nucl Med*. 1997;22(9):636–637.
- Ippolito E, Ricciardi Pollini PT, Falez F. Köhler's disease of the tarsal navicular: long-term follow-up of 12 cases. *J Pediatr Orthop*. 1984;4(4):416–417.
- Manusov EG, Lillegard WA, Raspa RF, et al. Evaluation of pediatric foot problems: part I. The forefoot and the midfoot. *Am Fam Physician*. 1996;54(2):592–606.
- Sharp RJ, Calder JDF, Saxby TS. Osteochondritis of the navicular: a case report. *Foot Ankle Int*. 2003;24(6):509–513.
- Stanton BK, Karlin JM, Scurran BL. Köhler's disease. *J Am Podiatr Med Assoc*. 1992;82(12):625–629.
- Williams GA, Cowell HR. Köhler's disease of the tarsal navicular. *Clin Orthop Relat Res*. 1981;(158):53–58.

CLINICAL PEARLS

- Although all patients eventually will have complete resolution of symptoms, immobilization in a cast for at least 8 weeks has shown to shorten the duration of symptoms.
- Sports may be resumed once symptoms have resolved.
- Long-term follow-up studies have found no increase in the rate of arthritis or other chronic foot problems in adults with a history of Köhler disease during childhood.

KYPHOSIS

Joseph Medellin, MD, MPH, MBA ▪ Mark E. Lavallee, MD, CSCS, FACSM, FAMSSM

BASICS

DESCRIPTION

- There are three general types of spine curvature disorders: kyphosis, scoliosis, and lordosis.
- Kyphosis is a fixed exaggerated anteroposterior (AP) curvature of the thoracic spine.
- Scoliosis is a fixed lateral curvature of the spine (>10 degrees by Cobb angle) and vertebral rotation.
- Lordosis is a fixed concave exaggerated AP curvature of the lumbar spine.
- Kyphoscoliosis is a combination of lateral and AP curvatures of the spine.
- Scheuermann juvenile kyphosis (SK) is osteochondrosis of the secondary ossification center of a vertebrae causing thoracic kyphosis.
- Synonym(s): curvature of the spine; hunchback; dowager's hump; postural round back

EPIDEMIOLOGY

- Most commonly seen in postmenopausal women who have osteoporosis
- Rare occurrence in skeletally maturing patients; occasionally seen in adolescents as they transition through their secondary growth spurt
- Females > males
- Kyphosis has an incidence of 1 in 1,000, whereas scoliosis is about 2 in 100.
- SK has been reported to be between 0.4% and 10% between ages 13 and 17 years and is more common in boys than girls.

ETIOLOGY AND PATHOPHYSIOLOGY

Genetics

- In 2007, CHD7 was identified as the first gene with polymorphisms associated with susceptibility to scoliosis; however, no genetic loci have been associated with adult kyphosis at this time.
- SK likely has a genetic etiology. Clinical and genetic investigations theorize an autosomal dominant inheritance associated with a mutant major gene, while also identifying candidate genes such as IHH, PAX1, and SOX9.

RISK FACTORS

- Female gender and remaining growth potential
- Family history is the primary risk. Inheritance patterns are still being actively elucidated.
- Myelodysplasia, Marfan syndrome, Ehlers-Danlos syndrome, osteogenesis imperfecta type 2, and achondroplasia have all been associated with kyphosis and/or scoliosis.

COMMONLY ASSOCIATED CONDITIONS

- Osteoporosis
- Vertebral fracture
- Scoliosis
- Marfan syndrome
- Ehlers-Danlos syndrome
- Osteogenesis imperfecta type 2
- Neurofibromatosis

DIAGNOSIS

HISTORY

- Upper back curvature, often painless
- Often noticed by an observer, such as a parent, partner, or spouse
- Cases of nonpainful, nontraumatic kyphosis are often discovered in school-based screenings, preparticipation examinations, or general wellness exams.
- A family history of kyphosis, scoliosis, connective tissue disorder, or neurologic disorder should be sought.

PHYSICAL EXAM

- Subtle findings, such as noticeable "hump" on back and/or hyperlordosis in lumbar spine (aka "swayback")
- Pain is not often a feature of idiopathic kyphosis; however, if present, other causes of kyphosis need to be evaluated.
- Check posture, leg length discrepancy, muscle tone, and assessment of reflexes.
- A complete neuro-orthopedic exam (i.e., cavus feet seen in Charcot-Marie-Tooth syndrome)
- Assess patient's ability to "correct" deformity with attempted thoracic hyperextension. Postural round back will improve, whereas true kyphosis will have minimal improvement.
- Marfanoid body habitus, hypermobile joints, or hyperextensible skin (i.e., Marfan or Ehlers-Danlos syndrome)
- Café-au-lait spots (i.e., neurofibromatosis)
- Adam forward bending test (to look for associated scoliosis): Patient stands with legs locked, bends at the waist, and arms toward feet. Examiner stands behind patient, lowers head, and views across patient's back, looking for elevated and rotated vertebral segments.
- A scoliometer may also be used to assess if patient has scoliosis. Measure the angle of trunk rotation (ATR). An ATR of 7 degrees or greater correlates (83% sensitivity, 86% specificity) to a clinically significant curve. The ATR multiplied by 3 estimates the curvature (Cobb angle).

DIFFERENTIAL DIAGNOSIS

- Congenital kyphosis: anomalies of vertebral segmentation and/or formation (Klippel-Feil syndrome; vertebral defects, anal atresia, cardiac defects, tracheoesophageal fistula, renal anomalies, and limb abnormalities [VACTERL] syndrome)
- Neuromuscular scoliosis: upper motor neuron (Friedreich ataxia, cerebral palsy, Charcot-Marie-Tooth syndrome, syringomyelia, muscular dystrophy) or lower motor neuron (poliomyelitis, spina bifida), spinal dysraphism (myelomeningocele)
- SK: pathognomonic Schmorl nodes on at least two consecutive levels
- Kyphosis secondary to bone demineralization (osteoporosis)
- Vertebral fractures/trauma
- Benign or malignant tumors (i.e., Paget disease of bone)
- Parkinson disease: "stooping posture"
- Spinal tuberculosis
- Rickets
- Marfan syndrome
- Osteogenesis imperfecta type 2
- Achondroplasia
- Ehlers-Danlos syndrome, especially kyphoscoliotic type
- Ankylosing spondylitis

DIAGNOSTIC TESTS & INTERPRETATION

- The initial imaging test for kyphosis is typically an AP and lateral chest x-ray. This allows for the assessment of degenerative joint disease, fractures, Schmorl nodes, and the angle of kyphosis. For a more comprehensive evaluation, a lateral standing radiograph of the entire spine is recommended.
- Schmorl nodes, which are protrusions of intervertebral disc cartilage through the vertebral body endplate of adjacent vertebrae, are characteristic of SK.
- If scoliosis is associated with kyphosis, standing posteroanterior (PA) and lateral radiographs of the entire spine are required. In children and adolescents, it is important to include the iliac crests and iliac apophyses in the radiographs to accurately assess the Risser score.
- If kyphosis or scoliosis is seen in a child, a bone age can be obtained to determine the best next steps in management. Hand and wrist x-rays are the gold standard to calculate bone age for a child.
- Indications for magnetic resonance imaging (MRI):
  - Age <10 years
  - Rapid progression of a curve
  - Abnormal neurologic examination
  - Atypical pain with inconclusive radiograph

TREATMENT

- Management options for kyphosis include observation, physical therapy, oral medications (for conditions like osteoporosis), bracing, and, in rare cases, surgical intervention (1)[C].
- Idiopathic kyphosis in adolescents and Scheuermann kyphosis seldom require surgery.
- When treating painful kyphosis, the first step is to identify the underlying cause.
- Observation: In young adolescents with a curvature of <50 degrees, no pain and no evidence of progression, observation may be sufficient.
  - Manage with serial radiographs every 4 to 6 months depending on skeletal maturity.
  - Skeletally mature with curves <40 degrees: Follow with history, physical exam, and occasional radiograph.
  - Consider lateral standing radiograph to include with observation imaging every 6 months.
  - Some clinicians advocate following juvenile patients with exaggerated kyphotic curves of >40 degrees at 4- to 6-month intervals until iliac crest growth plates close (2)[B].

- Oral medications: Check bone densitometry (dual energy x-ray absorptiometry) on patients with nontraumatic vertebral fracture and those with osteoporosis. Treatment of osteoporosis with bisphosphonates has been shown to improve kyphosis-related back pain. *Do not use bisphosphonates in women of reproductive age due to potential long-term teratogenic effects.*
- Physical therapy: Strengthening and stretching exercises for the abdominal, hamstring, and paraspinal muscles are recommended to prevent excessive lordosis and hamstring contractures.
  - Schroth physiotherapeutic scoliosis-specific exercise is a nonoperative treatment for scoliosis and kyphosis, used as a standalone or as an adjunct to bracing (3)[A].
  - Meta-analysis has indicated that using the Schroth method of physical therapy has led to statistically significant reductions in Cobb angle and improvements in quality of life; however, these changes did not reach a 5-degree threshold generally accepted as clinically significant and many of the studies have methodologic limitations (4)[A].
- Bracing: Painful curves between 50 and 70 degrees or progressive deformity >65 degrees may be braced (many associated with Scheuermann).
  - In immature with curve >60 degrees or in those who progress >10 degrees during observation to a curve >40 degrees, bracing should be considered.
  - The goal of bracing is to delay/prevent curve progression until skeletally mature.
  - More common rigid and soft bracing options include (5)[A]:
    - Milwaukee brace (for curves above T7) (rigid)
    - Thoracic lumbar sacral orthosis (TLSO) with an underarm rigid brace (if curve is below T7) (rigid)
    - Wood-Cheneau-Rigo de rotational brace (rigid)
    - Boston brace (rigid)
    - Lyon brace (very rigid)
    - Triac (low rigidity)
    - SpineCor (elastic)
    - ScoliSMART (soft suit)
    - Flexpine (semi-rigid)
  - Once the curve is supported, the patient should wear the brace 18 to 20 hours/d.
  - Outcomes of brace treatment are associated with how effectively the brace is worn. The development of force sensors and compliance monitors have been developed to monitor the quality of brace usage such as with the robotic spine exoskeleton (RoSE) dynamic brace (6)[B]. Brace use may be tapered to nighttime use once the progression of the curve is controlled. The Charleston brace and the Providence brace are two prominent nighttime braces that have been developed to reduce the wear time of rigid bracing and enhance the compliance of wearing braces (5)[A].
  - Contraindication to bracing: curves >80 degrees, extreme thoracic hypokyphosis, high thoracic or cervical curves
  - Standing radiograph images every 6 months (or 4 months if progressing and skeletally immature) should be performed.
  - Bracing juvenile/adolescent patients should be continued if there is no progression of curvature and vertical growth is still occurring. Generally, bracing continues until near skeletal maturity, such as Risser stage 4 for young women or Risser stage 5 for young men, or when other signs of growth cessation are present.
  - Spinal orthosis, especially dynamic hyperextension braces, seems effective in improving adverse outcomes associated with osteoporotic hyperkyphotic such as fatigue, back pain, and a reduction in back extensor strength (7)[A].
- Surgery: Literature supports surgical correction indicated at >75 degrees with SK and 60 degrees for congenital kyphosis.
  - Wedge osteotomies of the posterior aspect of the vertebrae have been done to correct those with severe kyphosis in skeletally mature patients without osteoporosis.
  - Vertebroplasty and balloon kyphoplasty are procedures available to patients who develop kyphosis related to osteoporosis or trauma-related collapse of thoracic vertebral body.
  - Once a curve reaches 80 degrees, it is assumed it is not controlled by bracing; operative correction with posterior instrumentation/fusion is recommended.
  - Upper thoracic kyphosis with curves >100 degrees cause significant restrictive lung disease.

ADDITIONAL THERAPIES

Postural "round back," not true kyphosis, has been shown to improve with physical therapy focused on postural control and core/shoulder girdle strengthening.

ONGOING CARE

FOLLOW-UP RECOMMENDATIONS

- Refer to orthopedic/spine specialist when there is a:
  - A thoracic curve that is too high for effective bracing (apex above T6)
  - Worsening curvature despite bracing
  - Curvature in the newborn and infant and any children <10 years old
  - Curvature associated with severe trauma/vertebral fracture
  - Curvature-associated malignancy
- Juvenile/adolescent kyphosis is often diagnosed or progresses during a sensitive time of life. Studies have demonstrated a negative effect on body image, self-esteem, and attitude with treatment. This may affect compliance. Treatment is time-consuming, confining, and can be uncomfortable all while the adolescent is faced with many lifestyle changes. Clinicians should be aware of the possible psychological impact from new demands on the patient and family. Discussions about patient's thoughts/feelings on treatment as well as support groups should be considered (8)[B],(9)[C].

REFERENCES

1. O'Donnell J, Wu W, Youn A, et al. Scheuermann kyphosis: current concepts and management. *Curr Rev Musculoskeletal Med*. 2023;16(11):521–530.
2. Weinstein SL, Dolan LA, Wright JG, et al. Effects of bracing in adolescents with idiopathic scoliosis. *N Engl J Med*. 2013;369(16):1512–1521.
3. Schreiber S. Whibley D, Somers EC. Schroth physiotherapeutic scoliosis-specific exercise (PSSE) trials—systematic review of methods and recommendations for future research. *Children (Basel)*. 2023;10(6):954.
4. Zhu Y, Zhu C, Song H, et al. Effectiveness of Schroth exercises for adolescent idiopathic scoliosis: a meta-analysis. *PeerJ*. 2025;13:e19639.
5. Ali A, Fontanari V, Fontana M, et al. Spinal deformities and advancement in corrective orthoses. *Bioengineering (Basel)*. 2020;8(1):2.
6. Park JH, Stegall PR, Roye DP, et al. Robotic spine exoskeleton (RoSE): characterizing the 3-D stiffness of the human torso in the treatment of spine deformity. *IEEE Trans Neural Syst Rehabil Eng*. 2018;26(5):1026–1035.
7. Sánchez-Pinto-Pinto B, Romero-Morales C, López- López D, et al. Efficacy of bracing on thoracic kyphotic angle and functionality in women with osteoporosis: a systematic review. *Medicina (Kaunas)*. 2022;58(6):693.
8. Bezalel T, Kalichman L. Improvement of clinical and radiographical presentation of Scheuermann disease after Schroth therapy treatment. *J Bodyw Mov Ther*. 2015;19(2):232–237.
9. Reichel D, Schanz J. Developmental psychological aspects of scoliosis treatment. *Pediatr Rehabil*. 2003;6(3–4):221–225.

ADDITIONAL READING

- Dolan LA, Haggerty KA, Weinstein SL, et al. Evaluation of TLSOS in the bracing in adolescent idiopathic scoliosis trial (BrAIST). *Scoliosis*. 2013;8(Suppl 1):048.
- Gao X, Gordon D, Zhang D, et al. CHD7 gene polymorphisms are associated with susceptibility to idiopathic scoliosis. *Am J Hum Genet*. 2007;80(5):957–965.
- Grossman DC, Curry SJ, Owens DK, et al. Screening for adolescent idiopathic scoliosis: US Preventive Services Task Force recommendation statement. *JAMA*. 2018;319(2):165–172.
- Jarvis J, Garbedian S, Swamy G. Juvenile idiopathic scoliosis: the effectiveness of part-time bracing. *Spine (Phila Pa 1976)*. 2008;33(10):1074–1078.
- Negrini S, Fusco C, Minozzi S, et al. Exercises reduce the progression rate of adolescent idiopathic scoliosis: results of a comprehensive systematic review of the literature. *Disabil Rehabil*. 2008;30(10):772–785.

CLINICAL PEARLS

- Sports and athletic activity are allowed and encouraged for all patients with nonpainful kyphosis in nonoperative treatment.
- Postoperative patients' return to play is at the discretion of the surgeon.
- Braces are used to prevent progression and are not intended to correct the curve. Compliance is essential to treatment success.
- Most studies support results with brace wear of 18 to 20 hours/d. Night-only braces have also been shown to have success.
- Braces for juvenile/adolescent patients should be worn until the Risser score is 4 (closed growth plates).
- Manipulation therapy has not been proven to help correct curvature of the spine.

LACERATIONS AND SOFT TISSUE INJURIES IN ATHLETES

Theodora L. Swenson, MD • Caitlyn C. Mooney, MD, FAAP, CAQSM

BASICS

DESCRIPTION

- Lacerations, contusions, hematomas, and abrasions are disruptions to the skin resulting from trauma.
- Soft tissue injuries include:
  - Friction blisters—pressure and repetitive shear forces causing delamination of the outermost epidermal skin layer causing fluid to accumulate between the separated layers
  - Chafing—repetitive skin irritation without separation of dermis from epidermis
  - Abrasions—superficial skin wounds mainly limited to the epidermis
  - Lacerations—full-thickness skin wounds involving the epidermis and dermis; may occur with injury to connective tissue, cutaneous nerves, and vasculature
  - Hematomas—blood extravasation outside of blood vessels into surrounding soft tissue
  - Seromas—clear serous fluid buildup that develops after surgery or injury
- Soft tissue injuries can occur on any part of the body:
  - Blisters generally occur at sites of friction.
  - Chafing most commonly occurs in areas of skin-to-skin contact (i.e., groin, axilla) or where clothes rub (i.e., "jogger's nipple").

EPIDEMIOLOGY

Nearly 11 million lacerations are treated in emergency departments yearly; this number does not include injuries treated in offices or on the sidelines.

ETIOLOGY AND PATHOPHYSIOLOGY

- Soft tissue injuries are most commonly caused by blunt trauma.
- Lacerations can also occur after contact with a sharp object, such as sporting equipment.

RISK FACTORS

- Athletes participating in contact sports and sports requiring sharp equipment are at highest risk for soft tissue injury.
- The most common preventable cause of skin trauma is improper equipment use and/or lack of use.
- Risk factors for friction blisters include poorly fitting footwear, moisture, heat/sweat, external load, and activity duration.

COMMONLY ASSOCIATED CONDITIONS

Associated symptoms can include:

- Bleeding
- Foreign body
- Paresthesia
- Loss of motor function
- Diminished vascularization

DIAGNOSIS

- First and foremost, observe standard universal precautions. In trauma, initially assess for limb- or life-threatening conditions via a primary and secondary survey and control bleeding.
- Diagnosis is made by visually examining the injury.

HISTORY

- Determine the time, mechanism, and circumstances surrounding the injury.
- Assess for additional injuries:
  - Tendon, muscle, vascular, or nerve injury; complaints of weakness, numbness, or tingling
  - Underlying fracture
- Obtain medication history:
  - Important medications to consider include aspirin, nonsteroidal anti-inflammatory drugs (NSAIDs), clopidogrel, direct-acting oral anti-coagulant (DOACs), Coumadin (warfarin), heparin, or other anticoagulant or antiplatelet medications and supplements
  - Consider allergies:
    - Latex, lidocaine, iodine, or pain medications
- Determine immunization status:
  - Assess if tetanus status is up-to-date.

PHYSICAL EXAM

- Physical exam should be focused to the site of injury.
- Visually inspect the wound and assess injury to underlying structures.
- Explore wound for foreign body.
- Note the location, size, shape, and estimate the amount of blood lost.
- Additional considerations, as below.
  - Vitals: Assess for hemodynamic stability.
  - Cardiovascular: Decreased peripheral pulses distal to the site of injury should initiate prompt referral.
  - Pulmonary: Unequal breath sounds after chest trauma necessitate evaluation for pneumothorax.
  - Head/eyes/ears/nose/throat: Assess for concussion and cranial nerves in cases of trauma.
  - Musculoskeletal: Deformities or concerns for fracture under an open wound should prompt referral or further evaluation.
  - Neurologic: Evaluate underlying nerve damage by performing a sensory exam distal to site of injury.
  - Skin: Patients with thin skin may require adapting the repair modality.
  - Psychological: Psychomotor agitation may make following universal precautions more challenging and may also signify underlying head trauma.

DIFFERENTIAL DIAGNOSIS

- Skin avulsion
- Contusion
- Abrasion
- Laceration
- Hematoma
- Seroma
- Rash/dermatitis

DIAGNOSTIC TESTS & INTERPRETATION

- Radiographs:
  - Useful for concerns of underlying fracture
  - May help to identify foreign bodies
- Computed tomography (CT):
  - May help to identify foreign bodies and underlying bony injuries
- Ultrasound (US):
  - Useful to identify foreign bodies with the same density as soft tissue (e.g., splinters) (1)
  - Provides real-time visualization
  - Can facilitate targeted foreign body removal, decreasing tissue destruction and patient discomfort (1)
  - Can facilitate the identification of fluid collections such as hematomas and seromas

TREATMENT

- Initial stabilization:
  - Manage airway, breathing, and circulation (ABCs).
  - Ensure hemostasis prior to further evaluation, treatment, or repair.
- Irrigation and preparation:
  - Gentle irrigation to dilute the wound's bacterial load with 50 to 100 mL of irrigation solution per centimeter of wound length (2).
  - Studies have shown clean gloves are not inferior to sterile gloves in terms of infection risk (3)[A].
  - Remove foreign bodies or contaminants in wound:
    - Nearly 1/3 of foreign bodies may be missed on initial exam (3).
    - Indications for removal of a foreign body include potential or actual injury to tendons, nerves, and vasculature; toxic substance or reactive agent; and source of pain.
    - Retained foreign bodies may result in "tattooing" of the skin.
  - Irrigate wound with clean tap water:
    - Multiple studies have shown that sterile saline is no more efficacious than tap water (1)[A].
    - A "rule of thumb" is to use 50 to 100 mL of irrigant per centimeter of laceration (1)[B].
  - Débride devitalized tissue and revise wound edges if necessary to achieve a good closure.
  - Clip hair near the wound but avoid shaving, because it may introduce bacteria into the wound.
  - Friction blisters:
    - Larger blisters can be drained to prevent expansion or epidermal "roof" can be left intact to act as a biologic dressing (4).
    - Blisters <1 cm can be left intact and covered with a protective dressing (4).
- Time to treatment:
  - Blisters, chafing, and abrasions can be treated immediately, and the athlete can return to play.
  - Lacerations may heal by primary closure, delayed primary closure, or secondary intention:
    - Close all "clean" wounds primarily, except puncture wounds not able to be adequately irrigated.
    - Delayed presentation, contaminated wounds, and noncosmetic animal bites should be irrigated, débrided, and bleeding should be controlled.
    - Delayed primary closure can be performed after 3 to 5 days to allow the patient's immune system to decrease the bacterial load.
    - Lacerations with delayed repair after 12 hours have no significant increased risk in infection compared to those repaired earlier (3)[B].
    - Healing by secondary intention is allowing a wound to heal by granulation. This is appropriate for partial-thickness avulsions, small and simple wounds, contaminated small wounds, and infected wounds (2).
- Analgesia:
  - Topical anesthesia:
    - Useful to treat abrasions, chafing, and blisters, as well as to further evaluate skin lacerations (5)
    - Most common options include 1% or 2% lidocaine jelly, LET (4% lidocaine, 0.1225% epinephrine, and 0.5% tetracaine), or EMLA (eutectic mixture of local anesthetics: 2.5% lidocaine and 2.5% prilocaine)
  - Local or regional anesthesia:
    - Preferred type of anesthesia for lacerations: amide agents (lidocaine and bupivacaine) and ester agents (procaine)

- Allergies to anesthetic:
  - Allergy to one group is not associated with allergy to anesthetic from another group.
  - Most allergies are caused by preservatives, so a pure agent, such as cardiac lidocaine, could be an alternative.
  - Intradermal diphenhydramine can be used for those patients allergic to the above anesthetics (3).
- Epinephrine increases local vasoconstriction to improve the duration of injected anesthetics (4):
  - Local anesthetic with epinephrine (up to 1:100,000) is safe for repair of the digits, including digital block (3)[B].
  - Reluctance to use epinephrine with lidocaine in distal tissues may be based on historic concern. Nevertheless, injected phentolamine can be used to reverse ischemia if this were to occur (2).
- Patient comfort can be increased by using a high-gauge needle, warming anesthetic to body temperature, injecting subcutaneously through the open wound, using a slower injection rate, and with adding sodium bicarbonate to the anesthetic (1:10 of total volume injected) (3).

- Modalities for closure:
  - Laceration location and differences in tissue tension determine the type of material used for closure.
  - Surgical tape:
    - Advantages: rapid application, patient comfort, least tissue reactivity, and low cost
    - Disadvantages: cannot apply to areas with hair, must remain dry, highest dehiscence rates, and low tensile strength
    - Application: Use benzoin tincture before applying tape onto dry skin edge.
  - Skin adhesives:
    - Advantages: rapid application, good cosmetic results, and excellent for children
    - Disadvantages: inadequate for moderate or heavy tension areas, can lose strength over time and dehiscence is possible
    - Application: Apply on dry skin edges, approximate skin edges.
  - Staples:
    - Advantages: rapid application, low tissue reactivity, low cost, and can be used in areas with a lot of hair
    - Disadvantages: does not provide meticulous closure, leaves more scarring, and removal can be painful
    - Application: Sterilize area, anesthesia, and roughly approximate edges.
  - Sutures:
    - Advantages: meticulous closure, most tensile strength, and lowest dehiscence rate
    - Disadvantages: anesthesia required, slow application, most tissue reaction
- Suture techniques:
  - The goal of suture repair is to bring the edges of the wound together to facilitate healing. Sutures that are too tight can result in pain, ischemia, necrosis, and wound dehiscence.
  - Use a needle driver to hold the needle and forceps to evert the skin edge. Needle enters the tissue at 90 degrees.
  - Start in the middle of the wound and bisect the laceration length with each subsequent suture to allow even tension distribution.
  - Suture technique: Simple interrupted is the easiest to master and can be applied to nearly every wound. Other techniques include horizontal mattress closure and vertical mattress closure.
  - Suture choice: There is no significant difference in cosmetic outcome, infection rate, or wound dehiscence between absorbable and nonabsorbable sutures (3).
    - Single versus multiple layer closure:
      - Single layer: performed with staples, adhesives, surgical tape, or sutures depending on location of laceration
      - Multiple layer: closes deep tissue dead space; lessens tension at the epidermal level, improving the cosmetic result
- Wound dressing:
  - Blisters: should be covered with a protective membrane or dressing, or a semipermeable membrane, or hydrocolloidal dressing if draining
  - Abrasions can be covered by a nonstick dressing, such as Telfa or Adaptic, then covered by an absorbent gauze dressing:
    - Alternative dressings include Tegaderm, zinc oxide–impregnated gauze, and occlusive hydrocolloidal dressings such as DuoDERM.
  - For hematomas, athletes can use a padded dressing for comfort.
  - Lacerations should be covered with a sterile gauze or nonadherent pad until the stitches or staples are removed.
    - If nonabsorbable sutures are used, apply ointment followed by dressing, and wound dressing should be changed daily.
- Scar-minimizing techniques: wound support, hydration, and optimizing scar maturity are thought to be beneficial for cosmetic outcome of scars.
  - Therapies to improve cosmesis include scar massage, vitamin E, onion extract preparations, adhesive tape support, and corticosteroids; however, evidence for some of these therapies is lacking (1).
  - Utilization of broad-spectrum sunscreen can improve cosmesis in scars.

MEDICATION

- Antibiotics:
  - Topical antibiotics also serve as a physical impediment for bacteria to enter the wound.
  - The roe of topical antibiotics for wounds remains controversial, as topical antibiotics are a common cause of allergic contact dermatitis, which can mimic cellulitis and infection. Petroleum-based ointments are an alternative.
  - Uncomplicated lacerations, abrasions, blisters, and chafing do not require systemic antibiotics:
    - A meta-analysis did not show benefit to prophylactic oral antibiotics for reducing wound infection in simple, nonbite wounds (5).
  - Open fractures, exposed tendon injuries, or exposed joint injuries typically require systemic antibiotics.
- Tetanus prophylaxis guidelines should be followed (6).
  - Patients who are pregnant or who have received 3 doses of tetanus toxoid should receive a dose of Tdap.
  - For clean wounds, a booster is given only if >10 years have elapsed since their last dose.
  - For contaminated or high-risk wounds, a booster is given if ≥5 years have passed since last dose.

ADMISSION, INPATIENT, AND NURSING CONSIDERATIONS

Admission criteria:

- Soft tissue injuries require hospitalization for:
  - Grossly contaminated wounds or wounds requiring extensive débridement
  - Open fractures
  - Hemodynamically unstable patient
  - Neurovascular compromise
  - Comorbid conditions such as a head injury or abdominal trauma
  - Wounds requiring ongoing intravenous (IV) antibiotics
- Eyelid lacerations should prompt a referral to an ophthalmologist.

ONGOING CARE

FOLLOW-UP RECOMMENDATIONS

Suture removal (3)

Wound Location	Timing (Days)
Face	3–5
Scalp	7–10
Arms	7–10
Trunk	10–14
Legs	10–14
Hands or feet	10–14
Palms or soles	14–21

REFERENCES

1. Rupert J, Honeycutt JD, Odom MR. Foreign bodies in the skin: evaluation and management. *Am Fam Physician*. 2020;101(12):740–747.
2. Silverberg B, Moyers A, Wainblat BI, et al. A stitch in time: operative and nonoperative laceration repair techniques. *Prim Care*. 2022;49(1):23–38.
3. Forsch RT, Little SH, Williams C. Laceration repair: a practical approach. *Am Fam Physician*. 2017;95(10):628–636.
4. Honsik KA, Romeo MW, Hawley CJ, et al. Sideline skin and wound care for acute injuries. *Curr Sports Med Rep*. 2007;6(3):147–154.
5. Cordoro KM, Ganz JE. Training room management of medical conditions: sports dermatology. *Clin Sports Med*. 2005;24(3):565–598.
6. Havers FP, Moro PL, Hunter P, et al. Use of tetanus toxoid, reduced diphtheria toxoid, and acellular pertussis vaccines: updated recommendations of the Advisory Committee on Immunization practices— United States, 2019. *MMWR Morb Mortal Wkly Rep*. 2020;69(3):77–83.

CLINICAL PEARLS

- Traumatic skin lesions are commonly seen in the athletic arena.
- Proper assessment and preparation will allow the best possible outcome for skin injuries and facilitate a safe return to play.
- Materials for treatment should be based on the location of the wound, the type of injury, and the experience of the treating provider.
- Return-to-play decisions should be based on the ability to adequately treat the injury, properly dress the wound, ability to limit infection, and the potential for exposure of bodily fluids.

LATERAL COLLATERAL LIGAMENT TEAR

Alexandra E. Warrick, MD, CAQSM ▪ Austin Jinwei Wang, DO ▪ Daniel C. Herman, MD, PhD, FAAPMR, FACSM, FISBS, CAQSM

BASICS

DESCRIPTION

- Partial or complete sprain of the lateral collateral ligament (LCL). The LCL is also known as the fibular collateral ligament (1).
- LCL consists of a cordlike fiber bundle (4 to 5 mm in width) that originates 1.4 mm proximal and 3.1 mm posterior to the lateral femoral epicondyle and inserts on the anterolateral aspect of the fibular head about 1 cm anterior to the apex: discrete extracapsular structure (2).
- Primarily prevents varus stress at the tibiofemoral joint. With the knee in extension, it is a secondary stabilizer to prevent tibial external rotation and posterior translation (2),(3).
- The LCL is a primary stabilizer of the posterolateral corner (PLC) of the knee in addition to the popliteal tendon and popliteofibular ligament (4).
- Mechanism of injury includes an acute varus force to the knee such as a direct blow to the medial knee; can also occur with noncontact knee hyperextension and varus stress (2)
- Injuries to the LCL may occur together with other knee pathology such as PLC, anterior cruciate ligament (ACL) injury, or posterior cruciate ligament (PCL) injury.
- Is in tension between 0 and 70 degrees of flexion, followed by slackening trend with deeper flexion

EPIDEMIOLOGY

- Least commonly injured knee ligament; LCL injuries account for 1.1% of all knee injuries (3).
- Isolated LCL injuries are rare (3).
- Infrequent site of overuse injury or rupture. If there is a grade 3 injury (complete LCL tear), it most commonly occurs at the fibular insertion, then midsubstance, and then femoral insertion (3).
- Associated with combat sports such as Brazilian jiu-jitsu as well as the noncontact sports of tennis and gymnastics (1),(2)
- Trauma may occur to the LCL outside of sports via motor vehicle accidents and falls.

RISK FACTORS

- Prior knee, ankle, or hip injury predisposes to increased injury rates
- Higher association with female gender, contact sports, and activities requiring pivoting and jumping
- PCL deficiency may increase risk of LCL injury.

DIAGNOSIS

HISTORY

- Acute lateral knee pain
- May hear/feel an associated "pop"
- Swelling to the lateral knee
- Mild disability with low-grade injury; difficult weight-bearing with high-grade injury/associated ligamentous injuries
- Instability with moderate- to high-grade injury
- Difficulty with cutting movements

PHYSICAL EXAM

- Ecchymosis to the lateral knee
- Swelling variable, effusion not common with isolated injuries; associated intra-articular injuries may cause significant effusion.
- Tenderness to palpation over the LCL; palpate in the "figure-of-4 position" with the knee bent and heel on the contralateral knee which allows the lateral compartment to open and intact LCL can be palpated (2).
- Laxity at 30 degrees flexion with varus stress test significant for isolated LCL injury (2)
- Classification of injury (2):
  - Grade 1 sprain—0 to 5 mm varus opening
  - Grade 2 sprain—6 to 10 mm varus opening
  - Grade 3 sprain—>10 mm varus opening
  - Compare to the contralateral knee.
- Laxity at zero degrees of flexion with varus stress test may indicate involvement of other ligaments such as ACL or PCL (2).
- Ligamentous evaluation of ACL (e.g., Lachman test)
- Ligamentous evaluation of PCL (e.g., posterior drawer test)
- Ligamentous evaluation of PLC (e.g., dial test, the posterolateral drawer test, recurvatum test) (2)
- Neurovascular evaluation including peroneal nerve sensory and motor function

DIFFERENTIAL DIAGNOSIS

- Proximal fibula avulsion fracture
- Biceps femoris strain
- Iliotibial band strain
- Popliteus strain/tear/tendinopathy
- ACL and/or PCL tears
- Lateral meniscus tear
- Lateral compartment chondral/osteochondral injury
- Tibial plateau fracture
- Proximal tibiofibular syndesmosis injury
- Associated loose body
- Peroneal nerve injury

DIAGNOSTIC TESTS & INTERPRETATION

- Plain radiographs to rule out fracture of lateral tibial plateau, lateral femoral condyle, or fibular head
- Magnetic resonance imaging (MRI) to assess integrity of LCL and associated knee structures (ACL, PCL, lateral meniscus, popliteus tendon, PLC)
- MRI may demonstrate medial compartment bruising if mechanism includes hyperextension/varus stress with injury to the LCL and PLC. Further bone bruises indicate additional ligamentous injury (2)[C].
- LCL injury grading and MRI findings (2)[C]:
  - Grade 1: mild injury, subcutaneous fluid around the LCL
  - Grade 2: partial tearing of the LCL; MRI demonstrates edema in and/or around the LCL.
  - Grade 3: complete tearing of the LCL with associated edema

TREATMENT

- Acute treatment includes rest, ice, and compression.
- Grade 1 and 2 LCL injuries are usually managed nonoperatively with early mobilization (2)[C].
- Mobilization and recovery time
  - Grade 1 injury: crutches as needed for pain; possible hinged knee brace; recovery time of 3 to 4 weeks
  - Grade 2: crutches and then hinged knee brace; recovery time of 8 to 12 weeks
  - Grade 3: immobilization with crutches and consultation with an orthopedic surgeon; hinged knee brace
- Grade 3 injuries are typically managed surgically; however, some results show that nonsurgically managed isolated grade 3 injuries were as likely as those with surgically managed injuries to return to play within a similar time period (2)[C].
- Analgesia:
  - Nonsteroidal anti-inflammatory drugs (NSAIDs), acetaminophen until acute pain subsides
  - Narcotics considered if needed for 24 to 72 hours for grade 2 or 3 injuries or combined ligamentous injuries after nonnarcotic medication

ADDITIONAL THERAPIES

- May consider more prolonged immobilization and bracing in varus knee, which is thought to increase stress on the injured ligament (3)[C]
- Quadriceps strengthening is important as quadriceps inhibition is common after knee injuries; start with isometric quadriceps strengthening and straight raise leg lifts.
- Exercise progression includes strength training, gait training, neuromuscular control exercises, and sport specific training.
- Postoperative rehabilitation involves an initial period of immobilization and non–weight-bearing with progression in range of motion and partial weight-bearing to full weight-bearing with a knee brace (5)[C].

SURGERY/OTHER PROCEDURES

- Surgery is considered for grade 3 LCL tears and combined ligamentous injuries such as PLC injuries and cruciate ligament injuries (3)[C].
- LCL surgery may include LCL repair or LCL reconstruction combined with PLC reconstruction as needed.
- Also indicated in acute LCL avulsion injuries that are unable to be reduced anatomically

ONGOING CARE

FOLLOW-UP RECOMMENDATIONS

- Consider referral to orthopedic surgery for nonreducible avulsion fracture or tibial plateau fracture, associated ligamentous injury or meniscal tear, or grade 3 injury that is not amenable to the initial 2 to 4 weeks of rehabilitation.
- Associated neurovascular injuries should be considered emergent, and appropriate surgical/radiographic consultations should be initiated and performed on the same day.
- Perform range of motion to prevent joint stiffness after initial immobilization.
- LCL sport prevention measures include strength and training programs, maintaining flexibility, warm-up exercises, and an emphasis on proper biomechanics/technique.

REFERENCES

1. Temponi EF, Saithna A, de Carvalho LH, et al. Nonoperative treatment for partial ruptures of the lateral collateral ligament occurring in combination with complete ruptures of the anterolateral ligament: a common injury pattern in Brazilian jiu-jitsu athletes with acute knee injury. *Orthop J Sports Med*. 2019;7(1):2325967118822450.
2. Grawe B, Schroeder AJ, Kakazu R, et al. Lateral collateral ligament injury about the knee: anatomy, evaluation, and management. *J Am Acad Orthop Surg*. 2018;26(6):e120–e127.
3. Dietrich G, Maeder B, Nyland J, et al. Isolated femoral LCL avulsion fracture in the adult knee: two patient cases and literature review. *Case Rep Orthop*. 2022;6507577.
4. Boksh K, Ghosh A, Narayan P, et al. Fibular—versus tibiofibular-based reconstruction of the posterolateral corner of the knee: a systematic review and meta-analysis. *Am J Sports Med*. 2023;51(14):3880–3892.
5. Levy BA, Stuart MJ, Whelan DB. Posterolateral instability of the knee: evaluation, treatment, results. *Sports Med Arthrosc Rev*. 2010;18(4):254–262.

ADDITIONAL READING

- Chahla J, Murray IR, Robinson J, et al. Posterolateral corner of the knee: an expert consensus statement on diagnosis, classification, treatment, and rehabilitation. *Knee Surg Sports Traumatol Arthrosc*. 2019;27(8):2520–2529.
- Haddad MA, Budich JM, Eckenrode BJ. Conservative management of an isolated grade III lateral collateral ligament injury in an adolescent multi-sport athlete: a case report. *Int J Sports Phys Ther*. 2016;11(4):596–606.
- Krukhaug Y, Mølster A, Rodt A, et al. Lateral ligament injuries of the knee. *Knee Surg Sports Traumatol Arthrosc*. 1998;6(1):21–25.
- Nannaparaju M, Mortada S, Wiik A, et al. Posterolateral corner injuries: epidemiology, anatomy, biomechanics and diagnosis. *Injury*. 2018;49(6):1024–1031.
- Shetty A, Prabhath S, Alappatt K, et al. Lateral collateral ligament and anterolateral ligament of the knee—a morphological analysis with orthopedic significance. *Knee*. 2021;28:202–206.

CLINICAL PEARLS

- Isolated LCL injuries are rare. Injuries to the LCL may occur together with other knee pathology such as PLC, ACL injury, or PCL injury.
- Grade 1 and 2 LCL injuries are usually managed nonoperatively, whereas grade 3 injuries are typically managed surgically.
- Return to play is greatly dependent on injury severity and the type of sport/activity.

LATERAL EPICONDYLITIS

Bryant Walrod, MD, CAQSM • Craig C. Young, MD

BASICS

DESCRIPTION

- Lateral epicondylitis, or lateral elbow tendinosis, is a degenerative overuse injury of the forearm and wrist extensor muscles, which causes pain at the lateral elbow.
- Synonym(s): tennis elbow, common extensor tendinopathy, epicondylalgia, lateral epicondylosis, lateral epicondyle tendinosis (LET)

EPIDEMIOLOGY

- Prevalence: 1–3% of general population
- Represents 20% of tennis injuries
- Accounts for ~90% of elbow epicondylitis
- Precipitated by tennis and other activities that require repetitive wrist extension, radial deviation, and forearm supination
- Occurs in dominant arm 75% of the time
- ~90% will have resolution or significant improvement within a year with all treatment options including clinical observation alone.

RISK FACTORS

- Age 40 to 60 years
- Smoking, obesity
- Improper equipment (e.g., inappropriate grip size, overstrung racquet, inappropriate-weight racquet)
- Poor technique (e.g., backhand with excessive wrist extension)
- Recreational tennis player
- Playing tennis for >2 hours daily
- Repetitive movement of >2 h/d

COMMONLY ASSOCIATED CONDITIONS

Posterior interosseous nerve entrapment (radial tunnel syndrome)

DIAGNOSIS

HISTORY

- Pain pattern: Patients typically report an insidious onset, but they will often relate a history of overuse without specific trauma. Pain can vary from mild (e.g., present only with aggravating activities like tennis or the repeated use of a hand tool), or it can be severe (e.g., holding a coffee cup will act as a trigger for the pain).
- Numbness or tingling: Radicular symptoms suggest nerve entrapment or radiculopathy.
- Backhand hitting style: Lateral epicondylitis is more common in players who hit with a one-handed backhand.
- Improper technique: hitting late in the backhand, improper positioning when striking the ball, or insufficient follow-through
- Equipment used, location, and frequency of play: Many cases of lateral epicondylitis are associated with improper equipment, old or wet tennis balls, racquets that are strung too tightly or too heavy, and fast surfaces. Shock-absorbing rubber vibration dampeners have not been shown to reduce risk.
- Poor conditioning: Poor general conditioning leads to fatigue of the core and shoulder muscles, which puts an overemphasis on the extensor muscles of the forearm.
- Scapular dyskinesis and poor rotator cuff control can lead to the development of lateral elbow pain.

PHYSICAL EXAM

- Pain at lateral elbow
- Pain with wrist and forearm movements
- Pain with gripping objects ("coffee cup sign") and shaking hands ("politician's sign")
- Decreased grip strength
- Localized tenderness over lateral epicondyle; also pain just distal and anterior to lateral epicondyle ~1 to 2 cm distal to the origin of the extensor carpi radialis brevis
- Tenderness with resisted wrist extension with wrist pronated and radially deviated
- Tenderness with resisted middle finger extension
- Tenderness with resisted supination
- Decreased internal rotation of ipsilateral shoulder causing compensatory excessive wrist flexion
- Scapular dyskinesia

DIFFERENTIAL DIAGNOSIS

- Posterior interosseous nerve entrapment
- Radial tunnel syndrome
- Osteoarthritis
- C7 radiculopathy
- Musculocutaneous nerve entrapment
- Chronic compartment syndrome of anconeus muscle
- Radiocapitellum osteochondritis dissecans (OCD) lesion (common in adolescents)
- Lateral collateral ligament strain
- Stress fracture
- Humeral fracture

DIAGNOSTIC TESTS & INTERPRETATION

Initial Tests (lab, imaging)

- Not usually needed for initial treatment
- Standard elbow radiography series (anteroposterior and lateral) should be obtained if other potential injuries are suspected (e.g., fracture, tumor, degenerative joint disease) or if injury is not responding to appropriate treatment.
- Up to 25% of cases have associated calcification in extensor aponeurosis; however, presence of these deposits does not affect initial treatment.
- Musculoskeletal (MSK) ultrasound (US) may reveal tendon thickening, partial tearing, calcifications, hypoechoic changes, and vascular ingrowth in the tendons.
- Magnetic resonance imaging (MRI) may reveal partial intrasubstance tears and tendinosis; MRI may assist with evaluation of other potential causes of lateral elbow pain like OCD lesions and stress fractures.

Diagnostic Procedures/Other

- A local anesthetic block may lead to symptom resolution and confirmation of the diagnosis.
- Pathologic findings:
  - Microscopic evaluation of the tendons does not show signs of inflammation but rather angiofibroblastic degeneration and collagen disarray.
  - Light microscopy reveals both an excess of fibroblasts and blood vessels that are consistent with neovessels or angiogenesis.
  - The tendons are relatively hypovascular near the tendon insertion. This hypovascularity may predispose the tendon to hypoxic tendon degeneration and has been implicated in the etiology of tendinopathies.
  - These findings support a failed healing response rather than a true inflammatory process.

TREATMENT

- Acute treatment:
  - Ice after activity
  - Relative rest: Limit activities that cause pain.
  - Oral analgesics
  - Anti-inflammatory medications: For control of symptoms, consider nonsteroidal anti-inflammatory drugs (NSAIDs), either topical or by mouth.
  - Air-filled counterforce bracing: can be effective in treating acute symptoms

- Wrist splints:
  - Use at night may decrease morning symptoms by stabilizing the wrist in a neutral position.
- Taping during activities may be useful.
- Corticosteroid injections may provide short-term relief of symptoms but do not appear to be effective for long-term management of chronic tendinopathies. There are also risks with corticosteroid injections into tendons (1)[B],(2)[A].
- Platelet-rich plasma injections may provide superior relief of symptoms of longer period of time when compared to cortisone but may have minimal effect on eventual outcome (1)[B], (3)[A],(4)[A].
- Modalities: Consider the use of US, phonophoresis, or iontophoresis. Some studies have shown them to be useful in returning an athlete to activity sooner, but they show no long-term benefit.

- Long-term treatment:
  - Watchful waiting: ~90% of patients symptom-free or nearly symptom-free at 1 year (5)[A]
  - Autologous blood, platelet-rich plasma, prolotherapy, botulinum toxin has demonstrated short-term effectiveness in small studies, but none have been shown to be significantly superior in the long term in meta-analysis or systematic reviews (2)[A], (3)[A],(5)[A].
  - Extracorporeal shock wave therapy may provide short-term relief of symptoms but may not be effective for long-term management of chronic tendinopathies (6)[A].
  - Acupuncture has demonstrated superior results when compared to other interventions.
  - More research is needed for newer interventions such as hyaluronic acid, bone marrow aspiration, and direct tenocyte injections.
  - US-guided percutaneous tenotomy procedure has been shown to be effective for chronic symptoms.
  - Surgical intervention has been shown to be useful in recalcitrant cases.
  - Physical therapy consisting of forearm stretching and strengthening program with progression to eccentric muscle strengthening of the common extensor tendon.
  - Blood flow restriction in physical therapy can also be considered.

ISSUES FOR REFERRAL

Consider referral for surgical intervention for individuals whose symptoms do not respond to a high-quality nonoperative treatment program for >6 months.

ADDITIONAL THERAPIES

- Technique modification: lessons from a professional instructor or coach about proper serve and backhand techniques
- Improve ergonomics in the work environment.
- Equipment: Ensure athlete is using properly sized, weighted, and strung racquet. Stretching and strengthening: Ensure athlete is on an appropriate conditioning program, preactivity warm-up, and postactivity cool-down programs.
- Evaluate and treat biomechanical risk factors such as scapular dyskinesis and rotator cuff weakness.

REFERENCES

1. Kamble P, Prabhu RM, Jogani A, et al. Is ultrasound (US)-guided platelet-rich plasma injection more efficacious as a treatment modality for lateral elbow tendinopathy than US-guided steroid injection? A prospective triple-blinded study with midterm follow-up. *Clin Orthop Surg*. 2023;15(3):454–462.
2. Lapner P, Alfonso A, Herbert-Davies J, et al. Position statement: nonoperative management of lateral epicondylitis in adults. *Can J Surg*. 2022:65(5):E625–E629.
3. Masiello F, Pati I, Veropalumbo E, et al. Ultrasound-guided injection of platelet-rich plasma for tendinopathies: a systematic review and meta-analysis. *Blood Transfus*. 2023;21(2):119–136.
4. Muthu S, Patel S, Gobbur A, et al. Platelet-rich plasma therapy ensures pain reduction in the management of lateral epicondylitis—a PRISMA-compliant network meta-analysis of randomized controlled trials. *Expert Opin Biol Ther*. 2022:22(4):535–546.
5. Ikonen J, Lähdeoja T, Ardern CL, et al. Persistent tennis elbow symptoms have little prognostic value: a systematic review and meta-analysis. *Clin Orthop Relat Res*. 2022;480(4):647–660.
6. Liu WC, Chen CT, Lu CC, et al. Extracorporeal shock wave therapy shows superiority over injections for pain relief and grip strength recovery in lateral epicondylitis: a systematic review and network meta-analysis. *Arthroscopy*. 2022;38(6):2018–2034.

ADDITIONAL READING

- Balevi ISY, Karaoglan B, Batur EB, et al. Evaluation of short-term and residual effects of Kinesio taping in chronic lateral epicondylitis: a randomized, double-blinded, controlled trial. *J Hand Ther*. 2023:36(1):13–22.
- ElMeligie MM, Gbreel MI, Yehia RM, et al. Clinical efficacy of high-intensity laser therapy on lateral epicondylitis patients: a systematic review and meta-analysis. *Am J Phys Med Rehabil*. 2023:102(1):64–70.
- Güngör E, Güngör ZK. Comparison of the efficacy of corticosteroid, dry needling, and PRP application in lateral epicondylitis. *Eur J Orthop Surg Traumatol*. 2022:32(8):1569–1575.
- Kaplan S, Sah V, Ozkan S, et al. Comparative effects of focused and radial extracorporeal shock wave therapies on lateral epicondylitis: a randomised sham-controlled trial. *J Coll Physicians Surg Pak*. 2023:33(5):554–559.
- Karanasios S, Korakakis V, Moutzouri M, et al. Low-load resistance training with blood flow restriction is effective for managing lateral elbow tendinopathy: a randomized, sham-controlled trial. *J Orthop Sports Phys Ther*. 2022;52(12):803–825.
- Kim CH, Park YB, Lee JS, et al. Platelet-rich plasma injection versus operative treatment for lateral elbow tendinosis: a systematic review and meta-analysis. *J Shoulder Elbow Surg*. 2022:31(2): 428–436.
- Sirico F, Ricca F, Di Meglio F, et al. Local corticosteroid versus autologous blood injections in lateral epicondylitis: meta-analysis of randomized controlled trials. *Eur J Phys Rehabil Med*. 2017;53(3):483–491.
- Zhou Y, Guo Y, Zhou R, et al. Effectiveness of acupuncture for lateral epicondylitis: a systematic review and meta-analysis of randomized controlled trials. *Pain Res Manag*. 2020:8506591.

CLINICAL PEARLS

- The lateral elbow serves as the origin of the forearm supination and wrist extensor muscles, and thus, elbow pain may result from repetitive use.
- Histologic biopsies of chronic lateral epicondylitis reveal no inflammation but rather signs of poor and disordered healing, a term called *angiofibroblastic degeneration*. Chronic lateral epicondylosis is not an inflammatory condition. Consider other treatments such as physical therapy and proinflammatory modalities in this case.
- Equipment modifications: appropriate racquet grip size; decrease racquet string tension; use only new, dry tennis balls; play on grass court if available
- When discussing the risks and benefits of the treatment options, make sure that you include the fact that clinical observation instead of active treatment will eventually lead to resolution in symptoms in most individuals.

LEGG-CALVÉ-PERTHES DISEASE

Christopher McGrew, MD, FACSM, CAQSM

BASICS

DESCRIPTION

- Juvenile idiopathic avascular necrosis of the capital femoral epiphysis of the femoral head
- Synonym(s): Perthes disease; aseptic necrosis of the femoral head

EPIDEMIOLOGY

- Incidence in general population 0.2 to 19.1/100,000 in children <15 years old, lowest in equatorial regions, higher incidence with increasing latitude (each 10 degrees latitude demonstrated 1.44 times increase in incidence) (1)
- Predominant age: affects children 3 to 12 years of age but is most common between the ages of 4 and 9 years; median age 7 years
- Predominant gender: male > female (4 to 5:1)
- Most prevalent among whites and Chinese; rare in blacks and Native Americans
- Bilateral hip involvement in 15–20% of patients

ETIOLOGY AND PATHOPHYSIOLOGY

Etiology of Legg-Calvé-Perthes disease (LCPD) is unclear, but the following has been proposed as a theoretical sequence of events:

- Blood supply to the capital femoral epiphysis is interrupted.
- Bone infarction occurs, especially in the subchondral cortical bone, whereas the articular cartilage continues to grow (articular cartilage receives its nutrients from synovial fluid).
- Revascularization occurs, and new bone ossification starts. At this point, a percentage of patients develop LCPD, whereas others have normal bone growth and development.
- LCPD is present when a subchondral fracture occurs. This is the result of normal physical activity, not direct trauma to the area.
- Changes to the epiphyseal growth plate occur secondary to the subchondral fracture.

RISK FACTORS

- Low birth weight (2)
- Short stature
- Delayed bone maturation
- Involved family member (after index sibling, incidence 1/35)
- Familial thrombophilia and hypofibrinolysis (controversial)
- Breech position at birth
- Preterm
- Hypercoagulability
- Exposure to second-hand smoke
- Attention-deficit hyperactivity disorder

DIAGNOSIS

HISTORY

Symptoms of LCPD usually have been present for weeks because the child often does not complain:

- Limp worsened by activity, usually most pronounced at end of day (may be painless)
- 60% present with pain and limp, 24% pain alone, 15% limp alone
- Hip or groin pain, which may be referred to the thigh
- Mild or intermittent pain in anterior thigh or knee
- Usually no history of trauma
- Inflammatory synovitis can mimic LCPD but usually resolves in 10 to 14 days.

PHYSICAL EXAM

- Examine the musculoskeletal system with a focus on the pelvis and lower extremities.
- Include range of motion (ROM) testing to evaluate for limited abduction and internal rotation and the presence or absence of hip flexion contracture.
- Evaluate for muscle atrophy of the thigh, calf, and buttocks, which may be seen in long-standing cases.
- Measure for possible leg-length discrepancy, which indicates advanced involvement of the femoral head.
- Evaluate gait. Up to 90% of patients demonstrate a limp (2). Trendelenburg gait is observed with abductor weakness.
- Perform log roll test of extended leg on examining table; painful and reduced ROM is observed compared with the opposite side.
- Short stature: Children with LCPD often have delayed bone age.

DIFFERENTIAL DIAGNOSIS

- Overuse/injury: Muscle strain/tendinopathy, apophysitis or apophyseal avulsion, stress fracture
- Inflammatory: transient synovitis, juvenile idiopathic arthritis, reactive arthritis
- Infectious: septic arthritis, osteomyelitis, pyomyositis
- Trauma: fracture
- Neoplasm: Ewing sarcoma, osteoid osteoma, acute leukemia, neuroblastoma
- Congenital: limb abnormality
- Developmental: hip dysplasia, slipped capital femoral epiphysis
- Sickle cell anemia, other hemolytic anemias, and hemophilia: osteonecrosis secondary to vascular infarcts
- Gaucher disease: osteonecrosis secondary to cerebroside and infarcts
- Certain genetic mutations (trisomy 21 and Klinefelter syndrome)
- Referred pain: knee or back etiology

DIAGNOSTIC TESTS & INTERPRETATION

- Complete blood count (CBC), erythrocyte sedimentation rate (ESR), and C reactive protein (CRP)
- Anteroposterior (AP) pelvis and bilateral frog-leg lateral views of the hip should be obtained but can appear normal early in course.
- Radiographic features:
  - Femoral head appears smaller and flatter than opposite head with a widened articular cartilage space and subchondral sclerosis (3).
  - If present bilaterally, typically will present at different stages on each side
  - With disease progression, a crescent-shaped radiolucent line may be seen in the central portion of the femoral head, especially on the lateral view.
  - Fracture, fragmentation, and resorption can occur.
- There are three major categories of radiographic classification: staging of disease, severity of presentation, and sphericity at maturity (3).
- Extent of femoral head involvement determines severity of disease. Radiographic changes can be divided into five distinct stages representing a continuum of the disease process, as follows:
  - Stage 1—cessation of femoral epiphyseal growth
  - Stage 2—subchondral fracture
  - Stage 3—resorption
  - Stage 4—reossification
  - Stage 5—healed or residual stage
- Bone scan and magnetic resonance imaging (MRI) can be used to evaluate and diagnose LCPD before radiographic changes are apparent.
- MRI may also be used to diagnose and evaluate disease progression and/or resolution over time if radiographs provide inadequate detail.
- Ultrasonography is useful to evaluate the presence of synovitis or effusion, which could be an early sign.

TREATMENT

GENERAL MEASURES

- The healing process involves revascularization of the femoral head, removal of necrotic bone, and replacement with viable bone. It is a biologic process that requires many months. No current interventions accelerate this process.
- Treatment is controversial; goal is to prevent a prearthrotic deformity and subsequent arthritis.
- Requires individual adaptations and close follow-up
- Treatment courses vary widely among patients.
- Nonsurgical treatment:
  - Treatment may involve simple observation, especially in children <6 years of age.
  - Analgesia: nonsteroidal anti-inflammatory drugs (NSAIDs) or acetaminophen
  - Activity restriction, crutches or wheelchair for non–weight-bearing, and abduction stretching exercises and occasionally bed rest. Abduction bracing/casting can be used for symptom relief and to hold the femoral head in the acetabulum.
  - Casting/bracing may be discontinued when there is radiographic evidence of subchondral reossification, usually after 12 to 18 months.

ADDITIONAL THERAPIES

- Both surgical and nonsurgical treatments are aimed at symptom reduction, prevention of capital femoral epiphysis destruction, and attainment of a spherical femoral head at healing.
- Rehabilitation:
  - Formal therapy program is recommended during and after bracing owing to extensive atrophy, contracture, and loss of motion.
  - A home stretching program is encouraged to maintain ROM.

SURGERY/OTHER PROCEDURES

- Goal is containment of femoral head to maintain or restore joint congruence during the period of biologic plasticity, leading to the restoration of a round femoral head. Results of surgical containment appear to be better than those of nonsurgical containment (orthosis). Surgical management typically involves either femoral osteotomy to redirect the involved portion within the acetabulum or a combined femoral and innominate osteotomy.
- In severe LCPD, a combined osteotomy showed the best outcomes for improving the spherical congruity of the hip joint (4)[A].
- Femoral osteotomy may cause shortening of the limb, leading to a chronic limp (5)[B].
- Techniques vary depending on age of child and severity of femoral head involvement.
- Advantages include less time required in a brace and earlier return to activity.
- Disadvantages include necessity of two operations.

ONGOING CARE

FOLLOW-UP RECOMMENDATIONS

All patients with suspected LCPD should be referred to a pediatric orthopedic surgeon promptly.

PROGNOSIS

- The younger the age of onset of LCPD (<6 years of age), the better is the prognosis.
- Children >10 years of age have a higher risk of complications including very high risk of developing osteoarthritis (6).
- Other factors for worse prognosis: girls, heavier weight, progressive loss of hip ROM, adduction contracture, longer duration from onset to completion of healing phase (3)
- Most patients have a favorable outcome.
- Prognosis is proportional to the degree of radiologic involvement as well as later age of onset, obesity, severely limited ROM, and female sex.

COMPLICATIONS

- Femoral head deformity (i.e., irregular contouring, flattening, or mushrooming of the head and shortening and broadening of the neck) along with flattening of the vertical wall of the acetabulum
- Degenerative joint disease (onset of severe arthritis varies from adolescence to more commonly in geriatric years)

REFERENCES

1. Perry DC, Machin DMG, Pope D, et al. Racial and geographic factors in the incidence of Legg-Calvé-Perthes disease: a systematic review. *Am J Epidemiol*. 2012;175(3):159–166.
2. Laine JC, Novotny SA, Tis JE, et al. Demographics and clinical presentation of early-stage Legg-Calvé-Perthes disease: a prospective, multicenter, international study. *J Am Acad Orthop Surg*. 2021;29(2):e85–e91.
3. Ng T, Liu R, Kulkarni VA. Legg-Calvé-Perthes disease: diagnosis, decision making, and outcome. *Curr Sports Med Rep*. 2024;23(2)45–52.
4. Adulkasem N, Phinyo P, Tangadulrat P, et al. Comparative effectiveness of treatment modalities in severe Legg-Calvé-Perthes disease: systematic review and network meta-analysis of observational studies. *Int Orthop*. 2022;46(5):1085–1094.
5. Wiig O, Terjesen T, Svenningsen S. Prognostic factors and outcome of treatment in Perthes' disease: a prospective study of 368 patients with five-year follow-up. *J Bone Joint Surg Br*. 2008;90(10):1364–1371.
6. Heesakkers N, van Kempen R, Feith R, et al. The long-term prognosis of Legg-Calvé-Perthes disease: a historical prospective study with a median follow-up of forty-one years. *Int Orthop*. 2015;39(5):859–863.

ADDITIONAL READING

- Berthaume MA, Perry DC, Dobson CA, et al. Skeletal immaturity, rostral sparing, and disparate hip morphologies as biomechanical causes for Legg-Calvé-Perthes' disease. *Clin Anat*. 2016;29(6):759–772.
- Gao H, Huang Z, Jia Z, et al. Influence of passive smoking on the onset of Legg-Calvé-Perthes disease: a systematic review and meta-analysis. *J Pediatr Orthop B*. 2020;29(6):556–566.
- Ibrahim T, Little DG. The pathogenesis and treatment of Legg-Calvé-Perthes disease. *JBJS Rev*. 2016;4(7):e4.
- Johansson T, Lindblad M, Bladh M, et al. Incidence of Perthes' disease in children born between 1973 and 1993. *Acta Orthop*. 2017;88(1):96–100.
- Leroux J, Amara SA, Lechevallier J. Legg-Calvé-Perthes disease. *Orthop Traumatol Surg Res*. 2018;104(Suppl 1):S107–S112.
- Lindblad M, Josefsson A, Bladh M, et al. Risk factors during pregnancy and delivery for the development of Perthes' disease: a nationwide Swedish study of 2.1 million individuals. *BMC Pregnancy Childbirth* 2020;20(1):192.

CLINICAL PEARLS

- Etiology of LCPD is unclear.
- Treatment courses vary widely among patients, and close follow-up is essential.
- Both surgical and nonsurgical treatments are aimed at symptom reduction, prevention of capital femoral epiphysis destruction, and attainment of a spherical femoral head at healing.
- Results of surgical containment appear to be better than those of nonsurgical containment (orthosis) in more advanced cases and in children >8 years of age.

L

LITTLE LEAGUE SHOULDER

Patrick J. Prazak, DO, CAQSM • Haris Vakil, MD

BASICS

DESCRIPTION

- Also known as thrower's shoulder
- Remodeling and deformation of the proximal humeral physis
- Overuse injury from recurrent, excessive torque placed on the growth plate during overhead activity
- Typically seen in overhead athletes, especially adolescent baseball pitchers
- First described in 1966 as osteochondrosis of the proximal humeral epiphysis and then reported again in 1974 as proximal humeral epiphysiolysis in adolescent baseball players.

EPIDEMIOLOGY

- Uncertain exact prevalence due to underreporting of pain with throwing
- Most common in male baseball players between ages of 11 and 16 years
- Has also been reported in swimming, volleyball, and cricket
- Can occur in any adolescent athlete involved in repetitive overhead rotational activities.

ETIOLOGY AND PATHOPHYSIOLOGY

- Unknown exact etiology
- Biomechanical studies have revealed shear stress arising from high torque during late cocking phase is large enough to lead to deformation of the proximal humeral growth plate.
- Other proposed mechanisms include stress leading to decreased blood supply or decreased bone mineralization.

Genetics

No known genetic disposition

RISK FACTORS

- Larger body size (height and weight)
- Lack of flexibility
- Period of rapid growth
- Muscular imbalance (1)
- The following risk factors are based on expert opinion:
  - Year-round pitching without 3 months of rest from throwing during the course of the year
  - Playing in multiple leagues at the same time
  - Inadequate rest between pitching outings
  - Throwing with a fatigued shoulder

GENERAL PREVENTION

Prevented by avoiding excessive, repetitive overhead activities, having adequate rest between outings, and not throwing with shoulder fatigue or pain

DIAGNOSIS

Diagnosis based on history, physical, and classic radiographic findings

HISTORY

- Patients typically complain of pain while throwing or with overhead activity but can also occur at rest.
- Pain with throwing is typically constant throughout throwing cycle.
- Most commonly presents with pain laterally over the proximal humeral physis but can present with diffuse pain all over shoulder or referred pain to upper arm
- Insidious onset of pain
- Patients may report recent increase in number of pitches thrown or recent change to playing on a larger field.

PHYSICAL EXAM

- Typical physical exam finding is tenderness to palpation over the proximal humeral physis without erythema, increased warmth, or soft tissue swelling.
- Can present with painful range of motion, including pain with abduction or forward flexion >150 degrees
- Can present with decreased strength of the rotator cuff musculature secondary to pain. Most common is reduced strength and pain with resisted external rotation.
- Can have reduced internal rotation of the shoulder due to posterior capsular tightness, but this finding can also be normal in an adolescent overhead athlete and is not pathognomonic for injury.

DIFFERENTIAL DIAGNOSIS

- Rotator cuff tendonitis/impingement
- Multidirectional instability
- Labral tear (usually superior labrum anterior posterior [SLAP] tear)
- Salter-Harris type I fracture of the proximal humeral physis
- Biceps tendonitis
- Osteochondral fragment of the glenoid

DIAGNOSTIC TESTS & INTERPRETATION

- Standard x-rays are the diagnostic gold standard, but ultrasound can be helpful to document tenderness at the physis or humeral retroversion.
- Anteroposterior x-rays of the affected shoulder in external rotation and internal with comparison films of the unaffected side are standard.
- Typical findings are widening of the affected growth plate, especially on the lateral side.
- May also see osteosclerosis, demineralization, cystic changes, metaphyseal calcification, or fragmentation (2)[C]
- Although not required for diagnosis, magnetic resonance imaging (MRI) will also show physeal widening on the T1-weighted images with periosteal and bone marrow edema and periosteal elevation (3)[A].

TREATMENT

GENERAL MEASURES

- Recommend rest from throwing for 1 month to 1 year (average of 4 months) with continued non-throwing athletic activities (3)[A].
- Treatment consists of rest from throwing and limited, as needed use of over-the-counter (OTC) pain medications such as acetaminophen or non-steroidal anti-inflammatory drugs (NSAIDs) for pain (4)[C].
- Physical therapy during rest period should focus on correcting kinetic chain abnormalities as well as flexibility and strength losses (5)[C].
- Recommended to complete an interval throwing program after finishing physical therapy

MEDICATION

Age-appropriate dose of any NSAID or acetaminophen can be used as needed for pain during initial period of rest.

SURGERY/OTHER PROCEDURES

No surgical correction required

ONGOING CARE

FOLLOW-UP RECOMMENDATIONS

- After 1- to 12-month rest and physical therapy to reassess exam and give guidance on starting an interval throwing program
- Should complete throwing program prior to returning to preinjury level of competition and throwing (5)[C]
- Repeat x-rays are not required because it can take up to a year for growth plate to return to normal.

PATIENT EDUCATION

- Patients, parents, and coaches should be educated on age-appropriate pitching recommendations, including pitch counts and age restrictions on throwing specialty pitches.
- Should also stress importance of not throwing with a fatigued arm or painful shoulder as this can lead to future injury

PROGNOSIS

Patients treated with appropriate rest and rehabilitation have an excellent long-term prognosis.

COMPLICATIONS

Alteration of throwing mechanics from throwing with pain may lead to other injuries, such as labral tears or injuries to the elbow of the same arm.

REFERENCES

1. Arnold A, Thigpen CA, Beattie PF, et al. Overuse physeal injuries in youth athletes. *Sports Health.* 2017;9(2):139–147.
2. Watkins RA, De Borja C, Ramirez F. Common upper extremity injuries in pediatric athletes. *Curr Rev Musculoskeletal Med.* 2022;15(6):465–473.
3. Bednar ED, Kay J, Memon M, et al. Diagnosis and management of Little League shoulder: a systematic review. *Orthop J Sports Med.* 2021;9(7):23259671211017563.
4. Shanley E, Thigpen C. Throwing injuries in the adolescent athlete. *Int J Sports Phys Ther.* 2013;8(5):630–640.
5. Myers NL, Kennedy SM, Arnold A, et al. A narrative review of Little League shoulder: proximal humeral physis widening is only one piece of the puzzle, it is time to consider posterior glenoid dysplasia. *JSES Int.* 2024;8(4):724–733.

ADDITIONAL READING

DiFiori JP, Benjamin HJ, Brenner JS, et al. Overuse injuries and burnout in youth sports: a position statement from the American Medical Society for Sports Medicine. *Br J Sports Med.* 2014;48(4):287–288.

CLINICAL PEARLS

- An adolescent should never throw with shoulder pain or fatigue.
- Loss of velocity or pitch control during an outing is a sign of shoulder fatigue.
- Pain with external rotation and pain along physis can indicate thrower's shoulder.

L

LITTLE LEAGUER'S ELBOW (MEDIAL EPICONDYLE APOPHYSITIS)

Connor Farrell, DO • Denice Praxidio, DO • Michael Prestgard-Duke, MD

BASICS

DESCRIPTION

- Medial epicondyle apophysitis (MEA)
- A chronic overuse injury due to repetitive valgus stresses/traction forces at the apophysis of the medial epicondyle
- Little League elbow (LLE), aka throwers elbow, specifically refers to MEA and should not be used to describe avulsion fractures, ulnar collateral ligament (UCL) injuries, or tendonitis.

EPIDEMIOLOGY

- It has been estimated that 20–40% of 9- to 12-year-old baseball players suffer from elbow pain, with 2/3 of symptoms occurring at the medial elbow.
- Among baseball/softball players, peak incidence of LLE is between the ages of 11 and 12 years (1), when prevalence is ~30% (2).
- X-ray screening of Little League Baseball regional and national championship contenders showed 57% had evidence of displacement of the medial epicondyle.
- Ultrasound (US) and magnetic resonance imaging (MRI) of youth baseball players have shown medial epicondyle abnormalities ranging from 10–50% on the throwing side (3).

ETIOLOGY AND PATHOPHYSIOLOGY

- The medial epicondyle is the site of attachment for the common flexor muscle origins and the UCL.
- There are six distinct secondary centers of ossification in the elbow: capitellum, radius, internal (medial) epicondyle, trochlea, olecranon, and external (lateral) epicondyle (CRITOE) ossification center to close, generally between ages 15 and 16 years in most individuals (1).
- Before ossification, repetitive valgus stresses to the elbow are more likely to injure the apophysis than the UCL, as the UCL and its attachment is 5 times stronger than the open apophysis. In late adolescence or adulthood, the same repetitive forces would be more likely to cause a UCL injury or avulsion fracture.
- In overhead athletes, LLE is caused by valgus stress forces placed on the elbow during late cocking and early acceleration phases of throwing.

RISK FACTORS

- Overuse and fatigue have the strongest contribution to risk (1).
- Position: shows magnitude of stress (pitcher > catcher > infielder > outfielder); playing pitcher and catcher on the same team
- Activity level: types of pitches, number of pitches, innings pitched, typical pitching rotation, increased pitch velocity, pitching through fatigue, pitching on multiple teams, pitching in multiple games on the same day or back to back days (1)
- Pitching >100 innings per year is associated with 3.5 times increased injury risk.
- Longitudinal study found a 35% increase in elbow pain in players aged 9 to 12 years who threw >75 pitches a game and a similar increase in pitchers who threw >600 pitches in a season.
- Fatigue: Pitchers who ignore fatigue and continue to pitch are at a >10 times risk for injury.
- Lack of physical conditioning has been associated with LLE.
- Family history of osteochondrosis
- Glenohumeral internal rotation deficit (GIRD) >25 degrees shown to increase shoulder and elbow pathology

GENERAL PREVENTION

- All pitchers should be taught to incorporate proper form and mechanics.
- Core strengthening and stretching exercises should be implemented, including yearlong general conditioning and proper warm-up.
- The most important factor is monitoring the number of competitive pitches in practice and games.
- Current recommendations for 8- to 14-year-olds include a maximum of 50 to 75 pitches per game, 75 to 125 per week, and 1,000 pitches for an entire season.
- The USA Baseball Medical and Safety Advisory Committee recommends the following:
  - Pitchers <13 years old only throw fastballs and changeups.
  - Ages 8 to 18 years should take at least 4 months off from throwing every year. 2 to 3 of those months should be continuous.
  - Avoid playing high-volume throwing positions such as pitcher and catcher until the fusion of apophysis.

COMMONLY ASSOCIATED CONDITIONS

- Flexion contracture
- If an avulsion fragment is incarcerated in the joint, it can severely damage the articular surface.
- UCL tear
- Ulnar nerve injury, cubital tunnel

DIAGNOSIS

HISTORY

- Age: important because of the different ages at which each growth center appears and/or closes
- Location: Most commonly, pain is located at the medial epicondyle; however, sometimes pain presents laterally or posteriorly.
- Duration (pain characteristics): The length of time that the athlete has had pain is usually an indirect measure of the severity of the problem. If the pain occurs during and after throwing, it is an ominous sign.
- Radiation: If pain or numbness radiates into the last two fingers, consider ulnar nerve involvement (neuritis).
- Mechanism (acute vs. chronic): Acute pain in the young athlete in the medial elbow is more consistent with avulsion fracture of the medial epicondyle. In chronic pain, athletes may complain of pulling, popping, giving out, or decreased velocity during throwing; pain accentuated during early and late cocking of throwing motion when there is maximum valgus stress on the medial elbow.

PHYSICAL EXAM

- Pain in the medial elbow
- Bilateral comparison of elbow appearance
- Inspection: Note the presence of swelling, muscle atrophy/hypertrophy, symmetry, and carrying angle (normal 5 to 10 degrees in males, 10 to 15 degrees in females); ecchymosis (rare) can be indicative of an avulsion.
- Palpation: medial/lateral epicondyles (point tenderness along medial epicondyle concerning for avulsion fracture), olecranon process, radial head collateral ligaments, ulnar nerve
- Range of motion: flexion/extension (flexion contracture >15 degrees consistent with avulsion fracture); supination/pronation usually normal; assess for UCL stability with valgus stress at 20 to 30 degrees of flexion (4)[C]
- Evaluation of the shoulder to assess for scapular dyskinesia, GIRD, and rotator cuff strength
- Neurologic: Check sensation along the ulnar nerve distribution; check Tinel sign at the cubital tunnel; check interosseous muscle strength in the hand.

DIFFERENTIAL DIAGNOSIS

- Medial epicondylitis
- Avulsion fracture
- UCL sprain/tear
- Osteochondritis dissecans (capitellum most common)
- Avascular necrosis/osteochondrosis of the capitellum (Panner disease) may have lateral pain.
- Neoplasms
- Referred pain: neck, shoulder, wrist

DIAGNOSTIC TESTS & INTERPRETATION

- Radiographs are useful to evaluate for widening of the medial epicondyle apophysis and humeral metaphysis with or without fragmentation, sclerosis, or thickening.
- Anteroposterior and lateral views of elbow
- Bilateral elbow images can be useful to compare medial epicondylar ossification centers.
- Appearance of growth centers: CRITOE:
  - Capitellum: appears at 1 to 2 years of age
  - Radial epiphysis (3 to 4 years)
  - Internal (medial) epicondyle (medial, 5 to 6 years)
  - Trochlea (9 to 10 years)
  - External (lateral) epicondyle (lateral, >10 years)
- Assess for the presence of anterior and especially posterior fat pad.
- Assess for displacement of epicondylar fragment (5)[C].
- Radiographs taken in early LLE may be normal up to 85% of the time.
- MRI, computed tomography (CT), or bone scan rarely indicated as the diagnosis is clinical but may be helpful if the athlete fails to show signs of improvement.
- MRI may show widening of the apophysis with varying levels of inflammation and bone marrow edema surrounding the apophysis.
- US has shown to have 88% positive predictive value and may demonstrate cortical discontinuity or fragmentation at the medial epicondyle in early LLE (3)[B].
- Either stress radiographs or US can assess for elbow instability defined as 3 mm or more of joint separation under valgus stress and UCL injury.

TREATMENT

- Acute treatment:
  - Ice and nonsteroidal anti-inflammatory drugs (NSAIDs) as needed
  - Typically 4 to 6 weeks of rest:
    - Athletes should work on general conditioning, endurance, and core-strengthening exercises during the initial period of rest from throwing.
    - Range-of-motion exercises, stretches, and strengthening with bands or light dumbbells focused on scapula retractor and posterior shoulder girdle can be beneficial.
  - A progression of a noncompetitive throwing program (i.e., The Thrower's Ten, Advanced Thrower's Ten) can begin after the initial rest period and if pain has resolved.
  - On average, total time to return to competition is 8 to 12 weeks.
- Long-term treatment is focused on prevention (4)[C]:
  - Pitch count guidelines (Major League Baseball [MLB] Pitch Smart):
    - Most recent guidelines updated in 2021
    - Ages <8 years (50 pitches per game), 9 to 10 years (75 pitches), 11 to 12 years (85 pitches), 13 to 16 years (95 pitches), 17 to 18 years (105 pitches), 19 to 22 years (120 pitches)
    - Guidelines also provide rest day rules, in-season recommendations for pitch count progressions, and annual inning limits.
    - These guidelines allow too many pitches per age group because they are not only based on the evidence but on a consensus with U.S. baseball.

ADDITIONAL THERAPIES

- Treatment depends on the amount of displacement of the medial epicondylar apophysis (5)[C],(6)[C].
- If a fragment is minimally displaced (2 to 5 mm):
  - Apply posterior splint until acute symptoms resolve (2 to 4 weeks).
  - Gradual active motion
  - Radiologic healing by ~6 weeks; at this time, start aggressive active motion.
  - When bony union is achieved, allow the patient to throw if pain free.
  - Allow return to competitive play when there is normal range of motion/strength/endurance while throwing and having completed throwing program, often up to 1 year after initial injury.
- If fragment is displaced >5 mm:
  - Open reduction and internal fixation Two cancellous screws to prevent rotation
  - Allow early gradual active motion.
  - After 6 weeks, aggressive rehabilitation program
  - Postsurgical treatment showed no difference in outcome between nonoperative versus operative with 25–75% fracture displacement.

ONGOING CARE

Closed reduction is associated with pseudoarthrosis, causing pain and instability as well as formation of double epicondylar epiphyses.

REFERENCES

1. DeFroda S, McGlone P, Levins J, et al. Shoulder and elbow injuries in the adolescent throwing athlete. *R I Med J (2013).* 2020;103(7):21–29.
2. Norton R, Honstad C, Joshi R, et al. Risk factors for elbow and shoulder injuries in adolescent baseball players: a systematic review. *Am J Sports Med.* 2019;47(4):982–990.
3. Watkins RA, De Borja C, Ramirez F. Common upper extremity injuries in pediatric athletes. *Curr Rev Musculoskelet Med.* 2022;15(6):465–473.
4. Leahy I, Schorpion M, Ganley T. Common medial elbow injuries in the adolescent athlete. *J Hand Ther.* 2015;28(2):201–210.
5. Zellner B, May MM. Elbow injuries in the young athlete—an orthopedic perspective. *Pediatr Radiol.* 2013;43(Suppl 1):S129–S134.
6. Cruz AI Jr, Steere JT, Lawrence JTR. Medial epicondyle fractures in the pediatric overhead athlete. *J Pediatr Orthop.* 2016;36(Suppl 1):S56–S62.

ADDITIONAL READING

- Axibal DP, Carry P, Skelton A, et al. No difference in return to sport and other outcomes between operative and nonoperative treatment of medial epicondyle fractures in pediatric upper-extremity athletes. *Clin J Sport Med.* 2020;30(6):e214–e218.
- Benjamin HJ, Briner WW Jr. Little League elbow. *Clin J Sport Med.* 2005;15(1):37–40.
- Holt JB, Pedowitz JM, Stearns PH, et al. Progressive elbow magnetic resonance imaging abnormalities in Little League baseball players are common: a 3-year longitudinal evaluation. *Am J Sports Med.* 2020;48(2):466–472.
- Mullaney M, Nicholas S, Tyler T, et al. Evidence based arm care: the throwers 10 revisited. *Int J Sports Phys Ther.* 2021;16(6):1379–1386.
- Osbahr DC, Chalmers PN, Frank JS, et al. Acute, avulsion fractures of the medial epicondyle while throwing in youth baseball players: a variant of Little League elbow. *J Shoulder Elbow Surg.* 2010;19(7):951–957.

CLINICAL PEARLS

- At present, baseball youth leagues have rules that limit the number of innings per week and length of time between pitching appearances. In addition, specific pitch count recommendations have been published and adopted by the Little League in conjunction with the MLB in a program called Pitch Smart (https://www.mlb.com/pitch-smart/pitching-guidelines/).
- Best prevention is to follow established pitching guidelines set forth by the Little League. An off-season conditioning program, including core and upper body strengthening along with a throwing program, may also be helpful. It is generally recommended to take 4 months off (at least 2 to 3 consecutive months) of throwing per year in adolescent athletes. If pain does begin to occur, the player should stop throwing and see a physician.

LOW BACK PAIN AND LUMBAR STRAINS

Diego Riveros, MD • John M. Kiel, DO, MPH

BASICS

DESCRIPTION

- Acute low back pain is pain of <3 months duration localized below the costal margin but above the inferior gluteal folds with or without leg pain.
- Synonym(s): lumbar strain; lumbar sprain; lumbago; low back syndrome
- Acute pain is felt in the low lumbar, lumbosacral, or sacroiliac region. It may be accompanied by sciatica, pain radiating down the distribution of the sciatic nerve.
- Chronic low back pain is the same unremitting pain that has been present for >3 months.

EPIDEMIOLOGY

- The total costs of low back pain in the United States exceed $100 billion per year from direct and indirect costs.
- Most common between the ages of 35 and 55 years
- ~1% of the U.S. population is chronically disabled because of back problems, and another 1% is temporarily disabled.

Incidence

- 90% of people experience low back pain in their lifetime; 5–10% will develop chronic back pain.
- Approximately 9.8% will develop sciatic nerve or radicular back pain.
- Various authors have reported incidences of 16–22% in populations 8 to 14 years of age.

Prevalence

- Annual prevalence in the U.S. population is 15–20%.
- Increases with age, peaking during the 6th decade of life

RISK FACTORS

- Age
- Activity
- Occupation
- Obesity
- Smoking
- Sedentary lifestyle
- Psychosocial factors
- Poor posture
- Chronic flexion injuries

GENERAL PREVENTION

- Exercise programs, posture training, body mechanics training, and weight loss have been advised.
- US Preventive Services Task Force has concluded that current evidence is not adequate to recommend for or against the routine use of interventions to prevent low back pain in adults.

DIAGNOSIS

HISTORY

- Initial history should focus on the patient's age and pain characteristics (onset, duration, severity, quality, radiation, aggravating factors, alleviating factors).
- Question patient about mechanism of injury and occupation.
- Determine if serious underlying conditions (red flags) are responsible for the back pain: fracture (steroid use, trauma, menopausal status); infection (fever, intravenous [IV] drug use, adenopathy, immunosuppression); cancer (weight loss, adenopathy, previous cancer); cauda equina syndrome (bowel or bladder incontinence, saddle anesthesia, major limb motor weakness).
- Assess psychological and socioeconomic problems.
- The patient should be assessed for the following red flags:
  - Is patient <20 or >55 years old with no prior history of back pain?
  - Known or previous cancer? Assume bone metastasis until otherwise proven.
  - IV drug abuse? Assume spinal abscess if tender.
  - Is pain increased or unrelieved by rest? Is low back pain relieved by bed rest?
  - Is pain associated with fever, chills, or weight loss? Look for infection or tumor.
  - Loss of bowel or bladder control and/or caudal anesthesia? Look for cauda equina syndrome.
  - TUNAFISH—Trauma, Unexplained weight loss, Neurologic symptoms, Age <20 or >55 years, Fever, Intravenous drug use (IVDU), Steroid use, History of cancer

PHYSICAL EXAM

- Tenderness to palpation located below the costal margin but above the inferior gluteal folds
- Possible radiation of pain to buttocks and lower extremity
- Pain aggravated by movement and alleviated by rest
- Limited range of motion of the lumbar spine
- True paraspinal muscular spasm is uncommon.
- Assess severity of pain by observing the patient's gait, posture, and demeanor.
- Prior to examining the back, check the temperature, weight.
- Consider checking skin, abdomen, pelvis, groin, peripheral pulses, and lymph nodes for pathology that may mimic spinal disease. A rectal exam should be performed to assess sphincter tone with bowel or bladder symptoms or inability to stand.
- With the patient standing, assess stance, spinal curvature, range of motion, heel-walk, toe-walk, and squat. Locate area of maximal pain.
- With patient sitting, assess patellar and Achilles deep tendon reflexes.
- With the patient supine, assess the straight-leg raise and contralateral straight-leg raise, ankle and great toe dorsiflexion, hip range of motion, sacroiliac joint stability, muscle strength testing, and sensory testing.
- If concern for lumbar spinal stenosis, consider a prone exam to perform a femoral stretch test.
- Pain in the low back is exacerbated by movement and is often accompanied by focal muscle spasm in the lumbar extensors.
- Patients prefer to stand in a semiflexed position and move slowly rather than sit motionless on the exam table.
- Walk on heels (L4–L5) and then toes (S1–S2).
- Assess back muscles for uncoordination or guarding (signs for spasm).

DIFFERENTIAL DIAGNOSIS

- Herniated disc
- Musculoskeletal sprains and strains
- Degenerative joint disease
- Posterior facet syndrome
- Spondylolisthesis
- Spinal stenosis
- Osteoporosis
- Ankylosing spondylitis
- Referred pain
- Tumor
- Infection
- Fracture
- Genitourinary
- Gynecologic
- Psychogenic
- 85% mechanical back pain (MBP)
- 5% symptomatic herniated disc
- 4% compression fracture
- 4% spondylolysis/spondylolisthesis
- 2% tumor, infection, rheumatologic disease, or referred pain

DIAGNOSTIC TESTS & INTERPRETATION

- In the absence of red flag symptoms, imaging can usually be delayed until 30 days after the initial assessment. This approach allows 90% of patients to recover spontaneously and avoids unneeded testing and procedures.
- If symptoms persist >30 days, consider plain radiographs.
- Depending on results of plain imaging and differential diagnosis, consider computed tomography (CT) scan, magnetic resonance imaging (MRI), and bone scan.
- If no red flags are identified in the history, then no imaging tests or laboratory tests are indicated.
- If a red flag is identified, then proceed with diagnostic testing as indicated.

TREATMENT

- Natural history of MBP, regardless of treatment: 33% resolve within 1 week, 70% resolve within 1 month, and 90–95% resolve within 3 months.
- Analgesia:
  - Acetaminophen for 2 weeks (as effective as nonsteroidal anti-inflammatory drugs [NSAIDs] if given on schedule)
  - NSAIDs <8 to 10 days can provide pain relief and allow early ambulation (caution for renal insufficiency, pregnancy, hypertension [HTN], gastrointestinal [GI] intolerance, history of gastric ulcers or bleeding).
  - Short-term tramadol can be considered.
  - Opioids have low-to-moderate evidence of short-term efficacy in chronic low back pain. The efficacy of long-term use remains unproven (1)[B]. Caution should be taken before initiating opioids for chronic back pain given risk of dependence and abuse.
  - Short-term (<2 weeks) centrally acting skeletal muscle relaxants are effective in the management of nonspecific low back pain, but due to adverse effects, they should be used with caution.

- Manipulative medicine:
  - Massage therapy may be effective for treatment of chronic back pain (1)[B].
  - Passive therapies, such as spinal manipulation therapy, muscle energy, and traction have no proven benefit.
  - Physical therapy modalities including muscle energy, low-level laser therapy, and ultrasound have no evidence to support their use.
  - Exercise therapy appears to be slightly effective at decreasing pain and increasing function in adults with chronic low back pain (2)[B].
  - The McKenzie method results in a decrease in and disability, but not pain, for acute low back pain (3)[A].
  - There is evidence that yoga results in small-to-moderate improvements in back-related function at 3 and 6 months; it may be slightly more effective for pain (2)[B].
  - Motor control exercise has low-to-moderate quality evidence that helps in chronic low back pain.
  - Combined chiropractic interventions slightly improved pain and disability for acute and sub-acute lower back pain.
  - Aquatic exercise appears to be beneficial in patients suffering from chronic back pain and pregnancy-related low back pain, but there is no evidence it is better than land-based exercise.
- Systemic corticosteroids: no proven benefit and significant potential harm (avascular necrosis of the hip) (4)[A]
- Antidepressants: There is no evidence that antidepressants are more effect than placebo in the management of nonspecific low back pain. There is some evidence that tricyclic antidepressants may be similar in effectiveness to gabapentinoids.
- Antiepileptic medications: Gabapentin and pregabalin use has shown nonsignificant improvement in pain compared to placebo. Topiramate is also slightly better than placebo for nonradicular back pain.
- Behavioral therapy: There is moderate-quality evidence that behavioral therapy can help individuals with chronic low back pain (5)[A].
- Herbal medicine: Low- to moderate-quality evidence shows that four topical herbal medicines may reduce pain in acute and chronic low back pain compared to placebo: cayenne, harpagoside, willow bark, and comfrey.
- Injection therapy: There is conflicting evidence regarding the efficacy of prolotherapy. When used alone, it is not an effective treatment; however, when combined with other modalities, it may improve chronic low back pain (1)[B]. There is insufficient evidence to support any specific drug for injection (NSAIDS, corticosteroids, etc.) or location (disc, muscles, etc.).
- Radiofrequency denervation: There is low-quality evidence supporting the use of radiofrequency denervation in patients with chronic low back pain (1)[C].
- Transcutaneous electrical nerve stimulation (TENS): There is no evidence from the small number of placebo-controlled trials to support the use of TENS (1)[A].
- Acupuncture: may have a favorable effect on self-reported pain and functional limitations in nonspecific chronic low back pain
- Insoles: There is strong evidence that insoles are ineffective for prevention of chronic back pain (6)[A].
- Lumbar support: There is moderate evidence that lumbar support is not more effective than no intervention in preventing low back pain.
- Long term:
  - Systematic review of the literature of chronic low back pain concluded that individualized exercise therapy programs that incorporated stretching or strengthening and supervision may improve pain and function in chronic nonspecific low back pain.
  - Cochrane review of the literature added that there is evidence that a graded activity program improves absentee outcomes in subacute low back pain. In acute low back pain, exercise therapy is as effective as either no treatment or other conservative treatments.

ISSUES FOR REFERRAL

Rapidly progressive neurologic deficits, symptoms of cauda equina syndrome or cord compression, acute vertebral collapse, suspicion of infection

ADDITIONAL THERAPIES

- Bed rest for 2 to 4 days may be required in patients with severe initial symptoms of sciatica. Prolonged bed rest (>4 days) should be avoided.
- Patients should be advised to stay active because this speeds recovery and reduces time away from work. It takes twice as long to regain conditioning as it does to lose it.
- Begin with low-stress aerobic activity such as walking, riding a bicycle, swimming, and eventually jogging.
- After [illegible]–2 weeks of general activity, specific conditioning exercises for trunk muscles may be helpful.
- Physical therapy may be helpful during the first month of symptoms. Goal of therapy is increasing function, not absence of pain.

SURGERY/OTHER PROCEDURES

- Considered only when serious spinal pathology or nerve root dysfunction due to a herniated lumbar disc is detected
- Patients with acute low back pain alone, without findings of serious conditions or significant nerve root compression, rarely benefit from surgery.
- Surgery has not been proven to help back pain without radiculopathy.

ONGOING CARE

FOLLOW-UP RECOMMENDATIONS

- Begin walking as soon as possible.
- Early osteopathic or chiropractic referral is often beneficial.
- Early orthopedic or physical therapy referral is rarely indicated.

REFERENCES

1. Foster NE, Anema JR, Cherkin D, et al. Prevention and treatment of low back pain: evidence, challenges, and promising directions. *Lancet*. 2018;391(10137):2368–2383.
2. Hayden JA, Ellis J, Ogilvie R, et al. Some types of exercise are more effective than others in people with chronic low back pain: a network meta-analysis. *J Physiother*. 2021;67(4):252–262.
3. Karlsson M, Bergenheim A, Larsson MEH. Effects of exercise therapy in patients with acute low back pain: a systematic review of systematic reviews. *Syst Rev*. 2020;9(1):182.
4. Migliorini F, Maffulli N. Choosing the appropriate pharmacotherapy for nonspecific chronic low back pain. *J Orthop Surg Res*. 2022;17(1):556.
5. Cherkin DC, Sherman KJ, Balderson BH, et al. Effect of mindfulness-based stress reduction vs cognitive behavioral therapy or usual care on back pain and functional limitations in adults with chronic low back pain: a randomized clinical trial. *JAMA*. 2016;315(12):1240–1249.
6. Chuter V, Spink M, Searle A, et al. The effectiveness of shoe insoles for the prevention and treatment of low back pain: a systematic review and meta-analysis of randomised controlled trials. *BMC Musculoskelet Disord*. 2014;15:140.

ADDITIONAL READING

- Baena-Beato PÁ, Artero EG, Arroyo-Morales M, et al. Aquatic therapy improves pain, disability, quality of life, body composition and fitness in sedentary adults with chronic low back pain. A controlled clinical trial. *Clin Rehabil*. 2014;28(4):350–360.
- Chou R, Baisden J, Carragee EJ, et al. Surgery for low back pain: a review of the evidence for an American Pain Society clinical practice guideline. *Spine (Phila Pa 1976)*. 2009;34(10):1094–1109.
- Macedo LG, Smeets RJ, Maher CG, et al. Graded activity and graded exposure for persistent nonspecific low back pain: a systematic review. *Phys Ther*. 2010;90(6):860–879.
- Vijan S, Manaker S, Qaseem A. Noninvasive treatments for acute, subacute, and chronic low back pain. *Ann Intern Med*. 2017;167(11):835–836.

CLINICAL PEARLS

- Acute low back pain is the most common musculoskeletal complaint seen by primary care providers associated with a significant morbidity, health care cost, and missed work.
- In the absence of red flags, imaging is generally not necessary on initial evaluation, and most patients will improve within 1 month.
- Red flags (TUNAFISH)—Trauma, Unexplained weight loss, Neurologic symptoms, Age <20 or >55 years, Fever, IVDU, Steroid use, History of cancer
- Initial conservative management includes minimal bed rest, nonopioid analgesia, muscle relaxants, and physical therapy.
- Discriminate use of opioid analgesia is needed due to risk for dependence and abuse.
- Alternative, evidence-based treatments include exercise therapy, yoga, chiropractic interventions, aquatic exercise therapy, behavioral therapy, and herbal medicine.
- There is no evidence supporting the use of corticosteroids, with increased risk of adverse events.

LUMBAR DISC DISEASE

Daniel C. Herman, MD, PhD, FAAPMR, FACSM, FISBS, CAQSM ▪ Kevin Nasre-Esfahani, DO, MS ▪ Alexandra E. Warrick, MD, CAQSM

BASICS

DESCRIPTION

- Any disease process that alters the normal anatomy of the disks between the vertebral bodies, causing various musculoskeletal and/or neurologic symptoms (low back pain, radiculopathy, urinary/bowel incontinence, etc.).
- It represents a broad spectrum of pathology, including disk herniations, disk space narrowing, disk desiccation, discogenic pain, and sclerosis of the end plates as well as many other lumbar spine abnormalities with various etiologies.
- Lumbar disk degeneration increases the risk of lumbar disk herniation.
- Lumbar disk herniations may cause compression on a spinal nerve root and associated radiating back and leg pain (1).
- Per North American Spine Society, disk herniation is defined as a localized displacement of disk material beyond the normal margins of the intervertebral disk space resulting in pain, weakness or numbness in myotomal, or dermatomal distribution (2).

EPIDEMIOLOGY

Incidence

- Approximately 3:1 male-to-female ratio
- Peak incidence is between the 4th and 6th decades of life.

ETIOLOGY AND PATHOPHYSIOLOGY

- Compromise in the integrity of the annulus fibrosus may allow herniation of the nucleus pulposus (3).
- Herniation of the nucleus pulposus of the disk may compress and irritate the adjacent nerve root.
- The disk herniates when the pressure within the nucleus pulposus increases from a torsional strain or compression, and it pushes against the outside ring of the annulus fibrosis and overcomes its tensile strength (3).
- The most common location of herniation is paracentral (as the posterior longitudinal ligament is weakest at this location), followed by central, and then foraminal (lateral).
- Different stages of herniation include protrusion, extrusion, and sequestration.
- Due to vertical anatomy of lumbar nerve roots, paracentral and foraminal disk herniation will affect different nerve roots.
- Most common site of herniation is L5–S1, affecting the S1 nerve root with a paracentral herniation and the L5 nerve root with a foraminal herniation (3).
- Second most common site of herniation is L4–L5, affecting the L5 nerve root with a paracentral herniation and the L4 nerve root with a foraminal herniation (3).
- Central herniation may present with back pain only, but the clinician should take caution for other possible red flags, such as cauda equina syndrome (see below).

RISK FACTORS

- Gradual age related decrease in the hydration of the disk, which decreases the cushioning effect, and increase in collagen content of the nucleus pulposus (3).
- Obesity, smoking, sedentary occupations, physical inactivity, lifting heavy loads, motor vehicle driving, and torsional stress (4)
- Family history of acquired spinal disorders, such as ankylosing spondylitis and degenerative arthritis
- Prior low back injuries or surgeries
- Recent studies have identified specific risk factors such as genetic markers and lifestyle factors such as prolonged sitting and poor ergonomic practices (4).

DIAGNOSIS

HISTORY

- May present with a history of multiple episodes of back pain that vary in severity and duration:
  - May present following an acute lifting or twisting injury
  - Acute disk herniation symptoms are worsened by coughing, sneezing, and Valsalva maneuver, as well as forward flexion.
- May present with pain originating in the low back and radiating to the buttock and down the posterior or lateral thigh to the ankle or foot:
  - More specific for disk herniation if the pain is greater in the leg than in the back or if the pain is worse with Valsalva maneuver
- Can present with back pain that does not radiate, but patient may note motor or sensory deficits
- Pay attention to patient history that may indicate alternate diagnosis such as history of malignancy, immunosuppression, drug use, etc.
- Red flag symptoms that may indicate an alternative diagnosis, including cauda equina syndrome, infection, or neoplasm (3):
  - Fecal incontinence
  - Loss of motor function
  - Perianal numbness
  - Radicular symptoms lasting >6 weeks
  - Saddle anesthesia
  - Urinary retention or incontinence
  - Unexplained fever, night sweats
  - Unintentional weight loss
  - No improvement with >6 weeks of conservative management

PHYSICAL EXAM

- A full physical exam of the back, pelvis, and lower extremities should be done, including a detailed neurologic exam:
  - Visual exam of the lower back and lower extremities and gait exam
  - Palpation of lower back, sacrum, and hips
  - Range of motion of lower back and lower extremities
  - Bilateral lower extremity strength, sensation, and reflex testing
- Provocative tests include:
  - Straight leg raise (SLR) of the ipsilateral limb to evaluate for nerve root compression (3)[C], performed with patient supine and passively raising the leg with hip flexed and knee extended. Symptoms are typically reproduced between 30 and 70 degrees of hip flexion.
  - Lasègue sign is positive with pain reproduced with knee extension during the SLR within the lumbosacral root distribution and resolution of pain with knee flexion.
  - Braggard sign involves lowering the leg just below pain threshold after SLR and causes symptoms with passive ankle dorsiflexion.
  - Bowstring sign: positive SLR, which is relieved with slight knee flexion and recreated by compression of the popliteal fossa
  - Crossed SLR involves performing SLR of the contralateral limb to evaluate for a nerve root compression with symptoms produced on the affected side (3)[C]. This test has a higher specificity for nerve root entrapment compared to SLR but low sensitivity.
  - Slump test: Patient in seated position is asked to slump forward in spinal flexion with chin flexed down to the chest; the knee is then passively extended; a positive test is reproduction of symptoms in the affected leg.
  - Femoral nerve tension test to assess for upper lumbar nerve root compression (L2–L4 nerve root impingement): Patient lies prone with passive hip extension and knee flexion with positive test resulting in reproduction of symptoms in the affected leg.
- Differentiate the findings of radiating leg pain from a lumbar or lumbosacral radiculopathy compared to tightness in the hamstrings.
- Compare to contralateral extremity.
- Other findings may include:
  - Decreased or loss of sensation, typically within a dermatomal distribution
  - Tendon reflex changes:
    - Diminished or absent patellar tendon reflex (predominantly L4 involvement, also L3)
    - Diminished or absent Achilles tendon reflex (S1 involvement)
  - Motor findings are often late findings. (Muscles receiving innervation from >1 spinal nerve root have the primary nerve root listed):
    - Weak hip flexion (L2 involvement)
    - Weak knee extension (L3 involvement)
    - Weak ankle dorsiflexion (L4 involvement)
    - Weak 1st toe extension (extensor hallucis longus [EHL]) or hip abduction (L5 involvement)
    - Weak ankle plantarflexion (S1 involvement)
- Waddell signs: to assess for possible nonorganic cause of back pain (psychological, socioeconomic, secondary gain, etc.) (3)[C]:
  - Tenderness:
    - Superficial tenderness with light palpation or tenderness on deep palpation but nonanatomic over a large area
  - Simulated tests:
    - Axial loading causes low back pain, or rotation of the hips and shoulders together causes low back pain.
  - Distraction:
    - Formal SLR is positive but when distracted, SLR does not produce pain.
  - Regional sensory or motor changes:
    - Glove and stocking sensation loss or nonanatomic muscular weakness (various muscles innervated by different nerve roots)
  - Overreaction:
    - Exaggerated response or emotions

DIFFERENTIAL DIAGNOSIS

- Cauda equina syndrome
- Referred pain (from other pelvic/hip disorders)
- Mononeuropathies or peripheral neuropathies (such as sciatica or meralgia paresthetica)
- Piriformis syndrome
- Sacroiliitis
- Spinal neoplasms
- Spinal stenosis
- Vascular insufficiency
- Vertebral fracture
- Spondylolisthesis
- Spondylolysis
- Infection/abscess

DIAGNOSTIC TESTS & INTERPRETATION

- Magnetic resonance imaging (MRI) is the preferred imaging modality; however, in the absence of red flag symptoms, MRI should be delayed for a 6-week trial of conservative treatment. If symptoms persist beyond 6 weeks, MRI may then be considered:
  - Important to note that imaging evidence of degenerative disk disease in asymptomatic individuals is very common and its prevalence increases with age (5)[C].
- Emergent imaging may be considered for red flag symptoms such as urinary retention, fecal incontinence, saddle anesthesia, progressive neurologic changes, and intractable pain.
- Plain radiographs may be beneficial to rule out osseous abnormalities (such as metastatic disease or fractures); in addition, they may demonstrate age-related degenerative changes.
- Computed tomography (CT) is also useful in evaluating osseous abnormalities and for those whom an MRI is contraindicated.
- CT myelogram can be useful for patient with MRI contraindications or with history of prior back surgeries (instrumentation can cause artifacts on MRI) (6)[C].

TREATMENT

GENERAL MEASURES

- Clinicians can reassure patients that most acute low back pain with or without sciatica symptoms generally has substantial improvement within the 1st month (6)[C].
- Most patients with acute/subacute low back pain improve over time regardless of treatment; therefore, nonpharmacologic treatment options are recommended first. These include superficial heat (moderate quality evidence), massage, acupuncture, and spinal manipulation (low quality evidence) (6)[C].
- Counsel regarding intradiscal pressure increasing with sitting and forward bending positions and is decreased with sitting and lying down (3)[C].
- Temporary bed rest has been debated and is not associated with better outcomes while increasing the risk for deconditioning. Activity as tolerated is recommended.
- Physical therapy and exercise-based interventions are recommended as first-line treatment along with medications for a 6-week conservative trial.
- After nonpharmacologic treatment, medications include nonsteroidal anti-inflammatory drugs (NSAIDs) or skeletal muscle relaxants while considering side effects and safety as muscle relaxants can cause sedation (6)[C]. Acetaminophen is associated with lower risk of adverse events compared to NSAIDs but demonstrated no significant benefit compared to placebo for the first 4 weeks of low back pain and was not evaluated for radicular low back pain (6)[C].
- For chronic low back pain, initial nonpharmacologic treatment is inclusive of exercise, tai chi, yoga, acupuncture, mindfulness-based stress reduction (6)[C].

MEDICATION

First Line

- Short-term NSAIDs or acetaminophen may be considered for low back pain.
- Although some have temporary relief of symptoms with oral steroids, the overall benefit remains inconclusive and is not standard of care.

Second Line

- For chronic low back pain, duloxetine was associated with a small improvement in function and pain intensity (6)[C].
- Opioids including tramadol are not standard of care given the risk for substantial harm, abuse, addiction, and side effect profile

SURGERY/OTHER PROCEDURES

- Epidural steroid injections can improve pain in the short term but do not provide long-term relief (2)[A].
- Surgical techniques for lumbar disk herniation include:
  - Open discectomy
  - Microdiscectomy
- Immediate indications for surgery include:
  - Cauda equina syndrome
  - Acute myelopathy
  - Severe motor deficits
  - Intractable pain
- Surgery may be considered with the failure of conservative therapy for lumbar disk herniation, and this may help with quicker improvement in pain; however, there has been no indication of an advantage with surgery compared to nonoperative treatment for midterm and long-term treatment (1)[A].
- For patients with lumbar disk herniation with radiculopathy whose symptoms warrant surgical intervention, discectomy may be considered; however, in patients with less severe symptoms; nonoperative treatment is effective for both short- and long-term relief (2)[C].

COMPLEMENTARY & ALTERNATIVE MEDICINE

- Modalities such as ultrasound and transcutaneous electrical nerve stimulation (TENS) do not have enough quality evidence to clearly assess their effectiveness (2)[C], although they may provide some short-term benefit.
- Traction produces conflicting evidence, and systemic reviews indicate that the results are inconsistent (2)[C].
- Aerobic conditioning and trunk muscle strengthening are important for good outcomes and preventing future injuries.

REFERENCES

1. Awadalla AM, Aljulayfi AS, Alrowaili AR, et al. Management of lumbar disc herniation: a systematic review. *Cureus*. 2023;15(10):e47908.
2. Kreiner DS, Hwang SW, Easa JE, et al. An evidence-based clinical guideline for the diagnosis and treatment of lumbar disc herniation with radiculopathy. *Spine J*. 2014;14(1):180–191.
3. Humphreys SC, Eck JC. Clinical evaluation and treatment options for herniated lumbar disc. *Am Fam Physician*. 1999;59(3):575–582, 587–588.
4. Ravichandran D, Pillai J, Krishnamurthy K. Genetics of intervertebral disc disease: a review. *Clin Anat*. 2022;35(1):116–120.
5. Sollman N, Fields AJ, O'Neill C, et al. Magnetic resonance imaging of the lumbar spine: recommendations for acquisition and image evaluation from the BACPAC spine imaging working group. *Pain Med*. 2023;24(Suppl 1):S81–S94.
6. Qaseem A, Wilt TJ, McLean RM, et al. Noninvasive treatments for acute, subacute, and chronic low back pain: a clinical practice guideline from the American College of Physicians. *Ann Intern Med*. 2017;166(7):514–530.

ADDITIONAL READING

- Brinjikji W, Luetmer PH, Comstock B, et al. Systematic literature review of imaging features of spinal degeneration in asymptomatic populations. *AJNR Am J Neuroradiol*. 2015;36(4):811–816.
- Greer S, Chambliss L, Mackler L, et al. Clinical inquiries. What physical exam techniques are useful to detect malingering? *J Fam Pract*. 2005;54(8):719–722.
- Peul WC, van Houwelingen HC, van den Hout WB, et al. Surgery versus prolonged conservative treatment for sciatica. *N Engl J Med*. 2007;356(22):2245–2256.
- Weinstein JN, Lurie JD, Tosteson TD, et al. Surgical vs nonoperative treatment for lumbar disk herniation: the Spine Patient Outcomes Research Trial (SPORT) observational cohort. *JAMA*. 2006;296(20):2451–2459.

CLINICAL PEARLS

- Obtaining a detailed and careful history and physical exam is the key for making proper diagnosis and treatment plan for any lumbar disk disease etiology.
- In the absence of red flag symptoms, conservative management may be attempted for 6 weeks prior to obtaining diagnostic imaging such as MRI.
- Conservative management may include NSAIDs and/or acetaminophen.
- Although some have temporary relief of symptoms with oral steroids, the overall benefit remains inconclusive.
- Epidural steroids may provide short-term relief but have not been shown to provide long-term relief.
- Clinicians can reassure patients that most acute low back pain with or without sciatica symptoms generally has substantial improvement within the first month.

LUNATE DISSOCIATION

Hirotaka Nakagawa, MD • Daniel C. Herman, MD, PhD, FAAPMR, FACSM, FISBS, CAQSM • Brandon Hassid, MD

BASICS

DESCRIPTION

- Dissociation or dislocation, is classified by the pattern of carpal collapse, either dorsal or volar in nature, after wrist trauma or injury.
- Although they have different meanings, dislocation is often used interchangeably with dissociation; a dislocated bone is always dissociated, but a dissociated bone is not always dislocated.
- Anatomy:
  - The carpal bones in the wrist are stabilized by multiple extrinsic and intrinsic ligaments. The scaphoid, lunate, and triquetrum have no tendon insertions and are described as an intercalated segment (motion depends on mechanical signals from ligamentously intact neighboring articulations) (1).
  - The dorsal component of the scapholunate interosseous ligament (SLIL) is the primary stabilizer of the lunate. Important secondary stabilizers include the intrinsic dorsal intercarpal (DIC) and extrinsic dorsal radiocarpal (DRC) ligaments (1),(2),(3).
  - Other secondary stabilizers include the scapho-trapezio-trapezoid (STT) ligamentous complex and radiolunate ligaments. The STT ligament complex plays a major role in preventing abnormal scapholunate (SL) rotation (1).
- Injury patterns:
  - Injury typically occurs when an extended wrist undergoes a forced axial load, such as in a fall on outstretched hand (FOOSH) with the hand in ulnar deviation (1).
  - Several injury patterns can occur with this mechanism, depending on several factors: position of the extremity at impact, quality of the bone, ligamentous strength, and direction of the force (2).
  - Isolated carpal dislocations are rare. Most information about them comes from case reports and surgical technique papers (2).
  - The terms *lunate dissociation*, *scapholunate dissociation (SLD)*, and *perilunate dissociation* and *dislocation* have overlapping features. Similarly, injury patterns to the lunate and adjacent structures have overlapping characteristics and nomenclatures.
  - Mayfield initially described four stages of perilunate instability in 1980 that have since been modified (2),(3):
    - Stage 1: disruption of scapholunate articulation
    - Stage 2: lunocapitate dislocation
    - Stage 3: lunotriquetral disruption
    - Stage 4: volar lunate dislocation
  - A four-stage classification system is used commonly to describe SLD (4):
    - Stage 1: Predynamic instability consists of the mildest form of SL injury and results from a stretched or partially torn SLIL. This may cause abnormal motion, synovitis, and wrist pain. Plain and stress radiographs are normal; arthroscopy may show attenuation of the SLIL or hemorrhage within the SL joint. Untreated, secondary stabilizers may become attenuated and progress to dynamic or static instability.
    - Stage 2: Dynamic instability is characterized by ligamentous tear of the palmar or dorsal aspect of the SLIL. Portions of the ligament may be still intact. Plain radiographs will be normal, but stress views show widening of the SL interval. An arthrogram may show abnormalities within the ligament.
    - Stage 3: Static instability occurs with complete tear to the SLIL and attenuation or attrition of the supporting wrist ligaments. Radiographic changes become evident (gap of 3 mm or greater between the lunate and scaphoid on AP x-ray (aka *Terry Thomas* sign) or an SL angle >60 degrees on lateral views). Dorsal intercalated segmental instability (DISI) is often present.
    - Stage 4: Scapholunate advanced collapse (SLAC) refers to progressive carpal misalignment, cartilage damage, and arthritis due to long-standing dissociation of the scaphoid and lunate. Changes begin at the radial styloid and can progress to the radioscaphoid fossa and eventually to the midcarpal joint.

EPIDEMIOLOGY

- Wrist injuries account for an estimated 3–9% of all athletic-related injuries.
- A 10-year study done at the Cleveland Clinic revealed that 14.8% of athletic participants <16 years old sustained upper extremity injuries, and of these, 9% involved the wrist.
- 10% of lunate dissociations present as open injuries, and 26% as polytraumas (3).
- Perilunate dislocations (PLDs) are the most common carpal dislocation (2).
- More common in men in the 2nd and 3rd decades of life; less common in the elderly (distal radius typically fractures before ligamentous injury occurs) and children (radial physis is weaker, resulting in Salter-Harris fractures) (2).
- SLD is more common in football than in any other sport.
- About 25% of the lunate dissociations are missed on initial examination (3).
- The incidence of lunate dissociation is uncommon, but failure to identify the injury results in long-term disability.

RISK FACTORS

- Any injury involving excessive wrist extension and ulnar deviation with intracarpal supination (typically a FOOSH injury)
- Chronic crutch-walkers, gymnasts, American football players, collision sports
- Increased ulnar negative variance

GENERAL PREVENTION

Controversy exists as to whether braces or wrist guards effectively prevent wrist injuries.

- One cadaveric model showed decreased carpal fractures, ligament, and capsular tears with bracing.
- In-line skating-type guards have not been shown to prevent wrist fractures.
- European studies of snowboarders show a significant decrease in the incidence of wrist fractures and injuries with wrist guards.
- Some are concerned that bracing/guards simply alter the area of force transmission.

COMMONLY ASSOCIATED CONDITIONS

- Scaphoid fractures occur with a similar mechanism of injury (FOOSH) and can co-occur.
- Failure to diagnose and treat lunate dissociation increases the risk of arthritic degeneration and development of SLAC wrist.
- 50% have associated median nerve symptoms (3).

DIAGNOSIS

HISTORY

- Obtain detailed mechanism (typically a FOOSH with extended and ulnar deviated wrist) and timing of injury.
- Patients often have pain with activities including pushing and gripping. It is often associated with painful popping or clicking with these activities (1).
- Evaluate for any concomitant injuries (elbow, forearm, etc.).

PHYSICAL EXAM

- Signs and symptoms:
  - 100% of patients have dorsal wrist pain, 91% have decreased grip strength, and 71% have decreased range of motion (ROM).
  - Clicking with wrist motion (nonspecific)
- Physical examination:
  - Inspect for swelling and deformity; compare with contralateral wrist.
  - Tenderness is typically on radial aspect of the wrist. There may also be tenderness just distal to Lister tubercle.
  - Scaphoid tenderness (anatomic snuffbox) is a scaphoid fracture until proven otherwise.

- Document wrist ROM and neurovascular status (pulses, sensation, particularly median nerve distribution because it can be diminished in severe dissociations owing to mechanical forces).
- Finger extension test: Hold wrist in flexion, and test active finger extension against resistance; causes pain over lunate
- Watson scaphoid test may be positive. The examiner places the thumb on the scaphoid tubercle, and the four fingers wrap around the distal radius. While the wrist is in ulnar deviation, pressure is directed dorsally with the thumb at the volar scaphoid. The wrist is then radially deviated. Pain is the hallmark of a positive test result, although a dramatic "clunk" may be felt or heard.
- Kleinman shear stress test for lunotriquetral instability: Wrist in neutral position, examiner's contralateral thumb is placed over dorsal lunate while ipsilateral thumb loads the pisotriquetral joint with a dorsally directed force. Pain is a positive test.
- The Reagan shuck test and Linscheid compression test are other maneuvers to determine lunotriquetral instability.

DIFFERENTIAL DIAGNOSIS

- Scaphoid fracture
- Colles fracture (or other distal radius fracture)
- Scaphoid impaction syndrome
- Tenosynovitis/tendinopathy of the wrist and finger extensors
- Dorsal wrist ganglion cyst
- Other carpal bone injury
- Osteoarthritis and rheumatoid arthritis (in more chronic cases)

DIAGNOSTIC TESTS & INTERPRETATION

Initial Tests (lab, imaging)

Radiographs: posteroanterior (PA), lateral, and oblique views of the wrist, clenched-fist view (obtain contralateral views for comparison):

- Gap of 3 mm on PA films ("Terry Thomas" or "Dave Letterman" sign, in reference to their gapped teeth) is classically used. However, Cautilli obtained PA radiographs on 100 normal wrists and found the mean gap in males was 4.0 mm, and in females, it was 3.6 mm. Zhu performed a similar study and found the mean gap to be 3.14 mm. Both studies revealed that gaps up to 5 mm were not necessarily indicative of carpal instability. Consequently, contralateral wrist films should be obtained for comparison.
- Clenched-fist view accentuates injury.
- Lateral views: Dorsal extension of the lunate is referred to as DISI and is highly suggestive of injury to the SLIL and at least one secondary stabilizer.
- SL angle is normally 30 to 60 degrees on lateral view; an angle >70 degrees is highly suggestive (1)[C].
- In PLD, "spilled teacup sign" may be seen on lateral x-ray; lunate is tipped anteriorly such that capitate is no longer sitting within the concave surface of the lunate.

Follow-Up Tests & Special Considerations

Magnetic resonance imaging (MRI) (1),(2)[C]:

- Modality of choice for evaluating SL ligament injury
- MRI should preferably be performed at centers with dedicated wrist ligament imaging protocols and specialized wrist coils.
- 3T MRI had a sensitivity of 76–89% and specificity of 97–100% in detecting SL ligament tear.
- Complete SLIL tears are characterized by distinct area of discontinuity within the ligament, outlined by fluid-like T2 hyperintensity, or by complete absence of the ligament. Fluid signal at attachments also can be seen.
- Computed tomography (CT) can also provide information about ligamentous injury and fracture pattern, if present.

Diagnostic Procedures/Other

Arthroscopic evaluation is the "gold standard" for identifying and grading SL injuries. Wrist arthroscopy combined with fluoroscopic evaluation allows dynamic anatomic and functional evaluation (1)[C].

TREATMENT

Acute treatment:

- Analgesia; nonsteroidal anti-inflammatory drugs (NSAIDs) short term 8 to 10 days max
- Reduction techniques:
  - Only for mild injuries (e.g., dynamic instability; see above)
  - Recommended for experienced providers only
- Immobilization:
  - Partial tears of SLIL can be treated conservatively with splinting in correct anatomic position. Symptoms guide management.
  - Patients with suspected ligamentous injury should be referred promptly to an orthopedist, preferably a hand specialist, because misdiagnosis can have significant consequences.

ISSUES FOR REFERRAL

- Immediate referral to hand surgeon if abnormal neurovascular status
- Timely referral to hand surgeon if any question in the diagnosis
- Once the diagnosis is made, surgical referral is prudent as operative repair is the standard of care. Pain, recurrent instability, and degeneration can occur without definitive management.

ADDITIONAL THERAPIES

- Prolonged immobilization for weeks to months after surgery is necessary to maintain carpal bone alignment and prevent SLAC wrist.
- Rehabilitation: physical therapy after immobilization to improve ROM and strength
- Typically considered a season-ending injury

SURGERY/OTHER PROCEDURES

- Standard of care typically involves immediate closed reduction followed by open reduction, ligament and/or bone repair, and internal fixation. Carpal tunnel release is often performed concomitantly (3)[C].
- As lunate dissociation progresses, open reduction and internal fixation (ORIF) and proximal row carpectomy (PRC) are considered (3)[C].
- Chronic injuries had worse functional outcomes compared with acute injuries for those who were treated with both ORIF and PRC (3)[C].
- In a single-center retrospective study involving 32 patients who underwent ORIF after either isolated PLD or fracture-dislocation, predictors of poor functional outcome were (i) magnitude of lunate dislocation and (ii) having undergone concomitant open carpal tunnel release (5)[B].

REFERENCES

1. Wessel LE, Wolfe SW. Scapholunate instability: diagnosis and management—anatomy, kinematics, and clinical assessment—part I. *J Hand Surg Am*. 2023;48(11):1139–1149.
2. Grabow RJ, Catalano L III. Carpal dislocations. *Hand Clin*. 2006;22(4):485–500.
3. Fisher ND, Bi AS, De Tolla JE. Perilunate dislocations: current treatment options. *JBJS Rev*. 2022;10(9).
4. Chim H, Moran SL. Wrist essentials: the diagnosis and management of scapholunate ligament injuries. *Plast Reconstr Surg*. 2014;134(2):312e–322e.
5. Garçon C, Degeorge B, Coulet B, et al. Perilunate dislocation and fracture dislocation of the wrist: outcomes and long-term prognostic factors. *Orthop Traumatol Surg Res*. 2022;108(5):103332.

ADDITIONAL READING

- Manuel J, Moran SL. The diagnosis and treatment of scapholunate instability. *Orthop Clin North Am*. 2007;38(2):261–277.
- Sauder DJ, Athwal GS, Faber KJ, et al. Perilunate injuries. *Orthop Clin North Am*. 2007;38(2):279–288.
- Slade JF III, Milewski MD. Management of carpal instability in athletes. *Hand Clin*. 2009;25(3):395–408.
- Young D, Papp S, Giachino A. Physical examination of the wrist. *Orthop Clin North Am*. 2007;38(2):149–165.

CLINICAL PEARLS

- Surgery results in ~35% loss of flexion and extension. This should still allow an athlete to return to activity in most cases.
- The ligament in the wrist has torn in this injury, and the bones have shifted, so they cannot heal correctly without surgery.
- Early detection and management are crucial to avoid long-term consequences.

MALLET FINGER

Rachel A. Coel, MD, PhD, FAAP, CAQSM • Quynh Hoang, MD, FAAP, CAQSM

BASICS

DESCRIPTION

- Mallet finger is defined as a stretching or tearing of the extensor tendon or a complete avulsion of the tendon insertion from the dorsal base of the distal phalanx with or without bony avulsion.
- The injury results in the inability to actively extend the distal interphalangeal (DIP) joint.
- It is most caused by sudden forced flexion of the fingertip while the DIP joint is actively extended.
- Less commonly, it can occur when the DIP joint is forcefully hyperextended with a resulting fracture at the dorsal base of the distal phalanx.
- Closed mallet finger is more common than open injury.
- Chronic mallet finger is defined as a mallet injury presenting >4 weeks after injury.

EPIDEMIOLOGY

- Usually occurs during sports participation when an extended finger is struck on the tip by a ball.
- Also occurs in the work environment or with minor household trauma.
- The most injured digit is the third (middle) finger of the dominant hand, although any digit, including the thumb, can be involved.
- Estimated prevalence is 5.6% of all hand and wrist tendon injuries (1)[A].

RISK FACTORS

Sports, especially those involving ball contact and hand-to-hand contact.

DIAGNOSIS

HISTORY

- Patient reports axial loading and/or hyperflexion of the DIP joint while the finger is held in extension. Classically, the extended finger is struck on the tip by a ball.
- Complaints of pain, swelling, and flexion deformity at the DIP joint of the affected finger as well as tenderness especially at the dorsal aspect, with inability to actively extend the DIP joint.

PHYSICAL EXAM

- There is tenderness to palpation over the dorsum of the DIP joint.
- Patient is unable to actively extend the DIP joint, although passive extension is possible.
- To effectively establish the diagnosis, hold the proximal interphalangeal (PIP) joint in a fixed position, and then have the patient extend at the DIP joint.
- An extensor lag at the DIP joint is present immediately after injury, but the deformity may be delayed by hours and even days or weeks.
- Also evaluate for open skin lesions, collateral stability, and digit rotation or angulation.
- There are three classification systems used to describe the type of mallet injury: Doyle, Wehbe and Schneider, and Burton classification (used for chronic mallet finger) (2)[C].
- Using the Doyle classification scheme, mallet finger injuries can be divided into four types:
  - Type I: closed injury ± small dorsal avulsion fracture
  - Type II: open injury with tendon laceration
  - Type III: open injury with deep abrasion, causing loss of skin, subcutaneous tissue, and tendon substance
  - Type IV: mallet fracture:
    - Transepiphyseal fracture in children
    - Hyperflexion injury with fracture involving 20–50% of articular surface
    - Hyperextension injury with fracture involving >50% of articular surface

DIFFERENTIAL DIAGNOSIS

- Tuft or distal phalanx fracture with deformity
- In the pediatric age group, injury to the epiphysis at the base of the distal phalanx may mimic a mallet finger.
- In the pediatric age group, consider Seymour fracture—an open physeal fracture involving the nail bed and germinal matrix.
- Dislocation of DIP joint

DIAGNOSTIC TESTS & INTERPRETATION

- Radiographs are recommended in all cases to evaluate for accompanying fracture or joint subluxation.
- Three views of the affected finger: posteroanterior, lateral, and oblique
- Three patterns: no avulsion fracture, small avulsion fracture (<30% articular surface), large avulsion fracture (>30% articular surface)
- Consider obtaining repeat radiographs at conclusion of continuous splinting to evaluate fracture healing.

TREATMENT

GENERAL MEASURES

- Restoring active DIP extension and maintaining flexion mobility is the goal of treatment. An untreated mallet finger can potentially lead to joint stiffness, osteoarthritis, or swan-neck deformity.
- Overall, there is insufficient evidence regarding when surgical intervention is indicated. Both surgical and nonsurgical treatment of either bony or tendinous mallet finger led to similar clinical outcomes (3)[A].
- Most mallet finger lesions can be managed nonoperatively with continuous finger splinting (1)[A].
- Injuries involving more than one-third of the DIP joint articular surface or those with subluxation or displacement have traditionally been treated with surgery. If subluxation cannot be reduced by splinting, surgery is advocated (3)[A],(4)[A].
- Surgical treatment may provide decreased residual extension lag compared to nonsurgical management, although the degree of extension lag has been shown to be clinically insignificant (3)[A],(4)[A].
- For nonoperative treatment, the involved finger should be splinted in full extension or slight hyperextension at the DIP joint.
- No flexion should occur at any time until treatment is complete.
- Splint continuously for at least 6 to 8 weeks with additional weeks of immobilization in cases of persistent lag (5)[A].
- If bony avulsion fracture: An extension splint should be applied for 6 weeks.
- If tendon injury without bone involvement: Splint in extension for at least 8 weeks.
- Although most studies recommend additional 2 to 4 weeks of nighttime splinting, the effectiveness of night splinting after initial treatment of mallet finger is unknown (5)[A].
- Compliance should be assessed at 2-week intervals until healing has occurred. Success rate of nonoperative treatment can be reduced if patients remove the splint or flex the DIP joint when changing splints during skin care.
- Monitor skin for signs of ulceration, maceration, or local allergic reactions due to splinting.
- Controversy exists regarding the optimal nonoperative treatment of each type of mallet finger with respect to the type of splint used and the length of immobilization.
- Regardless of the type of splint material or whether it is applied dorsally or volarly over the finger, any type of splint maintaining the DIP joint in extension is effective (6)[C].
- The most used is the Stack splint (plastic or custom-made thermoplastic), whereas aluminum/foam splints and Abouna metal splints are also often used.
- The last Cochrane systematic review (2009) concluded that there is insufficient evidence from existing studies to establish the relative effectiveness of distinct types of finger splints used versus the standard Stack splint. Additionally, there is insufficient evidence to determine when surgery is indicated.

ADDITIONAL THERAPIES

- DIP joint often is stiff after prolonged immobilization.
- After 6 to 8 weeks of continuous splinting, start DIP joint gentle active and passive range of motion (ROM) exercises.
- At the end of continuous immobilization, if a mallet deformity of >20 degrees recur, continue splinting for an additional 4 to 8 weeks.
- Consider extension splinting during athletic activities for an additional 4 to 8 weeks after continuous splinting has been completed.
- For chronic mallet finger injury, treatment includes initial trial of prolonged splinting (10 weeks). Surgery is considered if there is extensor lag of 40 degrees or if there is a functional deficit (6)[C].

SURGERY/OTHER PROCEDURES

ALERT
Although operative treatment is recommended for mallet fractures involving >30% of the articular surface or if there is volar subluxation of the distal phalanx, indications for surgical intervention remain controversial.

If a subluxation cannot be reduced by splinting, surgery is advocated. Other cited indications for surgery include open injuries, failure of nonsurgical treatment, cosmetic reasons, or patients requiring fine manual dexterity.

- Common surgical treatments include Kirschner wire (K-wire) extension block pinning, K-wire fixation, and absorbable bone anchor. A number of surgical techniques have been proposed but the most effective surgical method is still under debate. A recent meta-analysis comparing K-wire fixation versus suture anchor technique for mallet fingers showed no significant differences in clinical outcomes (1)[A].

ONGOING CARE

FOLLOW-UP RECOMMENDATIONS

- Regular physician assessment and diligent patient compliance are critical for successful nonoperative treatment.
- Assess compliance with continuous splinting at follow-up visits at 2-week intervals.
- If the splint is to be removed during the provider visit, the injured DIP joint should be always maintained in extension. To accomplish this, consider removing the splint with the palmar aspect of the hand and fingers resting on a firm flat surface, such as a table, then slide the splint off, inspect skin breakdown, and slide back on.
- For bony mallet injuries consider repeat radiographs at the conclusion of continuous splinting to assess for fracture healing.

PATIENT EDUCATION

- This injury requires careful patient compliance.
- The patient must understand the necessity of keeping the finger in extension for the entire duration of treatment, including during hygiene, splint changes, and skin care.
- The patient must monitor for skin damage from continuous splinting, including skin irritation, infection, allergic reaction, maceration, and ulceration.

COMPLICATIONS

ALERT
Patients may develop a slight extensor lag (5 to 10 degrees) with a mild loss of total motion, but it should not result in a functional deficit.

- A recent meta-analysis showed no clinically significant difference in outcomes between operative and nonoperative management of mallet finger (3)[A].
- The same meta-analysis showed no significant difference in complication rates between surgical and conservative treatment (3)[A].
- However, complications from surgical intervention are often more serious and long term. These include nail dystrophy or deformity, pin tract infection, osteomyelitis, skin necrosis, loss of reduction, arthritis, and skin necrosis.
- Complications from conservative treatment tend to be related to splinting and typically are short term. These include skin irritation, maceration, ulceration, superficial infection, splint-related pain, tape allergies, and dorsal bump.
- Other complications include permanent DIP joint stiffness, persistent flexion deformity, recurrence of mallet deformity, and, in cases of open injuries, osteomyelitis.
- Swan-neck deformity at the level of the PIP joint can occur if mallet finger injury is untreated or if there is poor patient compliance with splinting.

Pediatric Considerations

- Physeal and epiphyseal involvement at the base of the distal phalanx is common in pediatric mallet finger injuries.
- Children <12 years old are more likely to have a Salter-Harris type I or II fracture rather than a true mallet injury.
- In the pediatric age group, a nondisplaced mallet finger injury may be treated with continuous splinting of the DIP joint in extension or slight hyperextension for 4 to 6 weeks. Thereafter, the effect of additional nighttime splinting remains unknown.
- Extension splints should also be worn for sports activities for an additional 4 weeks after continuous treatment.
- Reduction is necessary for displaced fractures. If closed reduction is unsuccessful, then referral for surgical reduction and fixation is indicated.
- Extra attention should be considered to open fractures in pediatric patients, specifically Seymour fractures. A Seymour fracture is an open physeal fracture of the distal phalanx with associated injury to the nail bed of the finger. Evaluate the injured finger for nail bed laceration with possible germinal matrix interposition. Seymour fractures require surgery to reduce the entrapped germinal matrix at the fracture site. Complications include growth deformity of the nail or phalanx, flexion deformity, and osteomyelitis (6)[C].

REFERENCES

1. Huang Y, Wu K, Shi H, et al. Kirschner wire fixation versus suture anchor technique for mallet finger: a meta-analysis. *Medicine (Baltimore)*. 2021;100(11):e24996.
2. Bachoura A, Ferikes AJ, Lubahn JD. A review of mallet finger and jersey finger injuries in the athlete. *Curr Rev Musculoskelet Med*. 2017;10(1):1–9.
3. Peng C, Huang RW, Chen SH, et al. Comparative outcomes between surgical treatment and orthosis splint for mallet finger: a systematic review and meta-analysis. *J Plast Surg Hand Surg*. 2023;57(1–6):54–63.
4. Lin JS, Samora JB. Surgical and nonsurgical management of mallet finger: a systematic review. *J Hand Surg Am*. 2018;43(2):146.e2–163.e2.
5. Valdes K, Naughton N, Algar L. Conservative treatment of mallet finger: a systematic review. *J Hand Ther*. 2015;28(3):237–246.
6. Lamaris GA, Matthew M. The diagnosis and management of mallet finger injuries. *Hand (N Y)*. 2017;12(3):223–238.

ADDITIONAL READING

Handoll HHG, Vaghela MV. Interventions for treating mallet finger injuries. *Cochrane Database of Syst Rev*. 2004;(3):CD004574.

CLINICAL PEARLS

- The typical mechanism of injury is a "jamming" or axial load to the fingertip, resulting in the inability to actively extend the DIP joint.
- Without treatment, mallet finger may result in hyperextension (swan-neck) deformity at the PIP joint or osteoarthritis at the DIP joint.
- Controversy exists regarding optimal treatment of each type of mallet finger with respect to the type of splint used, the length of immobilization, and when surgery is indicated, which surgical technique should be considered.
- However, there is consensus that nonoperative management with splinting is the most common treatment of choice and is effective for most mallet finger injuries.
- After either operative or nonoperative treatment, a common complication of mallet finger injury is mild residual extension lag at the DIP joint.

MARFAN SYNDROME

Rebecca L. Carl, MD, MSCI

BASICS

DESCRIPTION

- An autosomal dominant genetic disorder of connective tissue
- System(s) affected: musculoskeletal, cardiovascular, ocular, skin/integument, endocrine/metabolic, pulmonary
- Genetics: autosomal dominant with high penetrance; 15–25% spontaneous mutation
- Incidence/prevalence in United States: 1/5,000 to 1/15,000
- Predominant age: genetic condition. Generally, clinical manifestations become apparent during late childhood or adolescence. There is a more severe early-onset form of this condition; affected individuals are generally diagnosed in the newborn period.
- Predominant gender: no gender predilection

ETIOLOGY AND PATHOPHYSIOLOGY

Genetic: ~75% of affected individuals have an affected parent; the remainder has a spontaneous mutation in the fibrillin-1 (*FBN-1*) gene.

RISK FACTORS

Advanced paternal age gives rise to a slightly increased risk only in cases that are not clearly familial.

GENERAL PREVENTION

Primary prevention: In families where an *FBN-1* gene mutation has been identified, preimplantation genetic diagnosis can be used to identify embryos without the mutation.

DIAGNOSIS

- Genetic testing, looking for mutations in the *FBN-1* gene, is available. Mutations can be identified in >90% of affected individuals (1)[A].
- The mainstay of diagnosis is clinical evaluation and application of established diagnostic criteria. These criteria, now known as the *Ghent nosology*, were revised most recently in 2010 (2)[C].
- The criteria for diagnosis in individuals with no family history include any of the following:
  - Pathologic *FBN-1* mutation and either ectopia lentis or aortic root dilatation (Z-score ≥2 points)
  - Ectopia lentis and aortic root dilatation (Z-score ≥2 points)
  - Aortic root dilatation (Z-score ≥2 points) and other systemic features (≥7 points)
- The criteria for diagnosis in individuals who have a first-degree relative with Marfan syndrome include any of the following:
  - Ectopia lentis
  - Systemic features (≥7 points)
  - Aortic root dilatation (Z-score ≥2 points or Z-score ≥3 points for individuals <20 years of age)
- Echocardiography, spine radiographs, and slit-lamp exam may be important in making the diagnosis.

PHYSICAL EXAM

- Features listed below with diagnostics points in parentheses (where applicable)
- Musculoskeletal (3)[C]:
  - Pectus carinatum (2 points)
  - Pectus excavatum (1 point)
  - Reduced upper segment to lower segment ratio with increased arm span: height ratio (>1.05) in the absence of scoliosis (1 point)
  - Positive thumb sign (thumb can protrude from ulnar side of a clenched fist) and/or wrist sign (thumb and 5th finger can encircle wrist and overlap) (3 points if both present, 1 point if one is present)
  - Decreased elbow extension (1 point)
  - Pes planovalgus (1 point, 2 points with medial displacement of the medial malleolus)
  - Protrusio acetabuli on radiographs (2 points)
  - Scoliosis of >20 degrees or thoracolumbar kyphosis (1 point)
  - High-arched palate with crowding of teeth
  - Three out of five characteristic facial features (1 point)
- Cardiovascular:
  - Mitral valve prolapse (1 point)
  - Dilatation of the main pulmonary aorta (age <40 years)
  - Calcification of the mitral valve annulus (age <40 years)
  - Dilatation or dissection of the descending or abdominal aorta (age <50 years)
- Ocular:
  - Myopia >3 diopters (1 point)
  - Flat cornea
  - Decreased miosis owing to hypoplastic iris or ciliary muscles
- Pulmonary (minor criteria only):
  - Spontaneous pneumothorax (2 points)
  - Apical blebs
- Skin/integument (minor criteria only):
  - Striae (1 point)
  - Recurrent hernia or hernia at an incision site
- Dura: lumbosacral dural ectasia (2 points)

DIFFERENTIAL DIAGNOSIS

- Loeys-Dietz syndrome
- Homocystinuria
- Marfanoid habitus
- Marfanoid skeletal and skin features (MASS) phenotype
- Ehlers-Danlos syndrome
- Beal syndrome (congenital contractural arachnodactyly)

DIAGNOSTIC TESTS & INTERPRETATION

- Targeted-gene genetic testing to look for *FBN-1* mutation (1)[A]
- Genomic sequencing may be indicated when clinical picture is less convincing for Marfan syndrome.
- Drugs that may alter lab results: N/A
- Disorders that may alter lab results: N/A
- Plain radiographs of the spine are useful prior to skeletal maturity to detect and quantify scoliosis.
- Initial diagnostic echocardiogram, followed by serial screening echocardiograms, is recommended beginning in adolescence to look for dilatation of the aorta and valvular changes.
- Pathologic findings:
  - Cystic medial necrosis of the aorta
  - Myxomatous degeneration of the cardiac valves

TREATMENT

- Long-term treatment
- Acute treatment: outpatient

MEDICATION

First Line

- No specific medical therapy is available. Medications may be used to treat manifestations of Marfan syndrome.
- β-Blockers and angiotensin II receptor blockers (ARBs) have been used to slow progression of aortic root dilatation (4)[A].
- Angiotensin-converting enzyme (ACE) inhibitors and calcium channel blockers have been used in patients who do not tolerate or fail to respond to β-blockers or ARBs.
- Contraindications for β-blockers: asthma, depression, Raynaud phenomenon
- Contraindications for ARBs: pregnancy
- Precautions: Refer to the manufacturer's profile for each drug.
- Significant possible interactions: Refer to the manufacturer's profile for each drug.

ISSUES FOR REFERRAL

- In addition to health supervision visits with primary care physicians, individuals with Marfan syndrome should have regular follow-up with cardiology and ophthalmology (5)[C].
- Geneticists are often involved in making the initial diagnosis.
- Orthopedic consultation is often helpful.
- In affected individuals, echocardiograms are typically performed every 12 months to screen for the presence of aortic root dilatation and worsening valvular insufficiency.

ADDITIONAL THERAPIES

- Antibiotic prophylaxis for endocarditis prior to medical and dental procedures is not uniformly recommended for Marfan patients with mitral valve prolapse (6)[C].
- Individuals with significant valvular regurgitation/insufficiency should consult their cardiologists about the necessity of infective endocarditis prophylaxis for their specific conditions (6)[C].
- Antibiotic prophylaxis should be given to individuals with a prior history of infective endocarditis or a history of valve replacement or repair of the aorta using graft material (6)[C].

SURGERY/OTHER PROCEDURES

Cardiac surgery is often required for people with Marfan syndrome who have aortic root diameter >5 cm, rapid rate of aortic root dilatation, or significant aortic valve regurgitation (6)[C].

ONGOING CARE

FOLLOW-UP RECOMMENDATIONS

- Athletes with Marfan syndrome can participate in low to moderate static/low-dynamic sports as long as they do not have moderate or severe mitral regurgitation, left ventricular dysfunction, and aortic root dilatation and have no family history of aortic root >50 mm, aortic dissection, or sudden death owing to Marfan syndrome (6)[C].
- Individuals with Marfan syndrome should not participate in contact sports or weight lifting (6)[C].

Patient Monitoring

- Routine health maintenance visits with a primary care physician
- Regular follow-up with cardiology; athletes should have screening echocardiograms every 6 to 12 months.
- Yearly ophthalmology follow-up owing to high rate of retinal detachment. Patients also have higher rates of myopia and glaucoma.

DIET

No special diet

PATIENT EDUCATION

Information is available from the National Marfan Foundation, 382 Main St., Port Washington, NY 11959; 800–8MARFAN, https://marfan.org.

PROGNOSIS

Life-threatening complications are cardiovascular. With the advancement of techniques to replace the aortic root, individuals with Marfan have a near-normal life span.

COMPLICATIONS

- Aortic dissection or aortic rupture
- Aortic valvular insufficiency owing to aortic root dilatation
- Mitral valve insufficiency, often associated with myxomatous change
- Bacterial endocarditis
- Spontaneous pneumothorax
- Retinal detachment

Pediatric Considerations

Early medical or surgical intervention may reduce the degree of scoliosis.

Pregnancy Considerations

Pregnant women with the Marfan syndrome need to be managed as high-risk patients, preferably with involvement of a cardiologist. The outcome is usually excellent.

REFERENCES

1. Faivre L, Masurel-Paulet A, Collod-Béroud G, et al. Clinical and molecular study of 320 children with Marfan syndrome and related type I fibrillinopathies in a series of 1009 probands with pathogenic FBN1 mutations. *Pediatrics*. 2009;123(1):391–398.
2. Loeys BL, Dietz HC, Braverman AC, et al. The revised Ghent nosology for the Marfan syndrome. *J Med Genet*. 2010;47(7):476–485.
3. Pollock L, Ridout A, Teh J, et al. The musculoskeletal manifestations of Marfan syndrome: diagnosis, impact, and management. *Curr Rheumatol Rep*. 2021;23(11):81.
4. Pitcher A, Spata E, Emberson J, et al. Angiotensin receptor blockers and β blockers in Marfan syndrome: an individual patient data meta-analysis of randomised trials. *Lancet*. 2022;400(10355):822–831.
5. Tinkle BT, Lacro RV, Burke LW; Council on Genetics. Health supervision for children and adolescents with Marfan syndrome. *Pediatrics*. 2023;151(4):e2023061450.
6. Braverman AC, Harris KM, Kovacs RJ, et al. Eligibility and disqualification recommendations for competitive athletes with cardiovascular abnormalities: Task Force 7: aortic diseases, including Marfan syndrome: a scientific statement from the American Heart Association and American College of Cardiology. *Circulation*. 2015;132(22):e303–e309.

CLINICAL PEARLS

- Clinicians should be on the lookout for the musculoskeletal manifestations of Marfan syndrome when performing preparticipation screening.
- Physicians should carefully evaluate individuals with increased arm span:height ratio (>1.05), characteristic facial features, and other stigmata of Marfan syndrome and consider referral to genetics, cardiology, and/or ophthalmology when appropriate.

MCP (METACARPOPHALANGEAL) COLLATERAL LIGAMENT SPRAIN

Rosalynn R. Z. Conic, MD, PhD, MPH ▪ Jason L. Zaremski, MD, CAQSM, FAAPMR, FACSM, FAMSSM

BASICS

DESCRIPTION

- Injury to the collateral ligaments of the metacarpophalangeal (MCP) joints; most commonly the MCP joint of the thumb
- An injury to the MCP ligament may result in a simple sprain to a complete tear of both proper and accessory ligaments.

EPIDEMIOLOGY

- Isolated injuries to collateral ligaments of the MCP joints are uncommon, except for those of the MCP joint of the thumb, which is the focus of this chapter.
- Ulnar collateral ligament (UCL) injuries of the MCP joint of the thumb (gamekeeper's thumb [chronic] or skier's thumb [acute]) occur more often than radial collateral ligament (RCL) injuries (1).
- UCL injury usually occurs distally, whereas RCL injury tends to be proximal (2).
- UCL sprain is the second most common injury encountered by skiers and most common ligamentous injury to the thumb.

Incidence

- UCL injury incidence is ~50/100,000 (1).
- Acute UCL injury is seen frequently in athletes including ball-handling athletes and other contact sports participants.

COMMONLY ASSOCIATED CONDITIONS

- Complete rupture of the collateral ligament (proper and accessory) and volar plate (1)
- Stener lesion occurs in 64–87% of complete UCL tears due to entrapment of the distal ruptured UCL in the intact adductor pollicis aponeurosis at its insertion into the base of the proximal phalanx, inhibiting healing (3).
- Three types of avulsion fractures: small fragment at the base of the proximal phalanx (~50% of injuries); a large, intra-articular fracture that involves at least 25% of the articular surface of the base of the proximal phalanx; and an avulsion fracture involving the volar plate (3)
- Dislocation of the thumb MCP joint

DIAGNOSIS

HISTORY

- MCP collateral ligament sprain is most commonly an acute injury related to trauma.
- Mechanism of injury to the UCL of the MCP joint of the thumb is sudden, forced, radial deviation (abduction) and extension resulting in partial or complete tear of the ligament.
- The mechanism of injury to the RCL of the MCP joint of the thumb is forced adduction or twisting of the flexed joint.
- Prompt diagnosis is the key to a good outcome.
- Chronic MCP collateral ligament sprain is usually secondary to a missed diagnosis from an earlier acute injury.

PHYSICAL EXAM

- A careful physical exam differentiates a sprain from a complete tear (1),(2).
- Always compare with asymptomatic thumb (1).
- Examine the joint for swelling, ecchymosis, and areas of tenderness.
- Hallmark symptoms of acute UCL injury are pain and swelling localized to the ulnar aspect of the MCP joint along the UCL.
- Acute injury: ecchymosis and pain over the ligament
- Chronic injuries may not be painful.
- A palpable mass may be present (possible Stener lesion).
- Thumb instability with diminished grip and pincer grasp may be noted (1).
- RCL injuries have pain and swelling localized to the radial aspect of the metacarpal head, and activities such as twisting to open a jar lid can exacerbate the symptoms.
- Anteroposterior (AP) and lateral radiographs should be obtained prior to stressing the joint because a nondisplaced fracture can be displaced as a result of the stress.
- If radiographs are negative, the stability of the ligament should be tested.
- Test the ligaments by applying radial stress (RCL) or ulnar stress (UCL) to the MCP joint in full extension and in 30 degrees of flexion.
- A collateral ligament injury should be suspected if during stress testing, a firm end point is lacking.
- Valgus stress of the flexed MCP joint with opening of ≥30 degrees or 15 degrees greater than the contralateral thumb indicates collateral ligament proper complete rupture; <30 degrees of laxity assume a partial tear (1).
- Valgus stress of the extended MCP joint with opening of ≥30 degrees suggest an accessory collateral ligament tear or volar plate tear (1).
- Grade 1 = ligament sprain without instability (1)
- Grade 2 = partial ligament tear with laxity but firm endpoint with valgus testing (1)
- Grade 3 = complete tear of collateral ligament (1)

ALERT

If unable to make a clear distinction on clinical exam, stress ultrasound (US) or magnetic resonance imaging (MRI) is indicated.

DIFFERENTIAL DIAGNOSIS

- Dislocation of the thumb MCP joint
- Fracture

DIAGNOSTIC TESTS & INTERPRETATION

- AP and lateral radiographs of the thumb to evaluate for a fracture.
- Stress radiographs are controversial because there is concern for displacement of nondisplaced ligaments or fractures (1),(3).
- Volar subluxation of the proximal phalanx seen on lateral view and radial deviation of the proximal phalanx seen on AP view ("Sag Sign") indicate complete ligament rupture.
- US may be used as an adjunct to the clinical exam for visualization of the ligament and determining further treatment (4).
- MRI is the best confirmatory test and used for surgical decision-making (4).

Pediatric Considerations

Stress films are contraindicated in children because of the risk of Salter-Harris fractures.

TREATMENT

GENERAL MEASURES

- Analgesia: nonsteroidal anti-inflammatory drugs (NSAIDs), ice
- Non–thumb-related collateral ligament sprains, depending on severity, can be splinted immobilized or "buddy taped" (2)[C].
- No detectable instability: immobilization (thumb spica splint) for 2 to 4 weeks dependent on severity (1)[C]
- Partial tear with stable joint: Thumb spica splint or cast for 4 to 6 weeks depending on severity of the injury (3)[C]; thumb is immobilized in slight flexion in the spica cast; the interphalangeal joint is not immobilized to allow active motion and prevent scarring of the extension mechanism.
- Avulsion fracture: Small avulsions that are not intra-articular can be treated nonoperatively; non-displaced fractures, thumb spica cast (application as above) for 4 to 6 weeks (3)[B]

ISSUES FOR REFERRAL

Prompt referral to an orthopedist or hand surgeon is indicated for all but uncomplicated injuries.

ADDITIONAL THERAPIES

When the cast is removed, range of motion (ROM) exercises are performed several times a day; a removable splint is worn for an additional time depending on the severity of injury.

SURGERY/OTHER PROCEDURES

- Complete tear: Repair surgically (3)[A].
- Avulsion fracture: Rotated, displaced, or large intra-articular fragments require surgical repair (3)[A].
- Surgical repair is necessary for Stener lesion; failure to recognize this injury or inadequate treatment can result in chronic instability (3)[A].

ALERT

Surgery is indicated for complete ligament tears; Stener lesions; and fractures that are displaced, rotated, or have significant articular involvement.

ONGOING CARE

- Sports participation: Protect the thumb for ~3 months with splinting (5).
- Returning to sport and play in a splint is dependent on sport-specific needs of the athlete (3),(6).
- Following surgery and recovery, >98% of athletes return to play at the same competitive level (6).

COMPLICATIONS

Inadequate treatment of UCL and RCL thumb injuries may result in chronic painful instability, weakness of pinch, and early onset osteoarthritis (2),(3).

REFERENCES

1. Avery DM III, Inkellis ER, Carlson MG. Thumb collateral ligament injuries in the athlete. *Curr Rev Musculoskelet Med.* 2017;10(1):28–37.
2. Robinson DM, Kakar S, Jelsing E. Acute thumb metacarpophalangeal joint ulnar collateral ligament injury: diagnosis, management, and return to sports considerations. *Curr Sports Med Rep.* 2023;22(6):238–244.
3. Forli A, Bentejac A, Lateur G, et al. Recent and chronic sprains of the first metacarpophalangeal joint. *Orthop Traumatol Surg Res.* 2022;108(1S):103156.
4. Rashidi A, Haj-Mirzaian A, Dalili D, et al. Evidence-based use of clinical examination, ultrasonography, and MRI for diagnosing ulnar collateral ligament tears of the metacarpophalangeal joint of the thumb: systematic review and meta-analysis. *Eur Radiol.* 2021;31(8):5699–5712.
5. Goldfarb CA, Puri SK, Carlson MG. Diagnosis, treatment, and return to play for four common sports injuries of the hand and wrist. *J Am Acad Orthop Surg.* 2016;24(12):853–862.
6. Allahabadi S, Kwong JW, Pandya NK, et al. Return to play after thumb ulnar collateral ligament injuries managed surgically in athletes: a systematic review. *J Hand Surg Glob Online.* 2023;5(3):349–357.

CLINICAL PEARLS

- Acute (thumb) UCL injuries are common injuries in all athletes.
- Timely diagnosis is important to determine the severity of the injury and immobilization timeframe.
- Stener lesion occurs in 64–87% of complete UCL tears due to entrapment of the distal ruptured UCL in the intact adductor pollicis aponeurosis.
- Non–thumb-related collateral ligament sprains, depending on severity, can be splinted immobilized or "buddy taped."
- If a displaced avulsion fracture and/or Stener lesion is present, prompt referral to an orthopedist or hand surgeon is recommended.

MCP (METACARPOPHALANGEAL) DISLOCATION

Griffin Elbert, DO, CAQSM • Catherine Carragee, MD

BASICS

- The metacarpophalangeal (MCP) joints are relatively stable joints, especially in flexion.
- Stability is provided by collateral ligaments on either side of the joint or the volar plate. The collateral ligaments are lax in extension and taut in flexion, thus most stable in flexion. The volar plate has a firm distal attachment to the proximal phalanx and a less stable proximal attachment to the metacarpal. It is the proximal attachment that is disrupted in a dislocation (1),(2).
- The index finger is most commonly affected, with the thumb and 5th finger also vulnerable to dislocations (3).

DESCRIPTION

- An MCP joint dislocation involves dislocation of the proximal phalanx in relation to the distal metacarpal.
- Dislocations may occur dorsally (most common), laterally (uncommon), or volarly (rare).
- The typical mechanism for a dorsal dislocation is hyperextension at the MCP joint:
  - In hyperextension, there is rupture of the proximal volar plate, and due to the anatomy of the joint, there is also proximal dorsal translocation of the base of the proximal phalanx over the distal metacarpal (3).
- The neurovascular bundle is located anterior to the lumbrical muscle and metacarpal head, placing it at risk for injury during traumatic dislocation (1).

ALERT

Classification of dislocations (1),(3):

- Simple dorsal: Articular surfaces are in partial contact, and there is no soft tissue interposed in the joint.
- Complex dorsal: The volar plate or other tissue is interposed between articular surfaces and is, by definition, an irreducible dislocation.
- Lateral: results from an injury to the ulnar or radial collateral ligament. The collateral ligaments of the thumb are more commonly injured than the collateral ligaments of the fingers (2),(4).
- Volar: rare, but may result from severe or repetitive blows to knuckle, leading to rupture of dorsal capsule with subsequent volar displacement of the proximal phalanx

EPIDEMIOLOGY

- MCP dislocations are much less common than proximal interphalangeal (IP) dislocations because of support from surrounding structures and protected position (1).
- Usually occurs in index finger, thumb, or 5th finger
- Nearly always a single digit but multiple digits may be involved.

RISK FACTORS

- Contact and ball-handling sports
- Prior history of injury or dislocation

DIAGNOSIS

HISTORY

- Complaints of pain, loss of function, and usually an obvious deformity
- Dorsal dislocation generally results from forced hyperextension of digit, as in striking the heel of an opponent while diving to make a tackle, or a fall on an outstretched hand (1)[C].

PHYSICAL EXAM

- Evaluate and document neurovascular status before and after reduction attempts.
- With dorsal dislocations, the metacarpal head is volarly displaced and will be easily palpable in the palm (1)[C].
- Simple dorsal: There is obvious deformity, with the phalanx resting at 60 to 90 degrees of hyperextension over the head of the metacarpal (5)[C].
- Complex dorsal: much more subtle deformity, with only slight hyperextension (10 to 15 degrees) of the phalanx; may find dimpling or puckering of the palmar aspect of the finger where the volar plate is caught between the ends of the bones (proximal phalanx and head of metacarpal). This is pathognomonic for a complex dislocation; slight ulnar deviation of the involved digit also may be noted (1),(5)[C].
- Lateral: swelling and tenderness along the ulnar or radial side of the MCP joint; assess for injury and laxity of the collateral ligaments by stressing the ligament with the MCP joint in flexion (4)[C].
- Volar: obvious deformity, with the phalanx positioned palmar to metacarpal

DIFFERENTIAL DIAGNOSIS

- Fracture of phalanx or metacarpal
- Tendon rupture
- Disruption of volar plate

DIAGNOSTIC TESTS & INTERPRETATION

- Anteroposterior (AP), lateral, and oblique views of involved digit (not the entire hand) generally show deformity, joint space widening, and any accompanying fracture (1)[C].
- Brewerton view (MCP joint flexed to 65 degrees, with the dorsum of the proximal phalanx flat against the film cassette and the beam angled 15 degrees ulnar to radial) helpful in identifying collateral ligament avulsion fractures and fractures of the metacarpal head

ALERT

- Presence of a sesamoid in the widened joint space of the involved digit is pathognomonic for a complex dorsal dislocation (because sesamoids are embedded in the volar plate) (1)[C].
- Evaluating the distance between the distal edge of the sesamoid of the thumb MCP compared to the MCP joint can aid diagnosis for dislocation as well as postreduction (4)[C].
- In skeletally immature patients, it is important to image the contralateral side to adequately evaluate for growth plate injuries.
- In skeletally mature patients, stress radiographs are sometimes used. Stress x-rays should only be done after static x-rays to prevent nondisplaced fractures from becoming displaced fractures. In the thumb, MCP joint laxity >30 to 35 degrees on stress x-rays is usually associated with a complete collateral ligament tear. Stress x-rays are not typically used in the skeletally immature patient because those patients are more likely to have a growth plate injury.
- Postreduction views: AP, lateral, and oblique to evaluate for joint congruity and/or fracture

ALERT

Up to 50% of MCP joint dislocations may have a concomitant fracture of the proximal phalanx base and/or the metacarpal head.

TREATMENT

- Anesthesia:
  - Various methods of anesthesia can be used for reduction, including local intra-articular, regional block, or intravenous (IV) sedation. Typically for intra-articular injections, a short-acting local anesthetic such as 1% lidocaine without epinephrine is used, although a longer acting agent such as bupivacaine may also be used. It is important to document neurovascular status prior to the administration of the anesthetic agent.
  - Usually not necessary for simple dislocations but intra-articular anesthesia or wrist block may facilitate reduction and prevent false conclusion that dislocation is complex if patient prevents reduction due to pain (2)[C].
  - For complex dislocations, digital block or general anesthesia in the operating room may be necessary if closed reduction is to be attempted.
  - Evaluate and document neurovascular status before and after reduction (2),(3),(4),(6)[C].

ALERT

- In general, reduction of dorsal MCP dislocations differs from most other dislocations in that distal traction should be avoided. By using traction, a simple dislocation can be converted to a complex one because the volar plate gets displaced and locked within the joint space (1),(3),(5)[C].
- Simple dorsal: First, relax flexors by placing wrist and IP joints into flexion; next, accentuate dislocation slightly by hyperextending proximal phalanx to 90 degrees (controversial), and then push base of proximal phalanx distally over the articular surface of the metacarpal into flexion while maintaining contact with metacarpal head to prevent entrapment of the volar plate (thus converting a simple dislocation into a complex one) (1),(3)[C].

- Reduction:
  - Complex dorsal: Attempt at closed reduction is warranted but usually not successful; reduction technique is similar to that of a simple dislocation (3)[C].
  - Lateral: Closed reduction is usually accomplished with gentle longitudinal traction, taking care not to interpose any soft tissue.

- Volar: Generally, reduction is performed open because of concomitant dorsal hood injury needs repair.
- Reasons for failed closed reductions: Volar plate is interposed in the joint space or metacarpal head has buttonholed through the palmar structures (1)[C].
- Evaluate tendon and ligament function. With thumb MCP dislocations, it is very important to assess the integrity and stability of the collateral ligaments, particularly the ulnar collateral ligament (UCL) (2)[C].
- Postreduction imaging: AP, lateral, and oblique radiographs of the involved digit to evaluate for joint congruity and/or fracture
- Simple dorsal: Dorsal blocking splint to prevent extension beyond neutral with the MCP joint in 50 to 70 degrees of flexion for 7 to 10 days if no evidence of significant instability; buddy taping also may be implemented. Active flexion exercises are permitted. With thumb MCP dislocations, a thumb spica splint is used for immobilization (1)[C].
- Complex dorsal: Postoperative immobilization is at the prerogative of the surgeon (ranges from buddy taping for 4 to 6 weeks to immobilization in 60 degrees of flexion). Early protective motion therapy with dorsal blocking splint initiated after the first week of injury or surgery to decrease joint stiffness (2)[C].
- Lateral: Majority of complete ligamentous injuries are splinted in 30 to 50 degrees of MCP flexion for 2 to 4 weeks followed by buddy taping; with significant instability especially of the border digits, primary surgical repair of the collateral ligament may be considered. Incomplete MCP collateral ligament injuries and complete tears in nonborder digits are usually treated with buddy taping and early range of motion (ROM) exercises (4)[C].
- Volar: Postoperative management varies and is at the prerogative of the surgeon.

MEDICATION

- Nonsteroidal anti-inflammatory drugs (NSAIDs) for pain relief
- If surgery is planned, may consider acetaminophen to avoid potential bleeding risks

ADDITIONAL THERAPIES

- PRICE: protection, rest, ice, compression, elevation
- In dislocations of the thumb, assessment of the UCL is essential. With a hyperextension/hyperabduction injury, a Stener lesion can result. A Stener lesion occurs when the adductor aponeurosis becomes interposed between the torn end of the UCL and its bony attachment on the proximal phalanx. Spontaneous healing cannot occur because the ligament is no longer in contact with its bony attachment (2).
- Occupational therapy may be indicated in more severe injuries.
- Dorsal dislocations that are stable postreduction need to be placed in a dorsal extension blocking splint to prevent extension beyond neutral and hyperextension. This position allows the volar plate to heal. Time frame is variable but typically 2 to 3 weeks. While in the extension blocking splint, active ROM is encouraged to prevent joint stiffness.
- Thumb MCP dislocations require immobilization in a forearm-based thumb spica splint or cast for 4 to 6 weeks (2).
- Initial therapy will focus on control of pain and swelling. General progression through rehab includes regaining full active ROM, followed by strengthening, and then function (activities of daily living and work-/sport-specific functions).
- If the injury can be properly protected in a splint or cast, an athlete may be able to return to activities immediately. Otherwise, after the injury has healed (3 to 6 weeks), an athlete can return to play with buddy taping for 1 to 3 more weeks for additional protection.

SURGERY/OTHER PROCEDURES

Surgery is often necessary for reduction, specifically for the complex dorsal and volar dislocations, as discussed above, and may be indicated for repair of severely damaged structures in other forms of dislocation (i.e., complete tear of UCL or RCL in lateral MCP joint dislocation) (3),(4)[C].

ONGOING CARE

FOLLOW-UP RECOMMENDATIONS

After successful closed reduction, most MCP dislocations should be followed up with an orthopedic surgeon or hand surgeon within a week.

PATIENT EDUCATION

Warn patients that finger and hand swelling can take months to resolve (3),(6).

PROGNOSIS

Prognosis of most MCP dislocations is good if identified early and managed appropriately.

COMPLICATIONS

- Joint stiffness and/or flexion contracture
- Degenerative/posttraumatic arthritis
- Avascular necrosis
- Osteochondral fracture
- Tendon adhesions/stiffness
- Ligamentous laxity
- Damage to the neurovascular bundle during open reduction, especially when using a volar approach
- Premature closure of the physeal plate (rare) (1),(2),(6)

REFERENCES

1. Dinh P, Franklin A, Hutchinson B, et al. Metacarpophalangeal joint dislocation. *J Am Acad Orthop Surg*. 2009;17(5):318–324.
2. Owings FP, Calandruccio JH, Mauck BM. Thumb ligament injuries in the athlete. *Orthop Clin North Am*. 2016;47(4):799–807.
3. Lourie GM, Hanson ZC. Finger metacarpophalangeal joint injuries in athletes: evaluation, diagnosis, treatment, and return to play. *J Am Acad Orthop Surg*. 2023;31(4):e177–e188.
4. Xu J, Han L, Zhang B, et al. The application of sesamoid position in diagnosing thumb metacarpophalangeal joint dorsal dislocation. *Orthop Surg*. 2024;16(4):984–988.
5. Schupp CM, Rand SE, Hanson TW, et al. Sideline management of joint dislocations. *Curr Sports Med Rep*. 2016;15(3):140–153.
6. Kabbani KT, Dimos K, Kosmas D, et al. Volar metacarpophalangeal dislocation of fingers: review of the literature. *J Hand Surg Glob Online*. 2021;3(4):228–232.

ADDITIONAL READING

- Lourie GM, Gaston RG, Freeland AE. Collateral ligament injuries of the metacarpophalangeal joints of the fingers. *Hand Clin*. 2006;22(3):357–364.
- Lee SJ, Montgomery K. Athletic hand injuries. *Orthop Clin North Am*. 2002;33(3):547–554.
- Rubin G, Orbach H, Rinott M, et al. Complex dorsal metacarpophalangeal dislocation: long-term follow-up. *J Hand Surg Am*. 2016;41(8):e229–e233.
- Rettig AC. Athletic injuries of the wrist and hand: part II: overuse injuries of the wrist and traumatic injuries to the hand. *Am J Sports Med*. 2004;32(1):262–273.
- Shah SS, Techy F, Mejia A, et al. Ligamentous and capsular injuries to the metacarpophalangeal joints of the hand. *J Surg Orthop Adv*. 2012;21(3):141–146.

SEE ALSO

MCP (Metacarpophalangeal) Collateral Ligament Sprain; Ulnar Collateral Ligament Injury of Thumb (Skier's Thumb)

CLINICAL PEARLS

- Dorsal dislocations are the most common type of MCP joint dislocations.
- When attempting to reduce a dorsal MCP joint dislocation, do not use distal traction; risk converting simple dislocation to a complex one
- In general, complex dorsal and volar MCP joint dislocations require surgery.

MEDIAL COLLATERAL LIGAMENT TEAR

Claudia Dal Molin, DO, RMSK, FAMSSM • Delmas J. Bolin, MD, PhD, FACSM

BASICS

Anatomy:
- The medial collateral ligament (MCL) has a single origin on the femur but two separate insertions on the tibia (1).
- The distal attachment of the superficial MCL is just >6 cm distal to the joint line (1).
- The superficial component is the primary restraint to valgus stress (1).
- The deep portion has a direct connection to medial meniscus (1):
  - It connects with the posteromedial corner (PMC) structures and is a secondary stabilizer in resisting external rotation and anterior-posterior translation of the knee (1).

DESCRIPTION
- Tension injury to the MCL occurs most commonly with a valgus stress (i.e., a blow to the lateral knee).
- Grade of injury classified by symptoms and physical exam by degree of joint opening with applied valgus stress at 0 degree and 30 degrees of flexion (1)
- I—minimal fiber tearing, localized tenderness, no instability (0 to 5 mm of laxity)
- II—greater degree of ligamentous tearing, slight to moderate abnormal motion (6 to 10 mm of laxity)
- III—complete tear, demonstrable instability (>10 mm of laxity)

EPIDEMIOLOGY
- MCL is the most frequently injured ligament of the knee (2).
- The most injurious sports are contact sports (e.g., wrestling, hockey, martial arts) (2).
- Intercollegiate athletes are at greater risk than intramural athletes (2).

COMMONLY ASSOCIATED CONDITIONS
- Medial meniscal tear
- Anterior cruciate ligament (ACL) tear
- Posterior oblique ligament (POL)/PMC injury
- Dislocation of the knee (rare)
- Patellar dislocation

DIAGNOSIS

HISTORY
- Mechanisms of injury:
  - Closed chain injury:
    - In contact/collision sports, an acute blow to the lateral aspect of the knee when the foot is planted results in valgus stress.
  - Open chain injury:
    - In kicking sports, the injury may be seen in players who are struck on the instep while passing the ball.
    - Skiers can injure the MCL by a noncontact valgus external rotation injury.
    - Overuse injuries to the MCL have been reported in breaststroke swimmers.
- History of a "pop" is concerning for an associated meniscal or ACL injury.
- Because the MCL is an extra-articular structure, the presence of an effusion is concerning for an associated intra-articular injury.
- Ask if the knee feels "loose" or if it is "moving in ways it wasn't intended to."

PHYSICAL EXAM
- Inspection: Note any antalgic gait, ecchymosis, swelling, effusion, presence of deformity. In pediatric patients, ecchymosis and swelling are concerning for a physeal injury.
- Palpation: Check for tenderness to palpation over the entire medial joint line and along the MCL from the adductor tubercle to its insertion on the anteromedial proximal tibia. Evaluate the entire knee to avoid missing concomitant injuries.
- Range of motion (ROM): Assess for any deficit of extension or flexion. ROM deficits or a locked knee can be a sign of a more serious concomitant injury (e.g., bucket handle meniscal tear).
- Ligamentous exam:
  - Valgus stress at 0 degree and at 20 degrees; laxity at 20 degrees alone indicates an isolated MCL injury. Laxity at both 0 degree and 20 degrees indicates an injury to the MCL and POL, knee capsule, and/or ACL (1).
  - Compare to the unaffected side.
  - Clinical grading: 1st degree = pain without laxity; 2nd degree = pain and laxity but firm endpoint; 3rd degree = no endpoint is present (1).
  - Estimate joint line opening—if >10 mm, coexisting intra-articular pathology (torn ACL or meniscus) will be present 80% of the time (1).
  - Assess for POL injury, which can lead to anteromedial rotatory instability (AMRI) and posterior horn meniscal tears. Estimate the amount of anteromedial tibial rotation by performing the anterior drawer test with the foot in both neutral and in 15 degrees of external rotation (1).
  - AMRI test is performed open-chain with tibia externally rotated, knee in 30 degrees flexion and valgus stress then applied; increased laxity (~10 mm medial joint opening) suggests injury to posteromedial capsule and POL.
  - Evaluate all other ligamentous structures (Lachman test, posterior drawer test, varus stress).
- Special tests: In addition to the above, McMurray/Thessaly tests should be used to evaluate for meniscal injury.
- Neurovascular exam: Popliteal nerve and artery injuries can occur with multiligament injuries and should not be missed.

DIFFERENTIAL DIAGNOSIS
- Medial meniscal tear
- Medial knee contusion (soft tissue or bony)
- Patellar instability (subluxation or dislocation)
- Fracture of the distal femoral or proximal tibial physis
- Tibial plateau fracture

DIAGNOSTIC TESTS & INTERPRETATION
- Radiography—standard weight-bearing knee series (anteroposterior [AP], notch, lateral, and sunrise views) are typically normal but can identify avulsions or osteochondral injuries. A Pellegrini-Stieda lesion is a calcification of the proximal MCL that can be seen in chronic injuries.
- Magnetic resonance imaging (MRI)—T2-weighted imaging is the gold standard for viewing edema and fiber continuity. Associated bone contusions (45% of MCL injuries) and concomitant injuries can also be seen.

TREATMENT

GENERAL MEASURES
- Grade I and II injuries:
  - PRICE (protection, rest, ice, compression, elevation) and nonsteroidal anti-inflammatory drugs (NSAIDs) are first line.
  - Weight-bearing as tolerated, with or without assistive devices based on comfort (1),(3)[C]
  - The clinical utility of bracing is unclear but may help with comfort. A hinged knee brace is often used for comfort and support. An extension block of 15 to 20 degrees in the first 1 to 2 weeks can potentially encourage healing in an anatomically shortened position. The brace can then be unlocked and weaned as tolerated if this mode of bracing is used. Braces can typically be discontinued in 3 to 12 weeks depending on the severity of the injury and clinical course (1),(3)[C].

- Active ROM is started immediately (1),(3)[C].
- Strengthening exercises are started immediately, progressing from static to dynamic as tolerated. Both open and closed chain exercises are used.
- Proprioception, agility, and sport-specific training can begin when full ROM and functional strength are regained (1),(3)[C].
- Athletes typically return to play in 1 to 4 weeks. Criteria include resolution of tenderness, full and pain free ROM and strength, and successful progression of sport-specific drills (1),(3)[C].

- Grade III injuries:
  - Isolated acute grade III injuries are often successfully treated nonoperatively. Operative consultation and treatment should be considered when complete ligament disruption is suspected, including intra-articular entrapment of the end of the ligament, a large bony avulsion injury, a tibial plateau fracture, a complete tibial side avulsion in athletes, or when AMRI is present (1),(3)[C].
  - Nonoperative management follows the same management principles outlined above in grade I and II injuries (1),(3)[C]:
    - A period of non–weight-bearing is used initially (1 to 3 weeks).
    - Early bracing may be preferred in order to reapproximate disrupted fibers and facilitate healing. Some providers lock the knee in extension, whereas others limit parts of ROM (90 degrees flexion block vs. terminal extension block at 20 degrees).
    - Avoid valgus and external rotation forces during the acute phase of healing (typically the first 3 to 4 weeks).
    - Strengthening exercises can begin once painless and full ROM is achieved. Progression to proprioceptive, agility, and sport-specific drills occurs similarly to grade I and II injuries.
    - Athletes typically return to play in 5 to 7 weeks.
- In patients who do not clinically improve with nonsurgical measures should be reevaluated for occult PMC injury with rotational instability. These patients may benefit from surgical reconstruction (4)[A].
- Experimental options:
  - Platelet-rich plasma (PRP) injections may be considered in injuries refractory to nonsurgical management when instability is not present. Most literature remains anecdotal (typically grades I and II with persistent pain) (5)[C].
  - Evidence for PRP injections in MCL injuries is limited to case studies and studies using animal models.
- Combined MCL/ACL injuries:
  - Early referral to orthopedics
  - MRI is helpful.
  - Surgical approach remains controversial, but most authors recommend ACL reconstruction after a period of rehabilitation to allow the MCL to heal. This approach has been shown to minimize postoperative arthrofibrosis. Initial rehabilitation mirrors that of grade III MCL injuries for the first 5 to 7 weeks while ACL reconstruction is typically delayed. Time is given for swelling to improve and for full ROM to be regained.
  - ACL/MCL reconstruction may be recommended for excessive valgus laxity. These patients typically require a more substantial initial period of non–weight-bearing.

MEDICATION

Short-term use of NSAIDs can help decrease pain and swelling. NSAID therapy can impair bone fracture healing and tendon-to-bone (enthesis) healing.

ONGOING CARE

COMPLICATIONS

The Pellegrini-Stieda lesion can be seen on radiographs. It represents calcification of the previously injured MCL.

REFERENCES

1. Stannard JP. Evaluation and treatment of medial instability of the knee. *Sports Med Arthrosc Rev*. 2015;23(2):91–95.
2. Roach CJ, Haley CA, Cameron KL, et al. The epidemiology of medial collateral ligament sprains in young athletes. *Am J Sports Med*. 2014;42(5):1103–1109.
3. Weber AE, Kopydlowski NJ, Sekiya JK. Nonsurgical management and postoperative rehabilitation of medial instability of the knee. *Sports Med Athrosc Rev*. 2015;23(2):104–109.
4. Varelas AN, Erickson BJ, Cvetanovich GL, et al. Medial collateral ligament reconstruction in patients with medial knee instability: a systematic review. *Orthop J Sports Med*. 2017;5(5):2325967117703920.
5. Yoshida M, Marumo K. An autologous leukocyte-reduced platelet-rich plasma therapy for chronic injury of the medial collateral ligament in the knee: a report of 3 successful cases. *Clin J Sport Med*. 2019;29(1):e4–e6.

ADDITIONAL READING

- D'Ambrosi R, Corona K, Guerra G, et al. Biomechanics of the posterior oblique ligament of the knee. *Clin Biomech (Bristol)*. 2020;80:105205.
- Madi S, Acharya K, Pandey V. Current concepts on management of medial and posteromedial knee injuries. *J Clin Ortho Trauma*. 2022;27:101807.
- Westermann RW, Spindler KP, Hettrich CM, et al. Outcomes following ACL and grade III MCL injuries: is there a role for MCL repair? *Orthop J Sports Med*. 2017;5(3 Suppl 3):2325967117S00126.

CLINICAL PEARLS

Common questions and answers:

- Q: How long until I can play again?
- A: For most sports, athletes with grade I injuries return in an average of 10 days. Those with grade II sprains may return in as little as 2 to 3 weeks. Grade III injuries can take 5 to 7 weeks for full recovery. Sport can influence speed of return: Soccer players may require more time because of the use of the instep to kick and pass the ball. Operative treatment of combined injuries can take 6 to 12 months.
- Q: Should I wear a brace?
- A: Bracing is typically used for all grades of MCL injuries. Grade III injuries can require a full year of bracing depending on the athlete and injury. Prophylactic bracing is controversial. Use has not demonstrated a clinically significant trend to MCL injury prevention.
- Q: Will I get early arthritis?
- A: A 10-year follow-up on isolated MCL injuries suggests that most patients have excellent function and no major radiographic evidence of arthritis.
- Q: Will it always bother me?
- A: After rehabilitation, most patients note only minor symptoms, if any at all. 10-year studies show most perform well with only minor decreases in physical ability.

M

MEDIAL EPICONDYLITIS

Craig C. Young, MD ▪ Yuka Kobayashi, DO

BASICS

DESCRIPTION

Medial epicondylitis is clinically defined as pain at the medial epicondyle due to repetitive flexion and pronation at the elbow. A more accurate term may be *medial epicondylosis* or *epicondylalgia*. It is usually an overuse injury that can affect both athletes and nonathletes. *Golfer's elbow* is a common term used for medial epicondylitis.

EPIDEMIOLOGY

- Diagnosed less often than lateral epicondylitis, a similar condition affecting the origin of the common extensor tendon on the lateral epicondyle
- Overall prevalence of up to 1% in general population but may be as high as 8% in occupational settings
- Diagnosis is most common in the 4th and 5th decades, although the condition has been seen in patients ranging from 12 to 80 years of age.
- Men and women are affected equally.
- The dominant hand is most often affected.
- Most patients will have resolution or significant improvement within a year with all treatment options including clinical observation alone.

ETIOLOGY AND PATHOPHYSIOLOGY

- Initially thought to be an inflammatory process, but histologic studies do not show inflammatory cells in chronic epicondylitis.
- Inflammation may play a role in the initial acute injury when microtearing of the tendon occurs.
- Histologic studies of chronic epicondylitis have shown abnormal collagen architecture due to a fibroblastic and immature vascular response, which causes incomplete tendon repair.
- Degenerative changes often seen in the pronator teres and flexor carpi radialis muscles and their tendons:
  - Palmaris longus, flexor digitorum superficialis, and flexor carpi ulnaris may also be involved.
- Common causes:
  - Activities that involve forceful and/or continuous wrist flexion and/or forearm pronation or a large amount of stabilization—especially with forearm supinated, such as racquet sports, swimming, swinging a golf club, throwing, playing tennis, waterskiing, or playing piano
  - Certain occupations (carpenters, plumbers, meat cutters, etc.) may be more at risk.

DIAGNOSIS

HISTORY

- Pain and tenderness along the medial elbow, extending into the forearm, which worsen with resisted forearm pronation or wrist flexion at 90 degrees of elbow flexion and/or full elbow extension
- Difficulty gripping without pain
- Decreased wrist strength
- Tightness/stiffness when stretching elbow and wrist

PHYSICAL EXAM

- Tenderness to palpation over the medial epicondyle, pronator teres, and flexor carpi radialis
- Local swelling and warmth may be present.
- Active and resisted range of motion may be full or limited depending on the severity of the injury.

DIFFERENTIAL DIAGNOSIS

- Entrapment neuropathy (i.e., cubital tunnel syndrome, carpal tunnel syndrome)
- Ulnar neuritis
- Ulnar collateral ligament (UCL) insufficiency
- Medial elbow apophysitis (i.e., "Little Leaguer's elbow")
- Inflammatory arthritis
- Ganglion cyst
- Cervical radiculopathy
- Thoracic outlet syndrome
- Myofascial pain

DIAGNOSTIC TESTS & INTERPRETATION

- Generally, not needed for initial evaluation
- In cases that are refractory to treatment or where the diagnosis is in question, elbow x-rays followed by ultrasound (US) or magnetic resonance imaging (MRI) may be considered.
- Musculoskeletal (MSK) US may reveal tendon thickening, calcifications, hypoechoic changes, and vascular ingrowth in the tendons.
- Calcification is most often in the flexor tendon and seems to be associated with a higher pain score as well as a history of steroid injection.

TREATMENT

- More studies are needed specifically on medial epicondylitis; most studies focus on treatment of lateral epicondylitis. Many of these treatments are used for medial epicondylitis as well.
- Initial treatment includes:
  - Relative rest: Limit activities that cause pain.
  - For control of symptoms consider ice, and acetaminophen or over-the-counter (OTC) nonsteroidal anti-inflammatory drugs (NSAIDs) as needed.
- The mainstay of treatment involves stretching and strengthening with progression to eccentric training exercise with or without formal physical therapy.
- Bracing may be helpful.
- If no improvement in 6 weeks, consider obtaining x-rays and initiating formal physical therapy.
- If still symptomatic, consider injection. Various techniques have been proposed, including dry needling of tendon, corticosteroid injection, botulinum toxin injection, prolotherapy, platelet-rich plasma injection, and autologous blood injection.
  - Corticosteroid injections may provide short-term relief of symptoms but do not appear to be effective for long-term management of chronic tendinopathies (1)[B].
- Platelet rich-plasma injections may provide superior relief of symptoms for longer periods of time when compared to cortisone but may have minimal effect on long-term outcome (1)[B].
- Modalities: Consider the use of US, phonophoresis, or iontophoresis. Some studies have shown them to be useful in returning an athlete to activity sooner, but they show no long-term benefit.
- If symptoms persist, consider advanced imaging with US or MRI to confirm diagnosis.
- Long-term treatment:
  - Watchful waiting: Most patients with epicondylosis will become symptom free or have significant improvement at 1 year.
  - Autologous blood, platelet-rich plasma, prolotherapy, botulinum toxin have demonstrated short-term effectiveness in small studies, but none have been shown to be significantly superior in the long term in meta-analysis or systematic reviews (1),(2)[B],(3)[A].
  - Extracorporeal shock wave therapy may provide short-term relief of symptoms but may not be effective for long-term management of chronic tendinopathies (4)[A].
  - US-guided percutaneous tenotomy procedure has been shown to be effective for chronic symptoms (5)[B].
- In patients with recalcitrant symptoms >6 months in duration, surgical intervention has been shown to be effective (6)[A].

ONGOING CARE

Home exercise program as follows:

- Strengthening:
  - Stay below the level of pain.
  - Perform two to three sets of 10 to 15 repetitions 2 to 4 times a week. Once three sets of 15 repetitions can be performed easily, increase the weight, reduce the repetitions to 10, and build back up to 15.
  - Wrist extension curls: With the forearm supported on a firm surface and the palm facing downward, lift and lower the weight.
  - Wrist flexion curls: With the forearm supported on a firm surface and the palm facing upward, lift and lower the weight.
  - Forearm pronation/supination: With the forearm supported on a firm surface, turn the palm up and then down while holding onto a weight.
  - Gripping: Gently grip a rubber ball, a towel, or putty and then advance to items with more resistance. Perform 10 to 30 repetitions, increasing in intensity once 30 repetitions can be performed.
  - Finger extension: Wrap a rubber band around the outside of all the fingers and thumb, gently extend the hand by opening the fingers, and then close the fingers. Perform 10 to 30 repetitions.
- Stretching:
  - Keep the stretch to a comfortable level.
  - Hold each stretch for ~30 seconds.
  - Repeat each stretch 3 to 6 times.

- Wrist flexion stretch: Bend the involved wrist down gently by grasping it with the other hand until a pulling sensation is felt. Keep the elbow straight.
- Wrist flexion stretch (advanced): same as for the wrist flexion stretch but with the addition of wrist movement toward the side of the little finger
- Wrist extension stretch: Bend the involved wrist up gently by grasping it with the opposite hand until a pulling sensation is felt. Keep the elbow straight.

REFERENCES

1. Kamble P, Prabhu RM, Jogani A, et al. Is ultrasound (US)-guided platelet-rich plasma injection more efficacious as a treatment modality for lateral elbow tendinopathy than us-guided steroid injection? A prospective triple-blinded study with midterm follow-up. *Clin Orthop Surg.* 2023;15(3):454–462.
2. Park HS, Jo SM, Dasari S, et al. Comparison of clinical outcomes of platelet-rich plasma for epicondylitis, elbow: simultaneous lateral and medial versus lateral versus medial. *Orthop Surg.* 2023;15(8):2110–2115.
3. Masiello F, Pati I, Veropalumbo E, et al. Ultrasound-guided injection of platelet-rich plasma for tendinopathies: a systematic review and meta-analysis. *Blood Transfus.* 2023; 21(2):119–136.
4. Liu WC, Chen CT, Lu CC, et al. Extracorporeal shock wave therapy shows superiority over injections for pain relief and grip strength recovery in lateral epicondylitis: a systematic review and network meta-analysis. *Arthroscopy.* 2022;38(6):2018.e12–2034.e12.
5. Boden AL, Scott MT, Dalwadi PP, et al. Platelet-rich plasma versus Tenex in the treatment of medial and lateral epicondylitis. *J Shoulder Elbow Surg.* 2019;28(1):112–119.
6. Arevalo A, Rao S, Willier DP III, et al. Surgical techniques and clinical outcomes for medial epicondylitis: a systematic review. *Am J Sports Med.* 2023;51(9):2506–2515.

ADDITIONAL READING

- Alzahrani WM. Platelet-rich plasma injections as an alternative to surgery in treating patients with medial epicondylitis: a systemic review. *Cureus.* 2022;14(8):e28378.
- Bae KJ, Park C, Ahn JM, et al. Magnetic resonance imaging evaluation of patients with clinically diagnosed medial epicondylitis. *Skeletal Radiol.* 2021;50(8):1629–1636.
- Balevi ISY, Karaoglan B, Batur EB, et al. Evaluation of short-term and residual effects of Kinesio taping in chronic lateral epicondylitis: a randomized, double-blinded, controlled trial. *J Hand Ther.* 2023;36(1):13–22.
- Bang JY, Hahn S, Yi J, et al. Clinical applicability of shear wave elastography for the evaluation of medial epicondylitis. *Eur Radiol.* 2021;31(9): 6726–6735.
- Barnes DE, Beckley JM, Smith J. Percutaneous ultrasonic tenotomy for chronic elbow tendinosis: a prospective study. *J Shoulder Elbow Surg.* 2015;24(1):67–73.
- Bohlen HL, Schwartz ZE, Wu VJ, et al. Platelet-rich plasma is an equal alternative to surgery in the treatment of type 1 medial epicondylitis. *Orthop J Sports Med.* 2020;8(3):2325967120908952.
- Ciftci YGD, Tuncay F, Kocak FA, et al. Is low-dose dextrose prolotherapy as effective as high-dose dextrose prolotherapy in the treatment of lateral epicondylitis? A double-blind, ultrasound guided, randomized controlled study. *Arch Phys Med Rehabil.* 2023;104(2):179–187.
- ElMeligie MM, Gbreel MI, Yehia RM, et al. Clinical efficacy of high-intensity laser therapy on lateral epicondylitis patients: a systematic review and meta-analysis. *Am J Phys Med Rehabil.* 2023;102(1):64–70.
- Güngör E, Güngör ZK. Comparison of the efficacy of corticosteroid, dry needling, and PRP application in lateral epicondylitis. *Eur J Orthop Surg Traumatol.* 2022;32(8):1569–1575.
- Hoogvliet P, Randsdorp MS, Dingemanse R, et al. Does effectiveness of exercise therapy and mobilisation techniques offer guidance for the treatment of lateral and medial epicondylitis? A systematic review. *Br J Sports Med.* 2013;47(17):1112–1119.
- Kang KB, Cheon SH, Lee HD. Radiologic evaluation and clinical effect of calcification in medial epicondylitis. *J Shoulder Elbow Surg.* 2022;31(2):375–381.
- Kaplan S, Sah V, Ozkan S, et al. Comparative effects of focused and radial extracorporeal shock wave therapies on lateral epicondylitis: a randomised sham-controlled trial. *J Coll Physicians Surg Pak.* 2023;33(5):554–559.
- Kim BS, Jung KJ, Lee C. Open procedure vs. arthroscopic débridement for chronic medial epicondylitis. *J Shoulder Elbow Surg.* 2023;32(2):340–347.
- Konarski W, Pobozy T, Kotela A, et al. Ultrasound in the differential diagnosis of medial epicondylalgia and medial elbow pain—imaging findings and narrative literature review. *Healthcare (Basel).* 2022;10(8):1529.
- Park H, Hahn S, Yi J, et al. Clinical assessments and MRI findings suggesting early surgical treatment for patients with medial epicondylitis. *Taehan Yongsang Uihakhoe Chi.* 2021;82(3):613–625.
- Pattanittum P, Turner T, Green S, et al. Nonsteroidal anti-inflammatory drugs (NSAIDs) for treating lateral elbow pain in adults. *Cochrane Database Syst Rev.* 2013;(5):CD003686.
- Placzek R, Drescher W, Deuretzbacher G, et al. Treatment of chronic radial epicondylitis with botulinum toxin A: a double-blind, placebo-controlled, randomized multicenter study. *J Bone Joint Surg Am.* 2007;89(2):255–260.
- Prabhakar G, Kanawade V, Ghali AN, et al. Medial elbow pain syndrome: current treatment strategies. *Orthopedics.* 2023;46(2):e81–e88.
- Saltychev M, Johansson J, Kemppi V, et al. Effectiveness of topical glyceryl trinitrate in treatment of tendinopathy—systematic review and meta-analysis. *Disabil Rehabil.* 2022;44(20): 5804–5810.
- Seidel DH, Ditchen DM, Hoehne-Hückstädt UM, et al. Quantitative measures of physical risk factors associated with work-related musculoskeletal disorders of the elbow: a systematic review. *Int J Environ Res Public Health.* 2019;16(1):130.
- Sirico F, Ricca F, Di Meglio F, et al. Local corticosteroid versus autologous blood injections in lateral epicondylitis: meta-analysis of randomized controlled trials. *Eur J Phys Rehabil Med.* 2017;53(3):483–491.
- Suresh SP, Ali KE, Jones H, et al. Medial epicondylitis: is ultrasound guided autologous blood injection an effective treatment? *Br J Sports Med.* 2006;40(11):935–939.
- Vukelic B, Abbey R, Knox J, et al. Which injections are effective for lateral epicondylitis? *J Fam Pract.* 2021;70(9):461–463.
- Zhu M, Rabago D, Chung VCH, et al. Effects of hypertonic dextrose injection (prolotherapy) in lateral elbow tendinosis: a systematic review and meta-analysis. *Arch Phys Med Rehabil.* 2022;103(11):2209–2218.
- Zwerus EL, Somford MP, Maissan F, et al. Physical examination of the elbow, what is the evidence? A systematic literature review. *Br J Sports Med.* 2018;52(19):1253–1260.

CLINICAL PEARLS

- Wrist splints are often more helpful than counterforce bracing if the patient has significant pain upon awakening. However, counterforce braces are often better tolerated during the day.
- Histologic biopsies of chronic epicondylitis reveal no inflammation, but rather signs of poor and disordered healing, a term called *angiofibroblastic degeneration*. Chronic epicondylosis is not an inflammatory condition. Consider other treatments such as physical therapy and proinflammatory modalities instead of anti-inflammatory agents.

MEDIAL GASTROCNEMIUS INJURY (TENNIS LEG)

Tammy Ng, MD • Glenn H. Sapp II, MD • Daniel C. Herman, MD, PhD, FAAPMR, FACSM, FISBS, CAQSM

BASICS

DESCRIPTION

Musculotendinous disruption of varying degrees in the medial head of the gastrocnemius muscle, resulting from sudden dorsiflexion of the foot during an eccentric loading (Athlete is actively plantarflexing as an outside force causes a sudden stretch/dorsiflexion moment).

RISK FACTORS

- Male
- 4th to 6th decades of life (1)
- Participation in sports involving quick accelerations, including racquet sports (tennis, squash), hill running, and track events involving jumping activities, but may also involve relatively low stress activities such as ascending stairs or occupational activities (1),(2)
- Muscles that have not been properly warmed up may be greater at risk.
- Participation during prolonged activities, as fatigued muscles with impaired coordination increases the risk of injury.
- Recurrent calf strains

DIAGNOSIS

- Audible pop or tearing sensation when injury to the medial calf occurs
- Pain in the calf region with radiation to the knee or the ankle
- Pain with range of motion (ROM) of the ankle, particularly dorsiflexion
- Swelling or bruising of the posterior calf

HISTORY

Athlete reports audible pop or experiencing tearing sensation at time of injury to the medial calf. The patient may complain of feeling like a stick struck the calf.

PHYSICAL EXAM

- Asymmetric calf swelling and increased circumference that can be serially measured. Swelling may be noted all the way to the ankle.
- Calf ecchymosis
- A visible or palpable defect may be present in the medial gastrocnemius muscle.
- Tenderness on palpation of the medial gastrocnemius muscle (more painful at the medial musculotendinous junction)
- Peripheral pulses should be normal.
- Pain with passive ankle dorsiflexion
- Pain with active resistance to ankle plantar flexion
- Palpation of the Achilles tendon demonstrates an intact tendon.
- Thompson test is negative: Thompson test should always be performed in the clinical setting of atraumatic, acute-onset pain in the posterior lower leg associated with an audible "pop."

DIFFERENTIAL DIAGNOSIS

- Baker cyst rupture
- Deep vein thrombosis (DVT)
- Plantaris tendon rupture
- Achilles tendon rupture
- Acute compartment syndrome after rupture of the medial head of the gastrocnemius
- Chronic exertional compartment syndrome (posterior)
- Posterior tibial tendon rupture or tendonitis
- Popliteal artery entrapment syndrome
- Anomalous gastrocnemius muscle rupture

DIAGNOSTIC TESTS & INTERPRETATION

- X-ray films of the tibia/fibula may be ordered to rule out an avulsion fracture or calcific tendinosis.
- Magnetic resonance imaging (MRI): the most sensitive and specific imaging method to show the area of disrupted soft tissue and surrounding structures (3)
- Ultrasound (US): will aid in ruling out a DVT or Achilles tendon rupture. The calf can also be serially imaged to assess the extent of injury and healing (3).
- A prognostic US classification based on connective tissue involvement has been proposed. Involvement of the free gastrocnemius aponeurosis on US has been associated with worse prognosis and longer return to play (4).
- Advanced imaging (MRI, US) is usually not necessary because the diagnosis is commonly made on clinical findings, although it may help inform return to play decisions for professional athletes.

TREATMENT

GENERAL MEASURES

- Prevention/reduction of swelling: elevation, compression dressing/sleeve, and ice for 20 minutes 3 to 4 times a day (1)[C]
- Early weight-bearing (may need crutches and/or bilateral heel lifts for normal gait)
- Ankle/foot bracing to keep the ankle in maximally tolerable dorsiflexion: In the early stages of treatment, using the splint at night may be helpful (2)[C].

MEDICATION

Nonsteroidal anti-inflammatory drugs (NSAIDs): Clinicians must carefully consider pain therapy in the initial 48 hours because decreased platelet activity may result in increased bleeding and larger hematoma formation with resultant effects on healing:

- Ibuprofen: adult: 600 mg PO q8h; children: 10 mg/kg PO q8h
- Naproxen: adult: 250 to 500 mg PO BID
- Ketorolac: adult: 30 mg intravenous (IV)/ intramuscular (IM) q6h or 10 mg PO q4–6h

ADDITIONAL THERAPIES

- Ice therapy for control of pain and swelling
- Active resistance dorsiflexion exercises until the athlete is pain free (2)[B]
- Apply compression dressing from the metatarsal heads to the gastrocnemius for the first 2 weeks (5)[B].
- Partial weight-bearing ambulation as soon as tolerable to maximize the contact of the sole of the foot to the ground (1),(2)[C]
- Stationary cycling, leg presses, and heel raises
- Proprioception and balance training
- Although nonsurgical treatment is first line, surgical fixation is a treatment option for patients who require forceful plantarflexion for their desired activities or occupation (6).

ONGOING CARE

PROGNOSIS

- Prognosis is excellent for the tennis leg sufferer to return to sports endeavors.
- Noncompliance can prevent players from returning to sports for 3 to 4 months.
- Early and aggressive rehabilitation allows most patients to recover within a few weeks.

REFERENCES

1. Fields KB, Rigby MD. Muscular calf injuries in runners. *Curr Sports Med Rep.* 2016;15(5):320–324.
2. Domeracki SJ, Landman Z, Blanc PD, et al. Off the courts: occupational "tennis leg." *Workplace Health Saf.* 2019;67(1):5–8.
3. Delgado GJ, Chung CB, Lektrakul N, et al. Tennis leg: clinical US study of 141 patients and anatomic investigation of four cadavers with MR imaging and US. *Radiology.* 2002;224(1):112–119.
4. Pedret C, Balius R, Blasi M, et al. Ultrasound classification of medial gastrocnemious injuries. *Scand J Med Sci Sports.* 2020;30(12):2456–2465.
5. Kwak HS, Lee KB, Han YM. Ruptures of the medial head of the gastrocnemius ("tennis leg"): clinical outcome and compression effect. *Clin Imaging.* 2006;30(1):48–53.
6. Cooper J, Arner JW, Peebles LA, et al. Surgical treatment of medial gastrocnemius tear. *Arthrosc Tech.* 2021;10(2):e519–e523.

ADDITIONAL READING

Millar AP. Strains of the posterior calf musculature ("tennis leg"). *Am J Sports Med.* 1979;7(3):172–174.

CLINICAL PEARLS

- Although the mechanism of injury is often during athletic events with quick or explosive motions, this injury may also occur during relatively minor activities.
- Considering the occasionally severe pain experienced at the time of the injury and subacutely, the patient should be counseled and reassured regarding the excellent prognosis of this injury.
- Weight-bearing and splints for maximizing tolerable ankle dorsiflexion early during treatment is key to functional progression and prevention of contractures and prolonged return to activities.
- Thompson test should be performed to rule out Achilles tendon rupture.

MEDIAL PLICA SYNDROME

Shane Geffe, MD ▪ Daniel C. Herman, MD, PhD, FAAPMR, FACSM, FISBS, CAQSM ▪
Sara N. Raiser, MD, FAAPMR, CAQSM

BASICS

DESCRIPTION

- Inflammation of the synovial lining forming an intra-articular band located over the medial aspect of the knee, resulting in fibrosis and persistent pain
- Cause of anterior knee pain, distinguishable from more common etiologies by snapping/clicking and/or palpable cord from the fibrotic plica

EPIDEMIOLOGY

Prevalence

- Medial plica may be found in up to 80% of knees undergoing arthroscopy, although the most reported range is 20–25% (1),(2).
- Most are asymptomatic, with 3–30% of medial plica resulting in persistent knee pain (3).
- Onset of symptoms usually occurs during 1st through 3rd decade.
- Gender:
  - Affects females more than males

ETIOLOGY AND PATHOPHYSIOLOGY

Four morphologic plicae exist which are differentiated by the degree of contact on the medial femoral condyle and patellar facet (3)[C]. Repetitive injury and inflammation of the medial synovium from the femur and/or the patella pinching tissue may occur with subsequent fibrosis, thickening, and loss of elasticity of the plica caused by:

- Repetitive knee flexion/extension (e.g., running, squatting)
- Direct trauma
- Underlying intra-articular abnormalities (e.g., foreign bodies, osteochondritis dissecans, or inflammatory arthritis)

Genetics

There is some evidence to suggest a genetic component due to the embryologic etiology of plica development, although this has not yet been established.

RISK FACTORS

- Congenital presence of plica
- Multiple injuries or surgeries over medial aspect of knee
- Poor structural mechanics, including weak quadriceps, tight hamstrings, and increased Q angle

GENERAL PREVENTION

Proper knee extension alignment and mechanics

COMMONLY ASSOCIATED CONDITIONS

- Knee valgus
- Heel valgus and midfoot pronation
- Patellofemoral chondromalacia

DIAGNOSIS

HISTORY

- Complaint of anterior and medial knee pain just proximal to medial joint line
- Pain is often unilateral.
- Often exacerbated by activity, including running, squatting, and ascending or descending stairs
- Patients commonly report popping, snapping, and catching with knee flexion.

PHYSICAL EXAM

- Palpable fibrotic cord located between medial border of the patella and medial femoral condyle
- Cord is painful with full knee extension or flexion (nonspecific).
- May have soft tissue swelling medial to patellar border
- Medial patellar plica (MPP) test: With patient supine, examiner applies pressure with thumb over inferior and medial aspect of the patellofemoral joint while passively flexing the knee from 0 to 90 degrees; positive test if pain in extension is relieved at 90 degrees of flexion

DIFFERENTIAL DIAGNOSIS

- Medial collateral ligament sprain
- Patellofemoral pain syndrome
- Patellar subluxation
- Osteochondritis dissecans
- Osteoarthritis
- Pes anserinus pain syndrome
- Medial meniscus tear

DIAGNOSTIC TESTS & INTERPRETATION

Initial Tests (lab, imaging)

- Initial diagnosis is usually clinical.
- Dynamic ultrasound (US) in office/training room may help establish diagnosis.

Follow-Up Tests & Special Considerations

Coupled with clinical suspicion, a noncontrast magnetic resonance imaging (MRI) (sensitivity 93%, specificity 81%) can be nearly as sensitive as knee arthroscopy for diagnosis as well as ruling out alternative etiologies (3)[C].

Diagnostic Procedures/Other

- Intra-articular injection of a local anesthetic can aid in diagnosis.
- Knee arthroscopy provides definitive diagnosis but is only indicated when conservative therapy fails.

TREATMENT

GENERAL MEASURES

- Acute phase:
  - Rest to reduce repetitive flexion/extension of the knee.
  - Ice
  - Compression knee sleeves or braces may be helpful to reduce swelling.
  - Elevating the knee above the level of the heart may help reduce swelling.
- Recovery phase:
  - Physical therapy (PT) or home exercise program (HEP) focusing on strengthening quadriceps, stretching of hamstring
  - Application of Kinesio tape with activity (1)[B]
  - Intra-articular corticosteroid injection

MEDICATION

Oral or topical nonsteroidal anti-inflammatory drugs (NSAIDs)

ISSUES FOR REFERRAL

Referral to orthopedic surgeon may be warranted if no improvement with conservative therapy, as the plica can cause cartilage damage to the patellofemoral joint.

ADDITIONAL THERAPIES

Orthotics to correct heel valgus if present

SURGERY/OTHER PROCEDURES

- Arthroscopic resection may be considered if conservative therapy fails after 6 months.
- Generally has high success rate (especially in those without chondral damage) (3)[C],(4)[A]
- Surgery is more successful in patients younger than age 30 years (5)[B].

ONGOING CARE

FOLLOW-UP RECOMMENDATIONS

Consider follow-up once monthly while patient is in recovery phase to evaluate for progress.

PATIENT EDUCATION

Patients should be counseled on the pathophysiology, conservative management options, and the potential complications if left unaddressed. In high-level athletes, surgery is potentially curative.

PROGNOSIS

Most patients respond to conservative therapy and rehabilitation.

COMPLICATIONS

Articular cartilage damage may develop as plica erosion into the cartilage surfaces of the femur and patella can create a sanding mark.

REFERENCES

1. Genc E, Duymaz T. Functional effects of kinesiology taping for medial plica syndrome: a prospective randomized control trial. *Physiother Theory Pract*. 2022;38(11):1581–1590.
2. Al-Hadithy N, Gikas P, Mahapatra AM, et al. Review article: plica syndrome of the knee. *J Orthop Surg (Hong Kong)*. 2011;19(3):354–358.
3. Erickson BJ, Campbell K, Cvetanovich GL, et al. Nonligamentous soft tissue pathology about the knee: a review. *Orthopedics*. 2016;39(1):32–42.
4. Gerrard AD, Charalambous CP. Arthroscopic excision of medial knee plica: a meta-analysis of outcomes. *Knee Surg Relat Res*. 2018;30(4):356–363.
5. Hufeland M, Treder L, Kubo HK. Symptomatic medial synovial plica of the knee joint: an underestimated pathology in young patients. *Arch Orth Trauma Surg*. 2019;139(11):1625–1631.

CLINICAL PEARLS

- Medial plica syndrome should be considered with a history of anterior knee pain after blunt trauma, twisting injury, or repetitive flexion/extension injury, especially with snapping, popping, or palpable fibrous band under the superior medial patellar facet.
- Diagnosis is typically clinical and only made when alternative pathologies are ruled out (usually by MRI).
- Treatment is primarily rehabilitation and avoidance of exacerbating activities.
- In severely symptomatic patients, intra-articular corticosteroids and appropriate Kinesio taping may serve as useful adjuncts to supervised PT and/or HEP.
- Arthroscopic plica excision is potentially curative and has Strength of Recommendation Taxonomy (SORT) A evidence for improved clinical outcomes in those that fail conservative management.

MEDIAL TIBIAL STRESS SYNDROME

Alecia Gende, DO, CAQSM, FACEP, FAAEM • Britt Marcussen, MD, FAAFP, CAQSM

BASICS

DESCRIPTION

- Typically, an overuse injury, with exercise-induced pain over the posteromedial border of the middle to distal 2/3 of the tibia
- Exact pathophysiology is unknown, thought due to traction on periosteum and repetitive loading across tibia (1).
- May be on a continuum with stress fracture
- Synonym(s):
  - "Shin splints"
  - Tibialis posterior myofasciitis
  - Soleus syndrome

EPIDEMIOLOGY

- 13.6–20% incidence in runners (1)
- 5.7% incidence and second most common musculoskeletal injury in military recruits (2)

RISK FACTORS

Risks for development of lower extremity overuse syndromes are a point of interest in literature. First four are considered higher risk (1),(3),(4):

- Female sex
- Higher body weight
- Navicular drop (an indicator of excessive pronation)
- Prior running injury
- Limited external/internal rotation of hip
- Limited ankle range of motion (ROM)
- Higher body mass index (BMI)
- Overall poor conditioning
- Limited core strength

GENERAL PREVENTION

Prevention methods are often encouraged; however, some systematic reviews show no statistical benefit from any prevention strategy (5)[C]:

- Shock-absorbing insoles/orthotics: most promising in studies (5),(6),(7)
- Pronation control insoles if navicular drop
- Replacing running shoes after 300 to 600 miles (8)
- Gradually increasing running programs

DIAGNOSIS

HISTORY

- Often insidious and progressive
- Temporally related to sudden increase in intensity/duration of activity, or change in playing/running surface from a softer surface to a harder surface such as concrete
- Early in course: Pain occurs during activity rather than at onset:
  - Sometimes relieved as activity continues
  - Often worse with toe off
  - Often aches after rest which is in contrast to chronic exertional compartment syndrome where pain is relieved quickly by rest
- Late in course: pain through full duration of activity:
  - Pain and aching continue after cessation of inciting activity.

PHYSICAL EXAM

- Tenderness to palpation along the middle to distal 2/3 of the tibia, along the posteromedial border
- Diffuse posteromedial pain with palpation is most sensitive finding (6).
- Lower extremity kinetic chain examination may reveal excessive pronation, navicular drop, or other alignment abnormalities, core weakness, and instability.
- Chronic cases: induration, soft tissue swelling, or nodularity
- Shoe examination reveals overpronation wear pattern, excessive age of shoes.

DIFFERENTIAL DIAGNOSIS

- Stress fracture
- Compartment syndrome
- Muscular strain
- Nerve entrapment
- Fascial defects
- Popliteal artery entrapment syndrome
- Effort-induced venous thrombosis

DIAGNOSTIC TESTS & INTERPRETATION

ALERT

- Overall, a clinical diagnosis, but imaging is needed to evaluate for other etiologies such as stress fracture.
- Plain films of anteroposterior and lateral tibia are often normal.
- Bone scan: Diffuse uptake along the posteromedial border of the tibia, often seen better on delayed images, involves radiation, shows whole body (if concern for bilateral or other associated areas of bony tenderness as in multiple stress fractures); sensitivity 74–84% (6)
- Computed tomography (CT): posteromedial cortical osteopenia, sensitivity 42–100%, specificity 82–100% in various studies, like bone scan involves radiation; may be useful in unclear clinical diagnosis; magnetic resonance imaging (MRI) is typically preferred over CT (6).
- MRI: Bone Marrow edema and periosteal signal may be seen, similar sensitivity and specificity to bone scan, no radiation (6).

TREATMENT

Acute treatment (5)[C]:

- Nonsteroidal anti-inflammatory drugs (NSAIDs) and ice most beneficial in acute stages
- Complete rest if possible
- Otherwise, graded running program, gradual increase in inciting activities
- Cross-training with nonimpact activities: swimming, water running, bicycling
- Low-energy extracorporeal shock wave therapy (ESWT) may provide some benefit (9).
- No benefit to immobilization
- Surgery rarely indicated

ADDITIONAL THERAPIES

- Special considerations (6)[C]:
  - Special taping techniques by athletic trainers may improve symptoms.
  - For very flat feet (pes planus), consider more supportive shoes or supportive inserts.
  - For very high-arched feet (pes cavus), consider increased cushioning in shoes or shock-absorbing inserts.
- Rehabilitation (6)[C]:
  - Target-specific stretching and strengthening exercises
  - Core strengthening
  - Towel calf stretches
  - Tracing alphabet with toes
  - Alternate heel/toe walking

SURGERY/OTHER PROCEDURES

- Generally limited success to fully return to level of presymptoms activity but more success with relief of pain
- Surgical procedures for recalcitrant cases (10):
  - Surgical release of the investing fascia around the soleus insertion on the posteromedial aspect of the tibia. Medial tibial stress syndrome is not a compartment syndrome, but releasing this fascia has helped with pain.
  - Surgical division of the insertion of the soleus on the periosteum can relieve associated periostitis.
  - Cauterization of the periosteum over the posteromedial tibia allows scarring and reattachment of the periosteum.

ONGOING CARE

- Changes in training techniques:
  - Increase rest days.
  - Add in cross-training days with non–weight-bearing activity such as swimming and biking.
  - Slow increase in training intensity/duration, with no more than a 10% increase per week
- Correct shoe type for foot type:
  - Some people may benefit from orthotics.

PATIENT EDUCATION

- Much education required
- Prolonged recovery course
- Gradual increase of training intensity (5),(6)[C]
- Rest sufficiently to overcome symptoms.
- Return slowly to avoid recurrence.
- New shoes every 3 to 6 months, 200 to 300 miles of wear (5)[C]

REFERENCES

1. Winkelmann ZK, Anderson D, Games KE, et al. Risk factors for medial tibial stress syndrome in active individuals: an evidence-based review. *J Athl Train*. 2016;51(12):1049–1052.
2. Sharma J, Greeves JP, Byers M, et al. Musculoskeletal injuries in British Army recruits: a prospective study of diagnosis-specific incidence and rehabilitation times. *BMC Musculoskelet Disord*. 2015;16:106.
3. Reinking MF, Austin TM, Richter RR, et al. Medial tibial stress syndrome in active individuals: a systematic review and meta-analysis of risk factors. *Sports Health*. 2017;9(3):252–261.
4. Hamstra-Wright KL, Bliven KCH, Bay C. Risk factors for medial tibial stress syndrome in physically active individuals such as runners and military personnel: a systematic review and meta-analysis. *Br J Sports Med*. 2015;49(6):362–369.
5. Craig DI. Medial tibial stress syndrome: evidence-based prevention. *J Athl Train*. 2008;43(3):316–318.
6. Reshef N, Guelich DR. Medial tibial stress syndrome. *Clin Sports Med*. 2012;31(2):273–290.
7. Naderi A, Bagheri S, Ahoor FR, et al. Foot orthoses enhance the effectiveness of exercise, shockwave, and ice therapy in the management of medial tibial stress syndrome. *Clin J Sports Med*. 2022;32(3):e251–e260.
8. Teyhen DS, Thomas RM, Roberts CC, et al. Awareness and compliance with recommended running shoes guidelines among U.S. army soldiers. *Mil Med*. 2010;175(11):847–854.
9. Garcia SG, Rona SR, Tinoco MCG, et al. Shockwave treatment for medial tibial stress syndrome in military cadets: a single-blind randomized controlled trial. *Int J Surg*. 2017;46:102–109.
10. Vogels S. Chronic recalcitrant medial tibial stress syndrome: is surgery an option? *Transl Sports Med*. 2021;4(4):508–517.

ADDITIONAL READING

- Korakakis V, Whiteley R, Tzavara A, et al. The effectiveness of extracorporeal shockwave therapy in common lower limb conditions: a systematic review including quantification of patient-rated pain reduction. *Br J Sports Med*. 2018;52(6):387–407.
- Lopes AD, Hespanhol LC Jr, Yeung SS, et al. What are the main running-related musculoskeletal injuries? A systematic review. *Sports Med*. 2012;42(10):891–905.
- Winters M, Eskes M, Weir A, et al. Treatment of medial tibial stress syndrome: a systematic review. *Sports Med*. 2013;43(12):1315–1333.

CLINICAL PEARLS

- Activity should be avoided until pain and tenderness resolve, followed by a slow, structured return to prior level of activity.
- There is no good evidence that special taping or an ACE bandage will shorten recovery, but it may help to improve symptoms.
- If time cannot be taken off from training, relative rest, with a 20–50% decrease in training intensity/duration. Work in cross-training days, with non–weight-bearing activity.
- Rehabilitation exercises should aim at stretching and strengthening involved musculotendinous units.
- Use a towel to pull your foot toward you and stretch your calf. Trace the alphabet with your feet. Alternate walking on toes and heels; "toe raises" to strengthen lower leg while standing on stairs or steps.

MENISCAL TEARS

Saif Usman, MD, FAMSSM, FAAFP

BASICS

DESCRIPTION

- Menisci are cartilaginous structures whose functions include distribution of joint fluid, shock absorption, deepening of the joint, nutrient distribution, load or weight-bearing, and joint stabilization especially in rotation.
- The peripheral 1/3 zone (red-red) has good vascular supply, central third zone (red-white) has limited vascular supply, whereas inner third zone (white) is avascular.
- The most common tear patterns are longitudinal, radial, horizontal, displaced, root, complex, and bucket-handle tears.
- Meniscal tears can disrupt knee biomechanics, causing varying degrees of symptoms and predisposing the knee to other short- and long-term sequelae, including quadriceps or hamstring inhibition, patellofemoral pain syndrome, altered gait, and osteoarthritis.
- Synonym(s): cartilage tear (common usage by patients for a meniscal tear)

EPIDEMIOLOGY

- One of the most common knee problems; annual incidence is 66/100,000 persons/y (1).
- Traumatic tears typically occur in ages 13- to 40-year-old individuals with activity-related injuries.
- Degenerative tears typically develop in patients aged >40 years.
- Vertical longitudinal tears are the most common types of tears.
- More common in males than females, with ratio between 2.5:1 and 4:1 (1)
- In athletic population, >1/3 are associated with anterior cruciate ligament (ACL) tears.

ETIOLOGY AND PATHOPHYSIOLOGY

- A meniscal tear may occur following twisting, shearing, or compressive forces from contact or noncontact mechanisms.
- Injury mechanism is typically a twisting moment through the knee in the flexed, weight-bearing position.

RISK FACTORS

- Male gender
- Abnormal mechanical axis
- Playing soccer or rugby (2)[A]
- Ligament deficiency
- Degenerative joint disease
- Discoid meniscus
- Poor quadriceps control
- Waiting >12 months between ACL tear and reconstruction surgery is a risk factor for medial meniscus tear (2)[A].

COMMONLY ASSOCIATED CONDITIONS

- ~1/3 of traumatic meniscal tears associated with ACL injury in athletes
- Tibial plateau and femoral shaft fractures

DIAGNOSIS

HISTORY

- Traumatic tears in the younger, athletic population are most frequently associated with a significant cutting/twisting injury, whereas degenerative tears in older patients usually lack identifiable trauma.
- Pain along joint line
- Pain with weight-bearing and twisting/turning of knee or squatting
- Degree of pain is variable, and patient may or may not be able to ambulate after acute injury.
- May be associated with slow onset of effusion over several hours
- Catching, locking, or clicking sensation
- Episodes of giving way
- Symptoms may wane but typically recur with resumption of activities.
- Subsequent intermittent effusions not uncommon

PHYSICAL EXAM

Exam findings suggestive of meniscal tear:

- Effusion/hemarthrosis may be a sign of meniscal, ligament, or osteochondral injury.
- Locked knee is suggestive of bucket-handle meniscal tear, ligament tear, or loose body.
- Valgus/varus instability suggestive of medial collateral ligament (MCL)/lateral collateral ligament sprain, which may have associated meniscal injury.
- Positive anterior/posterior drawer or Lachman test indicates cruciate ligament injury, which may have associated meniscal injury.
- An effusion combined with joint line tenderness is one of the most sensitive and reliable signs of a meniscal tear (3)[C].
- Positive McMurray test: palpable click and pain over joint line produced when meniscal fragment catches during test (diagnostic accuracy up to 63% when performed by skilled examiner) (4)[C]
- Positive Apley test: pain over the respective joint line with the patient prone and the knee flexed to 90 degrees, whereas the leg is internally and externally rotated under an axial load (diagnostic accuracy up to 58% when performed by skilled examiner) (4)[C]
- Positive Thessaly test: pain over the respective joint line with the patient standing on the affected leg at 5 and 20 degrees of knee flexion, followed by internal and external rotation of the leg and torso (diagnostic accuracy up to 59% when performed by skilled examiner) (4)[C]
- Atrophic quadriceps suggestive of chronic inhibition by pain or effusion
- May have decreased range of motion secondary to pain or effusion

DIFFERENTIAL DIAGNOSIS

- Knee osteoarthritis
- Synovitis
- Intra-articular loose body
- Articular cartilage defect (osteochondritis dissecans [OCD])
- Ligamentous injury, particularly ACL and/or MCL
- Patellar subluxation/dislocation
- Degenerative joint disease
- Chondromalacia patellae
- Tibial plateau fracture

DIAGNOSTIC TESTS & INTERPRETATION

- Standard weight-bearing anteroposterior/lateral/tunnel/patellar (sunrise, merchant) views to rule out other conditions such as loose body, arthritis, osteochondral defect, loose body, OCD, or fracture
- Ultrasound has some utility for superficial tears but limited ability to detect deep, internal structural abnormalities.

- Magnetic resonance imaging (MRI) useful to evaluate for concomitant structural damage when the diagnosis is in question or for operative planning
- Should be performed quickly for locking symptoms or suspicion for substantial injury; otherwise, is typically reserved for symptoms persisting >4 to 8 weeks in the otherwise healthy knee

TREATMENT

GENERAL MEASURES

- Initial treatment is rest, ice (20 minutes several times per day), compression, elevation (RICE)—and nonsteroidal anti-inflammatory drugs (NSAIDs).
- Immobilization is not recommended unless evaluating for fracture or major ligamentous injury; however, a hinged knee brace may offer support, protection, and symptom relief.
- Although infrequently required, crutches with partial weight-bearing may provide acute relief.
- Sports activity should be restricted until symptoms resolve or (if indicated) MRI is performed.
- Physical therapy to strengthen the muscles around the knee is a mainstay of current treatment.
- Further management decisions are based on patient's age, symptomatology, type of tear, and coexisting knee conditions.
- Younger patients with traumatic tears should be thoroughly evaluated and more aggressively treated.

ISSUES FOR REFERRAL

- Expedited surgical referrals should be made for:
  - Locked knee
  - Younger patients with meniscal tears (5)[C]
  - Locking symptoms, flap tears, and bucket-handle tears
  - Unstable radial tears posttraumatic especially in younger patients
  - Associated osteochondral defect, loose bodies, or fracture
  - Nonurgent referrals include tears treated nonoperatively but that continue to cause pain or disability.
- Individuals with degenerative joint disease will likely have meniscal tears, and the presence of one is not necessarily a cause for a surgical referral.

ADDITIONAL THERAPIES

- For discomfort persisting several weeks, intra-articular corticosteroid injections often provide significant relief.
- Stationary bicycle riding or a home exercise program/physical therapy addressing balance, quadriceps, and hamstring strength can reduce pain, increase range of motion, and help protect the knee from further injuries.
- Although surgery is not contraindicated, nonoperative interventions (including NSAIDs and corticosteroid injections) are appropriate initial treatment for:
  - Smaller central tears
  - Complex/degenerative tears
  - Tears in setting of degenerative joint disease

SURGERY/OTHER PROCEDURES

- Both partial meniscectomy and meniscal repair are outpatient-based procedures.
- Partial meniscectomy is frequently performed for flap and bucket-handle tears or for tears failing nonoperative treatment.
- Horizontal tears are typically degenerative tears and have a minimal chance of healing. Because they may progress to flap tears, they may be excised.
- Meniscal repair is indicated for all but the most complex tears in the pediatric population (5)[C].
- Occasionally, bucket-handle tears are amenable to repair.

ONGOING CARE

PROGNOSIS

- In the carefully chosen patient, meniscal repair is successful in up to 95% (5)[C].
- Successful repair compared to meniscectomy has a lower incidence of degenerative change and better functional scores at 10 years follow-up (6)[C].
- Total meniscectomy in previously normal knees results in significant arthrosis in 2/3 of patients by 15 years from surgery (6)[C].

COMPLICATIONS

- Injury to peroneal nerve possible with lateral meniscus repair
- Injury to infrapatellar branch of saphenous nerve possible with medial meniscus repair
- Repair could fail, resulting in repeat arthroscopy.
- Infection

REFERENCES

1. Morelli V, Braxton TM Jr. Meniscal, plica, patellar, and patellofemoral injuries of the knee: updates, controversies and advancements. *Prim Care*. 2013;40(2):357–382.
2. Snoeker BAM, Bakker EWP, Kegel CAT, et al. Risk factors for meniscal tears: a systematic review including meta-analysis. *J Orthop Sports Phys Ther*. 2013;43(6):352–367.
3. Bronstein RD, Schaffer JC. Physical examination of the knee: meniscus, cartilage, and patellofemoral conditions. *J Am Acad Orthop Surg*. 2017;25(5):365–374.
4. Blyth M, Anthony I, Francq B, et al. Diagnostic accuracy of the Thessaly test, standardised clinical history and other clinical examination tests (Apley's, McMurray's and joint line tenderness) for meniscal tears in comparison with magnetic resonance imaging diagnosis. *Health Technol Assess*. 2015;19(62):1–62.
5. Shi B, Stinson Z, Nault ML, et al. Meniscus repair in pediatric athletes. *Clin Sports Med*. 2022;41(4):749–767.
6. Lutz C, Dalmay F, Ehkirch FP, et al. Meniscectomy versus meniscal repair: 10 years radiological and clinical results in vertical lesions in stable knee. *Orthop Traumatol Surg Res*. 2015;101(Suppl 8):S327–S331.

ADDITIONAL READING

- Brelin AM, Rue JPH. Return to play following meniscus surgery. *Clin Sports Med*. 2016;35(4):669–678.
- Nguyen JC, De Smet AA, Graf BK, et al. MR imaging-based diagnosis and classification of meniscal tears. *Radiographics*. 2014;34(4):981–999.
- Persson F, Turkiewicz A, Bergkvist D, et al. The risk of symptomatic knee osteoarthritis after arthroscopic meniscus repair vs partial meniscectomy vs the general population. *Osteoarthritis Cartilage*. 2018;26(2):195–201.

CLINICAL PEARLS

- Not all meniscus tears require surgery.
- Younger patients with traumatic tears should be treated more aggressively.
- Patients with degenerative joint disease will likely have meniscal tears, and the presence of one is not necessarily a cause for a surgical referral.
- MRI is a good imaging modality for identifying tears and is more accurate and reliable than clinical assessment alone.

MENSTRUAL DISORDERS IN THE ATHLETE

Kayla Daniel, MD • Anastasia Fischer, MD, FAAFP, FACSM

BASICS

DESCRIPTION

- Menstrual dysfunction: a lack of regular menstrual periods 1 to 2 years after menarche (1):
  - Primary amenorrhea is the lack of spontaneous uterine bleeding:
    - By the age of 14 years without development of secondary sexual characteristics *or*
    - By the age of 15 years with otherwise normal development
  - Secondary amenorrhea is absence of menstruation for 3 consecutive months with previously regular menses.
  - Oligomenorrhea is when menstrual cycles occur >45 days apart (2).
  - Secondary amenorrhea and oligomenorrhea can be associated with functional hypothalamic amenorrhea.
  - Defined as chronic anovulation that is not attributable to organic causes and is often secondary to low energy availability (EA)
- Related conditions of menstrual dysfunction (3),(4):
  - Female athlete triad refers to the interrelationships among EA, menstrual function, and bone mineral density (BMD).
  - Relative energy deficiency in sport (RED-S) describes a syndrome of impairment in physiologic function, health, and athletic performance secondary to imbalance of dietary energy intake and energy expenditure:
    - Impairments in metabolic rate, menstrual function, bone health, immunity, protein synthesis, and cardiovascular health

EPIDEMIOLOGY

Prevalence

Prevalence of athlete menstrual dysfunction (5):

- High school 19–54%
- College 25–36%
- Professional 44–69%

ETIOLOGY AND PATHOPHYSIOLOGY

Functional hypothalamic amenorrhea is a low estrogen state, resulting from suppression of the hypothalamic-pituitary-ovarian axis due to energy deficit (1).

RISK FACTORS

- Misconceptions and lack of knowledge among females, caregivers, coaches, and medical providers regarding menstrual health
  - Common misconception that it is "normal" to skip a cycle or stop menstruating completely during high levels of activity (6)
- Low EA. EA is defined as energy intake minus exercise energy expenditure divided by kilograms lean body mass (LBM) (3).
  - In adult women, menstrual dysfunction presents when EA is <30 kcal/kg LBM per day.

COMMONLY ASSOCIATED CONDITIONS

- Altered BMD
- Nutritional deficiencies
- Decreased EA
- Disordered eating or eating disorders
- Psychiatric conditions (depression)
- Musculoskeletal injuries in sports

DIAGNOSIS

HISTORY

- Menstrual history:
  - Age of menarche, family history of menarche
  - Last menstrual period
  - Frequency and duration of menses
  - Longest time between menses
  - Changes in menstrual cycle with exercise
  - Previous or current use of hormonal therapy
- Diet history
- Exercise history:
  - Overtraining, history of sport-specific training
- Sexual history
- Changes in weight
- Psychosocial stressors
- History of stress fractures or sports-related injuries
- Medication use (including hormonal medications such as oral contraceptives)
- Symptoms of androgen excess, abnormal thyroid function, autoimmune and pituitary disorders:
  - Hair growth, acne
  - Temperature intolerance, palpitations, diarrhea, constipation, tremor, mood changes, dry skin
  - Headaches, visual changes, galactorrhea

PHYSICAL EXAM

- Vital signs and general appearance:
  - Height, weight, body mass index (BMI)
  - Heart rate, blood pressure, body temperature
  - Dysmorphic features such as webbed neck, short stature, low hairline
- Thyroid palpation
- Tanner stage
- Skin findings: acne, lanugo, hirsutism
- External genitalia exam:
  - Virilization, outflow tract obstruction, anomalies
- Pelvic examination:
  - Evidence of clitoromegaly, outflow tract obstruction, thin vaginal mucosa

DIFFERENTIAL DIAGNOSIS

- Hypothalamic dysfunction:
  - Functional hypothalamic amenorrhea:
    - Energy deficiency–related amenorrhea secondary to excessive exercise, weight loss, disordered eating
  - Primary gonadotropin-releasing hormone (GnRH) deficiency:
    - Congenital disorders such as Kallmann syndrome
  - Secondary/acquired GnRH deficiency:
    - Traumatic brain injury, brain tumor
- Physiologic:
  - Pregnancy
  - Hormonal contraception
  - Menopause
- Pituitary dysfunction:
  - Hyperprolactinemia
  - Prolactinoma
  - Cushing syndrome
  - Empty sella syndrome
  - Sheehan syndrome
  - Autoimmune disease
  - Medications
- Anatomic abnormality/outflow tract obstruction:
  - Congenital: müllerian agenesis, imperforate hymen, transverse vaginal septum, androgen insensitivity
  - Acquired: Asherman syndrome
- Primary ovarian insufficiency:
  - Congenital: gonadal dysgenesis, Turner syndrome
  - Acquired: ovarian neoplasm, ovarian destruction secondary to medications, radiation, autoimmune disorder
- Other endocrine gland dysfunction:
  - Thyroid dysfunction
  - Polycystic ovary syndrome (PCOS)
  - Adrenal dysfunction

DIAGNOSTIC TESTS & INTERPRETATION

- Initial labs:
  - Pregnancy test (human chorionic gonadotropin [hCG]), prolactin, thyroid-stimulating hormone (TSH)
  - If normal and workup for primary versus secondary amenorrhea is indicated, may consider other testing
- Progesterone challenge test:
  - If the patient has no menses following progesterone, confirm estrogen deficiency with estrogen challenge test.
  - Luteinizing hormone (LH), follicle-stimulating hormone (FSH) to evaluate for ovarian failure
- If evidence of hyperandrogenism and concern for PCOS, consider checking estradiol, testosterone (total and free), dehydroepiandrosterone sulfate (DHEA-S), and early morning salivary 17-hydroxyprogesterone.

- If structural abnormalities or an intrauterine device (IUD) maybe in place, pelvic ultrasound to evaluate for suspected anatomic abnormalities or polycystic ovaries
- Head magnetic resonance imaging (MRI) to look for pituitary abnormalities or space-occupying lesions in more severe cases
- Electrocardiogram (ECG) to evaluate for arrhythmia
- Electrolytes to evaluate for abnormalities from disordered eating
- Dual energy x-ray absorptiometry (DEXA) scan:
  - Indications:
    - One or more "high risk" triad factors
    - History of *Diagnostic and Statistical Manual of Mental Disorders*, 5th edition (*DSM-5*) diagnosed eating disorder
    - BMI:
      - Adults: BMI ≤17.5 kg/m^2, <85% estimated weight, or recent weight loss of 10% or more in 1 month
      - Adolescents: BMI <5% for age
    - Menarche at 16 years of age or older
    - Current or history of <6 menses >12 months
    - Two prior stress reactions/fractures, one high-risk stress reaction/fracture, or a low-energy nontraumatic fracture
    - Prior Z-score of < 2.0 (after at least 1 year from baseline DEXA)
  - Two or more "moderate risk" triad factors:
    - Current or history of disordered eating for 6 months or greater
    - BMI between 17.5 and 18.5, <90% estimated weight, or recent weight loss of 5–10% in 1 month
    - Menarche between ages 15 and 16 years
    - Current or history of 6 to 8 menses >12 months
    - One prior stress reaction/fracture
    - Prior Z-score between −1.0 and −2.0 (after at least 1-year interval from baseline DEXA) (7)[C]

TREATMENT

GENERAL MEASURES

Functional hypothalamic amenorrhea:

- Primary goal of treatment (+/− female athlete triad) is weight restoration or normalization of body weight through nutritional rehabilitation and exercise modifications with the goal of increasing EA (2),(7)[C].
- The expert panel on treatment and return to play of the female athlete concluded there is no evidence at this time to unequivocally recommend pharmacologic therapy in athletes with the female athlete triad disorders due to lack of evidence-based research in this population (7)[C].
- Combined oral or nonoral routes of contraceptive therapy create an exogenous ovarian steroid environment inducing withdrawal bleeding but do not restore spontaneous menses (5)[C].
- Combined oral contraceptive therapy is not associated with improved BMD in amenorrheic athletes (2),(7)[C].
- Transdermal estradiol cycling with oral progesterone can improve BMD in normal weight oligomenorrheic athletes over 12 months (8)[B].
- Consider pharmacologic therapy if there is a lack of response to nonpharmacologic management >1 year period and there is occurrence of a new clinically significant fracture during nonpharmacologic management (7)[C].
- Optimal calcium intake is between 1,000 and 1,300 mg/d and daily intake of 1,000 IU vitamin D for children <18 years and 600 to 2,000 IU for adults up to age 70 years; recommended that vitamin D levels be maintained between 32 and 50 ng/mL (7)[C]
- If a definitive cause of menstrual dysfunction is found, treatment targeting the disease is recommended (2)[C].

ADMISSION, INPATIENT, AND NURSING CONSIDERATIONS

Admission criteria specifically with suspected anorexia or bulimia:

- Bradycardia: heart rate <50 bpm in daytime or <45 bpm at night
- Tachycardia: >110 bpm
- Hypotension: systolic blood pressure (SBP) <90 mm Hg
- Postural tachycardia: >20 bpm differential
- Postural hypotension: >10 mm Hg differential
- Syncope
- Potassium <3.2 mmol/L
- Chloride <88 mmol/L
- QTc >430 milliseconds or evidence of arrhythmia
- Weight loss or failure to gain weight, which renders the patient at <75% of ideal body weight
- Refusal to eat or drink
- Intractable vomiting or hematemesis
- Suicide risk

REFERENCES

1. Gordon CM, Ackerman KE, Berga SL, et al. Functional hypothalamic amenorrhea: an Endocrine Society clinical practice guideline. *J Clin Endocrinol Metab*. 2017;102(5):1413–1439.
2. ACOG committee opinion no. 651: menstruation in girls and adolescents: using the menstrual cycle as a vital sign. *Obstet Gynecol*. 2015;126(6):e143–e146.
3. Nattiv A, Loucks AB, Manore MM, et al. American College of Sports Medicine position stand. The female athlete triad. *Med Sci Sports Exerc*. 2007;39(10):1867–1882.
4. Mountjoy M, Sundgot-Borgen J, Burke L, et al. The IOC consensus statement: beyond the female athlete triad—relative energy deficiency in sport (RED-S). *Br J Sports Med*. 2014;48(7):491–497.
5. Rauh MJ, Nichols JF, Barrack MT. Relationships among injury and disordered eating, menstrual dysfunction, and low bone mineral density in high school athletes: a prospective study. *J Athl Train*. 2010;45(3):243–252.
6. Armento A, VanBaak K, Seehusen CN, et al. Presence and perceptions of menstrual dysfunction and associated quality of life measures among high school female athletes. *J Athl Train*. 2021;56(10):1094–1099.
7. DeSouza MJ, Nattiv A, Joy E, et al. 2014 Female Athlete Triad Coalition consensus statement on treatment and return to play of the female athlete triad: 1st international conference held in San Francisco, California, May 2012 and 2nd International conference held in Indianapolis, Indiana, May 2013. *Br J Sports Med*. 2014;48(4):289.
8. Ackerman KE, Singhal V, Baskaran C, et al. Oestrogen replacement improves bone mineral density in oligo-amenorrhoeic athletes: a randomised clinical trial. *Br J Sports Med*. 2019;53(4):229–236.

CLINICAL PEARLS

- There is a correlation between BMD decline and number of missed menstrual cycles; loss of BMD is not fully reversible.
- Relative risk for stress fracture is 2 to 4 times greater in amenorrheic than eumenorrheic athletes.
- Indications for ordering a DEXA scan for BMD testing in a female athlete should follow the triad risk stratification guidelines.
- Treatment for menstrual dysfunction in the setting of functional hypothalamic amenorrhea should be focused on optimizing EA from a multidisciplinary team approach.
- Improving knowledge about menstrual health is essential in promoting female athlete well-being and safe participation in sports.

MERALGIA PARESTHETICA (MP)

Daniel C. Herman, MD, PhD, FAAPMR, FACSM, FISBS, CAQSM • Dayken Dawson, MD • Brandon Hassid, MD

BASICS

DESCRIPTION

- Entrapment or compression of the lateral femoral cutaneous nerve (LFCN), also known as the lateral cutaneous nerve of the thigh, typically occurring at the inguinal ligament causing anterolateral thigh pain and paresthesia
- The LFCN is a completely sensory nerve; thus, there are no motor effects.

EPIDEMIOLOGY

Incidence

- 4.3 cases per 10,000 patient-years in general population (1)
- 24.7 cases per 10,000 patient-years in those with diabetes mellitus (DM) (1)
- Males affected more commonly than females

ETIOLOGY AND PATHOPHYSIOLOGY

- Mechanical, metabolic, and iatrogenic causes
- Mechanical causes include tight garments, belts, body armor, direct trauma, and iliacus hematoma.
- Can be iatrogenic postoperatively after anterior approach for total hip arthroplasty or after lumbar spine surgery
- Infective/inflammatory conditions (2)

RISK FACTORS

- Tight garments, belts, and other items that may cause direct friction or pressure
- Weight gain: Patients with elevated body mass index (BMI) show an increased odds ratio of developing meralgia paresthetica (MP) ranging from 1.20 to 1.83 (2).

COMMONLY ASSOCIATED CONDITIONS

- DM
- Obesity
- Pregnancy

Pediatric Considerations

Children treated for osteoid osteoma of the hip may develop MP (3). MP has also been described with anterior superior iliac spine (ASIS) avulsion (3).

Pregnancy Considerations

Associated with pregnancy

DIAGNOSIS

HISTORY

- Burning, tingling, and/or numbness in anterolateral thigh
- May worsen with prolonged standing and walking and improve with sitting

PHYSICAL EXAM

- Diagnosis is often clinical.
- Overall, there is a paucity of clinically validated tests.
- Pelvic compression test—side lying with symptomatic side up. Examiner places downward pressure on pelvis for 45 seconds, considered positive if symptoms alleviated (1)[C],(4)[C]; small study with 20 patients confirmed by neurodiagnostic testing, sensitivity of 95% and a specificity of 93.3%.
- Neurodynamic testing—patient side lying with symptomatic side up and then extend and adduct hip to provoke symptoms (1)[C].
- Tinel sign—tapping over lateral inguinal ligament may cause symptoms (1)[C].

DIFFERENTIAL DIAGNOSIS

- Lumbar radiculopathy
- Lumbar stenosis
- Trochanteric bursitis

DIAGNOSTIC TESTS & INTERPRETATION

Initial Tests (lab, imaging)

- Consider pelvic x-ray to evaluate for bony tumor (1)[C].
- Nerve conduction studies may be used but are limited by body habitus because adipose can make exam difficult (1)[C]. Somatosensory evoked potentials have 81.3% sensitivity and sensory nerve conduction has 65.2% sensitivity (3)[C]. Ultrasound using LFCN cross-sectional area and comparison to the contralateral side may be helpful and easily obtainable (4)[C]. Note that there is a large amount of anatomical variation of the LFCN. A majority of cases exit as a single nerve, 1.9 cm medial to ASIS and inferior to inguinal ligament (4)[C].

Follow-Up Tests & Special Considerations

- Magnetic resonance neurography may assist in difficult causes but is not routinely used (3)[C].
- Consider appropriate imaging to evaluate for lumbar pathology.

Diagnostic Procedures/Other

- Diagnostic nerve block by landmark guidance: injection of 1% lidocaine 1 cm medial and 1 cm inferior to ASIS or at point of maximum tenderness; considered positive if immediate relief that lasts 30 minutes (2)[C],(3)[C]
- Diagnostic injection by ultrasound guidance is preferred because landmark-guided injection failure rate is as high as 60%. LFCN appears hypoechoic and swollen, with cross-sectional area >5 mm (3)[C],(5)[C].

TREATMENT

GENERAL MEASURES

- Objective evidence for treatment is weak.
- Weight loss
- Protect area
- Avoid compression activities or clothing.
- Physical therapy such as stretching exercises for the hip and abdominal core exercises

MEDICATION

First Line

Nonsteroidal anti-inflammatory drugs (NSAIDs) and/or tricyclic antidepressants or gabapentin (3)[C]

Second Line

Topical lidocaine, capsaicin, and transcutaneous electrical nerve stimulation (TENS) (1)[C],(2)[C]

ADDITIONAL THERAPIES

- Pulsed radiofrequency ablation (1)[C],(3)[C],(6)[C]
- Nerve block (1)[C],(3)[C]—small prospective study of 20 patients: 16 had relief after one injection, 4 patients had relief after two injections; however, follow-up was only for 3 months.

SURGERY/OTHER PROCEDURES

- Surgical options include neurolysis, neurolysis and transposition, or neurectomy (6)[C].
  - Success rates with neurolysis may be as low as 60% and patients may have reoccurrence (6)[C].
  - Neurectomy can provide symptom relief, but patients are likely to have permanent numbness (1)[C].
- Peripheral nerve stimulator—minimal case studies (2)[C]
- Spinal cord stimulator (2)[C]

COMPLEMENTARY & ALTERNATIVE MEDICINE

- Active release techniques (ART), mobilization of the pelvis, myofascial therapy for the abdominal musculature
- Acupuncture (3)[C]

ONGOING CARE

PROGNOSIS

According to a Cochrane data review, there are no randomized control trials (RCTs) to guide treatment or prognosis; however, some high-quality observational studies showed (5)[A]:

- 69% (20 of 29) of patients resolved spontaneously.
- 83% (130 of 157) of patients improved or resolved after perineural steroid injection.
- 88% (264 of 300) improved after surgical decompression and 94% (44 of 48) improved with neurectomy.
- 97% (99 of 102) of iatrogenic cases completely recovered.

REFERENCES

1. Cheatham SW, Kolber MJ, Salamh PA. Meralgia paresthetica: a review of the literature. *Int J Sports Phys Ther*. 2013;8(6):883–893.
2. Solomons JNT, Sagir A, Yazdi C. Meralgia paresthetica. *Curr Pain Headache Rep*. 2022;26(7):525–531.
3. Harney D, Patijn J. Meralgia paresthetica: diagnosis and management strategies. *Pain Med*. 2007;8(8):669–677.
4. Becciolini M, Pivec C, Riegler G. Ultrasound of the lateral femoral cutaneous nerve: a review of the literature and pictorial essay. *J Ultrasound Med*. 2022;41(5):1273–1284.
5. Khalil N, Nicotra A, Rakowicz W. Treatment for meralgia paraesthetica. *Cochrane Database Syst Rev*. 2012;12(12):CD004159.
6. Chakravorty A, Jaeger M. Surgical anatomy of the lateral femoral cutaneous nerve for meralgia paraesthetica: a simple technical guide for surgeons and trainees alike. *J Clin Neurosci*. 2022;101:52–56.

ADDITIONAL READING

Tagliafico A, Serafini G, Lacelli F, et al. Ultrasound-guided treatment of meralgia paresthetica (lateral femoral cutaneous neuropathy): technical description and results of treatment in 20 consecutive patients. *J Ultrasound Med*. 2011;30(10):1341–1346.

CLINICAL PEARLS

- LFCN impingement leads to sensory symptoms or paresthesias in the anterolateral thigh.
- Diagnosis is often clinical and based on history, but there is no strong evidence for current clinical examination maneuvers.
- There is great variability in nerve anatomy; and therefore, ultrasound-guided injections, rather than palpation-guided, are preferred.
- Based on a most recent Cochrane review in 2012, prognosis is good, including for those treated conservatively.

MOLLUSCUM CONTAGIOSUM

Steven K. Poon, MD, CAQSM • Kimberly G. Harmon, MD

BASICS

DESCRIPTION

Superficial pox virus skin infection

EPIDEMIOLOGY

- Prevalence 5.1–11.5% in pediatric age group
- Coinfection rate of 5–18% in HIV-positive patients (1)

ETIOLOGY AND PATHOPHYSIOLOGY

- Caused by the *Molluscipoxvirus* strain of the Poxviridae family
- Four major subtypes with molluscum contagiosum virus (MCV)-1 as the most common strain

RISK FACTORS

- Skin-to-skin contact
- Contact sports (i.e., wrestling)
- Sexual contact
- Autoinoculation
- Contaminated fomites (i.e., dirty towels) and community swimming pools

GENERAL PREVENTION

Avoid sharing used towels and sponges.

Pregnancy Considerations

Transmission to neonates can happen through skin-to-skin contact in the birth canal so treatment on active lesions should be considered prior to delivery.

DIAGNOSIS

- Characteristic rash that is usually asymptomatic but can become pruritic
- Located most frequently at the trunk, extremities, and face; can be in the perineum if sexually transmitted
- Typically, small (1 to 5 mm), smooth, pearly, flesh-colored papules with umbilication
- Can be larger in immunocompromised patients
- No associated prodrome, fever, or illness
- Not typically pigmented

HISTORY

- How long has it been there?
- Does it itch?
- Any blisters (usually more associated with herpetic lesions)?
- Do new lesions keep appearing?
- Sexually active or previous sexually transmitted disease (STD)?
- Contact sports participation?

PHYSICAL EXAM

Small, raised, 1- to 2-mm, flesh-colored (unpigmented) umbilicated lesions containing white core substance

DIFFERENTIAL DIAGNOSIS

- Atopic dermatitis
- Acne/ectopic sebaceous glands
- Warts
- Ingrown hairs
- Chicken pox
- Superficial or subepidermal cyst
- Benign skin tumor (i.e., acantholytic acanthoma)

DIAGNOSTIC TESTS & INTERPRETATION

- Diagnosis is almost always clinical.
- Polymerase chain reaction (PCR) and excision biopsy with histopathologic staining can be used for difficult diagnosis.

TREATMENT

GENERAL MEASURES

- Keep lesions covered.
- Avoid skin-to-skin contact with other individuals with lesions.
- Always use clean linens and towels.
- Acute treatment:
  - Watchful waiting for self-limited resolution with mean duration 6 to 13 months but can persist for longer
  - Mechanical removal (2),(3),(4),(5)[C]:
    - Cryotherapy
    - Curettage and deroofing
    - Pulsed dye laser therapy (less common)
  - Chemical therapy (2),(3),(4),(5)[C]:
    - Cantharidin
    - Salicylic acid gel or in combination products
    - Potassium hydroxide 5–10%
    - Podophyllotoxin
    - Retinoids
  - Immunomodulatory methods (2),(3),(4),(5)[C]:
    - Topical imiquimod
    - Oral cimetidine
    - Interferon-α for severely immunocompromised patients

Pregnancy Considerations

Some treatments such as podophyllotoxin cream is not recommended for pregnant women.

ONGOING CARE

PROGNOSIS

Most lesions are self-limiting and not associated with complications but can persist for months to years. Coexisting atopic dermatitis and immunodeficiency can lead to persistent lesions.

REFERENCES

1. Dohil MA, Lin P, Lee J, et al. The epidemiology of molluscum contagiosum in children. *J Am Acad Dermatol*. 2006;54(1):47–54.
2. Leung AKC, Barankin B, Hon KLE. Molluscum contagiosum: an update. *Recent Pat Inflamm Allergy Drug Discov*. 2017;11(1):22–31.
3. Forbat E, Al-Niaimi F, Ali FR. Molluscum contagiosum: review and update on management. *Pediatr Dermatol*. 2017;34(5):504–515.
4. Sterling J. Treatment of warts and molluscum: what does the evidence show? *Curr Opin Pediatr*. 2016;28(4):490–499.
5. Hebert AA, Bhatia N, Del Rosso JQ. Molluscum contagiosum: epidemiology, considerations, treatment options, and therapeutic gaps. *J Clin Aesthet Dermatol*. 2023;16(8 Suppl 1):S4–S11.

ADDITIONAL READING

- National Collegiate Athletic Association. Appendix C: skin infections in wrestling. *2017-18 and 2018-19 NCAA Wrestling Rules*. National Collegiate Athletic Association; 2017:96–99.
- Zinder SM, Basler RSW, Foley J, et al. National athletic trainers' association position statement: skin diseases. *J Athl Train*. 2010;45(4):411–428.

CLINICAL PEARLS

- Molluscum contagiosum can be contracted from another athlete via close contact, such as football or wrestling.
- Molluscum contagiosum is contagious, and it is spread by physical or sexual contact. Should keep them covered when participating; ideally, athletes should wait to resume contact sports for 24 to 48 hours after lesions are gone.
- Some regulatory bodies, such as the National Collegiate Athletic Association (NCAA), require that molluscum lesions are eradicated prior to any participation in contact/combat sports.

MONONUCLEOSIS

Rachel E. Chamberlain, MD, CAQSM • Christopher McGrew, MD, FACSM, CAQSM

BASICS

DESCRIPTION

- Acute viral syndrome classically, most commonly resulting from infection with the Epstein-Barr virus (EBV)
- EBV is a lymphotropic γ-herpesvirus that replicates in epithelial cells and B lymphocytes.
- Characterized by classic triad of fever, pharyngitis, and lymphadenopathy
- Synonym(s): "mono"; glandular fever

EPIDEMIOLOGY

- Peak incidence in the United States is between the ages of 15 and 19 years.
- Estimated prevalence 1–3% of adolescent/young adult population. U.S. incidence is estimated to be between 200 and 800 cases per 100,000 (1)[C].
- Evidence of infection via EBV antibody seroconversion occurs earlier in lower socioeconomic groups.
- In all populations, >90% seroconversion by the end of the 3rd decade of life, although many are not aware of having the disease
- No evidence to suggest that infectious mononucleosis (IM) is more or less prevalent in student athletes than among the general student population

ETIOLOGY AND PATHOPHYSIOLOGY

IM is caused by the EBV, which is a lymphotrophic γ-herpesvirus that replicates in epithelial cells and B lymphocytes (2)[B].

RISK FACTORS

- Transmission via passage of infected mucous membrane secretions, most commonly saliva ("the kissing disease"); incubation period typically 30 to 50 days (3)
- EBV also felt to be passed via respiratory tract secretions, blood, rectal, and potentially genital secretions, raising the possibility of sexual transmission. No aerosol transmission has been found.
- Lack of mononucleosis epidemics supports concept of low-level contagiousness.
- Relative risk of contracting EBV increased by factors negatively affecting the overall status of the immune system: baseline fatigue, overtraining, poor nutritional status

GENERAL PREVENTION

- General hand washing/hygiene measures
- Avoidance of sharing of water bottles, food, other utensils
- Proper rest/avoid overtraining
- Good nutrition
- Vaccines have been developed and tested, but none are currently approved.

COMMONLY ASSOCIATED CONDITIONS

Group A β-hemolytic streptococcal pharyngeal/tonsillar infection coexistent in up to 30% of cases

DIAGNOSIS

- IM remains a clinical diagnosis based on history, physical, and selected laboratory testing.
- Hoagland criteria are frequently cited for establishing diagnosis.
- Complete blood count (CBC) shows at least 50% lymphocytes, of which 10% are atypical (2)[B].
- Presence of fever, pharyngitis, and adenopathy
- Serologic confirmation
- Only 50% of patients with suggestive symptoms and serologic confirmation meet all of Hoagland criteria.
- The criteria are very specific but not sufficiently sensitive and may miss those acutely affected.

HISTORY

- Prodrome of malaise/fatigue followed by development of the classic triad of fever, sore throat, and enlarged lymph nodes
- Headache in many cases
- Patient often does not have known history of EBV exposure.
- Athlete may complain of poor exercise performance.
- Fatigue is often disabling, even for activities of daily living.

PHYSICAL EXAM

- Classic triad: fever, pharyngitis, and cervical lymphadenopathy (anterior and posterior), but presentation can be nonspecific (1)[B]
- Many patients manifest a prodrome of disabling fatigue/malaise.
- Pharyngitis characterized by yellow-gray tonsillar exudate and palatal edema
- Fevers of 39–40°C with evening peaks, typically for 10 to 14 days
- Abdominal pain
- Notable decline in exercise tolerance
- Fever often demonstrable
- Patient may appear fatigued and mildly to moderately ill but generally nontoxic.
- Exudative pharyngitis
- Palatal petechiae
- Periorbital edema
- Prominent anterior and posterior cervical lymphadenopathy (Lymphadenopathy may also involve axillary and inguinal regions.)
- Although splenomegaly is probably present in nearly all patients, peaking in the second and third week, physical exam for splenomegaly has poor sensitivity and specificity, and interexaminer reliability is poor.
- Overzealous abdominal exam may precipitate splenic injury in rare cases.
- With splenic rupture, may develop Kehr sign (patient supine, raise left leg, intra-abdominal blood tracks up to diaphragm, creates referred pain to left shoulder)
- Maculopapular, urticarial or petechial rash (Petechial rashes should raise suspicion for potential aplastic anemia, thrombocytopenia, or disseminated intravascular coagulation [DIC].)
- Maculopapular rash may often develop after antimicrobial administration: most commonly ampicillin or amoxicillin but has also been reported with the use of azithromycin, levofloxacin, and cephalexin.

DIFFERENTIAL DIAGNOSIS

- Primarily must be differentiated from nonspecific viral syndromes, lymphoma, leukemia, and *Streptococcus* pharyngitis.
- Concomitant *Streptococcus* infection is not uncommon.
- Many infectious agents may cause mononucleosis-like syndromes: cytomegalovirus, adenovirus, hepatitis A, human herpesvirus 6, HIV, rubella, toxoplasmosis.
- Medications causing mononucleosis-like syndromes: phenytoin, sulfa drugs

DIAGNOSTIC TESTS & INTERPRETATION

- Primary means of laboratory testing via nonspecific heterophile antibody studies (i.e., monospot qualitative agglutination slide test)
- Heterophile antibody (+) 60–70% at 1 week, 80–90% by 3 to 4 weeks (2)[B]
- Definitive diagnosis: EBV viral capsid antigen (VCA) immunoglobulin M (+) for acute infections, (−) for recent or past infections (2)[B]
- EBV VCA immunoglobulin G confirms past infection and generation of protective antibody.
- May use more specific EBV-associated antigens if necessary to determine exact phase of illness
- Classic hematologic findings include >10% atypical lymphocytes (Downey cell-activated cytotoxic suppressor [CD8] T lymphocytes), relative leukocytosis (up to 20,000), followed by mild neutropenia during week 2 of illness, mild hemolytic anemia, and mild thrombocytopenia (100,000 to 140,000/mm^3)
- Mild hepatitis (2- to 3-fold increase in liver function tests) may be seen in week 2 to 3 of illness.
- No routine imaging used for diagnosis or management of mononucleosis
- One-time imaging of the spleen for assessment of splenomegaly at the time of illness is not recommended because of the wide variability encountered in normal values (3),(4)[B].
- Contrasted abdominal computed tomography (CT) for concerns about splenic rupture (incidence of 1 to 2 per 1,000 cases of mononucleosis, often spontaneous)

TREATMENT

GENERAL MEASURES

- Care is primarily supportive/symptomatic.
- No effective treatment presently is available.
- Care should be taken to avoid splenic trauma; avoid exercise and activities with jarring movements.
- Athletes should avoid exercise for 2 weeks from onset of symptoms and be out of contact and vigorous activity for 3 to 4 weeks; shared decision-making should be used when making return to sport decisions (1),(5)[C].
- Use stool softeners to avoid increasing intra-abdominal pressure.
- Avoid alcohol and other liver toxins.

ISSUES FOR REFERRAL
Splenic rupture

ADDITIONAL THERAPIES
- Acyclovir/valacyclovir have been shown to decrease viral shedding but have no effect on the natural course of the illness, and no clinical benefit has been demonstrated (2)[B].
- Corticosteroids may be clinically indicated in cases with airway compromise, severe dysphagia, massive/painful spleen enlargement, myocarditis, or hemolytic anemia (6)[C].
- A Cochrane review evaluating the use of corticosteroids for symptom control in IM concluded that although symptoms were decreased for the first 12 hours, these benefits were lost at 2 to 4 days. Because there was no clear evidence on the effectiveness of steroids, and given the potential for adverse effects from the use of steroids, the Cochrane review recommended that corticosteroid use be avoided in uncomplicated cases (6)[A].

SURGERY/OTHER PROCEDURES
- Splenic rupture may be treated with either splenectomy or observation in selected situations (7)[A].
- Earlier return to play with splenectomy but must be weighed against risks of asplenia
- If splenectomy chosen, *Haemophilus influenzae*, pneumococcal, and meningococcal vaccination should be provided prior to splenectomy (2)[C].

COMPLEMENTARY & ALTERNATIVE MEDICINE
None

ONGOING CARE

DIET
No special recommendations other than balanced diet with adequate fluids and fiber to avoid constipation; avoid alcohol.

PROGNOSIS
- Most patients who contract IM have an uneventful clinical course with an unremarkable recovery.
- Athletes often kept out of noncontact activities for 2.5 to 3 weeks and contact activities for 3 to 4 weeks, although return to activity decision is individualized (3)[C].
- Some athletes may take as long as 3 months to return to their preillness levels of activity (8)[C].
- Adult form of mononucleosis is different from the disease in children and adolescents:
  - Most adults: pharyngitis or lymphadenopathy
  - Fever is often more prolonged.
  - Abnormal liver function more frequent
  - Lymphocytosis/presence of atypical lymphocytes less common

COMPLICATIONS
- A wide variety of complications can occur, involving virtually all organ systems:
  - Edema of Waldeyer ring, resulting in airway compromise and/or severe dysphagia
  - Splenomegaly: nearly universal in IM, so not truly a complication
  - Splenic rupture: reported in 0.1–2% of cases; most cases occur in first 3 to 4 weeks of illness; in one study, 50% nontraumatic. Splenic rupture can occur up to 8 weeks after onset of illness (5),(7),(9)[B].
  - Guillain-Barré syndrome
  - Cranial nerve palsies
  - Aseptic meningitis
  - Meningoencephalitis
  - Aplastic anemia
  - Hemolytic uremic syndrome
  - DIC
  - Jaundice
  - Acute acalculous cholecystitis
  - Myocarditis
- Conjecture that chronic fatigue syndrome may be associated with chronic EBV infection is not well supported in the literature.
- Immunocompromised (e.g., HIV, transplant patients, etc.): Lymphoma and other lymphoproliferative disorders are potential severe complications.

REFERENCES

1. Putukian M, McGrew CA, Benjamin HJ, et al. American Medical Society of Sports Medicine Position Statement: mononucleosis and athletic participation. *Clin J Sport Med.* 2023;33(4):359–367.
2. Dunmire SK, Verghese PS, Balfour HH Jr. Primary Epstein-Barr virus infection. *J Clin Virol.* 2018;102:84–92.
3. Putukian M, O'Connor FG, Stricker P, et al. Mononucleosis and athletic participation: an evidence-based subject review. *Clin J Sport Med.* 2008;18(4):309–315.
4. Hosey RG, Mattacola CG, Kriss V, et al. Ultrasound assessment of spleen size in collegiate athletes. *Br J Sports Med.* 2006;40(3):251–254.
5. Sylvester JE, Buchanan BK, Paradise SL, et al. Association of splenic rupture and infectious mononucleosis: a retrospective analysis and review of return-to-play recommendations. *Sports Health.* 2019;11(6):543–549.
6. Candy B, Hotopf M. Steroids for symptom control in infectious mononucleosis. *Cochrane Database Syst Rev.* 2006;(3):CD004402.
7. Bartlett A, Williams R, Hilton M. Splenic rupture in infectious mononucleosis: a systematic review of published case reports. *Injury.* 2016;47(3):531–538.
8. Becker JA, Smith J. Return to play after infectious mononucleosis. *Sports Health.* 2014;6(3):232–238.
9. Bartlett A, Williams R, Hilton M. Splenic rupture in infectious mononucleosis: a systematic review of published case reports. *Injury.* 2016;47(3):531–538.

ADDITIONAL READING

Shephard R. Exercise and the athlete with infectious mononucleosis. *Clin J Sport Med.* 2017;27(2):168–178.

CLINICAL PEARLS
- In most cases, athletes will not feel well enough to participate in activity for several weeks.
- In addition, although the risk for splenic rupture is extremely low, given that most of these occur within the first 3 weeks of illness, independent of spleen size, it is generally felt that it is safe to resume light activity 3 weeks from the onset of symptoms, as long as the athlete is afebrile, has a good energy level, and does not have any significant associated abnormalities. The risk of splenic rupture likely diminishes as more time progresses; therefore, delaying return to play should be considered if clinical features, lack of athlete readiness, and/or associated complications are present. Treatment must, therefore, be individualized to account for all of these issues (1),(5),(8),(9)[C].
- The appropriate time for safe return to contact play is unclear, although, given the risk for splenic rupture, a time frame of at least 3 weeks commonly is recommended. Return can occur only after the athlete has no remaining clinical symptoms, is afebrile, and has a normal energy level. The risk for splenic rupture likely decreases as more time passes, allowing for individualized return-to-play decisions, depending on the athlete, sport, and other factors (1),(8)[C].
- It is unclear what role exercise has on the natural history of IM disease. Although many athletes can self-regulate on return to ad lib activity if afebrile, it would appear that premature return to heavy exertion might prolong the duration of symptoms, most notably fatigue, and also be associated with a decrease in performance (1),(3)[C].
- Fortunately, because of the nature of transmission, epidemics of mononucleosis are uncommon. Care should be taken to avoid shared water bottles, utensils, and so forth. Teams that travel extensively together have greater potential contacts for transmission. As the incubation period is lengthy, identifying index cases is difficult. It is not practical or necessary to exclude infected teammates if appropriate measures are taken to avoid spread of the virus. Appropriate rest, proper nutrition, and avoiding overtraining may reduce susceptibility to IM.

MOREL LAVALLEE LESION

Arthur Davis Daniel, MD, CAQSM ▪ Kenneth S. Taylor, MD, FAAFP, CAQSM

BASICS

DESCRIPTION
- Closed soft tissue degloving injury
- Usually associated with high energy trauma or crush injuries
- Often missed on initial assessment potentially leading to difficulty with management and long-term morbidity

EPIDEMIOLOGY
- Not frequently seen in practice
- Prevalence of 8.2% has been noted with acetabular fractures (1).
- Male predominance at 2:1 male-to-female ratio, likely related to male predominance in polytrauma (1),(2)

ETIOLOGY AND PATHOPHYSIOLOGY
- Commonly with high energy trauma or crush injuries. 25% of patients with Morel Lavelle lesion (MLL) were involved in road traffic accidents (3).
- A subset of injuries has been described following a direct blow to the knee (1).
- Commonly associated with underlying fractures, such as acetabulum and pelvis.
- Areas most affected have mobile overlying skin and a tough underlying fascia (1).
- Thigh, hip, and pelvis are the most commonly associated locations. The greater trochanter represents >60% of cases (1).
- Characterized by separation of hypodermis from the underlying fascia due to a shearing force. This shearing force leads to disruption of lymphatic vessels, transaponeurotic capillaries, and locules of subdermal fat.
- Blood reabsorbed from the cavity overtime, leaving a hemosiderin layer. This layer causes inflammation in peripheral tissues forming a fibrous capsule, resulting in a chronic MLL (2).

DIAGNOSIS

HISTORY AND PHYSICAL EXAM
- Presents as painful, fluctuant swelling
- An important clinical feature is the presence of fluctuance and compression within the lesion.
- May be associated with decreased skin sensation and increased skin mobility
- May present within hours of injury, but up to 33% may appear days later (1)

DIFFERENTIAL DIAGNOSIS
- Abscess
- Bursitis
- Hematoma
- Fat necrosis
- Neoplasms

DIAGNOSTIC TESTS & INTERPRETATION
- Both magnetic resonance imaging (MRI) and ultrasound have been identified as imaging modalities of choice for MLL.
- Ultrasound is rapid, readily available, and provides dynamic evaluation of suspicious lesions.
- MRI provides high contrast resolution, multiplanar acquisition and greater anatomic detail.
- Role of ultrasound:
  - The majority of MLLs will demonstrate heterogeneous, hypoechoic appearance with internal septations and/or hyperechoic fat globules.
  - MLLs are compressible with the transducer and demonstrate no flow on color doppler.
  - 29% may be anechoic.
  - 38% may be homogeneous (3).
- Some studies cite ultrasound as the imaging modality of choice (4).

Test Interpretation
MRI classification of MLL (3),(4):
- Type I: seroma; hypointense on T1; hyperintense on T2
- Type II: subacute hematoma; hyperintense on both T1 and T2
- Type III: chronic organizing hematoma; hypointense on T1; hypointense/isointense on T2 with capsular formation
- Type IV: closed laceration; hypointense T1; hyperintense T2 with absence of capsule
- Type V: pseudonodular; variable T1 and T2 intensity
- Type VI: superimposed infection; thick enhancing capsule that can be associated with a sinus tract

TREATMENT

GENERAL MEASURES
- There are currently no established guidelines on management of MLL (1).
- Management options include supportive care with compression, aspiration, surgical débridement, or sclerodesis.
- Treatment is based on size and stage of the lesion.
- Compression bandage is only recommended in lesions with <50 mL of fluid.
- Aspiration alone has a high rate of recurrence if volume is >50 mL.
- Sclerodesis has shown an efficacy of 95.7% in acute or chronic lesions measuring up to 400 mL.

MEDICATION

First Line
- For small, acute lesions include compression, NSAIDs, physical therapy (3)
- Percutaneous drainage can be used for acute, larger lesions; may be used with sclerotherapy for chronic lesions (3)
- Open débridement is first-line therapy for acute lesions with underlying open fractures as well as chronic lesions with evidence of infections or tissue necrosis (3).

ADDITIONAL THERAPIES

- Sclerodesis
  - Efficacious in lesions up to 700 mL (2)
  - Sclerosing agents include doxycycline, erythromycin, bleomycin, vancomycin, absolute ethanol, tetracycline, and talc (2).
  - Majority of data is derived from use of doxycycline (2).
- Doxycycline sclerodesis procedure
  - Lesion first aspirated to evacuate the cavity; 100 mg of doxycycline reconstituted in 5 mL of sterile normal saline (20 mg/mL) is injected into the MLL; compressive bandage applied after procedure (5)

SURGERY/OTHER PROCEDURES

Chronic and large volume lesions are best treated with surgical débridement.

ONGOING CARE

PROGNOSIS

- Prognosis varies based on size and chronicity of lesions.
- Better prognosis with acute, smaller lesions

COMPLICATIONS

Complications can result from improper or untimely diagnosis and management (6). Complications include:

- Infected seroma
- Chronic cosmetic deformities
- Capsule formation
- Skin necrosis

REFERENCES

1. Agrawal U, Tiwari V. *Morel Lavallée Lesion*. StatPearls Publishing; 2023. Accessed August 14, 2025. https://www.ncbi.nlm.nih.gov/books/NBK574532/
2. Singh R, Rymer B, Youssef B, et al. The Morel-Lavallée lesion and its management: a review of the literature. *J Orthop*. 2018;15(4):917–921.
3. Diviti S, Gupta N, Hooda K, et al. Morel-Lavallée lesions—review of pathophysiology, clinical findings, imaging findings, and management. *J Clin Diagn Res*. 2017;11(4):TE01–TE04.
4. De Coninck T, Vanhoenacker F, Verstraete K. Imaging features of Morel-Lavallée lesions. *J Belg Soc Radiol*. 2017;101(Suppl 2):15.
5. Tejwani SG, Cohen SB, Bradley JP. Management of Morel-Lavallée lesion of the knee: twenty-seven cases in the national football league. *Am J Sports Med*. 2007;35(7):1162–1167.
6. Scolaro JA, Chao T, Zamorano DP. The Morel-Lavallée lesion: diagnosis and management. *J Am Acad Orthop Surg*. 2016;24(10):667–672.

ADDITIONAL READING

Neal C, Jacobson JA, Brandon C, et al. Sonography of Morel-Lavallée lesions. *J Ultrasound Med*. 2008;27(7):1077–1081.

CLINICAL PEARLS

- Closed traumatic soft tissue degloving injury due to a shearing force
- Most often in the peritrochanteric region
- Diagnosis requires a high index of suspicion and often missed at initial evaluation.
- Treatment is based on size of the lesion.
- Complications are a result of delayed or inaccurate diagnosis.

MYOFASCIAL PAIN AND TRIGGER POINTS

Navid Mahooti, MD, MPH, CAQSM

BASICS

DESCRIPTION

- Travell defined a myofascial trigger point (TrP) as "a hyperirritable spot in skeletal muscle that is associated with a hypersensitive palpable nodule in a taut band. The spot is painful on compression and can give rise to characteristic referred pain, referred tenderness, motor dysfunction, and autonomic phenomena."
- TrPs are the hallmark feature of myofascial pain (MP).
- The terms "trigger point," "tender point," and "acupuncture point" describe different entities that likely have overlapping features and often co-exist.
- *MP "syndrome"* implies the presence of widespread TrPs and/or unknown primary etiology.
- MP should not be conflated with fibromyalgia, chronic pain syndrome, polymyalgia, polyarthralgia, myositis.
- Myofascial TrP pain theory has been questioned by critics who point out various knowledge gaps.

EPIDEMIOLOGY

For adults presenting with pain, prevalence ranges from 30% to 85%. Lifetime prevalence is virtually 100%.

ETIOLOGY AND PATHOPHYSIOLOGY

Multifactorial development: biomechanical overload/overuse, structural, postural, posttraumatic, metabolic, and/or other abnormalities. No universally accepted definitions or diagnostic criteria. *Two basic pathophysiologic theories:*

- **Local/regional dysfunction: theories**
  - Simons' "integrated hypothesis": elevations of acetylcholine (ACh) at motor endplate sets off a cascade of events/positive feedback loop resulting in continued release of ACh which eventually leads to the release of myokines, inflammatory cytokines, and neurotransmitters
  - "Cinderella Hypothesis" by Hägg in 1991 posits that (mechanical overload) of muscle causes persistent, sustained activation of smaller type I (not type II) muscle fibers (i.e., "always working," like Cinderella).
  - Neuromuscular junction (NMJ) dysfunction: Active TrPs display miniature endplate potentials (MEPPs) and spontaneous electrical activity on electromyography.
  - Peripheral nerve compression (and neurogenic inflammation) → excess ACh
  - "Myofascial unit" (Stecco, 2002) places greater emphasis on the role of fascia to integrate the anatomical and functional components of movement.
    - Deep and superficial layers of musculoskeletal (MSK) fascia are highly organized: typed, identified, and described according to structure, function, and location.
    - Fascia plays important role in stability and mobility.
    - Deep fascia subdivided: epimysial or aponeurotic
      - Richly innervated: plays a role in proprioception and referred pain
      - Abundant in hyaluronate: facilitates smooth movements between fascial planes
    - Stecco distinguishes between a dermatome (exteroception) and fasciatome (proprioception).
    - Wang showed that ultrasound-guided injections of 0.5-mL saline into muscle and/or superficial and/or deep fascial planes overlying TrPs improved pain symptoms (implicates fascia alone in some cases).
- Central nervous system (CNS) dysfunction: theories
  - TrPs likely initiate and contribute to the persistence of central sensitization (CS), but TrPs do not cause CS.
  - Neurogenic inflammation, CS, and limbic system dysfunction all likely play a role in the initiation, amplification, and perpetuation of MP.

RISK FACTORS

Numerous: underlying structural abnormality (e.g., leg length discrepancy), biomechanical factors, postural, overuse, nerve entrapment, postsurgical, posttraumatic, nerve entrapment, ergonomics, stress, deconditioned muscle, fatigue, poor sleep, inactivity, prolonged sitting, infections, metabolic/hormonal disorders, and nutritional deficiencies

GENERAL PREVENTION

- Address and/or correct risk factors is most important.
- Regular exercise; customize dose and type.
- Optimize/improve core strength and flexibility.
- Optimize warm-up and cool-down routines; incorporate manual therapies/foam rolling.

COMMONLY ASSOCIATED CONDITIONS

- Virtually every traditional orthopedic diagnosis (Dx) has a TrP correlate that mimics typical symptoms; the temporal relationship between the two is unknown.
- MP is associated with certain nutritional deficiencies (e.g., iron, vitamin D and vitamin B_{12}, magnesium [Mg], selenium, zinc); gluten sensitivity; metabolic, visceral, endocrine (hypothyroid), infectious (parasitic infestation, recurrent vaginal yeast infections), and psychological conditions
- TrPs are prevalent across a wide range of MSK disorders and associated conditions, which further complicates Dx and treatment (Tx).

DIAGNOSIS

Dx is clinical, often an iterative process.

- The majority of patients who present with MSK problems have regional TrPs.
- Clinicians must determine whether the TrP is the *cause* of the presenting problem, or the *result* of it.
- Therapeutic needling (TN) techniques can serve as a diagnostic/therapeutic tool and help elucidate cause/effect relationships.

HISTORY

- Patients report regional symptoms, typically unilateral, that often resemble traditional orthopedic diagnoses.
- Descriptions may raise concern for a neurologic problem, resulting in an extensive, fruitless workup.
- Most common symptoms are pain and tightness.
- Other symptoms include instability, weakness, heaviness, burning, numbness, paresthesias, pruritus, imbalance, dysfunction, and vague descriptions.
- Patients may present asymptomatic (latent TrP) and have a pain-free, normal exam.
- Descriptions of symptoms may be nonspecific, migratory, temporally dependent, and even confusing to the clinician.
- Symptom onset can be acute (with or without injury/mechanism), subacute (can begin hours, days, or weeks after an inciting event), or insidious.
- Severity ranges from mild to excruciating, frequency from intermittent to persistent.
- Manual therapies (massage, foam rolling, percussive devices) and stretching often provide temporary relief.
- Patients with unrecognized MP often visit multiple health professionals and pursue numerous diagnostic tests and Txs, with no firm Dx.
- Patients with chronic, undiagnosed (or properly diagnosed but ineffectively treated) TrPs may be labeled with psychiatric diagnoses, fibromyalgia, etc.

PHYSICAL EXAM

- Palpation is the hallmark diagnostic tool: Clinicians must approach palpation systematically and meticulously to assess tissue tenderness, texture, asymmetries, restrictions, and reproduction of symptoms.
- Familiarity with TrP referral patterns aids in identification.
- 2018 Delphi Study concluded
  - *Active TrPs* must exhibit two of the following three features: (i) taut band, (ii) hypersensitive spot, (iii) referred pain upon palpation.
  - *Latent TrPs* are tender and associated with decreased range of motion; do not cause spontaneous pain (1)[C].

DIFFERENTIAL DIAGNOSIS

MP should be included on the differential Dx of every pain presentation; no body part is spared. Common TrP referral patterns are summarized below. Bold terms refer to the **painful area/traditional Dx** and arrow (→) points to the likely culprit muscle/myofascial complex.

- **Cervical radiculopathy** → cervical musculature (upper trap, levator, scalenes) infraspinatus, pectoralis muscles
- **Shoulder pain** → deltoid, rotator cuff *muscles*, pectorals, cervical muscles (trapezius, levator, rotator cuff muscles, latissimus dorsi)
- **Lateral/medial epicondylosis** → common extensors, supinator, brachioradialis, triceps, common flexors
- **Hand/wrist (carpal tunnel, ulnar neuropathy, general pain)** → dorsal or volar forearm
- **Costochondritis** → pectorals
- **Low back** → gluteals, vastus lateralis (VL), quadratus lumborum (QL), paraspinals, high flexors, lower trapezius
- **Buttocks, greater trochanteric pain (piriformis syndrome, "sciatica," sacroiliac dysfunction)** → gluteals, VL, hamstrings, tensor fascia lata (TFL), piriformis/abductors
- **Hip osteoarthritis**: adductors, quads, glutes
- **Meralgia paresthetica** → quadriceps (VL, vastus intermedius [VI], rectus femoris [RF])
- **Knee pain** → VL, vastus medialis obliquus (VMO), RF adductors, gastrocsoleus (GS), hamstrings
- **Lower leg pain** (chronic calf pain, shin splints, restless leg syndrome) → GS, lower leg muscles, VL
- **Plantar heel/arch pain, Achilles** → medial > lateral calf

DIAGNOSTIC TESTS & INTERPRETATION

No reliable diagnostic tests available. Promising emergent imaging modalities include higher resolution ultrasonography, ultrasound vibration elastography, magnetic resonance imaging (MRI) elastography, diffusion tensor imaging, and infrared thermography.

TREATMENT

GENERAL MEASURES

- Interventions and techniques that successfully release TrPs often achieve significant symptomatic relief of variable duration.
- Patients with significant short-term relief may schedule frequent visits and request (or insist upon) additional Txs.

- **Pitfall**: Clinicians' desire to relieve their patients' symptoms are at risk for:
  - Chasing TrPs with procedural interventions
  - Neglecting proper rehabilitation/physical therapy (PT)
  - Inadequate workup leading to delayed Dx/definitive Tx
- **To minimize risk of this pitfall**, the following comprehensive approach is suggested:
  - Identify and address risk factors/root causes (when practical/possible).
  - Select the most appropriate approach based on patient preferences/resources.
  - Patient education, maintenance Txs, home exercise program (HEP), addressing root causes
- Regional TrPs should be treated in the context of broader contributing factors. Most presentations are multifactorial and may require first- and second-line Txs, including image-guided procedures when appropriate.

MEDICATION

First Line

TN techniques and manual therapies have long been considered the most effective, evidence-based Txs for myofascial TrP.

- Mechanism of action of TN is unclear (anatomic/mechanical, physiological/biochemical, improved local blood flow and oxygenation, clearance of nociceptive substances are all potentially involved) (2)[A].
- TN generally not a stand-alone Tx. PT/HEP recommended as part of a comprehensive Tx plan.
- No universally accepted "best practice" regarding TN technique variables (needle length, bore, filiform vs. hypodermic, wet vs. dry) or which PT approach or modality is superior (active release, muscle energy, cupping. . .)
- TrP injections outperform dry needling (DN) (3)[A].
- Intramuscular electrical stimulation combined with DN no better than DN alone (4)[B]
- Patients with neck pain tend to feel better faster when DN is combined with standard PT versus standard PT alone, but no differences observed in mid to long term (5)[A].
- Multimodal, iterative Tx plan is often necessary, especially in chronic, complex problems: a series of TN Txs coupled with manual/PT, and other interventions to address associated risk factors/root causes.
- For patients who refuse PT (or previously did not respond), experienced clinicians may empirically treat with TN, provide guidance on home management strategies, and monitor response before prescribing formal PT and/or pursuing further workup.
- Observation and precise documentation of the patient's index symptoms, aggravators, and immediate response to TN helps identify culprit TrPs and informs both future Txs and/or additional workup.
- Assuming culprit TrPs are identified and needled properly:
  - If symptoms improve and return to baseline shortly after Txs, suggests the TrP is the *effect* of an underlying problem → further workup prudent
  - Significant, sustained, incremental improvement suggests a primary TrP etiology.
- Effective needling typically elicits local twitch responses (LTR) and immediate therapeutic benefit (2)[A].
- LTR may not be essential as some patients without LTR note benefit, and some patients with LTR note no benefit.
- If LTR is not elicited and no therapeutic benefit, suggests suboptimal palpation/needling technique, or misdiagnosis
- 5 to 15+ LTRs is typical per region treated; upward of 30+ is not unusual.
- Postprocedural discomfort is not uncommon.
  - Counsel: "It may get worse before it gets better."
  - Probably associated with needling technique, and number of TrPs treated/needle passes/LTRs
  - Although the role of an injectate (lidocaine, D5W) appears to have some benefit (decreased postprocedural pain, perhaps a therapeutic effect), ***corticosteroids have not been shown to improve outcomes, may cause harm, and are not recommended*** (6)[A].
  - Tx of postprocedural pain: ice, analgesics, and stretching, followed by manual therapies and PT
- Clinicians who skillfully perform TN often observe immediate resolution of symptoms in patients presenting with traditional orthopedic diagnoses or observe that TN outperforms standard interventions (e.g., steroid injection for knee osteoarthritis [OA] or lateral elbow pain). Possible explanations include:
  - Latent TrPs, which are subclinical/asymptomatic and may be present for an indefinite period → chronic asymmetric loads on bones, joints, tendons, and nerves → biomechanically inefficient movement patterns → short- and long-term clinical consequences:
    - Short term: development of persistent pain and tightness, increased risk of strains and injuries, unhelpful or even inappropriate Txs that focus on traditional orthopedic diagnoses
    - Long term: development of chronic conditions: tendinopathies, OA, nerve entrapments, etc.
  - Root causes are not always clearly identifiable.
  - Temporal, cause-and-effect relationship between TrPs and their purported root causes is not always straightforward.
  - Diagnostic/therapeutic injections can help tease it out.

Second Line

- Extracorporeal shock wave therapy (ESWT) is an emerging, promising modality for a variety of MSK conditions, including MP
  - Commonly used in Europe and Asia to treat various MSK problems and MP
  - Growing in popularity in the United States; however, not covered by insurance and not been shown to outperform "first-line" Txs
- Botulinum toxin: not consistently shown to outperform TN; insurance coverage variable
- Cupping: superior to no Tx, inferior to above
- Kinesio taping: temporary relief of cervical MP
- Weak evidence: common over the counter remedies (salves, balms, analgesics) and prescription medications (TCAs, muscle relaxants, benzodiazepines, opioids)

ONGOING CARE

PATIENT EDUCATION

- *Trigger Point Therapy Workbook* by Clair Davies
- National Association of Myofascial Physical Therapists (https://www.myofascialtherapy.org/)

PROGNOSIS

- Most cases improve with first-line Txs.
- If not responsive: broaden differential Dx and workup, consider regional diagnostic/therapeutic injections, optimize and/or investigate adherence with HEP/PT/manual therapy program, improve TN technique, consider second-line Tx options.

COMPLICATIONS

- TN techniques are generally safe but do carry risk: Vasovagal symptoms, postprocedural pain and bruising are not uncommon. Pneumothorax, cardiac tamponade, spinal epidural hematoma, abdominal visceral injury, as well nerve injuries have been reported.
- Anticoagulation: relative contraindication, very low risk of serious bleeding

REFERENCES

1. Fernández-de-Las-Peñas C, Dommerholt J. International consensus on diagnostic criteria and clinical considerations of myofascial trigger points: a Delphi study. *Pain Med*. 2018;19(1):142–150.
2. Kietrys DM, Palombaro KM, Azzaretto E, et al. Effectiveness of dry needling for upper-quarter myofascial pain: a systematic review and meta-analysis. *J Orthop Sports Phys Ther*. 2013;43(9):620–634.
3. Navarro-Santana MJ, Sanchez-Infante J, Gómez-Chiguano GF, et al. Dry needling versus trigger point injection for neck pain symptoms associated with myofascial trigger points: a systematic review and meta-analysis. *Pain Med*. 2022;23(3):515–525.
4. Brennan K, Elifritz KM, Comire MM, et al. Rate and maintenance of improvement of myofascial pain with dry needling alone vs. dry needling with intramuscular electrical stimulation: a randomized controlled trial. *J Man Manip Ther*. 2021;29(4):216–226.
5. Fernández-De-Las-Peñas C, Plaza-Manzano G, Sanchez-Infante J, et al. Is dry needling effective when combined with other therapies for myofascial trigger points associated with neck pain symptoms? A systematic review and meta-analysis. *Pain Res Manag*. 2021;2021:8836427.
6. Benzon HT, Elmofty D, Shankar H, et al. Use of corticosteroids for adult chronic pain interventions: sympathetic and peripheral nerve blocks, trigger point injections—guidelines from the American Society of Regional Anesthesia and Pain Medicine, the American Academy of Pain Medicine, the American Society of Interventional Pain Physicians, the International Pain and Spine Intervention Society, and the North American Spine Soc. *Reg Anesth Pain Med*. Published online March 12, 2025. doi:10.1136/rapm-2024-105593

ADDITIONAL READING

- Donnelly J, Fernández-de-Las-Peñas C, Finnegan M, et al. *Travell, Simons & Simons' Myofascial Pain and Dysfunction*. Lippincott Williams & Wilkins; 2019.
- Myers T. *Anatomy Trains*. Elsevier; 2020.
- PainScience.com: https://www.painscience.com/tutorials/trigger-points.php
- Stecco A, Giordani F, Fede C, et al. From Muscle to the myofascial unit: current evidence and future perspectives. *Int J Mol Sci*. 2023;24(5):4527.
- Stecco C, Pirri C, Fede C, et al. Dermatome and fasciatome. *Clin Anat*. 2019;32(7):896–902.
- Wang T, Vahdatinia R, Humbert S, et al. Myofascial injection using fascial layer-specific hydromanipulation technique (FLuSH) and the delineation of multifactorial myofascial pain. *Medicina (Kaunas)*. 2020;56(12):717.

CLINICAL PEARLS

- A common problem that mimics traditional MSK conditions and should be on the differential of every pain presentation
- Understanding the role of fascia and referred pain is essential to avoid misattribution/improper Txs.
- TN techniques largely considered first-line Tx, typically coupled with manual therapies and PT/rehabilitation exercises.
- Clinicians must seek to identify and address underlying risk factors/root causes.
- ESWT is growing in favor; access/costs are the challenges.

MYOSITIS OSSIFICANS

Alec Gabriel Contag, MD • Brianna Martinez, MD • Kenneth S. Taylor, MD, FAAFP, CAQSM

BASICS

DESCRIPTION

- Myositis ossificans (MO) is a localized, nonneoplastic, self-limiting heterotopic ossification that develops primarily in muscle from single or repetitive trauma as a result of aberrant tissue repair mechanisms (1),(2).
- Any extra skeletal soft tissue can be affected including striated muscle, subcutaneous fat, tendons, ligaments, nerves, aponeurosis, and fascia (1),(3),(4),(5).
- Horseback riders, weapon specialists in the military can present with MO due to repetitive trauma to large muscle groups (1).
- Anterior and proximal muscle groups of the thigh and arm are most frequently affected but may occur at any site or soft tissue (1).
- MO has three distinct phases (early, intermediate, and mature) based on clinical presentation, degree of calcification, and time from suspected or confirmed trauma (1),(3),(5).
- Average duration of symptoms can be weeks to months depending on size and stage of lesion.
- Synonym(s): MO traumatica (MOT), MO circumscripta, localized MO, posttraumatic myositis ossificans (PTMO), rider's bone, shooter's bone

EPIDEMIOLOGY

- MO is an acquired condition after injury and represents 60–75% of all MO (3).
- MO most frequently occurs in men in the 2nd or 3rd decade of life from a sport-related injury (2),(3),(4).
- This may be reflective of sport participation differences rather than genotypic or phenotypic differences in sex characteristics (1),(2).
- Vastus lateralis and brachialis are most affected, with higher proclivity to anterior and proximal structures than posterior or distal ones (4).
- Highest prevalence following a quadriceps muscle contusion
- Incidence increases with severity of injury.
- Is a rare finding in children (5)

ETIOLOGY AND PATHOPHYSIOLOGY

- No clear pathogenesis established
- It is postulated that after a muscle is crushed or torn, an inflammatory cascade recruits an influx of macrophages into the necrotic tissue. A prolonged macrophage invasion may lead to inappropriate differentiation and stimulation of mesenchymal cells into osteoblastic stem cells under anoxic conditions.
- A lesion matures over 3 to 6 months and forms an eggshell-like calcification on imaging.

RISK FACTORS

- Contact sports
- Aggressive physical therapy (PT) at onset of injury
- Reduced range of motion (ROM) of injured muscle
- Previous muscle injury
- Delay in treatment >3 days
- Adjacent joint effusion

GENERAL PREVENTION

- Minimize hemorrhage within the first 48 hours with rest, ice, compression, and elevation.
- Avoid aggressive PT within the first 48 hours of injury.
- Nonsteroidal anti-inflammatory drugs (NSAIDs) like indomethacin, if used within the 5 days post injury, may prevent heterotopic bone formation.

COMMONLY ASSOCIATED CONDITIONS

MO is a complication seen in 1 of 5 total hip arthroplasties and may occur in the joint capsule, adjacent tendon, ligament, or fascia. Given its relative rarity in children and the traumatic mechanism by which MO is formed, battered child syndrome is also associated with this condition in pediatric settings.

DIAGNOSIS

HISTORY

- Muscle contusion or strain becomes unresponsive to conservative therapy within the first 2 weeks.
- Symptoms intensify 2 to 3 weeks after trauma.
- Patient reports a rapidly growing, painful mass at the site of injury (3).
- Injured muscle becomes indurated and ROM progressively declines.
- Loss of ROM is seen in children (5).
- Night pain is often present.
- Symptoms slowly abate weeks to months later as the lesion matures (1).

PHYSICAL EXAM

- Initially may present with tenderness over palpable swelling or doughy, circumscribed mass at 1 to 2 weeks
- Persistent tenderness to palpation with local edema that fails to resolve on repeat exam
- Reduced ROM on exam that worsens 2 to 3 weeks after injury

DIFFERENTIAL DIAGNOSIS

- Early/intermediate conditions (1),(2),(3),(4),(5):
  - Muscle contusion
  - Tendon tear
  - Fracture
  - Compartment syndrome
  - Abscess
  - Rhabdomyolysis
  - Periosteal reaction
- Late/mature conditions:
  - Chronic avulsion injury
- Neoplasms:
  - Osteosarcoma, periosteal osteosarcoma, lymphoma, synovial sarcoma, bizarre periosteal osteochondromatous

DIAGNOSTIC TESTS & INTERPRETATION

Initial Tests (lab, imaging)

- There are no validated lab tests for MO (1)[C].
- Erythrocyte sedimentation rate (ESR), C-reactive protein (CRP), and alkaline phosphatase may be elevated but are nonspecific.
- Creatine phosphokinase (CPK) may be a future predictor of lesion development and severity (1)[C],(3)[C].
- Ultrasound (US): low cost, low radiation modality for early detection; can detect lesions before more advanced imaging; lesions have three zones: outer hypoechoic zone depicting traumatic or inflammatory fluid around the lesion, a middle hyperechoic zone representing the calcific rim, and an inner/central hypoechoic zone depicting fibroblastic stroma (1)[C],(4)[C].
- X-ray (XR): catches calcifications starting at 4 weeks but is poorly able to differentiate between neoplastic differentials (1)[C]; mature MO lesions are well-circumscribed, peripherally calcified masses, with a radiolucent center that has an eggshell-like appearance (2)[C]. Mature MO runs parallel to the shaft on XR and CT scan (1)[C].
- Computed tomography (CT) scan: Once MO is suspected clinically or on US, CT scan is the initial imaging of choice (1)[C]. CT scan best delineates the zonal pattern of calcification classic to MO (1)[C]. CT scan best differentiates between neoplastic pathologies (1)[C]. CT scan is most specific for calcifications (3)[C].
- Magnetic resonance imaging (MRI): Normally the lead study for soft tissue injuries, it is less able to observe calcification processes compared to XR or CT scan. MRI can detect swelling around calcification, which can help differentiate the lesion from sarcoma (4)[C].

Follow-Up Tests & Special Considerations

- Bone scan is not recommended (1)[C].
- A biopsy may be warranted for indeterminate lesions (1)[C].

TREATMENT

GENERAL MEASURES

- MO is often a self-limiting condition, in which clinical and radiologic follow-up will suffice without pharmacologic or surgical intervention (1)[C],(2)[C],(4)[C],(5)[A].
- Key is preventing hematoma formation in the early stages while maintaining function (1)[C],(2)[C],(5)[A].
- Rest, ice, compression, and elevation are universally recommended in the acute phase (1)[C],(6)[A].
- Aggressive PT should be avoided in the early stage, and recovery should focus on nonpainful ROM in first 2 to 3 days (1)[C],(6)[A].
- PT for recovery for the primary injured tissue is appropriate after an early period of rest and gentle ROM, but no trial data exists to support a specific rehabilitation protocol for MO (6)[A].

MEDICATION

- Most low-grade MO does not require NSAIDs.
- Current data on NSAIDs use is primarily focused on postoperative rather than traumatic MO, in which indomethacin is the most commonly used drug (2)[C].
- Current literature is divided on the efficacy of NSAIDs versus placebo for specific sites of injury.
- Given its low cost, a trial of NSAIDs to promote early symptomatic treatment and ROM is not unreasonable.

ADDITIONAL THERAPIES

- Preventive therapies:
  - Quad stretching has been proposed to dissipate contusions and reduce time to return to play (RTP) (2)[C].
  - Continuous passive motion therapy may be a promising modality in MO prevention in the early injury period (6)[A].
  - Radiation therapy is used postoperatively after hip replacement but is not used in traumatic cases (2)[C].
- Once heterotopic ossification develops:
  - Trials of bisphosphonate therapy has been used in case reports, but current data does not support its use.

SURGERY/OTHER PROCEDURES

- Surgical excision is rarely indicated and often not considered until the lesion is mature (~6 months) (1)[C],(2)[C],(3)[C],(4)[C],(5)[A],(6)[A].
- Surgery is contraindicated for immature lesions due to a high recurrence rate and otherwise self-limited nature (6)[A].
- Criteria for excision include lesion maturation complete, limited ROM and function, intractable pain resulting from mechanical irritation, neurovascular disturbance, and predisposition for further injury (1)[C],(4)[C],(5)[A].
- Biopsy should be considered only in cases of mature lesions with indeterminate morphology, where malignant diagnoses cannot be excluded (1)[C].

ONGOING CARE

PROGNOSIS

- Many athletes return to light physical activity within 3 months and full sport within 6 months.
- Symptoms related to MO may last longer than 6 months, but complete resorption of calcifications may take years or remain indefinitely.

REFERENCES

1. Walczak BE, Johnson CN, Howe BM. Myositis ossificans. *J Am Acad Orthop Surg*. 2015;23(10):612–622.
2. Meyers C, Lisiecki J, Miller S, et al. Heterotopic ossification: a comprehensive review. *JBMR Plus*. 2019;3(4):e10172.
3. Savvidou O, Papakonstantinou O, Lakiotaki E, et al. Post-traumatic myositis ossificans: a benign lesion that simulates malignant bone and soft tissue tumors. *EFORT Open Rev*. 2021;6(7):572–583.
4. Tyler P, Saifuddin A. The imaging of myositis ossificans. *Semin Musculoskelet Radiol*. 2010;14(2):201–216.
5. Cherry I, Mutschler M, Samara E, et al. Myositis ossificans in the pediatric population: a systematic scoping review. *Front Pediatr*. 2023;11:1295212.
6. Vasileiadis GI, Balta AA, Zerva A, et al. Role of kinesiotherapy in the prevention of heterotopic ossification: a systematic review. *Am J Phys Med Rehabil*. 2023;102(2):110–119.

ADDITIONAL READING

- Atwan Y, Abdulla I, Grewal R, et al. Indomethacin for heterotopic ossification prophylaxis following surgical treatment of elbow trauma: a randomized controlled trial. *J Shoulder Elbow Surg*. 2023;32(6):1242–1248.
- Cushner FD, Morwessel RM. Myositis ossificans traumatica. *Orthop Rev*. 1992;21(11):1319–1326.
- Łęgosz P, Otworowski M, Sibilska A, et al. Heterotopic ossification: a challenging complication of total hip arthroplasty: risk factors, diagnosis, prophylaxis, and treatment. *Biomed Res Int*. 2019;2019:3860142.
- Lempainen L, Mechó S, Valle X, et al. Management of anterior thigh injuries in soccer players: practical guide. *BMC Sports Sci Med Rehabil*. 2022;14(1):41.
- Simon T, Guillodo Y, Madouas G, et al. Myositis ossificans traumatica (circumscripta) and the return to sport: a retrospective series of 19 cases. *Joint Bone Spine*. 2016;83(4):416–420.

CLINICAL PEARLS

- MO can occur in the presence and absence of trauma and may mimic other benign or malignant pathology during its early stage.
- Early, accurate, multidisciplinary diagnosis of MO, and differentiation from malignant causes is essential to starting the right treatment and avoiding unnecessary tests.
- US is the most sensitive modality in early detection of MO, whereas CT scan is the imaging of choice for assessment of calcification.
- The presence of pain, reduced ROM after injury, and its classic calcification pattern over time help differentiate MO from other conditions.
- MO is a self-limited condition that allows most athletes to return to full, previous level of sport.
- Exceptionally symptomatic cases can be referred for surgical excision after the lesion has matured.

NASAL SEPTAL HEMATOMAS

Nicole L. Leonard, MD • Daniel C. Herman, MD, PhD, FAAPMR, FACSM, FISBS, CAQSM • Kevin J. Burnham, MD, CAQSM

BASICS

DESCRIPTION

- The nose is the most common injury site after facial trauma (1).
- Nasal bone fractures are the most common facial bone fracture in sports injuries (1).
- Nasal septal hematoma is a rare but serious complication of nasal trauma (1),(2),(3).
- Collection of blood under the mucoperichondrium or mucoperiosteum of nasal septal cartilage or bone
- Septal hematomas can occur bilaterally or unilaterally.
- Can occur within 24 hours of trauma, and if left untreated, can lead to irreversible destruction or deformity within 72 to 96 hours (3)

EPIDEMIOLOGY

- Exact incidence is unknown but reported to occur in 0.8–1.6% of patients with nasal injuries (2).
- Men are more commonly affected than women (2).
- Median time to diagnosis may be as long as 7 days (2).
- 90% of nasal fractures are associated with septal injury (3).

ETIOLOGY AND PATHOPHYSIOLOGY

- Trauma to the nasal septum can tear blood vessels adjacent to the septal cartilage, resulting in collection of blood between cartilage and perichondrium (3).
- In severe cases where the septal cartilage is fractured, blood can sweep to contralateral side resulting in a bilateral septal hematoma.
- Can be an ideal medium for bacterial proliferation and colonization, leading to a septal abscess

DIAGNOSIS

HISTORY

- Trauma most often caused by an inferior blow to the nose; this is because the supportive structure of the lower 2/3 of the nose is composed entirely of cartilage.
- Symptoms are mostly nonspecific. There should be a high index of suspicion if a patient presents with nasal pain or deformity after trauma. Nasal obstruction and pain are the most common symptoms(3)[C].

PHYSICAL EXAM

- Signs may include rhinorrhea, epistaxis, ecchymosis, nasal deformity, and swelling. The nose may be crepitant to palpation, usually from associated fracture (3)[C].
- Physical examination:
  - Must be performed with otoscope nasal speculum for better visualization (4)[B]
  - Control bleeding with direct pressure, topical decongestants, or cautery, as indicated for optimal visualization.
  - Sufficient lighting and suction are helpful.
  - Patient positioning: Drainage of blood from the nose is best achieved with the patient in a supine position with the head elevated.
  - Septal hematoma will appear as a bluish red bulge from the septum into the nasal vestibule or as an asymmetric mucosal fold (3)[C].
  - Septal hematomas do not shrink with use of decongestants (5)[C].
  - Ensure the absence of cerebrospinal fluid (CSF) leak: may present as clear rhinorrhea or patient may report a sweet taste (1)[C]
  - Direct palpation: Using a gloved finger or cotton tip applicator, gently palpate along the entire nasal septum, feeling for swelling, fluctuance, widening of the septum, or any other abnormalities.
  - Septal hematomas remain compressible with palpation via finger or cotton tip applicator (3)[C]:
    - In contrast, a deviated nasal septum will feel firm and concave on the contralateral side.
    - Blood clots adjacent to the nasal septum can falsely represent a septal hematoma and should be evacuated before examining the nasal septum.
    - Masses located deep within the nasal cavity, out of the reach of a gloved finger, may require palpation by a cotton swab, again, feeling for a soft mass as opposed to the firm cartilaginous septum.

DIAGNOSTIC TESTS & INTERPRETATION

- Clinical diagnosis, however, contrast-enhanced computed tomography (CT) may be in rare cases when the diagnosis is equivocal or to evaluate for abscess extension (5)[C]
- Delayed presentation to health care providers or failed drainage can lead to nasal septal abscess or deformity (3)[C].
- Purulent specimens should be sent for Gram stain and culture, both aerobic and anaerobic.
- If needed based on clinical concern, CSF leak can be evaluated using assays for β-2-transferrin or β-trace-protein.

TREATMENT

- The hematoma should be drained or incised urgently to avoid development of complications.
- Needle aspiration or sharp incision and drainage under local or general anesthesia followed by suction of the clot, if needed, and irrigation (5)[C]:
  - Mucosal incision should be made over the area of greatest fluctuance, with care taken not to damage the underlying cartilage.
  - Bilateral hematomas should be treated with staggered incisions to decrease risk of possible through-and-through perforation.
- Anterior nasal packing to approximate the perichondrium and prevent recurrence of the hematoma should be used; remove after 3 days (5)[C].
- Systemic antibiotic coverage with clindamycin or amoxicillin-clavulanic acid provides appropriate coverage against the most common abscess pathogens (6)[C], including:
  - *Staphylococcus aureus*
  - *Streptococcus pneumoniae*
  - Group A β-hemolytic *Streptococcus*
  - *Haemophilus influenzae*

ONGOING CARE

FOLLOW-UP RECOMMENDATIONS

- Patients and parents should be instructed on signs and symptoms of nasal septal hematoma because formation may be delayed (2)[B].
- Close follow-up is needed after diagnosis and drainage to monitor for failed drainage or recurrence.
- After immediate management, continue nasal packing and follow up with otolaryngologist in 3 days (5)[C].

COMPLICATIONS

- Reaccumulation of hematoma
- Nasal septal abscess
- Avascular necrosis
- Saddle nose deformity

REFERENCES

1. Leinhart J, Toldi J, Tennison M. Facial trauma in sports. *Curr Sports Med Rep*. 2017;16(1):23–29.
2. Ali HM, Zavala H, Chinnadurai S, et al. Nasal septal hematoma in children: time to diagnosis and resulting complications. *Int J Pediatr Otorhinolaryngol*. 2021;145:110734.
3. Sanyaolu LN, Farmer SEJ, Cuddihy PJ. Nasal septal haematoma. *BMJ*. 2014;349:g6075.
4. Sayin I, Yazici ZM, Abakay MA, et al. Nasal septal hematoma and abscess in children: an uncommon otorhinolaryngology emergency revisited. *J Craniofac Surg*. 2021;32(2):e125–e128.
5. Kass JI, Ferguson BJ. Videos in clinical medicine: treatment of hematoma of the nasal septum. *N Engl J Med*. 2015;372(22):e28.
6. Bartholomew RA, Mohan S, Keamy DG. Infected septal hematoma. *J Pediatr*. 2022;241:260–261.

ADDITIONAL READING

Kopacheva-Barsova G, Arsova S. The impact of the nasal trauma in childhood on the development of the nose in future. *Open Access Maced J Med Sci*. 2016;4(3):413–419.

CLINICAL PEARLS

- Minor trauma can lead to hematoma formation, even without signs of external injury. This can lead to delayed diagnosis.
- Any history of nasal trauma warrants intranasal examination.
- Delayed intervention can lead to abscess formation or irreversible nasal deformity.
- Nasal packing is left in place 3 days such that the mucosa can heal and reduce the risk of recurrence.
- After removal of packing, return to play is based on consideration of the associated nasal fracture and whether an infection is present.

NECK LACERATIONS AND PENETRATING INJURIES

Morgan Potter, MD • Laura Anderson, MD • Amie Kim, MD, CAQSM

BASICS

Pediatric Considerations

Aerodigestive and vascular injuries present with subtle findings and often lead to delayed diagnosis. The standard anatomic zones of the neck do not apply to infants and younger children. Computed tomography (CT) angiography is still the diagnostic study of choice.

ALERT

Quick things to know about treatment:

- Do not be fooled by the seemingly stable patient. These patients can decompensate rapidly and without warning.
- Airway tip—before attempting to secure the airway, have a surgical airway kit at the bedside.
- Circulation tip—occlusive dressings impregnated with petroleum jelly should be applied to lacerations over major veins to prevent air embolism with patients placed in Trendelenburg position.
- Disability tip—a cervical collar is only indicated if there is concomitant blunt trauma and a primary concern for cervical spine injury.
- Stable patients should be transferred to a trauma center.
- Unstable patients with penetrating neck trauma receive definitive care in the operating room (OR).
- Immediate surgical exploration is required in 15–20% of cases of penetrating neck injury (1).

DESCRIPTION

- Penetrating neck trauma is defined as a wound that violates the platysma muscle.
- Anatomic consideration: The neck is divided into *three zones* based on superficial landmarks and are numbered from most caudal to cephalad.
- It is important to note, just because the entrance wound is in one zone, does not preclude further damage to other zones or areas of the body.
  - Zone I extends from the top of the sternum to the sternal notch or cricoid cartilage:
    - Penetrating trauma in zone I carries the highest mortality due to injury to thoracic structures.
    - Isolated Horner syndrome may be the only presenting sign of injury to this zone.
    - Structures within zone I include the brachiocephalic vein, subclavian artery, common carotid artery, lung apices, trachea, thoracic duct, cervical nerve roots, and the esophagus.
  - Zone II extends from the cricoid cartilage to the angle of the mandible:
    - Zone II is the most common penetrating neck wound.
    - Zone II injuries are most easily identified. Treatment both in the emergency department (ED) and the OR is more often successful and carries the lowest mortality rates.
    - Structures within zone II include the pharynx, larynx, trachea, common carotid arteries, vertebral arteries, jugular veins, cervical spine, esophagus, thyroid.
  - Zone III extends cephalad from the angle of the mandible to the base of the skull:
    - Zone III is the least common penetrating neck wound.
    - Injuries to the distal carotid or vertebral arteries can mimic a stroke of the anterior or posterior circulation system, respectively.
    - Structures within this zone include cranial nerves IX to XII, hypopharynx, internal and external carotid arteries, vertebral arteries, jugular veins, and salivary glands.

EPIDEMIOLOGY

- Penetrating neck injuries: represent 5–10% of all trauma cases (2)
- Most common in young (mean age 30 years), males (>80%) (3)
- Mortality: 5% (3),(4),(5):
  - Exsanguination: 50% of mortality, most common cause of immediate death
- Concomitant injuries (5):
  - Aerodigestive tract injury (most common, ~10% per airway and digestive tract, respectively)
  - Vascular injury (9%): Carotid artery and internal jugular are the most commonly injured vessels.
  - Spinal cord injury: ≤3%
- 11% of patients require emergent intubation.

ETIOLOGY AND PATHOPHYSIOLOGY

- Globally, the most common mechanism of injury is stabbed wounds from violent assault, followed by gunshot wounds.
- Miscellaneous (self-harm, road traffic accident, glass shard, or metal fragment)

DIAGNOSIS

- Careful examination of the wound to determine integrity of the platysma
- Wounds should never be blindly probed, as this may dislodge a developing clot or prompt uncontrolled hemorrhage.
- Portable anteroposterior (AP) chest radiograph for suspected zone I injuries to detect hemopneumothorax, mediastinal air, or bleeding that extends into the upper mediastinum that may necessitate immediate intervention

PHYSICAL EXAM

- Physical exam findings must be divided into soft and hard signs. Any hard signs should prompt immediate transfer to the OR.
- Hard signs are associated with 90% rate of major injury.
- Vascular injury:
  - **Hard signs**:
    - Active hemorrhage/arterial bleed: expanding or pulsatile hematoma, shock, pulse deficits in either upper extremity, thrills or bruit at the neck
  - **Soft signs**: tracheal deviation, loss of normal anatomic landmarks, nonexpanding hematoma, venous oozing
    - Note: An intact pulse does not exclude a vascular injury.
- Laryngotracheal injury:
  - **Hard signs**: respiratory distress, crepitus, subcutaneous emphysema, air bubbling through wound
  - **Soft signs**: hoarseness, voice changes, stridor, hemoptysis, neck pain or tenderness, oropharyngeal blood, dyspnea, palpable deformity such as laryngeal fracture/crepitus
- Pharyngoesophageal injury: High index of suspicion required as obvious clinical signs are frequently absent.
  - **Hard signs**: hematemesis
  - **Soft signs**: dysphagia, odynophagia
- Neurologic injury:
  - **Hard signs**: central or peripheral nervous system deficits, Horner syndrome

DIFFERENTIAL DIAGNOSIS

- Vascular injury
- Pharyngoesophageal injury
- Laryngotracheal injury
- Peripheral or central nervous system injury
- Cervical spine injury: Note the absence of a neurologic deficit does not exclude a cervical spine injury.
- Associated head or thoracic trauma

DIAGNOSTIC TESTS & INTERPRETATION

No consensus on best diagnostic approach, and all decisions should be made in concert with the trauma service; typically divided by best test to evaluate each structural injury

- Aerodigestive:
  - CT with intravenous (IV) contrast of neck and chest with esophageal studies (contrast esophageal swallow or endoscopy, etc.)
  - Pneumothorax: chest radiograph, particularly in zone I injuries; point-of-care ultrasound (US) for lung sliding, lung point, and A-line reverberations
- Laryngotracheal injury: low threshold for CT neck and chest with IV contrast in stable patients without hard signs
- Vascular injury:
  - Stable patients without hard signs may be able to undergo multidetector helical CT angiography. The sensitivity and specificity of this approaches traditional angiography, which was the former gold standard (3)[B].
  - US with color flow Doppler combined with frequent, repeated physical exam is a fast, noninvasive therapeutic modality; however, this does not fully evaluate injuries to zone I or III, is operator-dependent, and can miss subtle findings.
- Pharyngoesophageal injury:
  - Always suspect esophageal injury in zone I injuries.
  - CT with contrast (CT+) is used to evaluate esophageal injury and in recent studies has been found to be 92% sensitive in ruling out aerodigestive injuries.
  - The addition of further testing is indicated if there is any concern for esophageal injury as 100% sensitivity is only reached with the addition of either esophagography or flexible endoscopy (4).
  - The chest x-ray can demonstrate nonspecific findings but does not rule out esophageal injury.

Initial Tests (lab, imaging)

- Baseline complete blood panel and chemistry panel
- Coagulation studies
- Type and cross-match
- Arterial or venous blood gas
- Human chorionic gonadotropin (hCG) or urine pregnancy if female
- Creatine phosphokinase (CPK)
- Troponin
- Consider ethanol (EtOH).

TREATMENT

- Initial stabilization: "C-ABCDE" approaches: C: circulation and hemorrhage control; "A" refers to airway management; "B" to breathing; "D" to disability or neurologic status; and "E" to exposure (undress) and environment (temperature control).
- If a patient is unstable or exhibits any hard signs, he or she should be stabilized airway, breathing, and circulation [ABCs] and emergently sent to the OR.
- Airway management:
  - Airway management should be done with the patient in cervical spine precautions if indicated.
  - Patients who are comatose or in respiratory distress require immediate intubation.

- Stable patients without evidence of respiratory distress may be aggressively managed with prophylactic intubation or closely observed with airway equipment at the bedside.
- Bag-valve mask can force air subcutaneously through fascial planes and should be done carefully.
- Orotracheal intubation with rapid sequence induction (RSI) is the method of choice for securing the airway. Ketamine and rocuronium are currently the recommended induction agents of choice.
- If any anticipation of need for intubation, the patient should be placed on nasal cannula or nonrebreather mask immediately for preoxygenation.
- Nasotracheal intubation is contraindicated with apnea, severe facial injury, or airway distortion for the risk of puncturing an expanding hematoma.
- Fiber-optic intubation is contraindicated with active bleeding that may obscure the scope.
- Percutaneous transtracheal ventilation may be useful when oral or nasotracheal intubation fails and should be used only as a temporizing measure until a more secure airway is obtained. It leaves the airway unprotected and is contraindicated in cases of upper airway obstruction, as it may cause barotrauma.
- If the trachea is exposed due to a complete or partial transection, the caudal end should be directly intubated.
- In all patients in whom intubation is attempted, there should be a surgical airway kit at the bedside. The physician must be prepared for a cricothyroidotomy or tracheostomy, as these are required in cases of severe facial injury, laryngotracheal injury, and uncontrolled upper airway hemorrhage.
- RSI can precipitate hemodynamic collapse. If possible, resuscitate, correct acidosis, and preoxygenate prior to intubation.
- An expanding hematoma has significant potential to occlude the airway over time.

- Breathing: Zone I injury can cause pneumothorax or subclavian vein injury and hemothorax, requiring needle decompression and tube thoracostomy. If immediate decompression is needed, finger thoracostomy is indicated prior to tube thoracostomy.
- Circulation:
  - Two large-bore IVs should be placed contralateral to the side of the injury to avoid ipsilateral venous injury.
  - If IV access cannot be obtained, consider placing an intraosseous (IO) access.
  - External hemorrhage should be controlled with direct pressure. Blind clamping of vessels is contraindicated due to the risk of further neurovascular injury.
  - If bleeding cannot be controlled, a Foley catheter can be inserted and inflated with saline to help tamponade bleeding.
  - Patients with uncontrolled bleeding or hemodynamic instability must go directly to the OR.
  - If possible, call ahead to the ED to activate a massive transfusion protocol to ensure the patient receives blood products on arrival.
  - Blood products are superior to fluid administration in the trauma patient, but fluids should be administered as a temporizing agent if blood is on delay.
  - Consider performing an extended focused assessment with sonography in trauma (FAST) US exam as part of the trauma secondary survey.
- Disability: Although penetrating neck trauma often does not involve the cervical spine, the cervical spine should be evaluated and cleared appropriately. Decision-making rules such as NEXUS criteria for C-spine imaging or Canadian C-spine Rule may be used.
- Exposure: It is essential to keep the hemorrhaging patient warm, as cooling can result in further disruption of coagulation.
- Prehospital:
  - Impaled objects should not be removed.
  - Gently suction to clear the airway of blood, secretions, or vomitus.
  - Lateral decubitus or prone positioning may be required to prevent aspiration.
  - The airway must be vigilantly monitored, as edema or expanding hematoma can progress to airway compromise.
  - Early oral intubation is indicated for clinical signs of respiratory distress, such as stridor, air hunger, or labored breathing, or if an expanding neck hematoma is present.
  - Cervical spine injury is uncommon in the context of low velocity penetrating injury and immobilization is not routinely advocated unless clinically suspected.
- ED treatment:
  - Alert and seemingly stable patients are known to rapidly decompensate; therefore, an airway setup should be at the bedside.
  - Nasogastric tube should not be placed due to risk of rupturing a pharyngeal hematoma.
  - Prophylactic antibiotics are recommended if a hollow viscus injury (such as pharyngoesophageal injuries) is suspected (5)[C]: (**cefoxitin or ceftriaxone**, **clindamycin**, **penicillin G** plus **metronidazole**). If concerns for or demonstrated skeletal fracture, cefazolin should be given within 1 hour prior to arrival in the ED.
  - Surgical consult for all wounds that penetrate the platysma muscle
    - Immediate surgical exploration is indicated in patients with "Hard signs," as itemized in "Physical Exam."
    - Selective approach in stable patients, especially in those with zone II injuries (1)[B]
  - Mandatory approach indicating surgical exploration in all cases of penetrating neck trauma is no longer widely practiced.
  - Tetanus prophylaxis with Tdap; if the wound is tetanus prone, consider the addition of tetanus immune globulin.
  - Traumatic arrest in patients with penetrating neck injury is an indication for ED thoracotomy.
  - Note for patients who are hemodynamically stable with vascular injuries that are operatively inaccessible, for example, a proximal zone III injury of the carotid, should be assessed by interventional radiologist (IR) or vascular for angiographic interventions such as embolization or stent.

GENERAL MEASURES

Aerodigestive and vascular injuries are subtle and often missed.

MEDICATION

- **Cefoxitin**: adult: 2 g IV within 1 hour of arrival to the ED and then q8h; pediatrics: 80 to 160 mg/kg/d divided q4–8h, max daily dose of 12 g/d
- **Ceftriaxone**: adult: 1 g IV and then q8h; pediatrics: 50 to 75 mg/kg/d divided q12–24h, max daily dose of 2 g/d
- **Clindamycin**: adult: 600 to 900 mg IV q8h; pediatrics: 25 to 40 mg/kg/d IV divided q6–8h *or*
- **Penicillin G**: adult: 24 million IU/d divided q4–6h; pediatrics: 150,000 to 250,000 IU/kg/d divided q4–6h *plus*
- **Metronidazole**: adult: 1 g load and then 500 mg IV q6h; pediatrics: 30 mg/kg/d IV divided q12h

ADMISSION, INPATIENT, AND NURSING CONSIDERATIONS

- Admission criteria:
  - All patients with penetrating neck trauma should be admitted and observed for at least 24 hours.
  - Observation must take place in a facility capable of providing definitive surgical care.
  - Patients with possible airway or vascular injury must be admitted to the intensive care unit.
- Discharge criteria: Asymptomatic patients who have negative studies may be discharged after at least 24 hours of observation.

REFERENCES

1. Kendall JL, Anglin D, Demetriades D. Penetrating neck trauma. *Emerg Med Clin North Am.* 1998;16(1):85–105.
2. Vishwanatha B, Sagayaraj A, Huddar SG, et al. Penetrating neck injuries. *Indian J Otolaryngol Head Neck Surg.* 2007;59(3):221–224.
3. Biffl WL, Moore EE, Rehse DH, et al. Selective management of penetrating neck trauma based on cervical level of injury. *Am J Surg.* 1997;174(6):678–682.
4. Arantes V, Campolina C, Valerio SH, et al. Flexible esophagoscopy as a diagnostic tool for traumatic esophageal injuries. *J Trauma.* 2009;66(6):1677–1682.
5. McConnell DB, Trunkey DD. Management of penetrating trauma to the neck. *Adv Surg.* 1994;27:97–127.

CLINICAL PEARLS

- The majority of penetrating neck injuries occur at zone II between the cricoid cartilage and the mandibular angle.
- Exsanguination is the most common cause of immediate death, so hemorrhage control is prioritized in the advanced trauma life support approach.
- A possible exception to the "Hard signs go to the OR rule" is that if a patient is stable and a thrill or bruit is identified, imaging over operative evaluation may be preferred because of the possibility of endovascular surgery.
- Cervical spine immobilization is not routinely recommended in low-energy injuries with the exception of blunt trauma or direct penetration of the spine.
- Surgical consultation should be obtained in all penetrating neck injuries.
  - It is important to note that despite Western Trauma Association guidelines, the use of neck zones as the ideal way to assess and triage a patient with penetrating neck injury is currently under debate.
  - The Eastern Association for the Surgery of Trauma supports the "no zone approach," which advocates for determination of operative management to be based on hemodynamic stability and the presence of hard signs.
  - Consider the use of topical hemostatic agents in the setting of uncontrollable bleeding. Commonly used agents include:
    - QuickClot
    - HemCon
    - Celox
    - WoundStat
    - TraumaStat
    - Combat gauze
    - Topical tranexamic acid preparation by soaking gauze in the IV formulation or into a topical paste with PO formulation

NONSTEROIDAL ANTI-INFLAMMATORY DRUG POISONING

Shane Hudnall, MD, CAQSM • Michelle A. Tedrowe, DO

BASICS

- Primary effect is competitive inhibition of cyclooxygenase (COX) enzyme, thus inhibiting production of prostaglandins, thromboxanes, and prostacyclin from arachidonic acid.
- There are two COX isoforms: COX-1 and COX-2.
- COX-1 is expressed in most tissues.
- COX-2 is induced more in inflammation and pain.
- Most adverse effects are attributed to COX-1 inhibition.
- Most are metabolized through the liver with urinary excretion.
- Class of drugs works as antipyretics, analgesics, and anti-inflammatory agents.
- Reduction of circulating prostacyclin and thromboxane results in platelet aggregation and vasodilation, respectively.
- Over-the-counter (OTC) nonsteroidal anti-inflammatory drugs (NSAIDs) include ibuprofen, naproxen, and aspirin.
- Classification:
  - Carboxylic acids:
    - Salicylates: aspirin, diflunisal
    - Propionic acids: ibuprofen, naproxen, ketoprofen
    - Acetic acids: indomethacin, etodolac, ketorolac, sulindac, diclofenac
    - Fenamates: meclofenamate, mefenamic acid
  - Enolic acids:
    - Oxicams: piroxicam, meloxicam
    - Pyrazolones: phenylbutazone
  - COX-2 inhibitors: celecoxib
- Meloxicam and etodolac have greater inhibition of COX-2 than COX-1 at low doses.

EPIDEMIOLOGY

Incidence

- >20 million Americans take NSAIDs on a regular basis.
- It is estimated that >30 billion OTC NSAIDs tablets are sold annually in the United States.
- ~70 million NSAIDs prescriptions are written each year in the United States.
- Acute NSAIDs poisoning is rare despite their extensive use.
- In most fatalities involving NSAIDs, patients ingested other pharmaceutical agents as well.
- Most poisonings are attributable to ibuprofen (>80,000 total yearly).

ETIOLOGY AND PATHOPHYSIOLOGY

- Toxicity:
  - Only a small percentage of overdoses (<0.5%) lead to serious harm (i.e., gastrointestinal [GI] bleeding, renal failure).
  - Most are asymptomatic or have nonspecific symptoms (nausea, vomiting, dizziness, somnolence).
  - There is some evidence to suggest topical NSAIDs are effective for pain relief in knee osteoarthritis (OA) with fewer systemic side effects compared to oral NSAIDs (1),(2).
- GI:
  - Most common adverse effects are GI related (i.e., vomiting, abdominal pain, dyspepsia, diarrhea, gastroesophageal reflux disease [GERD], constipation).
  - Gastric, duodenal, and large intestinal ulceration may occur (1–4% of users annually) likely secondary NSAIDs inhibition of prostaglandin synthesis leading to weakening of GI tract mucosal barrier. Use of misoprostol, H2-receptor antagonists, or proton pump inhibitor (PPI) can be protective to gastric mucosa.
  - 3 to 10 times more likely to have serious hemorrhage with NSAIDs
  - COX-2 inhibitors have been shown to delay ulcer healing in animal studies, but this has not been elucidated in humans.
  - Celecoxib is associated with fewer ulcers at 12 weeks and 6 months but no difference at 1 year (presence of ulcer or complications) compared to ibuprofen and diclofenac (3).
  - In patients requiring low-dose aspirin, celecoxib plus a PPI resulted in less recurrent bleeding and ulcers compared to naproxen plus a PPI (4).
  - Celecoxib may be associated with decreased colon adenomas, duodenal polyps, and cancer from inhibiting COX-2 and tumor growth, especially in those with familial adenomatous polyposis.
- Renal:
  - Second most common adverse effects
  - Inhibition of prostaglandins and thromboxane synthesis interferes with renal blood flow and glomerular filtration rate.
  - Leads to vasoconstriction (from blocking prostaglandin synthesis) and possibly acute renal failure or acute interstitial nephritis
  - Retention of sodium, potassium, and water may lead to congestive heart failure (CHF) exacerbation.
  - COX-2 inhibitors: adversely affect function in patients with volume depletion, underlying renal disease, heart failure, and cirrhosis
- Central nervous system (CNS):
  - About 30% of patients with NSAIDs overdose experience CNS toxicity.
  - Elderly particularly at risk
  - Can cause headache, confusion, delirium, psychosis, hallucinations, nightmares, tremor, seizures, tinnitus, transient hearing loss, and aseptic meningitis
- Cardiovascular:
  - Can raise blood pressure an average of 5 mm Hg and worsen control of hypertension (HTN) (5)
  - Increased risk of cardiovascular events in both nonselective NSAIDs and COX-2 inhibitors
  - Risk of bleeding and cardiovascular events further increased in patients on antithrombotic drugs concomitantly taking NSAIDs (6)
  - All are associated with increased risk of CHF exacerbation in those with a history of CHF.
- Pulmonary:
  - Asthmatics are at increased risk for bronchospasm owing to increased production of leukotrienes.
  - COX-2 inhibitors are much less likely to trigger bronchospasm.
  - Pulmonary infiltrates with eosinophilia are also possible.
  - Patients with clinical triad of asthma, nasal polyps, and allergic rhinitis are at increased risk for anaphylaxis to both salicylates and NSAIDs.
- Hepatic:
  - Possibility (although rare) of fulminant hepatic failure, hepatitis, elevated transaminases
  - Generally, this is reversible and only rarely fatal.
- Hematologic:
  - Aplastic anemia (now rare with decreased use of phenylbutazone and indomethacin), agranulocytosis, neutropenia, hemolytic anemia, thrombocytopenia possible
  - Decreased platelet aggregation may lead to increased GI bleeding.
  - COX-2 inhibitors have not been shown to decrease platelet function and are associated with a decreased risk of bleeding compared with nonselective NSAIDs.
- Skin: Toxic epidermal necrolysis and Stevens-Johnson syndrome are uncommon, but relative risk is increased slightly with NSAIDs use (including celecoxib) compared with placebo.
- Metabolic: may lead to anion gap metabolic acidosis

- Drug interactions:
  - Increased risk of GI bleeding when used with anticoagulants
  - Digoxin, lithium, sulfonylurea, and aminoglycoside levels are all increased with use of NSAIDs.
  - NSAIDs reduce antihypertensive effects of diuretics, β-blockers, and angiotensin-converting enzyme (ACE) inhibitors.
  - NSAIDs such as ibuprofen and naproxen can decrease renal clearance of methotrexate (5).
  - Celecoxib contains a sulfa moiety and may have cross reactivity in those allergic to sulfa antibiotics.

RISK FACTORS

- Suicidal ideation
- Untreated pain
- Patients unclear of maximum allowed dosage of NSAIDs

DIAGNOSIS

HISTORY

- Although significant symptoms may occur after 5 to 10 times the maximum dose has been ingested, there is a poor correlation between the amount ingested and toxic poisoning.
- Timing of ingestion
- Past medical history (i.e., peptic ulcer disease, chronic renal insufficiency)

PHYSICAL EXAM

- Airway, breathing, and circulation (ABCs)
- Vital signs: Monitor BP, respiratory rate, and oxygen saturation.
- Thorough neurologic examination (especially monitoring mental status)
- Rectal examination for gross or occult blood

DIAGNOSTIC TESTS & INTERPRETATION

- Complete blood count (CBC), comprehensive metabolic panel (CMP) (attention to transaminases), prothrombin time/partial thromboplastin time (PT/PTT); coagulation studies, arterial blood gas (ABG) (if patient has anion gap on CMP or altered mental status), fingerstick glucose (rule out hypoglycemia), pregnancy test (if child-bearing female)
- Consider salicylate and acetaminophen levels, but do not check serum or urine levels of other NSAIDs. Treat presumptively.
- Electrocardiogram (ECG) to look for prolongation of QRS or QTc
- Imaging generally not necessary unless concern for perforated ulcer is present.

TREATMENT

- Acute treatment:
  - Supportive measures:
    - Call poison control.
    - Secure the ABCs.
    - There is no antidote for NSAIDs poisoning.
    - Close monitoring is warranted for almost all patients, and usually, this is the only treatment necessary.
    - Consider giving intravenous (IV) fluids if there is any volume deficit clinically.
    - Benzodiazepines IV if patient has seizures
  - Decontamination:
    - Gastric lavage if patient presents within 1 hour of ingestion or patient has massive overdose.
    - Activated charcoal (1 g/kg adults, 0.5 to 1.0 g/kg in children) should be given to all patients with acute NSAIDs ingestion presenting within 2 hours unless contraindicated (i.e., bowel perforation).
    - Dialysis is unnecessary and ineffective for decontamination due to the nature of NSAIDs being highly protein bound.
- Long-term treatment: disposition:
  - Admit patient for any signs of toxicity (e.g., renal failure, vital sign changes, somnolence, electrolyte abnormalities).
  - Asymptomatic patients should be monitored for 4 to 6 hours to ensure that they do not have any signs of toxicity before discharging home (possibly longer for drugs such as naproxen and piroxicam that have longer half-lives).
  - Obtain psychiatric consultation for suicide attempts once medically stable.

REFERENCES

1. Zeng C, Wei J, Persson MSM, et al. Relative efficacy and safety of topical non-steroidal anti-inflammatory drugs for osteoarthritis: a systematic review and network meta-analysis of randomised controlled trials and observational studies. *Br J Sports Med*. 2018;52(10):642–650.
2. Zeng C, Doherty M, Persson MSM, et al. Comparative efficacy and safety of acetaminophen, topical and oral non-steroidal anti-inflammatory drugs for knee osteoarthritis: evidence from a network meta-analysis of randomized controlled trials and real-world data. *Osteoarthritis Cartilage*. 2021;29(9):1242–1251.
3. Silverstein FE, Faich G, Goldstein JL, et al. Gastrointestinal toxicity with celecoxib vs nonsteroidal anti-inflammatory drugs for osteoarthritis and rheumatoid arthritis: the CLASS study: a randomized controlled trial. Celecoxib long-term arthritis safety study. *JAMA*. 2000;284(10):1247–1255.
4. Chan FKL, Ching JYL, Tse YK, et al. Gastrointestinal safety of celecoxib versus naproxen in patients with cardiothrombotic diseases and arthritis after upper gastrointestinal bleeding (CONCERN): an industry-independent, double-blind, double-dummy, randomised trial. *Lancet*. 2017;389(10087):2375–2382.
5. Wongrakpanich S, Wongrakpanich A, Melhado K, et al. A comprehensive review of non-steroidal anti-inflammatory drug use in the elderly. *Aging Dis*. 2018;9(1):143–150.
6. Schjerning Olsen AM, Gislason GH, McGettigan P, et al. Association of NSAID use with risk of bleeding and cardiovascular events in patients receiving antithrombotic therapy after myocardial infarction. *JAMA*. 2015;313(8):805–814.

ADDITIONAL READING

- Hunter LJ, Wood DM, Dargan PI. The patterns of toxicity and management of acute nonsteroidal anti-inflammatory drug (NSAID) overdose. *Open Access Emerg Med*. 2011;3:39–48.
- Perazella MA, Tray K. Selective cyclooxygenase-2 inhibitors: a pattern of nephrotoxicity similar to traditional nonsteroidal anti-inflammatory drugs. *Am J Med*. 2001;111(1):64–67.
- Phillips RKS, Wallace MH, Lynch PM, et al. A randomised, double blind, placebo controlled study of celecoxib, a selective cyclooxygenase 2 inhibitor, on duodenal polyposis in familial adenomatous polyposis. *Gut*. 2002;50(6):857–860.
- Swan SK, Rudy DW, Lasseter KC, et al. Effect of cyclooxygenase-2 inhibition on renal function in elderly persons receiving a low-salt diet. A randomized, controlled trial. *Ann Intern Med*. 2000;133(1):1–9.

CLINICAL PEARLS

- There is no additional benefit to giving >1 dose of activated charcoal unless highly suspicious for overdose of sustained-release NSAIDs: naproxen, oxaprozin, or piroxicam.
- Ipecac has fallen out of favor for most acute ingestions and is not recommended for NSAID toxicity.

NURSEMAID'S ELBOW

John Munyak, MD

BASICS

DESCRIPTION

- Results from a traumatic subluxation of the radial head, which is produced by sudden forcible traction on the pronated hand or wrist with the relaxed elbow extended
- Subluxation of the radial head only occurs in pronation when the anteroposterior (AP) plane of the radial head diameter is narrowest.
- As the radial head subluxes, there is an interposition of the annular ligament in the radiocapitellar joint resulting in entrapment.
- Synonym(s): pulled elbow; radiocapitellar subluxation; subluxation of the head of the radius; subluxation of the radius by elongation; temper tantrum elbow; Malgaigne injury

EPIDEMIOLOGY

- One of the most common musculoskeletal injuries in children aged ≤4 years
- Uncommon in children >5 years of age because the distal attachments of the orbicular ligament are sufficiently strong to prevent occurrence
- Peak incidence is from age of 1 to 3 years old (1), with a predominance in females (2).

RISK FACTORS

- Frequently, the traction force occurs when the child suddenly attempts to pull away from a parent or drops to the ground.
- Pulling a child as he or she stumbles, lifting him or her up by the hand, or swinging the child by the hand(s) can also generate sufficient traction force.

DIAGNOSIS

- History alone is the basis for diagnosis in most cases.
- Consider prereduction radiographs if there is a history of trauma.
- Postreduction views are unnecessary.
- Consider x-rays if the child's arm does not return to normal function after performing appropriate reduction maneuvers.
- Consider additional imaging of the forearm, wrist, or humerus in young children.
- Point-of-care ultrasound (POCUS)—Educated clinicians used the POCUS on children in ages between 0 and 5 years who might have nursemaid's elbow which showed a diagnostic performance with a sensitivity of 100% and a specificity of 100%.
- Strong support for claims that the POCUS can be used as a replacement for x-rays and/or diminishes the excessive need for them in the first place as well as enhancement of care overall (3).

HISTORY

- In >80% of cases, there is a history of sudden longitudinal traction to a pronated, extended forearm (3),(4).
- Possible history of a "click" felt or heard by the person who pulled the child's arm
- May be a history of an incidental fall in which the arm, elbow, and forearm were impacted between the ground and the child's trunk (3),(4)
- Immediately following the injury, the child is usually tearful due to the pain and refuses to use the affected arm.
- Pain, if vocalized, may be referred toward the wrist.
- The child holds the forearm by his or her side, always in a pronated and partially flexed position (nursemaid's position).
- Often, there is no history of trauma and the parents may notice the affected extremity not being used.

PHYSICAL EXAM

- Child refuses to use the affected limb.
- The forearm is always pronated, and the elbow is partially flexed.
- The child typically holds the affected limb by his or her side, sometimes supporting the forearm with the other hand.
- The child may be tearful during physical exam.
- The child also may appear content and playful but declines to move the affected arm.
- Gentle palpation can reveal local tenderness over the anterolateral aspect of the radial head.
- By carefully avoiding movements involving the elbow and forearm, one can note painless range of motion of the wrist, hand, and shoulder.
- Typically, no obvious swelling or deformity
- There is minimal restriction to flexion and extension of the elbow, but supination of the forearm is markedly limited and resisted.
- Often, the appearance is that of a wrist injury with the wrist flexed and pronated.
- It is imperative to examine the joints above and below the suspected injury, as well as the clavicle, to increase the likelihood of identifying the primary injury site.

DIFFERENTIAL DIAGNOSIS

- Posterior elbow dislocation
- Distal radial buckle fracture (torus) or other radial fracture
- Ulnar fracture
- Supracondylar fracture or other fracture of the humerus
- Avulsion of the medial or lateral epicondyle
- Septic joint
- Synovitis

TREATMENT

GENERAL MEASURES

- Analgesia:
  - Not typically necessary for reduction
- Reduction techniques: flexion–supination and hyperpronation (4),(5)
- *Hyperpronation*:
  - Additional pressure is exerted to pronate the forearm further as the elbow is moved into full extension; if done correctly, may be more effective and less painful (5),(6)
- *Flexion–supination*:
  - The thumb is placed in the region of the radial head for palpation and the exertion of mild pressure (anterior to posterior).
  - The child's forearm is gently but firmly rotated into full supination.
  - The elbow is then flexed to 90 degrees by holding the child's forearm above the wrist and stabilizing the humerus and elbow with the other hand to prevent rotation of the shoulder. If any resistance is met, one should continue flexing the elbow to the point of maximal flexion.
  - As reduction is achieved, a palpable and sometimes audible "click" can be felt in the region of the radial head.
  - This maneuver will typically achieve instantaneous reduction of the radial head and instant relief of pain.
  - New literature stated that hyperpronation is much more beneficial and had solid evidence supporting this.
  - The "first-line reduction method" is hyperpronation (6).
  - "First attempt success" is 85% for hyperpronation and 53% for supination–flexion, as well as the "second attempt success" is 50% for hyperpronation and 23% for supination–flexion.
  - The "crossover outcome" success which is 100% for hyperpronation and 50% for supination–flexion.
  - Author's choice: "The way I do it with 33 years of experience" is direct pressure with the thumb on the radial head while hyperpronating with inline traction of the forearm and then flexing and extending to confirm the reduction while maintaining the radial head pressure, forearm inline traction, and hyperpronation.

- Postreduction evaluation:
  - Observation is necessary until there is a return of full function and use of the affected arm (often occurs immediately postmaneuver).
  - If function has not normalized in 15 minutes, a repeated attempt at reduction is recommended or obtain radiographs.
  - In some studies, the delay until normal use of the arm is achieved is longer when there has been a delay in treatment from the time of injury; therefore, near-normal function or significant improvement in function and postreduction may be sufficiently reassuring to continue observation at home with close follow-up within 24 hours.
  - If there is no evidence of recovery after several reduction attempts, the diagnosis must be reconsidered.
- Immobilization:
  - Immobilization is not necessary for the first occurrence of subluxation.
  - If reduction is delayed for >12 hours, consider immobilization in a sling and swath or with a posterior mold for 10 days with the elbow in 90 degrees of flexion and the forearm in full supination. Compliance is difficult in this age range.
  - For cases of multiple recurrences of nursemaid's elbow, some clinicians recommend a trial of immobilization of the upper limb in an above elbow cast or postmold for 2 to 3 weeks in conjunction with pediatric orthopedic consultation.

ADDITIONAL THERAPIES

- Special considerations:
  - In a child <6 months of age, consider abuse from a caretaker while evaluating the child. However, subluxation can occur while simply rolling over in this age group.
  - Recurrence of subluxation as a result of subsequent pulls occurs in ~5–40% of cases.
- Rehabilitation:
  - Prevention is key. The parent should be advised to avoid longitudinal traction strains on the arm by not pulling on the hand or wrist, but pick the child up by the trunk.
  - For the child who recovers fully after one or two reduction maneuvers, further therapy or intervention is unnecessary.

SURGERY/OTHER PROCEDURES

- Very rarely, the subluxed radial head may be irreducible by manipulation, especially in recurrent cases, requiring surgical intervention.
- The need for open reduction is extremely rare.

ONGOING CARE

FOLLOW-UP RECOMMENDATIONS

- Even when multiple attempts at closed reduction fail, spontaneous reduction almost always occurs.
- Usually no long-term sequelae
- Consider an occult fracture or cartilaginous injury if the response to treatment is not typical.

REFERENCES

1. Vitello S, Dvorkin R, Sattler S, et al. Epidemiology of nursemaid's elbow. *West J Emerg Med*. 2014;15(4):554–557.
2. Wong K, Troncoso AB, Calello DP, et al. Radial head subluxation: factors associated with its recurrence and radiographic evaluation in a tertiary pediatric emergency department. *J Emerg Med*. 2016;51(6):621–627.
3. Welch R, Chounthirath T, Smith GA. Radial head subluxation among young children in the United States associated with consumer products and recreational activities. *Clin Pediatr (Phila)*. 2017;56(8):707–715.
4. Krul M, van der Wouden JC, Kruithof EJ, et al. Manipulative interventions for reducing pulled elbow in young children. *Cochrane Database Syst Rev*. 2017;7(7):CD007759.
5. Bexkens R, Washburn FJ, Eygendaal D, et al. Effectiveness of reduction maneuvers in the treatment of nursemaid's elbow: a systematic review and meta-analysis. *Am J Emerg Med*. 2017;35(1):159–163.
6. Aksel G, Çorbacioğlu ŞK, Akoğlu H, et al. Comparative effectiveness of supination-flexion and hyperpronation maneuvers in radial head subluxation: a systematic review and meta-analysis. *Am J Emerg Med*. 2025;92:68–78.

ADDITIONAL READING

- McCreary DJ, Tambe N, Mullen N. What is the utility of point-of-care ultrasound for suspected pulled elbow? A single-centre case series. *J Paediatr Child Health*. 2024;60(11):698–702.
- Schunk JE. Radial head subluxation: epidemiology and treatment of 87 episodes. *Ann Emerg Med*. 1990;19(9):1019–1023.
- Spiegel R, Kleist S. Hyperpronation method for reduction of nursemaid's elbow. *Am Fam Physician*. 2018;97(10):Online.
- Ulici A, Herdea A, Carp M, et al. Nursemaid's elbow—supination-flexion technique versus hyperpronation/forced pronation: randomized clinical study. *Indian J Orthop*. 2019;53(1):117–121.

CLINICAL PEARLS

- Commonly occurring traction injury at age <4 years
- Educating families to avoid pulling or putting traction on the child's arm for several days following injury significantly decreases the risk of recurrence.
- "Herd immunity" can be obtained by telling all in your circle about the avoidance of pulling a child age <4 years by the hand.
- Long-term sequelae unlikely
- Evaluate returned usage of the elbow by making the child reach for a favorite object, parent's hand, or "eye candy."
- Consider fracture in the setting of antecedent trauma, significant swelling, deformity, or in cases of failed reduction attempts.

OBESITY AND WEIGHT MANAGEMENT

David Carfagno, DO, CAQSM ▪ Justin Rouintan, DO

BASICS

DESCRIPTION

- Body mass index (BMI) is a commonly used measure of obesity worldwide. It is defined as a person's weight in kilogram divided by the square of their height in meters (kg/m^2).
- Centers for Disease Control and Prevention (CDC) classifications for adults:
  - Underweight: BMI <18.5 kg/m^2
  - Healthy weight: BMI 18.5 to 24.99 kg/m^2
  - Overweight: BMI 25 to 29.99 kg/m^2
  - Obesity class I: BMI 30 to 34.99 kg/m^2
  - Obesity class II: BMI 35 to 39.99 kg/m^2
  - Obesity class III (severe): BMI >40 kg/m^2
- Waist circumference and risk of cardiometabolic disease:
  - At risk: >37 inches (94 cm) in men, >31.5 inches (80 cm) in women
  - Increased risk: >40 inches (102 cm) in men, >35 inches (88 cm) in women
- Obesity is caused by a complex interplay between biology, behavior, and environmental factors.
- Weight gain occurs when energy intake exceeds energy expenditure (i.e., positive energy balance).
- 1 lb of fat is equivalent to ~3,500 kcal of energy.

EPIDEMIOLOGY

According to data from the National Health and Nutrition Examination Survey (NHANES) during August 2021–August 2023:

- The prevalence of obesity in adults was 40.3%.
- The prevalence of severe obesity in adults was 9.4% (1).
- According to the World Health Organization (WHO) worldwide, 2.8 million people die each year secondary to being overweight or obese.
- The problem of obesity is growing in many developing countries. Obesity rates have tripled in the last 20 years in the developing world, with 18% of the world's children currently overweight or obese. The Middle East, Pacific Islands, Southeast Asia, and China are facing the greatest challenges.
- The effect of excess weight on mortality has been shown to boost the risk of death by anywhere from 22% to 91% according to a 2023 study that reevaluated BMI-mortality associations by accounting for biases in previous research (2).
- Extremely obese people—those who are ≥80 lb (36 kg) over a normal weight—live 3 to 12 years fewer than their normal-weight peers. ~6% of people are severely obese.
- The effect of severe obesity appears to be greater for men than women and for whites than blacks.

ETIOLOGY AND PATHOPHYSIOLOGY

- Several hormones regulate body weight. **Leptin**, from the hypothalamus, decreases appetite and increases metabolism, but people with obesity often develop resistance to it. In contrast, **ghrelin**, from the stomach, is an appetite-stimulating hormone that is high when the stomach is empty. Other hormones like adiponectin and peptide YY also play a role in appetite control.
- Metabolic syndrome comprises obesity, carbohydrate intolerance or type 2 diabetes, hypertension (HTN), dyslipidemia, and a prothrombotic inflammatory vascular environment:
  - It is more prevalent in males over females worldwide. Male accumulation of body fat is predominantly in the trunk and visceral rather than the subcutaneous fat. It is visceral fat that is the metabolically active fat, which produce adipokines, which increase insulin resistance.

COMMONLY ASSOCIATED CONDITIONS

- Obesity contributes to excess mortality from HTN, type 2 diabetes, coronary artery diseases, stroke, gallbladder disease, sleep apnea, and osteoarthritis.
- Cancers occurring more commonly in these individuals include endometrial, breast, prostate, colon, esophageal, and liver.
- Centripetal obesity, in which the waist-to-hip ratio is high, indicates a subset of individuals at much higher risk of cardiovascular diseases.
- Relative risk of HTN among obese adults aged 20 to 45 years is 5 to 6 times that of their nonobese counterparts.
- Relative risk of diabetes and of hypercholesterolemia is increased 2.9 and 1.5 times, respectively, in obese individuals.
- Several drugs are associated with weight gain of varying degree: amitriptyline, mirtazapine, atypical antipsychotics, gabapentin, pioglitazone, and sulfonylureas.
- Secondary causes of obesity include several endocrinopathies and syndromes, which result in abnormalities of systems regulating feeding behavior and/or energy expenditure (e.g., hypothyroidism, hypercortisolism, hypothalamic dysfunction, growth hormone deficiency, Prader-Willi syndrome, Bardet-Biedl syndrome, pseudohypoparathyroidism, polycystic ovary syndrome [PCOS], hypogonadism, insulinoma, menopause).

DIAGNOSIS

HISTORY

Obtain weight history, diet history, eating patterns, physical activity, and medications (past and current) and screen for sleep apnea. Ask about family history.

PHYSICAL EXAM

- Vital signs, including blood pressure (BP), heart rate, weight, height, waist circumference
- Appearance, including android (apple shaped/excess fat in abdomen) or gynoid (pear shaped/excess fat in thighs and buttock) fat deposition. Android has a higher predisposition to cardiovascular disease.
- In the office, BMI and waist-to-hip ratio are the most reliable methods to determine body fat. The gold standard test is the dual energy x-ray absorptiometry (DEXA) body composition.
- Oropharynx: Tooth enamel evaluation for chronic gastric reflux disease. Craniofacial abnormalities seen in conditions like Prader-Willi syndrome. A small posterior pharynx due to hypertrophic fat may be a clue for obstructive sleep apnea.
- Neck: Thyroid abnormalities, including asymmetrical or enlarged. Carotid bruits indicate atherosclerosis.
- Chest: Heart examination may reveal findings such as an enlarged heart, displaced point of maximal impulse, S3 and S4, all corresponding with cardiovascular disease and HTN. Atelectasis and bibasilar rales occur due to decreased lung compliance.
- Abdomen: appearance of subcutaneous and visceral fat deposition. Liver may be more prominent due to fatty liver.
- Musculoskeletal: Joint arthritis may be prevalent in obese patients. Careful to evaluate every joint, especially weight-bearing joints for effusion, range-of-motion abnormalities.
- Skin: maceration of the intertriginous skin folds. Acanthosis nigricans can be seen in Cushing, PCOS, and diabetes.

DIAGNOSTIC TESTS & INTERPRETATION

Initial Tests (lab, imaging)

- Complete metabolic panel, including glucose, liver function tests, lipid panel, thyroid-stimulating hormone, and HbA1c
- DEXA scan body fat composition: the gold standard test for determining body fat
- Other reliable tests include hydrostatic weighing, air displacement, skin calipers, body impedance.
- American College of Sports Medicine (ACSM) does not recommend routine exercise testing for all individuals with obesity. Instead, testing decisions are guided by the person's symptoms, medical history, and planned exercise intensity. Medical clearance is advised for those who are inactive, symptomatic, or have known cardiovascular, metabolic, or renal disease (3).

Diagnostic Procedures/Other

- Nocturnal pulse oximetry or formal sleep study
- Electrocardiogram, graded exercise treadmill Bruce ACSM protocol
- Exercise testing may be beneficial for obese patients. When performing standard exercise testing, the level of deconditioning typically observed in this population will necessitate a low initial workload (2 to 3 metabolic equivalents [METs]) and small workload increments per test stage (0.5 to 1.0 METs).
- Other comorbidities (e.g., HTN and other chronic diseases) or concerns (orthopedic limitations or elderly) may dictate modifications to the testing procedures.
- Use of leg or arm ergometry may enhance testing performance.
- Special attention to proper cuff size is necessary for accurate BP measurements.

TREATMENT

MEDICATION

- Pharmacologic therapy is appropriate for patients as an adjunct to lifestyle interventions to facilitate weight loss and prevent weight regain. Addition of exercise, resistance training, and adequate protein intake is paramount to successful treatment.
- Current criteria for the use of pharmacologic therapy for obesity are a BMI >30 kg/m^2 or a BMI >27 kg/m^2 in the presence of coexisting conditions (sleep apnea, coronary artery diseases [CADs], HTN, hyperlipidemia).

- There are several U.S. Food and Drug Administration (FDA)-approved medications for use in weight management. It is recommended to avoid all weight loss medications in pregnancy or breastfeeding (4).
- Orlistat (over-the-counter [OTC]: Alli; Rx: Xenical) inhibits gastric and pancreatic lipase, reducing fat absorption (4).
- Phentermine/topiramate (Qsymia)—phentermine is an adrenergic agonist promoting satiety via hypothalamic norepinephrine release and possibly leptin. Topiramate, a γ-aminobutyric acid (GABA) modulator used for seizures and migraines, may aid weight loss through glutamate inhibition and increased dopamine (5).
- Naltrexone/bupropion (Contrave)—naltrexone is an opioid antagonist; bupropion is a weak dopamine and norepinephrine reuptake inhibitor. Weight loss likely occurs via proopiomelanocortin (POMC) activation in the hypothalamus, reducing appetite and increasing energy use. Side effects include nausea, constipation, headache, vomiting, and dizziness; contraindicated in uncontrolled HTN, seizure disorders, eating disorders, drug/alcohol withdrawal, and MAOI use
- Liraglutide (Victoza/Saxenda) is a glucagon-like peptide-1 (GLP-1) receptor agonist approved for type 2 diabetes (Victoza) and chronic weight management (Saxenda).
- Semaglutide (once-weekly injection: Wegovy, Ozempic; or daily oral tablet: Rybelsus)—a GLP-1 receptor agonist approved for chronic weight management and type 2 diabetes. It activates GLP-1 receptors, which increases insulin secretion, decreases glucagon release, slows gastric emptying, and promotes satiety and reduced appetite.
- Tirzepatide (Zepbound), a once-weekly injectable, is approved for chronic weight management. It is a dual glucose-dependent insulinotropic polypeptide (GIP) and GLP-1 receptor agonist that boosts insulin, lowers glucagon, slows digestion, and promotes fullness, leading to significant weight loss.

ISSUES FOR REFERRAL

Ancillary services may be needed for a multidisciplinary approach, including psychologists, registered dietician, exercise physiologist, and physical therapy. Consider bariatric surgery consult (see below).

SURGERY/OTHER PROCEDURES

- Bariatric surgical treatments reduce calorie intake by restrictive or malabsorptive operations on the GI tract.
- The two main procedures are the Roux-en-Y bypass and the laparoscopic adjustable gastric banding, with similar weight loss outcomes.
- The National Institutes of Health guidelines for adults recommended the consideration of bariatric surgery with BMI at least 40 kg/m^2 or a BMI at least 35 kg/m^2 with significant obesity-related comorbidities.
- Bariatric surgery in adults improved diabetes (77% of patients), hyperlipidemia (83%), HTN (66%), and sleep apnea (88%).
- Adverse effects include perioperative complications, dehydration, bowel obstruction, anastomotic leaks, ulcers, cholelithiasis, and vitamin deficiencies.
- 30-day mortality rates are reported as 0.14% for bypass, 0.03% for gastric banding, and 0.08% for sleeve gastrectomy.

ONGOING CARE

DIET

For long-term weight maintenance, the U.S. Department of Agriculture's Dietary Guidelines for Americans recommends a healthy eating pattern focused on nutrient-dense foods (6). This includes a variety of vegetables, fruits, grains (with at least half being whole grains), low-fat dairy, and diverse protein sources. The guidelines also advise limiting daily intake of added sugars and saturated fats to less than 10% of total calories each, and consuming less than 2,300 mg of sodium. Alcohol should be avoided or consumed in moderation, defined as two drinks or less per day for men and one or less for women.

PATIENT EDUCATION

- Resting metabolic rate (RMR) is the energy your body expends at rest for essential functions like breathing and circulation, making it the largest part of your daily calorie use. You can measure it using indirect calorimetry or estimate it with formulas like Mifflin-St Jeor. RMR is crucial for calculating your total daily energy expenditure (TDEE) and planning calorie deficits.
- Calorie deficit guidelines:
  - Leading organizations like American Association of Clinical Endocrinologists (AACE), American Diabetes Association (ADA), ACSM, and International Society of Sports Nutrition (ISSN) recommend a 500- to 750-kcal/d deficit for weight loss. They advocate for personalized plans based on TDEE (RMR plus activity), stressing the importance of combining diet and exercise to preserve lean mass. They also endorse using RMR measurements or estimations to set personalized calorie goals.
- Exercise prescription is based on working on the model of frequency, intensity, and duration with goal in mind to encourage greater overall energy expenditure within the program for the obese individual.
- An effective exercise prescription for individuals with obesity aims to maximize overall energy expenditure. It should focus on aerobic activities using large muscle groups, performed 5 to 7 days per week for 45 to 60 minutes per session. Initially, the intensity should be moderate (40–60% of heart rate reserve), with an emphasis on increasing duration and frequency. The starting goal should be at least 150 minutes of moderate exercise weekly, with a long-term maintenance target of burning over 2,000 kcal per week. Due to a higher risk of orthopedic injury, lower-impact or non-weight-bearing activities may be necessary.
- The 2018 U.S. Department of Health and Human Services *Physical Activity Guidelines for Americans* (7):
- CDC strategies to prevent obesity (8):
  - The CDC suggests a multi-faceted approach to prevent obesity. This includes large-scale community media campaigns and small "point of decision" prompts to encourage active choices, like taking the stairs. Behavioral and social strategies teach people how to build physical activity into their daily lives. For youth, enhanced school-based physical education is key. Environmental and policy changes can increase access to places for physical activity and make communities more walkable. Finally, organized programs that promote active transport to school, such as walking or biking, are also effective.

REFERENCES

1. Emmerich SD, Fryar CD, Stierman B, et al. Obesity and severe obesity prevalence in adults: United States, August 2021–August 2023. NCHS Data Brief, no 508. National Center for Health Statistics; 2024. Accessed September 3, 2025. https://www.cdc.gov/nchs/data/databriefs/db508.pdf
2. Masters RK. Sources and severity of bias in estimates of the BMI–mortality association. *Popul Stud.* 2023;77(1):35–53.
3. Armstrong M, Paternostro-Bayles M, Conroy MB, et al. Preparticipation screening prior to physical activity in community lifestyle interventions. *Transl J Am Coll Sports Med.* 2018;3(22):176–180.
4. Yanovski SZ, Yanovski JA. Progress in pharmacotherapy for obesity. *JAMA.* 2021;326(2):129–130.
5. Johnson DB, Quick J. *Topiramate and Phentermine.* StatPearls Publishing; 2023. Updated March 27, 2023. Accessed August 29, 2025. https://www.ncbi.nlm.nih.gov/books/NBK482165
6. U.S. Department of Agriculture, U.S. Department of Health and Human Services. *Dietary Guidelines for Americans, 2020-2025.* 9th ed. U.S. Department of Agriculture and U.S. Department of Health and Human Services; 2020.
7. *Physical Activity Guidelines for Americans.* 2nd ed. U.S. Department of Health and Human Services; 2018.
8. Centers for Disease Control and Prevention. Strategies to Prevent Obesity and Other Chronic Diseases: *The CDC Guide to Strategies to Increase Physical Activity in the Community.* Department of Health and Human Services; 2011.

CLINICAL PEARLS

- Insulin resistance is most closely associated with visceral fat deposition and the release of adipokines and is poorly correlated with BMI.
- Obesity is associated with certain lifestyles but also has a genetic component. Certain alleles of the FTO gene have been strongly associated with obesity.
- Pharmacologic treatment is intended for those with a BMI >30 kg/m^2 or for those with a BMI >27 kg/m^2 and comorbidities. Surgery is indicated for patients with BMI >40 kg/m^2 or BMI >35 kg/m^2 with comorbidities, *per AACE and American Society for Metabolic and Bariatric Surgery (ASMBS) guidelines.*
- Treatment plans should be individualized and multifaceted. Diet and exercise are mainstays of treatment, but additional treatment options may be appropriate for some patients.

OCULAR TRAUMA, BLUNT

Arthur Davis Daniel, MD, CAQSM • Suraj A. Achar, MD, FAAFP, CAQSM

BASICS

DESCRIPTION

- Sports-related ocular injuries represent 1/3 of injuries leading to blindness in the United States.
- Traumatic ocular injuries are the leading cause of noncongenital blindness in persons <20 years old.
- Blunt ocular trauma makes up most sports-related eye injuries and the risk varies by sport.

EPIDEMIOLOGY

- 33% of ocular injuries resulting in blindness are related to sport.
- 11% of ocular injuries lead to long-term functional impairment.
- Majority of injuries are in athletes <18 years old.
- Males represent 81% of cases.
- Approximately 90% of these injuries are preventable with adequate eye protection.

ETIOLOGY AND PATHOPHYSIOLOGY

Blunt ocular trauma is classified based on whether the wall of the eyeball (the globe) has been broken. The two main categories are closed globe and open globe injuries.

- A closed globe injury occurs when the eye is struck by a blunt object, but the wall of the eye (the sclera and cornea) remains intact. Although the outer wall is not broken, the force of the impact can cause significant damage to the delicate structures inside the eye.
  - Pathophysiology: The injury happens from a rapid compression and expansion of the eyeball. Imagine a water balloon being squeezed and then released; this violent change in shape can tear blood vessels, dislocate the lens, and damage the retina.
  - Common causes: fists, airbags, and balls used in sports like baseball, basketball, or soccer
  - Resulting conditions: This type of trauma can lead to:
    - Traumatic hyphema: bleeding in the front chamber of the eye
    - Retinal detachment: The retina peels away from the back of the eye.
    - Macular hole: a small break in the macula, the part of the retina responsible for sharp, central vision
    - Orbital "blowout" fracture: a fracture of the thin bones that form the eye socket
- An open globe injury is more severe and is defined by a full-thickness breach of the cornea or sclera. The integrity of the eyeball has been compromised. This is an ophthalmologic emergency that typically requires immediate surgery to repair the globe and prevent permanent vision loss or loss of the eye itself.
  - Pathophysiology: These injuries are caused by an object that pierces, cuts, or ruptures the wall of the eye. They are subclassified based on the mechanism.
    - Rupture: caused by severe blunt trauma that causes the globe to burst at its weakest point
    - Laceration: a cut made by a sharp object
    - Penetrating injury: The object creates an entrance wound but does not exit the eye.
    - Perforating injury: The object creates both an entrance and an exit wound (passes through the eye).
    - Common causes: sharp objects like glass shards, metal fragments, knives, or high-velocity projectiles

RISK FACTORS

- Aged <18 years
- Low socioeconomic status
- Training >4 hours per day
- Inadequate or lack of eye protection (1),(2)

GENERAL PREVENTION

- 90% of ocular injuries are preventable with appropriate eye protection (3).
- Appropriate eye protection should be used in high-risk sports (3).
- Lenses should be made from a polycarbonate material or Trivex lens (3).

COMMONLY ASSOCIATED CONDITIONS

Orbital fracture is seen in 9.5% of sports-related ocular trauma.

DIAGNOSIS

HISTORY

- Mechanism of injury
  - Object type, size, and speed (e.g., ball, fist)
  - Use video replay if available to understand forces involved.
- Visual symptoms
  - Timing: Was vision loss immediate, delayed, or progressive?
  - Nature: Is it a complete blackout or a partial field cut?
  - Pattern: A "curtain" or "shadow" in the upper or lower visual field is highly suggestive of retinal detachment.
- Associated symptoms
  - Pain: Note any severe, deep ache (concern for increased intraocular pressure).
  - Diplopia (double vision): Is it present with gaze in a specific direction? (suggests orbital fracture with muscle entrapment)
  - Photopsias (flashes) or floaters: A sudden shower of floaters is a classic sign of a retinal tear or detachment.

PHYSICAL EXAM

- Begin with focused assessment to evaluate for any deformity, laceration, foreign body, proptosis, or erythema.
- Avoid any ocular pressure of contact with globe if there is concern for open globe injury.
- Assess visual acuity with a Snellen chart.
- Penlight exam can assess for anisocoria, hyphema, foreign bodies, and light reflexes.
- Check extraocular movement in all six cardinal positions to assess all ocular muscles.
- Slit lamp examination can be performed to better visualize the anterior and posterior segments as well as the retina.

DIFFERENTIAL DIAGNOSIS

- Commotio retinae
- Traumatic iritis
- Traumatic hyphema
- Orbital fracture
- Retrobulbar hematoma
- Traumatic macular hole
- Choroidal rupture

DIAGNOSTIC TESTS & INTERPRETATION

Initial Tests (lab, imaging)

CT scan: A noncontrast CT scan of the orbits and facial bones (with thin cuts) is the modality of choice for evaluating bony injuries. It is essential for identifying orbital fractures, such as a "blowout" fracture, and can reveal signs of muscle entrapment or a retrobulbar hematoma.

Follow-Up Tests & Special Considerations

- Further examination by an eye specialist should include tonometry to assess the intraocular pressures (1).
- Slit lamp examination improves visualization of the anterior and posterior segments of the eye (1).

TREATMENT

GENERAL MEASURES

- Sideline physicians should have a standard eye kit to include a penlight and Snellen chart.
- Visual acuity should be checked prior to penlight exam as bright light may affect acuity.

MEDICATION

- Cycloplegic agents are used to treat pain as they immobilize the ciliary body (4).
- Topical steroids can reduce ocular inflammation.

ADDITIONAL THERAPIES

For patients with traumatic hyphema, activity modification and bed rest are recommended to reduce the risk of rebleeding.

SURGERY/OTHER PROCEDURES

- **Lateral canthotomy and cantholysis**: A retrobulbar hematoma is an ophthalmologic emergency requiring immediate intervention. To prevent permanent vision loss from optic nerve ischemia, orbital decompression via lateral canthotomy and cantholysis should be performed within 2 hours of the injury.
- **Vitrectomy**: Traumatic macular holes may necessitate a vitrectomy to repair the macula. Surgical repair is most successful when performed within 3 months of the initial injury.

ONGOING CARE

FOLLOW-UP RECOMMENDATIONS

- Nearly all cases of ocular should include consultation or referral to an ophthalmologist.
- There are currently no established guidelines on return to play, but in general, patients should be pain free and has a good visual acuity.

REFERENCES

1. Toldi JP, Thomas JL. Evaluation and management of sports-related eye injuries. *Curr Sports Med Rep*. 2020;19(1):29–34.
2. Blanch RJ, Good PA, Shah P, et al. Visual outcomes after blunt ocular trauma. *Ophthalmology*. 2013;120(8):1588–1591.
3. Rodriguez JO, Lavina AM, Agarwal A. Prevention and treatment of common eye injuries in sports. *Am Fam Physician*. 2003;67(7):1481–1488.
4. Daniel AD, Achar S, Parikh M. Blunt ocular trauma in sport. *Curr Sports Med Rep*. 2023;22(11):375–379.

ADDITIONAL READING

- Dockery DM, Harrington MA, Gardiner MF, et al. A 5-year retrospective assessment of clinical presentation associated with sports injury in young people presenting to a tertiary eye center. *J Pediatr Ophthalmol Strabismus*. 2021;58(6):377–384.
- Gilani CJ, Yang A, Yonkers M, et al. Differentiating urgent and emergent causes of acute red eye for the emergency physician. *West J Emerg Med*. 2017;18(3):509–517.
- Haring RS, Sheffield ID, Canner JK, et al. Epidemiology of sports-related eye injuries in the United States. *JAMA Ophthalmol*. 2016;134(12):1382–1390.

CLINICAL PEARLS

- Sports-related ocular injuries represent 1/3 of eye injuries in the United States.
- Traumatic eye injuries are the leading cause of noncongenital blindness in persons <20 years old.
- Compression of the globe can result in a variety of injuries affecting both the anterior and posterior chambers of the eye.
- 90% of ocular injuries are preventable with proper eye protection.

OLECRANON BURSITIS

Alexei DeCastro, MD, FAAFP, CAQSM

BASICS

DESCRIPTION

Common condition, a superficial bursal or synovial-lined sack sits over the olecranon process of the ulna that fills with fluid

EPIDEMIOLOGY

- Bursitis (from all sources) accounts for approximately 2/10,000 hospitalizations a year (1).
- Annual incidence of 10/100,000 (1)
- Most common in males 18 to 88 years of age (1)
- 75% of cases are noninfectious and occur when repeated trauma or injuries

ETIOLOGY AND PATHOPHYSIOLOGY

- Direct injury/trauma
- Prolonged pressure (elbow leaning on table)
- Overuse
- Crystal induced (gout or pseudogout)
- Inflammatory rheumatoid or psoriatic arthritis,
- Infectious

RISK FACTORS

Favor Septic Bursitis	Favor Nonseptic Bursitis
• Immunocompromised	• Trauma
• Diabetes	• History of inflammatory conditions (inflammatory arthritis, gout)
• Systemic symptoms	

Warning: Patients with gout and rheumatoid arthritis may also have secondary infection of the bursa.

- Septic bursitis (1):
  - Altered immune system
  - Diabetes
  - Skin irritation or interruption around the area
  - Hematoma
- Noninfectious (1):
  - Trauma
  - Overuse
  - Any occupation in which elbow is flexed on regular basis or traumatized

GENERAL PREVENTION

- Infectious:
  - Care of overlying skin to prevent abrasions, lacerations
  - Good control of underlying medical conditions
- Noninfectious:
  - Soft pads not effective, hard or supported elbow pads, that is, like those worn by skateboarders
  - Avoid overuse.

COMMONLY ASSOCIATED CONDITIONS

- Rheumatoid arthritis—rheumatoid nodules
- Gout, pseudogout
- Repetitive flexion of elbow:
  - Direct trauma

DIAGNOSIS

HISTORY

- History of repetitive flexion of elbow (2)[A]
- History of trauma (2)[A]
- History of abovementioned systemic disease (2)[A]
- History of systemic inflammatory response syndrome (SIRS) criteria (2)[A]
- High risk of not only infection but also systemic involvement (1)[A]
- Temperature >38°C
- Heart rate (HR) >90 beats/min
- Respiratory rate (RR) >20 breaths/min
- White blood cell (WBC) >12,000/mL

PHYSICAL EXAM

- Posterior elbow bursal swelling
- Skin erythema and posterior elbow tenderness
- Should have normal range of motion (ROM) of elbow, if not, concern or joint involvement
- Overlying skin lesions, concern for infections
- Acute, may just be tendon over olecranon:
  - It is very difficult to distinguish between a septic and nonseptic arthritis when a patient does not have systemic symptoms (1),(3).

DIFFERENTIAL DIAGNOSIS

ALERT

A number of meta-analysis studies have attempted to develop algorithms for evaluating and treating olecranon bursitis, especially trying to separate out differentiating between septic and nonseptic bursitis and have failed.

- There are some general guidelines that can be followed.
- Chronic bursitis (>2 weeks) will produce a more thickened bursa and appear like "Popeye elbow."
- Bursitis with chronic drainage requires further investigation (i.e., imaging, aspiration, surgical removal of bursa with pathology and culture) to rule out chronic atypical infections (i.e., fungus or cancer).

DIAGNOSTIC TESTS & INTERPRETATION

- Historically, the bursa was drained and the fluid was analyzed to rule out septic bursitis.
- Recent meta-analysis revealed that glucose level, protein, and WBC content were not accurate in distinguishing between septic and infectious bursitis (1),(2),(3)[A].
- Gram stain was helpful with sensitivity approaching ≥90%.
- Radiographs may be useful in chronic cases to rule out tophi, spurs, foreign bodies, etc.

- The use of point-of-care ultrasound or magnetic resonance imaging (MRI) can be very useful in detecting fluid pockets but cannot differentiate between inflammation and infection.
- 75% of olecranon bursitis is noninfectious.
- Of the other 25%, systemic symptoms are the most accurate way to determine if the joint is septic, that is, inability to flex elbow and SIRS criteria.
- Open skin lesions, diabetes, and immunocompromised patients are of particular concern:
  - Meta-analysis of multiple studies found that aspiration did little to affect the course of the problem and that aspiration was associated with an increase in complications (3)[A].

TREATMENT

- For nonseptic bursitis, protection of the bursa from microtrauma with a stiff or hard type of elbow guard or pad has been useful (1)[A],(3)[A].
- Occupational modifications for repetitive work or elimination of microtrauma has been useful for nonseptic bursitis.

ALERT

- If the patient has no contraindication, nonsteroidal anti-inflammatory drugs (NSAIDs) can be used for pain. Caution should be used in patients with kidney disease or who are on disease-modifying antirheumatic drugs (DMARDs) for rheumatoid arthritis (2)[A].
- Recent literature shows that cases of noninfectious acute bursitis (75% of all cases of bursitis) do best with supportive management, no aspiration, or steroid injection. Protection of the bursa from continued microtrauma with a "hard" elbow protector and medication for pain relief. Be aware that chronic bursitis could be a sign of other pathology such as atypical infections or cancer and could be associated with other chronic conditions.
- A small number of patients with acute bursitis are septic. This condition can be more difficult to diagnose, and in these patients, aspiration of the bursa is the gold standard.
- *Staphylococcus aureus* is the most common pathogen from infected olecranon bursitis. Broad anterior treatment covering *S. aureus* is preferred. Intravenous (IV) antibiotic without systemic symptoms is not superior than treating the patient with oral (PO) antibiotics (1)[A],(3)[A].
- Any patient suspected of septic bursitis should have the bursa aspirated either in office with a large gauge needle or in the operating room (OR) with bursectomy.
- Synovectomy may be necessary to make the diagnosis or to treat the condition if nonsurgical treatment fails.
- Injection of doxycycline via ultrasound guidance has been shown to be effective in both aseptic and septic bursitis in short- and long-term case series, even after surgical failure or if surgical contraindications.
- Patients with chronic bursitis or chronic drainage should be referred to a surgeon for consideration of bursectomy (1)[A].

ONGOING CARE

PATIENT EDUCATION

- The care of patients with olecranon bursitis has changed over the years to a supportive approach.
- Unless septic bursitis is suspected, the bursa should not be aspirated or injected with corticosteroids.
- Chronic bursitis may require doxycycline injection versus surgical removal of the bursa if recurrent.

REFERENCES

1. Brown OS, Smith TO, Parsons T, et al. Management of septic and aseptic prepatellar bursitis: a systematic review. *Arch Orthop Trauma Surg*. 2022;142(10):2445–2457.
2. Nchinda NN, Wolf JM. Clinical management of olecranon bursitis: a review. *J Hand Surg Am*. 2021;46(6):501–506.
3. Reilly D, Kamineni S. Olecranon bursitis. *J Shoulder Elbow Surg*. 2016;25(1):158–167.

ADDITIONAL READING

- Baumbach SF, Lobo CM, Badyine I, et al. Prepatellar and olecranon bursitis: literature review and development of a treatment algorithm. *Arch Orthop Trauma Surg*. 2014;134(3):359–370.
- Blackwell JR, Hay BA, Bolt AM, et al. Olecranon bursitis: a systematic overview. *Shoulder Elbow*. 2014;6(3):182–190.
- Pangia J, Rizvi TJ. *Olecranon Bursitis*. StatPearls Publishing; 2024. Updated June 12, 2023. Accessed August 14, 2025. https://www.ncbi.nlm.nih.gov/books/NBK470291/
- Sayegh ET, Strauch RJ. Treatment of olecranon bursitis: a systematic review. *Arch Orthop Trauma Surg*. 2014;134(11):1517–1536.

CLINICAL PEARLS

- Current evidence favors treating nonseptic bursitis conservatively without drainage.
- Patients with an olecranon bursitis with any of the following are not only at higher risk of septic bursitis but also of systemic infection:
  - Fever
  - Immunocompromised
  - History of recent surgery
- Aspiration and the injection of corticosteroids into nonseptic olecranon bursa have been associated with an increased risk of complications (infection, chronic fistula, skin atrophy). Corticosteroid injection into the bursa is no longer recommended.
- Needle aspiration should not be done for symptomatic treatment. It should only be used to help diagnose infectious bursitis. Avoid risks of introducing infection by advancing a needle through cellulitis as well as avoiding intra-articular aspiration of the elbow joint.

ORAL LACERATIONS

Brent H. Messick, MD, MS, FAAFP, FASCM, CAQSM ▪ Kevin E. Burroughs, MD, CAQSM, FAMSSM

BASICS

DESCRIPTION

- Soft tissue injury in the orofacial area
- Typically results from a direct blow to the mouth resulting from a fall or impact by an opponent or object
- Lacerations may be an indirect result of an individual biting the cheek or lip.

EPIDEMIOLOGY

- Most common in contact sports not requiring face protection (basketball, soccer, baseball, wrestling)
- Other at-risk sports include bicycling, in-line skating, and gymnastics.
- Teenagers and children younger than age 10 years are most susceptible (1).

Incidence

As high as 1.06/100,000 athlete exposures (2)

Prevalence

The overall prevalence of dentofacial injuries among collective contact sports participants was approximately 30% (3).

RISK FACTORS

- Participation in collision or contact sports
- *Not* using a mouth guard during sports activity

COMMONLY ASSOCIATED CONDITIONS

- Fracture of the mandible, dental arch, palate
- Dental luxation or avulsion
- Tooth fracture
- Temporomandibular joint (TMJ) trauma
- Vessel injury
- Nerve transection
- Salivary gland duct injury

DIAGNOSIS

HISTORY

- Determine where and how the injury was sustained; common in sports but also seen as a result of fighting, assault, and abuse
- Determine areas of numbness or loss of muscle control to evaluate for nerve injury.
- Determine last tetanus immunization because wounds are often contaminated from the environment as well as from the oral cavity.
- Sensitivity of teeth (Assess for occult dental trauma.)

PHYSICAL EXAM

- Significant hemorrhage due to the abundant blood supply in the face and maxillofacial areas
- Visible defects with "through and through" lacerations (lacerations involving all layers: mucosa, muscular, subcutaneous [SC], and skin)
- Patient distress
- Head and neck examination for signs of neural injury
- Palpate over TMJ to evaluate for subcondylar mandibular fracture.
- Test mobility of jaw.
- Evaluate laceration for length and depth as well as for affected structures, including nerves and vessels (transected nerves need to be referred for surgical repair).
- Buccal lacerations need to be evaluated for parotid salivary flow from the Stensen duct. Parotid orifice is located opposite the maxillary 1st molar. Saliva should flow from the opening when the parotid gland is palpated (disruptions of the duct should be referred for repair).
- Evaluate for normal occlusion of the teeth. Dental examination should be performed to check for fractured, loose, or avulsed teeth.

DIFFERENTIAL DIAGNOSIS

- Contusion
- Abrasion
- Dental trauma (luxation, avulsion, fracture)

DIAGNOSTIC TESTS & INTERPRETATION

- If there is a clinical suspicion of a fracture or foreign body such as a tooth fragment, appropriate studies should be ordered: panoramic x-rays for teeth, plain radiographs for foreign bodies, or computed tomography (CT) for facial fractures, etc.
- Bone fixation/repair, if needed, should be performed before soft tissue closure.

TREATMENT

GENERAL MEASURES

- Most oral lacerations can be left to heal by secondary intention. Only those that are >1 cm, gapping at rest, or require hemostasis may need to be repaired (4).
- Copious irrigation of the wound to remove foreign debris and wound contaminants
- Clean with antiseptic scrub.
- Regional anesthesia via nerve block is preferred over local injection to minimize tissue distortion, making approximation easier (especially for the vermilion border).
- Infraorbital nerve block numbs the upper lip.
- Mental nerve block numbs the anterior lower lip and teeth.
- Maxillary nerve second division numbs the entire maxilla on the blocked side.
- Interrupted stitches using 3–0 chromic or similar absorbable suture material
- Inside-out and bottom-up technique; eliminating dead spaces helps prevent hematoma and subsequent infection.

- Muscular layer: 4–0 slow-absorbing suture; polyglactin suture breaks down more slowly than chromic suture, maintaining wound strength for ~30 days.
- Oral mucosa: 3–0 or 4–0 chromic or other absorbable suture material on a cutting needle
- Small intraoral lacerations may be left to heal by secondary intention.
- SC layer: 3–0 or 4–0 plain gut on a cutting needle
- Skin: 4–0 to 6–0 nylon
- Lip defects involving >33% usually require flap reconstruction (5).
- Suture orbicularis oris first (see above suture suggestions).
- Loosely approximate the vermilion border (very important for cosmetic appearance) with a suture at the junction with the skin and then proceed in layers as above.
- Most tongue lacerations can be treated conservatively and do not require sutures unless necessary for hemostasis (6).
- Lacerations involving the muscular layer or labial margin of the tongue require sutures.
- Lacerations involving the tip may require sutures to prevent a "forked tongue." Most can be left alone. Anterior tongue lacerations are rare and are often self-inflicted. Small ones can close, but large ones will require sutures. If the tongue heals "forked," it can also be corrected later if necessary.
- Repair in layers: 4–0 slow-resorbing polyglactin suture for the muscle and chromic suture for the mucosa.
- Small lacerations can be allowed to close by secondary intention if cosmetically acceptable.
- Hemorrhage typically from disruption of the muscular layer may require a stitch to obtain hemostasis.
- Large gaping lacerations can be repaired with one or two vertical sutures.

ADDITIONAL THERAPIES

- Tetanus immunization status
- Prophylactic antibiotics for severe or grossly contaminated laceration (Coverage for the oral flora includes amoxicillin, penicillin, clindamycin, or erythromycin.)
- Prophylactic antibiotic coverage for less severe lacerations can be considered due to an infection rate of 10% (6).
- If fracture is present, leave wound open until fixation is completed.

ADMISSION, INPATIENT, AND NURSING CONSIDERATIONS

Initial stabilization:

- Evaluate airway, breathing, and circulation (ABCs).
- Control hemorrhage.
- Protect the airway if compromised.

ONGOING CARE

FOLLOW-UP RECOMMENDATIONS

- Laceration associated with fracture or involving nerves or salivary ducts should be referred for definitive care as soon as possible.
- Refer dental trauma to a dentist or oral surgeon.
- Patients receiving antibiotics should be rechecked in 48 hours to ensure improvement and antibiotic susceptibility.

REFERENCES

1. Park HK, Park JY, Choi NR, et al. Sports-related oral and maxillofacial injuries: a 5-year retrospective study, Pusan National University Dental Hospital. *J Oral Maxillofacial Surg*. 2021;79(1):203.e1–203.e8.
2. Werlich MO, Honnef LR, Bett JVS, et al. Prevalence of dentofacial injuries in contact sports players: a systematic review and meta-analysis. *Dent Traumatol*. 2020;36(5):477–488.
3. Soto F, Murphy A, Heaton H. Critical procedures in pediatric emergency medicine. *Emerg Med Clin North Am*. 2013;31(1):335–376.
4. Marks M, Polecritti D, Bergman R, et al. Emergent soft tissue repair in facial trauma. *Facial Plast Surg Clin North Am*. 2017;25(4):593–604.
5. Katsetos SL, Nagurka R, Caffrey J, et al. Antibiotic prophylaxis for oral lacerations: our emergency department's experience. *Int J Emerg Med*. 2016;9(1):24.
6. Gonsalves CL, Zhu JW, Kim GY, et al. Surgical versus conservative management of tongue lacerations in the acute care setting: a systematic review of the literature. *Paediatr Child Health*. 2021;27(1):32–42.

ADDITIONAL READING

- Echlin P, McKeag DB. Maxillofacial injuries in sport. *Curr Sports Med Rep*. 2004;3(1):25–32.
- Echlin PS, Upshur REG, Peck DM, et al. Craniomaxillofacial injury in sport: a review of prevention research. *Br J Sports Med*. 2005;39(5):254–263.
- Labella CR, Smith BW, Sigurdsson A. Effect of mouthguards on dental injuries and concussions in college basketball. *Med Sci Sports Exerc*. 2002;34(1):41–44.
- Mark AM. Staying in the game with mouthguards. *J Am Dent Assoc*. 2022;153(6):592.
- Ranalli DN, Demas PN. Orofacial injuries from sport: preventive measures for sports medicine. *Sports Med*. 2002;32(7):409–418.

CLINICAL PEARLS

- Stitches placed inside the mouth will dissolve on their own. Sutures in the skin should be removed in 4 to 5 days to prevent significant scarring.
- Return to play depends on the severity of the injury, chance of reinjury, and availability/feasibility of protection for the wound.

OSGOOD-SCHLATTER DISEASE

Ayo Adu, MD, DC, CAQSM

BASICS

DESCRIPTION

- Traction apophysitis of the tibial tubercle at the insertion of the patellar tendon
- Overuse injury due to repetitive strain or microtrauma of the secondary ossification center of the tibial tubercle

EPIDEMIOLOGY

- One of the most common causes of knee pain in active adolescents
- More prevalent in male gender
- Prevalence among children between the ages of 12 to 15 years is 10% (1)[A].
- Age of onset coincides with growth spurts: males ages 10 to 15 years and females ages 8 to 13 years.

ETIOLOGY AND PATHOPHYSIOLOGY

- Chronic repetitive strain and microtrauma cause chronic avulsion of the secondary ossification center (2).
- The force is increased after periods of rapid growth.
- Chronic avulsion may cause separation of the patellar tendon insertion from the tibial tubercle, swelling, and enlargement.

RISK FACTORS

- Adolescents
- Male gender
- Sports that involve running and jumping
- Activities that involve direct contact with the knee (e.g., kneeling)
- Higher body weight
- Quadriceps muscle tightness (3)[B]
- History of Sever disease (4)[B]

DIAGNOSIS

HISTORY

- Anterior knee pain and swelling
- Symptoms are bilateral in 20–30% of patients.
- Pain begins as a dull ache that gradually increases with continued activity.
- Pain is worsened by running, jumping, direct trauma, kneeling, and squatting.
- Pain is improved with rest.

PHYSICAL EXAM

- Enlarged prominent tibial tubercle
- Tenderness of the proximal tibial tubercle at the patellar tendon insertion
- Poor flexibility of the quadriceps and hamstrings
- Able to maintain full, symmetric knee extension with active straight leg raise
- Inability to maintain symmetric knee extension with straight leg raise, especially in event of acute onset of pain at tibial tubercle, is highly suggestive for tibial tubercle avulsion fracture which requires imaging and likely temporary immobilization.
- Pain is exacerbated by knee extension against resistance, active or passive knee flexion, or by direct trauma to the tibial tubercle.

DIFFERENTIAL DIAGNOSIS

- Patellar tendonitis
- Sinding-Larsen-Johansson syndrome
- Tibial tubercle avulsion fracture
- Tibial plateau fracture
- Patellar fracture
- Osteochondritis dissecans
- Patellofemoral syndrome
- Pes anserine bursitis
- Patellar tendon rupture
- Patellar subluxation
- Chondromalacia patellae
- Hoffa disease (infrapatellar fat pad impingement)
- Osteomyelitis
- Tumor

DIAGNOSTIC TESTS & INTERPRETATION

- Osgood-Schlatter disease is a clinical diagnosis, and radiographs are not required for diagnosis. However, they may be helpful to evaluate for other conditions, such as acute tibial apophyseal fracture, osteomyelitis, and tumors (5)[A].
- X-ray:
  - Lateral view may show an elevated tibial tubercle with anterior soft tissue swelling, fragmentation of the tibial tubercle, or calcification and ossicle formation in the distal patellar tendon.

TREATMENT

GENERAL MEASURES

- Relative rest or activity modification is recommended.
- Activity as tolerated, including sports, is allowed as long as symptoms are tolerable and resolve within 24 hours.

- Pain control with hamstring stretching to reduce load on the tibial apophysis
- Protective pad may be worn over tibial tubercle to prevent direct trauma.
- Ice application especially after exercise
- Nonsteroidal anti-inflammatory drugs (NSAIDs) or acetaminophen can be used for up to 8 to 10 days as needed for significant pain not relieved by conservative measures.
- If significant symptoms, consider physical therapy consult.

ADDITIONAL THERAPIES

- Osgood-Schlatter disease is usually a benign and self-limited condition (6)[C] that resolves once growth plate closes at skeletal maturity, usually between the ages 14 and 18 years.
- Usual course is 6 to 18 months.
- Symptoms especially pain with kneeling may continue into adulthood despite conservative measures in 5–10% of patients.
- Recommended exercises include stretching of the quadriceps and hamstring and strengthening of the quadriceps.
- A subset of adolescents may experience prolonged pain associated with decreased sports-related function and quality of life (7)[B],(8)[B].

SURGERY/OTHER PROCEDURES

Surgical excision of the enlarged tibial tubercle and free ossicles may be considered in skeletally mature patients if conservative treatment has failed.

REFERENCES

1. Haines M, Pirlo L, Bowles KA, et al. Describing frequencies of lower-limb apophyseal injuries in children and adolescents: a systematic review. *Clin J Sport Med.* 2022;32(4):433–439.
2. Gholve PA, Scher DM, Khakharia S, et al. Osgood Schlatter syndrome. *Curr Opin Pediatr.* 2007;19(1):44–50.
3. Nakase J, Goshima K, Numata H, et al. Precise risk factors for Osgood-Schlatter disease. *Arch Orthop Trauma Surg.* 2015;135(9):1277–1281.
4. Watanabe H, Fujii M, Yoshimoto M, et al. Pathogenic factors associated with Osgood-Schlatter disease in adolescent male soccer players: a prospective cohort study. *Orthop J Sports Med.* 2018;6(8):2325967118792192.
5. Kabiri L, Tapley H, Tapley S. Evaluation and conservative treatment for Osgood-Schlatter disease: a critical review of the literature. *Int J Ther Rehabil.* 2014;21:91–96.
6. Ladenhauf HN, Seitlinger G, Green DW. Osgood-Schlatter disease: a 2020 update of a common knee condition in children. *Curr Opin Pediatr.* 2020;32(1):107–112.
7. Holden S, Olesen JL, Winiarski LM, et al. Is the prognosis of Osgood-Schlatter poorer than anticipated? A prospective cohort study with 24-month follow-up. *Orthop J Sports Med.* 2021;9(8):23259671211022239.
8. Guldhammer C, Rathleff MS, Jensen HP, et al. Long-term prognosis and impact of Osgood-Schlatter disease 4 years after diagnosis: a retrospective study. *Orthop J Sports Med.* 2019;7(10):2325967119878136.

CLINICAL PEARLS

- Athletes may participate in athletic activity as tolerated. Pain level should generally be tolerable, without a decrease in performance, and resolve within 24 hours of activity. If performance is decreased, the athlete should discontinue activity.
- Athlete should not "play through the pain." Instead, pain should be used as a measure of when to stop activity.
- Pain will resolve when the growth plate closes.
- Future complications can include persistent enlargement of the tibial tubercle, pain with kneeling, and possibly some limitation of activities.
- Prognosis is excellent, provided the athlete demonstrates good compliance with stretching recommendations.

OSTEITIS PUBIS

Shane Geffe, MD • Daniel C. Herman, MD, PhD, FAAPMR, FACSM, FISBS, CAQSM • Sara N. Raiser, MD, FAAPMR, CAQSM

BASICS

DESCRIPTION

- Inflammation of the pubic symphysis and surrounding tissue is often brought on by overuse in the athletic population.
- Should always be considered when treating athletes with groin pain
- Magnetic resonance imaging (MRI) is diagnostic modality of choice, but pubic symphyseal changes may be evident on radiographs.
- The condition is usually self-limited but may require a lengthy period of rest.
- Often coexists with femoroacetabular impingement

EPIDEMIOLOGY

- 5 to 80 cases per thousand in athletes (1)[C]
- Increased incidence in kicking sports, distance runners, and American football
- Males affected more than females

ETIOLOGY AND PATHOPHYSIOLOGY

- Histologic evidence supports the inflammatory paradigm, with increased marrow fibrosis and plasma cell content.
- Microtrauma to the pubic symphysis and surrounding tissues leads to inflammatory response.
- Several pathophysiologic theories exist—chronic inflammation secondary to trauma, infectious, reflex sympathetic dystrophic, microthrombotic, and avascular necrosis.
- Imbalance occurs between adductor muscles resulting in asynchronization and shearing of the symphysis.
- In patients with femoroacetabular impingement, compensatory alterations to the pelvic biomechanics can impart additional shear stress on the pubic symphysis.

RISK FACTORS

- Pregnancy
- Pelvic trauma
- Pelvic surgery
- Cutting sports, kicking sports, long-distance running
- Relative hip adductor weakness
- Increase in training intensity

GENERAL PREVENTION

- Intentional hip adductor strengthening and pelvic stabilization program
- Avoidance of over-training
- Early diagnosis and treatment

COMMONLY ASSOCIATED CONDITIONS

- Femoroacetabular impingement
- Rheumatoid arthritis

DIAGNOSIS

HISTORY

- Dull or achy pain localized to the pubic tubercle or more specifically the symphysis
- Indolent onset that progresses and may be associated with an increase in training load or venture into new sport/activity
- Exacerbation by shear forces on symphysis (navigation of stairs, long-distance running, rapid changes in lateral direction, rapid hip flexion/extension such as with kicking, side-lying, Valsalva)

PHYSICAL EXAM

- Tenderness to palpation over pubic tubercle/symphysis
- Pain with resisted hip adduction or sit-up maneuvers
- Single leg hop
- "Pubic spring test": Pressure over pubic tubercle with subsequent release causes pain at or near symphysis.
- Other conditions should be ruled out including:
  - Inguinal hernia
  - Core muscle origin/insertion injury
  - Pelvic inflammatory disease in females

DIFFERENTIAL DIAGNOSIS

- Adductor strain
- Core muscle injury (athletic pubalgia)
- Pubic bone stress injury
- Lumbar radiculopathy
- Inguinal hernia
- Pelvic inflammatory disease
- Femoroacetabular impingement

DIAGNOSTIC TESTS & INTERPRETATION

- Radiographs of the pelvis should be obtained on initial evaluation, including anteroposterior (AP) and "flamingo" views; characteristic findings on AP view include sclerosis, osteophytosis, or symphyseal widening; may be normal
- The "flamingo view":
  - Have patient stand on one leg while AP view of pelvis is taken.
  - If there is >2 mm of pubic tubercle displacement or pubic cleft measures >7 mm, this supports pelvic instability and thus osteitis pubis.
- MRI is more sensitive (100%) and thus the preferred modality. Characteristic findings include symphyseal or periarticular edema (2)[B]. However, symphyseal edema may be found in as high as 47% in asymptomatic athletes so results should be interpreted with caution (3)[B].

- Musculoskeletal ultrasound can detect articular/chondral abnormalities as well as the presence of periarticular edema but with reduced sensitivity as compared to MRI.
- Intrasymphyseal corticosteroid injection may provide symptom relief as well as aid in diagnosis (1)[C].

TREATMENT

GENERAL MEASURES

- Conservative treatment is best, with >90% of patients responding positively to nonoperative treatments albeit with variable treatment durations (1)[C].
- Rest from offending activity until pain-free with ambulation and light jogging, followed by abdominal and hip strengthening exercises allows almost all athletes to return to a normal life outside of sports.
- Duration of sport cessation is variable depending on sport, level of competition, position, and degree of pathology. Return to sport is typically on the order of months but can be as long as a year.

MEDICATION

Effective pharmacotherapy can include nonsteroidal anti-inflammatory drugs (NSAIDs), oral, or intrasymphyseal corticosteroids.

ISSUES FOR REFERRAL

Referral to orthopedic surgeon may be necessary if failure of conservative measures after 6 months.

SURGERY/OTHER PROCEDURES

- <10% of patients require surgery (5)[C].
- Curettage of necrotic tissue (most common surgical intervention)
- Arthrodesis
- Pubic resection
- Addressing femoroacetabular impingement with arthroscopy can result in significant improvement in athletes with comorbid osteitis pubis (6)[B].

COMPLEMENTARY AND ALTERNATIVE MEDICINE

- Bisphosphonates demonstrated safe and mildly effective response in a small cohort (1)[C]
- Platelet-rich plasma
- Extracorporeal shock wave therapy has been shown to shorten return-to-play time (4)[A].
- Insertional abdominus rectus percutaneous tenotomy

ONGOING CARE

FOLLOW-UP RECOMMENDATIONS

Reasonable to follow up sparingly in relative rest period, with monthly reevaluation after progression into rehabilitation

PATIENT EDUCATION

- Patients should be counseled on average return-to-play times, as they can be lengthy.
- Addressing biomechanics of training and position-related fundamentals is paramount.

PROGNOSIS

- >90% of cases resolve with conservative therapy.
- Up to 25% of cases can recur (3)[B].
- The extension of edema from the bone into the surrounding structures on MRI imaging is associated with a worse prognosis and delayed return to activity (1)[C].
- 30% of athletes that failed conservative treatment and underwent pubic curettage did not return to previous level of activity (5)[B].

COMPLICATIONS

- Avascular necrosis of the pubic bone
- Stress fracture
- Infection
- Chronic pain

REFERENCES

1. Amer ML, Omar K, Malde S, et al. The challenges in diagnosis and management of osteitis pubis: an algorithm based on current evidence. *BJUI Compass*. 2022;3(4):267–276.
2. Koh E, Boyle J. Pubic apophysitis in elite Australian rules football players: MRI findings and the utility of VIBE sequences in evaluating athletes with groin pain. *Clin Radiol*. 2020;75(4):293–301.
3. Paajanen H, Hermunen H, Ristolainen L, et al. Long-standing groin pain in contact sports: a prospective case-control and MRI study. *BMJ Open Sport Exerc Med*. 2019;5(1):e000507.
4. Rhim HC, Shin J, Kang J, et al. Use of extracorporeal shockwave therapies for athletes and physically active individuals: a systematic review. *Br J Sports Med*. 2024;58(3):154–163.
5. Athanasiou V, Ampariotou A, Lianou I, et al. Osteitis pubis in athletes: a literature review of current surgical treatment. *Cureus*. 2022;14(3):e22976.
6. Saito M, Utsunomiya H, Hatakeyama A, et al. Hip arthroscopic management can improve osteitis pubis and bone marrow edema in competitive soccer players with femoroacetabular impingement. *Am J Sports Med*. 2019;47(2):408–419.

ADDITIONAL READING

Yax J, Cheng D. Osteomyelitis pubis: a rare and elusive diagnosis. *West J Emerg Med*. 2014;15(7):880–882.

CLINICAL PEARLS

- This diagnosis should be considered in any patient with groin pain.
- High comorbidity with femoroacetabular impingement, which may alter pelvic biomechanics
- No evidence-based guideline for treatment of this condition exists, and the majority of these patients improve with rest.
- Conservative and surgical management of this condition often results in extensive rest and meticulous, precise, and very attentive to detail rehabilitation.

OSTEOARTHRITIS

Kevin deWeber, MD, FAMSSM, FAAFP, FACSM, RMSK

BASICS

DESCRIPTION
A predominantly noninflammatory, slowly progressing, degenerative condition of articular cartilage, sometimes known as "degenerative joint disease"

EPIDEMIOLOGY

Incidence
Exact incidence depends on the definition or technology used to identify. Knee or hip replacement for osteoarthritis (OA) is performed on ~1/3 of Americans.

Prevalence
- Radiographic prevalence exceeds symptomatic prevalence.
- Symptomatic prevalence significantly increases with age and varies with affected joint, with highest prevalence in the knee and hand, followed by hip, glenohumeral, foot/ankle, and acromioclavicular (1).

ETIOLOGY AND PATHOPHYSIOLOGY
- OA is caused by an imbalance between breakdown and repair of joint tissue:
  - Cartilage matrix (collagen, water, proteoglycans) slowly degrades.
  - Chondrocytes slowly die off; those that remain are unable to maintain adequate repair.
  - Mechanical forces contribute to progressive cartilage loss.
- Early stages: cartilage fibrillation (fine fraying)
- Middle and late stages: formation of extra subchondral bone and cysts and osteophytes (usually at joint margins)
- Predominantly noninflammatory but occasional inflammatory clinical flares

RISK FACTORS
- Systemic risk factors (1) contribute to development of OA by creating an environment where the joint is vulnerable:
  - Age: strongest risk factor—10-fold increase between ages 30 and 65 years
  - Obesity: linear increase in risk with rising body mass index (BMI); increases risk in hand, knee, and hip, so metabolic as well as biomechanical factors involved
  - Gender: females with higher severity and prevalence
  - Nutritional factors: no conclusive data on diet, vitamins, or minerals
  - High bone mineral density increases risk.
- Joint biomechanical risk factors (1) cause direct trauma to articular cartilage:
  - Joint injury (fractures, dislocations, ligament and meniscal ruptures, articular surface damage)
  - Occupations involving high physical demands: repetitive use of joints, heavy lifting, frequent squatting
  - Sports: knee OA associated with elite-level impact sports; hip OA associated with elite-level impact sports, especially handball, soccer, and hockey; competitive running is associated with more knee and hip OA compared to recreational running (2)[A].
  - Abnormal joint biomechanics (dysplasia [hip OA], leg length inequality [knee OA], malalignment, instability, abnormal innervation). Cam-type femoral-acetabular impingement predisposes to hip OA.

Genetics
- OA has a genetic component, especially in women, and comprises 30–65% of risk.
- 21 genes identified to contribute (1)

GENERAL PREVENTION
- Avoidance of joint trauma or extremes of joint activity (immobilization or gross overuse)
- Weight reduction

COMMONLY ASSOCIATED CONDITIONS
- Degenerative meniscal tears in knee OA
- Labral tears in hip OA
- Calcium pyrophosphate deposition disease (CPPD)—unsure if causes OA or associated with it

DIAGNOSIS
- OA is diagnosed primarily through history and physical examination and confirmed by plain films. It can be classified as primary or secondary.
  - Primary OA (idiopathic): related to systemic risk factors mentioned earlier; may be particular or generalized
  - Secondary OA: Causes include previous trauma/internal derangement and inflammatory or deposition joint diseases (e.g., gout, rheumatoid arthritis [RA], CPPD).
- Most commonly affected joints include the distal interphalangeal (DIP) and proximal interphalangeal (PIP) joints of the hands; carpometacarpal (CMC) joint of the thumb; and the 1st metatarsophalangeal (MTP), hips, knees, cervical spine, and lumbar spine.

HISTORY
- Insidious onset over months to years is typical.
- Most common symptoms are pain (especially after excessive activity), crepitus or grinding, and noninflammatory joint swelling.
- There is typically short-lived (<30 minutes) stiffness after immobilization, improving with mobilization.
- Some patients experience muscular weakness in the surrounding soft tissue and pseudo instability.
- There may be a personal history of prior joint trauma or a family history of OA.

PHYSICAL EXAM
- Joint line tenderness is common in hands and knees.
- Joints may have crepitus, decreased range of motion (ROM), effusion, and atrophy of surrounding muscles.

- In knees, involved compartments include medial (most common), patellofemoral, and/or lateral. Effusion and trace joint warmth are common in acute flares.
- In hands, may see nodules in the DIP and PIP joints, termed *Heberden* and *Bouchard nodes*, respectively
- In hips, decreased and painful internal rotation are early signs, and tenderness over the anterior joint line is a later finding.
- Severely affected joints may appear misshapen or deformed due to osteophytes or malalignment.

DIFFERENTIAL DIAGNOSIS

- RA
- Collagen vascular diseases
- Crystal deposition disease (gout, CPPD)
- Meniscal or labral tears

DIAGNOSTIC TESTS & INTERPRETATION

Initial Tests (lab, imaging)

Plain films are the modality of choice for diagnosis, severity assessment, and monitoring progression (3):

- Hip: weight-bearing anteroposterior (AP) best
- Knee: Weight-bearing AP in 20 to 45 degrees of flexion (Rosenberg view) is most sensitive; sunrise and lateral views helpful for patellofemoral joint.
- Shoulder: true glenohumeral AP (Grashey) best
- Thumb CMC joint: Three views of wrist are adequate.
- Hands: AP and lateral
- X-ray characteristics include osteophytes, joint space narrowing, subchondral sclerosis, and cyst formation.
- Radiographic severity is quantified using the Kellgren-Lawrence scale but may not correlate with symptoms.
  - Grade 1: equivocal osteophytes
  - Grade 2: definite osteophytes
  - Grade 3: joint space narrowing
  - Grade 4: bone-on-bone appearance
- Diagnostic ultrasound can detect effusion, synovitis, meniscal extrusion and degeneration, joint space narrowing, osteophytes.
- Computed tomography (CT) and magnetic resonance imaging (MRI) should only be considered if other conditions are suspected. MRI is sensitive in detecting OA of the knee, but there is a high rate of false-positive findings that may not correlate with signs and symptoms.

Diagnostic Procedures/Other

- Arthrocentesis and joint fluid examination are not routinely necessary but is useful when infection or crystal deposition are being considered.
- Serology is only used to rule out other disorders, if clinically suspected:
  - Rheumatoid factor and antinuclear antibody titers are normal.
  - Inflammation markers (erythrocyte sedimentation rate, C-reactive protein) usually are normal.

TREATMENT

GENERAL MEASURES

- The "core set" of treatments for all patients should include patient education, weight loss if overweight/obese, and an exercise program (4),(5)[A].
- Patient education is important and effective (5),(6),(7)[A]:
  - Set reasonable expectations on outcome (pain reduction, increased function, not cure).
  - Modify of activities to minimize pain and risk of joint trauma.
  - Importance of nonpharmacologic therapies
- Weight reduction of 5% or more improves knee and hip pain (4),(5),(6),(7)[A].
- Exercise and weight reduction of 11.4% is associated with no pain at 18 months in 38% of patients. Exercise has an immediate beneficial effect.
- Aquatic and low-impact land-based aerobic exercise, strength training, mind-body exercise (yoga, tai chi etc.), and ROM exercise are all beneficial; programs involving all types may be most beneficial (4),(5),(6),(7)[A].
- Walking aids for knee and hip OA (cane, crutch in contralateral hand; walkers for bilateral OA) (5),(6),(7)[A]
- Optimal management requires a combination of modalities (7)[A].
- Surgical replacement is best reserved for patients with severe pain that affects quality of life or activities of daily living who have failed multiple conservative measures (7)[C].

MEDICATION

No disease-modifying agents are yet available.

First Line

- Oral glucosamine sulfate (not hydrochloride [HCl]) 1,500 mg/d and/or chondroitin sulfate 1,200 mg/d modestly reduce pain in hip/knee/hand OA (4),(6),(7)[A] but probably have no disease-modifying effect.
- Topical nonsteroidal anti-inflammatory drugs (NSAIDs) are effective; onset of pain reduction 1 to 2 weeks and work as well as oral NSAIDs (4),(5),(6),(7)[A]
- Older studies show that topical capsaicin is effective for knee OA; high incidence of local irritation (4),(5),(6),(7)[A]

Second Line

- Oral NSAIDs effective but have higher risks; reserved for short-term therapy (4),(5),(6),(7)[A]:
  - Cyclooxygenase-2 (COX-2) inhibitors are not more effective; less gastrointestinal (GI) toxicity but not without risks
  - Discourage chronic use of NSAIDs; if necessary, add gastroprotection with a proton pump inhibitor (4),(5) or misoprostol.
- Intra-articular injection of platelet-rich plasma (PRP) improves pain and function in knee OA up to 12 months after single injection, with greater efficacy than hyaluronate (8)[A].

- Intra-articular injections with corticosteroids are effective for 2 to 4 weeks or more (4),(5),(6),(7)[A]:
  - Reserve for patients not responding to oral medications or for inflammatory flares.
  - Limit to 3 to 4 injections per year per joint.
  - No long-term adverse effect on diabetic control
  - Intra-articular hyaluronate injections may modestly reduce pain and improve function for 1 to 6 months (4),(5),(6),(7), but they are not routinely recommended by the American College of Rheumatology (ACR) or the American Academy of Orthopaedic Surgeons (AAOS).

Third Line

- Duloxetine (a pain-modulating serotonin and norepinephrine reuptake inhibitor [SNRI]) reduces chronic pain in knee or multijoint OA, especially in those who catastrophize (4),(5),(6)[A].
- Weak opioids (e.g., tramadol, codeine) can be considered for short-term refractory pain; those requiring long-term use may benefit from maximization of nonpharmacologic therapies and/or surgery (4),(5),(6),(7)[A]. Long-term use and stronger opioids should be avoided because research now shows no improved pain scores at 1 year compared to acetaminophen or NSAIDs and greater risks. Opioids if given within 2 years of total knee arthroplasty (TKA) worsen long-term outcomes after surgery.
- Extracorporeal shock wave therapy (ESWT) may show some improvement in pain reduction and function but still needs further study (9).

ISSUES FOR REFERRAL

- A multidisciplinary approach may help patients make the most of available therapies: physical therapy, personal exercise training, health care education, nutrition, complementary and alternative medicine, etc.
- Surgical referral when cartilage has thinned to "bone-on-bone" status and pain/dysfunction are severe despite conservative therapies.

ADDITIONAL THERAPIES

- Valgus bracing for isolated medial knee OA with varus malalignment improves stability and reduces pain in some patients (4),(5),(6),(7)[A]. Ideal patients are not obese and are younger and more physically active.
- Soft braces (sleeves) for knee OA can improve pain and function (4),(5),(6)[A].
- Wedge insoles for isolated medial or lateral knee OA may be effective; evidence is conflicting (4),(6)[A].
- Thermal therapies (heat, cold) may be effective (6)[A].
- Walking aids (e.g., cane) reduce pain in hip/knee OA (4),(5),(6),(7)[A].

COMPLEMENTARY & ALTERNATIVE MEDICINE

- Acupuncture reduces pain briefly/slightly in knee OA (7)[A].
- Massage therapy improves pain and function (7)[A].
- Balneotherapy (spa, mineral baths; common in Europe) may improve pain/function in knee OA (6)[A].
- Traditional Chinese medications are likely effective in improving pain in knee OA (10)[A].
- Therapies with no proof of efficacy include static magnets and neuromuscular electric stimulation.

SURGERY/OTHER PROCEDURES

- Indicated in patients with recalcitrant pain and interference with activities of daily living despite maximizing conservative management (5)[B]
- Arthroscopic débridement for mechanical symptoms (catching, giving out) not effective, even for partial meniscal tears (6)[A]
- Medial or compartment knee OA:
  - Wedge osteotomy may be effective (5)[B].
  - Unicompartmental arthroplasty (replacement) effective (6)[B]
  - Interposition arthroplasty (joint spacer insertion): no data on safety/efficacy
- TKA: very effective (4)[C]:
  - Hardware durable 10 to 15 years
  - Try to delay TKA until after 55 years by maximizing other treatments.
  - Rate of hardware failure <10 years is 3 times higher in age <55 versus >70 years.
- Total hip arthroplasty or joint resurfacing is effective in hip OA (6)[B].
- Glenohumeral OA: total shoulder arthroplasty more effective/durable than humeral head replacement
- Cartilage replacement techniques for severe focal defects are gaining in popularity and evidence:
  - Autologous cartilage implantation: Arthroscopy harvests patient's cartilage, chondrocytes are replicated in culture, and second arthroscopy fills cartilage defect with cells.
  - Osteoarticular cartilage transplant: Cartilage from patient's non–weight-bearing surface in knee joint is placed into defect.
  - Cadaver cartilage allografts to fill large defects

ONGOING CARE

FOLLOW-UP RECOMMENDATIONS

- Follow-ups to monitor and adjust treatment plan may improve outcomes by building a trusting patient-provider relationship.
- Reassessment of radiographic severity can be helpful every 2 to 4 years in patients with clinical worsening to assist in planning surgical referral.

PATIENT EDUCATION

- See "Treatment" or "General Measures."
- Public education materials: https://www.webmd.com/osteoarthritis/default.htm

PROGNOSIS

OA is a progressive arthropathy with highly variable course.

REFERENCES

1. Vina ER, Kwoh CK. Epidemiology of osteoarthritis: literature update. *Curr Opin Rheumatol* 2018;30(2):160–167.
2. Alentorn-Geli E, Samuelsson K, Musahl V, et al. The association of recreational and competitive running with hip and knee osteoarthritis: a systematic review and meta-analysis. *J Orthop Sports Phys Ther.* 2017;47(6):373–390.
3. American College of Radiology. ACR Appropriateness Criteria. Accessed August 25, 2025. https://acsearch.acr.org/list
4. Bruyère O, Honvo G, Veronese N, et al. An updated algorithm recommendation for the management of knee osteoarthritis from the European Society for Clinical and Economic Aspects of Osteoporosis, Osteoarthritis and Musculoskeletal Diseases (ESCEO). *Semin Arthritis Rheum*. 2019;49(3):337–350.
5. Bannuru RR, Osani MC, Vaysbrot EE, et al. OARSI guidelines for the non-surgical management of knee, hip, and polyarticular osteoarthritis. *Osteoarthritis Cartilage*. 2019;27(11):1578–1589.
6. Rillo O, Riera H, Acosta C, et al. PANLAR consensus recommendations for the management in osteoarthritis of hand, hip, and knee. *J Clin Rheumatol.* 2016;22(7):345–354.
7. Zhang W, Nuki G, Moskowitz RW, et al. OARSI recommendations for the management of hip and knee osteoarthritis: part III: changes in evidence following systematic cumulative update of research published through January 2009. *Osteoarthritis Cartilage*. 2010;18(4):476–499.
8. Filardo G, Previtali D, Napoli F, et al. PRP Injections for the treatment of knee osteoarthritis: a meta-analysis of randomized controlled trials. *Cartilage*. 2021;13(Suppl I):364S–375S.
9. Chen L, Ye L, Liu H, et al. Extracorporeal shock wave therapy for the treatment of osteoarthritis: a systematic review and meta-analysis. *Biomed Res Int*. 2020;1907821.
10. Lin Z, Zheng J, Chen M, et al. The efficacy and safety of Chinese herbal medicine in the treatment of knee osteoarthritis: an updated systematic review and meta-analysis of 56 randomized control trials. *Oxid Med Cell Longev*. 2022;6887988.

CLINICAL PEARLS

- OA is a degenerative disorder of joints and is predominantly noninflammatory but can have inflammatory flares.
- Core treatments for all types include patient education on goals and self-management, multimodal exercise, and weight reduction for those overweight.
- Multidisciplinary treatment—providers, physical therapists, nutritionists, fitness trainers, nurse educators, complementary/alternative therapists—can optimize outcomes.
- Topical NSAIDs, exercise, and weight loss are first-line therapies.
- Oral NSAIDs should be limited to 8 to 10 days and corticosteroid injection; PRP injections have limited long term data.
- Opioids should be avoided.

OSTEOCHONDRITIS DISSECANS

Holly J. Benjamin, MD, FAMSSM, FACSM ▪ Melissa Faubert, DO, CAQSM ▪ Sujith Kochat, MD

BASICS

DESCRIPTION

- Osteochondritis dissecans (OCD) defined as a focal idiopathic alteration of subchondral bone with risk for instability and disruption of adjacent articular cartilage that may result in premature osteoarthritis
- It is classified into juvenile and adult forms, depending on the presence or absence of immature physes.
- Most commonly occurs at the posterolateral aspect of medial femoral condyle, talar dome, and humeral capitellum but can occur in all large joints

EPIDEMIOLOGY

- Incidence estimated to be 15 to 30/100,000 person-years
- Predominantly males > female (4:1)
- Juvenile form is the most common form.
- Knee is the most common location.
- Occurs typically in ages 12 to 19 years, rarely occurs in older individuals

ETIOLOGY AND PATHOPHYSIOLOGY

- Multiple hypotheses as to etiology—likely multifactorial (biologic and mechanical factors), no consensus exists currently
- Most accepted hypothesis is repetitive microtrauma leads to microfractures.
  - Results in focal ischemia and subsequent growth impairment which leads to cartilage separation and fragmentation
- Other hypotheses include single traumatic episode, genetic causes, inflammatory causes, and vascular abnormalities (1).

RISK FACTORS

ALERT
OCD in one joint is a risk factor for contralateral involvement; 20–30% of patients with OCD of the knee have bilateral involvement.

- Sports involving jumping, pivoting, cutting movements
- Sports with repetitive loading of the elbows, such as baseball and gymnastics, are specific risk factors for OCD of the elbow.

GENERAL PREVENTION

- Using proper mechanics and avoiding overload, especially with the elbow and capitellum in adolescent throwers
- Strength and joint stability training

DIAGNOSIS

HISTORY

- Insidious onset of symptoms
- Vague, poorly localized joint pain
- Varying levels of pain and stiffness
- May or may not report joint swelling
- May have sensation of locking or catching or giving way

PHYSICAL EXAM

- Effusion may be present.
- Decreased or painful range of motion (ROM)
- Poorly localized joint line tenderness
- Mild antalgic gait in lower extremity OCDs
- In knee OCD, ipsilateral quad atrophy is occasionally seen but is not specific.

DIFFERENTIAL DIAGNOSIS

- Fracture
- Ligamentous or cartilage injury
- Tendinosis
- Inflammatory arthropathy
- Mechanical issue (i.e., patellofemoral pain syndrome)
- Juvenile: apophyseal injury
- Adult: osteoarthritis

DIAGNOSTIC TESTS & INTERPRETATION

Initial Tests (lab, imaging)

- X-ray is first line for diagnosis due to radiographs being inexpensive and readily available.
- Characteristic appearance on x-ray is a well-circumscribed lucent defect in subchondral bone that may or may not contain an internal bone density (1)[A]:
  - In children, these findings may reflect normal development of ossification centers (magnetic resonance imaging [MRI] can differentiate, whereas x-ray often cannot).
- MRI is preferred method for characterizing and staging OCD lesions.
- T1-weighted sequences allow lesion size measurement, and T2-weighted sequences provide information on articular cartilage integrity, reactive marrow edema, and fluid or cystic changes around the edge of the lesion.
- MRI staging classification (2)[A]:
  - Stage I: subchondral lesion of low signal intensity indicating subchondral compression fracture; stable
  - Stage II: hypointense rim on images indicating demarcation with or without partial separation of lesion; stable
  - Stage III: high signal intensity and underlying cystic changes indicative of instability with detached, nondisplaced fragment; unstable
  - Stage IV: complete dislocation of osteochondral fragment into the joint space; loose body may or may not be seen; CT scans can evaluate lesion size, location, loose bodies, and healing after fixation, but due to radiation exposure and inability to obtain soft tissue contrast, it is not commonly used.
- Ultrasound has been shown to be comparable to MRI and arthroscopy in detecting OCD lesion stability in the capitellum when using an ultrasound classification system. Due to operator-dependent skill and interpretation, MRI is still recommended over ultrasound for diagnosis and staging (1)[A].

Diagnostic Procedures/Other

- Arthroscopy is the gold standard for assessing OCD lesions (size, staging, stability, etc.) (3)[A]:
  - Grade I: stable lesions with continuous but softened area with intact cartilage
  - Grade II: lesions with partial discontinuity that are stable when probed
  - Grade III: lesions with complete discontinuity but not dislocated
  - Grade IV: empty defect, displaced or unstable fragment
- However, arthroscopy is rarely performed as a diagnostic procedure but rather as a therapeutic procedure (see below).

TREATMENT

GENERAL MEASURES

- Early recognition of condition is important; if not treated, can lead to degenerative osteoarthritis
- Skeletal maturity and lesion stability drive treatment decisions.
- Nonoperative treatment is recommended first line for patients with open physes, stable lesions, and minimal symptoms (4)[A].
  - Immediate cessation of impact activities is recommended, but there is no consensus on immobilization, offloading, and level of activity that may be acceptable (3)[A].
  - Physical therapy is generally initiated after an initial period of rest from sport.
  - Counsel patients that recovery may take 3 to 6 months.
- Operative treatment is offered to patients with closed physes, unstable lesions, mechanical symptoms, and/or failure of 3 to 6 months of nonoperative treatment.
- There are numerous surgical techniques which may include reduction and fixation, subchondral bone drilling, bone grafting, osteochondral transplantation (autograft or allograft), and autologous chondrocyte implantation (ACI/matrix-induced ACI [MACI]) (1)[A].

ISSUES FOR REFERRAL

Orthopedic referral is indicated for all patients with unstable OCD lesions, for adults with OCD, and for those juvenile or adult patients who fail conservative treatment.

ADDITIONAL THERAPIES

- Physical therapy may be initiated for conservatively managed patients. Stretching, ROM exercises, conditioning exercises, and strengthening are beneficial.
- Postoperative physical therapy can be tailored to the procedure and sport.

SURGERY/OTHER PROCEDURES

- Patients with larger lesions, greater skeletal maturity, and high signal on MRI likely will do better with surgery.
- Arthroscopy has better outcomes than open procedures.
- Surgical options include (2)[B]:
  - Débridement, loose body removal, with or without marrow stimulation
  - Fixation, with or without bone grafting
  - Transarticular/retroarticular drilling
  - ACI
  - Osteochondral autograft/allograft transplantation
- An area of future interest and potential treatment options is regenerative medicine involving platelet-rich plasma (PRP) or stem cell/bone marrow aspirate treatments.

ONGOING CARE

PROGNOSIS

- All patients with OCD lesions have increased risk for osteoarthritis, but risk decreases with proper healing.
- Sclerosis on x-ray and synovial fluid behind the lesion on MRI correlate with poor prognosis.
- Groups who underwent fixation of OCD lesion had lower rates of osteoarthritis at 30 years old follow-up compared to drilling and allografts (4)[A].

REFERENCES

1. Chau MM, Klimstra MA, Wise KL, et al. Osteochondritis dissecans: current understanding of epidemiology, etiology, management, and outcomes. *J Bone Joint Surg Am.* 2021;103(12):1132–1151.
2. Bruns J, Werner M, Habermann C. Osteochondritis dissecans: etiology, pathology, and imaging with a special focus on the knee joint. *Cartilage.* 2017;9(4):346–362.
3. Andriolo L, Candrian C, Papio T, et al. Osteochondritis dissecans of the knee—conservative treatment strategies: a systematic review. *Cartilage.* 2019;10(3):267–277.
4. Chau MM, Tompkins MA. Osteochondritis dissecans of the knee in young athletes. *Clin Sports Med.* 2022;41(4):579–594.

ADDITIONAL READING

Carey JL, Grimm NL. Treatment algorithm for osteochondritis dissecans of the knee. *Orthop Clin North Am.* 2015;46(1):141–146.

CLINICAL PEARLS

- Juvenile OCD patients with stable lesions require a significant period of restriction from strenuous activity.
- Patients should be pain free before return to sports.
- MRI is gold standard for staging and guides treatment plan.
- Juvenile unstable lesions or stable lesions that do not progress toward healing should be referred for surgical consultation and potential arthroscopy.
- All skeletally mature lesions should be referral for surgical consultation and potential arthroscopy.
- Juvenile OCD has a good potential for full recovery if treated appropriately but still may lead to early degenerative joint disease.
- Adult forms tend to be more complicated and often lead to early degenerative joint disease.

OSTEOMYELITIS

Wikien Hung Pinto, MD • Caitlyn C. Mooney, MD, FAAP, CAQSM

BASICS

DESCRIPTION

- Infection of the bone by microbes
- Classifications are based on pathogenesis:
  - Hematogenous osteomyelitis (HOM): caused by microorganisms seeding from the blood
  - Nonhematogenous osteomyelitis (OM): develops adjacent to contiguous infection or after direct inoculation
  - Native bone versus orthopedic implant-associated infection
  - Commonly categorized based on duration: Acute infections develop over days to weeks.
  - Subacute infections present within 1 to several months of disease onset; often vague and lack of systemic symptoms
  - Chronic infections: months to years; often occur by direct contamination

EPIDEMIOLOGY

- ~22 cases per 100,000 person-years
- Incidence increases with age.
- Acute OM occurs in ~8 of 100,000 children/y.
- Hematogenous dissemination is more common in infants, children, and immunocompromised.
- HOM most commonly occurs in the long bones of the upper and lower extremities.
- Contiguous spread of infection from ulcers, local trauma, and periprosthetic joint infections are more common in older adults with comorbid conditions.
- The recurrence rate of chronic OM is 10–30%.
- Hip and knee periprosthetic joint infection incidence is 2.1% and 2.3%, respectively, and the risk is highest in the early postoperative period (1).
- Infectious complications occur in 5% of traumatic/orthopedic implants during the lifetime of the implant.
- Vertebral infections are the most common location of hematogenous spread in adults and represent 4–10% of cases (2).
- 4% lifetime risk of foot OM in diabetic patients
- Morbidity significant: chronic pain, disability, amputation, infection extension, and sepsis

ETIOLOGY AND PATHOPHYSIOLOGY

- Infectious agents include bacteria, mycobacteria, and fungi; they may be monomicrobial or polymicrobial. Normal bone is highly resistant to infection unless it results from a very large inoculum, trauma, or the presence of a foreign body.
- Pathophysiology in brief:
  - Routes of infection include hematogenous (bloodstream), contiguous (nearby infections), and direct inoculation (penetrating trauma, fracture, orthopedic procedures).
  - Hematogenous: Microbes travel to the vascular metaphysis of the long bones via the blood. The sluggish blood supply at the metaphysis allows the microbes to colonize the bone. The immune response causes lysis of the surrounding bone, increased pressure, and decreased oxygen to promote infection. The interruption of the blood supply results in necrosis of the bone.
  - Chronic infection is characterized by an involucrum, a sheath of new bone surrounding a sequestrum of dead bone. This not only walls off the infection but also isolates the area from the immune system.
  - Biofilm: a sticky layer of microorganisms that adhere to surfaces; virulence factor that contributes to chronic OM/implant-associated infection
- Bacterial OM:
  - Age and inoculation methods are important factors in species prevalence.
  - *Staphylococcus aureus*: most common pathogen of HOM (adults and pediatrics) and implant-associated OM
  - Methicillin-resistant *S. aureus* (MRSA) is increasingly common.
  - Group A *Streptococcus*, *Streptococcus pneumoniae*, and *Kingella kingae* are the next most common pathogens in children.
  - Newborns: *S. aureus* and group B *Streptococcus*
  - *Pseudomonas* species: intravenous (IV) drug use and puncture through rubber sole
  - *Salmonella* species predominate in sickle cell disease patients.
  - Consider anaerobes if a "fight bite" injury.
- Vertebral OM:
  - Primarily in adults
  - Focal neck or back pain with fever
- Fungal and mycobacterial infections are rare and more common in immunosuppressed patients.
  - Mycobacterial OM:
    - Most commonly by mycobacterium tuberculosis
    - Any bone can be involved, frequently in the lower thoracic spine (Pott disease).
    - Typically, insidious onset, presenting as a "cold abscess" with swelling, erythema, pain, and mild or no local warmth
  - Fungal OM: coccidioidomycosis, blastomycosis, cryptococcosis, candidiasis, or sporotrichosis
  - Usually associated with indwelling catheters, intravenous drug use (IVDU), prolonged neutropenia, or trauma
- Subacute OM: Brodie abscess is rare; 2% of all patients with OM
  - Cavitary lesion in epiphysis or metaphysis characterized by small, localized lucency surrounded by reactive, dense-appearing bone
- Chronic OM most likely *Staphylococcus epidermidis* or *S. aureus*, *Pseudomonas*, *Serratia*, *Escherichia coli*

RISK FACTORS

- Open fracture
- Surgical manipulation (orthopedic, colorectal, genitourinary procedures)
- IV drug use
- Immunocompromise
- Peripheral vascular disease/peripheral neuropathy
- Sickle cell disease
- Bacteremia
- Presence of orthopedic implant
- Age: young children and elderly

GENERAL PREVENTION

- Timely diagnosis and treatment of primary infections to avoid seeding of bone
- Use of prophylactic antibiotics with injury or manipulative surgery; ideally within 6 hours
- Appropriate wound management

DIAGNOSIS

HISTORY

- Children with acute hematogenous osteomyelitis (AHO) may present with abrupt-onset high fever, chills, fatigue, irritability, lethargy, refusal to walk, pseudoparalysis, restricted motion and local pain, edema, erythema, and tenderness.
- Most adults present with vague complaints, nonspecific pain of the involved limb, minimal fever, or constitutional symptoms.
- OM, due to contiguous focus, often presents with painful or unstable joints and little or no fever.
- Subacute OM presents with insidious onset of mild, possibly intermittent, poorly localized pain, minimal or no fever, and few constitutional symptoms.
- In chronic OM, there is local bone loss and may present with persistent drainage through fistulas or sinus tracts, nonhealing ulcers, recurrent pain, possibly low-grade fever, and mild systemic symptoms.
- Diabetic patients with foot ulcer larger than 2 × 2 cm or exposed bone, OM is highly likely.

PHYSICAL EXAM

- Fever (temperature >100.4°F) but not always present
- Swelling, erythema of involved area
- Local warmth, fluctuance, or tenderness to palpation
- Decreased use of extremity, refusal to bear weight
- Limited movement of adjacent joint
- Other possible foci of infection
- Sinus tract drainage
- Passive range of motion tolerated, unlike septic arthritis

DIFFERENTIAL DIAGNOSIS

- Acute leukemia
- Acute rheumatic fever
- Rheumatoid arthritis (adult or juvenile)
- Acute gout, pseudogout
- Cellulitis
- Malignant bone tumors (Ewing sarcoma, osteosarcoma)
- Septic arthritis
- Multiple myeloma (elderly)
- Sepsis
- Deep vein thrombosis, thrombophlebitis
- Intervertebral disk disorders
- Fracture
- Aseptic bone infarction
- Neuropathic joint disease (Charcot arthropathy)
- Transient synovitis
- Venous insufficiency
- Chronic recurrent multifocal OM

DIAGNOSTIC TESTS & INTERPRETATION

- Laboratory investigations can be helpful but generally lack specificity for OM:
  - Complete blood count may reveal leukocytosis with neutrophilia in acute OM.
  - C-reactive protein (CRP) and erythrocyte sedimentation rate (ESR) almost always elevated
  - Changes in CRP detected sooner
  - CRP and procalcitonin levels correlate with clinical response to therapy and may be used to monitor treatment.
  - In chronic OM, leukocytosis is uncommon; the ESR and/or CRP may be elevated or normal.
- High pretest probability, positive probe-to-bone test, and plain radiography can be enough to diagnose OM in patients with diabetic foot ulcers.
- Blood culture positive in ~3% of cases
- Bone aspiration and/or bone biopsy are essential to guide antibiotic therapy.
  - Send for Gram stain and culture (aerobic, anaerobic, mycobacterial, and fungal) and histopathology.
  - False-negative blood or biopsy cultures are common in patients on empiric antibiotic therapy.
- If OM is suspected in patients with at least 2 weeks of symptoms, the initial imaging of choice is conventional radiographs.
- Radiographs:
  - Osseous changes usually appear 14 days after symptom onset.
  - 80% have normal radiographs in the first 2 weeks.
  - Features include periosteal elevation and/or destruction of bone with radiolucency, fading cortical margins, and no surrounding reactive bone.
  - Chronic OM demonstrates sequestrum (a focal sclerotic lesion with a lucent rim).
- Magnetic resonance imaging (MRI):
  - MRI is the test of choice in patients with <2 weeks of symptoms, normal radiographs, or suggestive radiographs without definitive features.
  - MRI is effective in early detection (3 to 5 days of disease onset) and localization.
  - Reported 90% sensitivity
  - Bone marrow edema is the earliest pathologic finding.
- Computed tomography (CT):
  - If MRI is not available, CT is an appropriate alternative test.
- Ultrasonography:
  - It may show periosteal thickening and elevation, soft tissue abscess, or fluid collection; provides direction for aspiration; cannot evaluate bone cortex.
- Nuclear studies:
  - Radioisotope bone scan (triple phase with technetium-99m) sensitivity is comparable to MRI, but the specificity is poor; only to be used if metal hardware precludes MRI or CT
  - When combined with CT, positron emission tomography has the highest sensitivity and specificity (>90%) but is not widely available and is expensive.

TREATMENT

- Multidisciplinary approach including but not limited to orthopedics, infectious disease, microbiology, pharmacist
- Treatment options include both surgical management and antimicrobial therapy.
- Empiric treatment is guided by the age of the patient, severity of disease, and suspected organism(s).
- Delaying antibiotics is recommended if clinically possible until microbial culture and sensitivity are available.
- Recommend broad-spectrum coverage and narrowing based on cultures.
- In AHO in children, surgical intervention is generally required to débride foci of infection, excise sequestra, drain subperiosteal, intramedullary, or soft tissue abscess or failure to improve after a trial of antimicrobial therapy.
- Empiric regimens for AHO in children (3)[A]:
  - Local MRSA rates <10%: oxacillin/nafcillin or cefazolin
  - Local MRSA rates 10–20%: clindamycin or vancomycin
  - Severe illness: vancomycin with or without protein synthesis-inhibiting antibiotic (e.g., clindamycin)
  - Antibiotic resistance, allergy, or poor tolerability: daptomycin and linezolid
  - Suspected *K. kingae* (e.g., preschool age, epiphyseal OM) anti-MRSA + β-lactam with or without β-lactamase inhibitor or cephalosporin

- Empiric regimens for OM in adults (4)[A]
  - OM without retained implant: ceftriaxone + vancomycin (high MRSA prevalence, colonization, prior positive cultures, health care exposure) or oxacillin, cloxacillin, nafcillin, cefazolin if MRSA coverage is deemed unnecessary
  - Diabetic foot OM: β-lactam with or without β-lactamase inhibitor or ceftriaxone +/− metronidazole +/− vancomycin
  - *Pseudomonas aeruginosa* coverage: chronic wounds with prior courses of antibiotics; prior positive cultures, gangrenous wounds; recent surgical procedure, sites of infection associated with pseudomonas (e.g., malignant otitis externa)
  - OM with retained implant: <3 months: antipseudomonal β-lactam + vancomycin; >3 months: ceftriaxone + vancomycin
- Antibiotic selection:
  - In methicillin-susceptible *S. aureus* (MSSA), suspected first-line options include parenteral β-lactam antibiotics (nafcillin, oxacillin) or cefazolin; alternatives, ceftriaxone and vancomycin
  - Coagulase-negative staphylococci should be treated with vancomycin.
  - Addition of rifampin may reduce relapse of OM, mainly in infections with retained implant.
  - Gram-negative organisms, fluoroquinolones are the drug of choice.
  - For diabetic foot infections or penicillin allergies, fluoroquinolones are an alternate option for staphylococcal infections.
  - Sickle cell patients use fluoroquinolones except in the pediatric population. An alternative is 3rd-generation cephalosporin.
- Antibiotic duration in children (5)[A]:
  - Initial parenteral antibiotics followed by oral antibiotics for a total of 2 to 4 weeks
  - Vertebral OM, especially with *S. aureus*, is immunocompromised for a longer course.
- Antibiotic duration in adults:
  - The optimal duration of therapy is not certain; the total duration (IV and step-down to oral) is usually 6 weeks.
  - Recommend treatment with IV antibiotics 6 weeks from last débridement.
  - For chronic OM, a total treatment period of 4 to 8 weeks of IV antibiotics followed by oral antibiotics
  - Long-term oral therapy (3 to 6 months) may be warranted for infected orthopedic hardware.
- Surgery:
  - Indications for surgery include antibiotic failure, infected surgical hardware, and chronic OM with necrotic bone and soft tissue; impending sinus formation, drainage into a synovial joint, and signs of subperiosteal pus or synovitis (indicating an acute component).
- Hyperbaric oxygen and negative pressure wound therapy may be useful adjunctive therapy.
- OM following trauma:
  - Initial management includes irrigation, débridement, administering antibiotics (ideally within 6 hours), tetanus immunization.
  - Duration of prophylactic antibiotics: Closed fractures require a single dose, whereas open fractures require antibiotics for 24 to 72 hours.
  - Consider removal of hardware and additional débridement as needed.
- Subacute OM:
  - Brodie abscesses respond well to surgical curettage of the abscess, cancellous bone grafting, and antibiotic therapy.
- Chronic OM:
  - Remove infected prosthetic devices and hardware.
  - Treatment can be palliative or curative.
  - Curative: Débridement of all devitalized bone and soft tissue is essential for cure, amputation or reconstruction.
  - Palliative: débridement and drainage followed by antibiotics and analgesics

ONGOING CARE

- Initial protection of extremity including splinting, protected weight-bearing, and protected range of motion until partial healing.
- Closely monitor for signs of response to treatment (clinical and laboratory); weekly serum inflammatory markers (CRP, ESR) can be useful.
- Radiologic healing is slower than clinical healing and usually occurs within 3 to 12 months.
- The purpose of follow-up after a year is to assess bone growth and alignment.

PROGNOSIS

Variable but markedly improved with timely diagnosis and aggressive treatment

COMPLICATIONS

- Include bone abscess, bacteremia, fracture, loosening of hardware, overlying cellulitis, and draining soft tissue tracts.
- Sinus tract formation may be associated with neoplasms, especially with long-standing infections:
  - Squamous cell carcinoma (Marjolin ulcer) is the most common tumor associated with chronic OM.
  - Recalcitrant infection should prompt biopsy evaluation for malignancy.
- Growth disturbances are exceedingly rare in children.
- The most common complication is recurrence. The recurrence rate of OM in adults is ~30% at 12 months, and it is 50% for *P. aeruginosa* infections.

REFERENCES

1. Patel R. Periprosthetic joint infection. *N Engl J Med*. 2023;388(3):251–262.
2. Conan Y, Laurent E, Belin Y, et al. Large increase of vertebral osteomyelitis in France: a 2010–2019 cross-sectional study. *Epidemiol Infect*. 2021;149: e227.
3. Woods CR, Bradley JS, Chatterjee A, et al. Clinical practice guideline by the Pediatric Infectious Diseases Society and the Infectious Diseases Society of America: 2021 guideline on diagnosis and management of acute hematogenous osteomyelitis in pediatrics. *J Pediatric Infect Dis Soc*. 2021;10(8):801–844.
4. Spellberg B, Aggrey G, Brennan MB, et al. Use of novel strategies to develop guidelines for management of pyogenic osteomyelitis in adults: a WikiGuidelines group consensus statement. *JAMA Netw Open*. 2022;5(5):e2211321.
5. Huang CY, Hsieh RW, Yen HT, et al. Short- versus long-course antibiotics in osteomyelitis: a systematic review and meta-analysis. *Int J Antimicrob Agents*. 2019;53(3):246–260.

ADDITIONAL READING

- Li HK, Rombach I, Zambellas R, et al. Oral versus intravenous antibiotics for bone and joint infection. *N Engl J Med*. 2019;380(5):425–436.
- Nabizadeh N, Crawford CH III, Glassman SD, et al. Severity and outcome of neurologic deficits in patients with pyogenic spondylodiscitis: a systematic review. *Orthop Clin North Am*. 2022;53(1):105–112.

CLINICAL PEARLS

- The most common pathogen implicated in the development of OM in both children and adults is *S. aureus* (MRSA, MSSA).
- Often, abrupt high fever presents with AHO. It is not uncommon to have no fever or a low-grade fever with the other forms of the disease.
- Initial imaging of choice is plain radiographs; if <2 weeks from the onset of symptoms, MRI can detect changes within 3 to 5 days and is superior to CT and bone scan.
- Optimal treatment should be provided by multidisciplinary teams.

OSTEOPOROSIS

Julie M. Kerr, MD, CAQSM

BASICS

DESCRIPTION

- Systemic disorder characterized by decreased bone mass and microarchitectural deterioration of bone leading to bone fragility and increased susceptibility to fractures of the femoral neck, total hip, and lumbar spine
- World Health Organization (WHO) definitions:
  - Osteopenia (low bone mass):
    - Bone mineral density (BMD) defined as T-score between −1.0 and −2.5 standard deviation (SD) below the mean of a young adult reference population on dual-energy x-ray absorptiometry (DEXA)
  - Osteoporosis (decreased bone mass):
    - BMD T-score ≤2.5 SD below the mean of a young adult reference population
  - Severe osteoporosis: BMD T-score ≤2.5 SD below the mean of a young adult reference population with a history of fracture
  - In adolescents and young adults, definition is based on <2 SD below the mean Z-score based on age, *not* T-score.
- Classifications:
  - **Primary:** age-related (postmenopausal estrogen deficiency, age-related vitamin D deficiency)
  - **Secondary:** (drug or concurrent medical condition etiology)

EPIDEMIOLOGY

- Prevalence of osteoporosis will increase as the population ages.
- 10.2 million Americans have osteoporosis and 43.4 million have osteopenia. Lifetime risk of osteoporosis fracture is 1 of every 2 Caucasian women and 1 in 5 men; osteoporosis less frequent in African Americans, but those with osteoporosis have same elevated fracture risk as Caucasians.

RISK FACTORS

- Female sex
- Race:
  - Non-Hispanic Caucasian race
  - Asian race
- Parental history of osteoporotic hip fracture
- Personal history of fracture—presence of a single spine fracture increases risk of subsequent vertebral compression fracture by 5-fold and risk of hip and other fractures 2- to 3-fold.
- Age ≥65 years
- Low body weight (<58 kg [128 lb])
- Diet low in calcium; low in vitamins C, D, and K; and decreased copper, manganese, and zinc mineral content
- Estrogen deficiency: postmenopausal or premenopausal secondary to overexercising and/or eating disorder
- Sedentary lifestyle, lack of weight-bearing exercise
- History of falls
- Female athlete triad: low energy availability (EA) (with or without disordered eating), menstrual dysfunction, low BMD
- Medications: glucocorticoids, anticonvulsants, cancer chemo drugs, thyroid replacement drugs, proton pump inhibitors (PPIs)
- Excessive alcohol (>4 drinks/d; >2 drinks/d women) and active or passive tobacco use
- Other diseases: diabetes, hyperparathyroidism, hyperthyroidism, multiple myeloma, rheumatoid arthritis
- Impaired absorption of calcium, phosphate, and vitamin D from the gastrointestinal (GI) tract, as in inflammatory bowel disease, gastrectomy, celiac disease, jejunoileal bypass, or pancreatic insufficiency

GENERAL PREVENTION

- Identification and treatment of risk factors/secondary causes of osteoporosis (1)[A]
- Reports of calcium with or without vitamin D supplementation and cardiovascular (CV) risk, but conflicting data
- Bone Health & Osteoporosis Foundation (BHOF) and Institute of Medicine (IOM) recommend 1,000 mg/d for men aged 19 to 70 years and women aged 19 to 50 years; 1,200 mg/d women 51 and older and men 71 and older.
- Increasing dietary calcium is first line.
- Calcium supplements should be taken if dietary intake cannot meet recommended levels.
- Current evidence supports the use of calcium plus vitamin D to reduce fracture risk in community-dwelling and institutionalized middle-aged to older adults (2)[A].
- BHOF recommends daily intake of 800 to 1,000 U of vitamin D.

DIAGNOSIS

HISTORY

- General risk factor assessment
- Low trauma fracture at age 50 years and above
- Historical height loss: peak height age 20 years—current height ≥4 cm
- Prospective height loss: previously documented height—present height ≥2 cm
- Evaluate Fracture Risk Assessment Tool (FRAX) 10-year fracture risk calculation for hip fracture and major osteoporotic fracture of spine, forearm, hip, and shoulder (https://www.bonehealthandosteoporosis.org/ and https://www.fraxplus.org/).

PHYSICAL EXAM

Silent disease, that is, not evident on exam unless advanced stage and subsequent fracture. Those with undiagnosed compression fractures may have tenderness to palpation in the midline of the spine.

DIAGNOSTIC TESTS & INTERPRETATION

- Assessment of biochemical markers of bone turnover: osteocalcin, total and bone-specific alkaline phosphatase useful in monitoring response to treatment
- Serum type I collagen propeptide, pyridinoline levels in blood and urine, and plasma tartrate-resistant acid phosphatase levels are markers used in research settings.
- DEXA measures bone mineral content of lumbar spine, femoral neck, and distal radius yielding BMD (g/cm^2) and is the basis of definition for osteoporosis according to WHO criteria.
- Vertebral fracture assessment (VFA) uses central DEXA of the thoracic and lumbar spine to assess for compression fractures; lower cost and radiation than plain radiographs of the spine
- Thoracic and lumbar spine films can be useful for identification of fracture and determination of significant arthritis that might falsely elevate T-score.

TREATMENT

Osteoporosis treatment reduces fracture risk and is recommended by the BHOF for women and men with a personal history of a hip or vertebral fracture, a T-score ≤−2.5, or a combination of low bone mass (T-score −1.0 to −2.5) and a 10-year probability of hip fracture of at least 3% or any major fracture of at least 20% as calculated by FRAX fracture assessment tool (2)[A].

MEDICATION

First Line

- Bisphosphonates: most prescribed therapy for the prevention and treatment of osteoporosis; inhibit both osteoblast and, to a greater extent, osteoclast activity, thus decreasing bone turnover and increasing BMD; decrease vertebral fracture 41–70%:
  - Adverse effects: GI: nausea, vomiting, abdominal pain, dyspepsia, esophagitis, reflux, atypical femur fractures (AFF)
  - Risk of osteonecrosis of jaw a rare complication that can occur in the setting of invasive dental procedures such as tooth extraction or implantation:
    - Alendronate (Fosamax):
      - Decreases spine and hip fracture 50% over 3 years
    - Risedronate (Actonel):
      - Reduced incidence of vertebral fractures by 39%, hip fractures by 27%, and nonvertebral fractures by 22%
    - Ibandronate (Boniva):
      - Has antifracture effectiveness in the spine only; reduces incidence of vertebral fractures by 33–50% over 3 years; intravenous (IV) 3 mg every 3 months increases BMD or oral

- Zoledronic acid (Reclast):
  - Reduces incidence of vertebral fractures by 62–70%, hip fractures by 41%, and nonvertebral fractures by 21–25%
  - Once yearly IV, obtain calcium and vitamin D levels prior and correct insufficiencies.
  - Cost for IV medications is high but may be indicated in high-risk women who cannot tolerate or are noncompliant with oral therapy due to pre-dose and post-dose fasting and posture requirements.
- Estrogen-related therapies
- Selective estrogen receptor modulators: raloxifene (Evista):
  - Estrogen agonist activity in bone tissue and on lipids, with antagonist activity in breast and uterine tissue; especially useful in women at elevated risk for breast cancer
  - Decreases vertebral and nonvertebral fracture 30–50%
  - No hip fracture prevention
- Estrogen therapy (ET)/hormone therapy (HT)
  - FDA approved for prevention of osteoporosis and relief of vasomotor symptoms and vulvovaginal atrophy
  - Women with hysterectomy are treated with ET.
  - Women with intact uterus require HT.
  - Biliary issues, breast cancer (with HT), endometrial hyperplasia (with ET)
  - Analysis of Women's Health Initiative (WHI) substudy data showed no increase in CV disease in women starting treatment using HT, within 10 years of menopause.
- Conjugated estrogen/bazedoxifene (Duavee)
- Estrogen with estrogen agonist/antagonist
  - Females who have not undergone hysterectomy
  - Reduces risk for endometrial hyperplasia
  - Increases mean lumbar and hip BMD
- Parathyroid hormone:
  - Teriparatide (Forteo), Abaloparatide (Tymlos):
    - Recombinant human parathyroid hormone with bone anabolic activity stimulating bone formation and inhibiting resorption
    - 20 μg subcutaneous (SC) daily for 2 years
    - Indicated for postmenopausal women with severe bone loss, men with osteoporosis at elevated risk of fracture, and in persons not improved with bisphosphonate therapy
    - Decreases vertebral fracture 65–69%
    - Decreased nonvertebral fracture 35–40%
    - No hip fracture prevention (2)[A]
- Denosumab (Prolia):
  - Human monoclonal antibody inhibiting osteoclast bone resorption
  - Reduces risk of vertebral, nonvertebral, and hip fractures
  - SC every 6 months
  - High-risk women
  - Rebound increase in bone resorption and increase in vertebral fracture after discontinuation of treatment for 12 months.
- Romosozumab (Evenity): human monoclonal antibody
  - FDA approved for postmenopausal women at high risk for fracture, poor response, intolerance to other therapies
  - Reduces fractures and increases BMD in lumbar spine and total hip
  - Reduced risk of vertebral fracture by 73%
  - Monthly SC injection for 1 year
  - May increase risk for CV events (boxed warning)

Second Line

Calcitonin (Miacalcin, Fortical)

- Antiresorptive treatment via osteoclast inhibition
- Decreases occurrence of vertebral compression fractures by 30% but not nonvertebral or hip fractures
- Women 5 years postmenopausal if alternative treatments not suitable
- 100 IU SC/intramuscular (IM) daily or every other day
- 200 IU intranasal spray daily with 1,000 mg calcium and 400 IU vitamin D
- Significantly reduces acute fracture pain
- Association between malignancy and calcitonin-salmon use with increased risk of 4.1% compared with placebo 2.9% reevaluate periodically (1)[A],(2)[A].

ALERT

When ET/HT use is intended solely for fracture prevention, FDA recommends approved non-estrogens be considered first.

COMPLEMENTARY & ALTERNATIVE MEDICINE

- Physical therapy and rehabilitation can reduce disability, improve strength, improve function of activities of daily living (ADLs), and decrease risk of falls.
- Weight-bearing exercise with additional resistance training can maintain bone mass and can help prevent falls when coupled with adequate dietary calcium and vitamin D intake.
- Fall prevention addressing vision deficits, balance and gait abnormalities, cognitive impairment, dizziness, and home safety assessment

ONGOING CARE

FOLLOW-UP RECOMMENDATIONS

Patient Monitoring

- Changes in BMD levels indicative of real biologic change can be measured after 1 year of treatment with serial DEXA.
- Changes in bone turnover marker levels in treated patients can be observed within 3 months of treatment initiation. Suppression of bone turnover markers after 3 to 6 months of treatment and increases after 1 to 3 months of anabolic therapy have been predictive of BMD responses and fracture risk reduction (1)[A].
- T-score targets of >-2.5 reasonable in assessing efficacy of initial drug therapy or changing therapy but may not be applicable to all patients.

REFERENCES

1. Foessl I, Dimai HP, Obermayer-Pietsch B. Long-term and sequential treatment for osteoporosis. *Nat Rev Endocrinol.* 2023;19(9):520–533.
2. LeBoff MS, Greenspan SL, Insogna KL, et al. The clinician's guide to prevention and treatment of osteoporosis. *Osteoporos Int.* 2022;33(10):2049–2102.

ADDITIONAL READING

- Ebeling PR, Nguyen HH, Aleksova J, et al. Secondary Osteoporosis. *Endocr Rev.* 2022;43(2):240–313.
- Watts N. Postmenopausal osteoporosis: a clinical review. *J Womens Health (Larchmt).* 2018;27(9):1093–1096.

CLINICAL PEARLS

- U.S. Preventive Services Task Force (USPSTF) recommends DEXA screening for women aged >65 years and men aged ≥70 years regardless of clinical risk factors.
- USPSTF recommends screening for postmenopausal women aged <65 years at increased risk of osteoporosis, determined by clinical risk assessment tool.
- Osteoporosis treatment reduces fracture risk and is recommended for those with personal history of fracture and those at elevated risk as defined by the BHOF.
- Drug holiday after 5 years of oral and 3 years of IV bisphosphonate in patients no longer at high risk for fracture (T-score >-2.5, no new fractures)

OVERTRAINING SYNDROME

W. Scott Black, MD, MS • Srikanth Nithyanandam, MBBS, MS, CAQSM

BASICS

DESCRIPTION

- Overreaching:
  - The accumulation of training and/or nontraining stress resulting in a short-term decrease in performance capacity, with or without related physiologic and psychological symptoms. It can take several days to several weeks for the recovery of performance capacity and resolution of psychological symptoms to occur.
  - States of overreaching exist along a spectrum, ranging from functional (planned) overreaching where the expected outcome is a positive adaptation or improvement in performance, to nonfunctional overreaching (NFOR) where the balance between training stress and recovery is disrupted.
  - In cases of NFOR, a restoration of performance may occur after several days to weeks of rest (1)
- Overtraining:
  - The accumulation of training and/or nontraining stress, which results in a long-term decrease in performance capacity with or without related physiologic and psychological symptoms. Recovery of performance capacity and resolution of psychological symptoms can take several weeks to several months to occur. When being used to describe a clinical entity, this is often referred to as "overtraining syndrome" (OTS).
  - The distinction between NFOR and OTS lies in the time required for performance restoration. As a result, diagnosing OTS often becomes possible only in retrospect.
  - Synonym(s) include "unexplained underperformance syndrome," "staleness," and "burnout" (1).

EPIDEMIOLOGY

- Functional overreaching is common and may be intentionally induced as part of a training regimen (1).
- The prevalence of NFOR and OTS is difficult to estimate given the vague nature of the symptoms and the lack of a widely accepted diagnostic test. Nevertheless, some studies have suggested a rate of NFOR/OTS of about 10% in athletes coming out of an intense training cycle (1). Other studies have noted a lifetime incidence of 30–60% in nonelite and elite endurance athletes, respectively (1).

ETIOLOGY AND PATHOPHYSIOLOGY

- Currently, there is no universally accepted hypothesis as to the cause of OTS.
- OTS represents the final common result of persistent, repetitive, or excessive activation of various allostatic mechanisms.
- Multiple pathophysiologic mechanisms have been proposed as causes for OTS: dysfunction of the autonomic nervous system (sympathetic or parasympathetic forms of OTS), hypothalamic dysfunction (hypothalamic–pituitary–adrenal axis and hypothalamic–pituitary–gonadal axis), muscle trauma with resulting cytokine-mediated systemic inflammation, reduced blood glutamine levels, decreased blood levels of branched-chain amino acids, low dietary intake of nutrients, and glycogen depletion (1),(2).

RISK FACTORS

- Highly motivated athletes who respond to poor athletic performance by increasing training loads.
- Athletes are subjected to generic overload stimuli, without individualized training.
- Additional "nonathletic" stressors (social, economic, scholastic, relationship, etc.)
- Nutritional deficiency/reduced energy availability.

GENERAL PREVENTION

- Consensus currently is that there is no effective treatment for OTS other than rest and recovery. Therefore, the emphasis should be on prevention (1),(2).
- Daily training logs:
  - Helpful in determining the cumulative strain involved with training
  - To be useful in early detection of OTS, systematic documentation of subjective and objective factors must be completed at baseline (when the athlete has no signs or symptoms) and reevaluated regularly.
  - Although small daily variations occur in athletes, training logs can identify an individual athlete's abnormal response to training at an early stage.
  - Once identified, interventions can be made to prevent further deterioration of performance and normalization of subjective and objective criteria.
  - Training logs should include:
    - Daily workout schedule (including intensity, duration, and mode of training)
    - Rating of perceived exertion (RPE) for the *entire* training session on a specific day. This can be done using the modified (category ratio) Borg scale, which rates perceived effort from 0 (nothing at all) to 10 (almost maximal).
    - The product of the session RPE and session duration can be recorded and represents an objective measurement of daily "training load."
    - Some general description of sense of fatigue or overall state of well-being of the athlete
- Proper coaching and training techniques:
  - Recognize overtraining early and intervene.
  - Avoid monotony in training.
  - Avoid punishing poor training performance with higher levels of training.
  - Training goals should be formulated on a week-to-week basis during times of increased training.
  - Training loads should display day-to-day variability.
  - Alternate hard day/easy day and include 1 rest day per week (hard day = RPE >5; easy day = RPE <5)
  - If athlete begins to show strain (performance decrements, increasing RPE at low-level training), reduce training to a lower level.
- Ensure adequate recovery:
  - Athletes should have no less than one passive rest day each week.
  - All athletes should be assessed for adequacy of sleep. Significant individual differences exist in the amount of sleep necessary for adequate recovery, so it is best to simply inquire if athletes feel well rested and energetic each day.
  - Screen for negative energy balance in athletes with signs/symptoms suggestive of NFOR/OTS.
  - Ensure adequate glycogen replenishment.

DIAGNOSIS

- There is no single diagnostic test or pathognomonic finding indicative of OTS. Diagnostic process should consider common biopsychosocial factors that may contribute to athlete underperformance (2)[C].
- An algorithm to aid in the diagnosis of OTS in athletes has been proposed (1)[C].
- A three-step diagnostic tool has been created to help establish the diagnosis of OTS. Its authors report 100% accuracy in distinguishing OTS-affected athletes from healthy athletes (3)[B].
- Research supports the use of psychological testing in the evaluation of possible cases of OTS (1)[B].
- Profile of Mood States questionnaire is the most studied and is part of the three-step diagnostic tool mentioned above.
- Several additional sport-specific psychological evaluation tools are currently available: (i) Standardized Overtraining Questionnaire from the French Society for Sports Medicine, (ii) Recovery-Stress Questionnaire for Athletes (RESTQ-Sport), and (iii) Daily Analysis of Life Demands in Athletes (DALDA).
- Overlap between OTS and relative energy deficiency in sport (RED-S) is significant. An evaluation of OTS should include careful screening for RED-S (4).

- Measurements of psychomotor speed (e.g., Stroop test) may show decrements from baseline early in NFOR (1)[B].
- A two-bout training optimization (TOP) exercise test in which adrenocorticotropic hormone (ACTH) and prolactin are measured following two sequential maximum graded exercise tests separated by 4 hours has shown promise in being able to distinguish NFOR from OTS (5),(6)[B].
- Reduced performance on speed-endurance or short, high-intensity exercise tests (decreased performance on time trials) is consistently found (1),(2)[B].
- VO_2max may be reduced, but unchanged values are not unusual.
- Blood lactate at submaximal steady-state exercise and at maximal exercise may be reduced from baseline.
- Performance decrements may be seen when evaluating maximum sport-specific performance with increased perceived exertion at a given workload.
- Decreased coordination may be observed.

HISTORY

- Review training logs and performance results if possible.
- Consider:
  - Is there objective evidence of persistent decreased performance?
  - Current training load: intensity, frequency, duration, and/or mode of training
  - Historical training load over past several months
  - Any changes in "nonathletic" stressors (e.g., financial problems, family illness, relationship problems, scholastic concerns)
  - Any changes in sleep pattern
  - Recent exposure to infection
  - Changes in menstruation
  - Nutritional assessment

PHYSICAL EXAM

- Because OTS is a spectrum of diseases, the clinical presentation varies among individual athletes.
- Document temperature to help identify systemic infection.
- Evaluate resting heart rate and blood pressure (BP), including orthostatic assessment.
- Height, weight, BMI, and body composition assessment may help identify chronic energy deficiency.
- Head/eyes/ears/nose/throat exam to evaluate possible upper respiratory infection/infectious mononucleosis
- Neck exam for adenopathy or thyroid abnormalities
- Chest auscultation to evaluate for cardiopulmonary disease
- Abdominal examination to evaluate spleen and liver
- Neurologic examination to evaluate neuromuscular disease

DIFFERENTIAL DIAGNOSIS

- Major depression or other psychological disorder
- RED-S infectious disease (e.g., mononucleosis, COVID-19, or other infections)
- Adverse effects of drugs (including drug abuse or misuse)
- Micronutrient deficiencies (e.g., iron-deficiency anemia)
- Cardiopulmonary disease (e.g., asthma, cardiomyopathies)
- Concussion
- Less common causes of athlete underperformance (e.g., diabetes, thyroid disease, inflammatory autoimmune conditions, myalgic encephalomyelitis, cancer, neuromuscular disease)

TREATMENT

- Optimal treatment may best be accomplished through collaboration with nutrition and psychology practitioners, exercise scientists, and the patient's athletic trainers and coaches.
- The primary treatment for OTS is relative or absolute rest, depending on the severity of overtraining (1)[C].
- During the rest period, the clinician should evaluate and manage any conditions that might be interfering with adequate recovery (sleep disturbance, nutritional deficiency, etc.).
- Mild cases may improve with a relative decrease in training load (frequency and/or intensity), an increase in rest between training sessions, and/or an increase in training variety (cross-training).
- More severe cases may need weeks to months of absolute rest. Occasionally, athletes never return to their previous level of function.

REFERENCES

1. Meeusen R, Duclos M, Foster C, et al. Prevention, diagnosis, and treatment of the overtraining syndrome: joint consensus statement of the European College of Sport Science and the American College of Sports Medicine. *Med Sci Sports Exerc.* 2013;45(1):186–205.
2. Lewis NA, Collins D, Pedlar CR, et al. Can clinicians and scientists explain and prevent unexplained underperformance syndrome in elite athletes: an interdisciplinary perspective and 2016 update. *BMJ Open Sport Exerc Med.* 2015;1(1):e000063.
3. Cadegiani FA, da Silva PHL, Abrao TCP, et al. Diagnosis of overtraining syndrome: results of the endocrine and metabolic responses on overtraining syndrome study: EROS-DIAGNOSIS. *J Sports Med (Hindawi Publ Corp).* 2020;2020:3937819.
4. Stellingwerff T, Heikura IA, Meeusen R, et al. Overtraining syndrome (OTS) and relative energy deficiency in sport (RED-S): shared pathways, symptoms, and complexities. *Sports Med.* 2021;51(11):2251–2280.
5. Meeusen R, Nederhof E, Buyse L, et al. Diagnosing overtraining in athletes using the two-bout exercise protocol. *Br J Sports Med.* 2010;44(9):642–648.
6. Buyse L, Decroix L, Timmermans N, et al. Improving the diagnosis of nonfunctional overreaching and overtraining syndrome. *Med Sci Sports Exerc.* 2019;51(12):2524–2530.

ADDITIONAL READING

- Cadegiani FA, Kater CE. Hormonal aspects of overtraining syndrome: a systematic review. *BMC Sports Sci Med Rehabil.* 2017;9:14.
- Foster C. Monitoring training in athletes with reference to overtraining syndrome. *Med Sci Sports Exerc.* 1998;30(7):1164–1168.
- Kreher JB. Diagnosis and prevention of overtraining syndrome: an opinion on education strategies. *Open Access J Sports Med.* 2016;7:115–122.
- Meeusen R, Duclos M, Gleeson M, et al. Prevention, diagnosis, and treatment of the overtraining syndrome. *Eur J Sport Sci.* 2006;6(1):1–14.

CLINICAL PEARLS

- Consensus presently is there is no effective treatment for OTS other than relative or absolute rest from physical activity depending on the severity while addressing nutritional, sleep, and stress levels to promote recovery.
- Emphasis should always be on prevention.
- There is no single diagnostic test for OTS.
- An algorithm to aid in the diagnosis of OTS in athletes has been proposed.

PAGET-SCHROETTER SYNDROME

Chris Koutures, MD, FAAP

BASICS

DESCRIPTION

- Paget-Schroetter syndrome (PSS) is venous thrombosis resulting from chronic compression of the subclavian vein (1). Compression in an anatomically normal extremity occurs in extremes of shoulder abduction or external rotation (1).
- Thrombosis occurs within a triangular space bordered by the 1st rib, clavicle, and subclavius muscle/ costoclavicular ligament (2).
- PSS is a subset of the venous thoracic outlet syndrome (VTOS) (1).
- Synonyms: effort thrombosis (1); primary VTOS (3)

EPIDEMIOLOGY

Incidence

- Rare syndrome that has been estimated to be about 1 to 2/100,000 people per year, which would translate to 3,000 to 6,000 incidences in the United States yearly (4)
- Mean age of presentation is early in the 3rd decade, and the male to female ratio is 2:1 (4).

ETIOLOGY AND PATHOPHYSIOLOGY

- PSS results from chronic or repeated compression of the subclavian vein within the thoracic outlet (2).
- Compression occurs inside of a triangular space (the venous thoracic outlet) formed by the 1st rib, clavicle, and the subclavius muscle or costoclavicular ligament (2).
- A narrow thoracic outlet for the subclavian vein increases the chances of compression of the vein, which can lead to stasis of venous blood flow as well as decreased mobility of the vein and subsequent increased susceptibility to trauma with arm use (5).
- A narrow venous thoracic outlet is further compressed when the arm is in abduction and/or external rotation (1).
- Repeated trauma to the vein leads to a cycle of endothelial injury causing intimal hyperplasia, inflammation, fibrosis, worsening stasis and compression of the vein (5), and increasing risk of thrombosis. Stretching of the vein as the arm moves can also cause small tears and further damage (3).

RISK FACTORS

- Anatomic variations of the size and position of the costoclavicular ligament or anterior scalene or subclavius muscle that cause a narrow outlet (2)
- Athletes who perform repeated overhead movement of the upper extremity such as throwing, swimming, and weight lifting (2)
- Occupations requiring repeated overhead movement (2)
- The role of thrombophilia is debated (2).

GENERAL PREVENTION

Early recognition of symptoms and detection of possible intermittent obstruction without thrombosis, which can increase risk of thrombus development (2)

COMMONLY ASSOCIATED CONDITIONS

43% of patients with VTOS had either occult 1st rib fracture, irregular costochondral calcification, and/or osteophytic degeneration of the anterior portion of the 1st rib (6).

DIAGNOSIS

HISTORY

- Classic presentation: abrupt painful and swollen upper extremity with blue hue in a young athletic male (2)
- Symptoms typically occur within 24 hours of vigorous or heavy upper extremity activity (1).

PHYSICAL EXAM

- Visual inspection reveals asymmetric swelling and superficial venous engorgement of the upper arm (1),(2).
- Axillary vein may be palpated as a hard, linear structure, which may represent extension of clotted vein (1).
- There are no specific physical exam tests to confirm diagnosis (1).

DIFFERENTIAL DIAGNOSIS

- Neurologic or arterial thoracic outlet syndrome
- Tumors of the head, neck, or arm, including Pancoast tumor
- Complex regional pain syndrome
- Lymphedema
- Secondary causes of thrombosis such as presence of central line, pacemaker lead, or thrombophilia.

DIAGNOSTIC TESTS & INTERPRETATION

Initial Tests (lab, imaging)

- Urgent venous duplex ultrasound is recommended for initial diagnostic purposes because thrombolysis is optimal if performed within 2 weeks of symptom onset (3)[B].
- If no thrombus is identified and concern for intermittent occlusion, arm should be placed in abduction with assessment of flow through the subclavian and axillary veins (2)[C].
- There may be a role for computed tomography angiography (CTA) or magnetic resonance angiography (MRA) if ultrasound is limited due to patient body habitus.

Follow-Up Tests & Special Considerations

Contrast venography is indicated for those with abnormal initial ultrasound and plans for endovascular intervention (2)[C].

TREATMENT

GENERAL MEASURES

- Anticoagulation, symptomatic treatment, and relief of extrinsic compression (2)
- Symptom relief requires pain control and compression (2).
- Catheter-directed thrombolysis provides short-term benefits (2).
- First rib resection and scalenectomy (FRRS) for complete decompression of the thoracic outlet (2)[C]

MEDICATION

Anticoagulation alone is not recommended due to a high rate of disability and recurrent thrombosis, and prolonged anticoagulation is lifestyle limiting (2)[B]. However, temporary anticoagulation will be necessary.

ISSUES FOR REFERRAL

Patients with suspected PSS should be referred immediately to a vascular specialist as rate of successful thrombolysis after 14 days or more of symptoms decreases significantly (2)[B].

SURGERY/OTHER PROCEDURES

- Currently, decompression of the thoracic outlet via 1st rib resection after thrombolysis or anticoagulation is generally considered the treatment of choice; however, some studies have disputed the need (4)[C].
- Multiple approaches to this have been developed (2).
- The infraclavicular approach allows complete resection of the anterior first rib, subclavius muscle, and costoclavicular ligament. This eliminates the extrinsic compression that precipitated the initial thrombotic event, with excellent long-term patency rates (7)[A].

ADMISSION, INPATIENT, AND NURSING CONSIDERATIONS

Inpatient management may be required for patients with severe symptoms, particularly if anticipating thrombolytic or surgical therapy.

ONGOING CARE

FOLLOW-UP RECOMMENDATIONS

- After surgical decompression, patients discharged on therapeutic anticoagulation, typically weight-based low-molecular-weight heparin (2).
- Follow-up venography should be performed 2 to 3 weeks postoperatively (2)[C].
- Anticoagulation may be continued if vein has reoccluded or until patency achieved, up to 6 months (2)[C].
- Anticoagulation for 3 to 6 months after thrombolysis and decompression is recommended, although some studies have advocated for limiting anticoagulation to 3 months (4)[C].
- Passive range of motion should be initiated during anticoagulation to prevent stiffness (1). Angioplasty may be recommended for those with persistent intrinsic defects of the vein or those with chronic occlusion (2)[C].

Patient Monitoring

There is no standardized method of monitoring. Some monitor with ultrasound or venography postoperatively, with repeat ultrasound if there is any recurrence of symptoms (3),(4)[C].

PATIENT EDUCATION

Recurrence is possible, some may argue, more commonly without decompressive surgery. Patients should be educated to return with any signs of recurrence.

PROGNOSIS

- The majority of literature regarding outcomes after treatment of PSS is based on uncontrolled, single-center series, making definitive data difficult to extrapolate (4).
- Prompt thrombolysis and 1st rib resection has been reported to lead to better outcomes (2)[C].
- For young athletes, return to play has been noted to be quicker with earlier intervention (1).

COMPLICATIONS

- Pulmonary embolism
- Postthrombotic syndrome
- Recurrent thrombosis (5)

REFERENCES

1. Mall NA, Van Thiel GS, Heard WM, et al. Paget-Schroetter syndrome: a review of effort thrombosis of the upper extremity from a sports medicine perspective. *Sports Health*. 2013;5(4):353–356.
2. Moore R, Lum YW. Venous thoracic outlet syndrome. *Vasc Med*. 2015;20(2):182–189.
3. Hangge P, Rotellini-Coltvet L, Deipolyi AR, et al. Paget-Schroetter syndrome: treatment of venous thrombosis and outcomes. *Cardiovasc Diagn Ther*. 2017;7(Suppl 3):S285–S290.
4. Illig KA, Doyle AJ. A comprehensive review of Paget-Schroetter syndrome. *J Vasc Surg*. 2010;51(6):1538–1547.
5. Alla VM, Natarajan N, Kaushik M, et al. Paget-Schroetter syndrome: review of pathogenesis and treatment of effort thrombosis. *West J Emerg Med*. 2010;11(4):358–362.
6. Sheng GG, Duwayri YM, Emery VB, et al. Costochondral calcification, osteophytic degeneration, and occult first rib fractures in patients with venous thoracic outlet syndrome. *J Vasc Surg*. 2012;55(5):1363–1369.
7. Samoila G, Twine CP, Williams IM. The infraclavicular approach for Paget-Schroetter syndrome. *Ann R Coll Surg Engl*. 2018;100(2):83–91.

CLINICAL PEARLS

- PSS is venous thrombosis of the subclavian/axillary vein caused by compression of the venous thoracic outlet in conjunction with chronic injury to the vein by repeated overhead arm activity.
- Definitive treatment of choice is still debated but currently consists of anticoagulation or thrombolysis, followed by decompressive surgery.
- Prognosis and treatment outcomes would best be assessed by prospective randomized trials which are lacking.

PANNER DISEASE AND OCD OF ELBOW CAPITELLUM

Kevin Machino, DO ▪ Holly J. Benjamin, MD, FAMSSM, FACSM

BASICS

DESCRIPTION

- Panner disease (osteochondrosis) and osteochondritis dissecans (OCD) of the capitellum are conditions of the elbow seen in children and adolescents, respectively. They occur in young athletes who perform repetitive upper extremity exercises such as throwers, weight lifters, and gymnasts.
- Both conditions are overuse injuries of the elbow that involve disordered endochondral ossification of the humeral capitellum. They are generally considered different pathologic entities but may be a continuum of disordered endochondral ossification.

EPIDEMIOLOGY

- Most commonly unilateral (<10% are bilateral) and occur in the dominant arm in both (1)
- Boys are affected more often than girls in both.
- Panner disease occurs in children:
  - More common before the age of 10 years
- OCD of the capitellum occurs in adolescents:
  - Average patient age is between 12 and 17 years.
- OCD lesions of the capitellum are most common, but disorders of the radial head, trochlea, olecranon, and olecranon fossa are also described.

ETIOLOGY AND PATHOPHYSIOLOGY

- Precise etiology is not well established for both (2).
- Panner disease:
  - Involves the entire ossific center of the capitellum
  - Repetitive valgus loading across the radiocapitellar joint causes microvascular trauma leading to ischemic injury of the capitellum.
  - Articular chondrocyte viability may be compromised by repetitive compressive loading.
  - Ossific nucleus of capitellum has a tenuous blood supply, which may be vulnerable to stresses at the elbow.
- OCD of the elbow capitellum:
  - Involves a portion of the capitellum
  - Disrupted growth of articular cartilage and subchondral bone results in spontaneous avascular osteonecrosis and formation of osteochondral fragments
  - Histopathologic examination has failed to demonstrate an inflammatory process despite nomenclature ("osteochondritis").
  - OCD is likely a result of repetitive compressive forces exerted across the radiocapitellar joint during a time of epiphyseal vulnerability.
- Genetics
  - A genetic predisposition has been hypothesized.

RISK FACTORS

- Valgus stress results in lateral compression and shear forces applied to the radiocapitellar joint during the late cocking and early acceleration phases of throwing and racquet sports.
- Increased weight-bearing and axial impact loads across the upper extremity are seen in young gymnasts and weight lifters.
- Repetitive compressive forces may compromise vulnerable blood supply to capitellum and result in articular cartilage breakdown and fragmentation of subchondral bone.
- Initially articular surface softens, followed by subchondral collapse. This may lead to fragmentation in Panner disease or formation of loose bodies in OCD (loose bodies not seen in Panner).

GENERAL PREVENTION

- Proper throwing technique in overhead throwing athletes
- Adequate rest from activities that cause repetitive microtrauma to the lateral elbow including pitch counts for pitchers
- Early evaluation of elbow pain in high-risk patients

DIAGNOSIS

HISTORY

- Often associated with history of repetitive valgus stress to the elbow (sports-related activities)
- Insidious onset of elbow pain with activity:
  - Acute, sudden onset is rare.
- Most common presenting symptoms are pain, swelling, and limited range of motion.
- Pain is exacerbated by activity and relieved with rest. Pain is often lateral, but diffuse pain can occur.
- Other symptoms: stiffness, clicking, catching, grinding, locking

PHYSICAL EXAM

- Tenderness over radiocapitellar joint
- Loss of extension; 15 to 30 degrees is common:
  - Loss of flexion less common
  - Pronation, supination usually unaffected
- Effusion may be present.
- Crepitus may be present with active or passive pronation and supination.
- Pain with radiocapitellar compression test:
  - Arm actively pronated and supinated with elbow fully extended, while applying axial load.

DIFFERENTIAL DIAGNOSIS

- Trochlear lesions (avascular necrosis, OCD of the elbow trochlea)
- Distal humerus fracture
- Epicondylar avulsion fracture
- Posterolateral elbow impingement
- OCD of the radial head
- Angular deformity of the radial neck
- Ulnar collateral ligament (UCL) injury
- Tendinopathy

DIAGNOSTIC TESTS & INTERPRETATION

Initial Tests (lab, imaging)

- Labs are not indicated unless other underlying etiology is suspected (e.g., infectious, endocrine)
- Plain radiographs (3)[C],(4)[B]:
  - Obtain anteroposterior and lateral elbow radiographs:
    - May be compared to contralateral elbow to detect subtle changes of capitellum
    - Able to demonstrate interval healing
  - Panner disease:
    - Changes in morphology (decreased size), contour irregularities (epiphysis with fissuring), flattened articular surface, fragmentation and collapse, radiolucency, sclerosis of the capitellum
  - OCD of capitellum:
    - Low sensitivity (44–47%) to detect OCD
    - Similar appearance to Panner disease; however, loose bodies and capitellar flattening more common in OCD
    - Focal lucency in subchondral bone in anterolateral capitellum
    - Minami radiographical classification of capitellar OCD:
      - Grade 1: radiolucency or localized flattening
      - Grade 2: nondisplaced fragment
      - Grade 3: displaced fragment or loose bodies
- Magnetic resonance imaging (MRI):
  - Imaging modality of choice
  - Capable of detecting early lesions not visible on plain radiographs (bone edema)
  - Useful for lesion characterization of size and extent
  - Allows assessment of lesion stability and integrity of articular cartilage
  - MRI also able to demonstrate interval healing and lesion resolution
  - There are several staging or classification systems that have been used for elbow OCD lesion with MRI (i.e., Itsubo, Bruns, and DiPaola classifications).
  - Itsubo MRI classification of capitellar OCD:
    - Stage 1: normal shaped capitellum, spotted areas of high signal intensity (lower than normal cartilage)
    - Stage 2: stage 1 + several spotted areas of high signal intensity (higher than cartilage)
    - Stage 3: stage 2 + discontinuity and noncircularity of chondral surface signal of capitellum + no high signal interface between lesion and floor
    - Stage 4: lesion separated by high intensity line
    - Stage 5: capitellar lesion is defected or displaced from floor
- Computed tomography (CT) arthrography:
  - Useful for confirming presence of intra-articular loose bodies
  - Depicts cartilage integrity and fissuring
- Ultrasound (US):
  - Able to assess subchondral bone and overlying cartilage integrity
  - Can assess joint stability
  - Operator-dependent imaging modality
- Radionuclide bone scan:
  - Very sensitive but nonspecific for Panner disease and OCD of the capitellum
  - Limited usefulness in the diagnosis and staging of these conditions

Diagnostic Procedures/Other

Elbow arthroscopy allows direct visualization of the articular cartilage surface for staging:

- May fail to identify changes of the capitellum not evident at joint surface

TREATMENT

MEDICATION

Analgesics and nonsteroidal anti-inflammatory drugs (NSAIDs) may be used as necessary for pain relief.

ISSUES FOR REFERRAL

- Panner disease:
  - Persistent pain or symptoms despite appropriate conservative care
- OCD of the capitellum:
  - Persistent pain or symptoms despite appropriate conservative care
  - Symptomatic loose bodies
  - Articular cartilage fracture
  - Unstable, loose, or displaced osteochondral lesion

ADDITIONAL THERAPIES

Little evidence exists for duration of treatment, bracing, or physical therapy for these conditions:

- Panner disease:
  - Rest from offending activities and avoidance of radiocapitellar joint loading for 3 to 6 months.
  - Nonoperative treatment provides excellent long-term prognosis.
  - Surgery rarely necessary
  - Similar natural history to Perthes disease in the hip
- OCD of the capitellum:
  - Skeletal maturity and lesion stability are considered the most important factors for clinical decision-making
    - Nonoperative treatment for early, intact, and stable lesions in skeletally immature patients is recommended.
    - In skeletally mature patients with symptomatic OCD, early referral for surgical consultation is preferred.
    - Patients with stage 3 to 5 lesions on MRI, particularly in the presence of a loose body, is an indication for early surgical referral.
  - Nonoperative management:
    - Rest from offending activities and avoidance of radiocapitellar joint loading for 3 to 6 months.
      - Some advocate for hinged unloader elbow brace to avoid excessive valgus stress.
    - Conservative monitoring with serial radiographs is reasonable in skeletally immature patients, often with successful resolution of stable OCD lesions over a period of weeks to months.

SURGERY/OTHER PROCEDURES

- Operative management is indicated for the following reasons (5)[C]:
  - Failure of appropriate conservative management
  - Mechanical symptoms
  - Intra-articular loose bodies
  - Unstable lesions
- Operative techniques vary, include the following:
  - Loose body or unstable fragment removal
  - In situ fixation of unstable osteochondral fragment
  - Chondroplasty
  - Autologous chondrocyte implantation
  - Osteochondral autograft transplantation system (OATS)
  - Subchondral drilling (microfracture)
  - Closing wedge osteotomy of the lateral epicondyle

ONGOING CARE

FOLLOW UP RECOMMENDATIONS

Patient Monitoring

Return to activity:

- Gradual progressive return to activity and sports can begin after a period of rest when patient is asymptomatic.
- Physical therapy may begin when symptoms improve:
  - Range of motion, stretching, and gentle strengthening while avoiding radiocapitellar stress
- Evidence of healing should be seen on follow-up radiographs or MRI before return of elbow loading:
  - Serial radiographs performed at 6-week intervals are useful to document healing or progression.
  - MRI follow-up 6 months after initiation of conservative management to document lesion healing; consider imaging at 1 year.
- Athlete should be monitored closely by health care team during return to sport:
  - Progress activity as tolerated, gradually increasing weight-bearing and load across lateral elbow.
  - Rest and resumption of activity avoidance if symptoms return
- For pitchers, recommend strict adherence to established pitch count recommendations.
- It is important to establish good core strength to improve sport mechanics and potentially decrease loading of the radiocapitellar joint.

PATIENT EDUCATION

- Instruct patients on importance of proper sport biomechanics and technique.
- Strict adherence to pitch counts upon return to pitching
- Reevaluation is necessary for return of elbow symptoms after return to sport.
- Consider activity modification to decrease elbow loading following recovery.

PROGNOSIS

- Favorable prognostic factors (6)[C]:
  - Open capitellar physis
  - Age <10 years
  - Normal elbow range of motion
  - Absence of mechanical symptoms
  - Stable lesion with radiographic findings of subchondral lucency or flattening
- Poor prognostic factors:
  - Closed capitellar physis
  - Age >10 years for Panner disease and skeletally mature elbow for OCD
  - Loss of elbow extension
  - Mechanical symptoms
  - Unstable lesion or loose bodies (stage 4/5)
  - Large fragment involving >50% of capitellum

COMPLICATIONS

- Many patients will have persistent loss of extension despite good clinical outcome with return to sport.
- Early degenerative joint disease and continued symptoms of pain and stiffness are more likely in advanced cases.
- Some athletes have difficulty returning to high-risk weight-bearing or throwing sports.

REFERENCES

1. Chavda S, Abeid KA, Alhajri KK, et al. Osteochondrosis of humeral capitellum, diagnosis and treatment—a case report. *J Orthop Case Rep*. 2021;11(7):74–77.
2. Chau MM, Klinistra MA, Wise KL, et al. Osteochondritis dissecans: current understanding of epidemiology, etiology, management, and outcomes. *J Bone Joint Surg Am*. 2021;103(12):1132–1151.
3. Bruns J, Werner M, Habermann CR, et al. Osteochondritis dissecans of smaller joints: the elbow. *Cartilage*. 2021;12(4):407–417.
4. van den Ende KIM, Keijsers R, van den Bekerom MPJ, et al. Imaging and classification of osteochondritis dissecans of the capitellum: x-ray, magnetic resonance imaging or computed tomography? *Shoulder Elbow*. 2019;11(2):129–136.
5. Baker CL III, Romeo AA, Baker CL Jr. Osteochondritis dissecans of the capitellum. *Am J Sports Med*. 2010;38(9):1917–1928.
6. Kobayashi K, Burton KJ, Rodner C, et al. Lateral compression injuries in the pediatric elbow: Panner's disease and osteochondritis dissecans of the capitellum. *J Am Acad Orthop Surg*. 2004;12(4):246–254.

ADDITIONAL READING

- Churchill RW, Munoz J, Ahmad CS. Osteochondritis dissecans of the elbow. *Curr Rev Musculoskeletal Med*. 2016;9(2):232–239.
- Claessen FM, Louwerens JK, Doomberg JN, et al. Panner's disease: literature review and treatment recommendations. *J Child Orthop*. 2015;9(1):9–17.
- Edmonds EW, Polousky J. A review of knowledge in osteochondritis dissecans: 123 years of minimal evolution from König to the ROCK study group. *Clin Orthop Relat Res*. 2013;471(4):1118–1126.
- Greiwe RM, Saifi C, Ahmad CS. Pediatric sports elbow injuries. *Clin Sports Med*. 2010;29(4):677–703.

CLINICAL PEARLS

- Panner disease and OCD of the elbow capitellum are common causes of elbow pain and disability in young adolescent athletes.
- Repetitive overuse of the elbow, such as in throwing sports, gymnastics, and weight lifting, is a known risk factor.
- Clinical suspicion warrants evaluation with plain radiographs and MRI.
- Early, stable lesions that are treated with prompt rest and nonoperative treatment have favorable results and return to activity in skeletally immature patients.
- Patients with advanced unstable lesions, loose bodies, mechanical symptoms, or failed conservative management are candidates for operative treatment as well as OCD patients who are skeletally mature.

PARONYCHIA

Holly J. Benjamin, MD, FAMSSM, FACSM ▪ Rachel Danzig, MD, FAAP

BASICS

DESCRIPTION
- Inflammation of the folds of skin surrounding the fingernail or toenail
- Disrupts the barrier between nail and nail fold
- May be acute (<6 weeks) or chronic (>6 weeks)
- Typically infectious but can be noninfectious
- System(s) affected: skin/exocrine
- Genetics: no known genetic pattern
- Synonym(s): eponychia; perionychia (1)

EPIDEMIOLOGY
- Incidence/prevalence in United States: common
- Predominant age: all ages
- Predominant gender: female > male (3:1)
- Risks: occupation and work environment

ETIOLOGY AND PATHOPHYSIOLOGY
- Acute: <6 weeks; usually painful, purulent infection from skin flora such as *Staphylococcus aureus*, *Streptococcus pyogenes*; oral flora such as *Eikenella corrodens*; anaerobic bacteria; viruses such as herpes simplex
- Chronic: >6 weeks; usually primarily related to mechanical and chemical irritants, *Candida albicans* secondary; less frequently, bacteria
- Acute flare on chronic: *Pseudomonas* spp (2).

RISK FACTORS
- Acute: trauma to skin surrounding nail, nail biting, finger sucking, manicures, retained foreign body, ingrown nails
- Chronic: frequent immersion of hands in water, diabetes mellitus, artificial nail placement
- Reported to be an adverse effect of certain drugs: antiretrovirals, systemic retinoids, epidermal growth factor receptor inhibitors, and cytotoxic chemo (1)
- May be considered work related in bartenders, waitresses, nurses, and others who often wet their hands

GENERAL PREVENTION
- Use moisturizing lotion after washing hands; avoid prolonged exposure to irritants; avoid nail trauma; keep nails short, square cut.
- Avoid nail trauma, biting, picking, and manipulation, and finger sucking.
- Chronic: Avoid frequent wetting of hands. Wear rubber gloves with a cloth liner; keep nails trimmed and square cut.
- Good diabetic control

COMMONLY ASSOCIATED CONDITIONS
- Diabetes mellitus (1)
- May be associated with atopic dermatitis or psoriasis

DIAGNOSIS

- Special tests: digital pressure test to look for abscess
- Diagnostic procedures: none typically needed
- Optional: ultrasound to look for abscess, x-ray for underlying fracture or osteomyelitis; or magnetic resonance imaging (MRI) if atypical and severe (3)

PHYSICAL EXAM
- Separation of nail fold from nail plate
- Erythematous, painful swelling of skin around nail plate
- Purulent; less likely fluctuant
- Abscess may be present
- Deformity of nail plate
- Green discoloration in nail (*Pseudomonas*) (2)

DIFFERENTIAL DIAGNOSIS
- Herpetic whitlow
- Felon (finger pulp infection)
- Psoriasis (nail)
- Eczema
- Reiter syndrome
- Dermatomyositis
- Onychomycosis
- Pyogenic granuloma
- Squamous cell carcinoma (chronic and rare)
- Melanoma (3)

DIAGNOSTIC TESTS & INTERPRETATION
- None usually needed or required
- Gram stain, culture and sensitivity if abscess drained
- Potassium hydroxide preparation plus fungal culture if indicated

TREATMENT

GENERAL MEASURES

- Treatment depends on severity of inflammation and abscess formation.
- Acute: (mild) warm compresses with warm water or antiseptic soaks and a topical antibiotic (triple antibiotic ointment)
- Chronic: Avoid irritants; keep fingers dry (4).
- Base antibiotic treatment on local resistance patterns and culture, if applicable.
- Incision and drainage (I&D) (definitive and therapeutic); is usually indicated
- Limited need for oral antibiotics after successful abscess drainage (1),(2)[B]

MEDICATION

First Line

- Acute (minimal inflammation; no abscess):
  - Frequent soaks with warm water, aluminum acetate, vinegar, dilute povidone-iodine solution, or chlorhexidine
  - Topical antibiotics may be added (gentamicin, mupirocin, bacitracin).
- Acute (inflammation with no response to soaks, topical antibiotics, or abscess drainage):
  - Amoxicillin-clavulanate 875/125 mg q12h
  - Clindamycin 300 to 450 mg q6h
  - Doxycycline 100 mg q12h
  - Trimethoprim-sulfamethoxazole 160 mg/800 mg q12h
    Dicloxacillin 250 to 500 mg q6h
  - Cephalexin 500 mg q6–8h
  - Ciprofloxacin 500 to 750 mg q12h
- Chronic:
  - Topical corticosteroids q12–24h
  - Tacrolimus topical q12h
  - Fungus: topical imidazoles (clotrimazole, ciclopirox)
- Systemic (multiple fingers or toes):
  - Fluconazole (Diflucan) 200 mg/wk
  - Oral corticosteroids short course
- Viral: acyclovir 400 mg q8h
- Contraindications: medication allergy

Second Line

Antipseudomonal medications

SURGERY/OTHER PROCEDURES

- I&D of abscess, if present (5)[B],(6)[B]
- Partial or complete nail removal if ingrown nail present
  - Insert no. 11 scalpel blade under lateral eponychial fold until pus drains or 22-gauge needle, bevel up
  - Anesthesia (local) rarely needed
  - Add oral medication only if abscess or cellulitis.

ONGOING CARE

FOLLOW-UP RECOMMENDATIONS

Routine follow-up until healed, activity as tolerated, follow prevention guidelines

DIET

- No special diet
- Zinc 20 mg daily supplementation may be helpful (4).

PATIENT EDUCATION

Follow general prevention guidelines.

PROGNOSIS

Good, if properly identified and treated appropriately

COMPLICATIONS

- Acute: subungual abscess
- Chronic: secondary ridging, thickening, nail dystrophy, discoloration of nail, nail loss

REFERENCES

1. Leggit JC. Acute and chronic paronychia. *Am Fam Physician*. 2017;96(1):44–51.
2. Relhan V, Bansal A. Acute and chronic paronychia revisited: a narrative review. *J Cutan Aesthet Surg*. 2022;15(1):1–16.
3. Marin JR, Dean AJ, Bilker WB, et al. Emergency ultrasound-assisted examination of skin and soft tissue infections in the pediatric emergency department. *Acad Emerg Med*. 2013;20(6):545–553.
4. Biesbroeck LK, Fleckman P. Nail disease for the primary care provider. *Med Clin North Am*. 2015;99(6):1213–1226.
5. Shafritz AB, Coppage JM. Acute and chronic paronychia of the hand. *J Am Acad Orthop Surg*. 2014;22(3):165–174.
6. Ritting AW, O'Malley MP, Rodner CM. Acute paronychia. *J Hand Surg Am*. 2012;37(5):1068–1070.

CLINICAL PEARLS

- Acute paronychia is usually bacterial, whereas chronic paronychia is usually due to irritants.
- Diagnosis is based on history and physical.
- Treatment should start with warm compresses and I&D if an abscess is present.
- Antibiotics should cover methicillin-resistant *S. aureus* (MRSA) and be chosen based on local resistance patterns.
- Topical corticosteroids or tacrolimus are first line for chronic paronychia.

PARSONAGE-TURNER SYNDROME (PTS)

Soroosh Amanat, MD • Kenneth S. Taylor, MD, FAAFP, CAQSM

BASICS

DESCRIPTION

- A condition of the peripheral nervous system involving a form of brachial plexopathy characterized by acute pain, muscle weakness, and muscle atrophy
- Also known as neuralgic amyotrophy

EPIDEMIOLOGY

Incidence

- Earlier literature studies estimated the annual reported incident is approximately 2 cases per 100,000 people.
- Now believed to be much higher due to underdiagnosis
- Based on one study of primary care physicians after education on the condition, the annual incidence was measured to be 1 case per 1,000 individuals (1)[C].
- Gender differences: men > women; 2.5:1 ratio
- Limb involvement: upper limb > lower limb
- Age of onset: between ages of 30 and 70 years, with average age of onset of 40 years old

ETIOLOGY AND PATHOPHYSIOLOGY

- There is no well-established etiology or pathophysiology.
- Most commonly presumed to be an inflammatory autoimmune response to a precipitating condition or trigger
- Alternative hypotheses for the pathophysiology of Parsonage-Turner syndrome (PTS) have been reported.

Genetics

- Septin-9 protein (SEPT9) gene has been identified as a causal gene for hereditary brachial plexus neuropathy (1)[C].
- This is inherited in an autosomal dominant pattern. It has similar clinical presentation as neuralgic amyotrophy and often with recurrent attacks (1)[C].

RISK FACTORS

- A precipitating factor is identified in approximately half of PTS cases (1)[C].
- The most common antecedent event is an infectious prodrome. Second most common is surgical procedures (1)[C].
- Other triggers including immunizations, pregnancy, and strenuous physical activity.

DIAGNOSIS

HISTORY

- Although there are clinical variants of PTS, the classic presentation for PTS is defined by three phases:
  - Phase 1: painful phase
  - Phase 2: weakness, atrophy, and sensory phase
  - Phase 3: recovery phase
- Most commonly, individuals experience onset of abrupt, unilateral shoulder and/or arm pain with associated weakness (1)[C].
- The onset is common to occur at night and with worsening pain in the evenings (1)[C].
- Pain is usually described as constant, severe neuralgic pain.
- Subsequently, there is usually onset of muscle weakness and atrophy as well as often numbness and tingling.
- Recovery phase generally starts 1 month after onset of symptoms.
- Most common nerves affected include the suprascapular, long thoracic, musculocutaneous, radial, and/or anterior interosseous nerves (1)[C].
- Clinical presentation can be diverse including bilateral in presentation (2)[C].
- Nerves outside of brachial plexus can also be affected. Phrenic nerve can also be involved and presents with shortness of breath and orthopnea (2)[C].

PHYSICAL EXAM

- Weakness of the affected muscle groups
- Some patients may have complete paralysis and also limited by pain.
- Winged scapula is very common finding.
- Muscle wasting and atrophy of affected muscle groups
- Deep tendon reflexes are usually normal.

DIFFERENTIAL DIAGNOSIS

- Rotator cuff tendinopathy or subacromial bursitis
- Cervical radiculopathy or myelopathy
- Adhesive capsulitis
- Entrapment neuropathy
- Thoracic outline syndrome
- Myofascial pain syndrome
- Pancoast tumor

DIAGNOSTIC TESTS & INTERPRETATION

Initial Tests (lab, imaging)

- Should maintain a high clinical suspicion based on history
- Labs can be performed to exclude potential alternative causes.
- Imaging studies can be used to support a diagnosis of PTS. Other studies such as magnetic resonance imaging (MRI) cervical neck can rule out other causes.
- Electrodiagnostic testing include electromyography (EMG) and nerve conduction studies (NCS) have traditionally been considered first-line diagnostic tests to support diagnosis (2)[C].

Diagnostic Procedures/Other

- Nerve conduction and EMG studies can demonstrate patchy axonal damage of a peripheral nerve.
- EMG studies may not reflect muscle denervation for 4 weeks after onset of symptoms.
- NCS: can assist in determining lesion location and exclude common mononeuropathies (2)[C]
- EMG: used to confirm and document the pattern of denervation; however, often take up to 4 weeks for EMG to reflect denervation (2)[C]

- Routine MRI of the shoulder may show atrophy and edema of affected muscle groups supportive of presumed diagnosis.
- Recent advancements in imaging now include magnetic resonance (MR) neurography and high-resolution ultrasound (HRUS).
- Ultrasound findings include thickening and edema of nerves, followed by hourglass constrictions and possible nerve torsion (3)[B].
- MR neurography findings include edema and atrophy of muscles with focal nerve segment changes including hourglass constrictions (1)[C].

TREATMENT

GENERAL MEASURES

- Treatment of PTS primarily involves conservative management and is based on the phase at time of diagnosis.
- The evidence for treatment for neuralgic amyotrophy is lacking (4)[A].
- In the primary painful phase of the condition, initial primary treatment is focused on pain management.
- In the later stages of weakness and atrophy, a rehabilitation program involving physical and occupational therapy is the mainstay of treatment.

MEDICATION

- Medications are the primary management strategy during the painful phase though effectiveness can be limited due to severity of pain
- Common medications used include nonsteroidal anti-inflammatory drugs (NSAID), and acetaminophen, and patients with severe pain may require opioids (1)[C].
- Other medications include gabapentinoids antidepressants (1)[C].
- Anecdotal evidence and one case series suggest early corticosteroids may improve pain and recovery (4)[A].

ADDITIONAL THERAPIES

- Majority of patients have limitations in daily living due to pain, fatigue, and weakness which is treated with a rehabilitation program including physical and occupational therapy.
- Evidence that a multidisciplinary rehabilitation program is more beneficial for functional capability than usual care (5)[B].
- Specific rehabilitation programs focus on training motor control, particularly scapular dyskinesia, and combined self-management strategies (5)[B].

SURGERY/OTHER PROCEDURES

- Surgical procedures can include neurolysis, nerve transfers, and tendon transfers (6)[B].
- In patients with chronic weakness not responsive to conservative therapy and hourglass constrictions, microsurgical neurolysis can provide significant improvement (6)[B].

ONGOING CARE

FOLLOW-UP RECOMMENDATIONS

Patient Monitoring

- Should have regular visits as part of rehabilitation program to monitor progress in motor control and strength
- Can have repeat EMG/NCS to monitor nerve involvement

PROGNOSIS

- The majority of patients show good to complete recovery (approximately 75%).
- However, recovery process is considered slow and usually requires between 1 and 3 years from onset of condition.

REFERENCES

1. Meiling JB, Boon AJ, Niu Z, et al. Parsonage-Turner syndrome and hereditary brachial plexus neuropathy. *Mayo Clin Proc*. 2024;99(1):124–140.
2. Gstoettner C, Mayer JA, Rassam S, et al. Neuralgic amyotrophy: a paradigm shift in diagnosis and treatment. *J Neurol Neurosurg Psychiatry*. 2020;91(8):879–888.
3. Wang T, Qi H, Wang Z, et al. The role of ultrasonography in diagnosis of neuralgic amyotrophy. *Skeletal Radiol*. 2023;52(7):1305–1311.
4. van Alfen N, van Engelen BGM, Hughes RAC. Treatment for idiopathic and hereditary neuralgic amyotrophy (brachial neuritis). *Cochrane Database Syst Rev*. 2009;2009(3):CD006976.
5. Janssen RMJ, Lustenhouwer R, Cup EHC, et al. Effectiveness of an outpatient rehabilitation programme in patients with neuralgic amyotrophy and scapular dyskinesia: a randomised controlled trial. *J Neurol Neurosurg Psychiatry*. 2023;94(6):474–481.
6. Krishnan KR, Sneag DB, Feinberg JH, et al. Outcomes of microneurolysis of hourglass constrictions in chronic neuralgic amyotrophy. *J Hand Surg Am*. 2021;46(1):43–53.

CLINICAL PEARLS

- PTS is classically characterized by acute onset of unilateral, severe painful phase most commonly affected the shoulder. This is followed by muscle weakness and atrophy.
- PTS has traditionally been diagnosed by clinical presentation and NCS/EMG studies, but advancements in imaging now include MR neurography and ultrasound.
- Management is often conservative including rehabilitation program and anecdotal evidence for corticosteroids.
- The majority of patients fully recover.

PATELLAR DISLOCATION AND INSTABILITY

Keenan Wheeler, DO • Aaron D. Gray, MD

BASICS

DESCRIPTION

- Patellar instability is defined as hypermobility of the patella in either the medial or lateral direction.
- Medial instability is extremely rare.
- Complete dislocation and subluxation represent variations in severity of instability.
- Acute dislocation typically occurs with a twisting injury and strong contraction of the quadriceps; rarely, it is due to direct trauma to the medial aspect of the patella.

EPIDEMIOLOGY

- Incidence of initial lateral patellar dislocation: 23.2 per 100,000 person-years
- Increased incidence in adolescents aged 14 to 18 years of 147.7 per 100,000 person-years (1)
- Recurrence rate reported to range 15–80% after initial dislocation and >50% after a second dislocation (2)

RISK FACTORS

- Prior history of subluxed or dislocated patella
- Recurrence rate 15–50% after initial dislocation
- Adolescent age
- Patella alta ("high-riding patella")
- Trochlear dysplasia
- Excessive genu valgum
- Excessive tibial torsion
- Lateralized tibial tuberosity
- Risk factors associated with developmental dysplasia (firstborn girl, high birth weight, deliver by cesarean section, breech delivery)

COMMONLY ASSOCIATED CONDITIONS

- Avulsion fracture of the superior medial pole of the patella
- Osteochondral fractures of the lateral femoral condyle or posterior patellar articular surface
- Tear of the medial patellofemoral ligament (MPFL)
- Concomitant major ligamentous or meniscal injury
- Cartilage injuries to the patellofemoral joint expected in 70–96% of acute or recurrent dislocation (2)

DIAGNOSIS

Prehospital:

- Patient has severe pain and may have heard a pop at time of dislocation.
- Knee is usually held in 20 to 30 degrees of flexion, and patella is palpable laterally.
- Hemarthrosis causing an acutely swollen knee
- Tenderness to palpation over the medial edge of patella
- Tenderness at the medial femoral epicondyle, the origin of the MPFL
- Consider subluxation if:
  - History is consistent with a dislocation, but pain and examination findings have resolved.
  - Presence of patella alta (high-riding patella) or laterally displaced patella

HISTORY

- Mechanism of injury?
- Initial or recurrent?
- History of previous knee injury or patellofemoral pain syndrome?
- Does your patella feel like it is slipping or moving laterally on certain movements (sense of instability)?
- Do you have swelling?

PHYSICAL EXAM

- Moving patellar apprehension test is the most sensitive and specific for patellar instability.
- "J" sign: Seated patient extends the knee; the patella tracks from midline to lateral in terminal extension.
- Screen for hypermobility with Beighton score.
- Lateral patellar glide of >3 quadrants with apprehension is consistent with patellar hypermobility.
- Immediately after dislocation, patella may remain dislocated laterally with notable bony prominence medially due to uncovered medial femoral condyle (3).
- Obvious effusion
- Tenderness most apparent over the medial edge of patella and lateral femoral condyle
- Patients fear of redislocation when knee is flexed.
- Assess for concomitant ligamentous and meniscal injuries.

DIFFERENTIAL DIAGNOSIS

- Subluxation versus dislocation
- Although history of patellar dislocation is classic, consider other entities that cause early effusions or hemarthrosis (e.g., anterior cruciate ligament [ACL] tear, meniscal tear, and tibial plateau fractures).

DIAGNOSTIC TESTS & INTERPRETATION

- Anteroposterior, lateral (30-degree flexion), and axial patellar views (merchant or sunrise)
- An axial patellar view is necessary to evaluate the presence of associated osteochondral fractures. Avulsion fracture or calcification along the medial edge of the patella is considered pathognomonic for patellar dislocation. Assesses patellar tilt, subluxation, and trochlear dysplasia.
- Lateral view identifies trochlear morphology and evidence of dysplasia (cross-over sign, double contour, supratrochlear spur), and patella alta.
- Cross-sectional imaging is reserved for recurrent dislocations, suspected concomitant soft tissue injury, confirmed osseous injury, hemarthrosis, and/or when operative management is decided (2).
- Magnetic resonance imaging (MRI) finding of medial patellar facet contusion combined with lateral femoral condyle contusion is pathognomonic for patellar dislocation (3).
- Musculoskeletal ultrasound is comparable to MRI in identifying MPFL complete or partial rupture (4) or functional impairment with dynamic testing.

TREATMENT

- If not reduced spontaneously, may require conscious sedation for pain control and muscle relaxation
- Alternatively, local anesthetization with intra-articular instillation of lidocaine and/or bupivacaine
- Patellar reduction requires extension of the leg with simultaneous gentle pressure on patella directed lateral to medial. Addition of hip flexion can further reduce tension from the quadriceps.
- Postreduction radiographs shoulder be obtained to confirm reduction and evaluate for fractures.
- After reduction, rest, ice, focal compression, and elevation are indicated for the first 24 to 48 hours.
- Protected weight-bearing with advancement as tolerated is recommended; partial for 0 to 2 weeks, >50% by 3 to 4 weeks, and discontinuation by 6 weeks
- Compressive cryotherapy in the first 72 hours postinjury reduces swelling and pain symptoms (5).

P

MEDICATION
- Acetaminophen
- Trial of nonsteroidal anti-inflammatory drugs in the absence of identified acute fractures or after initial fracture healing phase

ISSUES FOR REFERRAL
Orthopedic referral indicated if:
- Osteochondral lesion or fracture noted on either plain radiographs or cross-sectional imaging
- Recurrent patellar dislocations despite adequate rehabilitation, especially in younger patients (<14 years old), in whom recurrence rates can reach 60%
- Evidence of joint locking
- High-risk athlete participates in activities involving pivoting (e.g., field and court sports, dancing) and is at increased risk of recurrent patellar dislocation.

ADDITIONAL THERAPIES
- A significant number of patients develop large hemarthrosis. Aspiration may be considered after 48 to 72 hours, both to relieve pain and to check for fat globules, which might help diagnose an occult osteochondral fracture.
- Patellar stabilizing braces are recommended as use maintains neutral patellar alignment and allows early mobilization. Taping is not recommended.
- Range of motion exercises are initiated as soon as tolerated with goal of full range of motion by 6 weeks.
- Combination proximal and multijoint exercises improve pain and joint function compared to isolated knee rehabilitation alone. Isometric quadriceps exercises are initiated as soon as possible, although it is often difficult and painful for the athlete to produce a contraction that involves the vastus medialis oblique (VMO).

SURGERY/OTHER PROCEDURES
- Evidence supports nonoperative treatment for initial episodes of acute lateral patellar dislocation (3),(4).
- Operative treatment for patellar instability is reserved for nonoperative treatment failure after approximately 6 months, for recurrent instability, and for concomitant ipsilateral injury requiring operative management.
- Surgical management includes MPFL reconstruction, proximal extensor mechanism realignment alone, or combined proximal and distal realignment.
- MPFL reconstruction restores the medial restraining forces providing improved short and long-term outcomes for recurrent dislocations (3).
- Distal realignment procedures performed for recurrent instability result in low dislocation rates with good to excellent patient satisfaction (2).
- Isolated lateral retinacular release has no long-term benefit for patellar instability.

REFERENCES

1. Sanders TL, Pareek A, Hewett TE, et al. Incidence of first-time lateral patellar dislocation: a 21-year population-based study. *Sports Health*. 2018;10(2):146–151.
2. Weber AE, Nathani A, Dines JS, et al. An algorithmic approach to the management of recurrent lateral patellar dislocation. *J Bone Joint Surg Am*. 2016;98(5):417–427.
3. Previtali D, Milev SR, Pagliazzi G, et al. Recurrent patellar dislocations without untreated predisposing factors: medial patellofemoral ligament reconstruction versus other medial soft-tissue surgical techniques—a meta-analysis. *Arthroscopy*. 2020;36(6):1725–1734.
4. Zhang GY, Zheng L, Ding HY, et al. Evaluation of medial patellofemoral ligament tears after acute lateral patellar dislocation: comparison of high-frequency ultrasound and MR. *Eur Radiol*. 2015;25(1):274–281.
5. Watson R, Sullivan B, Stone AV, et al. Lateral patellar dislocation: a critical review and update of evidence-based rehabilitation practice guidelines and expected outcomes. *JBJS Rev*. 2022;10(5).

ADDITIONAL READING

- Iobst CA, Stanitski CL. Acute knee injuries. *Clin Sports Med*. 2000;19(4):621–635.
- Knutson T, Bothwell J, Durbin R. Evaluation and management of traumatic knee injuries in the emergency department. *Emerg Med Clin North Am*. 2015;33(2):345–362.

CLINICAL PEARLS

- Patellar dislocation is a common diagnosis in an adolescent with knee effusion after twisting injury. Tenderness of the medial patella in this situation can suggest patella dislocation. Tenderness at the medial femoral epicondyle can suggest concomitant MPFL injury.
- Return to sports: There should be evidence of adequate healing (absence of sensations of instability, lack of effusion, and absence of pain on patellofemoral compression) and adequate function (able to perform rotational movements such as pivoting, cutting, and twisting without evidence of instability) for return to sports. Athlete may need a patellar stabilizing braces to accomplish this.

PATELLAR/QUADRICEPS TENDINOPATHY

Jackson Bagby, DO, MS • Scott Goodsell, DO • Natalie Ronshaugen, MD, CAQSM

BASICS

DESCRIPTION

- Overuse syndrome of the patellar and/or quadriceps tendons/knee extensor mechanism complex
- Anterior knee pain worsened by activity such as jumping or running
- Also termed "jumper's knee"

EPIDEMIOLOGY

Prevalence

- Commonly seen in athletes who participate in sports with excessive jumping or running (volleyball, basketball, soccer, track and field)
- Prevalence is estimated to be 40–50% among high-level volleyball players and 35–40% among elite basketball players.
- Affects males and females equally

RISK FACTORS

- Participation in a sport with excessive jumping movements (volleyball, basketball), as well as rapid acceleration and deceleration
- Risk increases with training volume and intensity.
- Poor flexibility of quadriceps and hamstrings
- Anatomic variants that can lead to abnormal repetitive biomechanical stresses such as patella alta, patella baja, or patellar malalignment/maltracking
- Use of a fluoroquinolone antibiotic within the past 90 days, although symptoms have appeared as late as 6 months after last exposure
- Underlying connective tissue disease such as rheumatoid arthritis or ankylosing spondylitis

ETIOLOGY AND PATHOPHYSIOLOGY

- Histopathology shows (1):
  - Collagen degeneration and disorganization/disruption of normal parallel arrangement of fibrils
  - Microscopic to macroscopic intrasubstance tendon tears can occur.
  - Increase in mucoid ground substance
  - Fibroblast proliferation
  - Neovascularization
  - Intratendinous calcifications with gritty toothpaste-like consistency can occur.
- More accurately termed tendinopathy which includes the full spectrum of disease from tendinitis (early stage lasting about 1 week when inflammatory cells are present) to tendinosis (end stage after months to years when tendon is thickened and has central mucoid degeneration)

DIAGNOSIS

HISTORY

- Anterior knee pain with insidious onset, exacerbated by activity or by prolonged knee flexion (2)
- Participation in a sport with excessive jumping
- A progressive condition of anterior knee pain (Blazina classification):
  - Phase 1: pain after activity
  - Phase 2: pain during and after activity not affecting performance
  - Phase 3: pain during and after activity impeding performance

PHYSICAL EXAM

- Patellar tendinitis: localized tenderness at the patellar tendon origin (inferior pole of the patella), patellar tendon midsubstance, and/or patellar tendon insertion (tibial tubercle)
- Quadriceps tendinitis: localized tenderness at the quadriceps tendon and/or quadriceps tendon insertion (superior pole of the patella)
- Both: pain reproduced with extension of the knee against resistance and/or pain with maximal stretching of the quadriceps
- Both: poor flexibility of the quadriceps and hamstrings

DIFFERENTIAL DIAGNOSIS

- Patellofemoral pain syndrome
- Hoffa disease (fat pad impingement)
- Osgood-Schlatter disease
- Sinding-Larsen-Johansson syndrome
- Chondromalacia patella/patellofemoral osteoarthritis
- Osteochondral lesions
- Patellar subluxation/dislocation
- Patellar stress fracture
- Patellar tendon rupture (partial or complete)
- Quadriceps tendon rupture (partial or complete)
- Prepatellar bursitis
- Lumbar radiculitis/radiculopathy involving the L3 and/or L4 nerve roots

DIAGNOSTIC TESTS & INTERPRETATION

- Patellar/quadriceps tendinitis remains a clinical diagnosis, and routine imaging is neither required nor recommended.
- Plain film radiographs may show occasional intratendinous calcification.
- Magnetic resonance imaging (MRI) may reveal increased signal within the patellar or quadriceps tendon and/or at the junction with the patella (1).
- Ultrasound (US) may reveal focal hypoechoic areas in the patellar or quadriceps tendon and/or neovascularization on color Doppler flow (1).
- The study of choice and relevance of abnormalities remain somewhat controversial.

TREATMENT

MEDICATION

- Conservative measures typically include relative rest (reduction in amount or intensity of training to achieve pain-free state), ice, acetaminophen, and/or nonsteroidal anti-inflammatory drugs (NSAIDs).
- NSAIDs are commonly used as analgesics and may be beneficial for acute symptoms; however, there is a lack of evidence showing benefits in chronic cases.
- Topical nitroglycerin patches provide no significant pain relief versus placebo (3),(4)[A].

ADDITIONAL THERAPIES

- Mainstay of treatment is stretching and strengthening exercises for the quadriceps to improve flexibility and stimulate tendon tissue repair (3)[C],(5)[C].
- Eccentric strengthening exercises of the quadriceps and/or progressive tendon-loading exercise therapy improves pain (5).
- Combination of static quadriceps stretching and eccentric quadriceps strengthening provided better outcomes than either treatment alone (1)[C].

- Correction of biomechanical abnormalities (if possible) and/or training errors
- Wearing a patellar tendon strap has been shown to decrease localized tendon strain forces and may help reduce symptoms during sports participation (1)[C].

SURGERY/OTHER PROCEDURES

- Iontophoresis/phonophoresis
- Percutaneous interventions for those who fail conservative therapy for >6 months (under US guidance):
  - Needle tenotomy
  - Platelet-rich plasma (PRP) injections
  - Prolotherapy
  - Tendon hydrodissection, where the peritenon/fat pad is separated from the tendon, disrupting the neovessels and nerves
  - Ultrasonic tenotomy
- Extracorporeal shock wave therapy (ECSWT) directed at areas of tendinopathy
- Open surgical tenotomy may be considered for patients who fail to respond to 6 months of conservative measures and/or who fail to respond to the aforementioned less invasive procedures.
- No randomized trials have been able to clearly demonstrate superior efficacy of one procedure or surgical technique over others.

ALERT

Steroid injections into a tendon should be avoided due to the risk of tendon rupture (6),(7).

ONGOING CARE

- Corticosteroid injections into the patellar tendon or quadriceps tendon should be avoided due to the theoretical increased risk of tendon rupture (6),(7).
- Patellar tendinopathy has a high rate of recurrence, with athletes in volleyball having the highest rate.
- Symptoms can last from months to years, and physical rehabilitation programs will need to include a prolonged course and often be maintained.

REFERENCES

1. Rosen AB, Wellsandt E, Nicola M, et al. Clinical management of patellar tendinopathy. *J Athl Train*. 2022;57(7):621–631.
2. Kane SF, Olewinski LH, Tamminga KS. Management of chronic tendon injuries. *Am Fam Physician*. 2019;100(3):147–157.
3. Llombart R, Mariscal G, Barrios C, et al. The best current research on patellar tendinopathy: a review of published meta-analyses. *Sports (Basel)*. 2024;12(2):46.
4. Loescher J, Waclawski P, Guthmann R. Topical nitroglycerin for lower extremity tendinopathy. *Am Fam Physician*. 2022;105(2):196–197.
5. Breda SJ, Oei EHG, Zwerver J, et al. Effectiveness of progressive tendon-loading exercise therapy in patients with patellar tendinopathy: a randomised clinical trial. *Br J Sports Med*. 2021;55(9):501–509.
6. Kamel SI, Rosas HG, Gorbachova T. Local and systemic side effects of corticosteroid injections for musculoskeletal indications. *AJR Am J Roentgenol*. 2024;222(3):e2330458.
7. Brinkman JC, Reeson E, Chhabra A. Acute patellar tendon ruptures: an update on management. *J Am Acad Orthop Surg Glob Res Rev*. 2024;8(4):e24.00060.

ADDITIONAL READING

- Bahr R, Fossan B, Løken S, et al. Surgical treatment compared with eccentric training for patellar tendinopathy (jumper's knee). A randomized, controlled trial. *J Bone Joint Surg Am*. 2006;88(8):1689–1698.
- Blazina ME, Kerlan RK, Jobe FW, et al. Jumper's knee. *Orthop Clin North Am*. 1973;4(3):665–678.
- Everhart JS, Cole D, Sojka JH, et al. Treatment options for patellar tendinopathy: a systematic review. *Arthroscopy*. 2017;33(4):861–872.
- Hall MM, Finnoff JT, Smith J. Musculoskeletal complications of fluoroquinolones: guidelines and precautions for usage in the athletic population. *PM R*. 2011;3(2):132–142.
- Lian OB, Engebretsen L, Bahr R. Prevalence of jumper's knee among elite athletes from different sports: a cross-sectional study. *Am J Sports Med*. 2005;33(4):561–567.
- Matschke V, Jones JG, Lemmey AB, et al. Patellar tendon properties and lower limb function in rheumatoid arthritis and ankylosing spondylitis versus healthy controls: a cross-sectional study. *ScientificWorldJournal*. 2013;2013:514743.
- Peers KHE, Lysens RJJ. Patellar tendinopathy in athletes: current diagnostic and therapeutic recommendations. *Sports Med*. 2005;35(1):71–87.
- Schwartz A, Watson JN, Hutchinson MR. Patellar tendinopathy. *Sports Health*. 2015;7(5):415–420.

CLINICAL PEARLS

- Patellar/quadriceps tendinopathy remains a clinical diagnosis, and the mainstay of treatment is strengthening of the quadriceps muscles through exercises such as one-legged squats emphasizing the eccentric (negative) phase for a prolonged period of time (6 months to 1 year) which promotes the slow and gradual process of microscopic tendon repair via mechanotransduction.
- If the diagnosis is in question or if the patient is not responding to an appropriate course of conservative measures including eccentric quadriceps strengthening exercises, then patellar/quadriceps tendinopathy can be confirmed by either MRI or US.
- If the patient is not responding to an appropriate course of conservative measures after 6 months and patellar/quadriceps tendinopathy is confirmed by either MRI or US, then ECSWT or minimally invasive US-guided procedures (percutaneous needle tenotomy [PNT], PRP, prolotherapy, or ultrasonic tenotomy) or open surgical tenotomy can be considered.

PATELLAR/QUADRICEPS TENDON RUPTURE

Rathna R. Nuti, MD, CAQSM, FAAFP

BASICS

DESCRIPTION

- Partial or complete rupture of the patellar or quadriceps tendon
- Synonym(s): extensor mechanism disruption

EPIDEMIOLOGY

- Quadriceps tendon ruptures are uncommon with an estimated 1.37 cases per 100,000 people/y (1).
- Quadriceps tendon ruptures tend to occur most commonly in the 6th and 7th decade with a male preponderance of 4 to 8:1, and ethnically with >10-fold increased risk of major tendon rupture in black American men (1),(2).
- Quadriceps tendon ruptures are twice as common in the nondominant limb, with bilateral ruptures reported at around 6–12% of all ruptures (1),(2).
- The mechanism of rupture can be direct or indirect with the most common causes being simple fall, fall down stairs, and sporting activities.

ETIOLOGY AND PATHOPHYSIOLOGY

- Males aged <40 years typically occur from sudden eccentric overload, often in the form of a sudden quadriceps contracture with the knee flexed at around 60 degrees (1),(2).
- Patellar tendon ruptures usually are complete, occurring most commonly at the osteotendinous junction in athletic trauma versus midsubstance in those with systemic disease (2).
- Quadriceps tendon ruptures usually occur within 1 to 2 cm from the superior patellar pole in a relatively hypovascular zone. Patients aged <40 years having midsubstance tears and those >40 years of age rupturing at the tendon-bone junction (2).
- Chronic tendinosis, corticosteroids, fluoroquinolones, and systemic disease change tendon structure, decreasing its failure point.

RISK FACTORS

- Trauma
- High-power sports (e.g., high jump, basketball, weightlifting)
- Previous total-knee arthroplasty, anterior cruciate ligament (ACL) reconstruction using patellar autograft or excision of tendinosis
- Steroid injection in the patellar or quadriceps tendon
- Fluoroquinolone use in previous 6 months
- Degenerative tendon changes (i.e., fatty infiltration, collagen alteration, vascular deficiency)
- Advanced age
- Preexisting/chronic renal disease
- Microvascular damage due to diabetes mellitus, hyperparathyroidism, systemic lupus erythematosus
- Autoimmune inflammatory diseases (rheumatoid arthritis, gout)
- Osteogenesis imperfecta
- Uremia
- Obesity
- Tumors

COMMONLY ASSOCIATED CONDITIONS

- Jumper knee/tendinopathy
- Patellar spurs
- Quadriceps injury

DIAGNOSIS

HISTORY

- Mechanism of injury: specifically jumping, stumbling, or slipping
- Hearing or feeling "pop" or tearing sensation
- Immediate, disabling pain
- Difficulty straightening or bearing weight on affected extremity
- Acute onset of swelling
- History of chronic patellar or quadriceps tendinosis
- History of steroid injection in tendon
- Recent fluoroquinolone use

PHYSICAL EXAM

- Classic triad
  - Acute anterior thigh/knee pain
  - Inability to actively extend the knee (particularly versus resistance), or have extension lag. Patient may be able to hold in extension particularly if internal leg rotation.
  - Palpable suprapatellar defect (may be masked by swelling acutely, or by scar tissue in chronic presentation)
- Diffuse swelling or effusion
- Ecchymosis, possible hemarthrosis
- Audible sensation of crepitus
- Patella alta in complete patellar tendon rupture
- Patella baja in complete quadriceps tendon rupture
- Tenderness to palpation over patellar poles, retinaculum, or tibial tuberosity
- Absence of or altered patellar tendon reflex
- Altered gait if able to bear weight
- Quadriceps atrophy (in chronic cases)

DIFFERENTIAL DIAGNOSIS

- Fracture
- Muscular strain (grade I or II)
- Patellar subluxation/dislocation
- Meniscal or ligamentous pathologies
- Osgood-Schlatter disease
- Sinding-Larsen-Johansson syndrome

DIAGNOSTIC TESTS & INTERPRETATION

- Laboratory studies are rarely indicated but depending on history and physical exam may be performed to evaluate for associated risk factors.
- Diagnosis typically based on clinical presentation and physical exam findings; however, imaging is commonly used to confirm the diagnosis.
- Plain radiographs:
  - Obtain anteroposterior, lateral, tunnel, and patellar (sunrise or merchant) views.
  - Contralateral films allow comparison of patellar height/position.
  - In this clinical setting, superior or inferior patellar migration without fracture is conclusive for rupture; Insall-Salvati index <0.8 for patella baja and quadriceps rupture (3), conversely an index of >1.2 would indicate patella alta and likely patellar tendon rupture
  - Avulsion fractures may occur at the superior or inferior patellar poles or the tibial tuberosity.
  - Obliteration of the quadriceps shadow, suprapatellar soft tissue defect, or joint effusion
  - Rule out tumor or fracture.
- Ultrasound (US):
  - Normal tendon 6 to 11 mm thick
  - High-resolution US shows hypoechogenicity to anechoic area in acute tears, tendon thickening, and heterogeneous echotexture in chronic tears (1),(4).
  - Dynamic evaluation is more useful.
  - Highly user dependent
  - Inexpensive and high sensitivity
- Magnetic resonance imaging (MRI):
  - Considered the gold standard with high sensitivity and specificity and a positive predictive value (PPV) of 1.0 (1)
  - May be performed if diagnosis cannot be made by clinical and radiographic examination or clinically obtuse patient
  - Findings include increased T2 signal in the tendon, wavy and discontinuous tendon fibers with associated edema or hemorrhage.
  - In-depth information regarding the extent of the rupture and evaluation of concomitant intra-articular pathology
- Pathologic findings:
  - Pathologic changes usually are degenerative, including hypoxic degenerative tendinopathy, mucoid degeneration, tendolipomatosis, and calcifying tendinopathy.
  - Can identify comorbid injury with anterior cruciate tear, medial and then lateral meniscus pathology most frequently involved (1)

TREATMENT

GENERAL MEASURES

- Immobilization of knee with straight-leg immobilizer, ice, elevation, and crutch-assisted ambulation in the immediate setting
- Immobilization and crutch use should be continued until evaluation and, if indicated, surgical intervention are completed.
- **Incomplete tendon ruptures:**
  - Partial-thickness or incomplete ruptures can be managed with nonsurgical treatments.
  - Initial treatment when extensor mechanism intact is immobilization in full extension with progression to weight-bearing as tolerated in a hinged knee brace (locked out) (1),(2),(4)[C].

- Following this, treatment can be divided into three stages:
  - Acute phase
  - Rehabilitation phase
  - Return-to-activity phase
- In the acute phase, the goal is to restore motion progressively stretching. When patient can do a straight-leg raise without pain, he or she can initiate isometric activity and can initiate progressive knee flexion. When at 90-degree flexion without pain, patient can advance to knee extension exercises through a 30-degree arc of motion and advance as tolerated.
- Rehabilitation and return-to-activity phases are integrated and last 3 to 6 months (1),(4).
- Therapeutic aspiration can be considered for evacuation of hematoma if present in partial tears to decrease chance for quadriceps inhibition (1).
- Surgery is indicated for complete ruptures or for incomplete ruptures failing to respond to nonoperative treatment (2).

ISSUES FOR REFERRAL

Patients should be referred for orthopedic evaluation as soon as a patellar/quadriceps tendon rupture is suspected to decrease complications (2)[B].

SURGERY/OTHER PROCEDURES

- Surgery is necessary for all complete ruptures to restore the extensor mechanism of the knee; it is also indicated for partial ruptures failing nonoperative treatment (2).
- Repair should occur as soon as possible, preferably within 1 week but 24 hours to 1 month is acceptable (1)[C]. Delays >6 weeks complicate surgical intervention and lead to poorer outcomes (2)[B].
- The exact surgical intervention depends on which portion of the extensor mechanism was disrupted and the acuity of the injury.
- If ruptures are several months old, semitendinosus tendon or synthetic graft may be used in the repair.
- Historically, most surgeons have used a postoperative protocol as outlined (2),(5)[C]:
  - Strict immobilization for 4 to 6 weeks, followed by a further period of passive motion and eccentric exercises prior to allowing concentric exercises, aiming for full recovery by 4 to 6 months (2)
  - Immediate start of isometric quadriceps exercises
  - Weeks 0 to 3: 0 to 45 degrees of active flexion and passive extension
  - Weeks 4 to 6: progression to 0 to 90 degrees of active flexion and passive extension
  - 6 weeks onward: straight-leg raise exercises
  - 8 weeks onward: stationary biking and water running
  - 3 months onward: progressive quadriceps exercises
  - 4 months onward: jogging
  - 9 months onward: Jumping and contact sports permitted comprehensive physical therapy program should be completed before return to athletics.
- More recent studies have shown that prolonged immobilization leads to stiffness, persistent pain, weakness, reductions in bone and muscle mass, impairment in patellar mobility, and suboptimal cartilage nutrition (1)[B].
- No specific protocols have been validated in randomized controlled trials (RCTs) so are presented as expert opinion, but early motion and functional rehabilitation have been shown to be safe. One such protocol is outlined:
  - Phase I (0 to 6 weeks): brace locked in full extension; weight-bearing as tolerated; range of motion (ROM): flexion to 30 degrees (0 to 2 weeks), 60 degrees (2 to 4 weeks), and 90 degrees (4 to 6 weeks)
  - Phase II (6 to 12 weeks): brace unlocked to 45 to 60 degrees of flexion at week 6 and 90 degrees at week 7; straight-leg raises and closed kinetic chain strengthening; ROM: progress to full ROM by week 12.
  - Phase III (12 to 16 weeks): Advance to open and closed kinetic chain strengthening exercises. Limit active knee extension.
  - Phase IV: (16 to 20 weeks): Advance to strengthening and functional drills; leg extensions from 30 to 0 degree; progress as tolerated.
  - Phase V: (20 to 24 weeks): plyometric drills; multidirectional drills, increase strengthening exercises, and progressively advance to running and sprinting programs as appropriate; return-to-play testing and decisions.

ONGOING CARE

PATIENT EDUCATION

- Reasonable function can be obtained in most individuals, especially in the acute tendon rupture that is repaired immediately.
- Most patients can return to their previous occupation, but many have difficulty returning to their preinjury athletic level, particularly with quadriceps tendon ruptures.

PROGNOSIS

- Outcome after repair is closely related to the length of time between injury and repair, the quality of the preexisting tissues, and the tendon healing at the proper length and tension.
- If the tendon is repaired immediately, most patients experience nearly full return of knee motion.

COMPLICATIONS

- Loss of flexion is common after quadriceps tendon rupture.
- Extensor mechanism weakness
- Postoperative infection
- Degenerative change at the patellofemoral joint

REFERENCES

1. Arnold EP, Sedgewick JA, Wortman RJ, et al. Acute quadriceps tendon rupture: presentation, diagnosis and management. *JBJS Rev.* 2022;10(2):e21.00171.
2. Pengas IP, Assiotis A, Khan W, et al. Adult native knee extensor mechanism ruptures. *Injury.* 2016;47(10):2065–2070.
3. Ni Fhoghlu C, Ellanti P, Moriarity A, et al. MRI features of a quadriceps tendon rupture. *BMJ Case Rep.* 2015;2015:bcr2015209942.
4. Brinkman JC, Reeson E, Chhabra A. Acute patellar tendon ruptures: an update on management. *J Am Acad Orthop Surg Glob Res Rev.* 2024;8(4):e24.00060.
5. Ibounig T, Simons TA. Etiology, diagnosis and treatment of tendinous knee extensor mechanism injuries. *Scand J Surg.* 2016;105(2):67–72.

ADDITIONAL READING

- Gao X, Shao Z, Liu S, et al. A case report of spontaneous rupture of the quadriceps tendon. *Clin Case Rep.* 2017;5(9):1477–1481.
- Greis PE, Holmstrom MC, Lahav A. Surgical treatment options for patella tendon rupture, part I: acute. *Orthopedics.* 2005;28(7):672–679.
- Ilan DI, Tejwani N, Keschner M, et al. Quadriceps tendon rupture. *J Am Acad Orthop Surg.* 2003;11(3):192–200.
- Kannus P, Józsa L. Histopathological changes preceding spontaneous rupture of a tendon. A controlled study of 891 patients. *J Bone Joint Surg Am.* 1991;73(10):1507–1525.
- Perfitt JS, Petrie MJ, Blundell CM, et al. Acute quadriceps tendon rupture: a pragmatic approach to diagnostic imaging. *Eur J Orthop Surg Traumatol.* 2014;24(7):1237–1241.
- Phillips K, Costantino TG. Diagnosis of patellar tendon rupture by emergency ultrasound. *J Emerg Med.* 2014;47(2):204–206.
- White DW, Wenke JC, Mosely DS, et al. Incidence of major tendon ruptures and anterior cruciate ligament tears in US Army soldiers. *Am J Sports Med.* 2007;35(8):1308–1314.

CLINICAL PEARLS

- Rupture of the extensor mechanism is an uncommon yet disabling injury requiring prompt diagnosis and early surgical management.
- Suspect patellar or quadriceps tendon rupture in any patient with acute knee pain and inability to actively extend the knee.
- Do not forget to evaluate for other intra-articular knee injuries.
- Early ROM and functional mobilization with weight-bearing after surgery has shown to be a safe form of rehabilitation.

PATELLOFEMORAL PAIN (PFP)

Michael Prestgard-Duke, MD • Vihangi Hindagolla, DO

BASICS

DESCRIPTION

- Overuse injury with pain located around or behind the patella
- Multifactorial with contribution from intrinsic anatomic structure and extrinsic training. These factors cause biomechanical changes resulting in abnormal alignment of the patella.
- Synonyms:
  - Chondromalacia patella (term frequently used in older literature; a subset of anterior knee pain related to softening/damage to the articular cartilage)
  - Runner's knee
  - Patellar tracking dysfunction

EPIDEMIOLOGY

- Anterior knee pain represents 20–40% of all knee problems.
- Most common running injury presenting to sports medicine clinic.
- Heterogenous incidence of patellofemoral pain (PFP) is 10%.
- Incidence rate for amateur runners in general population is 1,080.5/1,000 person-years.
- Annual prevalence is 22.7% in the general adult population, and 28.9% in the adolescent population.
- More common in females (~2:1)

RISK FACTORS

- Recent increase or change in training/activity
- Increased joint overload with activities (i.e., running, squats, lunges)
- Family history of patellofemoral or anterior knee pain
- Early sports specialization
- Static anatomic malalignment (i.e., increased femoral anteversion, inward-looking patella, leg length discrepancy of >1 cm, external tibial torsion, pronated feet, valgus/varus deformities of the lower leg
- Dynamic biomechanical deviations (i.e., excessive or insufficient foot pronation, knee abduction impulses, patellar hypermobility or hypomobility)
- Strength imbalances in quadriceps (i.e., vastus medialis oblique [VMO] deficit relative to vastus lateralis), hamstrings, and hip musculature
- Gluteus medius inhibition or dysfunction; leads to decreased hip control and greater femoral adduction and/or internal rotation
- Elevated body mass index (BMI) is correlated with PFP in adults, but not adolescents. However, it is not considered to be a risk factor for developing PFP in either group.
- Increased Q-angle has not been found to be a risk factor for future development of PFP.

COMMONLY ASSOCIATED CONDITIONS

- Chondral injury (common with history of blunt trauma)
- Increased residual laxity or tearing of the medial patellar stabilizers with lateral dislocation of the patella
- Patellofemoral compartment osteoarthritis

DIAGNOSIS

HISTORY

- Recent changes in activity frequency, type, or intensity
- Changes to current exercise footwear, or increase in duration of wear
- Anterior knee pain after prolonged sitting ("theater sign"), squatting, running, climbing/descending stairs
- Insidious onset of anterior knee pain with activity
- Perceived instability with "buckling" of the knee secondary to pain and not due to ligament/tendon injury or subluxation.
- History of subluxation/dislocation episodes or direct trauma to the knee
- Prior treatments, including nonsteroidal anti-inflammatory drugs (NSAIDs), taping, physical therapy, orthotics, injections, or surgery raise suspicion for PFP

PHYSICAL EXAM

- Physical examination tests have been reported to have sensitivities <50%, although specificity for some tests have ranged from 72% to 100% (1)[A].
- Evaluate gait (Trendelenburg gait, quadriceps avoidance) and overall limb alignment as mentioned in "Risk Factors."
- Dynamic testing with single- and double-leg squats to assess patellar motion
- Evaluate lumbar spine, core strength, and hips.
- Evaluate neurologic system.
- Note any atrophy of the lower extremity, especially VMO and vastus lateralis.
- Assess strength of gluteus medius using Trendelenburg test or side-lying hip abduction test.
- Examine flexibility of quadriceps and hip (Thomas test), iliotibial band (Ober test), hamstring (popliteal angle test), and gastrocsoleus (ankle range of motion).
- Assess for presence of J-sign (abrupt lateral motion of patella with full extension) during active flexion and extension of the knee.
- Assess for patellar height: patella alta, patella baja, squinting patella, or grasshopper eyes (proximal and lateral patellar rotation).
- Rule out patellar and quadriceps tendinopathy, ligamentous instability, and meniscal pathology.
- Evaluate the prepatellar, infrapatellar, and pes anserine bursae and for presence of joint effusion. Note that knee effusion is not a typical finding of PFP; its presence is likely related to other pathology.
- Examine for patellar facet and retinacula tenderness; tenderness over lateral retinaculum is present in 90% of patients.
- Evaluate patellar glide and apprehension:
  - Divide patella into four quadrants.
  - If unable to move >1 quadrant laterally or medially, this is suggestive of a tight medial or lateral retinaculum.
  - If able to translate >3 quadrants medially or laterally, suggestive of hypermobile patella; hypermobility usually seen with positive patellar apprehension as the patient senses impending patellar dislocation
- Perform patellar tilt test: With knee in full extension or 30 degrees of flexion, press posteriorly on medial aspect of patella. Lateral patella should translate anteriorly; if examiner cannot get the lateral border of patella to horizontal with posterior pressure on medial edge, suggestive of a tight lateral retinaculum.
- Note that crepitus is minimally helpful for diagnosis as many healthy people also have crepitus on exam.

DIFFERENTIAL DIAGNOSIS

- Patellar or quadriceps tendinopathy
- Patellofemoral osteoarthritis
- Patellar instability with subluxation or dislocation
- Osteochondral defect of the trochlear or patellar surface
- Osteochondritis dissecans
- Iliotibial band syndrome
- Infrapatellar fat pad inflammation or impingement
- Synovial plica
- Retinacular strain
- Osgood-Schlatter apophysitis (proximal anterior tibia)
- Sinding-Larsen-Johansson apophysitis (inferior patellar pole)
- Referred pain from the hip, often affecting the anterior distal thigh and knee
- Multiple other sources of knee pain and arthritis (e.g., gout, infection, reflex sympathetic dystrophy, neuroma, or sickle cell disease)
- Pigmented villonodular synovitis

DIAGNOSTIC TESTS & INTERPRETATION

- Imaging studies are not required for an accurate diagnosis of PFP syndrome. Multiple studies have evaluated sulcus angle, patellar height (determined by Insall-Salvati index), patellar tilt (determined by Laurin angle), and patellar displacement (determined by Merchant angle) and have found no significant difference between symptomatic and asymptomatic patients (1)[A].
- Imaging studies are only recommended if there is clinical suspicion of another diagnosis, or if a patient has failed 1 to 2 months of initial conservative management. Most radiographs will appear normal. Any structural abnormalities may need to be addressed when determining the appropriate care plan for an individual patient.
- Computed tomography (CT), magnetic resonance imaging (MRI), or bone scintigraphy may be considered to determine presence of alternative pathology causing anterior knee pain or to assist with surgical options when conservative management has failed.
- Plain radiographs:
  - Anteroposterior bilateral standing: may show varus or valgus orientation of femur, knee, or tibia
  - Lateral view of affected knee: Evaluate for patellar height with Insall-Salvati ratio (patellar tendon length to patella length); ratio <0.8 consistent with patella baja; ratio >1.2 consistent with patella alta
  - Merchant view of bilateral patellofemoral joints to evaluate for shallow sulcus angle, subluxation degree, and femoral condyle appearance. Standing, loaded Merchant view is more accurate representation of joint kinematics.
  - Tunnel view if osteochondral defect is suspected

- CT:
  - Useful to evaluate patellofemoral relationships (e.g., tilt and subluxation), especially in patients with suspected subluxation at <30 to 45 degrees of flexion that is poorly visualized on plain film.
  - Useful to evaluate intraosseous lesions and to plan selective surgical realignment procedures
- MRI:
  - Useful in evaluation of soft tissue, including patellofemoral cartilage, other articular cartilage, tendinopathy, and retinacula
  - Stages III and IV chondromalacia can be evaluated reliably with accuracy of 89%.

TREATMENT

GENERAL MEASURES

- There is no evidence that a single treatment modality works for all patients with patellofemoral syndrome. Limited evidence shows that some treatment modalities may work for some subgroups of patients with PFP (likely dependent on etiology) (2)[A].
- Because PFP is typically multifactorial in origin, adequate treatment should address multiple facets of care and include an emphasis on education:
  - 80% of patients respond to conservative management.
  - Reduce activities that may have led to onset of symptoms, such as resistance training (lunges or full squats), increased mileage with running, or plyometric exercises.
  - Encourage relative rest using alternate exercises (i.e., pool running, bicycling, swimming, or using an elliptical trainer).
  - Evaluate footwear with focus on excessive deterioration, inadequate support, or excessive support.
  - Ice, compression, and elevation can help with acute pain control.
- Physical therapy should focus on the findings or deficits seen for each individual patient (e.g., strength training for those with muscle weakness and flexibility training for those with decreased range of motion):
  - Strength training with focus on knee and hip exercises; especially knee extension, hip abduction, and external rotation
  - Flexibility training should address the hamstrings, quadriceps, hip flexors, iliotibial band, and gastrocsoleus.
  - Open versus closed kinetic chain training programs can lead to good functional outcomes.
  - Isokinetic exercise (variable resistance applied so movement remains at a constant speed) has positive effects on knee joint position sense, which in turn increases strength and work capacity.
- Physical therapy can reduce pain in short, medium, and long terms and improve function in medium and long terms (3)[A].
- Knee joint mobilization/manual therapy, when used as part of comprehensive approach, has shown to be effective compared to control group (4)[A].

MEDICATION

- Medication management should focus on pain control, not inflammation control.
- Acetaminophen or NSAIDs may be used initially to provide pain relief during daily activities.
- Steroid injections are of limited value.
- Topical analgesics may be helpful for those with superficial hypersensitivity.

ADDITIONAL THERAPIES

- Education in combination with a physical treatment (exercise, orthoses or patellar-taping/mobilization is more likely to reduce symptoms at 3 months. At 12 months, education alone is comparable to education combined with physical treatments (5)[A].
- Orthotics: Off-the-shelf foot orthoses improve pain in the short term, but long-term benefits are uncertain (3)[A].
- Unproven and ineffective therapies:
  - There is low-level evidence that patellofemoral braces and running technique retraining may reduce the risk of PFP. Further studies are needed (6)[A].
  - Patellar taping likely only has a placebo effect and, if used, should be combined with proven therapies as above (2)[A],(3)[A].
  - Acupuncture or dry needling to trigger points have uncertain effects (3)[A].
  - Electrophysical agents (e.g., ultrasound, phonophoresis, and laser therapy), although once widely used, are inappropriate and unproven (3)[A].
  - Hyaluronic acid injections have no clinically meaningful effect on pain or functional outcomes.

SURGERY/OTHER PROCEDURES

- Considered if identifiable lesion seen on imaging and if patient has not shown improvement after >6 months of adequate conservative therapy
- Isolated lateral retinacular release of the patella has not been shown to provide long-term benefit for treatment of patellar instability but may be used along with proximal or distal realignment of the extensor mechanism.
- Patients with Q-angles >20 degrees plus abnormal congruence angles may undergo distal realignment procedures such as an anterior medial tibial tubercle transfer.
- Patients with dislocations may be appropriate for surgery if symptoms of patellofemoral instability were present before their dislocation.
- Patellectomy and derotational osteotomies are last resorts.

REFERENCES

1. Haim A, Yaniv M, Dekel S, et al. Patellofemoral pain syndrome: validity of clinical and radiological features. *Clin Orthop Relat Res.* 2006;451:223–228.
2. Saltychev M, Dutton RA, Laimi K, et al. Effectiveness of conservative treatment for patellofemoral pain syndrome: a systematic review and meta-analysis. *J Rehabil Med.* 2018;50(5):393–401.
3. Collins NJ, Barton CJ, van Middelkoop M, et al. 2018 consensus statement on exercise therapy and physical interventions (orthoses, taping and manual therapy) to treat patellofemoral pain: recommendations from the 5th International Patellofemoral Pain Research Retreat, Gold Coast, Australia, 2017. *Br J Sports Med.* 2018;52(18):1170–1178.
4. Jayaseelan DJ, Scalzitti DA, Palmer G, et al. The effects of joint mobilization on individuals with patellofemoral pain: a systematic review. *Clin Rehabil.* 2018;32(6):722–733.
5. Winters M, Holden S, Lura CB, et al. Comparative effectiveness of treatments for patellofemoral pain: a living systematic review with network meta-analysis. *Br J Sports Med.* 2020;55(7):369–377.
6. Culvenor AG, van Middelkoop M, Macri EM, et al. Is patellofemoral pain preventable? A systematic review and meta-analysis of randomised controlled trials. *Br J Sports Med.* 2020;55:378–384.

ADDITIONAL READING

- Brushøj C, Hölmich P, Nielsen MB, et al. Acute patellofemoral pain: aggravating activities, clinical examination, MRI and ultrasound findings. *Br J Sports Med.* 2008;42(1):64–67.
- Gulati A, McElrath C, Wadhwa V, et al. Current clinical, radiological, and treatment perspectives of patellofemoral pain syndrome. *Br J Radiol.* 2018;91(1086):20170456.
- Hart JM, Kuenze C, Norte G, et al. Prospective, randomized, double-blind evaluation of the efficacy of a single-dose hyaluronic acid for the treatment of patellofemoral chondromalacia. *Orthop J Sports Med.* 2019;7(6):2325967119854192.
- Lattermann C, Toth J, Bach BR Jr. The role of lateral retinacular release in the treatment of patellar instability. *Sports Med Arthrosc Rev.* 2007;15(2):57–60.
- Lester JD, Watson JN, Hutchinson MR. Physical examination of the patellofemoral joint. *Clin Sports Med.* 2014;33(3):403–412.
- Logan CA, Bhashyam AR, Tisosky AJ, et al. Systematic review of the effect of taping techniques on patellofemoral pain syndrome. *Sports Health.* 2017;9(5):456–461.
- Neal BS, Lack SD, Lankhorst NE, et al. Risk factors for patellofemoral pain: a systematic review and meta-analysis. *Br J Sports Med.* 2019;53(5):270–281.
- Smith BE, Selfe J, Thacker D, et al. Incidence and prevalence of patellofemoral pain: a systematic review and meta-analysis. *PLoS One.* 2018;13(1):e0190892.
- Smith TO, Drew BT, Meek TH, et al. Knee orthoses for treating patellofemoral pain syndrome. *Cochrane Database Syst Rev.* 2015;(12):CD010513.
- Thijs Y, Van Tiggelen D, Roosen P, et al. A prospective study on gait-related intrinsic risk factors for patellofemoral pain. *Clin J Sport Med.* 2007;17(6):437–445.

CLINICAL PEARLS

- Return to activity:
  - If patient has PFP during, immediately following, or the day after exercising:
    - Decrease activity. Avoid strength training exercises such as full squats and lunges.
    - Consider alternate activities, such as an elliptical trainer, bicycling, or swimming.
    - For runners who need to maintain running-specific conditioning, use a floatation belt for pool running.
- Education and physical therapy with a focus on knee and hip strength and lower extremity flexibility are proven effective and are mainstays of treatment.
- Foot orthoses can reduce short-term pain; patellar taping and knee bracing are unproven.
- 80% of patients respond to a nonoperative therapy, most within 4 weeks; complete resolution of symptoms may take longer.

PECTORALIS MAJOR TENDON RUPTURE

Alexandra E. Warrick, MD, CAQSM • Corey T. Gatewood, MD •
Daniel C. Herman, MD, PhD, FAAPMR, FACSM, FISBS, CAQSM

BASICS

DESCRIPTION

- Pectoralis major (PM) is a powerful adductor and internal rotator and contributes to flexion of the humerus.
- Main source of power to the torso during strenuous activity
- Two heads:
  - Superior/clavicular: originates at medial clavicle and upper sternum
  - Inferior/sternal: originates at distal sternum, external oblique fascia, costal cartilage of first 6 ribs
- Clavicular and sternal head tendons converge and rotate to form a U-shaped tendon laterally that includes the anterior and posterior tendon layer that inserts laterally to the bicipital groove on the humerus (1).
- Inferior portion of the sternal head which inserts as the superior part of the posterior tendon layer is most typically involved during a partial tendon injury (1).
- Tears most commonly refer to complete avulsion of the pectoralis tendon at the humeral insertion. Full-thickness tears include both the anterior and posterior layers of the tendon.
- Bony avulsion, muscle origin injury, and muscle belly injury occur at lower incidence (1).
- Innervation: medial and lateral pectoral nerves
- Blood supply: pectoral branch of thoracoacromial artery, lateral thoracic artery, and branches of the internal mammary artery
- Associated with weight lifting (bench press) mostly but possible with sports-related injuries, falls, and direct trauma to the tendon (2)

EPIDEMIOLOGY

- Between 1822 and 2010, 365 cases of PM tears have been reported, with >75% occurring after 1990. Increasing incidence is attributed to increased popularity of weight lifting and contact sports (2).
- Men 20 to 40 years old are more likely to sustain a PM injury than women; elderly are also at higher risk (2).

ETIOLOGY AND PATHOPHYSIOLOGY

- Stretching of the PM muscle during active eccentric contraction (1)
- Weight lifting (bench press specifically) is a common mechanism (1). Electromyogram (EMG) studies demonstrate maximal activation at the beginning of the ascent phase of the lift.
- Direct trauma to the muscle independently or with sports-related activity (wrestling, rugby, boxing, judo, wakeboarding, skiing, ice hockey, handball, mountain climbing, parachuting, rodeo competition, football, windsurfing, rock climbing, and kabaddi)
- Falls and manual transfers have also been reported (3).

RISK FACTORS

- Medications:
  - Anabolic steroids can cause muscle strength to increase disproportionately to tendon strength, making tendons more susceptible to injury. Additionally, anabolic steroids decrease tendon elasticity, leading to reduced elongation under submaximal stress and collagen dysplasia (2).
  - Antibiotics: Fluoroquinolones can weaken tendons and disrupt collagen synthesis, resulting in increased susceptibility to rupture (3).
- Systemic diseases: connective tissue disorders, collagen vascular disease, diabetes
- Advanced age
- Disuse atrophy
- Tobacco use

DIAGNOSIS

HISTORY

- Men 20 to 40 years of age (4)
- Usually report a pop or tearing in the shoulder (4)
- Complain of pain/weakness in chest or shoulder (2)

PHYSICAL EXAM

- Swelling and ecchymosis in anterior shoulder/chest most common; ecchymosis localized to the anterior arm is relatively specific for distal humeral attachment rupture as opposed to musculotendinous junction rupture (5).
- Loss of pectoralis contour, palpable defect, and deformity of the anterior axillary fold
- Shoulder motion limited by pain
- Weakness in adduction and internal rotation
- Dropped nipple sign (where the affected side's nipple appears lower than the uninjured side)

DIFFERENTIAL DIAGNOSIS

- Long head biceps subluxation
- Proximal humerus fracture
- Glenohumeral dislocation
- Rotator cuff tear
- Subscapularis muscle tear
- Medial pectoral nerve entrapment

DIAGNOSTIC TESTS & INTERPRETATION

- Plain radiographs initially to rule out bony avulsions, fracture, or dislocations (4)[C]
- Characteristic finding on x-ray is soft tissue swelling and loss of PM shadow (4)[C].
- Ultrasound (US) can serve as a valuable supplement to clinical examination when there is uncertainty in diagnosis, whereas magnetic resonance imaging (MRI) can be used if diagnosis remains equivocal or as a useful aid to surgical planning (4)[C].
- US findings will depend on location and time from injury, ranging from muscle fiber disruption that is hypoechoic with a mixed echogenic hematoma when acute to an anechoic fluid collection when chronic (1)[C]. Additionally, there may be a gap between the deltopectoral groove and coracobrachialis muscle.
- MRI is optimal. It assesses grade, muscle retraction, acuity, and presence of adhesions in chronic tears (4)[C]. Findings associated with PM and tendon injuries included edema in the muscle belly, intramuscular hematoma, and fluid gaps (2)[C].
- Standard MRI alone will not suffice; a dedicated sequence is necessary, including axial slices that extend from superior to the quadrilateral space and inferior to the deltoid tuberosity, along with coronal oblique cuts (4)[C]. In acute injury, T1-weighted axial imaging has been found to be most effective in determining tears, whereas T2-weighted imaging has been found to be most effective for evaluating chronic injuries.

TREATMENT

- Acute treatment:
  - Nonsteroidal anti-inflammatory drugs (NSAIDs) and acetaminophen
  - Ice
  - Sling immobilization: 2 to 3 weeks with passive range of motion (ROM)
  - Majority of acute PM tendon ruptures are treated surgically.
- Long-term care:
  - Tear type, patient age, activity level, and cosmetic desires determine care (4)[C].
  - Most partial tears, sternoclavicular tears, and muscle belly tears are treated nonsurgically (4)[C].
  - Complete sternal tears require surgical repair to restore function and strength (4)[C].
  - Nonsurgical treatment may be adequate in elderly/inactive population irrespective of type of tear (4)[C].
  - Gradually return to strength training with incorporation of maximum strength exercises after 6 months. Patients are advised not to lift >50% of their one repetition maximum until 6 months after PM repair (6)[C].

P

ONGOING CARE

- Nonsurgical treatment:
  - Begin shoulder mobilization and gentle stretching/strengthening when tolerated (4)[C].
  - At 3 to 6 weeks, progress to active ROM.
  - At 6 to 12 weeks, incorporate resistance bands, isometric exercises, and gradually increase to muscle strength and endurance (6)[C].
  - Unrestricted activity at 2 to 3 months after injury (4)[C]
- Surgical management:
  - Acute PM repair has greater improvement in functional outcomes, pain, satisfaction, cosmesis, and return to sport when compared to chronic repair (5)[A].
  - Chronic PM repair led to improvements in functional outcomes, strength (isokinetic/isometric), cosmesis, and resting deformity when compared with nonoperative treatment (5)[A].
  - Chronic PM repairs are accompanied by increased difficulty due to muscle retraction and adhesions, requiring the use of autograft or allograft to augment PM tendon repair (5)[A].
  - There is no consensus on superiority in graft type (autograft and allograft) or surgical technique: transosseous tunnels (TT), cortical button, or suture anchor (SA). However, studies have demonstrated regardless of repair technique, PM tendon repairs are weaker than the native tendon.

COMPLICATIONS

Nonoperative: persistent weakness, cosmetic deformity, hematoma, risk for abscess formation, myositis ossificans (2)[C]

- Operative: neuropathy, rerupture, hematoma, hypertrophic scar formation, and infection (5)[A]
- Failure of PM tendon repair was reported to be more common in patients with body mass index of >30 kg/m^2 and greater amount of time between the injury and surgery pre versus post 1.5 months (2)[C].

REFERENCES

1. Chiavaras MM, Jacobson JA, Smith J, et al. Pectoralis major tears: anatomy, classification, and diagnosis with ultrasound and MR imaging. *Skeletal Radiol*. 2015;44(2):157–164.
2. Brown SM, Cole WW III, Provencher MT, et al. Pectoralis major injuries: presentation, diagnosis, and management. *JBJS Rev*. 2021;9(5).
3. Magone K, Ben-Ari E, Gyftopoulos S, et al. Pectoralis major tendon tear: a critical analysis review. *JBJS Rev*. 2021;9(8).
4. Butt U, Mehta S, Funk L, et al. Pectoralis major ruptures: a review of current management. *J Shoulder Elbow Surg*. 2015;24(4):655–662.
5. Bodendorfer BM, Wang DX, McCormick BP, et al. Treatment of pectoralis major tendon tears: a systematic review and meta-analysis of repair timing and fixation methods. *Am J Sports Med*. 2020;48(13):3376–3385.
6. Manske RC, Prohaska D. Pectoralis major tendon repair post surgical rehabilitation. *N Am J Sports Phys Ther*. 2007;2(1):22–33.

ADDITIONAL READING

- Elliott BC, Wilson GJ, Kerr GK. A biomechanical analysis of the sticking region in the bench press. *Med Sci Sports Exerc*. 1989;21(4):450–462.
- Elmaraghy AW, Devereaux MW. A systematic review and comprehensive classification of pectoralis major tears. *J Shoulder Elbow Surg*. 2012;21(3):412–422.
- Giordano JR, Klein B, Hershfeld B, et al. A review of chronic pectoralis major tears: what options are available? *Clin Shoulder Elb*. 2023;26(3):330–339.
- Kowalczuk M, Elmaraghy A. Pectoralis major rupture: evaluation and management. *J Am Acad Orthop Surg*. 2022;30(7):e617–e627.
- Kowalczuk M, Rubinger L, Elmaraghy AW. Pectoralis major ruptures: tear patterns and patient demographic characteristics. *Orthop J Sports Med*. 2020;8(12):2325967120969424.
- Mirzayan R, Andelman SM, Sethi PM, et al. Acellular dermal matrix augmentation significantly increases ultimate load to failure of pectoralis major tendon repair: a biomechanical study. *J Shoulder Elbow Surg*. 2020;29(4):728–735.
- Stringer MR, Cockfield AN, Sharpe TR. Pectoralis major rupture in an active female. *J Am Acad Orthop Surg Glob Res Rev*. 2019;3(10):e19.00030.

CLINICAL PEARLS

- Usually, a complete avulsion of PM tendon at humerus
- Most commonly occurs during weight lifting, specifically bench press.
- Patients may report a pop and present with swelling, ecchymosis, and palpable tendon deformity.
- MRI is gold standard for diagnosis.
- Type of tear, patient age, and activity level dictate treatment with surgery providing superior outcomes in the acute versus chronic time period.
- Surgical repair provides best outcomes in terms of strength, return to play, and patient satisfaction.

PERIORBITAL AND ORBITAL CELLULITIS

Bernadette Pendergraph, MD • John Cheng, MD

BASICS

DESCRIPTION

- Periorbital (preseptal) cellulitis (1):
  - Infection or inflammatory process of the orbicularis oculi muscle and/or dermis anterior (superficial) to the orbital septum
  - Rarely progresses to orbital cellulitis
- Orbital (postseptal) cellulitis (1):
  - Severe infection or inflammatory process of the fat and muscles posterior (deep) to the orbital septum

EPIDEMIOLOGY

- More common in children than adults, based on retrospective cohort studies
- Periorbital cellulitis:
  - Predominantly in children <5 years old
  - Incidence is roughly equal in males and females.
- Orbital cellulitis:
  - Children up to 16 times more likely than adults to be affected (1.6/100,000 vs. 0.1/100,000) (2)
  - Incidence is roughly 2:1 male-to-female ratio.

ETIOLOGY AND PATHOPHYSIOLOGY

- Children: tend to be monobacterial (3):
  - *Staphylococcus aureus*, methicillin-sensitive (MSSA) (26.3%)
  - Various streptococcal species—*intermedius, pyogenesis, pneumoniae* (40%)
  - *Anaerobes* (13%)
  - *Staphylococcus aureus*, methicillin-resistant (MRSA) (5%)
  - *Haemophilus influenzae* (4%)
- Adults: tend to be polymicrobial (1):
  - *Staphylococcus*. Methicillin sensitive from 23% to 72%; methicillin resistance increasing over time
  - *Streptococcus*
  - Mixed *aerobes* and *anaerobes*
- Periorbital cellulitis (4):
  - Progression of preexisting infections:
    - Conjunctivitis
    - Hordeolum (stye)
    - Dacryocystitis or dacryoadenitis (infection or inflammation of lacrimal duct or gland, respectively)
    - Upper respiratory infection
  - Superficial trauma:
    - Insect bite
    - Impetigo
    - Acne
    - Penetrating injury
  - Hematogenous dissemination: especially in children 3 to 36 months old due to pneumococcal bacteremia
- Orbital cellulitis (1),(4):
  - Typically occurs by one of the following:
    - Spread of organisms from sinuses (especially ethmoid) to orbital cavity (i.e., sinusitis); most common cause
    - Hematogenous dissemination
    - Direct/traumatic inoculation: less common than periorbital cellulitis
      - Surgical procedures

RISK FACTORS

Periorbital and orbital cellulitis precursors include:

- Upper respiratory tract infections:
  - Sinusitis or sinus disease (acute or chronic)
- Dental disease or surgery.
- Previous eye surgery.
- Trauma:
  - Scratches
  - Insect bites
- Compromised immunity (1),(4)

GENERAL PREVENTION

- Avoiding periorbital skin trauma is important for prevention:
  - Protective goggles or other American National Standards Institute–approved eyewear may decrease risk.
- Vaccine coverage of common causative organisms:
  - Children who receive at least two *Haemophilus influenzae* type b (Hib) immunizations are unlikely to have Hib-related infection.

DIAGNOSIS

- Clinical diagnosis is based on history, signs and symptoms, and neurologic exam. Early identification of orbital cellulitis is essential, as disease progression can lead to blindness, meningitis, or death.
- Predictive accuracy of history and physical for orbital cellulitis is 82% (1).

HISTORY

- Periorbital cellulitis:
  - Pain
  - Conjunctivitis
  - Epiphora (excessive tearing)
  - Blurred vision
  - Fever
  - Recent or current upper respiratory infection
- Orbital cellulitis:
  - Above, plus:
    - Painful or decreased eye movement, diplopia
    - Facial or dental surgery
    - Recent sinusitis
    - Other systemic infections

PHYSICAL EXAM

- Periorbital cellulitis:
  - Periorbital swelling, erythema, warmth, and tenderness
  - Normal vision
  - Full and painless extraocular muscle (EOM) range of motion
  - No proptosis
  - No afferent pupillary defect (4)
- Orbital cellulitis (1):
  - Eyelid swelling (does not extend beyond orbital rim)
  - Proptosis (anterior bulging of eye from orbit)
  - Chemosis (swelling of conjunctiva)
  - Ophthalmoplegia (limited ocular motility)
  - Painful EOM
  - Decreased visual acuity
  - Presence of one or more of the following has a 76% sensitivity and 76% specificity for orbital cellulitis:
  - Motility limitation
    - Proptosis
    - Moderate-severe chemosis
  - Temperature > 100.4°F within 24 hours of presentation

DIFFERENTIAL DIAGNOSIS

- Periorbital cellulitis:
  - Allergic reaction
  - Edema:
    - Hypoproteinemia or congestive heart failure
  - Orbital trauma
  - Dermoid cyst
  - Thyroid-associated ophthalmopathy
  - Herpes simplex
  - Chalazion
- Orbital cellulitis:
  - Cavernous sinus thrombosis
  - Orbital trauma
  - Thyroid-associated ophthalmopathy
  - Orbital myositis
  - Granulomatosis with polyangiitis → systemic vasculitis
  - Idiopathic orbital inflammatory syndrome
  - Tumor: rhabdomyosarcoma, lymphoma, or leukemia

DIAGNOSTIC TESTS & INTERPRETATION

- Laboratory testing has limited utility in distinguishing between periorbital and orbital cellulitis (1)[C].
- CRP and ESR are more likely to be elevated in orbital cellulitis compared to periorbital cellulitis (1)[C].
- Complete blood count (CBC): Leukocytosis is more common with orbital cellulitis (1)[C].
- Blood culture if sepsis suspected but less likely positive in adults than children
- Ocular or nasal swabs are less specific than blood cultures (1)[C].
- Gram stain and culture of tissue aspirate or draining purulent material: Surgical aspirates often have the best results.
- Lumbar puncture/cerebrospinal fluid evaluation if athlete appears markedly ill, has insufficient Hib immunization, or meningitis must be ruled out.
- CT of brain, orbits with and without IV contrast is recommended imaging modality (1)[C] (91–100% accurate) (5)[C]:
  - If clinical features cannot differentiate between periorbital and orbital cellulitis
  - If unable to perform complete physical exam secondary to patient discomfort or periorbital edema
  - Signs or symptoms of ocular compartment syndrome
    - Decreased or double vision
    - Limited eye movement
    - Pain with eye movement
    - Proptosis
    - Relative afferent pupillary defect
  - Signs or symptoms of CNS involvement (1)[C]
  - Clinical deterioration or failure to improve following 24 to 48 hours of parenteral antimicrobial therapy
- Magnetic resonance imaging (MRI) of brain and orbits, with and without contrast (1)[C]:
  - Better than CT for soft tissue involvement, even without gadolinium contrast. Lack of radiation is preferable, especially in pediatric patients. However, increased imaging time and less access to MRI
  - May be needed to detect smaller abscesses
  - Suspicion for intracranial complications (e.g., altered mentation, persistent fever)
  - MR with venography or angiography to detect cavernous sinus thromboses
- Ultrasound:
  - A systemic review of ultrasound accuracy in diagnosing orbital cellulitis revealed low-quality evidence that ultrasound may assist in diagnosis of orbital cellulitis (6)[B].

TREATMENT

Emergency department (5)[C]:

- Establish intravenous (IV) access, administer oxygen for serious complications, including sepsis, meningitis, and cavernous sinus thrombosis.
- Consider vancomycin in geographic areas with prevalent penicillin-resistant pneumococci or MRSA.
- Children with orbital cellulitis require:
  - CT scan
  - Start parenteral antibiotics after imaging confirmation; initiate antibiotics immediately if toxic appearance.
  - Recommend pediatric ophthalmologic and otolaryngology (ear, nose, and throat [ENT]).
  - Prompt surgery may be necessary.

MEDICATION

First Line

- Periorbital cellulitis (1)[C]:
  - There is no evidence that IV antibiotics are generally better than oral antibiotics.
  - Suspected MSSA or streptococcal spp:
    - Dicloxacillin or cephalexin
      - Adults: 500 mg PO 4 times daily
      - Pediatrics: 25 to 50 mg/kg/d PO in 4 divided doses daily
  - Suspected MRSA:
    - Clindamycin:
      - Adults: 600 mg IV q8h OR 300 to 450 mg PO QID
      - Pediatrics: 25 to 40 mg/kg/d IV divided TID *or* 30 to 40 mg/kg/d PO divided TID
    - Bactrim (trimethoprim and sulfamethoxazole):
      - 8 to 12 mg/kg/d (trimethoprim component) IV in 4 divided doses
      - 8 to 12 mg/kg/d (trimethoprim component) PO in in 2 divided doses

- Orbital cellulitis:
  - A retrospective review of pediatric patients in the United States showed heterogeneity of antibiotic treatment. Generally, empiric treatment will target *Staphylococcus aureus* (MSSA and MRSA), *Streptococcus*, gram-negative organisms, and *anaerobes* (3)[C].
  - Hospitalize patients with suspected orbital cellulitis.
  - IV antibiotics:
    - Adults (1)[C]:
      - Vancomycin 15 to 20 mg/kg IV q8–12h *plus*
      - One of the following:
        - Piperacillin-tazobactam
        - Ampicillin-sulbactam
        - Ceftriaxone
        - Cefotaxime *and* Metronidazole
    - Pediatrics (1)[C]:
      - Same as above dosed appropriately
    - Penicillin allergy (1)[C]:
      - Adults:
        - Vancomycin (at above dose) *plus*
        - Ciprofloxacin 400 mg IV twice daily, or 500 to 750 mg orally twice daily, *or*
        - Levofloxacin 500 to 750 mg IV or orally once daily

ALERT

Fluoroquinolones have black box warning for tendinopathy/tendon rupture and are not considered first-line therapy in pediatrics due to potential for arthropathy. Consider infectious disease consultation before use in athletes or pediatric population.

- Several reviews and meta-analyses show statistically shorter hospital stays when systemic corticosteroids are used with IV antibiotics. A Cochrane review showed insufficient evidence to draw conclusions due to heterogeneity in dosing, timing, and duration. Different regimens have been documented, with insufficient data to suggest advantages or disadvantages:
  - Penicillin allergy:
    - Type 1 anaphylaxis, urticarial, or Stevens-Johnson syndrome:
      - Avoid all β-lactams.
    - Nonurticarial rash to penicillin:
      - Cephalosporin in controlled environment
  - Optimal duration of therapy not determined (1)[C]:
    - One study revealed 14 (±3) days of IV antibiotics for periorbital cellulitis and 17 (±5) days for orbital cellulitis.
    - Typical course of 10 to 21 days, transition to oral therapy as symptoms resolve
  - Complicated or no response to antibacterial regimen (1)[C]:
    - Prompt evaluation by ophthalmology or ENT for surgery
  - Symptomatic treatments (1)[C]:
    - Sinus decongestion
    - Nasal sprays
    - Oral decongestants
    - Oral antihistamines

ISSUES FOR REFERRAL

Multidisciplinary management:

- Orbital cellulitis:
  - Adults: infectious disease, ENT, and ophthalmologist
  - Pediatrics: infectious disease, ENT, ophthalmologist, and pediatrician

SURGERY/OTHER PROCEDURES

- Periorbital cellulitis:
  - Based on retrospective reviews, surgical intervention rarely needed; procedures include functional endoscopic sinus surgery, I&D of abscess or fluid collection (5)[C].
- Orbital cellulitis:
  - Retrospective reviews show that 77–100% of pediatric cases are successfully treated without surgery (5)[C].
- Subperiosteal or other orbital abscess may need surgery with:
  - Visual impairment
  - Progressive ophthalmoplegia
  - Abscess size >3.8 mL on CT
  - Lack of clinical improvement following 24 to 48 hours of antibiotics
- Cavernous sinus thrombosis:
  - Generally, requires endoscopic drainage of involved sinus(es) (5)[C]

ADMISSION, INPATIENT, AND NURSING CONSIDERATIONS

- Most patients with orbital cellulitis should be admitted for IV antibiotics:
  - With significant clinical improvement, can transition to oral antibiotics, although significant numbers may need outpatient parenteral antibiotics (3)[C]
  - No improvement, repeat CT scan and surgical intervention
- Initial stabilization (1)[C]:
  - Adequate fluid resuscitation:
    - 500 mL or 20 mL/kg bolus for dehydration, sepsis, or hypotension

- Admission criteria (1)[C]:
  - Any signs of orbital cellulitis:
    - Outpatient treatment should only be attempted if the eye is at least 50% open and very close outpatient follow-up can be guaranteed.
  - Toxicity or systemic illness
  - Incomplete physical exam of eye
  - Clinical deterioration on oral antibiotics
  - Uncertainty that patient can get adequate care at home
- Discharge criteria:
  - No more than modest swelling, tolerating oral antibiotics well with progressive improvement, nontoxic appearance, and reliable caregivers
  - Monitor for progressive swelling, irritability, increased fever, or vision changes.

ONGOING CARE

FOLLOW-UP RECOMMENDATIONS

Return-to-play guidance:

- Athlete and medical personnel must be able to demonstrate the following:
  - Asymptomatic with normal physical exam
  - Must pass sport-specific functional assessment
- Closely observe the athlete's performance in practice prior to clearing for competition.
- With any complications noted below, athlete should be cleared by appropriate specialist.

Patient Monitoring

Repeat imaging in patients with orbital cellulitis if there is any question about resolution following treatment.

COMPLICATIONS

- Blindness
- Cavernous sinus thrombosis
- Meningitis
- Subdural empyema
- Brain abscess

REFERENCES

1. Pelletier J, Koyfman A, Long B. High risk and low prevalence diseases: orbital cellulitis. *Am J Emerg Med.* 2023;68:1–9.
2. Kornelsen E, Mahant S, Parkin P, et al. Corticosteroids for periorbital and orbital cellulitis. *Cochrane Database Syst Rev.* 2021;4(4):CD013535.
3. Anosike BI, Ganapathy V, Nakamura MM. Epidemiology and management of orbital cellulitis in children. *J Pediatric Infect Dis Soc.* 2022;11(5):214–220.
4. Gordon AA, Phelps PO. Management of preseptal and orbital cellulitis for the primary care physician. *Dis Mon.* 2020;66(10):101044.
5. Wong SJ, Levi J. Management of pediatric orbital cellulitis: a systematic review. *Int J Pediatr Otorhinolaryngol.* 2018;110:123–129.
6. Anwar MR, Mahant S, Agbaje-Ojo T, et al. Diagnostic test accuracy of ultrasound for orbital cellulitis: a systematic review. *PLoS One.* 2023;18(7):e0288011.

CLINICAL PEARLS

- Orbital cellulitis is any infection/inflammatory process posterior to orbital septum and can be life-threatening, whereas periorbital cellulitis is anterior to orbital septum.
- Prompt consideration of orbital cellulitis if any painful/restricted eye movements, diplopia (resolves with eye closure), photophobia, change in color vision, proptosis, or afferent pupillary defect
- Most common causative organisms currently are *Staphylococcus* and *Streptococcus* spp.
- If clinically unable to differentiate, obtain CT of brain and orbits with and without contrast; MRI warranted if additional questions or extension of infection to brain, possible cavernous sinus thrombosis
- Treatment of orbital cellulitis includes hospital admission and empiric IV antibiotics for 3 to 5 days, followed by oral course of antibiotics.
- Close outpatient follow-up for orbital cellulitis with clearance by appropriate specialists prior to return to play

PERONEAL TENDON DISLOCATION/SUBLUXATION

Holly J. Benjamin, MD, FAMSSM, FACSM ▪ Claire Gross, MD, CAQSM

BASICS

DESCRIPTION

- The lateral compartment of the ankle contains the peroneus longus (PL) and peroneus brevis (PB) tendons.
- The tendons lie posterior to the lateral malleolus in the retromalleolar groove within a single tendon sheath and are fixed in place by the superior peroneal retinaculum (SPR).
- The actions of PB and PL are ankle eversion and ankle plantarflexion and contribute to dynamic ankle stability.
- There are two categories of peroneal tendon subluxation/dislocation:
  - Anterior dislocation:
    - Disruption of the SPR allows the peroneal tendons to sublux or dislocate anteriorly.
    - Avulsion of the SPR from the lateral malleolus can occur during an acute, traumatic injury or from repetitive overuse.
  - Intrasheath subluxation:
    - The PB and PL tendons reverse positions within the common sheath, usually occurring with ankle circumduction, causing a snapping sensation.

EPIDEMIOLOGY

- Generally considered a rare injury in sports
- May be a missed injury in up to 40% of cases (1), can be misdiagnosed as a lateral ankle sprain
- Associated with calcaneal fractures (2)

ETIOLOGY AND PATHOPHYSIOLOGY

- Acute avulsion of the SPR is usually due to contraction during dorsiflexion of an everted foot or inversion of a dorsiflexed ankle.
- Forceful contraction of the peroneal tendons within the sheath can tear the SPR (1).
- Chronic, atraumatic subluxation can also occur, related to anatomic variants and/or generalized ligamentous laxity.
- Originally described in ballet dancers
- Classically seen in sports such as skiing, football, ice skating, soccer, basketball rugby, and gymnastics

RISK FACTORS

- Anatomic variations may increase susceptibility:
  - A low-lying PB muscle belly intruding under the SPR
  - Presence of a peroneal quartus muscle, an accessory muscle, which, if present, lies within the retromalleolar groove with the peroneal tendons
  - Shallow, flat, or concave retromalleolar groove (up to 18% prevalence)
  - Excessive calcaneal varus
  - Pes cavus
  - Developmental absence of the SPR
- Generalized ligamentous laxity
- Contact sports
- Excessive push off and jump landing

COMMONLY ASSOCIATED CONDITIONS

- Conditions predisposing to hindfoot varus such as Charcot-Marie-Tooth
- Chronic ankle instability
- Calcaneal fractures (14% of calcaneal fractures) (2)

DIAGNOSIS

HISTORY

- Snapping or popping at time of injury over lateral ankle
- High index of suspicion after trauma with lateral ankle pain
- Most common mechanism is contraction during dorsiflexion of an everted foot or inversion of a dorsiflexed ankle.
- History and initial physical exam may be indistinguishable from a lateral ankle sprain.
- Lateral ankle pain that localizes posterior or inferior to the lateral malleolus
- Lateral snapping or popping with walking or ankle circumduction, with or without history of ankle trauma
- May report prior history of lateral ankle sprain (1)
- May report recent corticosteroid or fluoroquinolone use

PHYSICAL EXAM

- Acute injury may present with lateral ankle swelling and pain, resembling lateral ankle sprain or occurring in conjunction with an ankle sprain.
- Swelling and/or ecchymosis posterior to the lateral malleolus and may track along path of the tendons
- Tenderness to palpation over the tendons
- Resisted ankle dorsiflexion and eversion of ankle or circumduction while compressing the tendons may reproduce subluxation or snap/click.
- Chronic ankle instability
- Excessive calcaneal varus in standing
- Generalized ligamentous laxity (1)[C]

DIFFERENTIAL DIAGNOSIS

- Peroneal strain, tendonitis, or tear
- Lateral ankle sprain
- Lateral ankle instability
- Ankle fracture
- Achilles tendinopathy
- Tarsal coalition
- Sinus tarsi syndrome
- Talar osteochondral lesion
- Sural neuritis

DIAGNOSTIC TESTS & INTERPRETATION

Initial Tests (lab, imaging)

- Radiographs:
  - Assess for associated fracture.
  - "Fleck sign" shows the avulsion of cortical bone from the lateral aspect of the lateral malleolus, indicative of SPR avulsion (1)[C].

- Computed tomography (CT):
  - May be obtained to evaluate the size and shape of the retromalleolar groove and for presurgical planning (1),(2)[C]
- Ultrasound (US):
  - Dynamic real-time imaging can reveal the integrity of the SPR and can demonstrate subluxation out of the groove or intrasheath reversal of the peroneal tendons (positive predictive value [PPV] 100%).
  - Can see presence of the SPR if intact (3)[C]
- Magnetic resonance imaging (MRI):
  - Evaluates the integrity of the SPR
  - Elucidates the size and shape of the retromalleolar groove
  - Tendons will be out of place if frankly dislocated and not reduced but may appear to be in proper position if subluxation is not occurring at the time the image is obtained (1)[C].

Diagnostic Procedures/Other

- Not commonly performed
- Tendoscopy of the peroneal tendons
- Performed for diagnostic and therapeutic purposes
- Findings at time of tendoscopy include:
  - SPR tear
  - Low-lying PB muscle belly
  - Peroneus quartus tendon
  - Tendinosis
  - Split tendon tears (4)[C]

TREATMENT

- Acute treatment:
  - Rest, ice, compression, and elevation (RICE)
  - Nonsteroidal anti-inflammatory drugs (NSAIDs)
  - Limit weight-bearing if painful; off-load as needed for pain-free ambulation.
  - Ankle bracing to limit the excursion of the foot and may decrease the episodes of painful subluxation
  - Activity modification to reduce the occurrence of subluxation in certain patients if the subluxation is activity specific
  - If symptoms are minimal, can try a J-shaped compression pad and lateral heel wedge.
- Conservative treatment (5)[C]:
  - Immobilization 5 to 6 weeks with below-knee casting or bracing with ankle in slight plantarflexion
  - Although this is the initial intervention, there is up to 50% failure of nonsurgical treatment with persistent pain, instability, and recurrent dislocation.
  - Physical therapy for biomechanical evaluation and ankle stabilization
  - Regenerative medicine techniques such as platelet-rich plasma (PRP) injection for chronic tendinopathy with or without instability has shown promise in case reports.
  - Early referral for surgical evaluation is appropriate for athletes.
  - Recurring symptoms after a trial of conservative treatment are indications for surgical referral.

SURGERY/OTHER PROCEDURES

- Surgical intervention is commonly required due to high incidence of recurrence with nonoperative treatment (1)[C].
- Many techniques exist; there are no studies comparing techniques (4),(5)[C]:
  - Primary repair or reconstruction of the SPR and/or tendons
  - Deepening of the retromalleolar groove may be performed if required.
  - Resection of low-lying PB muscle belly or peroneus quartus (accessory muscle) may be performed if present.
  - Procedure may be open or tendoscopic.

ONGOING CARE

PROGNOSIS

- Good overall with both conservative and surgical
- Postoperative return to sport 87–98%
- Recurrence rate 50–75% after conservative treatment (1)
- Recurrence is rare after surgical intervention (4),(6).
- Return to sport rate 47–100% with mean time to return 51 months (6)[A].

REFERENCES

1. Bahad SR, Kane JM. Peroneal tendon pathology. *Orthop Clin North Am.* 2020;51(1):121–130.
2. Park CH, Gwak HC, Kim JH, et al. Peroneal tendon subluxation and dislocation in calcaneus fractures. *J Foot Ankle Surg.* 2021;60(2):233–236.
3. Lugo-Pico JG, Kaiser JT, Sanchez RA, et al. Peroneal tendinosis and subluxation. *Clin Sports Med.* 2020;39(4):845–858.
4. Danna NR, Brodsky JW. Diagnosis and operative treatment of peroneal tendon tears. *Foot Ankle Orthop.* 2020;5(2):2473011420910407.
5. van Dijk PAD, Kerkhoffs GMMJ, Chiodo C, et al. Chronic disorders of the peroneal tendons: current concepts review of the literature. *J Am Acad Orthop Surg.* 2019;27(16):590–598.
6. Di Santo P, Basciani S, Papalia GF, et al. Return to sport after surgical treatment for dislocation of the peroneal tendon: a systematic review of the current literature. *Appl Sci.* 2023;13:7685.

ADDITIONAL READING

- Dallaudière B, Pesquer L, Meyer P, et al. Intratendinous injection of platelet-rich plasma under US guidance to treat tendinopathy: a long-term pilot study. *J Vasc Interv Radiol.* 2014;25(5):717–723.
- Golshani A, Zhu L, Cai C, et al. Incidence and association of CT findings of ankle tendon injuries in patients presenting with ankle and hindfoot fractures. *AJR Am J Roentgenol.* 2017;208(2):373–379.
- Pesquer L, Guillo S, Poussange N, et al. Dynamic ultrasound of peroneal tendon instability. *Br J Radiol.* 2016;89(1063):20150958.

CLINICAL PEARLS

- Peroneal subluxation can either be from SPR disruption leading to tendon dislocation over the lateral malleolus (anterior dislocation) or the two tendons subluxing over each other within the sheath (intrasheath dislocation).
- Lateral ankle pain due to acute peroneal dislocation is frequently misdiagnosed as a lateral ankle sprain.
- Conservative treatment is generally attempted initially, but recurrence rate is high, and surgical intervention is commonly required.

PES ANSERINE BURSITIS

Alecia Gende, DO, CAQSM, FACEP, FAAEM • Britt Marcussen, MD, FAAFP, CAQSM

BASICS

DESCRIPTION

- Acute or chronic inflammatory condition that affects the medial aspect of the knee, specifically area of pes anserine bursa and pes anserine tendons
- The pes anserine bursa, located on anteromedial proximal tibia, buffers insertion of pes anserine tendon, a conjoining tendon of sartorius, gracilis, and semitendinosus muscles.
- Sartorius, gracilis, and semitendinosus are responsible for knee flexion and internal rotation of tibia and protect the knee against valgus and rotary stress.
- Initially thought of as a bursitis but may be better understood as a tendinopathy because pes anserine tendon can be pain generator.
- The pes anserine bursa, which is deep to the tendon, typically does not communicate with the knee joint.

EPIDEMIOLOGY

- Exact incidence and prevalence are unknown.
- Pes anserine bursitis is rare with a reported prevalence of < 2.5% in patients with medial knee pain (1).
- In patients with knee pain or swelling and history of osteoarthritis (OA), the prevalence of pes anserine bursitis is slightly increased (2).

ETIOLOGY AND PATHOPHYSIOLOGY

Exact etiology is unclear, but tendinopathy, friction on the bursa from repetitive stressors, valgus forces, or direct trauma to bursa maybe be causative.

RISK FACTORS

- Female
- Obesity
- Knee OA
- Knee malalignment
- Type 2 diabetes mellitus
- Long-distance runners

COMMONLY ASSOCIATED CONDITIONS

- Medial collateral ligament (MCL) pathology
- OA
- Obesity
- Pes planus
- Valgus knee deformity

DIAGNOSIS

HISTORY

- Gradual onset of symptoms
- May present with vague medial knee pain
- Tenderness +/− acute swelling within localized area of the tendon and bursa along the medial tibia
- Exacerbated by rising from a seated position; ascending or descending a flight of stairs or lying in bed with one knee pressing on the other

PHYSICAL EXAM

- Assess knee alignment—check for valgus or varus deformity.
- Tenderness at the insertion of the pes anserine tendon at the proximal medial tibia, ~2 to 5 cm below the anteromedial joint line of the knee
- Pain occasionally is reproduced with resisted external rotation of the tibia and flexion of the knee or with McMurray test confusing picture of a meniscus pathology.
- Pain may also be reproduced when a valgus stress is applied. This may make it difficult to distinguish this problem from an MCL injury; however, MCL injuries are typically superior and posterior to this type of bursitis.
- Hamstring-popliteal angle can be measured to assess hamstring flexibility. Have the patient flex the hip to 90 degrees and then passively extend the leg. The angle is formed by a perpendicular line to the femoral shaft and the tibial shaft.
- Chronic cases are marked by local pain, swelling, and fullness at the site of the bursa.
- Rarely, crepitus of the bursa is palpated; more commonly the bursa is edematous.

DIFFERENTIAL DIAGNOSIS

- Stress fracture
- MCL injury
- OA
- Medial meniscus tear or cyst
- Tendinosis of sartorius, gracilis, or semitendinosus
- Medial plica and discoid medial meniscus
- Patellofemoral pain syndrome
- Regional tumors, including villonodular synovitis, osteochondromatosis, and synovial sarcoma.
- Prepatellar bursitis

DIAGNOSTIC TESTS & INTERPRETATION

Initial Tests (lab, imaging)

- Typically, a clinical diagnosis; plain films are done to evaluate bony pathology or OA.
- Musculoskeletal (MSK) ultrasound (US) when skilled MSK ultrasonography available; demonstrates enlarged bursa and possible loculated fluid collection within bursa
- Magnetic resonance imaging (MRI) is performed to evaluate other knee pathology (meniscus and MCL injuries) and may confirm diagnosis in refractory cases.

Diagnostic Procedures/Other

- Aspiration of the bursa is not indicated.
- In difficult cases, a local anesthetic block may be used to confirm the diagnosis. Relief of pain with the injection is diagnostic.

TREATMENT

The mainstay of treatment for patients with pes anserine bursitis is to reduce pain and inflammation through the following (3)[C]:

- Activity modification
- Hamstring stretching
- Closed kinetic chain quadriceps strengthening.
- Short-term anti-inflammatory medications
- Ice massage
- Use of a pillow between knees at night
- Address gait abnormalities.
- Older patients and those with chronic pain should be encouraged to maintain activity levels to prevent disuse atrophy.
- Weight loss

MEDICATION

First Line

Topical nonsteroidal anti-inflammatory drugs (NSAIDs) should be tried before oral NSAIDs if possible; short-term use of nonselective NSAIDs as first line and the selective cyclooxygenase-2 (COX-2) inhibitors if there are tolerance issues (3)[C]

Second Line

Corticosteroid injections are traditionally used as second-line treatment. Injection may be done by palpation or preferably US guided.

ALERT

Take caution to exclude medial tibial plateau stress fractures as etiology of pain prior to corticosteroid injections. Masking stress fracture pain with injection may lead to adverse outcome.

ADDITIONAL THERAPIES

Modalities such as US, Kinesio taping, and ice massage can be helpful in relieving pain in patients with pes anserine bursitis.

SURGERY/OTHER PROCEDURES

- Extracorporeal shock wave therapy is another alternative to injection.
- Surgery is a rare option in chronic cases and includes tendon débridement, bursectomy, and/or excision of bony exostoses.

ONGOING CARE

- In general, patients experience success with conservative treatments:
  - Hamstring strengthening
  - Quadriceps strengthening
  - Activity modification
  - Topical NSAIDs or short-term oral NSAIDs
  - Ice massage
- Most patients will experience alleviation of pain within 6 to 8 weeks but may persist for several months.

FOLLOW-UP RECOMMENDATIONS

Patients may return to their activities based on their level of pain and function.

PATIENT EDUCATION

- The following recommendations can be made to the patient:
  - Minimize the use of stairs and climbing.
  - Eliminate squatting.
  - Prevent direct pressure on the bursa by using a pillow between the legs at night.
  - Avoid crossing the legs.
- Patients and their coaches should be counseled on the gradual increase in activity based on symptoms.

PROGNOSIS

Pes anserine bursitis is usually a self-limiting condition, with few complications if the individual decides to participate through the pain. In general, pain resolves after 6 to 8 weeks of conservative treatment (3)[C].

REFERENCES

1. Rennie WJ, Saifuddin A. Pes anserine bursitis: incidence in symptomatic knees and clinical presentation. *Skeletal Radiol.* 2005;34(7):395–398.
2. Uysal F, Akbal A, Gökmen F, et al. Prevalence of pes anserine bursitis in symptomatic osteoarthritis patients: an ultrasonographic prospective study. *Clin Rheumatol.* 2015;34(3):529–533.
3. Helfenstein M Jr, Kuromoto J. Anserine syndrome. *Rev Bras Reumatol.* 2010;50(3):313–327.

ADDITIONAL READING

- Khosrawi S, Taheri P, Ketabi M. Investigating the effect of extracorporeal shock wave therapy on reducing chronic pain in patients with pes anserine bursitis: a randomized, clinical-controlled trial. *Adv Biomed Res.* 2017;6:70.
- Saggini R, Di Stefano A, Dodaj I, et al. Pes anserine bursitis in symptomatic osteoarthritis patients: a mesotherapy treatment study. *J Altern Complement Med.* 2015;21(8):480–484.
- Sapp GH, Herman DC. Pay attention to the pes anserine in knee osteoarthritis. *Curr Sports Med Rep.* 2018;17(2):41.
- Sarifakioglu B, Afsar SI, Yalbuzdag SA, et al. Comparison of the efficacy of physical therapy and corticosteroid injection in the treatment of pes anserine tendino-bursitis. *J Phys Ther Sci.* 2016;28(7):1993–1997.

CLINICAL PEARLS

- Pes anserine bursitis and/or tendinopathy may be a cause of medial-sided knee pain.
- Diagnosis can be made with local tenderness over the bursa, located 2 to 5 cm distal to the joint line; a negative valgus stress test; and negative radiographs.
- Treat any underlying gait abnormalities; use activity modification, ice, NSAIDs, and steroid injection to decrease pain and inflammation. Consider stress fractures prior to any injection.

PHALANGEAL INJURIES

Jeffrey C. Leggit, MD, CAQSM

BASICS

- Frequently dismissed as minor injuries and therefore may present as subacute or chronic injuries
- All finger injuries require radiographic evaluation.
- Attempt to reduce dislocations immediately if neurovascular compromise is suspected.

DESCRIPTION

- Typically, due to direct trauma (i.e., crushing injury to the distal phalanx with high likelihood of concomitant soft tissue injury such as nail bed trauma)
- Dislocations are inherently associated with ligament and tendon injuries.

EPIDEMIOLOGY

Prevalence

- Hand fractures represent 19–28% of all fractures.
- Account for 10–15% of all sports-related injuries
- Phalangeal fractures are the most common sports-related fractures in adolescents and adults.
- 50% of all hand fractures are distal phalanx fractures.
- 49% of all hand injuries are dislocations or subluxations and the most frequent dislocation in the hand is a dorsal dislocation of the proximal interphalangeal (PIP) joint.

ETIOLOGY AND PATHOPHYSIOLOGY

Usually low-energy mechanism: fall, twisting or crush injury, or direct trauma

RISK FACTORS

Middle finger and thumb are the most commonly affected digits because they tend to be more exposed than the other digits.

COMMONLY ASSOCIATED CONDITIONS

- Soft tissue injury
- Nail bed trauma
- Tendon injuries:
  - Mallet finger, also known as "baseball finger": injury of the terminal portion of the common extensor tendon
  - Jersey finger: injury of the flexor digitorum profundus from the insertion on the distal phalanx. 75% of jersey finger injuries affect the ring finger.
- Central slip injuries
- Collateral ligament injuries
- Flexor pulley ruptures
- Dislocations—high risk for concomitant ligamentous injuries/disruptions

DIAGNOSIS

HISTORY

- Hand dominance
- Occupation and/or athletic position
- Environment surrounding injury (risk of infection)
- Mechanism of injury and hand position at time of injury:
  - Forceful flexion of distal phalanx suggests a mallet injury.
  - Forceful hyperextension of an actively flexed digit, such as while grabbing a player jersey, suggests a jersey finger injury.
- Palpable or audible pop at the time of injury
- Associated symptoms of numbness or tingling suggest associated nerve injury.
- Swelling and ecchymosis suggest serious injury such as fracture, dislocation, or tendon rupture.

PHYSICAL EXAM

- Pain, swelling, focal tenderness, and ecchymosis are common findings.
- Subungual hematoma frequently encountered with distal phalanx fracture; presence of a subungual hematoma should prompt radiographic imaging.
- Gross deformity, such as a mallet deformity or evidence of open fracture
- Malrotation (flex distal interphalangeal [DIP] and PIP while keeping metacarpophalangeal [MCP] extended; all fingertips should point toward scaphoid tubercle; if they do not, malrotation is present)
- Scissoring (overlapping digits during midrange of active flexion/extension. Digits may realign in full flexion. Malformation is typically associated.)
- Interphalangeal joints allow flexion and extension with normal arc of motion from 0 to 120 degrees of extension. Thorough assessment of range of motion can help identify ruptured tendons.
- Volar plate provides block to hyperextension, and collateral ligaments provide lateral stability.
- Assess collateral ligament stability with stress testing in extension and 20 to 30 degrees of flexion:
  - Laxity >10 degrees in extension or >15 degrees in flexion is pathologic.
- Assess integrity of flexor and extensor tendons:
  - Inability to actively flex the distal phalanx at the DIP with the PIP joint in extension suggests a jersey finger injury.
  - Inability to actively extend the distal phalanx at the DIP, with passive extension at the DIP intact, suggests a mallet injury.
- Assess neurovascular status.

DIAGNOSTIC TESTS & INTERPRETATION

Initial Tests (lab, imaging)

- True posteroanterior (PA), lateral, and oblique radiographs of fingers (not just hands) before and after reduction
- Lateral radiographs are used to assess joint alignment. "Dorsal V sign" indicates subtle but significant subluxation of the joint (1).
- Oblique radiographs aid with diagnosis of phalangeal head fractures (2).
- Oblique or spiral fractures may be associated with shortening (3)[C].
- Ultrasound can assess tendon and ligamentous injuries both statically and dynamically.

Diagnostic Procedures/Other

Inspection of nail bed for suspected laceration or hematoma

TREATMENT

- Hand:
  - Nondisplaced extra-articular fractures:
    - Buddy tape nondisplaced fractures: Never leave 5th finger isolated and unprotected (remember to place absorptive padding between digits).
    - Drain subungual hematoma by trephination of the nail if >50% nail bed is involved and repair nail bed if lacerated as long as there is not a concomitant fracture (could create an open fracture).
    - Splint PIP joints in 45 to 60 degrees of flexion (2)[C]
    - Allow range of motion to prevent stiffness.
    - Oral analgesics
    - Pain decreases over 2 to 3 weeks.
  - Displaced intra-articular fractures of interphalangeal joint:
    - Closed reduction with longitudinal traction within 7 to 10 days following injury (4)[C]
    - Acceptable reduction is <2 mm of displacement or shortening, <15 degrees of angulation, and no rotational deformity (2)[C].
    - Refer to hand surgeon if >30% of volar intra-articular surface is involved (2)[C].
    - If unstable after closed reduction, then open reduction internal fixation is required (2)[C].

- Interphalangeal joint dislocations:
  - Digital or wing block anesthesia
  - Reduction of dorsal dislocations: Apply an extension force along with longitudinal traction followed by gentle downward pressure on distal phalanx while stabilizing the proximal phalanx.
  - Reduction of volar dislocations: Apply a flexion force along with longitudinal traction followed with gentle upward pressure on the distal phalanx while stabilizing the proximal phalanx.
  - Volar and rotatory dislocations may not be reducible as the middle phalanx can "buttonhole" through the extensor mechanism (4).
  - Buddy tape to next digit for 3 to 4 weeks (caution with 5th finger) (5)[C]
  - Immediate protected return to play is recommended for stable PIP joint dislocations.
  - Reduce and splint PIP fracture dislocation with dorsal subluxation in 30-degree flexion to block extension (6)[C].
  - Unstable reductions require surgical management.
- Extensor tendon injury: mallet finger:
  - Conservative management is preferred in almost all cases (6)[C].
  - Splint with the DIP joint in full extension for 6 to 8 weeks at all times for both bony and soft tissue mallet injuries. Daily splint changes to assess skin integrity. DIP should not be allowed to flex at any time. Splinting during sports participation should continue for an additional 6 to 8 weeks (6)[C].
  - Surgical management with reduction and fixation of the DIP is reserved for irreducible displaced injuries or injuries with significant joint incongruity, typically those involving >1/3 of the articular surface (2),(6)[C]. Surgery may be considered for early return to activity on a case-by-case basis.
- Flexor digitorum profundus injury: jersey finger:
  - Always require surgical repair.
  - Urgency of repair depends on degree of tendon retraction. Type I injuries, in which the tendon retracts to the level of the distal palmar crease, should be surgically repaired within 1 week. Tendon repair in type II or III injuries with lesser degree of tendon retraction can occur up to several weeks from the time of injury (5)[C].
  - Return to play typically between 2 and 3 months

• Foot:
- Nondisplaced fracture:
  - Hard-sole shoe for toe fractures and weight-bearing as tolerated with crutches
- Displaced fractures:
  - Short leg walking cast with toe platform

Pediatric Considerations

Seymour fractures—distal phalanx fracture through the physis with concomitant nail bed trauma that occurs in the skeletally immature. It is an open fracture despite an often-benign appearance. It is typically irreducible and requires open fracture reduction and nail bed repair. Skeletally immature athletes should not return to play until healing is certain due to risk to the growth plate.

SURGERY/OTHER PROCEDURES

- Unstable fractures
- Irreducible dislocations
- Condylar fractures of the proximal and middle phalanges
- Consider surgical referral for intra-articular fractures >30% surface area or fractures with >2-mm displacement.
- Flexor tendon injuries
- Open fractures other than nail bed or tufts
- Early surgical repair considered for those who must return to activity early

ONGOING CARE

- Buddy tape/splint simple fractures continuously for a minimum of 2 weeks; protected return to play with splinting during sporting activities for another 4 weeks
- For persistent mallet injuries with a deformity of >20 degrees, an additional 6 weeks of splinting may be needed.
- Chronic mallet injuries can be successfully managed with up to 3 months of splinting (6)[C].
- Consider occupational therapy consult for those who present late or have ongoing stiffness.
- Soft shoe or splint for comfort for toe phalangeal fracture

FOLLOW-UP RECOMMENDATIONS

Patient Monitoring

- Fractures that required reduction should be seen within 1 week, and repeat radiographs should be obtained to check for fracture stability.
- Subungual hematoma: 24 hours

PROGNOSIS

Most heal well within 4 weeks but may develop stiffness.

COMPLICATIONS

- Chronic pain
- Chronic deformity: Even with ideal management of a mallet injury, a 5- to 10-degree extensor lag may persist. Untreated mallet injuries can lead to swan-neck deformity
- Stiffness and loss of range of motion. The PIP joint is especially prone (4).

REFERENCES

1. Williams CS IV. Proximal interphalangeal joint fracture dislocations: stable and unstable. *Hand Clin*. 2012;28(3):409–416.
2. Wahl EP, Richard MJ. Management of metacarpal and phalangeal fractures in the athlete. *Clin Sports Med*. 2020;39(2):401–422.
3. Miller EA, Friedrich JB. Management of finger joint dislocation and fracture-dislocations in athletes. *Clin Sports Med*. 2020;39(2):423–442.
4. Rosenbaum YA, Aman HM. Acute hand injuries in athletes. *Phys Sportsmed*. 2017;45(2):151–158.
5. Yeh PC, Shin SS. Tendon ruptures: mallet, flexor digitorum profundus. *Hand Clin*. 2012;28(3):425–430.
6. Salazar Botero S, Hidalgo Diaz JJ, Benaïda A, et al. Review of acute traumatic closed mallet finger injuries in adults. *Arch Plast Surg*. 2016;43(2):134–144.

ADDITIONAL READING

- Cheah AE, Yao J. Hand fractures: indications, the tried and true and new innovations. *J Hand Surg Am*. 2016;41(6):712–722.
- Rettig AC. Athletic injuries of the wrist and hand. Part I: traumatic injuries of the wrist. *Am J Sports Med*. 2003;31(6):1038–1048.
- Soubeyrand M, Biau D, Jomaah N, et al. Penetrating volar injuries of the hand: diagnostic accuracy of US in depicting soft-tissue lesions. *Radiology*. 2008;249(1):228–235.
- Wang T, Qi H, Teng J, et al. The role of high frequency ultrasonography in diagnosis of acute closed mallet finger injury. *Sci Rep*. 2017;7(1):11049.

CLINICAL PEARLS

- Obtain radiographs in all finger injuries before and after reduction.
- Mallet injuries are the most common closed tendon injury in the athlete, particularly baseball and softball athletes.
- Jersey finger injuries must be diagnosed early because all jersey finger injuries require surgical repair.
- Seymour fractures may appear benign but are open fractures and need to be recognized as such.
- Have a high suspicion for concomitant soft tissue injury; all dislocations have associated ligament and tendon injuries.
- Early mobilization is critical to reduce stiffness and loss or range of motion.

P

PHOTODERMATITIS

Jayson Loeffert, DO • Daniel Schlegel, MD, MHA • Matthew L. Silvis, MD, FAMSSM

BASICS

- Photodermatitis is an abnormal skin reaction to light or ultraviolet (UV) rays.
- The reaction may be acute or chronic, allergy mediated, or irritative and often is associated with substances or conditions that create an increase in photosensitivity.

DESCRIPTION

- Light-induced eruptions seen in a pattern of photodistribution on the skin
- Exogenous:
  - Phototoxic reactions (nonallergic): result of acute toxic effect on skin by UV light alone (sunburn) or together with a photosensitizing substance; occurs in 100% of individuals if exposed to enough of the agent and light
  - Photoallergic eruptions (allergic, delayed hypersensitivity): a form of allergic dermatitis resulting from combined effects of a photosensitizing substance (drugs or chemical) plus UV light
- Endogenous:
  - Porphyria cutanea tarda: defect in uroporphyrinogen decarboxylase, inherited, and acquired types
  - Erythropoietic protoporphyria: autosomal dominant deficiency in ferrochelatase, diagnosed in childhood
- Idiopathic and immunologic:
  - Polymorphous light eruption: chronic, intermittent light-induced eruption with erythematous papules, urticaria, or vesicles owing to a certain threshold of UV light; presents in 20s and 30s; spring and summer most common
  - Chronic actinic dermatitis: lichenified papules or plaques on sun-exposed areas; pruritic; older adults
  - Solar urticaria: immunoglobulin E (IgE) formation with mast cell degranulation; urticaria minutes after sun exposure; disappears within hours
- Photoaggravated conditions:
  - Lupus erythematosus
  - Dermatomyositis
  - Atopic dermatitis
  - Seborrheic dermatitis
- UV radiation:
  - Both UVA and UVB are responsible for photodermatitis (light-induced eruptions); therefore, both UVA and UVB should be blocked during outdoor sport activities.
  - UVA range 320 to 400 nm: penetrates skin deepest; can penetrate window glass; 360-nm wavelength is peak for many photosensitizing drugs.
  - UVB range 290 to 320 nm: penetrates skin superficially; responsible for most acute skin erythema

EPIDEMIOLOGY

- Can affect patients from all backgrounds and races who are exposed to UV light
- Most frequently identified photoallergens by photopatch testing: medications, sunscreen agents, fragrances, and antiseptics

Incidence

Up to 29.7% of persons who use sensitizing agents will get a reaction.

Prevalence

Estimated 25% of Caucasians in the United States are Fitzpatrick skin type I or II and have an increased risk of sunburn with limited exposure.

ETIOLOGY AND PATHOPHYSIOLOGY

- Exogenous photosensitizers (over 300 drugs known):
  - Antiarrhythmics
  - Nonsteroidal anti-inflammatory drugs (NSAIDs)
  - Phenothiazines
  - Diuretics
  - Quinolones
  - Tetracyclines
  - Thiazides
  - Sulfonamides
  - Sulfonylureas
  - Oral contraceptives
  - Topicals: psoralens, coal tars, photoactive dyes (e.g., eosin, acridine orange)
- Phytophotosensitizing agents:
  - Citrus fruits (Rutaceae): lemon, lime, grapefruit; furocoumarins are more concentrated in the peel.
  - Fig (Moraceae)
  - Cayenne pepper, paprika, chili, tabasco (Solanaceae)
  - Nettle (Urticaceae)
- Photoallergens:
  - Antiseptics
  - Fragrances
  - Medications
  - Sunscreen filters

Genetics

- Skin types I and II will exceed sunburn threshold tolerance in 10 to 20 minutes of noontime summer sunlight.
- Other genetic conditions increase risk (e.g., xeroderma pigmentosa, porphyrias).

RISK FACTORS

Fitzpatrick skin types:

- Type I: never tan, always burn
- Type II: occasionally tan, usually burn
- Type III: usually tan, occasionally burn
- Type IV: easily tan, rarely burn
- Type V: brown skin
- Type VI: black skin

GENERAL PREVENTION

- Avoid sun from 10 AM to 2 PM when 2/3 of total daily UV radiation reaches the earth.
- Avoid being outdoors during high UV index days.
- Avoid indoor tanning beds.
- Use protective clothing: long sleeves, wide-brim hats, sunglasses. Consider UV protective clothing.
- Use tinted glass windows.
- Identify and avoid sun-sensitizing drugs and agents (see under "Etiology and Pathophysiology").
- Sunscreens:
  - No. 30 sun protection factor (SPF) or greater recommended
  - Apply 30 minutes before exposure and every 2 hours, especially after sweating and swimming.
  - 1 oz to cover whole body
  - Physical blocking agents: zinc oxide, titanium dioxide, iron oxide, kaolin
  - Sunscreen with ingredients that filter out both UVA and UVB rays recommended.
- UVB filters:
  - Para-aminobenzoic acid (PABA) derivatives
  - Cinnamates
  - Salicylates
  - Octocrylene
- UVA filters:
  - Benzophenones
  - Avobenzone (Parsol 1789)
  - Anthranilates
- Physical blocking agents:
  - Iron oxide
  - Kaolin
  - Titanium dioxide
  - Zinc oxide
  - UV protective factor (UPF) clothing

DIAGNOSIS

HISTORY

- History of previous sun or UV light exposure
- Exposure to, or ingestion of, the many sun-sensitizing agents
- Family history of similar disorders
- Type of sunscreen and how the sunscreen has been used prior to reaction

PHYSICAL EXAM

- Phototoxic:
  - Erythema
  - With increasing severity: vesicles and bullae
  - Classic example: sunburn
  - Nails may exhibit onycholysis.
  - Chronic: epidermal thickening, elastosis, telangiectasia, and pigmentary changes
  - Sharp lines of demarcation between involved and uninvolved skin (sunlight exposure)
  - Phototoxic eruption owing to topicals: area of application
  - Usually develops minutes to hours after sun exposure
  - Hyperpigmentation may follow resolution.
  - Pain
- Photoallergic:
  - Papules with erythema and occasionally vesicles
  - Area exposed to light with less distinct borders
  - Usually delayed: 24 hours or more after exposure
  - May spread to unexposed areas
  - Pruritus
- Polymorphous light eruption:
  - Erythematous papules
  - Occasionally urticaria or vesicles
  - Scattered over sun-exposed areas with normal skin in between
  - Can spread to nonexposed areas
  - Often flares in spring or early summer
  - Desensitization affect (less over the course of the summer)
  - Burning or pruritus may precede lesions.
- Chronic actinic dermatitis:
  - Lichenified papules on sun-exposed areas in older person
  - Usually pruritic
  - Biopsy and phototesting confirm diagnosis.
- Solar urticaria:
  - Urticaria within minutes of UV exposure
  - Unidentified photosensitizing agent
  - Wheals itch and burn and disappear within hours

- Porphyria cutanea tarda:
  - Skin fragility
  - Blisters, crusts, milia
  - Mottled skin pigmentation
  - Hypertrichosis on periorbital area
- Erythropoietic protoporphyria:
  - Presents by age 2 years
  - Child cries or screams in pain when exposed to sun.
  - Burning feeling, induration, and purpura
  - Waxy thickening of skin on knuckles

DIFFERENTIAL DIAGNOSIS

- Phototoxicity
- Photoallergic reaction
- Cellulitis
- Pityriasis rosea
- Viral exanthem
- Drug eruption
- Polymorphous light eruption
- Chronic actinic dermatitis
- Solar urticaria
- Porphyria
- Atopic dermatitis
- Seborrheic dermatitis
- Dermatomyositis
- Systemic lupus erythematosus
- Stevens-Johnson syndrome

DIAGNOSTIC TESTS & INTERPRETATION

Initial Tests (lab, imaging)

- Antinuclear antibody and other rheumatologic tests when systemic lupus erythematosus and dermatomyositis are suspected
- Check serum, urine, and stool porphyrin if porphyria is suspected.
- Drugs that may alter lab results: N/A
- Disorders that may alter lab results: N/A

Diagnostic Procedures/Other

- Photopatch test: Test a small patch of a potentially photosensitive substance on the skin to find out if this is the substance that caused the reaction. Examples of substances tested include medications, sunscreens or other lotions, fragrances, antiseptics, and plant products.
- Phototest: Test the skin for a photoreaction to UV light after normal diet and/or after ingestion of a possible photosensitizing agent such as an NSAID, a sulfa drug, a diuretic, or an oral contraceptive pill.
- Skin biopsy: used to determine the type of skin inflammation and the potential disease process or malignancy
- Pathologic findings:
  - Lymphohistiocytic dermal infiltrates and spongiosis seen in the more common condition of phototoxicity.

TREATMENT

GENERAL MEASURES

- Avoid sunlight/limit exposure.
- Protective clothing/sunscreens
- Ice packs/cold water compresses

MEDICATION

- Drugs of choice for phototoxic and photoallergic reactions (1),(2),(3):
  - NSAIDs, topical or oral (e.g., diclofenac gel or oral 75 mg BID, ibuprofen)
  - Oral and topical corticosteroids have not been shown to be effective in mild or severe injury.
  - Antihistamines for pruritus (e.g., hydroxyzine 25 to 50 mg QID)
  - Sunscreens for prevention: Use broad-spectrum sunscreen to block both UVA and UVB.
- Treatment for polymorphous light eruption:
  - Desensitization with UVB or UVA (psoralen UVA [PUVA]) phototherapy for 15 minutes 2 to 3 times per week during the spring
  - Antimalarial drugs for protections during the spring and summer
  - Topical or oral steroids once the outbreak has occurred, continue 3 to 7 days.
- Treatment for chronic actinic dermatitis:
  - Topical and oral corticosteroids
  - Topical tacrolimus
  - Low-dose PUVA
  - Mycophenolate mofetil
  - Cyclosporine
  - Azathioprine
- Treatment for solar urticaria:
  - Antihistamines
  - Low-dose PUVA
- Treatment for porphyria cutanea tarda:
  - Phlebotomy
  - Avoid hepatotoxins and iron.
  - Antimalarial drugs
- Treatment for erythropoietic protoporphyria:
  - β-Carotene
  - Narrowband UVB
  - PUVA
- Contraindications: Refer to manufacturer's profile for each drug.
- Precautions: PABA, benzophenones, and cinnamates may cause contact dermatitis. Also, if allergic to benzocaine, procaine, paraphenylenediamine, or sulfonamides, one may have allergy to PABA. Refer to manufacturer's profile for each drug.
- Significant possible interactions: Refer to manufacturer's profile for each drug.

ADDITIONAL THERAPIES

Long-term treatment:

- Sun and light radiation protection and avoidance
- Identification and avoidance of photo enhancing, sensitizing, and allergic substances

ONGOING CARE

FOLLOW-UP RECOMMENDATIONS

Avoid sunlight.

Patient Monitoring

Monitor as necessary for persistence or recurrence.

DIET

No special diet

PATIENT EDUCATION

- Avoidance of sunlight
- Avoidance of photosensitizing drugs
- Protective clothing, wide-brimmed hat
- Use sunglasses that wrap around and absorb UVA and UVB rays.
- Use lip balm sunscreens.
- Sunscreens:
  - SPF 30 or greater with both UVA and UVB protection
  - Apply 15 to 30 minutes before exposure.
  - Reapply generously every 1 to 2 hours and especially after swimming or sweating.
  - Stress application to be sure to cover neck and ears (one study showed that 60% of people miss these areas).
  - Children:
    - Avoid midday sun.
    - For those <6 months of age, use titanium dioxide, which is less likely to irritate the skin.
- Fingernail protection can prevent subungual damage.
- Photocontact allergy to sunscreen has been reported.

PROGNOSIS

Good with avoidance/protection measures

COMPLICATIONS

Geriatric Considerations

More likely to experience adverse reactions to causative drugs.

REFERENCES

1. Bowers JM, Hamilton JG, Lobel M, et al. Sun exposure, tanning behaviors, and sunburn: examining activities associated with harmful ultraviolet radiation exposure in college students. *J Prim Prev*. 2021;42(5):425–440.
2. Faurschou A, Wulf HC. Topical corticosteroids in the treatment of acute sunburn: a randomized, double-blind clinical trial. *Arch Dermatol*. 2008;144(5):620–624.
3. Fernandez-Ruiz J, Montero-Vilchez T, Buendia-Eisman A, et al. Knowledge, behavior, and attitudes related to sun exposure in sportspeople: a systematic review. *Int J Environ Res Public Health*. 2022;19(16):10175.

ADDITIONAL READING

- Drucker AM, Rosen CF. Drug-induced photosensitivity: culprit drugs, management and prevention. *Drug Saf*. 2011;34(10):821–837.
- Fitzpatrick TB, Johnson RA, Polano MK, et al. *Color Atlas and Synopsis of Clinical Dermatology: Common and Serious Diseases*. 2nd ed. McGraw-Hill; 1992:210–213.
- Martina E, Rosa L, Postacchini V, et al. Photoprotection and photodermatitis: a case. *Contact Dermatitis*. 2017;76(1):54–55.
- McKee PH, Calonje E, Granter SR. *Pathology of the Skin: With Clinical Correlations*. Vol 1. 3rd ed. Elsevier Mosby; 2005:630–633.
- Scalf LA, Davis MDP, Rohlinger AL, et al. Photopatch testing of 182 patients: a 6-year experience at the Mayo Clinic. *Dermatitis*. 2009;20(1):44–52.
- Tyring SK, Lupi O, Hengge UR. *Tropical Dermatology*. Elsevier; 2006:441–443.
- Wolf ST, Kenney LE, Kenney WL. Ultraviolet radiation exposure, risk, and protection in military and outdoor athletes. *Curr Sports Med Rep*. 2020;19(4):137–141.

CLINICAL PEARLS

- Use sunscreens that block UVA and UVB rays.
- Consider phototoxic, photoallergic, or polymorphous light eruption as a diagnosis for any rash in sun-exposed areas.

PHYSEAL INJURIES IN CHILDREN: SALTER-HARRIS CLASSIFICATION

Rachel A. Coel, MD, PhD, FAAP, CAQSM

BASICS

DESCRIPTION

- In pediatric bone, the primary areas of growth include the physis and the epiphysis.
- Physeal injuries may occur in the skeletally immature population from acute trauma as well as from chronic overuse and repetitive loading, infections, tumors, ischemia, iatrogenic injury, or postoperative trauma.
- In 1963, Salter and Harris described a classification scheme for acute injuries to the physis (1)[C].
- Although most physeal fractures heal well, growth plate injuries can lead to complications including avascular necrosis, premature growth arrest, or angular deformities.

EPIDEMIOLOGY

- Occurs most commonly after 10 years of age but can be seen in any skeletally immature patient
- Typical age range: 10 to 16 years of age; median age: 13 years (peak incidence: boys 14 years, girls 11 years)
- Predominant gender: boys > girls (~2:1)
- Most common time frame: spring through summer months (more outdoor playtime and sports)
- Most common bone location: distal radial physis
- Most common reported type of physeal injury: Salter-Harris type II (75%) (Underdiagnosis of type I injuries is a likely explanation for preponderance of type II injuries.)

Prevalence

Current estimates suggest that from 15% to 30% of all pediatric fractures involve the physis (2)[C],(3)[C].

ETIOLOGY AND PATHOPHYSIOLOGY

- There are two types of epiphyses: traction epiphyses (apophyses), where major tendons originate or insert into bone, and pressure epiphyses, at the ends of long bones.
- Traction epiphyses shape and strengthen bone but do not add longitudinal growth; hence, their injury typically does not cause longitudinal growth arrest.
- Pressure epiphyses add longitudinal growth to long bones and are susceptible to compression, shear, and tensile forces.
- The physis, located between the epiphysis and the metaphysis of long bones, serves as the area of rapid longitudinal bone growth.
- Injury to the physis or pressure epiphyses may result in growth disturbance.
- The active physis consists of four zones of cells separated by cartilage matrix; the third zone (hypertrophic zone) is the area most susceptible to injury and cleavage.
- The epiphysis provides the nutrient blood supply to the physis; epiphyseal injury can cause disruption of normal growth and maturation owing to compromised vascular supply.
- Injured physeal cells may be repaired with a bridge, or bar, of bone or fibrous cells between the epiphysis and metaphysis, which can lead to growth disturbance.
- The physis is surrounded peripherally by the groove of Ranvier and the ring of LaCroix, which add growth, strength, and stability to the growth plate (2)[C],(3)[C].

RISK FACTORS

- Skeletal immaturity
- Falls, especially while running or playing
- Competitive organized sports, especially contact sports
- Recreational sports, such as skiing/snowboarding, skateboarding, trampolining, scooters, and bicycling
- Overuse training activities that cause repetitive loading and stress, such as gymnastics, cheerleading, throwing, and running
- Invasive pathology, including osteomyelitis, septic arthritis, burns, and tumors (4)[C]
- Iatrogenic injury, such as operative trauma, chemotherapy/irradiation
- Health conditions, such as metabolic disorders, malnutrition, Blount disease

GENERAL PREVENTION

- Monitor training demands, especially in young athletes during periods of heightened growth.
- Cross-training to avoid overuse and repetition
- Overtraining prevention: Alternate periods of heavy training with designated periods of rest.
- Protection from falls or impact: wrist braces, knee and elbow pads for skating, cycling, and contact sports

DIAGNOSIS

Salter-Harris classification of epiphyseal plate injuries (1)[C]:

- Type I: injury including complete separation of epiphysis from metaphysis without bone fracture
- Type II: Separation occurs partially along physis and exits through an associated metaphyseal bone fracture.
- Type III: intra-articular epiphyseal fracture extending out through partially separated physis
- Type IV: intra-articular epiphyseal fracture extending through the full thickness of physis and out through metaphyseal bone fracture
- Type V: severe crush injury at one area of physis
- Although cited less frequently, Peterson, Rang, and Ogden have subsequently proposed additional classifications of Salter-Harris fractures (2)[C],(3)[C].

HISTORY

- Fall onto an outstretched hand (FOOSH) is a common mechanism of distal radius growth plate injury (5)[C].
- Abduction, adduction, and twisting mechanisms are especially common in tibial physeal injuries and other lower extremity growth plate injuries (1)[C],(5)[C].
- Severe abduction or adduction mechanisms in the ankle or knee can cause type V crush injury to the physis (1)[C],(5)[C].
- Patient often reports "sprain" of a joint.
- Chronic stress injuries to the physis may present with a history of intense training with minimal rest or with overuse repetitive motion, such as baseball pitchers or gymnasts. Patients complain of focal pain at the area of the physis (5)[C],(6)[C].

PHYSICAL EXAM

- Swelling
- Angular or rotational deformity
- Ecchymosis
- Focal tenderness to palpation
- Limited range of motion due to pain or deformity
- Refusal to bear weight
- Salter-Harris type I injuries are often a clinical diagnosis owing to the radiolucent nature of physis on radiographs.

DIFFERENTIAL DIAGNOSIS

- Bone fractures
- Sprains: physeal injuries commonly mistaken for sprains
- Ligamentous rupture
- Dislocation
- Infection (abscess, osteomyelitis, septic arthritis)
- Tumor
- Renal failure
- Hypothyroidism
- Steroid treatment or chemotherapy
- Genetic disorder (achondroplasia)
- Blount disease—traction injury to proximal tibial physis

DIAGNOSTIC TESTS & INTERPRETATION

- Initial approach:
  - Plain x-ray trauma series: typically three to four views of injured joint (anteroposterior [AP], lateral, and oblique) (3)[C],(6)[C]
  - Type I fractures and chronic stress injuries may appear as physeal widening, epiphyseal displacement, or irregularity and sclerosis at the metaphysis; however, no radiographic abnormality is common (3)[C],(6)[C].
  - Comparative plain films of the opposite side may be helpful (3)[C],(6)[C].
  - Stress radiography may worsen physeal injury and should be used with caution (5)[C],(6)[C].
  - Type II to IV fractures are usually evident on plain x-rays and demonstrate associated bone fracture lines or bone fragmentation (Thurstan Holland sign) (1)[C],(2)[C],(4)[C].
  - Evaluate fractures for angulation and displacement.
- Follow-up:
  - Growth recovery lines, or Park-Harris lines, appear in the metaphysis on plain films typically 12 weeks after trauma (3)[C],(6)[C].
  - If they are parallel to the epiphysis and extend entirely across the metaphysis, future growth disturbance is unlikely.
  - If they are angled, curved, or highly irregular, subsequent growth disturbance is more likely.
- Special considerations:
  - If growth plate injury is suspected but plain radiographs are negative, advanced diagnostic measures may be employed, such as computed tomography (CT) or magnetic resonance imaging (MRI) (2)[C],(3)[C]. Another option includes ultrasound (US) (2)[C]. US can be helpful to differentiate ligamentous versus physeal injury.
  - Advanced imaging typically is advocated only if initial management of the injury seen on x-rays will be altered by determination of definitive radiographic alignment (5)[C].
  - MRI: can identify intact versus separated growth plate, physeal bridging, growth arrest, and avascular necrosis as well as cartilage, ligamentous/tendinous, and soft tissue imaging (3)[C],(4)[C],(6)[C]

- CT scan: useful in further defining known physeal injuries and aids in treatment planning, such as alignment and displacement of fractures at the articular surface, growth arrest, physeal bridging, and surgical planning (2)[C],(3)[C],(4)[C],(6)[C]
- Lower extremity limb length discrepancy may be evaluated with CT scanogram or full-length hips-to-ankles standing AP x-ray (4)[C].

TREATMENT

Emergency department (ED) treatment:

- Nondisplaced or minimally displaced type I and II fractures: splint immobilization, ice, elevation, and sports medicine or pediatric orthopedics referral (5)[C]
- Type III and IV fractures: Obtain orthopedic consultation in ED owing to intra-articular fracture (5)[C].
- If diagnosed in ED, type V fractures require orthopedic consultation (5)[C].

MEDICATION

Pain management should be addressed (over-the-counter [OTC] vs. prescription pain medications).

ADDITIONAL THERAPIES

- Diagnosed type I fractures: closed reduction and rigid immobilization (cast vs. brace) for 3 to 4 weeks
- Suspected type I fractures: immobilization for 1 to 2 weeks and then reexamination and repeat radiographs for periosteal reaction. If healing reaction is evident, immobilize for 1 to 2 more weeks. Alternatively, MRI, CT, or US imaging may be obtained to definitively identify physeal versus soft tissue injury (2)[C],(3)[C].
- Type II fractures: typically closed reduction and rigid immobilization with casting for 3 to 4 weeks; if unstable, refer to orthopedic surgery (2)[C],(3)[C].
- Type III and IV fractures: Refer to orthopedic surgery; often require open reduction and internal fixation to ensure stability and joint surface congruity (1)[C],(3)[C].
- Diagnosed type V fractures: non–weight-bearing cast for 3 to 4 weeks followed by another 2 to 3 weeks of weight-bearing casting; refer to orthopedic surgery (1)[C],(3)[C].
- Late-diagnosis type V fractures: frequently missed diagnosis acutely and diagnosed after growth disturbance has occurred; refer to orthopedic surgery (4)[C].
- Multiple attempts at reduction and reductions performed 7 days after the date of injury are not recommended owing to increased risk of physeal injury (1)[C],(3)[C],(4)[C].
- Consider bracing for sports activity for another 3 to 4 weeks after initial rigid immobilization is complete and while the patient is in rehabilitation.
- Consider physical therapy prior to return to play for ankle and knee physeal injuries.

SURGERY/OTHER PROCEDURES

- May be required for significantly displaced or unstable type I or type II fractures or, more commonly, for intra-articular type III and IV fractures
- Operative techniques may be necessary to produce anatomical reduction and fixation of the fracture. Care is taken to minimize further trauma to the physis and surrounding blood supply (2)[C],(3)[C].
- Intra-articular fractures require anatomic alignment to maintain joint surface congruity. Surgical techniques should be considered if anatomic alignment cannot be obtained or maintained with nonsurgical measures (2)[C],(3)[C],(4)[C].
- Surgery may also be indicated for growth complications after Salter-Harris fracture, including physeal bar or growth arrest leading to limb length discrepancy or angular deformity. CT scanning can be helpful for surgical planning. Effective surgical techniques may include epiphysiodesis (fusion of the growth plate), corrective osteotomy, physeal bone bar resection, lengthening, grafting, and use of spacers (3)[C],(4)[C].

ONGOING CARE

FOLLOW-UP RECOMMENDATIONS

Consider bracing for sports activity for another 3 to 4 weeks after initial rigid immobilization is complete.

ALERT

Patients, especially those with high-risk type II to V injuries, should be monitored for growth disturbance or deformity every 6 months for the 1st year after physeal injury (2)[C]. The majority of clinically significant growth disturbances occur within the first 2 years after injury (2)[C]. Some recommendations suggest patients should be reevaluated annually until skeletal maturity owing to risk of growth disturbance complications until adolescent growth spurt has been completed (4)[C].

PATIENT EDUCATION

Patients and their parents should be informed of the risk of complications with growth plate injury, including late-onset avascular necrosis, growth arrest, or deformity.

PROGNOSIS

- Several studies suggest that Salter-Harris classification is not a reliable predictor of outcome (2)[C],(4)[C].
- Fracture displacement, nonanatomic reduction, location of injury, high-energy mechanism of injury, associated soft tissue injury, older age, and iatrogenic injury may be the best predictors of physeal growth disturbance (2)[C],(4)[C].
- Physeal injury to the distal femur and proximal and distal tibia have increased risk of clinically significant growth disturbance (2)[C],(4)[C].
- Estimates range from 30% to 75% of all physeal injuries lead to some type of growth disturbance or angular deformity (1)[C],(2)[C],(4)[C],(6)[C].
- However, current estimates predict only 1–10% of these patients demonstrate significant functional deficits requiring surgical intervention (3)[C],(6)[C].

ALERT

Typically, Salter-Harris type I and II fractures have a good to excellent prognosis. Types III and IV have a poorer prognosis, and type V injury invariably results in growth disturbance with the worst prognosis (1)[C],(2)[C],(4)[C],(5)[C],(6)[C].

- Older children have a worse prognosis owing to shorter duration of remaining growth that may allow for remodeling (2)[C],(4)[C].
- Decreased remodeling potential exists in older children nearing skeletal maturity (4)[C].
- Other indicators of poor prognosis include compromised epiphyseal blood supply, repeated or forceful manipulation of physis during reduction, and open physeal fracture (1)[C],(2)[C],(4)[C].

COMPLICATIONS

- Entrapment of periosteum within fracture site
- Partial or complete growth arrest/limb length discrepancy
- Fibrous bone bar/physeal bridging
- Angular deformity
- Avascular necrosis
- Arthritis after intra-articular Salter-Harris III to IV fracture
- Regardless of age of onset of physeal injury, growth disturbances may not manifest until the adolescent growth spurt (5)[C].
- Risk of complications (3)[C],(4)[C],(5)[C]:
  - Greatest risk in early adolescence (pubescence) during periods of rapid growth
  - Increases with higher grade acute Salter-Harris injury (types III to V) (Type V has nearly 100% focal growth arrest rate.)
  - Increases with high-velocity, high-energy injury
  - Increases in lower extremity injury, especially distal femur (52% growth disturbance rate), proximal tibia, and distal tibia (43%) (2)[C],(4)[C]
  - Also may occur with chronic repetitive stress injury to physis

REFERENCES

1. Salter RB, Harris WR. Injuries involving the epiphyseal plate. *J Bone Joint Surg Am*. 1963;45(3):587–622.
2. Singh A, Mahajan P, Ruffin J, et al. Approach to suspected physeal fractures in the emergency department. *J Emerg Trauma Shock*. 2021;14(4):222–226.
3. Singh V, Garg V, Parikh SN. Management of physeal fracture: a review article. *Indian J Orthop*. 2021;55(3):525–538.
4. de Pablos J, Arenas-Miquelez A, Arbeloa-Gutierrez L. Update on premature physeal closure: diagnosis and treatment. *Curr Opin Pediatr*. 2021;33(1):79–89.
5. Perron AD, Miller MD, Brady WJ. Orthopedic pitfalls in the ED: pediatric growth plate injuries. *Am J Emerg Med*. 2002;20(1):50–54.
6. Nguyen JC, Markhardt BK, Merrow AC, et al. Imaging of pediatric growth plate disturbances. *Radiographics*. 2017;37(6):1791–1812.

SEE ALSO

Osgood-Schlatter Disease; Sever Disease/Calcaneal Apophysitis

CLINICAL PEARLS

- The Salter-Harris classification system of physeal injuries in children describes growth plate injuries by the level of involvement of the physis, the bone, and the joint.
- Growth plate injury can occur from both acute trauma and chronic stress, as well as from infection or tumor.
- Although most physeal injuries have a favorable prognosis, up to 10% may result in significant growth arrest, angular deformity, or avascular necrosis.
- There are numerous prognostic indicators, such as age at onset of injury, location of injury, severity of injury, accuracy of reduction, and iatrogenic injury.
- Orthopedic surgery consultation is recommended for unstable, displaced, or angulated fractures and for growth complications.

PIP JOINT DISLOCATIONS

Jarrod Yamanaka, MD, CAQSM ▪ Jennifer Oberstar, MD, CAQSM

BASICS

DESCRIPTION

- The proximal interphalangeal (PIP) joint is a hinge joint allowing flexion and extension with little lateral movement because collateral ligaments are tight through entire range of motion (ROM) (1).
- Dislocations may be dorsal (most common), ventral, or rotary subluxation where the twisting injury to the finger causes buttonholing of the head of the proximal phalanx through a tear in the central slip and lateral band (2).
- Synonym(s): finger dislocation

EPIDEMIOLOGY

- 10% of all dislocations (2)
- Most commonly injured joint in the hand (3)

RISK FACTORS

Playing sports, particularly contact and ball sports

GENERAL PREVENTION

Wear appropriate sport-specific padding and safety equipment when participating in sports or activities.

DIAGNOSIS

HISTORY

- Ascertain the direction of dislocation if already reduced.
- Determine mechanism: Dislocated finger may be due to forced hyperextension or hyperflexion of digit from traumatic athletic injury, entrapment of finger between objects, or a fall.

PHYSICAL EXAM

- Swelling and deformity at the PIP joint
- Deformity will indicate direction of dislocation.
- Careful palpation about the joint to locate the most tender area can help to differentiate between injuries:
  - Volar tenderness: volar plate
  - Lateral joint line tenderness: collateral ligaments
  - Dorsal tenderness: central slip injury
- Neurologic examination before and after reduction: Check sensation in distal finger (radial and ulnar sides).
- Check extensor tendon function: Have patient actively extend PIP and distal interphalangeal (DIP) joints.
- If able to extend DIP but not PIP joint, consider central slip rupture, which may lead to a boutonnière deformity. Extended DIP and flexed PIP with late loss of DIP flexion is the most disabling problem.
- Check flexion:
  - Have patient actively flex PIP joint with other fingers held in extension.
  - Check DIP flexion with PIP held in extension.
  - If unable to flex DIP joint, consider flexor digitorum profundus rupture, which requires surgical consultation.
- Check collateral ligaments:
  - Apply radial and ulnar stress with PIP joint in full extension and 30 degrees of flexion.
  - Look for increased laxity; compare with contralateral hand.
- Check volar plate:
  - Excessive hyperextension is consistent with volar plate injury.
  - If volar plate is unstable and not treated properly, it will lead to hyperextension of the PIP joint and flexion of DIP joint—a swan-neck deformity.

DIFFERENTIAL DIAGNOSIS

- Fracture-dislocation: Large dorsal fracture-dislocations can be missed, with the volar fracture involving >50 of joint surface with dorsal subluxation of the remaining portion of the middle phalanx (1)[C].
- Central extensor tendon rupture (boutonnière injury) of central slip allows lateral bands to slip below PIP joint and cause PIP flexion with DIP extension. (See "Central Slip Avulsion and Pseudoboutonnière Deformities.")

DIAGNOSTIC TESTS & INTERPRETATION

- X-rays: two views, including anteroposterior and lateral, before reduction if possible
- Oblique view if initial x-rays are negative but high suspicion of fracture
- May see small volar avulsion fracture
- With rotary subluxation, will see true lateral view of middle phalanx with oblique view of proximal phalanx, or vice versa

TREATMENT

- Determine stability: generally, fractures involving joint <30% stable, 30–50% borderline, >50% unstable
- If stable, can proceed nonoperatively
- Dorsal dislocation reduction:
  - If reduced before onset of swelling, reduction is easier.
  - Reduce with longitudinal traction and gentle pressure to the dorsal aspect of the midphalanx.

- Postreduction evaluation:
  - X-rays: two views if not already obtained
  - Rule out dorsal fracture-dislocation.
  - Check collateral ligament stability after reduction.
- Immobilization (2)[C]:
  - If dorsally dislocated and stable, simple, and reduced quickly, patient can continue sporting activity after "buddy taping" fingers if injury is to nondominant hand.
  - Stable: Splint for 1 to 2 weeks in 15 to 20 degrees of flexion with a figure-of-eight (also may use extension block splint) until pain free; often have volar plate injury; if so, consider splint in flexion for 4 to 5 weeks.
  - Splint should include only PIP joint; may be dorsal or volar
  - "Buddy tape" for an additional 3 to 4 weeks
  - Can treat with "buddy taping" alone for 3 to 6 weeks if no volar plate injury
- Volar dislocation reduction (2)[C]:
  - Partial flexion, distal translation
  - Closed treatment if minimally displaced avulsion fracture
  - Avulsion fracture reduces with full extension.
- Postreduction evaluation (2)[C]:
  - X-rays: two views
  - Check collateral ligament stability after reduction.
- Immobilization (2)[C]:
  - Splint PIP joint in full extension for 6 weeks (dorsal or volar splint) because central slip is often involved, DIP and metacarpophalangeal joints free.
  - Need to actively and passively flex DIP joint
  - Night splint for an additional 3 to 4 weeks
  - Splint until full active extension of PIP joint and active flexion of DIP joint.
- Rotary subluxation reduction:
  - Sometimes difficult to reduce closed
  - Closed reduction:
    - Digital block
    - Gentle traction with metacarpophalangeal and PIP joints at 90 degrees of flexion
    - Dorsiflex wrist (relaxes extensor mechanism)
    - Apply gentle rotatory and traction force.
- Postreduction evaluation:
  - X-rays: two views
  - Check collateral ligament stability after reduction.
- Immobilization: "buddy tape" after closed reduction

ADDITIONAL THERAPIES

Rehabilitation (2)[C]:

- Hand therapy within 1 to 3 days for both operatively and nonoperatively managed injuries (1)
- Dorsal dislocation: Work on ROM when out of splint.
- Volar dislocation: Work on ROM of DIP and metacarpophalangeal joints while in splint.
- Rotary subluxation: Start active and passive ROM when out of splint; add resisted ROM when pain free, active and passive ROM.
- Refer to hand therapy if persistent stiffness.

SURGERY/OTHER PROCEDURES

- Indication: inability to reduce the dislocated digit
- Dorsal fracture-dislocation carries significant risk of long-term disability if treated improperly.
- Volar dislocation with significant avulsion fracture or fracture does not reduce with extension and carries high risk of disability if treated improperly (2)[C].

REFERENCES

1. Miller EA, Friedrich JB. Management of finger joint dislocation and fracture-dislocations in athletes. *Clin Sports Med*. 2020;39(2):423–442.
2. Saitta BH, Wolf JM. Treating proximal interphalangeal joint dislocations. *Hand Clin*. 2018;34(2):139–148.
3. Joyce KM, Joyce CW, Conroy F, et al. Proximal interphalangeal joint dislocations and treatment: an evolutionary process. *Arch Plast Surg*. 2014;41(4):394–397.

ADDITIONAL READING

- Itadera E, Okamoto S, Miura M. Ratio of dislocation types of the proximal interphalangeal joint of the fingers: a new classification system for initial therapy. *J Orthop Sci*. 2019;24(6):1042–1046.
- Pang EQ, Yao J. Anatomy and biomechanics of the finger proximal interphalangeal joint. *Hand Clin*. 2018;34(2):121–126.
- Skelley NW, McCormick JJ, Smith MV. In-game management of common joint dislocations. *Sports Health*. 2014;6(3):246–255.

CLINICAL PEARLS

- PIP dislocations are common athletic injuries that can often be reduced on the sidelines.
- Return to play can be immediate with "buddy taping" or if able to play in splint.
- Volar slip fracture involving >20% of the joint's articular surface are unstable and may require a referral to an orthopedist for further treatment.
- Recurrent dorsal dislocations occasionally can result in pseudoboutonnière deformity. Treat with dynamic splinting.
- Early mobilization is key to preventing long-term stiffness.

PIRIFORMIS SYNDROME

Douglas Comeau, DO, FAAFP, FAMSSM ▪ *David J. Cormier, DO, DPT, CAQSM, FAAPMR* ▪
Angelene M. Elliott, DO

BASICS

DESCRIPTION

- Sciatic nerve irritation as it courses underneath or through the piriformis muscle causing buttock pain with or without radiation into the leg
- The piriformis muscle acts as an external rotator in hip extension and an abductor in hip flexion.
- Piriformis muscle spasm or hypertrophy can occur in certain motions, such as running downhill or repetitive motions.
- Direct irritation of the sciatic nerve may be caused by inflammatory agents released from an injured piriformis muscle.
- Anatomic anomalies causing compression such as tumor or gluteal artery aneurysm
- Synonym(s): piriformis syndrome; sciatica; sciatic neuritis; "hip pocket neuropathy"; "wallet neuritis"; "pelvic outlet syndrome"; "deep gluteal syndrome"; "pseudo sciatica"

EPIDEMIOLOGY

Incidence

- 6/100 cases of sciatica; 2.4 million cases per year (1)
- Mean age: 38 years old
- Predominant gender: female > male (6:1 in some trials)
- The incidence of piriformis syndrome is skewed secondary by the lack of evidence-based guidelines. The ratio is likely higher.

ETIOLOGY AND PATHOPHYSIOLOGY

- The piriformis muscle originates at the S2–S4 vertebrae, sacrotuberous ligament, and upper margin of the greater sciatic foramen.
- The piriformis muscle then passes through the greater sciatic notch, inserting on the greater trochanter.
- It is innervated by L5, S1, and S2.
- In hip extension, the piriformis serves as an external rotator.
- In hip flexion, it serves as a hip abductor.

RISK FACTORS

- In roughly 20% of the population, the sciatic nerve passes through the piriformis muscle, which may irritate the nerve and cause pain.
- Leg length discrepancy may predispose a patient to development of symptoms.
- A Morton foot can predispose a patient from the change in ambulation.

GENERAL PREVENTION

- Maintaining an appropriate lumbar core stabilization can decrease the recurrence of symptoms.
- A core stabilization program includes the anterior pelvis, posterior back, and buttocks.

COMMONLY ASSOCIATED CONDITIONS

- Sciatica
- Gluteal strain

DIAGNOSIS

HISTORY

- Trauma to the gluteal region is seen in <50% of patients.
- Chronic pain in the buttock and hip area
- Pain when getting out of bed
- Inability to sit for a prolonged time
- Sitting on hard surfaces exacerbates pain.
- Location of referred pain; can be L5 or S1 dermatome
- Complaint of pain with movements that cause external hip rotation
- Women may complain of dyspareunia.

PHYSICAL EXAM

- Cramping or aching pain in the buttock ± pain radiating into the hamstrings
- Sensation of "tight hamstrings"
- Point tenderness to deep palpation over any part of the piriformis muscle
- Pain increased with sitting
- Full range of motion and 5/5 strength in active and passive forward flexion and extension
- Negative stork test
- Negative straight leg raise and negative flexion, abduction, and external rotation
- Buttock pain ± radiation to hamstrings produced by combination of hip flexion, adduction, and internal rotation (FAIR); this maneuver stretches the piriformis muscle.
- Pace sign: weakness in resisted abduction and external rotation
- FAIR with palpation to pain over piriformis
- Beatty test: deep buttock pain produced by the side-lying patient holding a flexed knee several inches off the table
- Freiberg test: forceful internal rotation of the extended thigh
- Tenderness to palpation over the piriformis muscle
- Sciatic notch tenderness
- Usually normal neurologic examination
- Pelvic and/or digital rectal examination elicits pain ipsilaterally proximal to the ischial tuberosity.
- A proposed clinical scoring system using history and exam may be helpful with sensitivity of 96.4% and specificity of 100% (2).

DIFFERENTIAL DIAGNOSIS

- Lumbar facet arthropathy
- Lumbar spondylolysis and spondylolisthesis
- Lumbosacral radiculopathy
- Myofascial pain
- Achilles tendinitis
- Cord tumor
- Spinal stenosis
- Aneurysm of the inferior or superior gluteal artery
- Fibrotic band around the sciatic nerve
- Hematoma
- Gluteal abscess
- Hamstring origin tendinopathy
- Hip spine syndrome
- Gluteal tendinopathy
- Gluteal trigger points
- Pelvic tumor
- Endometriosis and other pelvic diseases
- Bursitis: obturator internus, trochanteric or ischial

DIAGNOSTIC TESTS & INTERPRETATION

Initial Tests (lab, imaging)

- No laboratory tests are recommended in the workup.
- Diagnostic imaging is rarely helpful in confirming the diagnosis.
- Clinical history and physical examination are keys to diagnosing piriformis syndrome.
- Further diagnostic tests may be needed to rule out other potential diagnoses.
- Magnetic resonance imaging (MRI) and computed tomography (CT) scanning can be used if history and physical examination are not conclusive; two case reports supporting the use of magnetic resonance neurography to confirm the diagnosis and verify the effect of treatment (3).
- Atrophy or fibrous tissue replacement of the piriformis muscle on MRI or CT scan supports the diagnosis.
- Musculoskeletal ultrasound (US) demonstrating hypertrophy of the muscle is a newer radiologic technique that may be used in difficult cases.

Diagnostic Procedures/Other

Electromyography (EMG) findings of peronei and/or tibial H reflex prolongation in the adducted, internally rotated, flexed hip strongly anecdotally support the diagnosis in some studies; however, EMG is typically normal and not a recommended diagnostic tool.

TREATMENT

Emergency department (ED) treatment:

- Low back pain is one of the top 10 causes of acute emergency visits.
- Typically, a lumbar spine film will be taken and is negative.
- The patient should be treated with nonsteroidal anti-inflammatory drugs (NSAIDs) and muscle relaxants and sent for primary care and/or sports medicine follow-up.

MEDICATION

First Line

- NSAIDs for 4 to 10 days
- Short course of analgesics and/or muscle relaxants may be beneficial (4)[C].
- Ice
- Acetaminophen

ADDITIONAL THERAPIES

- Relative rest for a short period but should begin piriformis stretch and physical therapy as soon as possible.
- Physical therapy incorporating stretching and strengthening of the piriformis muscle; also should incorporate correction of pelvic obliquities and leg length discrepancies (4)[A]
- Deep muscle massage with US
- Long-term treatment:
  - Continued lumbar stabilization program
  - Continued piriformis stretching
- Injections:
  - With no improvement after conservative therapy, consider local injection of anesthetic (1–2% lidocaine hydrochloride ± bupivacaine 4 to 6 mL) with or without steroids (mixed evidence for use of steroids) under fluoroscopic or US guidance into the tender area within the piriformis muscle.
  - Botulinum toxin has shown benefit in randomized, double-blind, controlled trials (5)[A] and nonrandomized controlled trials (6)[C]. The mechanism of action would be decreasing the piriformis spasm by injecting botulinum.
- Surgery as indicated earlier for recalcitrant cases of piriformis syndrome

SURGERY/OTHER PROCEDURES

- If conservative treatment fails, surgical release of the piriformis muscle around the sciatic nerve should be used as a last resort. In these cases, surgery has a favorable outcome in the majority of cases (7).
- Patients with documented EMG nerve impairment have the best outcome after surgical release.

COMPLEMENTARY & ALTERNATIVE MEDICINE

- Osteopathic manipulative treatment (OMT) may be used in conjunction with physical therapy.
- Techniques include muscle energy technique and myofascial release to help with piriformis strengthening and stretching.

ADMISSION, INPATIENT, AND NURSING CONSIDERATIONS

A patient typically is admitted only if preoperative for surgical correction.

ONGOING CARE

FOLLOW-UP RECOMMENDATIONS

Patient Monitoring

- Initially, a patient should follow up with primary care or sports medicine 6 to 8 weeks after starting physical therapy (8).
- On follow-up, close interaction should be maintained to ensure compliance with the home exercise program (lumbar stabilization).

PATIENT EDUCATION

- Patient education may include home exercise program handouts to ensure compliance.
- Showing the patient a diagram of the piriformis and its closeness to the sciatic nerve may help in patient recognition.

PROGNOSIS

- Prognosis is predicated on compliance with home exercise program and core stability.
- Although compliance with core stabilization cannot guarantee lifelong relief of symptoms, a stronger core can decrease the chance of recurrence.

COMPLICATIONS

- Complications typically occur without early diagnosis and treatment.
- Chronic low back pain may be debilitating and multifactorial.

REFERENCES

1. Siddiq MAB, Hossain MS, Uddin MM, et al. Piriformis syndrome: a case series of 31 Bangladeshi people with literature review. *Eur J Orthop Surg Traumatol*. 2017;27(2):193–203.
2. Michel F, Decavel P, Toussirot E, et al. Piriformis muscle syndrome: diagnostic criteria and treatment of a monocentric series of 250 patients. *Ann Phys Rehabil Med*. 2013;56(5):371–383.
3. Yang HE, Park JH, Kim S. Usefulness of magnetic resonance neurography for diagnosis of piriformis muscle syndrome and verification of the effect after botulinum toxin type A injection: two cases. *Medicine (Baltimore)*. 2015;94(38):e1504.
4. Rouzier P. Piriformis syndrome. In: *The Sports Medicine Patient Advisor*. McKesson; 2004:123–125.
5. Fishman LM, Wilkins AN, Rosner B. Electrophysiologically identified piriformis syndrome is successfully treated with incobotulinum toxin A and physical therapy. *Muscle Nerve*. 2017;56(2):258–263.
6. Kirschner JS, Foye PM, Cole JL. Piriformis syndrome, diagnosis and treatment. *Muscle Nerve*. 2009;40(1):10–18.
7. Han SK, Kim YS, Kim TH, et al. Surgical treatment of piriformis syndrome. *Clin Orthop Surg*. 2017;9(2):136–144.
8. Jankovic D, Peng P, van Zundert A. Brief review: piriformis syndrome: etiology, diagnosis, and management. *Can J Anaesth*. 2013;60(10):1003–1012.

CLINICAL PEARLS

- Prevention: a strong core stabilization program to increase strength and range of motion, including a hip mobility program
- Any activities that involve prolonged sitting (i.e., biking) should be avoided.
- Return to play: Weight-bearing as tolerated 5 to 10 days after surgery with gradual return to full activity; avoidance of prolonged sitting for 4 to 6 weeks after surgery is recommended.

PLANTAR FASCIITIS

Nicole Madrilejo, MD

BASICS

DESCRIPTION

- Degeneration and irritation of the plantar fascia origin at the medial calcaneal tuberosity on the anteromedial side of the heel and surrounding perifascial structures
- Synonym(s): enthesopathy of plantar fascia; plantar fasciosis

EPIDEMIOLOGY

- Plantar fasciitis accounts for 80% of patients with plantar heel pain.
- Occurs bilaterally in up to 33% of patients
- Estimated prevalence up to 10% of the general population
- Nearly 2 million patients receive treatment each year in the United States.
- In the running population, plantar fasciitis accounts for 10% of running injuries.
- Peak age of incidence is between 40 and 60 years but can occur in adults of all ages.

ETIOLOGY AND PATHOPHYSIOLOGY

- Likely multifactorial
- ~50% of patients with plantar fasciitis will have heel spurs. Up to 19% of patients without plantar fasciitis will also have heel spurs. Heel spurs can occur with plantar fasciitis, but they are not the cause.
- Histologic findings include myxoid degeneration, microtears in the fascia, collagen necrosis, and angiofibroblastic hyperplasia.

RISK FACTORS

- Female sex
- Excessive torsion and hyperpronation with poor supporting footwear
- Poor shock dissipation with cavus foot
- Hindfoot valgus with pronation deformity
- Limited ankle dorsiflexion
- Varus knee alignment in runners
- Obesity
- Diabetes
- Prolonged standing on hard surfaces
- Spiked athletic shoes

DIAGNOSIS

HISTORY

- Insidious and progressive pain in the inferior heel that can radiate across the medial side and less so to the lateral aspect
- Pain can involve both feet.
- Pain can be described as throbbing, searing, or piercing.
- Worst with first few steps out of bed in the morning
- Pain tends to lessen with gradually increased activity and worsens at the end of the day.
- Worsens after periods of prolonged standing or inactivity
- Pain exacerbated with walking barefoot, on toes, in dress shoes, on hard surfaces, or upstairs

PHYSICAL EXAM

- Tenderness localized to anteromedial aspect of the heel with palpation
- Tight Achilles heel cord
- Pes planus or pes cavus foot deformity
- Passive range of motion: hypermobility of subtalar joint, midtarsal joint, and first ray
- Pain with passive dorsiflexion of toes
- Gait evaluation: calcaneus everted at heel lift
- Palpable defect or loss of arch height may be seen if complete tear has occurred.

DIFFERENTIAL DIAGNOSIS

- Skeletal:
  - Calcaneal stress fracture
  - Bone contusion
  - Subtalar arthritis
  - Inflammatory arthropathies
  - Infections (osteomyelitis/subtalar pyarthrosis)
  - Neoplasm
- Soft tissue:
  - Intrinsic muscle strain (abductor hallucis, flexor digitorum brevis, quadratus plantae)
  - Plantar fibromatosis
  - Plantar fascia rupture
  - Achilles tendinitis
  - Posterior tibial tendonitis
  - Retrocalcaneal bursitis
  - Fat pad atrophy
- Neurologic:
  - Entrapment of branches of the posterior tibial nerve usually at or after passage through the posterior tarsal tunnel: medial plantar nerve, lateral plantar nerve, or medial calcaneal nerve
  - Radicular symptoms of L4–S1 (sciatic nerve)
  - Abductor digiti quinti nerve entrapment
  - Peripheral neuropathy

DIAGNOSTIC TESTS & INTERPRETATION

- Imaging is not routinely needed. Radiographic evaluation would be appropriate in patients who fail to improve with appropriate treatment in a reasonable amount of time or if patient presents with an atypical history or physical exam.
- X-rays may show calcifications in the soft tissues around the heel or osteophytes on the anterior calcaneus (i.e., heel spurs).

- Ultrasound (US) may show >4 mm, hypoechoic echotexture, and perifascial edema. Reduced plantar fascia elasticity during real-time sonoelastography could be suggestive of plantar fasciitis (1). Shear wave elastography (SWE) emerging as a novel approach to quantify fascial stiffness (2).
- Triple-phase bone scan can differentiate between plantar fasciitis and a calcaneal stress fracture. A bone scan or magnetic resonance imaging (MRI) should be ordered when heel pain has not improved after 4 to 6 months of nonsurgical treatment.

TREATMENT

- Initial treatment is conservative and consists of pain control, activity modifications, exercise therapy, shoe modifications, and weight loss.
- Avoidance of activities causing or exacerbating pain
- Avoid flat shoes and barefoot walking.
- Nonsteroidal anti-inflammatory drugs (NSAIDs) for analgesic effect
- Early morning stretching of heel cord as well as throughout the day
- Night splinting
- Ice massage and deep friction massage of the arch and insertion
- Shoe inserts: prefabricated insoles (i.e., soft heel pads/Silastic), custom orthotics, or medial heel wedges
- Arch taping during athletic activities
- Motion-control shoes with rigid heel counters
- Posterior-tension night splints
- Supination strap
- Physical therapy with plantar fascia: specific stretching and Achilles tendon stretching programs
- High-load eccentric strength training has potential to improve symptoms faster than stretching (3)[B].
- Platelet-rich plasma (PRP) injections appear to have superior outcomes compared to corticosteroid injections in the medium and long term, with fewer associated risks such as fat pad atrophy (4)[B].
- Dexamethasone (Decadron) or acetic acid iontophoresis
- Extracorporeal shock wave therapy as second-line therapy (5)[A]
- Walking cast
- Conservative therapy should be used for a minimum of 6 months and, preferably, for 12 months as >90% of patients respond positively to nonsurgical management.

SURGERY/OTHER PROCEDURES

- Surgery can be considered after failure of extensive conservative therapy, even up to 2 years: operative release of proximal fascia of deep abductor fascia
- Plantar fasciotomy can be either partial or complete and is a common surgical procedure for treating recalcitrant cases of plantar fasciitis.
- Postoperative recovery includes splint for 2 weeks, mild stretching and ambulation with crutches and walking boot, pool running for 3 weeks, and return to activity in 3 to 4 months.

COMPLEMENTARY & ALTERNATIVE MEDICINE

- Acupuncture
- Direct myofascial release

REFERENCES

1. Sconfienza LM, Silvestri E, Orlandi D, et al. Real-time sonoelastography of the plantar fascia: comparison between patients with plantar fasciitis and healthy control subjects. *Radiology*. 2013;267(1):195–200.
2. Gatz M, Betsch M, Quack V, et al. Shear wave elastography for treatment monitoring of plantar fasciitis. *J Sports Med Phys Fitness*. 2020;60(8):1137–1147.
3. Rathleff MS, Mølgaard CM, Fredberg U, et al. High-load strength training improves outcome in patients with plantar fasciitis: a randomized controlled trial with 12-month follow-up. *Scand J Med Sci Sports*. 2015;25(3):e292–e300.
4. Hohmann E, Tetsworth K, Glatt V. Platelet-rich plasma versus corticosteroids for the treatment of plantar fasciitis: a systematic review and meta-analysis. *Am J Sports Med*. 2021;49(5):1381–1393.
5. Charles R, Fang L, Zhu R, et al. The effectiveness of shockwave therapy on patellar tendinopathy, Achilles tendinopathy, and plantar fasciitis: a systematic review and meta-analysis. *Front Immunol*. 2023;14:1193835.

ADDITIONAL READING

- Clanton TO, Porter DA. Primary care of foot and ankle injuries in the athlete. *Clin Sports Med*. 1997;16(3):453–466.
- Koc TA Jr, Bise CG, Neville C, et al. Heel pain—plantar fasciitis: revision 2023. *J Orthop Sports Phys Ther*. 2023;53(12):CPG1–CPG39.
- Lemont H, Ammirati KM, Usen N. Plantar fasciitis: a degenerative process (fasciosis) without inflammation. *J Am Podiatr Med Assoc*. 2003;93(3):234–237.
- Neufeld SK, Cerrato R. Plantar fasciitis: evaluation and treatment. *J Am Acad Orthop Surg*. 2008;16(6):338–346.
- Tafur M, Bencardino JT, Roberts CC, et al. ACR appropriateness criteria chronic foot pain. *J Am Coll Radiol*. 2020;17(Suppl 11):S391–S402.
- Trojian T, Tucker AK. Plantar fasciitis. *Am Fam Physician*. 2019;99(12):744–750.
- Williams SK, Brage M. Heel pain—plantar fasciitis and Achilles enthesopathy. *Clin Sports Med*. 2004;23(1):123–144.

CLINICAL PEARLS

- Initial treatment is conservative, focusing on high-load eccentric strength training.
- There is moderate evidence to suggest that PRP injections are superior to corticosteroid injections in the management of plantar fasciitis, providing medium- and long-term relief of symptoms. In addition, the risks associated with corticosteroid injection likely outweighs the benefits of corticosteroid injection.
- Surgery should only be considered after exhaustive conservative treatment of at least 6 months to 1 year has failed.

PLANTAR FIBROMATOSIS

Brandan Mayer-Blackwell, MD

BASICS

DESCRIPTION

- Fibrotic nodule(s) on the plantar aspect of the foot
- Insidious onset of plantar pain, often worse with walking
- Also known as Ledderhose disease after the German physician Georg Ledderhose who characterized the disease in 1987

EPIDEMIOLOGY

- 2:1 more common in males than females
- Bilateral in 25% of patients
- Effects <200,000 people in the United States (1)
- Greatest prevalence in middle age
- Juvenile onset often portends more aggressive disease with local infiltration into tissues beyond the plantar fascia.

ETIOLOGY AND PATHOPHYSIOLOGY

- The defining characteristic of plantar fibromatosis is fibroblast hyperactivity and over proliferation.
- There is no definitive cause but increased cytokine signaling has been documented (including platelet derived growth factor, transforming growth factor β, interleukin-1α, and interleukin-1β).
- Plantar fibromatosis follows three stages.
  - Stage 1, proliferative phase: increased fibroblast activity; histology shows plump immature spindle cells in a background of fascial fibrosus
  - Stage 2, involutional phase: nodule formation; histology shows increased type III collagen and maturation of fibroblasts
  - Stage 3, residual phase: scar and contracture formation; histology shows reduced collagen and myofibroblasts

Genetics

Genetic predisposition, including one indel on chromosome 5 and one SNP on chromosome 16 (2)

RISK FACTORS

- Family history
- Alcohol or nicotine use
- Diabetes
- Epilepsy

GENERAL PREVENTION

No prevention strategy has been shown to be effective.

COMMONLY ASSOCIATED CONDITIONS

- Dupuytren contracture (15% comorbidity)
- Peyronie disease

DIAGNOSIS

HISTORY

- Patients present for plantar foot pain or painful nodules on the plantar aspect of their feet.
- Pain is usually worse with standing or walking.
- Restrictive shoes or walking barefoot may exacerbate symptoms.
- Onset of symptoms is usually slow and insidious.

PHYSICAL EXAM

- Exam will show subcutaneous nodules (with or without tenderness to palpation) on the plantar aspect of the foot.
- Nodules are most often located in the medial or central slip of the plantar aponeurosis.
- Nodules will almost never be present in the proximal third of the fascia, and if they are, it should raise concern for a plantar fascia tear rather than fibromatosis.
- Nodules are generally 0.5 to 3 cm in size.

DIFFERENTIAL DIAGNOSIS

- Plantar fasciitis or plantar fascia rupture
- Subcutaneous cyst or fat necrosis
- Desmoid tumor
- Foreign body
- Malignant tumor: epithelioid sarcoma, rhabdomyosarcoma, or liposarcoma

DIAGNOSTIC TESTS & INTERPRETATION

Initial Tests (lab, imaging)

- Physical exam is often adequate for diagnosis.
- X-ray and CT scans are low yield other than ruling out other disease processes.
- Ultrasound is first line in diagnosis given its speed and cost.
- Magnetic resonance imaging (MRI) can be used for additional diagnostic accuracy and surgical planning.
- On T1-weighted MRI, the nodules will have low signal intensity corresponding to dense collagen fibers.
- On T2-weighted MRI, the nodules will have low signal intensity during the residual phase and intermediate signal intensity during the active phase.

Follow-Up Tests & Special Considerations

Although infrequently used, a biopsy with histologic and immunohistochemistry analysis can provide the most definitive diagnosis.

- Ultrasound interpretation
  - Ultrasound will show single or multiple fusiform nodules in the plantar aponeurosis.
  - The nodules do not invade adjacent tissues (except rarely in the more aggressive type of plantar fibromatosis seen in juveniles).
  - The nodules can be isoechoic or hypoechoic but frequently have mixed echogenicity. They will be visible against the background of the striated, homogenous, hyperechoic plantar aponeurosis.
  - Cohen et al. found 65% of nodules have posterior acoustic enhancement and 80% have little to no vascularity on doppler (3)[C].
  - Larger lesions can demonstrate the comb sign, where the hypoechoic nodule is interrupted by hyperechoic alternating fibrous collagen bands, creating the appearance of a comb.

TREATMENT

GENERAL MEASURES

- Treatment should start with conservative measures, even though they are not disease modifying, because nonconservative treatments for plantar fibromatosis confer significant risks.
- All patients should wear supportive, cushioned footwear to decrease tension on the plantar fascia.
- Off-loading pads surrounding the plantar nodules can reduce pain.

MEDICATION

First Line

- Ultrasound-guided intralesional steroid injections can decrease cytokine production leading to reduced collagen and fibroblasts.
- Steroid injections for Dupuytren contracture have shown 97% success in reducing the size of lesions with 50% recurrence rates at 3 years (4)[B]. Although less well studied, similar results have been seen with plantar fibromatosis. Injection protocols often require up to 3 to 5 rounds of injections with 15- to 30-mg triamcinolone, given at 4 to 6 weeks intervals.
- Frequent steroid injections increase the risk for plantar fascia rupture.
- Extracorporeal shock wave (ECSW) therapy is a low-risk treatment option. Shockwave therapy has been studied and used for Peyronie disease and Dupuytren contracture. A small cohort study examining ECSW in plantar fibromatosis showed improved pain and function as well as reduced nodule thickness (5)[C].

Second Line

- Verapamil is thought to decrease collagen production and increase collagenase activity.
- Topical 15% verapamil can be used alone or in conjunction with steroid injections.
- Topical verapamil is applied twice daily for 9 months.
- Intralesional verapamil injections have also been used for Peyronie disease, but there are no studies demonstrating their efficacy for plantar fibromatosis.
- Radiation treatment has been shown to be an effective modality for decreasing nodule size and symptoms. Five sessions of local radiation therapy resulted in 78% patient satisfaction (6)[B].
- Significant side effects of radiation include local skin reactions as well as a theoretical risk of soft tissue sarcoma and skin cancer.

EXPERIMENTAL THERAPIES

- Collagenase treatment with clostridium histolyticum is used for Peyronie disease and Dupuytren contracture, but the only study investigating it for plantar fibromatosis showed no benefit. This may be due to the nodular rather than cord architecture of the plantar lesions. However, individual case studies have reported success.
- Tamoxifen is not recommended at this time. Tamoxifen has been shown to have in vitro activity at reducing fibroblast growth but has never been shown effective in vivo studies.

SURGERY/OTHER PROCEDURES

- Surgical removal can be used for refractory cases; local excision is typically avoided due to a high recurrence rate.
- Local excision has a recurrence rate of 60–100%.
- Wide local excision (removing a 2- to 3-cm margin around the nodule) has a recurrence rate up to 60%.
- Complete plantar fasciectomy is the most aggressive surgical option and has a recurrence rate up to 25% (1)[C].

ONGOING CARE

FOLLOW-UP RECOMMENDATIONS

Patient Monitoring

Patients frequently have recurrence of nodules and symptoms after treatment, so additional follow-up is often required to maintain symptom control.

DIET

Weight loss can help off-load the plantar fascia, so a healthy diet is encouraged for symptom relief.

REFERENCES

1. Meyers AL, Marquart MJ. *Plantar Fibromatosis*. StatPearls Publishing; 2023. Updated February 28, 2024. Accessed August 20, 2025. https://www.ncbi.nlm.nih.gov/books/NBK557674
2. Kim SK, Ioannidis JPA, Ahmed MA, et al. Two genetic variants associated with plantar fascial disorders. *Int J Sports Med*. 2018;39(4):314–321.
3. Cohen BE, Murthy NS, Mckenzie GA. Ultrasonography of plantar fibromatosis: updated case series, review of the literature, and a novel descriptive appearance termed the "Comb Sign." *J Ultrasound Med*. 2018;37(11):2725–2731.
4. Ketchum LD, Donahue TK. The injection of nodules of Dupuytren's disease with triamcinolone acetonide. *J Hand Surg Am*. 2000;25(6):1157–1162.
5. Hwang JT, Yoon KJ, Park CH, et al. Follow-up of clinical and sonographic features after extracorporeal shock wave therapy in painful plantar fibromatosis. *PLoS One*. 2020;15(8):e0237447.
6. De Haan A, van Nes JGH, Werker PMN, et al. Radiotherapy for patients with Ledderhose disease: long-term effects, side effects and patient-rated outcome. *Radiother Oncol*. 2022;168:83–88.

CLINICAL PEARLS

- Physical exam will typically show 1- to 2-cm subcutaneous nodules on the plantar aspect of the foot, most often in the distal aspect of the medial or central plantar fascia.
- Ultrasound and MRI are the most effective diagnostic modalities.
- Conservative measures such as cushioned footwear and off-loading pads are first-line treatment. Ultrasound-guided intralesional steroid injections and ECSW therapy are reasonable next treatment options if conservative care fails.

PNEUMOTHORAX AND HEMOTHORAX

Nicole L. Leonard, MD • Daniel C. Herman, MD, PhD, FAAPMR, FACSM, FISBS, CAQSM

BASICS

DESCRIPTION

- Air (pneumothorax), blood (hemothorax), or both (hemopneumothorax) in the pleural space between the lung and chest wall
- Classification of pneumothorax (1)
  - Spontaneous: no obvious precipitating factor present; further divided into:
    - Primary spontaneous pneumothorax (PSP): no apparent underlying pulmonary disease
    - Secondary spontaneous pneumothorax (SSP): clinically apparent underlying disease
  - Nonspontaneous or traumatic: caused by trauma; can be further divided into:
    - Iatrogenic: secondary to a medical procedure or intervention
    - Noniatrogenic: secondary to blunt or penetrating injuries
  - Tension pneumothorax: Progressive accumulation of air in the pleural space causing compression of mediastinal structures (i.e., heart) and restricting venous return in the contralateral lung which can lead to cardiorespiratory collapse.
- Synonym(s): collapsed lung

EPIDEMIOLOGY

- PSP is one of the most common thoracic diseases affecting adolescents and young adults.
- Male predominance
- Older patients more likely to have SSP due to an underlying disorder
- Peak incidence at ages 16 to 25 years for males, uniform for females (2)
- High recurrence rate, 25–54% (2)

Incidence

- Male: 12.3 per 100,000
- Female: 2.2 per 100,000 (2)
- Exercise and sport accounts for <10% of reported cases of pneumothoraces (3)
- 80% of penetrating chest injuries present with pneumothorax (4).

ETIOLOGY AND PATHOPHYSIOLOGY

- PSP:
  - Theorized to be caused by the rupture of subpleural blebs
  - Rupture caused by increased intrathoracic pressure or shear force (coughing, straining, vomiting).
- SSP:
  - Associated with primary lung disease and/or systemic conditions with lung involvement
- Iatrogenic pneumothorax:
  - Tear in visceral pleura from a procedure resulting in air leak into the pleural space (e.g., transthoracic needle aspiration/biopsy, subacromial injections, tracheostomy, central venous catheter insertion, barotrauma)
- Noniatrogenic pneumothorax:
  - Penetrating or blunt trauma, rib fracture, diving
- Hemothorax: caused by virtually any disruption of the tissues of the chest wall and pleura with subsequent bleeding into pleural space
- Precipitating factors may include atmospheric pressure changes and exposure to loud music.

RISK FACTORS

- Tall, thin, young, males
- Smoking (i.e., tobacco, cannabis)
- Substance use such as heroin, ecstasy, speed, and cocaine
- Congenital apical lung blebs
- Underlying lung disease (e.g., chronic obstructive pulmonary disease [COPD], cystic fibrosis, tuberculosis [TB])
- Connective tissue disorder (Marfan)
- Homocystinuria
- Trauma, especially rib fractures (most commonly first 4 and last 2, multiple, or flail segments) or scapular fractures; can be acute with the fracture or can happen when returning to play prior to fracture healing (5)
- Preparticipation recommendations:
  - SCUBA contraindicated if history of spontaneous pneumothorax.

GENERAL PREVENTION

- Avoid smoking and substance use.
- If history of pneumothorax, avoid SCUBA, contact sports, and trauma.

COMMONLY ASSOCIATED CONDITIONS

- COPD
- Cystic fibrosis
- Asthma
- Marfan syndrome
- Lung malignancy
- Lung infections (i.e., pneumonia, TB)

DIAGNOSIS

- Clinical diagnosis with radiologic confirmation
- Mechanism of injury is vital and often provides an early foundation for diagnosis (4).
- Initial evaluation should include vital sign assessment and auscultation in a quiet setting.

HISTORY

- Trauma to thoracic wall
- Persistent pain at injury site
- Shortness of breath
- Localized chest pain, especially pleuritic, frequently present: may radiate to neck, shoulder, back, or abdomen
- Dyspnea and/or tachypnea frequently present
- Up to 25% of patients may be asymptomatic, especially if small.

PHYSICAL EXAM

- Hypoxia, tachypnea, and possibly tachycardia
- Decreased or absent breath sounds on affected side
- Decreased tactile fremitus on side of pneumothorax
- Asymmetric lung expansion
- Hyperresonance to percussion in the case of pneumothorax; dullness to percussion in the case of hemothorax
- In tension pneumothorax, tracheal deviation away from site of pneumothorax, neck vein distension, and laterally displaced cardiac impulse all may be present.
- Crepitation or subcutaneous (SC) emphysema may be present, especially in traumatic pneumothorax.
- Possible pallor or cyanosis (usually with tension pneumothorax)

DIFFERENTIAL DIAGNOSIS

- Acute aortic dissection
- Chest wall/rib contusion
- Lung contusions
- Rib fracture
- Myocardial infarction
- Pulmonary embolism
- Esophageal rupture
- Aspiration, bacterial, or viral pneumonia

DIAGNOSTIC TESTS & INTERPRETATION

Initial Tests (lab, imaging)

- Chest x-ray (CXR): White visceral pleural line defines the interface of the lung and pleural air:
  - Inspiratory and expiratory films have equal sensitivity in detecting pneumothoraces, so a standard inspiratory chest radiograph is sufficient in most cases (4).
  - Studies have shown CXR to have poor sensitivity due to easy interference and mimics of visceral pleura.
  - Portable CXR should be obtained early in conjunction with primary and secondary trauma surveys as it provides a quick snapshot.
- Ultrasound: absence of lung sliding, comet-tail artifact (B-lines), and presence of lung point for pneumothorax; hemothorax shows anechoic area in pleural space (4):
  - Superior to CXR with sensitivity of 81%, specificity of 98%, LR + of 67.9, and LR − of 0.18.
  - Dependent on user skill level and availability
- Computed tomography (CT) scan remains gold standard given visual clarity but requires more radiation, time, and effort.

Diagnostic Procedures/Other

- Electrocardiogram (ECG) often demonstrates right-axis deviation, decreased QRS amplitude, precordial T-wave inversion, and tachycardia.
- If hemodynamically unstable and findings are consistent with a pneumothorax (most likely tension pneumothorax), may consider emergency needle aspiration, which is both diagnostic and therapeutic
- Diagnosis is confirmed by rapid gush of air coming through the needle.

TREATMENT

GENERAL MEASURES

- Acute treatment:
  - Determine if patient is hemodynamically stable because primary job is to stabilize.
  - Airway, breathing, and circulation (ABCs) of basic life support, especially airway management
  - Semi-Fowler position; supine, head of bed at 30 to 45 degrees
  - Supplemental oxygen
  - If unstable and/or findings consistent with a tension pneumothorax, emergency needle decompression followed by insertion of thoracostomy tube should be performed.
  - Needle decompression is performed by inserting a large-caliber needle (usually 14 to 16 gauge), preferably with a catheter over needle, into the 2nd intercostal space at the midclavicular line just above the 3rd rib.
  - If catheter over needle, then remove needle and leave plastic sheath; may attach a syringe
  - Thoracostomy tube typically placed above rib in 5th intercostal space anterior to midaxillary line.
  - Flail chest may accompany rib fractures; if present, stabilize flail segment with manual pressure or a bulky dressing to the segment.

- Foreign body should not be removed until transferred to emergency room.
- If open pneumothorax, cover wound with three-sided occlusive dressing to create flap valve, prohibiting air entrance but allowing air to escape during exhalation.

- Emergency personnel:
  - Supplemental oxygen
  - Intravenous (IV) line placement
  - Transport to emergency facility
- Further treatment depends on patient characteristics and clinical circumstances:
  - When pneumothorax is small, tension-free pneumothorax (no mediastinal shift) and patient is hemodynamically stable without dyspnea, treat expectantly without chest tube and with supplemental oxygen and observation only (6):
    - Must be observed in the emergency department (ED) for 4 to 6 hours with repeat radiographs
    - Exception is when associated with underlying lung disease; requires urgent and immediate treatment
  - When pneumothorax is large (>20%) and clinically stable, treat initially with either needle decompression or pleural aspiration (6):
    - If aspiration fails, treat with closed thoracostomy chest tube insertion.
  - If patient is clinically unstable, he or she should undergo chest tube insertion:
    - If the chest tube insertion is delayed, decompression can be performed as a bridge.
    - The chest tube can be connected to a water-seal device or suction. No specific data indicating which strategy is superior (6).
  - In cases of recurrent PSP, definitive management is recommended with video-assisted thoracoscopic surgery (VATS) after chest tube insertion.
- Chest tube size recommendations based on systematic reviews:
  - Small-bore chest tubes (<14 gauge) are preferred due to similar success rates with decreased cadence of complications (6).
  - Large-bore chest tubes indicated in some instances (i.e., large air leak present or viscous fluid needs to be drained)
- Hemothorax with even a small pneumothorax requires a chest tube to preclude development of "trapped lung," which eventually may require decortication.

MEDICATION

- Lidocaine (Xylocaine) 1% for chest tube insertion
- Oral or IV medication prior to chest tube insertion and after as needed for comfort
- May consider Tylenol #3 or other narcotic for oral use, especially around time of chest tube insertion

ISSUES FOR REFERRAL

Should refer to cardiothoracic surgeon in cases of persistent air leak or recurrent pneumothorax requiring further intervention

ADDITIONAL THERAPIES

Avoid chest binders, taping, and so forth, which tend to compromise deep inspiration and may contribute to the development of atelectasis.

SURGERY/OTHER PROCEDURES

- VATS: resection of any abnormal lung parenchyma:
  - Should consider, along with chest tube placement, if pleural aspiration alone is unsuccessful
  - Should perform in cases of recurrent PSP after chest tube insertion
  - Consider in patients being managed with a chest tube who have a persistent air leak.
- Pleurectomy: removal of parietal pleura
- Pleurodesis:
  - Mechanical: physical pleural abrasion
  - Chemical: agents delivered either via procedure or chest tube
  - Remains controversial

ADMISSION, INPATIENT, AND NURSING CONSIDERATIONS

- Admission criteria:
  - Hemodynamically unstable
  - Tension pneumothorax and/or chest tube placement
  - Pneumothorax with >15–20% lung volume loss
  - All patients with SSP
- Discharge criteria:
  - Removal of chest tube; depends on indication of tube
  - Repeat x-ray after removal of chest tube (prior to discharge) to check for recurrence.

ONGOING CARE

FOLLOW-UP RECOMMENDATIONS

Patient Monitoring

- Advise patient that pain likely will be present for at least 6 weeks, especially if rib fracture produced the pneumothorax.
- Follow up recommended even when managed conservatively.
- Recheck CXR in 4 to 6 weeks.
- No clear consensus on return to play, but studies have shown an average of 3 to 4 weeks from a resolved pneumothorax (7).

PATIENT EDUCATION

- Counsel on high risk of recurrence if spontaneous pneumothorax: For traumatic pneumothorax, there is no increased risk of recurrence compared with other types.
- Counsel against smoking.
- Air travel recommendations (5),(6):
  - Commercial air travel is contraindicated in the presence of an acute, unresolved pneumothorax.
  - For commercial travelers, no travel for 2 to 3 weeks after radiographic resolution of pneumothorax.
  - May restrict air travel in persons with a history of pneumothorax with underlying lung disease
- SCUBA diving absolute contraindications:
  - A history of a spontaneous pneumothorax
  - Diving within 3 months after any type of nonspontaneous pneumothorax
  - Expert divers with recurrent pneumothorax following a pleurectomy

PROGNOSIS

- Depends on type and extent: Small (<20%) usually resolves on own without treatment.
- When associated with underlying disease, even when small, is more serious and higher morbidity rate (6)
- Recurrence rate is ~40% for both primary and secondary pneumothoraces (2).
- Most recurrences occur within 1.5 to 2 years; recurrence is at its highest likelihood in the first few months after the initial pneumothorax.
- For traumatic pneumothorax, there are no data to suggest that there is an increased risk of recurrence with or without return to play.
- Recurrence rate increases with each recurrence.
- Most recurrences are seen on the same side but not always.

COMPLICATIONS

Recurrence: If it occurs, consider VATS pleurodesis or thoracotomy.

REFERENCES

1. Huan NC, Sidhu C, Thomas R. Pneumothorax: classification and etiology. *Clin Chest Med.* 2021;42(4):711–727.
2. Olesen WH, Titlestad IL, Andersen PE, et al. Incidence of primary spontaneous pneumothorax: a validated, register-based nationwide study. *ERJ Open Res.* 2019;5(2):00022-2019.
3. Tschopp JM, Bintcliffe O, Astoul P, et al. ERS task force statement: diagnosis and treatment of primary spontaneous pneumothorax. *Eur Respir J.* 2015;46(2):321–335.
4. Tran J, Haussner W, Shah K. Traumatic pneumothorax: a review of current diagnostic practices and evolving management. *J Emerg Med.* 2021;61(5):517–528.
5. Doscas ME, Achar S. Professional soccer player with shortness of breath: a case of hemothorax in sport. *Curr Sports Med Rep.* 2023;22(5):161–163.
6. DeMaio A, Semaan R. Management of pneumothorax. *Clin Chest Med.* 2021;42(4):729–738.
7. Espinoza D, Sisk T, Chiampas G, et al. Return to play in asthma and pulmonary conditions. *Return to Play in Football.* 2017:771–781.

ADDITIONAL READING

- Baumann MH, Strange C, Heffner JE, et al. Management of spontaneous pneumothorax: an American College of Chest Physicians Delphi consensus statement. *Chest.* 2001;119(2):590–602.
- Bobbio A, Dechartres A, Bouam S, et al. Epidemiology of spontaneous pneumothorax: gender-related differences. *Thorax.* 2015; 70(7):653–658.
- Plojoux J, Froudarakis M, Janssens JP, et al. New insights and improved strategies for the management of primary spontaneous pneumothorax. *Clin Respir J.* 2019;13(4):195–201.
- Staub LJ, Biscaro RRM, Kaszubowski E, et al. Chest ultrasonography for the emergency diagnosis of traumatic pneumothorax and hemothorax: a systematic review and meta-analysis. *Injury.* 2018;49(3):457–466.
- Vuong NL, Elshafay A, Thao LP, et al. Efficacy of treatments in primary spontaneous pneumothorax: a systematic review and network meta-analysis of randomized clinical trials. *Respir Med.* 2018; 137:152–166.

CLINICAL PEARLS

- Various classifications based on etiology and pathophysiology.
- Clinical diagnosis with radiologic confirmation; US with highest sensitivity, but CT scan remains the gold standard.
- Return to activity:
  - Return to play: 3 to 4 weeks, greater if fractures
  - Air travel: contraindicated until 2 to 3 weeks after chest tube removal (only if repeat x-ray shows resolution of pneumothorax)
  - SCUBA diving: contraindicated if history of spontaneous pneumothorax

POPLITEAL (BAKER) CYST

Samuel J. Galloway, MD, CAQSM

BASICS

DESCRIPTION

- Cystic enlargement of the *gastrocnemius-semimembranosus bursa*, located on the medial side of the popliteal fossa between the medial head of the *gastrocnemius* and the *semimembranosus* tendon:
  - Primary cysts arise with no communication into the joint (more common in children).
  - Secondary cysts are associated with communication between the bursa and joint capsule (more common in the adult population).
- Originally reported by Robert Adams in 1840, described in detail and named by William Baker in his article published in 1877

EPIDEMIOLOGY

Prevalence

- Most prevalent cyst/soft tissue mass in the posterior knee
- In adults, prevalence has been reported with ranges from 5% to 19% of patients presenting with knee problems (1).
  - Varies depending on type of imaging used and population sampled
  - Peak age in adults is 35 to 70 years, whereas in pediatrics is 4 to 7 years (1).
- No consistent significant gender difference

ETIOLOGY AND PATHOPHYSIOLOGY

- Cysts usually are associated with intra-articular pathology, such as osteoarthritis or meniscus tears.
- In children, they are often associated with rheumatic joint disease as degenerative changes are less common in this population.
- Result from communication between the *gastrocnemius-semimembranosus bursa* and joint capsule (in secondary cysts)
- A valve-like structure between the joint space and bursa results in one-way flow of synovial fluid into the bursa, leading to cyst formation:
  - Valve is open when the knee is in flexion and closed when the knee is in extension due to tension from *semimembranosus* and *gastrocnemius*.
- Intra-articular knee pressure is negative during partial flexion (minus 6 mm Hg) and positive during extension (16 mm Hg) (1).
- Intra-articular knee pathology results in increased production of synovial fluid, which accumulates in the bursa leading to popliteal cyst.
- Intra-articular bodies may make their way into the cyst.

Genetics

No known genetic factors; consider underlying causes (e.g., rheumatoid arthritis).

RISK FACTORS

- Intra-articular knee pathology
- History of trauma

GENERAL PREVENTION

Avoid knee trauma.

COMMONLY ASSOCIATED CONDITIONS

- In adults, most commonly associated with intra-articular pathology of the knee, resulting from increased production of synovial fluid:
  - Meniscal pathology (most commonly tears of the posterior horn of medial meniscus)
  - Osteoarthritis/rheumatoid arthritis
  - Anterior cruciate ligament tear
  - Other joint disease: infectious arthritis, pigmented villonodular synovitis
- In pediatrics, cysts are most commonly a primary process and do not communicate with the joint space and are not associated with intra-articular pathology.

DIAGNOSIS

HISTORY

- Most are small, asymptomatic, and discovered incidentally on imaging.
- Symptoms, if present, include posterior knee pain, swelling, palpable mass, or knee stiffness.
- Patients may only present with symptoms of associated intra-articular knee pathology.
- Patients may present with leg swelling, calf pain, and positive Homans sign due to compression of adjacent structures or cyst rupture.

PHYSICAL EXAM

- May or may not have palpable medial popliteal mass depending on size
- Knee should be examined from full extension to at least 90 degrees of flexion.
- Tense cyst with knee in extension softens or decreases in size with knee flexion (Foucher sign):
  - Change in findings related to knee position helps to differentiate popliteal cyst from solid masses.
- May have physical findings of cyst compression on surrounding structures (see "Complications")

DIFFERENTIAL DIAGNOSIS

- Deep vein thrombosis (DVT)
- Popliteal artery aneurysm
- Solid tumors (lipoma, sarcoma, etc.)
- Other cystic structures (ganglion cyst, meniscal cyst, myxoid tumors)

DIAGNOSTIC TESTS & INTERPRETATION

Initial Tests (lab, imaging)

- Ultrasonography is the initial imaging modality of choice (2)[C]:
  - Visualization of localized collection of anechoic or hypoechoic fluid
  - Meta-analysis found ultrasound has a sensitivity of 94% and specificity of 100% (3)[A].
  - Inexpensive, noninvasive, no radiation exposure, and can be performed in the office
  - Can reliably detect cysts >1 to 2 cm in size
  - Can differentiate cyst from solid mass
  - Doppler can help to differentiate from popliteal artery aneurysm or other vascular structures.
  - Allows for good visualization of cyst in relation to surrounding structures
- Plain radiographs are often helpful to evaluate for other associated joint pathology:
  - May be able to see loose bodies in cyst if present
- Magnetic resonance imaging (MRI) is the gold standard for diagnosis and can better delineate the cyst as well as evaluate internal derangement of the knee that is not able to be visualized with ultrasound (2)[C].

Diagnostic Procedures/Other

Arthrography with contrast or contrast + air can be useful for diagnosis; however, less common now with availability of MRI (1):

- Can be helpful for visualizing ruptured cyst with tracking of leaked contrast
- May result in false positive due to distension of the joint capsule or enlargement of a normal bursa due to injection of fluid volume (1)

Test Interpretation

Fluid aspirate can be sent for cellular studies to rule out infectious, inflammatory, or gouty causes.

P

TREATMENT

GENERAL MEASURES

- Management of underlying joint pathology, if present, is necessary; otherwise, there is a very high rate of cyst recurrence.
- Asymptomatic cysts that were an incidental finding on evaluation of the knee for other reasons do not require any treatment (1)[C].
- When symptomatic and without vascular or neural compression, initial treatment should be nonoperative for >6 weeks; rehab directed toward maintaining knee flexibility (2)
- Intra-articular corticosteroid injections have been shown to decrease the size and symptoms associated with cysts.
- Direct cyst aspiration and corticosteroid injection were found to be superior to intra-articular approach, but both can be beneficial (4)[A].
- If the cyst contains septations/loculations, then fenestration prior to corticosteroid injection improves response to treatment (4)[A].
- If the cyst does not communicate directly with the joint space, direct aspiration and injection of corticosteroid is necessary.
- Platelet-rich plasma (PRP) injection may be beneficial; more studies are needed (5)[C].

ISSUES FOR REFERRAL

Symptomatic cysts not improved with conservative measures or cysts with multiple recurrences should be referred for surgical management (4).

SURGERY/OTHER PROCEDURES

- Surgical excision should be reserved for cases resistant to initial therapy that continue to be symptomatic or limit mobility:
  - Also should be considered initially for cysts compressing surrounding structures (2)[C]
- Intra-articular knee pathology should be addressed during surgical management of cyst; if this is not corrected, recurrence rates have been reported at 63% (6)[A].
- Several different surgical approaches have been described, with success rates of 85–98% (6)[A]:
  - Cyst either fully excised or communication with knee joint surgically closed
  - Some studies have shown enlargement of the cyst opening rather than closure may be superior (4)[A].

ONGOING CARE

FOLLOW-UP RECOMMENDATIONS

Monitor for symptom improvement after treatment initiated; follow up as needed if cyst recurs.

PATIENT EDUCATION

- Discuss pathophysiology of cyst formation and options for management, including both conservative and surgical.
- Educate patients on the potential for cyst recurrence and need for further treatment.

PROGNOSIS

- Many cysts are asymptomatic, discovered incidentally, and do not require any intervention.
- Most cysts in pediatrics do not require intervention and resolve spontaneously.
- Most will improve with treatment of underlying joint pathology.
- Cysts have been shown to decrease in size and symptoms with corticosteroid injection.
- Cysts often recur in patients with underlying joint pathology that is not adequately treated.
- Surgery is very effective, but not definitive, and cysts may recur despite full excision.

COMPLICATIONS

- Cyst rupture or dissection can cause calf pain, swelling, and/or ecchymosis that extends distally
- Enlarged cyst may compress adjacent vein, resulting in pseudothrombophlebitis or thrombophlebitis with symptoms of leg swelling and erythema.
- Compression of tibial nerve may result in neuropathy, plantar foot numbness, or gastrocnemius atrophy.
- Compression of popliteal artery may lead to limb claudication or ischemia.
- Compartment syndrome may result from cyst rupture, which requires emergent management.

REFERENCES

1. Handy JR. Popliteal cysts in adults: a review. *Semin Arthritis Rheum*. 2001;31(2):108–118.
2. Frush TJ, Noyes FR. Baker's cyst: diagnostic and surgical considerations. *Sports Health*. 2015;7(4):359–365.
3. Liu K, Li X, Weng Q, et al. Diagnostic accuracy of ultrasound for the assessment of Baker's cysts: a meta-analysis. *J Orthop Surg Res*. 2022;17(1):535.
4. Van Nest DS, Tjoumakaris FP, Smith BJ, et al. Popliteal cyst a systematic review of non-operative and operative treatment. *JBJS Rev*. 2020;8(3):e0139.
5. Song B, Yeh PC, Jayaram P. Leukocyte-rich platelet-rich plasma application in post-traumatic osteoarthritis with popliteal cyst: a case report. *Regen Med*. 2020;15(6):1695–1702.
6. Zhou X, Li B, Wang J, et al. Surgical treatment of popliteal cyst: a systematic review and meta-analysis. *J Orthop Surg Res*. 2016;11:22.

ADDITIONAL READING

- Acebes JC, Sánchez-Pernaute O, Díaz-Oca A, et al. Ultrasonographic assessment of Baker's cysts after intra-articular corticosteroid injection in knee osteoarthritis. *J Clin Ultrasound*. 2006;34(3):113–117.
- Angoules AG. Baker's cyst rupture may mimics deep vein thrombosis. *Emerg Med*. 2012;2:e108.
- Hayashi D, Roemer FW, Dhina Z, et al. Longitudinal assessment of cyst-like lesions of the knee and their relation to radiographic osteoarthritis and MRI-detected effusion and synovitis in patients with knee pain. *Arthritis Res Ther*. 2010;12(5):R172.
- Tessier S, Murphy RJ, Peake KN, et al. Baker's cyst: a harbinger of systemic joint disease in children. *Clin Pediatr (Phila)*. 2024;63(3):419–422.

CLINICAL PEARLS

- Many cysts are asymptomatic and discovered incidentally on imaging. These can be managed expectantly.
- In adults, most popliteal cysts are associated with intra-articular joint pathology. In pediatrics, most cysts are primary and not related to any underlying pathology.
- Ultrasound is the initial imaging modality of choice; MRI is the gold standard for diagnosis.
- Initial treatment for symptomatic popliteal cysts should be conservative treatment options or cyst aspiration and/or knee arthrocentesis with corticosteroid injection.
- Cysts that do not respond to conservative measures should be referred for surgical management.

POPLITEAL ARTERY ENTRAPMENT SYNDROME

Timothy Tiu, MD, FAAPMR, CAQSM • Sandra de Mel, MD

BASICS

DESCRIPTION

- Anatomic abnormality in popliteal artery entrapment syndrome (PAES) was first described in 1879 by Anderson Stuart, a medical student, during anatomy dissections (1).
- Arterial insufficiency from external compression of the popliteal artery by surrounding musculotendinous structures (1):
  - Can have concurrent compression of popliteal vein and/or tibial nerve (1)

EPIDEMIOLOGY

- True incidence unknown with prevalence thought to range from 0.6% to 3.5% (1)
- Occurs bilaterally in approximately 30–67% of cases (2),(3)
- Most frequently occurs in individuals with well-developed muscles (e.g., athletes, military) (2).
- Male:female ratio ranges from 2:1 to 15:1 (1).
- Average age: 46 years in anatomic PAES and 26 years in functional PAES (3)

ETIOLOGY AND PATHOPHYSIOLOGY

- Classified into anatomic and functional PAES (1):
  - Anatomic variations:
    - Congenital deviation of popliteal artery
    - Embryologic anomaly of musculotendinous structures surrounding popliteal artery
  - Functional entrapment:
    - Popliteal artery compression demonstrated with stress maneuvers in symptomatic individuals but without any apparent anatomic abnormalities
    - Associated with hypertrophy of the medial gastrocnemius, plantaris, and soleus
- Long-term sequalae develop as progressive neovascularization, inflammatory cell infiltration, and vessel wall disruption lead to arterial wall fibrosis (3):
  - Begins in arterial adventitia (stage 1), then the media (stage 2), and finally the intima (stage 3)
  - Progressive fibrosis of arterial wall leads to intraluminal stenosis, poststenotic dilation, and true aneurysm formation.
  - Intimal fibrosis results in thrombogenic flow surface, causing formation of mural thrombus.
  - Development of arterial occlusion in the diseased vessels occurs in a slow and chronic nature, allowing for the creation of collateral vessels (2).

RISK FACTORS

- Active individuals, without any atherosclerotic risk factors, who participate in activities involving excessive ankle dorsiflexion and plantarflexion (e.g., football, basketball, soccer, running on inclines, marching up/down hills) (4)
- Functional entrapment typically affects young, athletic women (average age 26 years) (3).
- Anatomic entrapment typically affects middle-aged men (average age 46 years) (3).

DIAGNOSIS

HISTORY

- Leg (calf or anterolateral compartment) and foot pain/claudication (deep ache or cramping) (5):
  - Symptoms are related to the degree of popliteal artery compression (5).
- Pain typically occurs suddenly after intense exercises involving the lower limbs and resolves quickly once activity ceases (3),(4),(5).
- Claudication may occur paradoxically with walking, rather than running, due to prolonged gastrocnemius contraction with walking (5).
- Paresthesia of foot occurs sometimes (4):
  - Repeated injury of tibial nerve during ankle dorsiflexion can cause paresthesia.
  - Paresthesia is more common in PAES than chronic exertional compartment syndrome.
- Other symptoms: coldness, blanching, and numbness of the calf/foot (4)
- Must ascertain details of training regimen, surface conditions, and shoe wear to rule out other common causes of leg/foot pain (4)

PHYSICAL EXAM

- If patent popliteal artery, generally will have normal physical exam at rest (5)
- Exam components (5):
  - Palpation of bones and soft tissues of the leg/foot for tenderness:
    - May elicit tenderness in calf only after exercise
  - Evaluation for localized or diffuse edema
  - Palpation of bilateral dorsalis pedis and posterior tibial artery pulses for reduction in pulse volume between limbs
    - Must be performed in neutral position and with stress maneuvers
    - Stress maneuvers:
      - Passive ankle dorsiflexion with knee extended
      - Active plantarflexion with knee extended
      - Mechanism: causes tension on gastrocnemius and induces external compression

DIFFERENTIAL DIAGNOSIS

- Chronic exertional compartment syndrome
- Muscle strains (gastrocnemius, soleus, plantaris)
- Tendinopathy
- Medial tibial stress syndrome
- Stress fracture
- Nerve entrapment (common peroneal nerve, superficial peroneal nerve, saphenous nerve)
- Arteritis (Buerger disease)
- Neurogenic claudication

DIAGNOSTIC TESTS & INTERPRETATION

Initial Tests (lab, imaging)

- Stress ankle brachial index (ABI):
  - Comparative ratio of ankle blood pressure to upper extremity blood pressure
  - May be normal at rest
  - Decrease in ABI >30% during plantarflexion or postexercise may be indicative of vascular pathology (1).
- Duplex ultrasound (DUS): commonly used for initial investigation alongside ABI (1),(3):
  - Allows for anatomic evaluation with B-mode images as well as provides analysis of arterial flow during dynamic/stress maneuvers
  - Initial imaging of artery done with leg in neutral position to evaluate for intimal changes, stenosis, or aneurysm and to evaluate velocity/waveform of arterial flow
  - Repeat evaluation to be done after stress maneuvers with ankle plantarflexed against resistance:
    - Repeated plantarflexion until patient symptomatic may be needed
    - All portions of popliteal artery must be assessed (above knee joint to below knee joint).
  - Diagnostic sonographic finding: obstruction of flow within the popliteal artery.
  - Concurrent popliteal vein entrapment can be evaluated by squeezing calf to evaluate for normal venous flow.
  - Drawbacks: can overdiagnose occlusion (2)[C]
- Magnetic resonance imaging (MRI) and magnetic resonance angiogram (MRA):
  - Combination of stress positional T2-weighted MRI and MRA useful for visualization of anatomy in popliteal fossa and providing accurate arterial imaging (3)[C]
  - Dynamic MRI/MRA imaging has been attempted but may result in motion artifact:
    - Patient asked to dorsiflex and plantarflex ankle with maximal exertion while axial images across popliteal region is obtained
    - Patient to dorsiflex and plantarflex until pain is reproduced and then asked to maximally plantarflex while contrast MRA performed
  - Drawbacks:
    - False-negative results can occur with <50% stenosis due to decreased spatial resolution of MRA.
    - Expensive
    - Dynamic MRI/MRA imaging may result in motion artifact due to difficulty in maintaining muscle contraction during imaging.
- Computed tomography angiography (CTA):
  - Alternative diagnostic modality to MRA:
    - Less costly than MRI/MRA
  - Drawback: exposure to ionizing radiation (3)[C]
- Arteriography:
  - Gold standard test for PAES (2),(3),(5)
  - Can confirm diagnosis if PAES suspected on MRI/MRA (4)
  - Should be performed bilaterally after exercise or with provocative maneuvers (may be normal when ankle in neutral position) (5)[C]
  - Drawbacks:
    - Invasive: involves placement of catheter and injection of radiopaque contrast into artery of interest
    - Exposure to ionizing radiation (5)[C]
- Bone scans and radiography can be used to rule out stress fractures (5)[C].

Follow-Up Tests & Special Considerations

1/3 to 1/2 of asymptomatic individuals can demonstrate popliteal artery narrowing or occlusion with resisted ankle dorsiflexion or plantarflexion (4).

Test Interpretation

PAES classification (1):

- Type I: Popliteal artery aberrantly passes medially to the normal medial head of gastrocnemius.
- Type II: Medial head of gastrocnemius inserts more laterally than usual resulting in the normally oriented popliteal artery to pass medial to the muscle.
- Type III: Medial head of gastrocnemius has accessory slip arising laterally, which compresses the popliteal artery.
- Type IV: Popliteal artery is compressed by running deep to popliteus muscle or by anomalous fibrous band.
- Type V: entrapment of popliteal vein
- Type VI: functional entrapment without any anatomic abnormality

TREATMENT

SURGERY/OTHER PROCEDURES

- Surgery is advised in all cases of anatomic PAES to prevent long-term arterial damage (2).
- Severely symptomatic functional PAES requires surgical evaluation (2).
- Entrapment types I to V:
  - If undamaged popliteal artery and stage 1 (early) disease:
    - Surgical exploration with division and resection of entrapment mechanism (medial head of gastrocnemius, abnormal muscle slips or tendinous bands) to restore normal arterial flow provides excellent outcomes (5)[C]
    - The three commonly used surgical approaches are posterior, medial, and Turnipseed approach. These provide various access points to the different muscles/tendons contributing to PAES (2)[C].
  - Whereas the posterior and medial surgical approaches often involve resection of the medial head of the gastrocnemius, the Turnipseed approach resects distal plantaris muscle plus fascia of the soleus/gastrocnemius, which is hypothesized to provide relief without significant muscle compromise in higher level athletes (2)[C].
    - For intermittent occlusion, timely musculotendinous release of popliteal artery has superior outcomes (2),(4)[C].
  - If any occlusion, stenosis, or aneurysm: Placement of saphenous vein graft with division of any entrapment mechanism is recommended (4),(5)[C].
- Functional entrapment (type VI):
  - In the case of severe and repetitive symptoms, surgical treatment is indicated. Asymptomatic functional PAES does not require immediate surgical evaluation.
  - Botulinum toxin A injections under ultrasound guidance to the medial head of the gastrocnemius and plantaris muscles have been shown to be a possible alternative to surgery (2),(6).
    - It is hypothesized that the toxin acts to paralysis the muscle involved in vessel compression and causes localized muscle atrophy (6).
    - With functional PAES having a lower surgical success rate than anatomic PAES, this is a viable option for this population with preliminary evidence of long-term benefits (6).
  - If there is evidence of arterial degeneration, vascular reconstruction is needed (5)[C].

ONGOING CARE

PROGNOSIS

- PAES is generally considered progressive if left untreated (4):
  - Can result in eventual complete obstruction of popliteal artery causing risk of severe leg ischemia, disability, or limb loss (1),(2)
  - Distal embolization of mural thrombus to peripheral vessels can occur, causing acute ischemia (3),(4).
- Rate of arterial wall degeneration may depend on degree of compression and magnitude of compression rather than duration of compression (4).
- Poor medium-term patency if popliteal occlusion is treated with thrombolysis, angioplasty, or thrombectomy with patching (4)
- With acute occlusion, thrombolysis, and angioplasty alone have high risk of reocclusion and will not be effective without addressing underlying cause of entrapment:
  - Once thrombosis or aneurysm has occurred, arterial degeneration is severe and the artery not salvageable (4).
- Excellent 10-year patency with aneurysm repair or treatment of occlusion with saphenous vein bypass graft (4).
- Excellent results with myotomy for type VI entrapment (4)

REFERENCES

1. Grimm NL, Danilkowicz R, Shortell C, et al. Popliteal artery entrapment syndrome. *JBJS Reviews*. 2020;8(1):e0035.
2. Lovelock T, Claydon M, Dean A. Functional popliteal artery entrapment syndrome: an approach to diagnosis and management. *Int J Sports Med*. 2021;42(13):1159–1166.
3. Levien L. Popliteal artery entrapment syndrome. *Semin Vasc Surg*. 2003;16(3):223–231.
4. Edwards PH Jr, Wright ML, Hartman JF. A practical approach for the differential diagnosis of chronic leg pain in the athlete. *Am J Sports Med*. 2005;33(8):1241–1249.
5. Joy S, Raudales R. Popliteal artery entrapment syndrome. *Curr Sports Med Rep*. 2015;14(5):364–367.
6. Shultz M, Isner-Horobeti ME, Lecocq J. Botulinum toxin: a new treatment for functional popliteal artery entrapment syndrome? Five patients relieved more than one year. *Ann Phys Rehabil Med*. 2018;61(1):8–12.

ADDITIONAL READING

- Clemens MS, Scott DJ, Watson JDB, et al. A diagnostic evolution: surgical experience with popliteal artery entrapment syndrome at a military tertiary referral center. *Ann Vasc Surg*. 2015;29(6):1078–1083.
- Hislop M, Brideaux A, Dhupelia S. Functional popliteal artery entrapment syndrome: use of ultrasound guided Botox injection as a non-surgical treatment option. *Skeletal Radiol*. 2017;46(9):1241–1248.
- Isner-Horobeti M, Muff G, Masat J, et al. Botulinum toxin as a treatment for functional popliteal artery entrapment syndrome. *Med Sci Sports Exerc*. 2015;47(6):1124–1127.
- Kwon Y, Kwon T, Gwon J, et al. Anatomical popliteal artery entrapment syndrome. *Ann Surg Treat Res*. 2018;94(5):262–269.
- Lejay A, Delay C, Georg Y. Five year outcomes of surgical treatment for popliteal artery entrapment syndrome. *Eur J Vasc Endovasc Surg*. 2016;51(4):557–564.
- Shahi N, Arosemena M, Kwon J, et al. Functional popliteal artery entrapment syndrome: a review of diagnosis and management. *Ann Vasc Surg*. 2019;59:259–267.
- Skeik N, Thomas TM, Engstrom BI, et al. Case report and literature review of popliteal artery entrapment syndrome. *Int J Gen Med*. 2015;8:221–225.

CLINICAL PEARLS

- Sudden onset of claudication symptoms in young adult with no atherosclerotic risk factors is highly suggestive of PAES (4).
- Isolated popliteal artery aneurysm or occlusion in young and physically active individuals should be considered due to PAES or cystic adventitial disease unless otherwise proven (4).
- If diagnosed early, PAES is the most common surgically correctable cause of leg claudication in young adults.
- No current evidence to suggest that surgical intervention is needed for asymptomatic patients with "functional entrapment" noted only on imaging studies without any anatomic abnormalities, given this likely represents a physiologic rather than pathologic finding (2)
- Botox is emerging as a viable alternative to surgery in patients with functional PAES (6).

POPLITEAL TENDONITIS

Laura J. Lintner, DO, CAQSM ▪ Jack Keeley, MD

BASICS

DESCRIPTION

- The popliteus muscle originates at the lateral condyle and travels underneath the biceps femoris tendon and lateral collateral ligament (LCL). It inserts on the posteromedial surface of the tibia and forms the floor of the popliteus fossa (1).
- Often, a popliteofibular ligament is also present. This anchors the early popliteus tendon to the proximal aspect of the fibula (2).
- The femoral origin of the popliteus is consistently anterior and distal to the femoral attachment of the LCL.
- The primary function of the popliteus muscle is internal rotation and stabilization of the tibia on the femur while walking (3).
- May help prevent forward translation of the femoral condyle relative to the lateral tibial plateau during downhill running
- Popliteal tendonitis is a cause of posterolateral knee pain due to inflammation of the popliteus tendon that connects the lateral femoral condyle to the proximal tibia.

EPIDEMIOLOGY

Rare, uncommon

ETIOLOGY AND PATHOPHYSIOLOGY

- May occur as overuse injury or acutely in case of trauma
- Popliteus tendonitis occurs due to repetitive stress on the popliteal tendon from training on declined surfaces. Downhill running places stress on the popliteal tendon as it attempts to prevent forward displacement of the femoral condyle relative to the lateral tibial plateau.
- Mechanism of injury can be due to direct stretch or when overused to maintain posterolateral stability (3).
- There have been rare cases reported of acute calcific tendinopathy of the popliteus tendon.
- Case report of a cyamella (sesamoid bone) within the popliteus muscle causing popliteal tendonitis (4)

RISK FACTORS

- May be associated with pes planus due to increased external rotation of the tibia
- Long distance runners, especially those training on declined surfaces
- Quadriceps weakness

GENERAL PREVENTION

- Appropriate warm-up before sports participation
- Avoid overtraining and running on de/incline or uneven surfaces.
- Consider foot orthoses for pes planus.
- Maintain good quadriceps strength.

COMMONLY ASSOCIATED CONDITIONS

True rupture of the popliteus tendon commonly occurs in combination with other posterior lateral corner injuries (3).

DIAGNOSIS

HISTORY

- Commonly presents with lateral knee pain when the knee is partially flexed 15 to 30 degrees while weight-bearing or when sitting cross legged
- Severe lateral knee pain accompanied by swelling
- Pain during the initial swing phase of the gait (3)
- History of running or walking downhill (often with subsiding pain after 2 days of activity cessation) (5)
- May describe trauma to the knee (hyperextension or direct force to anteromedial knee)

PHYSICAL EXAM

- Tenderness to palpation of posterolateral knee, often with localization to lateral knee upon flexion at 15 to 30 degrees (5)
- Gait analysis with posterior knee pain reported in initial swing phase
- Stable ligamentous exam with hemarthrosis could indicate rupture of the popliteus tendon (3).
- Posterolateral knee pain with resisted internal and external rotation of the tibia
- Figure-4 position: Have the patient flex, abduct, and externally rotate their hip so the ankle on the side of their affected knee rests on the contralateral knee (cross-legged position). Tenderness elicited particularly around the tendon insertion on the lateral femoral condyle may suggest popliteal tendonitis.
- Test the strength of the popliteal muscle by having the patient actively externally rotate their lower leg against examiner resistance with their knee flexed at 90 degrees (Garrick test). Pain elicited with this maneuver suggests popliteal pathology.

DIFFERENTIAL DIAGNOSIS

- Posterior cruciate ligament (PCL) injury
- Posterolateral corner injury
- Popliteal (Baker) cyst
- Hamstring strain
- Semimembranosus tendinopathy

DIAGNOSTIC TESTS & INTERPRETATION

- Can be a clinical diagnosis or diagnosis of exclusion
- X-rays are usually normal but may demonstrate calcifications on the lateral aspect of the knee (in the case of acute calcific popliteal tendinopathy).
- Ultrasound may demonstrate tendon hypoechogenicity, swelling, and increased Doppler signal.
- Magnetic resonance imaging (MRI) may demonstrate inflammation and edema surrounding the popliteus muscle.
- Arthroscopy alone may be inadequate for diagnosis due to poor visualization of the musculotendinous junction and femoral insertion (3); however, this can be valid diagnostic option in recalcitrant cases.

TREATMENT

GENERAL MEASURES

- Treatment plan for isolated popliteal tendon rupture has not been formalized (3)[C].
- Usually conservative with ice, rest, and nonsteroidal anti-inflammatory drugs (NSAIDs) for pain
- Avoid activity that aggravates pain (walking/running downhill) for at least 6 weeks.
- Gradual return to activity
- Due to the rarity of an isolated popliteal tendon avulsion, consensus is not clear on conservative versus surgical management, as both have demonstrated success.

MEDICATION

- Encourage patient to purchase shoes with good support.
- Orthotics may provide benefit to those with hyperpronation.

ISSUES FOR REFERRAL

- Ruptured tendon or calcific tendonitis
- Failed conservative treatment

ADDITIONAL THERAPIES

- Physical therapy, including shock wave therapy, ultrasonography, dry needling, and massage are additional treatment options.
- Physical therapy may provide benefit through hamstring stretching and eccentric quadriceps strengthening (6)[C].

SURGERY/OTHER PROCEDURES

- Corticosteroid injections have shown benefit to those who do not respond to conservative therapy.
- Surgery may be performed for an avulsed tendon or if with failure to respond to conservative therapy for >6 months.

Geriatric Considerations

In elderly patients, surgery is indicated only when the knee is locked; potentially, this could be accomplished with simple resection (3).

ONGOING CARE

FOLLOW-UP RECOMMENDATIONS

- Treatment plan has not been formalized for isolated popliteal tendonitis (3).
- Consider follow-up after initial 6-week conservative management for overuse popliteal tendonitis.
- Consider more immediate follow-up and management for acute popliteal pathology.

PATIENT EDUCATION

- Counsel on need for rest and compliance with physical therapy treatment.
- If recalcitrant, may require more invasive treatment options

PROGNOSIS

With proper treatment, activity adjustments, and biomechanical adjustments, the prognosis of popliteal tendonitis should follow a general pattern of healing for inflammatory tendon injury.

COMPLICATIONS

- Acute calcific tendonitis
- Tendon rupture

REFERENCES

1. Zabrzyński J, Huri G, Yataganbaba A, et al. Current concepts on the morphology of popliteus tendon and its clinical implications. *Folia Morphol (Warsz)*. 2021;80(3):505–513.
2. Grassi A, Pizza N, Lucidi GA, et al. Anatomy, magnetic resonance and arthroscopy of the popliteal hiatus of the knee: normal aspect and pathological conditions. *EFORT Open Rev*. 2021;6(1):61–74.
3. English S, Perret D. Posterior knee pain. *Curr Rev Musculoskelet Med*. 2010;3(1–4):3–10.
4. Rehmatullah N, McNair R, Sanchez-Ballester J. A cyamella causing popliteal tendonitis. *Ann R Coll Surg Engl*. 2014;96(1):91E–93E.
5. Farrell C, Kiel J, Seemann L, et al. Popliteus tendon injuries. *Orthopedics*. 2023;46(4):e193–e198.
6. Nyland J, Lachman N, Kocabey Y, et al. Anatomy, function, and rehabilitation of the popliteus musculotendinous complex. *J Orthop Sports Phys Ther*. 2005;35(3):165–179.

ADDITIONAL READING

- Petsche TS, Selesnick FH. Popliteus tendinitis: tips for diagnosis and management. *Phys Sportsmed*. 2002;30(8):27–31.
- Tennent TD, Goradia VK. Arthroscopic management of calcific tendinitis of the popliteus tendon. *Arthroscopy*. 2003;19(4):E35.

CLINICAL PEARLS

- Popliteal tendonitis is a rare cause of posterolateral knee pain most likely to occur in long distance runners or hikers (especially after significant downhill activity).
- Popliteal tendonitis rarely occurs in isolation, often coinciding with injury to surrounding structures including the ACL, PCL, medial/lateral menisci, as well as surrounding musculature.
- In the case of acute pain over the posterolateral knee, acute calcific popliteal tendonitis or popliteal tendon rupture should be considered.
- The general treatment for popliteal tendonitis is rest, ice, anti-inflammatory medication, and avoidance of painful activity. Physical therapy for proper knee function, and lower extremity flexibility and strengthening, can assist in improvement.
- Gradual return to activity
- Recalcitrant cases could benefit from advanced imaging and possible cortisone injection or arthroscopic evaluation.

POSTERIOR CRUCIATE LIGAMENT (PCL) TEAR

Briana Beach, DO ▪ Christopher Mariano, DO ▪ Priscilla Tu, DO, FAOASM, FAAP, FAAMA, FACOFP

BASICS

DESCRIPTION

Rupture of any or all parts of the posterior cruciate ligament (PCL) of the knee (anterolateral portion and posteromedial portion)

EPIDEMIOLOGY

Incidence

- All knee injuries in general population 3% (1)
- Knee injuries in trauma patients 37% (1)
- Knee injuries in athletes <2%, although may be underreported and/or underdiagnosed (1)
- Of all PCL injuries, 45% are vehicular trauma and 40% from sport (2).
- 48% of patients will have combined ligament injuries (2) and >60% will have an additional capsuloligamentous injury of which the posterolateral corner is most common (3).

RISK FACTORS

- Contact sports, especially American football
- Other sports, specifically soccer, skiing, ice hockey, and wrestling
- Improper personal positioning when riding in vehicles

COMMONLY ASSOCIATED CONDITIONS

- Anterior cruciate ligament (ACL) tear
- Lateral or medial collateral ligament tears
- Meniscal derangement
- Posterolateral corner injury
- Tibial plateau fractures
- Bony avulsions at the insertions of the cruciate ligament
- Avulsion fracture at the tibial tubercle
- Fibular head fracture
- Chondral injury
- Posterior knee subluxation or dislocation caused by hamstring force in the PCL-deficient knee

DIAGNOSIS

HISTORY

- "Dashboard injury": traumatic injury often seen in motor vehicle accidents, with posteriorly directed force to the anterior proximal tibia in a flexed knee (1)
- Similar mechanism to preceding in sports, particularly in American football and wrestling, resulting from an opponent hit to lower leg driving tibia backward and rupturing PCL (2)
- Often in sports, fall onto flexed knee, particularly with foot plantarflexed
- Less commonly, cutting, twisting, and hyperextension injury in sports; often accompanied by other ligament injuries
- Unlike ACL injuries, often do not report hearing or feeling a "pop" or "tear" (4)
- Acute injuries:
  - Pain in the posterior knee
  - Pain with kneeling
  - Feeling of instability
- Chronic injuries:
  - Vague anterior knee pain
  - Pain with or inability to descend inclines/stairs, deceleration, or running at full stride

PHYSICAL EXAM

- Rapid onset (within few hours) of swelling and tenderness in knee
- May have difficulty walking or walk with slight limp
- Anterior patellar contusions may be seen.
- Posterior knee or popliteal ecchymosis may be found.
- Neurovascular examination:
  - Perform neurovascular examination before other provocative tests.
  - Important to determine and document associated nerve damage or vascular injury (particularly popliteal artery injury)

ALERT

If combined with an ACL injury, assume vascular injury, perform ankle-brachial index (ABI), and, if low stat, refer to vascular surgeon. However, even with normal ABI, there are case reports of delayed popliteal occlusions, so repeat neurovascular examinations should be considered.

- Comprehensive knee examination:
  - Rule out dislocation.
  - Rule out other ligament or meniscus injuries.
- Posterior drawer test:
  - 90% sensitive and 99% specific for diagnosing PCL tears (4)
  - Perform with the patient supine and knee flexed at 90 degrees and hip flexed at 45 degrees.
  - Examiner stabilizes foot.
  - A posteriorly directed force is applied to the proximal tibia to elicit abnormal posterior tibial translation.
  - Posterior translation of 0 to 5 mm (grade 1), 5 to 10 mm (grade 2), and >10 mm (grade 3)
  - A secondary grading scale of the amount of posterior translation of the tibial plateau in relation to femoral condyles can also be used:
    - Grade A: plateau anterior to condyle
    - Grade B: plateau flush to condyle
    - Grade C: plateau posterior to condyle (4)
- Posterior sag test:
  - Perform with the patient supine and knee flexed at 90 degrees and hip flexed at 45 degrees.
  - Examiner stabilizes both heels.
  - Observe the knee from lateral perspective.
  - Normally, the tibial plateau sits ~1 cm anterior to the femoral condyles.
  - An abnormal contour, or sag, of the tibial plateau in relation to the femoral condyles is consistent with PCL deficiency.
- Quadriceps active test:
  - Perform with the patient supine and knee flexed at 90 degrees and hip flexed at 45 degrees.
  - Examiner stabilizes the foot, and the patient attempts to extend the knee while the examiner applies a counter force against the ankle.
  - Patient also may be asked to activate quadriceps by sliding foot down the table.
  - In a PCL-deficient knee, the posteriorly subluxed tibia will translate anteriorly with quadriceps activated.
- Dynamic posterior shift test:
  - Patient is supine with knee and hip flexed at 90 degrees.
  - Examiner slowly extends knee.
  - With a PCL tear, there will be "clunk" near full extension when the posteriorly subluxed tibia is reduced.

DIFFERENTIAL DIAGNOSIS

- ACL tear
- Patellar subluxation
- Tibial or fibular fracture
- Medial or lateral collateral ligament tear/sprain
- Meniscal derangement
- Posterolateral corner injury
- Knee dislocation

DIAGNOSTIC TESTS & INTERPRETATION
- Radiographic evaluation with anteroposterior (AP), lateral, sunrise, and tunnel views to rule out bony avulsions, other fractures, or patellar subluxations
- Oblique views are sometimes helpful to evaluate for tibial plateau fractures.
- Flexion weight-bearing posteroanterior and patellar radiographs can help to distinguish early degenerative changes from chronic PCL deficiencies.
- Stress radiographs: 8 mm or more posterior tibial translation is indicative of complete PCL tear.
- Magnetic resonance imaging (MRI):
  - Reported to be up to 100% sensitive and specific in evaluating an acute complete PCL rupture
  - The healing process in chronic PCL injuries may mask the degree of tear on MRI.
  - No specific bone bruising pattern with PCL tears on MRI, but medial compartment bruising is associated with PCL–posterolateral corner injuries (5).
  - Also can evaluate other soft tissue pathology of the affected knee

TREATMENT

GENERAL MEASURES
- Acute treatment:
  - Ice
  - Compression
  - Elevation
- Immobilization:
  - Partial weight-bearing
  - Possible immobilization in full extension for grade 3 lesions

ISSUES FOR REFERRAL
- Early orthopedic referral except in uncomplicated, isolated grade 1 and 2 lesions
- Early physical therapy referral may be beneficial because loss of proprioception and sprint speed are major problems with return to play.

ADDITIONAL THERAPIES
- Physical therapy
- No one protocol has been proven to have better outcomes than another (4)[B].
- General concepts of nonoperative rehab programs:
  - Multiphase with time-specific and objective finding–related phases
  - Progressive weight-bearing
  - Quadriceps strengthening
  - Immobilization initially, with progressive addition of flexion until full range of motion (ROM) achieved
  - Functional PCL brace may be useful but not proven effective (4)[B].
  - Sport-specific therapy protocol should be developed for optimal return to play (3)[C].

SURGERY/OTHER PROCEDURES
Indications include (6):
- Associated bony avulsion fractures
- Multiple ligament injuries
- Persistent pain in grade 3 lesions
- Chronic symptomatic instability with activities of daily living or with sports
- Acute grade 3 injury in young, active patient

ONGOING CARE

COMPLICATIONS
- Nonoperative:
  - Chronic PCL laxity
  - Progressive medial compartment and patellofemoral degenerative changes
  - Increased risk of meniscal tears, articular cartilage injury with chronic PCL insufficiency
  - Increased risk of future total knee arthroplasty (TKA) and osteoarthritis than those surgically repaired within 1 year (6)[B]
- Operative:
  - Most common: residual laxity
  - Iatrogenic neurovascular injury (especially of the popliteal artery)
  - Loss of motion
  - Infection
  - Medial femoral condyle osteonecrosis
  - Anterior knee pain
  - Painful hardware

REFERENCES

1. Wind WM Jr, Bergfeld JA, Parker RD. Evaluation and treatment of posterior cruciate ligament injuries: revisited. *Am J Sports Med*. 2004;32(7):1765–1775.
2. McAllister DR, Petrigliano FA. Diagnosis and treatment of posterior cruciate ligament injuries. *Curr Sports Med Rep*. 2007;6(5):293–299.
3. Kumar A, Sinha S, Arora R, et al. The 50 top-cited articles on the posterior cruciate ligament: a bibliometric analysis and review. *Orthop J Sports Med*. 2021;9(11):23259671211057851.
4. Kew ME, Cavaunaugh JT, Elnemer WG, et al. Return to play after posterior cruciate ligament injuries. *Curr Rev Musculoskelet Med*. 2022;15(6):605–615.
5. LaPrade CM, Civitarese DM, Rasmussen MT, et al. Emerging updates on the posterior cruciate ligament: a review of the current literature. *Am J Sports Med*. 2015;43(12):3077–3092.
6. Wang SH, Chien WC, Chung CH, et al. Long-term results of posterior cruciate ligament tear with or without reconstruction: a nationwide, population-based cohort study. *PLoS One*. 2018;13(10):e0205118.

ADDITIONAL READING

- Ahn JH, Lee SH, Choi SH, et al. Evaluation of clinical and magnetic resonance imaging results after treatment with casting and bracing for the acutely injured posterior cruciate ligament. *Arthroscopy*. 2011;27(12):1679–1687.
- Li YS, Lin KC, Chen CY, et al. Popliteal artery occlusion concomitant with a tibial plateau fracture and posterior cruciate ligament avulsion fracture. *J Int Med Res*. 2020;48(2):300060519869073.
- Petrigliano FA, McAllister DR. Isolated posterior cruciate ligament injuries of the knee. *Sports Med Arthrosc Rev*. 2006;14(4):206–212.

CLINICAL PEARLS
- Posterior drawer is the most sensitive and specific test for PCL. If it shows >10 mm of posterior translation, have a high suspicion for posterolateral corner injury (4).
- In isolated grades 1 and 2 PCL tears, uncomplicated patients may be able to return to play with knee brace within 2 to 4 weeks depending on the sport.
- In grade 3 injuries, uncomplicated patients may take up to 3 months of rehabilitation before return to play.
- MRI is the imaging of choice for acute injuries, but stress radiographs may be more beneficial for chronic injuries.
- If concerned for neurovascular injury despite a normal ABI, consider serial examinations or if combined ACL and PCL injury consider magnetic resonance angiography (MRA) or computed tomography (CT) angiogram.

POSTERIOR INTEROSSEOUS NERVE SYNDROME

Carly Morgan, DO, ATC • Richard A. Okragly, MD, FAMSSM

BASICS

DESCRIPTION

- A peripheral nerve syndrome occurring in the extensor compartment of the forearm secondary to extrinsic compressive or intrinsic inflammatory processes
- Presenting as a painful insidious weakness of the extensor muscles supplied by the posterior interosseous nerve (PIN) without sensory deficits

EPIDEMIOLOGY

- Incidence reported as approximately 3 per 100,000 people annually (1)
- Dominant arm is involved twice as much as the nondominant arm.
- More common in manual laborers, body builders, racquet sports, orchestra musicians
- Male > female (2:1)
- Most common compressive neuropathy of radial nerve (1)

RISK FACTORS

- Microtrauma from overuse/repetitive pronation and supination (usually strenuous activity)
- Trauma (Monteggia or radial head fractures)
- Autoimmune inflammatory disease (rheumatoid synovitis, Parsonage-Turner syndrome)
- Space-occupying lesions (lipoma, neuroma, ganglion, fibroma)
- Iatrogenic (elbow/forearm surgery)

ALERT

Extracorporeal compression (tight arm bands, e.g., holding a rifle sling wrapped around the forearm for prolonged periods, as seen in military recruits)

ETIOLOGY AND PATHOPHYSIOLOGY

- The PIN is a deep motor branch off of the radial nerve originating just proximal to the lateral epicondyle, coursing along the dorsal surface of the radius/interosseous membrane under the arcade of Frohse entering the forearm between the two heads of supinator and eventually dividing into medial and lateral branches innervating extensor carpi ulnaris, extensor digitorum communis, extensor digitorum minimi and abductor pollicis longus, extensor pollicis longus, extensor pollicis brevis, and extensor indicis proprius, respectively.
- Potential sites of extrinsic mechanical compression include the extensor carpi radialis brevis (ECRB), fibrous tissue anterior to radial head, arcade of Frohse (fibrous arch formed by the superficial proximal supinator 3 to 5 cm distal to the lateral epicondyle), leash of Henry (recurrent radial vessels fanning out across the PIN at the level of the radial neck), and proximal > distal edge of the supinator.
- Result from either extrinsic or intrinsic compression is a swollen nerve with demyelination and possible axonal injury of the nerve.

GENERAL PREVENTION

Avoidance of preventable risk factors

DIAGNOSIS

HISTORY

- Identifiable risk factor related to overuse usually present
- Progressive weakness of thumb, fingers, and wrist extension
- Pain in the forearm/wrist dependent on site of PIN pathology
- No sensory deficits
- May have concurrent Monteggia fracture or radial head fracture/dislocation

PHYSICAL EXAM

- In severe/chronic cases, forearm atrophy may be present.
- Sensation intact
- Tinel sign may or may not be positive depending on etiology
- Weakness/inability to extend wrist in neutral or ulnar deviation. There is preservation of wrist extension in radial deviation owing to ECRB/extensor carpi radialis longus (ECRL), which are not innervated by PIN.
- Weakness/inability to extend fingers/thumb at the metacarpophalangeal joint
- Tenderness on deep palpation along proximal radius
- Resisted wrist supination or middle finger extension can provoke pain.

DIFFERENTIAL DIAGNOSIS

- Other radial nerve pathology:
  - Radial nerve palsy
  - Radial tunnel syndrome (lateral forearm pain only without neurologic deficits)
  - Wartenberg syndrome (sensory only, no motor)
- Cervical (C7) radiculopathy
- Lateral epicondylitis (tennis elbow)
- Forearm extensor tendon rupture
- Peripheral neuropathy
- Brachial plexus compression

DIAGNOSTIC TESTS & INTERPRETATION

Initial Tests (lab, imaging)

- Plain radiographs: obtained to exclude osseous pathology, not commonly needed to diagnose
- Ultrasound (US, preferred imaging): can identify structural changes to the PIN including pathologic enlargement, site of entrapment with dynamic testing, increased nerve vascularity, nerve hypoechogenicity; also can identify space-occupying lesions; can be used for bilateral comparison (2)[C]
- Magnetic resonance imaging (MRI): not always indicated but can demonstrate PIN neuritis, muscular denervation, space-occupying lesions, and other pathology helpful in the event surgical intervention needed

Diagnostic Procedures/Other

Electromyography (EMG)/nerve conduction velocity studies (NCVS): used to identify anatomical location of nerve injury, injury severity, and exclude cervical radiculopathy, brachial plexopathy, or other polyneuropathy; findings:

- Normal sensory nerve action potentials (SNAPs)
- Slowed conduction velocity, prolonged distal latency, reduced amplitude compared to unaffected side
- Needle examination reveals membrane instability/abnormal spontaneous activity with positive sharp waves and fibrillations.
- Triceps, anconeus, brachioradialis, and ECRB/ECRL are spared.
- Can use to compare preoperative and postoperative measurements to trend recovery

TREATMENT

- Guided by etiology
- Conservative management almost always first line (3):
  - Rest/activity modification/physical therapy
  - Anti-inflammatory medication
  - Immobilization with wrist splint

MEDICATION

First Line

Nonsteroidal anti-inflammatory drugs (NSAIDs) (3)[C]:

- Helpful in pain control

Second Line

Corticosteroid injection (3)[C]:

- Placement dependent on location of pathology

ISSUES FOR REFERRAL

- Refractory cases (3 months without improvement)
- Progressive symptoms despite conservative treatment
- Severe symptoms

ADDITIONAL THERAPIES

Physical therapy that includes:

- Range of motion exercises that increase strength, endurance, and postural awareness
- Progressive strengthening and modified work-simulated tasks
- Application of heat and/or US
- Massage
- If severe, a dynamic splint is needed to hold the fingers in extension.
- Occupational therapy
- US-guided hydrodissection (4)[B]
  - Using an injectate such as glucose water to separate nerve from surrounding tissue to relieve compression

SURGERY/OTHER PROCEDURES

Surgical decompression may be necessary in refractory cases or if an identifiable compressive lesion is present to avoid irreversible nerve/muscle damage. Outcome after surgery is generally positive (3).

ONGOING CARE

FOLLOW-UP RECOMMENDATIONS

Follow-up and early physical therapy postoperatively to prevent contractures and stiffness

PROGNOSIS

Prognosis for full recovery is generally good with mean duration of symptoms around 3 to 4 months. After surgical decompression, it may take up to 12 months to fully recover (5).

REFERENCES

1. Węglel A, Karauda P, Zielinska N, et al. Radial nerve compression: anatomical perspective and clinical consequences. *Neurosurg Rev*. 2023;46(1):53.
2. Xiao TG, Cartwright MS. Ultrasound in the evaluation of radial neuropathies at the elbow. *Front Neurol*. 2019;10:216.
3. Mansuripur PK, Deren ME, Kamal RO. Nerve compression syndromes of the upper extremity: diagnosis, treatment, and rehabilitation. *R I Med J*. 2013;96(5):37–39.
4. Chen S, Wang Y. Dynamic ultrasonography for supinator syndrome: a case report. *Can J Neurol Sci*. 2018;45(1):126–127.
5. McGraw I. Isolated spontaneous posterior interosseous nerve palsy: a review of aetiology and management. *J Hand Surg Eur Vol*. 2019;44(3):310–316.

ADDITIONAL READING

Wheeless CR III. Posterior interosseous nerve compression syndrome. Wheeless' Textbook of Orthopaedics. Updated July 22, 2020. Accessed September 12, 2023. http://www.wheelessonline.com

CLINICAL PEARLS

- History of repetitive forearm pronation/supination with key exam findings of forearm pain, extensor weakness, and normal sensation
- Good prognosis with activity modification and conservative management; surgery rarely needed

POSTEROLATERAL CORNER INJURY

Tanner Craig Eiben, DO, CAQSM ▪ James M. Daniels, MD, MPH, PhD, RMSK, FAAFP, FACOEM, FACPM, FAMSSM ▪ Cesar S. Arguelles, MD, CAQSM

BASICS

DESCRIPTION

- Posterolateral corner (PLC) injury of the knee can be defined as damage to an area of complex anatomic structure that is primarily stabilized by the lateral (fibular) collateral ligament (LCL), the popliteus tendon (PT), and popliteofibular ligament (PFL).
- PLC was once referred to as "the dark side of the knee" due to the limited understanding of the structures and how to treat them (1).
- "PLC injury" does not have a universally accepted definition among orthopedists and currently lacks a classification system for the many variations of PLC injuries.
- PLC injuries are often overlooked yet clinically important because it can complicate the treatment of other ligament injuries—anterior cruciate ligament (ACL) and posterior cruciate ligament (PCL) (2).
- An isolated injury of PLC is rare (3).
- PLC laxity following injury is more common than initially believed as it is associated with cruciate ligament injuries (missed diagnosis is a common cause of ACL reconstruction failure) (2).
- There are 10 main anatomic structures that make up the PLC of the knee. The first three listed below are the primary structures:
  - Static structures:
    - LCL
    - PT
    - PFL
    - Lateral capsule with its thickened anterolateral ligament (ALL)
    - Arcuate ligament (variable)
    - Fabellofibular ligament and fibula (variable)
  - Dynamic structures:
    - Biceps femoris (long and short heads)
    - Popliteus muscle
    - Iliotibial (IT) tract
    - Lateral head of gastrocnemius
- More information on the primary stabilizers of the PLC:
  - LCL: originates from the lateral femoral condyle and inserts onto the anterior aspect of the fibula. It is the most lateral structure of the PLC. It serves as the primary varus stabilizer of the knee.
  - PT: Its femoral attachment is the most anterior aspect of the PLC. Before this, it courses through a sulcus which includes a small tunnel through the lateral meniscus. It becomes the popliteus muscle which inserts into the posterior aspect of the tibia. This structure is the primary resistor to external rotation of the tibia and secondary restraint to posterior and varus translation. It is the "key of the knee" because it causes external femoral rotation and knee flexion, "unlocking" the knee.
  - PFL: This ligament acts like a sling to hold the popliteus muscle-tendon complex down against the posterolateral portion of the tibia. It restrains posterior translation and provides posterolateral and external rotatory stability. It has two divisions: the anterior and the more robust posterior. They wrap around the musculotendinous junction of the popliteus muscle/tendon and then insert onto the fibular styloid process.

EPIDEMIOLOGY

- Most PLC injuries are associated with ACL or PCL injuries. Only 28% of PLC occur in isolation. An isolated injury is one of the least common traumatic problems of the knee (<2% of all ligament injuries to the knee). Yet, a PLC injury is present in almost 16% of all knee injuries.
- The main reason this injury has to be considered is that failure to diagnose a PLC injury in patients with ACL and/or PCL injuries can lead to graft failure and/or premature arthritis of the knee.

ETIOLOGY AND PATHOPHYSIOLOGY

- Associated with an acute episode of injury; if this is not part of the history, doubt the diagnosis of PLC injury.
- High-velocity injury:
  - Falls, landing on fully extended lower extremity
  - Knee then "fails" in varus, hyperextended position and buckles.
- Any knee hyperextension injury (contact or noncontact)
- Knee dislocation
- High-velocity varus blow to anteromedial aspect of knee
- Twisting injury with involvement of multiple ligaments
- Given the high-energy mechanisms typically associated with these injuries and surrounding anatomic structures, a neurovascular exam in these patients is *essential* (see "Physical Exam").

RISK FACTORS

- Female gender
- Sports competition (vs. practice)
- Contact sports
- American football
- Prior knee or ankle injury

COMMONLY ASSOCIATED CONDITIONS

- ACL tears
- PCL tears
- Knee dislocation
- Lateral meniscus tear
- Common fibular (peroneal) nerve injury
- Vascular injury to popliteal or geniculate arteries
- Bone contusion

Geriatric Considerations

PLC injuries can be associated with tibial plateau fractures in osteopenic elderly patients. They may be weight-bearing despite severe injury and knee effusion. In this group of patients with these clinical findings, the clinician should have an increased index of suspicion. Even if x-ray is negative, a computed tomography (CT) will often show the fracture.

Pediatric Considerations

Salter-Harris (SH) fracture of tibia can occur. The definition of type I SH fracture is tenderness over physis and "negative" original radiograph. PLC injuries are more posterior than SH injuries with palpation.

DIAGNOSIS

HISTORY

- Not as common in pediatric or geriatric population
- Any injury that may hyperextend, externally rotate, or force the tibia into varus angle can injure the PLC (1)[A].
- A posterolateral blow to the anteromedial portion of the tibia (1)[A]
- Contact and noncontact; low or high velocity (1)[A]
- Important to obtain the mechanism of injury to a hyperextended knee or knee dislocation (1)[A]
- Difficult to make diagnosis without some type of history of trauma (1)[A]
- Chronic injury may present with gait issues or difficulty using stairs (1)[A].
- Often have instability symptoms with full knee extension (1)[A]
- Often associated with other injuries; most common is with ACL and then PCL; may also injure common fibular nerve or blood supply from geniculate artery

PHYSICAL EXAM

- Neuro: Common fibular (peroneal) nerve injury has effect on great toe extension, ankle dorsiflexion, and sensory of the anterolateral lower leg and dorsum of the foot
- Vascular: 2-second capillary refill and palpation of both dorsalis pedis and posterior tibial arteries
- Effusion/pain has a big effect on musculoskeletal (MSK) exam. Do serial exams if early in presentation.
- Watch for varus thrust gait (varus alignment with weight-bearing, neutral alignment during non–weight-bearing).
- Ottawa Knee Rules for radiographic evaluations are very helpful; if the patient passes Ottawa Knee Rules, very low chance of acute PLC injury:
  - Ottawa Knee Rules: Obtain radiographs if:
    - 55 years old or older
    - Isolated tenderness over patella
    - Tenderness over head of fibula
    - Inability to flex knee to 90 degrees
    - Inability to bear weight four steps both immediately after injury and in acute care setting
- Because PLC injuries rarely occur in isolation, other injuries should be evaluated. If no end point on any ligament test or if more than one ligament is lax, assume knee dislocation and treat as such:
  - *ACL*—Lachman, pivot shift, anterior drawer test
  - *PCL*—prominent tibial plateau, posterior sag test, quad active flexion test, posterior drawer test
- Use of point-of-care ultrasound (POCUS) allows more precise measurement of joint gapping (3)[C].
  - Tests more specific for PLC: These maneuvers are not well studied, but when used in an additive fashion (all negative or positive), they are useful in evaluating a PLC injury (3)[C].
  - *Varus stress test of LCL*—varus force applied to knee in full extension. If increased gapping occurs as compared to contralateral knee, suspect both PLC and one or both cruciate ligament injury. If gapping only occurs at 30 degrees of flexion, suspect LCL only (2)[C].

– *Dial test*: Patient is in prone position. The examiner grabs the patient's forefoot while allowing the heels to touch. The knees are flexed to 30 degrees and then the tibias are externally rotated by the examiner. The knees are then flexed 90 degrees and the same maneuver is repeated. If there is >10 degrees difference compared to the contralateral knee at either position, the result is a positive test. If the difference exists only at 30 degrees of flexion, it implicates the PLC. If the difference is 90 degrees of flexion, it implicates both the PLC and the PCL are injured (1)[B],(4)[B],(5)[B].
– *Reverse pivot shift test*: essential component of the PLC evaluation, positive predictive value 68%, and negative predictive value 89%. Patient should be in supine position with knee flexed to 90 degrees. The lateral joint line is palpated, and the knee is slowly extended while the examiner places a valgus force and external rotation on the tibia. At approximately 30 to 40 degrees of flexion, if the knee subluxes, it indicates a positive test (1)[B].
– *Posterolateral drawer test*: a difficult test to learn; only positive with high-grade PLC injury. Patient supine with knee flexed 90 degrees, foot flat on table. Examiner places a posterior, external rotation force on the proximal tibia. If the tibial tuberosity rotates in reference to the femur, it is a positive test (1)[B].
– *Posterior drawer test*: Patient setup is the same as posterolateral drawer test, except all force is aimed posteriorly at the proximal tibia without rotational forces. Look for increased posterior translation of the tibia beneath the femur as compared to the contralateral side. If the test is positive with >12 mm difference as compared to the contralateral knee, additional injury to the PLC is highly probable (2)[B].

DIFFERENTIAL DIAGNOSIS

- ACL tear
- PCL tear
- Knee dislocation
- Tibial plateau fracture
- Growth plate injury
- Bone contusion
- Lateral meniscus tear
- IT band subluxation at knee
- Fibular nerve injury
- Vascular injury to geniculate artery system (3),(4)[B]

DIAGNOSTIC TESTS & INTERPRETATION

- Ottawa or Pittsburgh Knee Rules
- Anteroposterior (AP), lateral, sunrise views
- Bilateral varus stress views with physician-applied force at 20 degrees of flexion are helpful in acute and chronic cases for demonstrating increased gapping (6)[C].
- POCUS; some authors routinely scan all of their ACL injuries to rule out injury to popliteus and LCL. The PFL is more difficult to scan.
- Magnetic resonance imaging (MRI) is the gold standard for diagnosis of PLC injury. It also evaluates cruciate ligament injuries and helps with presurgical planning (6)[C].

ALERT

Look for arcuate sign on radiographs. This is an avulsion fracture for the fibular head associated with PLC injury and ACL injury. Also look for the Segond fracture, an avulsion fracture from lateral tibial plateau associated with ACL injury.

TREATMENT

- Because an isolated injury of the PLC is extremely rare and most PLC injuries are associated with multiple ligament injuries to the knee, some clinicians promote treating all of these injuries as grade III with immobilization, non–weight-bearing, and close (within 48 hours) follow-up with an orthopedic surgeon (1),(3)[C].
- The following table describes the grades of injury using the Hughston classification and suggested correlating treatments.

Grade	Definition	Treatment
Grade I: minimal ligament disruption	0–5 mm of lateral opening	Hinge brace Crutches Allow knee flexion Exercise, weight-bearing 4–5 wk
Grade II: moderate ligament disruption	5–10 mm of lateral opening	Crutches Knee immobilizer Non–weight-bearing × 3 wk Then treat like grade I
Grade III: severe ligament disruption (no end point)	>10 mm of lateral opening	Immobilizer Non–weight-bearing Crutches Orthopedic referral

ALERT

Grading can be difficult without experience and POCUS. A good working relationship (or phone consult) with an experienced orthopedic surgeon is very helpful. It is perfectly fine to treat all of these injuries as a grade III, especially if other injuries (i.e., ACL, PCL, meniscus), are suspected.

SURGERY/OTHER PROCEDURES

- Although consensus on diagnosis and treatment algorithms for PLC injuries have not been well defined, there is evidence that reconstruction of the damaged structures of the three primary PLC structures has better outcomes than repair of existing tissue structure (1)[B],(3)[B],(5)[B],(6)[C]. Primary repair can be performed to damaged secondary structures (hybrid approach).
- Surgery is ideally performed within 2 to 3 weeks after the time of injury (6)[C]. PLC reconstruction is used for most grade III injuries and failed conservatively treated lower grade injuries (1)[B],(3)[B],(6)[C].
- Rehabilitation should emphasize mobilization as early as postoperative day 1 and athletes should not return to play earlier than 9 months following their surgery. No specific rehab protocols have been defined otherwise (6)[C].
- Chronic injuries typically require high tibial osteotomy to correct varus malalignment prior to proceeding to PLC reconstruction (6)[C].

ONGOING CARE

COMPLICATIONS

- Fibular nerve injury
- Vascular injury
- Physical injury
- Multiple ligamentous injury
- If ACL or PCL is repaired and PLC injury is missed, early arthritis and graft failure are highly likely.
- Arthrofibrosis (1)[B],(3)[B],(4)[B]

REFERENCES

1. Chahla J, Moatshe G, Dean CS, et al. Posterolateral corner of the knee: current concepts. *Arch Bone Jt Surg*. 2016;4(2):97–103.
2. Swinford ST, LaPrade R, Engebretsen L, et al. Biomechanics and physical examination of the posteromedial and posterolateral knee: state of the art. *J ISAKOS*. 2020;5:378–388.
3. Pacheco RJ, Ayre CA, Bollen SR. Posterolateral corner injuries of the knee: a serious injury commonly missed. *J Bone Joint Surg Br*. 2011;93(2):194–197.
4. Schweller EW, Ward PJ. Posterolateral corner knee injuries: review of anatomy and clinical evaluation. *J Am Osteopath Assoc*. 2015;115(12):725–731.
5. Figueroa F, Figueroa D, Putnis S, et al. Posterolateral corner knee injuries: a narrative review. *EFORT Open Rev*. 2021;6(8):676–685.
6. Chahla J, Murray IR, Robinson J, et al. Posterolateral corner of the knee: an expert consensus statement on diagnosis, classification, treatment, and rehabilitation. *Knee Surg Sports Traumatol Arthrosc*. 2019;27(8):2520–2529.

ADDITIONAL READING

- Arthur A, LaPrade RF, Agel J. Proximal tibial opening wedge osteotomy as the initial treatment for chronic posterolateral corner deficiency in the varus knee. *Am J Sports Med*. 2007;35(11):1844–1850.
- Geiger D, Chang E, Pathria M, et al. Posterolateral and posteromedial corner injuries of the knee. *Radiol Clin North Am*. 2013;51(3):413–432.
- LaPrade R. Posterolateral knee injuries. Robert LaPrade MD, PhD: Complex Knee and Sports Medicine Specialist. Accessed August 26, 2025. https://drrobertlaprademd.com/posterolateral-knee-injuries-posterolateral-corner-knee-injury-outside-of-knee-pain-twin-cities-minnesota/
- Sekiya JK, Swaringen JC, Wojtys EM, et al. Diagnostic ultrasound evaluation of posterolateral corner knee injuries. *Arthroscopy*. 2010;26(4):494–499.
- Stiell IG, Greenberg GH, Wells GA, et al. Prospective validation of a decision rule for the use of radiography in acute knee injuries. *JAMA*. 1996;275(8):611–615.
- Stoller DW. The knee. In: *Stoller's Atlas of Orthopaedics and Sports Medicine*. Wolters Kluwer/Lippincott Williams & Wilkins; 2008:261–424.
- Vinson EN, Major NM, Helms CA. The posterolateral corner of the knee. *AJR Am J Roentgenol*. 2008;190(2):449–458.
- Weiss S, Krause M, Frosch KH. Posterolateral corner of the knee: a systematic literature review of current concepts of arthroscopic reconstruction. *Arch Orthop Trauma Surg*. 2020;140(12):2003–2012.

CLINICAL PEARLS

- Be thorough with every patient. PLC injuries are easily overlooked and are often associated with other ligamentous and neurovascular injuries. Clinicians should not let themselves be distracted by torn cruciate ligaments.
- Look for Segond and arcuate fractures on radiographs.
- Evaluate whole knee (i.e., Ottawa Knee Rules are a good start when looking for other pathology).
- Because this injury is often associated with multiligament pathology, some clinicians consult orthopedic surgery on every suspected case.
- Definitive algorithms for more precise diagnosis and treatment are still being developed.

PREGNANCY IN SPORTS

David E. Olson, MD, CAQSM, FACSM ▪ Nardos Dawit, MD ▪ Rebekah Fiers, MD

BASICS

American College of Obstetricians and Gynecologists (ACOG) 2020 recommendations for exercise in pregnancy:

- People without contraindications should and can safely participate in aerobic and strength exercise when pregnant.
- In the absence of either medical or obstetrical complications, pregnant people should participate in at least 150 minutes of moderate-intensity aerobic activity per week. There is no evidence that this is detrimental to the pregnant person or fetus if the pregnancy is uncomplicated.
- A thorough clinical evaluation should be performed prior to the initiation of any exercise program. In the absence of contraindications, regular and moderate intensity exercise is advised and has been shown to benefit most people. Pregnant people should be counseled on warning signs of when to stop exercise.
- Avoid activities with a high risk of falling or trauma such as hockey, soccer, basketball, gymnastics, horseback riding, downhill skiing, vigorous racquet sports, and scuba diving. Pregnant people should avoid exercises where they will be in the supine position or exposed to prolonged motionless standing.
- Pregnant people who plan to exercise at altitudes of >6,000 feet should be made aware of signs of altitude sickness.
- Recommended exercises include walking, hiking, jogging/running, aerobic dance, swimming, cycling, rowing, cross-country skiing, and dancing.
- Athletes participating in National Collegiate Athletic Association (NCAA) or professional sports may continue to participate in sports during the early phases of pregnancy. However, they should be made aware of the risks and benefits of continued participation in high-level sports, and they should be monitored more closely.
- As pregnancy progresses, athletic performance tends to decline. The physical demands of high-intensity training should be balanced with close monitoring of body temperature, hydration status, and weight. Patients engaged in high-intensity training should be seen more frequently than their routine prenatal visits.
- Gradual resumption of exercise in the postpartum period is advised.
- Return to physical activity after pregnancy has been associated with decreased incidence of postpartum depression and postpartum recovery time (1),(2),(3).

ETIOLOGY AND PATHOPHYSIOLOGY

- Thermoregulation:
  - In active nonpregnant people, exercise can elevate body temperature >103°F (39.2°C). Current recommendations are that core body temperature should not rise >1.5°C above resting temperature or >38.9°C during exercise in pregnancy (2),(4),(5).
  - Studies show that pregnant people appear well protected against hyperthermia even during prolonged exercise when the intensity is low. However, nearly all previous studies have been performed in pregnant people who trained prior to the study, and no prospective trials exist that focus primarily on the risk of elevated temperatures. Also, no human study has elicited an increase of >1.1°C in maternal core temperature during pregnancy in response to exercise (4),(6),(7),(8).
- Metabolic changes:
  - Utilization of glucose is of potential concern for the fetus. However, no studies have shown an actual decrease in fetal growth during exercise because there is likely increased glucose delivery after exercise, and pregnant people who exercise may have an increased placental size. Regular aerobic exercise has been shown to lower fasting and postprandial glucose concentrations in several small studies of previously sedentary individuals with gestational diabetes mellitus (GDM) (2),(7),(9),(10),(11).
- Lower back and pelvic pain:
  - These symptoms are commonly associated with hormonal change and shift in the point of gravity. The increased levels of estrogen and relaxin in pregnancy lead to ligamentous laxity associated with back and pelvic pain.
  - Symptoms may be exacerbated with weight-bearing and activity.
  - Sitting, rest, and recumbency often ameliorate symptoms, and good results have been seen following acupuncture and use of a pelvic binder.
  - Hyperlordosis of pregnancy is associated with ligamentous laxity and contributes to low back pain.
  - Pubic symphysis pain is caused by widening of the pubic symphysis due in part to the effects of relaxin:
    - Rupture of the pubic symphysis is a rare complication.
    - Treatment is generally conservative.
    - Consideration of operative intervention is needed if diastasis is >4 cm (1),(2).
- Cardiopulmonary changes:
  - Cardiac output may increase up to 45% by as early as 24 weeks' gestation.
  - After 20 weeks' gestation, cardiac output is greatly influenced by body position. Specifically, a recumbent position may decrease cardiac output due to aortocaval compression by the uterus causing decreased venous return.
  - Decreased splanchnic blood flow may result from the effects of exercise potentially compromising uterine or umbilical artery blood flow:
    - Doppler ultrasound (US) has shown no change in perfusion to either artery.
    - An increase in fetal heart rate (FHR) by 10 to 30 beats/min may occur during or after maternal exercise.
    - A small percentage of fetuses have developed bradycardia or decelerations in response to maternal exercise. Episodes of bradycardia resolved within 2 minutes and were not thought to be substantial enough to result in fetal hypoxia. Additionally, there were no identifiable adverse birth outcomes (1),(2).
    - Iron supplementation is advised. It is not uncommon for a pregnant female to have a hemoglobin of 12.5 mg/dL or less due to increased plasma volume and hemodilution (2),(7).

GENERAL PREVENTION

- Warning signs to terminate exercise while pregnant (1),(3),(4):
  - Vaginal bleeding
  - Dyspnea prior to exertion
  - Dizziness
  - Headache
  - Chest pain
  - Muscle weakness affecting balance
  - Calf pain or swelling
  - Regular painful contractions
  - Decreased fetal movements
  - Amniotic fluid leakage
- Absolute contraindications to exercise in pregnancy (1),(2),(3),(4),(12):
  - Incompetent cervix/cerclage
  - Fetal growth restriction (FGR)
  - Multiple gestations (more than triplets)
  - Persistent 2nd- or 3rd-trimester bleeding
  - Placenta previa after 25 to 28 weeks' gestation
  - Severe preeclampsia
  - Premature labor during current pregnancy
  - Premature rupture of membranes

COMMONLY ASSOCIATED CONDITIONS

- Orthopedic considerations during pregnancy include:
  - Soft tissue swelling in the 2nd and 3rd trimesters; this may manifest as carpal tunnel syndrome (CTS):
    - Elevated prolactin, fluid retention, and hand positioning during nursing may worsen symptoms.
  - de Quervain tenosynovitis and meralgia paresthetica, neuropathy of the lateral femoral cutaneous nerve, are often seen.
  - Symptoms from nerve compression syndromes typically resolve after pregnancy and should be treated conservatively.
  - Night splints can relieve CTS, and steroid injections are useful in patients with recalcitrant symptoms. Similar treatments are recommended for de Quervain patients. For patients with meralgia paresthetica, loose-fitting clothes, positional changes, and activity modification often relieve symptoms.
- In late pregnancy and after delivery, transient changes in cortisol and clotting factors can lead to femoral head osteonecrosis:
  - Symptoms can include antalgic gait, pain at rest, and painful range of motion.
  - Treatment consists of restricted weight-bearing; avoid surgery until after delivery.

- Transient osteoporosis of pregnancy should be suspected in any patient with an antalgic gait and complaints of pain with activity, with minimal pain at rest (5),(6),(9):
  - Usually presents in the 3rd trimester and plain anteroposterior (AP) radiographs with appropriate shielding often show diffuse osteopenia of the pelvis:
    - Magnetic resonance imaging (MRI) may show high-intensity signal in the bone marrow on T2 images.
  - Treatment consists of protected weight-bearing. Use of calcitonin is controversial but may shorten the duration of symptoms; bisphosphonate exposure during gestation may lead to decreased fetal bone growth.
  - Transient osteoporosis of pregnancy usually results in a self-limited course with no long-term sequelae; however, failure to properly diagnose could lead to fracture.
  - Serial exams are important to distinguish between these conditions. The clinician should try to avoid unnecessary radiographs because hip pain is common in pregnancy.

ONGOING CARE

Specific sport recommendations include (1),(2):

- Stationary upright cycling is recommended by the Society of Obstetricians and Gynecologists of Canada (SOGC) and American College of Sports Medicine (ACSM):
  - FHR and maternal temperature are not negatively affected. However, there may be more variability of FHR and maternal temperature with higher intensity and longer duration exercise.
  - No negative fetal outcomes have been reported.
  - Cycling for 30 minutes at a maternal heart rate around 140 beats/min or exercising for 15 minutes at a rate of 155 beats/min is recommended.
- Swimming is an optimal exercise during pregnancy due to buoyant effects and the thermally conductive properties of water. It is recommended by ACOG, SOGC, and ACSM:
  - Baseline FHR may be less affected by swimming than cycling (1),(3),(10).
- Many pregnant women use walking as a primary means of exercise throughout pregnancy:
  - Walking is recommended by ACOG, SOGC, and ACSM. It increases maternal sense of well-being and decreases physical complaints.
  - It has not been shown to have a negative effect on maternal weight gain or on labor outcomes (1),(2).
- Weight-training exercises and physical therapy have been recommended by ACOG to help maintain posture and prevent low back pain:
  - No incidents of adverse effects have been reported with light to moderate weight training with free weights or weight machines.
  - Moderate strength conditioning has been shown to be safe in a healthy pregnancy with no obvious positive or negative effects; minimal FHR changes from baseline may be noted; fetal wakefulness is increased.
  - Avoid weight training in the supine position late in gestation (1),(2).
- SCUBA diving is not endorsed by the ACOG:
  - Those who dive frequently and professionally are at 3 to 6 times greater risk for spontaneous abortion, FGR, and fetal malformation (1).
- High-altitude exercise: Few cases of injury have been reported with exercises such as skiing, hiking, mountain biking, and running:
  - Pregnancy complications such as low birth weight occur at a higher rate at altitudes >10,000 feet. SOGC has suggested to modify or avoid mountain climbing all together. Cycling with short bursts of moderate to high intensity at altitude levels of 6,000 and 7,300 feet have been reported without injury to mother or fetus (10). Most studies have looked at sedentary pregnant individuals, more research is needed in elite athletes (13).
  - Sports with abdominal trauma risk from contact or falling such as downhill skiing, water skiing, horseback riding, road cycling, surfing, basketball, vigorous racquet sports, ice hockey, soccer, and gymnastics are discouraged (3).
- Running can become uncomfortable later in gestation:
  - Jogging is supported by ACOG. It may enhance placental growth, indicating a healthy pregnancy outcome (14).
- People who continue to exercise throughout pregnancy generally maintain their training regimens and level of fitness. Among these pregnant people, cardiovascular risk level generally continues well below levels among the general populace and pregnant people who temporarily stopped exercise during pregnancy (10),(14).

REFERENCES

1. Committee on Obstetric Practice. Physical Activity and Exercise During Pregnancy and the Postpartum Period. Committee Opinion Number 804. 2020. Accessed August 16, 2025. https://www.acog.org/clinical/clinical-guidance/committee-opinion/articles/2020/04/physical-activity-and-exercise-during-pregnancy-and-the-postpartum-period
2. Artal R, O'Toole M. Guidelines of the American College of Obstetricians and Gynecologists for exercise during pregnancy and the postpartum period. *Br J Sports Med.* 2003;37(1):6–12.
3. Kramer MS, McDonald SW. Aerobic exercise for pregnant people during pregnancy. *Cochrane Database Syst Rev.* 2006;(3):CD000180.
4. Olson DA, Sikka RS, Hayman J, et al. Exercise in pregnancy. *Curr Sports Med Rep.* 2009;8(3):147–153.
5. Ritchie JR. Orthopedic considerations during pregnancy. *Clin Obstet Gynecol.* 2003;46(2):456–466.
6. Artal R, Fortunato V, Welton A, et al. A comparison of cardiopulmonary adaptations to exercise in pregnancy at sea level and altitude. *Am J Obstet Gynecol.* 1995;172(4 Pt 1):1170–1178.
7. Clapp JF III. Exercise during pregnancy: a clinical update. *Clin Sports Med.* 2000;19(2):273–286.
8. Soultanakis-Aligianni HN. Thermoregulation during exercise in pregnancy. *Clin Obstet Gynecol.* 2003;46(2):442–455.
9. Borg-Stein J, Dugan SA, Gruber J. Musculoskeletal aspects of pregnancy. *Am J Phys Med Rehabil.* 2005;84(3):180–192.
10. Clapp JF III. Long-term outcome after exercising throughout pregnancy: fitness and cardiovascular risk. *Am J Obstet Gynecol.* 2008;199(5):489.e1–489.e6.
11. Magro-Malosso ER, Saccone G, Di Tommaso M, et al. Exercise during pregnancy and risk of gestational hypertensive disorders: a systematic review and meta-analysis. *Acta Obstet Gynecol Scand.* 2017;96(8):921–931.
12. Meah VL, Davies GA, Davenport MH. Why can't I exercise during pregnancy? Time to revisit medical 'absolute' and 'relative' contraindications: systematic review of evidence of harm and a call to action. *Br J Sports Med.* 2020;54:1395–1404.
13. McManis BG. Integrative review of exercise at altitude during pregnancy. *Int J Environ Res Public Health.* 2021;18(17):9272.
14. Guerra JJ, Steinberg ME. Distinguishing transient osteoporosis from avascular necrosis of the hip. *J Bone Joint Surg Am.* 1995;77(4):616–624.

ADDITIONAL READING

- Cunningham FG, Gant NF, Leveno KJ, et al, eds. *Williams Obstetrics.* 21st ed. McGraw-Hill; 2001
- Drinkwater B, Artal R. Heat stress and pregnancy. In: Mittlemark R, Drinkwater B, eds. *Exercise in Pregnancy.* Williams and Wilkins; 1991.

CLINICAL PEARLS

- Positive effects of exercise during pregnancy include potential risk reduction for development of GDM, pregnancy-induced hypertension (HTN), and preeclampsia; decreased rate of cesarean section and operative deliveries; also, a decrease in postpartum depression symptoms and decreased incidence of urinary incontinence (1),(11).
- Exercise during pregnancy does not increase the risk for preterm birth.
- The cardiovascular benefits of exercise are the same for pregnant people as they are for nonpregnant people.
- Exercise in morbidly obese pregnant people may have a preventative effect on the development of GDM.
- All pregnant people should be evaluated for medical and/or obstetrical contraindications prior to beginning an exercise regimen (1),(3),(4).
- Recreational and competitive athletes with uncomplicated pregnancies should remain active. They should be monitored by regular prenatal visits unless participating in high-intensity exercise.
- Sedentary individuals without contraindications should be encouraged to begin exercising for the health benefits.
- Pregnant people participating in higher intensity sports should be monitored closely throughout their pregnancy.

PRIMARY BONE AND SOFT TISSUE TUMORS

William Andrew, DO, CAQSM

BASICS

DESCRIPTION

Heterogenous group of neoplasms of the skeleton and nonepithelial extraskeletal supportive tissue that may mimic a variety of sports injuries making early recognition and diagnoses crucial (1)

EPIDEMIOLOGY

- Rare—<1% of newly diagnosed malignancies worldwide (2),(3)
- Bone tumors
  - Malignant
    - Osteosarcoma (37%)
    - Chondrosarcoma (23.6%)
    - Ewing sarcoma (12.2%)
- Soft tissue tumors
  - Lower extremity: 45%
  - Upper extremity: 15%
  - Head and neck: 10%
  - Retroperitoneum: 15%
  - Chest and abdomen: 15%
  - Viscera, connective tissue: rare

Incidence

- Primary bone tumors
  - Approximately 3,970 cases (2,160 in males; 1,810 in females) are projected to be diagnosed in the United State in 2023.
  - Bimodal: peak in 2nd decade of life (osteochondroma, osteosarcoma, Ewing sarcoma) and increasing after 5th decade of life (chondrosarcoma, chondroma, Paget, and radiation-induced sarcomas)
  - Majority of benign bone tumors arise in the 1st and 2nd decade of life (solitary and aneurysmal bone cysts, nonossifying fibromas, fibrous cortical defects, enchondromas, osteoblastoma, osteoid osteoma, chondroblastoma, Langerhans cell histiocytosis).
- Soft tissue tumors
  - Approximately 13,400 cases (7,400 in males; 6,000 in females) are projected to be diagnosed in the United State in 2023.
  - Slow increase until a sharp increase after 6th decade of life

Prevalence

- Primary bone tumors
  - <1% of newly diagnosed malignancies worldwide (2),(3)
  - Most common overall is osteosarcoma, followed by chondrosarcoma, and Ewing sarcoma.
    - In adults, the most common is chondrosarcoma, osteosarcoma, and chordomas.
    - In children and teens, the most common is osteosarcoma, Ewing sarcoma, and chondrosarcoma.
- Primary soft tissue tumors
  - <1% of all malignant solid tumors in adults (2)
  - Most common overall is undifferentiated pleomorphic sarcoma, followed by liposarcoma, and leiomyosarcoma.

ETIOLOGY AND PATHOPHYSIOLOGY

- Variable
  - Tumors with specific translocations (Ewing sarcoma, aneurysmal bone cyst, mesenchymal chondrosarcoma)
  - Gene mutations or amplifications or deletions (chondrosarcoma, fibrous dysplasia, chordoma osteochondroma)
  - Genetic instability with complex karyotypes (osteosarcoma)
- Soft tissue tumors
  - Mostly sporadic mutations
  - Less commonly syndromic causes, radiation, carcinogens, or chronic lymphedema

Genetics

- Majority occurs de novo.
- Although there are multiple genetic syndrome associations
  - Neurofibromatosis, Li-Fraumeni syndrome, retinoblastoma
  - Other hereditary cancer syndromes

RISK FACTORS

- Strong evidence
  - Radiation (2)
  - HHV8 infection (Kaposi sarcoma)
- Suggestive evidence
  - Hernias (pediatric sarcomas)
  - Adolescent growth factors (pediatric sarcomas)
  - Occupational exposure (adult sarcomas)
  - Herbicides and chlorophenol exposure (soft tissue tumors)
  - Place of residence/industrial emissions (soft tissue tumors)

DIAGNOSIS

HISTORY

- Pain and/or local swelling that may pre-date any injury
- Pain is more common in bony tumors, less in soft tissue tumors (1),(2),(4).
- Concerning symptoms include (1),(2),(4):
  - Pain of or proportion
  - Longer than expected duration of pain
- Unreliable symptoms include (1),(2),(4):
  - Night pain without improvement with rest (neither sensitive nor specific)
  - Constitution symptoms (not sensitive)

PHYSICAL EXAM

- Thoroughly palpate local and adjacent bony and soft tissue structures and assess range of motion and gait (1),(2),(4).
- May or may not have an appreciable mass; however, concerning features include (1),(2),(4)):
  - Fixed
  - >4 cm diameter
  - Deep to subcutaneous tissue

DIFFERENTIAL DIAGNOSIS

- Metastatic disease
  - Assess for concomitant malignancy.
  - Advanced imaging may help distinguish from primary lesions (1),(2),(4).
  - Most common: prostate, breast, kidney, thyroid, and lung (1),(2),(4)
  - Less common: colorectal, stomach, bladder (1),(2),(4)
  - Axial metastases more common than appendicular due to presence of red bone marrow (1),(2),(4)
- Hematomas
  - Be sure to distinguish from a soft tissue sarcoma that has additional internal hemorrhaging.
    - Magnetic resonance imaging (MRI) may show soft tissue swelling and subcutaneous ecchymosis that would *not* be present in sarcomas (1),(2),(4).
    - Soft tissue sarcoma capsules usually contain hemorrhage, so superficial ecchymosis may be more suggestive of a hematoma (1),(2),(4).
- Stress fractures
  - Assess for new strenuous activity, relative energy deficiency in sport (RED-S).
  - May have similar x-ray findings (sclerosis, reactive bone with periosteal elevation) (2),(4)
  - Consider MRI if refractory to rest.

- Compartment syndrome
  - Distinguish with acuity and evidence of neurovascular compromise.
- Exertional compartment syndrome
  - Activity association may distinguish from tumor.
- Venous thromboembolism
  - Assess risk factors.
  - Evaluate with sonogram.

DIAGNOSTIC TESTS & INTERPRETATION

- Radiography
  - Soft tissue processes and calcification/mineralization (5)
  - Include adjacent joints if there is concern for referred pain (5).
  - 30–50% of trabecular bone needs to be destroyed before a lesion is visible on x-ray (5).
  - Tumor pattern may distinguish between benign and aggressive behavior (5).
- CT
  - May help characterize extent of bony lesions and percutaneous image-guided biopsy planning if indicated (5)
- MRI
  - Generally the imaging modality of choice
  - Always get MRI with and without contrast if concerned about cancer (5).
    Can help characterize malignant features, lesion size/extension
  - Can help rule out for similarly presenting pathology, for example, hematoma, stress fracture
- Biopsy
  - Required for definitive diagnosis, although only done if there is concern for malignant process in which case wide margin excision is usually performed

Initial Tests (lab, imaging)

- See above for initial imaging.
- May consider the following labs (2):
  - Comprehensive metabolic panel (CMP)
  - γ-Glutamyl transferase (GGT)
  - Complete blood count (CBC)

Follow-Up Tests & Special Considerations

Prompt referral to orthopedic or surgical oncology

Diagnostic Procedures/Other

Per oncology

- Generally excisional biopsy

Test Interpretation

Per pathology

TREATMENT

GENERAL MEASURES

- Per oncology
- May initiate supportive care if symptomatic
  - Relative rest, activity modification, protection, topical modalities such as heat/ice, over-the-counter analgesics
  - Reasonable to consider prescription pain medications including cautious use of opioids for severe pain

MEDICATION

Pain control as above

First Line

Per oncology

ISSUES FOR REFERRAL

See above.

ADDITIONAL THERAPIES

Per oncology

SURGERY/OTHER PROCEDURES

Per oncology

COMPLEMENTARY & ALTERNATIVE MEDICINE

- Supportive care (See above.)
- Massage
- Acupuncture
- Osteopathic manipulation

ADMISSION, INPATIENT, AND NURSING CONSIDERATIONS

Per oncology

ONGOING CARE

FOLLOW-UP RECOMMENDATIONS

Per oncology

Patient Monitoring

Per oncology

PROGNOSIS

Variable with factors including:

- Tumor size and depth
- Histology and stage
- Genetic profile

COMPLICATIONS

- Variable
- Mostly involving mass effect and postoperative sequelae

REFERENCES

1. Krych A, Odland A, Rose P, et al. Oncologic conditions that simulate common sports injuries. *J Am Acad Orthop Surg*. 2014;22(4):223–234.
2. Ferguson JL, Turner SP. Bone cancer: diagnosis and treatment principles. *Am Fam Physician*. 2018;98(4):205–213.
3. Mirabello L, Troisi RJ, Savage SA. International osteosarcoma incidence patterns in children and adolescents, middle ages and elderly persons. *Int J Cancer*. 2009;125(1):229–234.
4. Green NM, Abas S, Sajid S, et al. Presentation of bone tumours: clinical findings and initial management of patients. *Orthop Trauma*. 2021;35(3):108–114.
5. Bestic JM, Wessell DE, Beaman FD, et al. ACR Appropriateness Criteria® primary bone tumors. *J Am Coll Radiol*. 2020;17(5S):S226–S238.

ADDITIONAL READING

Conrad EU III, ed. *Orthopedic Oncology: Diagnosis and Treatment*. Thieme; 2009.

CLINICAL PEARLS

- Early diagnosis and expedited referral are key to management.
- Suspect if symptoms not related to activity or if there is a delay in expected recovery.
- Low threshold for early imaging, at a minimum radiographs with preference for MRI with and without contrast
- Appropriate specialty care includes orthopedic oncology (if available) or surgical oncology and may include medical oncology and general orthopedics.

PRONATOR SYNDROME

Kevin E. Burroughs, MD, CAQSM, FAMSSM • Chadwick C. Nabors, DO, CAQSM

BASICS

Median nerve compression, typically by the pronator teres (PT) muscle, leading to a combination of symptoms including volar forearm pain with varied median neuropathy symptoms such as weakness and sensory changes, usually provoked by repetitive activity.

DESCRIPTION

- Pronator syndrome (PS) is a collective term for conditions that cause a compressive neuropathy of the median nerve at the elbow and proximal forearm.
- Classically, and most commonly, it involves entrapment of the proximal median nerve between the humeral and ulnar heads of the PT muscle, although other pathologic sites of median nerve compression at the elbow and forearm must be considered.
- Other primary pathologic sites of compression include:
  - The lacertus fibrosus (LF) or bicipital aponeurosis
  - A fibrous arch of the flexor digitorum superficialis (FDS) also called the sublimis arch
  - Ligament of Struthers (1),(2)
- An accessory head of the flexor pollicis longus (FPL) also called the Gantzer muscle (1)
- Synonym(s): lacertus fibrosus syndrome; pronator teres syndrome; sublimis bridge syndrome

EPIDEMIOLOGY

- Relatively uncommon but should be considered in any patient with median neuropathy including those with carpal tunnel symptoms or volar hand numbness
- Carpal tunnel syndrome (CTS) is responsible for >90% of cases of median nerve entrapment neuropathies (1).

Prevalence

- Usually presents in a gradual onset of symptoms in the 4th and 5th decade and 4 times more common in women (1),(2)
- Delay in diagnosis ranging from 9 months to 2 years
- Sudden onset of symptoms is more likely to occur in younger and more active population as a result of sports or weightlifting injuries.

ETIOLOGY AND PATHOPHYSIOLOGY

- The median nerve receives contributions from C5 to C8 and part of T1 at the level of the brachial plexus.
- The PT muscle is the most common site of compression of the proximal median nerve.
  - The PT usually has both humeral (superficial) and ulnar (deep) heads, but the deep head can be absent in up to 45% of people and be replaced with a fibrous structure.
  - The median nerve typically courses between the two heads of the PT, but it can run deep to both heads or pierce either head.
- LF or bicipital aponeurosis is a fascial extension of the distal biceps tendon that extends across the antecubital fossa obliquely. It may compress the median nerve as it crosses over it.
- The FDS comprises of two heads and either one or both heads may form fibrous arches, sublimes arch, that overly the median nerve as a potential site of compression.
- Compression can also occur proximally as it passes under the ligament of Struthers which is a fibrous arch extending from the supracondylar process at the medial aspect of the distal 1/3 of the humerus (approximately 3 to 6 cm proximal to the medial epicondyle) to the medial epicondyle. This occurs in only 1–2% of the population.
- Another site of compression can be due to an accessory muscle of the FPL also known as the *Gantzer muscle* which is present in 20–75% of individuals.
- Compression between the heads of the PT muscle is the most common etiology, with the sublimis arch being the second most common (1).

RISK FACTORS

- Repetitive occupational pronation/supination (i.e., carpenters)
- Acute forceful pronation or wrist flexion
- Weight lifters with hypertrophied pronator-flexor mass

DIAGNOSIS

HISTORY

- Typically, patients complain of an aching or fatigue-like pain in proximal forearm. Other symptoms may include occasional hand pain, dysesthesias of the radial 3 1/2 digits, and cramping in the hand (writer's cramp).
- Many report an increase in pain with exercise or an increase in activity, especially with pronation and gripping.
- Frank hand weakness occurs only in long-standing or severe cases.
- Motor and sensory symptoms can be poorly defined.
- Onset typically is insidious, but a specific event may cause a sudden increase in pain.
- Typically, pain does not occur at night, as it would with CTS.

PHYSICAL EXAM

- Thickened or hypertrophied pronator muscle mass
- Tenderness or positive Tinel sign proximal and lateral to the proximal edge of the pronator muscle typical.
- Pronator compression testing involves applying pressure over the PT (approximately 6 cm distal to the elbow crease and 4 cm lateral to the medial epicondyle in adults), and in the course of the median nerve for 30 seconds and is positive if paresthesias are provoked. This can be accentuated by resisted pronation with the elbow flexed 0 to 45 degrees.
- Compression at this site causes pain or paresthesias radiating to the palm and/or radial 3 1/2 digits within 30 seconds of compression.
- May have weakness or atrophy of the hand intrinsics innervated by the median nerve (LOAF muscles): lumbricals (first two on radial side of hand), opponens pollicis, abductor pollicis brevis, and flexor pollicis brevis
- May have weakness of the extrinsic finger flexors, wrist flexors, and pronator quadratus

ALERT

PS should not have a Tinel sign at the wrist nor reproduction of symptoms with nerve compression testing at the wrist.

- Tests of spinner can determine location of median nerve entrapment (1):
  - Pain or paresthesia reproduced with resisted flexion of the forearm in a position of >120 degrees of elbow extension, maximal supination: lacertus entrapment of median nerve
  - Reproduction of pain or paresthesia with resisted pronation (forearm in neutral) as the elbow is extended: pronator entrapment of median nerve.
  - Reproduction of symptoms with resisted proximal interphalangeal (PIP) joint flexion of the middle finger with forearm fully supinated and elbow extended: FDS entrapment of median nerve (caution, can be present with CTS as well)

DIFFERENTIAL DIAGNOSIS

- CTS (common): *Double crush phenomena* can occur where both CTS and PS appear in same arm.
  - Consider possibility in those who have failed CTS surgery.
  - Although there is data to suggest that patient's with and without double crush phenomena have similar clinical benefit after carpal tunnel release (3)
  - The prevalence of PS among patients with CTS is 6–11.5% (2).
- C6 or C7 radiculopathy (common)
- Anterior interosseous syndrome (Kiloh-Nevin syndrome) (uncommon, motor function affected, *not sensory symptoms*)
- Thoracic outlet syndrome (rare)
- Neuralgic amyotrophy (brachial neuritis, Parsonage-Turner syndrome) (rare)

DIAGNOSTIC TESTS & INTERPRETATION

The diagnosis of PS is best made through history and physical exam, although other diagnostic modalities may help to confirm the diagnosis and can exclude other conditions (1).

Initial Tests (lab, imaging)

- Plain radiographs of the elbow rule out bone involvement such as a *supracondylar process* (exostosis that attaches to ligament of Struthers).
- Magnetic resonance imaging (MRI)

ALERT

The median nerve often is poorly depicted at the elbow due to the minimal amount of perifascial fat in this region; *MRI is not indicated* for the diagnosis of PS but may be used for excluding other etiologies. The nerve can look normal at the site of entrapment.

- On MRI, the PT and other muscles innervated by the median nerve distal to the site of the lesion may show abnormally high signal intensity on T2-weighted, fat-suppressed, short tau inversion recovery (STIR), or T1-weighted images, or atrophy in more advanced cases (4).

Diagnostic Procedures/Other

Electrodiagnostic testing:

- Needle electromyography (EMG) can be helpful in confirming the diagnosis but cannot be completely relied upon as majority (69–93%) of cases of PS have negative electrodiagnostic testing (1).
- On EMG, a positive test may show slow motor conduction in the forearm with normal distal motor latency (1).

ALERT

In the electrodiagnostic evaluation of CTS, EMG of muscles innervated by the median nerve proximal to the wrist should also be performed to decrease unnecessary carpal tunnel surgeries.

TREATMENT

GENERAL MEASURES

- Small studies show a wide range of improvement in nonsurgical interventions, but no randomized trials have been performed; up to 3 to 6 months of conservative treatment is recommended (2),(5)[C].
- Rehabilitation is the initial treatment and can be summarized using the acronym APORIM:
  - *Activity modification*: avoidance of provocative activities
  - *Protection* from external compression
  - *Orthoses*: Night splints to prevent excessive elbow flexion and pronation can be considered.
  - *Rehabilitation*: Assess proximal and distal kinetic chain (shoulder girdle and wrist) for strength, flexibility, and movement; forearm flexor muscle stretching, nerve-gliding exercises
  - *Injections* can be considered at point of compression, but exercise caution to avoid direct injection into nerve bundle.
  - *Medication*: nonsteroidal or steroid anti-inflammatory medications
- Ultrasound-guided nerve hydrodissection with saline or dextrose has been described in small case series.

SURGERY/OTHER PROCEDURES

- Surgical management is controversial unless there is a clear compressive area discovered.
- If conservative measures fail, or if muscle atrophy or denervation occurs, one should consider exploration and release of all potential sites of entrapment.
- For a proven supracondylar process, excision of the bone prominence and release of the ligament of Struthers should provide resolution.
- Surgical approaches vary, but most recommend complete decompression of the median nerve in the upper forearm:
  - In retrospective studies, approximately 80% of patients, there was complete or partial resolution of symptoms with open surgical decompression within 6 weeks (1)[B].
  - Endoscopic release continues to be a growing treatment option and has shown to be an effective option for patients with PS (6).

ONGOING CARE

Postsurgical intervention, active range of motion as early as postoperative day 2, with full return to activity by 6 to 8 weeks (1)

REFERENCES

1. Adler JA, Wolf JM. Proximal median nerve compression: pronator syndrome. *J Hand Surg Am*. 2020;45(12):1157–1165.
2. Binsaleem S. Median nerve entrapment neuropathy: a review on the pronator syndrome. *JSES Rev Rep Tech*. 2024;5(1):70–78.
3. Hansen LM, Jiang EX, Hodson NM, et al. Patients with and without double crush syndrome achieve similar rates of clinical improvement following carpal tunnel release. *Hand (N Y)*. 2025;20(4):549–554.
4. Ku V, Cox C, Mikeska A, et al. Magnetic resonance neurography for evaluation of peripheral nerves. *J Brachial Plex Peripher Nerve Inj*. 2021;16(1):e17–e23.
5. Boyd CJ, Singh NP, Robin JX, et al. Compression neuropathies of the upper extremity: a review. *Surgeries*. 2021;2(3):320–334.
6. Barnett SA, Shah SA, Ahmad RI. Endoscopic proximal median nerve decompression: an alternative treatment for pronator syndrome. *J Hand Surg Glob Online*. 2021;3(4):210–214.

ADDITIONAL READING

- Balcerzak AA, Ruzik K, Tubbs RS, et al. How to differentiate pronator syndrome from carpal tunnel syndrome: a comprehensive clinical comparison. *Diagnostics (Basel)*. 2022;12(10):2433.
- Bencardino JT, Rosenberg ZS. Entrapment neuropathies of the shoulder and elbow in the athlete. *Clin Sports Med*. 2006;25(3):465–487, vi–vii.
- Chang KV, Wu WT, Hsu PC, et al. Ultrasonography in pronator teres syndrome: dynamic examination and guided hydrodissection. *Pain Med*. 2022;23(1):219–220.
- Löppönen P, Hulkkonen S, Ryhänen J. Proximal median nerve compression in the differential diagnosis of carpal tunnel syndrome. *J Clin Med*. 2022;11(14):3988.
- Tetro AM, Pichora DR. High median nerve entrapments. An obscure cause of upper-extremity pain. *Hand Clin*. 1996;12(4):691–703.
- Werner CO, Rosén I, Thorngren KG. Clinical and neurophysiologic characteristics of the pronator syndrome. *Clin Orthop Relat Res*. 1985;(197):231–236.

CLINICAL PEARLS

- Tinel test and other compression tests of the median nerve at the wrist level should be absent.
- Symptoms of PS typically do not occur at night. Also, wrist splints typically do not improve symptoms.
- Surgical intervention is typically reserved for failure of conservative treatment.
- Prognosis usually depends on the severity of median neuropathy; worse prognosis with extensive axon loss and atrophy. Expect some reinnervation of distal musculature once the median nerve is free from compromising structures.
- Postsurgical recovery is expected in 6 to 8 weeks.

PROTEINURIA IN SPORTS

Mario Gutierrez, MD, CAQSM

BASICS

DESCRIPTION

- Proteinuria is defined as the excretion of >150 mg/d of urinary protein (1).
- Macroalbuminuria implies a loss of >300 mg/d and microalbuminuria a loss of 30 to 300 mg/d (2).
- Exercise-induced proteinuria (3):
  - Transient increase in urine protein following exercise; resolves over 24 to 48 hours
  - Relatively common, benign finding
  - Proteinuria related more to exercise intensity than duration
  - Due to increased glomerular permeability and decreased tubular resorption of protein as a result of reversible physiologic change in the kidney
  - May also be due to a decrease in the intravascular volume from acute dehydration in athletes partaking in severe or extreme exercise
  - No known long-term sequelae

EPIDEMIOLOGY

- Proteinuria is common, as glomerular filtration rate (GFR) declines the prevalence can range from 6.0% to 23% (1).
- In the athletic population, prevalence between 18% and 100%, depending on type of activity and intensity (3)
- Seen in activities with higher exercise intensity, such as boxing, wrestling, gymnastics, football, and rowing
- Also seen in long-distance running and swimming

ETIOLOGY AND PATHOPHYSIOLOGY

- Factors underlying exercise-induced proteinuria include local vascular changes, local hypoxia, lactate accumulation, oxidant stress, hormonal changes, and a general septic reaction (2),(4).
- Proteins seen in the urine include:
  - Plasma proteins such as albumin, transferrin, kappa, and lambda chains
  - Tubular proteins such as secretory immunoglobulin A (IgA), Tamm-Horsfall protein
- Three categories of proteinuria (3):
  - Glomerular:
    - Increased filtration of macromolecules across the glomerular capillary wall
    - Permeability affected by increased organic acid production, renin-angiotensin system, prostaglandins, and catecholamine activation
    - Urine protein components similar to plasma proteins
    - Seen with mild-to-moderate exercise
  - Tubular:
    - Decreased resorption of filtered proteins
    - Presence of low-molecular-weight proteins
    - Due to saturation of reabsorbing mechanisms caused by a higher quantity of proteins filtered at the glomerular level
    - Seen in strenuous exercise in combination with glomerular proteinuria
  - Overflow:
    - Increased production of low-molecular-weight proteins (e.g., multiple myeloma)
    - Unless preexisting condition is present, not seen in exercise-induced proteinuria

DIAGNOSIS

The history and physical are important to differentiate benign and transient exercise-induced proteinuria from pathologic causes of proteinuria.

HISTORY

- Exercise type, intensity, and duration
- Prior history of renal disease
- Underlying conditions that may cause proteinuria
- History of recent illness
- Family history of renal disease

PHYSICAL EXAM

Identifying signs of underlying renal disease or process, including (5)[C]:

- Elevated blood pressure (BP)
- Peripheral edema
- Flank pain
- Abdominal bruits

DIFFERENTIAL DIAGNOSIS

- Transient proteinuria:
  - Orthostatic proteinuria:
    - Elevated protein excretion in upright position, with normal excretion in recumbent position
    - Most common cause of proteinuria in children (6)
    - Diagnosis is made by collecting urine throughout the day and then again in the morning after recumbent all night. If orthostatic proteinuria is present, protein level in overnight sample will be within normal limits. Elevated protein in overnight sample should prompt workup for persistent proteinuria (5)[C].

- Fever
- Stress
- Pregnancy
- Seizures
- Glomerular causes (e.g., minimal change disease, membranous glomerulonephritis)
- Tubular causes (e.g., hypertensive nephrosclerosis)
- Overflow (e.g., multiple myeloma, hemoglobinuria)
- Postrenal causes in patients with inflammation of the urinary tract (e.g., urinary tract infection [UTI], nephrolithiasis, tumors)

DIAGNOSTIC TESTS & INTERPRETATION

- Urinalysis/dipstick:
  - Inexpensive, quick screening test for proteinuria
  - Standard dipstick test measures albumin concentration via a colorimetric reaction.
  - False-positive results seen with alkaline urine; highly concentrated urine; gross hematuria; presence of certain medications (penicillin, sulfonamides, tolbutamide); and the presence of pus, semen, or vaginal secretions
  - False-negative results seen with dilute urine or when urine proteins are nonalbumin or low-molecular-weight
  - In exercise-induced proteinuria, dipstick may become positive within 30 minutes of onset of exercise and is positive for 24 to 48 hours.
  - Usually not >2+ on dipstick
  - For dipstick-positive proteinuria lasting >48 hours after a period of rest, further workup is required (3),(5)[C].
- Further workup (3),(5)[C]:
  - Blood urea nitrogen and creatinine
  - Complete blood count (CBC)
  - 24-hour urine collection for creatinine and total protein or spot protein-to-creatinine ratio
- Imaging not routinely used in exercise-induced proteinuria
- For persistent proteinuria or suspicion of renal parenchymal disease, a renal ultrasound (US) should be performed (5)[C].
- Dimercaptosuccinic acid (DMSA) scan is the preferred study to detect renal scarring (6)[C].

TREATMENT

GENERAL MEASURES

- Exercise-induced proteinuria is transient and self-limited; no specific therapy indicated
- For underlying renal disease, treatment aimed at specific cause
- Screening for proteinuria during sports preparticipation physical examination (PPE) is not recommended.

ISSUES FOR REFERRAL

Evaluation by nephrologist should be considered for:

- Persistent proteinuria, especially in patients >30 years old
- Elevated serum creatinine
- Evidence of underlying medical disease or glomerular process

ONGOING CARE

PROGNOSIS

There is no evidence that suggests these athletes are at increased risk for chronic renal disease or have any reason to limit physical activity.

REFERENCES

1. Waheed S. Assessment of proteinuria. BMJ Best Practice. Updated August 7, 2025. Accessed August 16, 2025. https://bestpractice.bmj.com/topics/en-us/875
2. Shephard RJ. Exercise proteinuria and hematuria: current knowledge and future directions. *J Sports Med Phys Fitness*. 2016;56(9):1060–1076.
3. Bellinghieri G, Savica V, Santoro D. Renal alterations during exercise. *J Ren Nutr*. 2008;18(1):158–164.
4. Saeed F, Naga Pavan Kumar Devaki P, Mahendrakar L, et al. Exercise-induced proteinuria? *J Fam Pract*. 2012;61(1):23–26.
5. Burroughs K, Spittler J. Renal and genitourinary problems. In: Madden CC, Putukian M, McCarty EC, et al. *Netter's Sports Medicine*. 2nd ed. Elsevier; 2018:222.
6. Leung AKC, Wong AHC, Barg SSN. Proteinuria in children: evaluation and differential diagnosis. *Am Fam Physician*. 2017;95(4):248–254.

CLINICAL PEARLS

- Exercise-induced proteinuria is transient, lasting 24 to 48 hours.
- Repeat testing in 48 hours after a period of rest to ensure clearance of protein.
- Persistent proteinuria requires workup for underlying renal disease.

PSEUDOANEMIA

Amity Clow, MD

BASICS

DESCRIPTION

- Dilutional phenomenon in endurance athletes leading to hemoglobin and hematocrit values that are lower than normal
- Technically, not a true "anemia" because athletes tend to have increased total mass of red blood cells in circulation, compared to sedentary individuals (1)
- Caused by plasma volume expansion by 10–20% with little change in red cell numbers (i.e., oxygen-carrying capacity) (2)
- Contributing factors include:
  - Exercise-induced release of aldosterone, renin, and vasopressin
  - Increased size of vascular bed owing to muscle hypertrophy
  - Retention of crystalloids and colloids governed by hormones
  - Oxidative stress and release of chemical factors that alter red blood cell structure and function (3)
- Theoretically, this increased blood volume decreases viscosity, thereby maximizing stroke volume, cardiac output, and subsequent oxygen delivery (4).
- Hemodilution occurs over the 48 hours after every episode of endurance exercise and may persist for as long as 1 week after discontinuing training (2).
- If training continues, red cell mass will catch up with plasma volume expansion over the span of few weeks, causing hemoglobin and hematocrit values to normalize.
- Synonym(s): sports anemia; athletes' pseudoanemia; dilutional pseudoanemia

EPIDEMIOLOGY

Incidence

- Elite athletes involved in endurance training
- Previously sedentary individuals starting an exercise program
- Athletes increasing intensity of training

DIAGNOSIS

HISTORY

Check exercise schedule, type of training activity, and occurrence of any symptoms.

PHYSICAL EXAM

- Hemoglobin levels 13 to 14 g/100 mL in men and 11 to 12 g/100 mL in women; dose-response relationship between amount/intensity of exercise and hemoglobin drop (5)
- Elite endurance athletes have a greater degree of dilutional pseudoanemia than amateur endurance athletes.
- Females are more likely than males to have iron deficiency anemia with sports ± presence of pseudoanemia.
- No particular symptoms or physical findings
- Laboratory studies are performed if etiology is unclear or symptoms are present.
- Normal mean corpuscular volume

- No hematuria or hemoglobinuria on urinalysis
- Normal bilirubin and haptoglobin
- Ferritin may be lower in endurance athletes, owing to the same relative dilutional effect; values often $<60\ \mu g/L$, occasionally $<30\ \mu g/L$, but $<15\ \mu g/L$ = iron deficiency (6)

DIFFERENTIAL DIAGNOSIS

- Iron deficiency anemia
- Gastrointestinal (GI) bleeding
- Hematuria
- Foot-strike hemolysis
- Hemolysis due to muscle contraction compressing capillaries (7)

TREATMENT

- Rule out iron deficiency anemia.
- Self-limited condition; indices return to pretraining levels after training is discontinued.
- Normal physiologic response; no treatment required

REFERENCES

1. Mairbäurl H. Red blood cells in sports: effects of exercise and training on oxygen supply by red blood cells. *Front Physiol*. 2013;4:332.
2. Eichner ER. Sports medicine pearls and pitfalls: nature's anticoagulant. *Curr Sports Med Rep*. 2009;8(1):2–3.
3. Liu CH, Tseng YF, Lai JI, et al. The changes of red blood cell viscoelasticity and sports anemia in male 24-hr ultra-marathoners. *J Chin Med Assoc*. 2018;81(5):475–481.
4. El-Sayed MS, Ali N, El-Sayed Ali Z. Haemorheology in exercise and training. *Sports Med*. 2005;35(8):649–670.
5. Chatard JC, Mujika I, Guy C, et al. Anaemia and iron deficiency in athletes. Practical recommendations for treatment. *Sports Med*. 1999;27(4):229–240.
6. Bärtsch P, Mairbäurl H, Friedmann B. Pseudo-anemia caused by sports. *Ther Umsch*. 1998;55(4):251–255.
7. Chiu YH, Lai JI, Wang SH, et al. Early changes of the anemia phenomenon in male 100-km ultramarathoners. *J Chin Med Assoc*. 2015;78(2):108–113.

ADDITIONAL READING

- Balaban EP. Sports anemia. *Clin Sports Med*. 1992;11(2):313–325.
- Raunikar RA, Sabio H. Anemia in the adolescent athlete. *Am J Dis Child*. 1992;146(10):1201–1205.
- Watts E. Athletes' anaemia. A review of possible causes and guidelines on investigation. *Br J Sports Med*. 1989;23(2):81–83.
- Weight LM, Darge BL, Jacobs P. Athletes' pseudoanemia. *Eur J Appl Physiol Occup Physiol*. 1991;62(5):358–362.

CLINICAL PEARLS

With pseudoanemia, iron supplementation does not affect occurrence or improve lab values, nor is it necessary unless there is a coexisting iron deficiency anemia.

PULMONARY CONTUSION

Douglas Comeau, DO, FAAFP, FAMSSM • Christina Kim, MD, CAQSM, FAAFP

BASICS

- The clinical syndrome, following blunt chest trauma of chest pain and respiratory difficulty, with or without hemoptysis, confirmed by findings on chest radiographs (CXRs) or other imaging:
  - Specific symptoms may include persistent and progressive shortness of breath, tachypnea, or decreasing pulse oximetry.
  - CXR or computed tomography (CT) demonstrates focal or diffuse infiltrates that *do not conform* to pulmonary lobes or segments.
  - Typically, manifests within hours of injury, peak at 72 hours, and resolves within 7 days (1)
- Although rarely reported in sports, the true incidence is not well-known:
  - Several case studies since 1997 (2),(3),(4),(5),(6)
  - Most of the literature reviews severe trauma and injury, such as motor vehicle accidents, that generally require more intervention than those reported in sports.
- Although pulmonary contusion is dramatic in presentation, athletes appear to recover and return to play within 1 week limited primarily by chest wall pain rather than respiratory status.

DESCRIPTION

- Blunt trauma to the chest causing disruption of alveolar capillary interface, resulting in collection of blood, edema, and protein in the interstitium and alveoli
- Clinical diagnosis is suggested by hemoptysis or progressive respiratory distress and confirmed by imaging.
- Synonym(s): bruised lung

EPIDEMIOLOGY

- In contact sports, chest wall contusions occur frequently and are managed by athletic trainers without being reported.
- There are several sport-reported cases of pulmonary contusion in the literature since 1997 (2),(3),(4),(5),(6).
- In all comers to an emergency department (ED) during the 1990s (7):
  - 26% of rib fractures are associated with pulmonary contusion.
  - 32% are associated with hemothorax/pneumothorax.

ETIOLOGY AND PATHOPHYSIOLOGY

Blunt trauma to the chest causing disruption of alveolar capillary interface, resulting in collection of blood, edema, and protein in the interstitium and alveoli which can lead to bronchospasm, increase in production and decrease of clearance of mucus, and decrease in production of surfactant, resulting in possible pulmonary dysfunction like ventilation/perfusion mismatch, increase in intrapulmonary shunt, increase in lung fluid, and loss of lung compliance. This results in damaged lung that is unable to exchange gas effectively in respiration.

RISK FACTORS

- Collision/contact sports
- Sports with high speeds or where the athlete is airborne:
  - Cycling, equestrian, winter sports, auto and motorcycle racing, and extreme sports

GENERAL PREVENTION

Use protective equipment and padding appropriate for the activity, such as seat restraints in motor sports to prevent ejection:

- Padding may diffuse force on impact.
- Padding after the injury can decrease pain of subsequent impacts.

COMMONLY ASSOCIATED CONDITIONS

- Chest wall contusion
- Rib fracture
- Pneumothorax
- Hemothorax
- Hemopneumothorax
- If high-velocity trauma, intra-abdominal organ injury may occur.

DIAGNOSIS

Diagnosis is suspected when an athlete sustains a blunt trauma to the chest and has respiratory difficulty:

- Hemoptysis after an injury is highly suggestive of a pulmonary contusion.

HISTORY

- Blunt nonpenetrating trauma
- Chest wall contusion is often the initial diagnosis.
- Hemoptysis may be present, but its absence does not rule out a contusion.
- Pain in the shoulder or scapular angle suggests abdominal or diaphragmatic injury.
- If a fever is present, consider infectious differential.
- Consider pulmonary parenchymal contusion when dyspnea is progressive over hours or days or if hemoptysis occurs.
- Nasal or facial trauma supports consideration of epistaxis as possible etiology of bleeding instead of pulmonary injury in the absence of obvious chest trauma.
- High-energy/velocity injuries should increase suspicion for associated injuries.

PHYSICAL EXAM

- High-velocity/energy injuries should prompt full trauma evaluation:
  - Both primary and secondary surveys should be performed.
- Dyspnea or tachypnea must be present for diagnosis, unless hemoptysis occurs.
- Palpable and pleuritic chest wall pain are present due to the impact force required to produce a pulmonary contusion.
- Arm or trunk movement may worsen chest pain.
- Dyspnea may persist after rest.
- Tender chest wall region
- Ecchymosis will not be present initially, but crepitus or more severe point tenderness is present when ribs are fractured.
- Auscultation is generally normal:
  - Consider hemopneumothorax if abnormal lung sounds are present.
  - Rales may be present.
- Inspect and record naso-oropharyngeal findings, as hemoptysis may be reported later:
  - Note any evidence of bleeding in the nose or mouth.
  - Evaluate nose and posterior pharynx for sites of bleeding, as nasal trauma or bites of cheeks or tongue are more common than pulmonary contusion as the source of blood in suspected hemoptysis.
- Evaluate for cervical (C)-spine and abdominal injuries in the presence of significant blunt trauma to the chest.
- Record serial vital signs/exams if athlete is unable to return to play to observe for deterioration:
  - Pulse oximetry <91% suggests contusion with arteriovenous (AV) shunting.
- Abdominal examination for tenderness or guarding is critical:
  - Penetrating injury occurring anteriorly at 5th rib interspace or below may penetrate the abdomen.
- Observe the chest closely for paradoxical movement of a segment of ribs indicative of flail chest.

DIFFERENTIAL DIAGNOSIS

- Pulmonary embolus
- Traumatic pneumothorax or hemothorax
- Diaphragmatic, splenic, or hepatic injury
- Pulmonary laceration or hematoma
- Spontaneous pneumothorax
- Rib fracture or contusion
- Naso-oropharyngeal trauma
- Epistaxis

DIAGNOSTIC TESTS & INTERPRETATION

Initial Tests (lab, imaging)

- Decreasing pulse oximetry (<91%) suggests pulmonary contusion with AV shunting:
  - Consider pneumothorax with low pulse oximetry.
- Posterior, anterior, and lateral CXR:
  - Rib films may not contribute to management in absence of pulmonary symptoms or clinical flail fracture.
  - Clinically significant hemopneumothorax and pneumothorax can generally be evaluated with negative radiographs; however, additional imaging should be considered based on the mechanism of injury and clinical findings, as normal radiographs do not definitively exclude underlying lung injury or rib fracture.
- Posterior, anterior, and lateral CXR reveals peripheral infiltrate in area of trauma when significant contusion occurs:
  - Generally seen within 6 hours but may take up to 48 hours for radiographic changes
  - The infiltrate may not correlate to lobular architecture.
  - Enlargement in x-ray in first 24 hours is generally a poor prognostic finding.
- CT and other imaging will be guided by the clinical picture:
  - CT may be useful to determine the need for mechanical ventilation and likelihood of pneumonia or acute respiratory distress syndrome (ARDS).
  - Ventilation/perfusion scan may show matched ventilation/perfusion defect, unlike pulmonary embolus, which shows ventilation/perfusion mismatch.
- Chest ultrasound (US) may be comparable to CT for pulmonary contusion.
- Follow-up imaging guided by clinical symptoms and severity of injury:
  - Isolated contusion in the athlete generally does not require repeat radiographs.
  - Consider if symptoms are not resolving over 5 to 7 days or worsen.

Diagnostic Procedures/Other

If hemoptysis is recurrent over >48 hours, bronchoscopy may be considered, depending on clinical status (8):

- Hemoptysis should generally clear within 1 week.

P

TREATMENT

- Prehospital:
  - Primary on-field concerns:
    - Multiple sites of trauma in motor sports or high-velocity sports should be stabilized and transported immediately by emergency services to a designated trauma center:
      - Primary concerns with severe trauma are airway, breathing, and circulation.
      - Evaluate for C-spine injury; immobilize as indicated.
      - Expose by removing equipment as needed.
      - Report any increase in dyspnea; may need support, oxygen, and ventilation
  - Mild to moderate injuries may be observed on site and reevaluated frequently for signs of decompensation.
  - Transport for worsening symptoms:
    - Dyspnea and tachypnea are the most important signs of deterioration.
- ED treatment:
  - In cases of multiple trauma due to motor vehicle accident or high-velocity impact, general trauma protocols should be followed.
  - In contact sports, trauma with isolated pulmonary contusion may be treated with observation and minimal support as needed:
    - Pain medication
    - Oxygen
  - Penetrating injuries and flail chest are associated with a much higher risk of complications, including the need for mechanical support.

MEDICATION

- Acetaminophen and nonsteroidal anti-inflammatory drugs (NSAIDs) can be used as first line for mild to moderate pain:
  - Consider avoiding NSAIDs in patients with hemoptysis.
- Short course <5 days of opioid pain medications may be considered in more severe cases:
  - Monitor use closely, as these may cause respiratory depression.

ADDITIONAL THERAPIES

- Isolated pulmonary contusion in stable patients does not require additional treatment:
  - Rest from strenuous exercise as needed to allow pulmonary healing.
- Additional supportive and treatment measures will be dictated by the severity of injuries:
  - Pulmonary toilet
  - Chest tube may be required emergently if hemopneumothorax is present.
- Light exercise or walking promotes deep breathing and reduces atelectasis.
- When asymptomatic, begin stepwise return to play as tolerated by symptoms.
- Rib taping and other attempts at immobilization are generally not effective and should be used with caution, as they could possibly increase the risk of atelectasis and pneumonia.

ADMISSION, INPATIENT, AND NURSING CONSIDERATIONS

- Admission criteria:
  - Traumatic injuries requiring stabilization and support
  - Patient with respiratory difficulty, tachycardia and oxygen saturations <95%
  - Patients with uncontrolled pain
- Special considerations:
  - Rib fractures can be associated with severe blunt trauma, but these cases generally involve high-energy mechanism.
  - Flail chest is a rare but serious complication requiring hospitalization to observe for pulmonary deterioration and need for intubation with respiratory support.
  - Pulmonary laceration:
    - Transfer of energy from the chest wall; shear forces often are generated that can tear the lung.
    - Most lacerations heal without complications, but elastic recoil of the lung may extend the laceration to form a pulmonary pseudocyst, which may result in infection, abscess, hemoptysis, air leak, adult respiratory distress syndrome, and death.
  - Airway avulsion or rupture:
    - Most common site is within 2.5 cm of the carina between tracheal rings.
    - Findings include subcutaneous emphysema and hemoptysis.
  - Isolated pneumothorax is uncommon with blunt trauma due to dense fibroconnective tissue surrounding carina and mainstem bronchi.
- Discharge criteria:
  - Stable patients can be discharged home with observation and instructions to return for worsening symptoms:
    - Pain controlled
    - No significant dyspnea
    - Stable oxygen saturation on room air:
      - No consensus but generally >90% for an otherwise healthy individual

ONGOING CARE

Return to play (2),(3)[C]:

- Sideline diagnosis with hemoptysis or persistent pain precludes return to that contest.
- Athlete may return to full activity at 1 week if they tolerate progressive training without dyspnea, hemoptysis, or limited performance after the last episode.
- After strenuous exercise is tolerated for 48 hours and athlete is able to perform at a level appropriate for contact sports, return to play in contact sports may be allowed.

FOLLOW-UP RECOMMENDATIONS

- Report any deterioration in performance or dyspnea.
- Pulmonary consultation for bronchoscopy if hemoptysis persists

PROGNOSIS

- Most isolated pulmonary contusions will resolve without complication.
- Chest wall pain usually persists for 6 weeks but generally will not interfere with function.
- Isolated pulmonary contusion in young, healthy patients is not associated with mortality.

COMPLICATIONS

- Posttraumatic empyema
- ARDS (strong association if thoracic trauma severity score at admission >13) (9)[C]
- Pneumonia
- Factors associated with a poor outcome in severe pulmonary contusion (multiple traumas/motor vehicle accident):
  - Poor outcome = death, prolonged hospitalization >7 days, severe complications (pneumonia, empyema, atelectasis requiring bronchoscopy or bronchopleural fistula):
    - Pulmonary contusion on admission CXR
    - Three or more rib fractures
    - Chest tube insertion
    - Hypoxia on admission (PO_2 <70 torr)

REFERENCES

1. Cohn SM, Dubose JJ. Pulmonary contusion: an update on recent advances in clinical management. *World J Surg*. 2010;34(8):1959–1970.
2. Lively MW, Stone D. Pulmonary contusion in football players. *Clin J Sport Med*. 2006;16(2):177–178.
3. Meese MA, Sebastianelli WJ. Pulmonary contusion secondary to blunt trauma in a collegiate football player. *Clin J Sport Med*. 1997;7(4):309–310.
4. Gillespie H, Sisson R, DiFiori JP. Pulmonary contusion in a football player. *Curr Sports Med Rep*. 2013;12(2):57–58.
5. Milne LW. Thoracic trauma in polo: two cases and a review of the literature. *J Emerg Med*. 2011;40(4):410–414.
6. Lively MW. Pulmonary contusion in a collegiate diver: a case report. *J Med Case Rep*. 2011;5:362.
7. Ziegler DW, Agarwal NN. The morbidity and mortality of rib fractures. *J Trauma*. 1994;37(6):975–979.
8. Bidwell JL, Pachner RW. Hemoptysis: diagnosis and management. *Am Fam Physician*. 2005;72(7):1253–1260.
9. Daurat A, Millet I, Roustan J, et al. Thoracic trauma severity score on admission allows to determine the risk of delayed ARDS in trauma patients with pulmonary contusion. *Injury*. 2016;47(1):147–153.

ADDITIONAL READING

- Dubinsky I, Low A. Non-life-threatening blunt chest trauma: appropriate investigation and treatment. *Am J Emerg Med*. 1997;15(3):240–243.
- Kuo K, Kim AM. *Rib Fracture*. StatPearls Publishing; 2025. Accessed August 16, 2025. https://www.ncbi.nlm.nih.gov/books/NBK541020/
- Matsuak ME, Yau CC, Fibel KH. Medical sports injuries in American football players. *HSS J*. 2023;19(3):277–284.

CLINICAL PEARLS

- Blunt thoracic trauma with high-energy mechanism should always prompt a thorough evaluation, as pulmonary contusions and rib fractures are commonly associated with significant internal injuries:
  - This is in contrast to most sports-related injuries, which are usually lower energy and are generally associated with good outcomes.
- Significant morbidity in clinically stable patients has not been reported. One episode of hemoptysis in an asymptomatic athlete will likely not recur and imaging is not required. Pulmonary dysfunction associated with a contusion may take 24 to 48 hours to develop as fluid accumulates in the air spaces. Serial reevaluations daily may be needed to detect worsening tachypnea and tachycardia. Get emergency follow-up evaluation if delayed deterioration occurs rapidly.
- Future ability to play is only as limited by chest wall pain. Return to peak conditioning depends on ability to reach maximum exertion effort. Involuntary guarding of pleuritic pain during healing may delay recovery to peak form for up to 6 weeks.

QUADRICEPS CONTUSION

Kinshasa Morton, MD, CAQSM • Jason P. Womack, MD

BASICS

DESCRIPTION

- The quadriceps extends the knee and stabilize the pelvis and patella during the gait cycle. The muscles also work with the hamstrings to coordinate the movements of kicking, jumping, and running (1),(2).
- Quadriceps contusions occur when traumatic thigh injury causes muscle fiber damage and capillary rupture that causes bleeding within the quadriceps muscle tissue (1). These are common sports-related injuries, seen most frequently in high-impact sports, such as rugby, soccer, or football (3),(4).
- Recurrent quadriceps contusions predispose to more severe injury and development of complications (2),(4).
- Delay in onset of therapy leads to a higher percentage of complications and delay in recovery (1),(2).
- Synonym(s): thigh bruise; dead leg; quadriceps hematoma

EPIDEMIOLOGY

- Thigh injuries account for 14% of all lower extremity sports-related injuries in high school sports (3),(5).
- Muscle contusion injuries are second only to strain injuries as a major cause of morbidity in the modern athlete (1),(2).
- Incidence varies by sport, with contact sports having higher incidence of these injuries (3).
- Quadriceps strains and contusions account for approximately 40% of all injuries in high-level soccer players (3).

RISK FACTORS

- Direct trauma to the middle portion of the quadriceps muscle belly, given the increased vascularity at that point (1),(5)
- Inappropriately sized, thinly cushioned, or nonuse of thigh pads (1)
- Associated medical problems that increase the risk of bleeding (such as liver disease, coagulopathies, etc.) increase the risk of quadriceps contusion (3),(5).

COMMONLY ASSOCIATED CONDITIONS

- Quadriceps strain
- Femur or patellar fracture
- Myositis ossificans traumatica (MOT)
- Acute compartment syndrome (ACS) of anterior thigh

DIAGNOSIS

HISTORY

- Patient or athlete will often describe a distinct injury or trauma to the thigh occurring during a high-impact collision with opponent or sports equipment (1).
- Pain and/or swelling may be immediate or delayed and may not limit the athlete until after the completion of competition (1).

PHYSICAL EXAM

- Inspection:
  - May ambulate with antalgic gait or has reluctance to bear weight (1),(5)
  - May have area of ecchymosis at trauma site (1),(5)
  - Swelling in the anterior thigh, which may extend to proximal knee (5):
    - Patients with severe quadriceps contusions may get knee effusion without intra-articular pathology.
- Palpation:
  - Tense and tender to palpation over area of direct injury; most commonly anterior lateral thigh (1),(5)
- Range of motion (ROM):
  - Reduced ability to actively flex the knee (1),(5)
- Strength:
  - Reduced ability to perform straight leg raise (1),(5)
  - Reduced ability to perform knee extension against resistance (1),(5)
- Sensation:
  - Sensation deficits along anterolateral thigh may occur but are rare. If present, must consider ACS (1),(5)
- Grading of contusions:
  - Mild: normal gait, localized tenderness, active range of motion (AROM) knee flexion >90 degrees (1)
  - Moderate: antalgic gait, swollen and tender mass in quadriceps, AROM knee flexion 45 to 90 degrees (1)
  - Severe: severely antalgic gait, visibly swollen and tender mass, AROM knee flexion >45 degrees (1)

ALERT

ACS: Elevated pressure within the anterior thigh compartment due to bleeding causes impaired blood flow to tissues and eventually ischemia (6):

- Can occur from similar mechanisms to quadriceps contusion (6)
- Surgical emergency and must be quickly identified by rapid swelling, pain out of proportion to exam, decreased sensation and pulses (6)
- If there is concern, athlete needs to be evaluated in emergency department (ED) with compartment testing (6).

DIFFERENTIAL DIAGNOSIS

- Femur fracture or contusion
- Quadriceps tendon rupture
- Quadriceps strain or muscle tear
- Patellar fracture
- ACS of the thigh
- Morel-Lavallée lesion

DIAGNOSTIC TESTS & INTERPRETATION

- Diagnosis can typically be made clinically with a thorough history and physical exam (1),(2),(4).
- Radiographs:
  - Rarely needed acutely unless concern for femur fracture (1),(2)
  - May be more help in cases of delayed recovery in diagnosis of the development of MOT (1),(2)
- Musculoskeletal (MSK) ultrasound:
  - Can be used to diagnose hematomas and rule out associated muscle tears or tendon ruptures (2),(4),(6)
  - Contusions appear as a focal loss of muscle fibrillary architecture with a heterogenous region of increased echogenicity, which may cross fascial boundaries (2),(4),(6).
  - Serial ultrasounds can assess size of resolving contusion at future visits (2),(6).
  - Can aid in making the diagnosis when an athlete presents subacutely without known mechanism of injury
  - Ultrasound may provide a clearer assessment of injury severity and prognosis than clinical classification (7).
- Magnetic resonance imaging (MRI):
  - Rarely needed acutely but can be used if point-of-care ultrasound is not available or inconclusive (2),(4),(5)
  - Can reliably detect and grade quadriceps contusions (2),(4),(5)

TREATMENT

GENERAL MEASURES

- Acute treatment (first 24 hours):
  - RICE therapy—rest, ice, compression, and elevation to limit the severity of contusion (1),(4),(5):
    - Rest reduces retraction of ruptured myofibrils, preventing large gaps in the muscle (4).
    - Icing associated with smaller hematoma formation, less inflammation, and early muscle regeneration (4)
    - Compression reduces intramuscular bleeding (4).
    - Elevation reduces interstitial fluid accumulation (swelling) (4).

- Immobilization—initially, the knee should be immobilized in an elastic wrap or hinged knee brace at 120 degrees of flexion for 24 hours to limit hematoma formation (1),(4).
- Subacute treatment (after first 24 hours):
  - Discontinue immobilization and begin stretching (1):
    - Passive flexion with goal of 120 degrees of pain-free flexion (1),(5)
    - Begin active quadriceps stretching and strengthening exercises once pain decreases and motion improves (1).
  - Strengthening should progress from isometric to isotonic to isokinetic training (4).
- Long-term treatment/rehabilitation:
  - May return to sports-specific training when:
    - ROM on injured quadriceps side and uninjured side are equal (1),(4).
    - Use of injured quadriceps is pain free with basic movement (1),(4).
  - Prior to return to sport, player should be fitted for oversized quadriceps pad (1):
    - Helps to protect from recurrent injury, which could lead to MOT
    - Wear for 3 to 6 months or until end of season.

MEDICATION

- Nonsteroidal anti-inflammatory drugs (NSAIDs) can be used depending on the severity of the injury (1),(4).
- Use is typically delayed for 48 hours after initial injury to avoid interference with coagulation and the development of hematoma (8).
- For severe injuries, NSAIDs may prevent development of MOT, although further studies need to be done to determine the most appropriate dose and choice of NSAID (1).

ISSUES FOR REFERRAL

Isolated quadriceps contusions rarely require referral. Indications for referral include complications such as myositis ossificans, tendon rupture, fracture, or compartment syndrome (1),(4),(5).

SURGERY/OTHER PROCEDURES

- Aspiration should be reserved for large hematomas or those that clearly restrict motion. If indicated, aspiration should be performed within the first week of injury (2),(4),(6).
- Steroid injections are not recommended for treatment of these injuries (1),(4).
- Surgery is rarely, if ever indicated (1),(4).

COMPLEMENTARY & ALTERNATIVE MEDICINE

Massage and muscle manipulation should be avoided in the acute phase because these can worsen underlying injury (4),(5).

ONGOING CARE

FOLLOW-UP RECOMMENDATIONS

- Athletes should follow up approximately every 2 weeks to assess ongoing ROM and strengthening (2).
- Serial ultrasounds can also be performed at these visits to document resolution of hematoma and early signs of MOT (2).

PROGNOSIS

- Quadriceps contusions typically resolve over the course of 3 to 10 weeks, depending on severity (1). With appropriate rehabilitation, patients and athletes can expect to regain full strength and ROM (1).
- Athletes should adhere to a functional progression of sport-specific activities as part of their rehabilitation. They should have symmetric, pain-free ROM and at least 85% strength recovery prior to return to sport (1).

COMPLICATIONS

MOT: Benign heterotopic calcification of the traumatic hematoma (4):

- Suspect MOT when lesions persist >2 weeks or get worse over time (1),(4).
- Early signs of myositis ossificans may be identifiable on MSK ultrasound (1). At later stages, it can be seen on radiographs and MRI.
- Risk increases with larger contusions (1).
- Athletes with MOT who have persistent pain and limited motion may have the heterotopic bone removed when it has matured, at least 12 months after the initial injury (1),(4).

REFERENCES

1. Kary J. Diagnosis and management of quadriceps strains and contusions. *Curr Rev Musculoskelet Med.* 2010;3(1–4):26–31.
2. Pasta G, Nanni G, Molini L, et al. Sonography of the quadriceps muscle: examination technique, normal anatomy, and traumatic lesions. *J Ultrasound.* 2010;13(2):76–84.
3. Fernandez WG, Yard EE, Comstock RD. Epidemiology of lower extremity injuries among U.S. high school athletes. *Acad Emerg Med.* 2007;14(7):641–645.
4. Järvinen TA, Järvinen TL, Kääriäinen M, et al. Muscle injuries: optimizing recovery. *Best Pract Res Clin Rheumatol.* 2007;21(2):317–331.
5. Trojian TH. Muscle contusion (thigh). *Clin Sports Med.* 2013;32(2):317–324.
6. Purohit NB, King LJ. Ultrasound of lower limb sports injuries. *Ultrasound.* 2015;23(3):149–157.
7. Torres RJL, Hattori S, Kato Y, et al. Ultrasonography and return to play of the different clinical grading of quadriceps contusions: a case series. *J Med Ultrason (2001).* 2018;45(2):375–380.
8. Haws BE, Luo TD, Al'Khafaji IM, et al. Definitive management of thigh contusions in athletes: but how definitive? A systematic review. *J ISAKOS.* 2017; 2(2):67–74.

ADDITIONAL READING

- Aronen JG, Garrick JG, Chronister RD, et al. Quadriceps contusions: clinical results of immediate immobilization in 120 degrees of knee flexion. *Clin J Sport Med.* 2006;16(5):383–387.
- Diaz JA, Fischer DA, Rettig AC, et al. Severe quadriceps muscle contusions in athletes. A report of three cases. *Am J Sports Med.* 2003;31(2):289–293.
- How MI, Lee PK, Wei TS, et al. Delayed presentation of compartment syndrome of the thigh secondary to quadriceps trauma and vascular injury in a soccer athlete. *Int J Surg Case Rep.* 2015;11:56–58.
- Lempainen L, Mechó S, Valle X, et al. Management of anterior thigh injuries in soccer players: practical guide. *BMC Sports Sci Med Rehabil.* 2022;14(1):41.
- Weiss NA, Johnson JJ, Anderson SB. Morel-Lavallée lesion initially diagnosed as quadriceps contusion: ultrasound, MRI, and importance of early intervention. *West J Emerg Med.* 2015;16(3):438–441.

CLINICAL PEARLS

- Quadriceps contusions are caused by blunt trauma to the quadriceps muscle belly and area graded according to size and loss of function.
- Point-of-care ultrasound is the imaging modality of choice for diagnosis as well as ongoing assessment.
- Initially, the knee should be immobilized with an elastic wrap or hinged knee brace in 120 degrees of flexion for 24 hours. After that, athlete can proceed with graduated flexibility and strengthening protocol.
- Suspect MOT when a quadriceps contusion is not improving as expected over 2 to 3 weeks.

QUADRICEPS TEAR

Jason P. Womack, MD ▪ Kinshasa Morton, MD, CAQSM

BASICS

Quadriceps strains and tears are graded based on the degree of injury:

- Grade I: stretch injury of muscle fibers
- Grade II: partial tearing of muscle fibers
- Grade III: complete tear of muscle fibers:
  - Grade III tears most commonly involve the distal rectus femoris muscle.
  - Grade III tears may involve complete rupture of the extensor mechanism if the distal quadriceps tendon is involved (1).
  - Proximal ruptures may involve avulsion of anterior inferior iliac spine (AIIS).

EPIDEMIOLOGY

- Rectus femoris is the most common location of clinically significant quadriceps strains.
  - Majority of injuries around the muscle body along the central tendon, with distal and proximal injuries being rare (2)
- Represents 10% of injuries to soccer players
- Proximal rupture/avulsion is rare:
  - More commonly seen in adolescent, kicking athletes
- Distal quadriceps rupture is a rare event:
  - 88% of ruptures occur in those >40 years of age.

ETIOLOGY AND PATHOPHYSIOLOGY

- Commonly affects athletes with repetitive functional overloading of the extensor mechanism in an eccentric fashion:
  - The dominant kicking leg is at risk for quadriceps strain (3).
- National Collegiate Athletic Association (NCAA) injury surveillance saw highest rates in men's and women's soccer from 2009 to 2015 (3).

RISK FACTORS

- Quadricep muscle strain (3),(4)
  - No age correlation
  - Female sex
  - Dominant kicking leg
  - Greater in competition versus training
- Distal tendon rupture (5):
  - Age >40 years
  - Hemodialysis patients
  - Anabolic steroid use
  - Diabetes
  - Gout
  - Hyperparathyroidism
  - Hypocalcemia

DIAGNOSIS

HISTORY

- Strain to quadriceps muscle is most commonly associated with kicking, jumping, sprinting, or change in direction.
- Pain is often immediate.
- May lead to local pain and swelling
- Strains are a noncontact injury. History of contact leads to diagnosis of quadriceps contusion.

PHYSICAL EXAM

- Appearance:
  - There may be swelling and possibly ecchymosis around the area of injury.
- Palpation:
  - Tenderness, spasm, or both at the area of muscle injury
  - A defect in the muscle tissue may be felt in grade III strains.
  - In distal quadriceps ruptures, the intercondylar notch may be palpated because the quadriceps tendon is not present.
- Range of motion:
  - The extensor mechanism must be evaluated in all knee and quadriceps injuries.
  - Inability of any active extension of the knee is concerning for quadriceps rupture.
  - Strains show pain with active extension and passive knee flexion.

ALERT

Lack of active extension of the knee should raise concern of complete tendon rupture that requires prompt diagnosis and surgical consultation.

- Strength exam:
  - Weakness and/or painful knee extension secondary to the injured muscle tissue is common.
- Neurologic exam:
  - Sensation and reflexes are intact:
    - No reflex will be present in complete rupture.

DIFFERENTIAL DIAGNOSIS

- Quadriceps tendonitis
- Quadriceps contusion
- Patellar tendinitis
- Patellofemoral pain syndrome
- Patellar dislocation/subluxation
- Sinding-Larsen-Johansson disease
- Myositis ossificans

DIAGNOSTIC TESTS & INTERPRETATION

- Plain radiographs:
  - Not helpful in the diagnosis of acute quadriceps strain
  - A history of an old quadriceps strain with reaggravation may suggest myositis ossificans that would be visualized on plain radiographs.
  - Radiographs should be obtained in the skeletally immature with proximal pain to rule out avulsion fracture.
  - Complete ruptures may show patella baja on lateral views.
- Magnetic resonance imaging (MRI):
  - Not necessary in quadriceps strain, but will show edema and possible defects in the musculature
  - Proximal ruptures may show avulsion of the AIIS and degree of retraction from the pelvis.
- Ultrasound (US):
  - Partial tearing:
    - Hypoechoic cleft seen in the muscle belly adjacent to the central tendon
    - Scanning in the long and short axis helps to determine the extent of the strain.
  - Complete rupture:
    - Complete discontinuity noted on scanning in the long axis

TREATMENT

GENERAL MEASURES

- Grade I and II injuries are treated in a similar fashion with rest, ice, compression, and pain control.
- Gentle stretching as permitted to maintain range of motion
- Early surgery is indicated for complete distal rupture:
  - Proximal rupture/avulsion may be treated nonoperatively.
  - Recovery of range of motion with stretching
  - Exercise to regain strength of the quadriceps and hamstring tendons.
  - Padding could be worn to protect the injured portion of the quadriceps musculature.

MEDICATION

Nonsteroidal anti-inflammatory drugs (NSAIDs):

- NSAIDs may be used acutely to help with pain.
- Controversy exists as to whether NSAIDs delay healing and collagen formation.

ALERT

If there is a suspected quadriceps contusion with hematoma, be aware that NSAIDs use could theoretically increase bleeding. Conversely, early use of indomethacin in high-risk quadriceps contusions may reduce the risk of myositis ossificans.

ISSUES FOR REFERRAL

Prompt surgical referral and surgery is indicated for quadriceps rupture at the patellar insertion.

ADDITIONAL THERAPIES

- If hematoma is discovered, aspiration can be considered to decrease pain and promote early range of motion; may also decrease risk of development of myositis ossificans (6)
- Platelet-rich plasma injections are often considered for improved recovery and healing, but evidence is limited to case reports and expert opinion.

SURGERY/OTHER PROCEDURES

- Acute rupture of the distal quadriceps tendon:
  - Requires prompt surgical repair
  - Time from injury to repair is the greatest determinant of outcome in athletes with quadriceps tendon ruptures. Repair within 2 to 3 weeks yields significantly better outcomes (1)[C].
  - End-to-end repairs and tendon-to-bone repairs are used, depending on the level of the rupture.
- Proximal avulsion of the AIIS:
  - Vast majority are successfully treated nonoperatively.
  - Surgery to reattach the avulsed AIIS may be successful treatment if there is continued pain, disability, or both after conservative measures have failed.
- Intrasubstance rectus femoris grade III strains:
  - Removal of the tear may benefit those who continue to have pain or dysfunction after physical therapy.
  - Case reports suggest a role for PRP in the treatment of intrasubstance tears of the rectus femoris.

ONGOING CARE

Return to play:

- When quadriceps has 120 degrees of flexion
- No signs of quadriceps weakness
- May take days to months based on the degree of injury

COMPLICATIONS

- Myositis ossificans—rare after noncontact injury but has been reported and can lead to prolonged pain or dysfunction
- Missed distal ruptures can lead to complicated surgical procedure and complicated postsurgical courses.

REFERENCES

1. Ibounig T, Simons TA. Etiology, diagnosis and treatment of tendinous knee extensor mechanism injuries. *Scand J Surg*. 2016;105(2):67–72.
2. Brukner P, Connell D. 'Serious thigh muscle strains' beware the intramuscular tendon which plays an important role in difficult hamstring and quadriceps muscle strains. *Br J Sports Med*. 2016;50(4):205–208.
3. Eckard TG, Kerr ZY, Padua DA, et al. Epidemiology of quadriceps strains in National Collegiate Athletic Association Athletes, 2009–2010 through 2014–2015. *J Athl Train*. 2017;52(5):474–481.
4. Pietsch S, Pizzari T. Risk factors for quadriceps muscle strain injuries in sport: a systematic review. *J Orthop Sports Phys Ther*. 2022;52(6):389–400.
5. Gao X, Shao Z, Liu S, et al. A case report of spontaneous rupture of the quadriceps tendon. *Clin Case Rep*. 2017;5(9):1477–1481.
6. Yoon ES, Lin B, Miller TT. Ultrasound of musculoskeletal hematomas: relationship of sonographic appearance to age and ease of aspiration. *AJR Am J Roentgenol*. 2021;216(1):125–130.

ADDITIONAL READING

Kary JM. Diagnosis and management of quadriceps strains and contusions. *Curr Rev Musculoskelet Med*. 2010;3(1–4):26–31.

CLINICAL PEARLS

- Quadriceps strains are common in sports with kicking and other eccentric quadriceps loads.
- Be sure to rule out quadriceps tendon rupture by examining an intact extensor mechanism.

Q

RADIAL TUNNEL SYNDROME

Katherine M. Pohlgeers, MD, MS, CAQSM

BASICS

DESCRIPTION

- Radial tunnel syndrome (RTS) is an entrapment neuropathy which leads to chronic and oftentimes vague symptoms of lateral forearm and elbow pain. For this reason, it was initially thought to be a resistant form of lateral epicondylitis because of a seemingly large overlap in physical examination findings. It is unclear whether RTS and posterior interosseous nerve (PIN) syndrome are two separate entities or a continuum of the same condition:
  - The presence of weakness is common with PIN.
  - In contrast, RTS typically presents as a pure pain syndrome without any objective clinical muscular weakness (1).
- RTS was first discovered when physicians were unable to relieve discomfort in patients with lateral epicondylitis. These two syndromes may also exist concurrently, in which case they are often confused and misdiagnosed, with patients presenting with epicondylitis that can exacerbate symptoms of RTS (2).

EPIDEMIOLOGY

Incidence

Over the past five decades, the diagnosis of RTS has become increasingly accepted in the field. It is now thought to be the cause of up to 2% of peripheral entrapment neuropathies in the upper extremity, affecting as many as 8 in 100,000 people (3).

ETIOLOGY AND PATHOPHYSIOLOGY

Anatomically, the radial nerve originates from the posterior cord of the brachial plexus with contributions from C5–C8. The posterior cord divides into the axillary and radial nerves anterior to the subscapularis; the latter then travels along the spiral groove on the posterior aspect of the humerus and reaches the lateral intermuscular septum approximately 12 cm proximal to the lateral epicondyle. The radial nerve then splits into the PIN and superficial branch approximately 3 cm distal to the lateral epicondyle under the brachioradialis (BR) (3),(4). The PIN then enters the radial tunnel, which is approximately 5 cm in length, starting at the radiocapitellar joint bounded medially by the biceps tendon and brachialis and laterally by the BR and extensor carpi radialis brevis (ECRB) and extensor carpi radialis longus, with a proximal roof formed by the fibrous bands of these muscles along with the superficial head of the supinator (4). Compression can occur at the following sites (5):

- The arcade of Frohse (most common area of compression)
- Leash of Henry (an arcade of anastomosing branches of the recurrent radial artery)
- Fibrous bands at the humeroradial joint and the radial head
- Tendinous superomedial margin of the ECRB

RISK FACTORS

- Repetitive pronation and supination of the forearm (5)
- Repetitive use of force and static work with the elbow extended
- Repetitive use of the index and middle fingers during activities (e.g., computer mouse use)
- Other causes include idiopathic entrapment, lipomas, cysts, or rheumatoid synovitis.

DIAGNOSIS

HISTORY

- For the past several decades, history and physical examination findings have been the benchmark to diagnose RTS. Patients with RTS usually complain of chronic, aching pain to the lateral and dorsal forearm (5). Of note, most do not experience constant and specific motor deficits, which can be seen with PIN nerve entrapment outside the radial tunnel, such as weakness of wrist and finger extension (5).
- Typically, do not have paresthesias, but instead, characteristic pain at the area of entrapment pain often worsens with rotational movements of the forearm (6).

PHYSICAL EXAM

- Often, provocative maneuvers that can be used to aid in the diagnosis of RTS are also positive in patients with lateral epicondylosis, which is a closely associated differential diagnosis.
- Pressure that is applied over a patient's lateral forearm approximately 3 to 5 cm distal to the elbow (over the supinator muscle) with the wrist in full supination should reproduce pain (pronation during this maneuver should relieve the pain) (6).
- Positive Tinel sign at the radial tunnel (1)
- Patients typically have tenderness to palpation at the mobile wad, distal to the lateral epicondyle, pain recreated at the site of compression with resisted supination, and pain recreated at the site with resisted middle finger extension (5).

DIFFERENTIAL DIAGNOSIS

- Lateral epicondylitis
- PIN syndrome
- Osteoarthritis and/or synovitis of the radiocapitellar joint
- A muscle tear of the ECRB
- Posterior plica impingement (6)

DIAGNOSTIC TESTS & INTERPRETATION

Initial Tests (lab, imaging)

- Not usually needed for initial treatment
- Standard elbow radiographs (anteroposterior and lateral) are sufficient if other sources of pain or injury are suspected (fracture, degenerative joint disease [DJD], tumor, calcific tendinopathy, etc.).
- Shoulder and cervical radiographs can be helpful to exclude other pathologies causing radiation of symptoms to the elbow.
- Magnetic resonance imaging (MRI) can show radial nerve entrapment or other soft tissue pathology such as tendon thickening, partial intrasubstance tendon tearing, or articular cartilage injury.
- Ultrasound is another useful diagnostic tool to demonstrate hyperechoic thickening, tearing hypoechoic changes, or vascular ingrowth.

Diagnostic Procedures/Other

Electrodiagnostic studies lack specific findings for RTS and often are normal in patients with RTS. Patients with conductive slowing of the radial nerve likely have associated motor findings, thereby precluding a diagnosis of RTS. However, abnormal findings on electrodiagnostic studies may elucidate other causes of pain, such as cervical radiculopathy (6). Local anesthetic injection into the radial tunnel can be used to differentiate RTS from epicondylitis (2)[C].

TREATMENT

- Nonoperative approaches are first-line treatment (3)[C]:
  - Immobilization of the wrist with splinting or casting
  - Physical therapy which may include nerve-gliding exercises, ultrasonographic therapy, heat/cold modalities (6).
  - Short term anti-inflammatory medication
  - Corticosteroid injections ideally ultrasound guided
- Operative treatment should be considered in patients that have failed conservative treatments for at least 3 months (2)[C]:
  - The decompression is performed for the radial nerve and both of its branches: the PIN and superficial branch of the radial nerve (SBRN).
  - Studies have suggested that patients with isolated RTS and no concurrent compressive neuropathy or tendinopathy have more favorable outcomes compared with patients with isolated RTS who have associated conditions (6).
  - Good outcomes have been reported in 86% of patients with isolated RTS compared with 43% of patients with concomitant lateral epicondylosis and 57% of patients with other compressive neuropathies (6). The surgical goal is complete decompression of the PIN within the radial tunnel. Areas of focus for decompression include the arcade of Frohse, the leading edge of the proximal ECRB, and the compressive fascia of the distal supinator (6).

ONGOING CARE

- Return to activity should be undertaken slowly as symptoms improve.
- Rehabilitation program should be continued for both nonoperative and postoperative patients.

REFERENCES

1. Kane SF, Lynch JH, Taylor JC. Evaluation of elbow pain in adults. *Am Fam Physician*. 2014;89(8):649–657.
2. Kaswan S, Deigni O, Tadisina KK, et al. Radial tunnel syndrome complicated by lateral epicondylitis in a middle-aged female. *Eplasty*. 2014;14:ic44.
3. Hulkkonen S, Lampainen K, Auvinen J, et al. Incidence and operations of median, ulnar and radial entrapment neuropathies in Finland: a nationwide register study. *J Hand Surg Eur*. 2020;45(3):226–230.
4. Levina Y, Dantuluri PK. Radial tunnel syndrome. *Curr Rev Musculoskelet Med*. 2021;14(3):205–213.
5. Wolf JM, Patel R, Ghosh K. Radial tunnel syndrome: review and best evidence. *JAAOS*. 2023;31(15):813–819.
6. Strohl AB, Zelouf DS. Ulnar tunnel syndrome, radial tunnel syndrome, anterior interosseous nerve syndrome, and pronator syndrome. *J Am Acad Orthop Surg*. 2017;25(1):e1–e10.

CLINICAL PEARLS

- Entrapment of the deep branch of the radial nerve within the radial tunnel
- Diagnosis is based primarily on clinical examination, leading to some skepticism of the actual prevalence.
- Advanced imaging may be of benefit diagnostically
- No motor deficits
- Often misdiagnosed as lateral epicondylitis
- Nonoperative treatment is preferred (nonsteroidal anti-inflammatory drugs [NSAIDs], physical therapy, injections); however, surgery is a viable option for those who are refractory to conservative measures.

RELATIVE ENERGY DEFICIENCY IN SPORTS

Diana Filtz, MD, FAAP, CAQSM • Mackenzie Erdmann, MD

BASICS

DESCRIPTION

- In 2014, the International Olympic Committee defined a new condition called relative energy deficiency in sports (REDs) as a more comprehensive and inclusive term to replace what was previously identified as the female athlete triad ("triad") (1).
- The triad is a condition found in female athletes that refers to low energy availability (with or without disordered eating), menstrual dysfunction, and low bone mineral density (BMD) (1).
- REDs refers to impaired physiologic and/or psychological functioning caused by low energy availability that can occur in all athletes, not strictly female. These physiologic impairments can include metabolic, menstrual, bone health, immunity, mental health, gastrointestinal (GI), and cardiovascular health dysfunction and more (2).

EPIDEMIOLOGY

Prevalence

- Prevalence of REDs ranges from 22–63% in athletic populations, with higher prevalence in sports emphasizing leanness, endurance, or weight categories. Both males and females are affected (3).
- REDs is common and often under-recognized, with most athletes presenting with at least one symptom consistent with REDs in some cohorts (4).

ETIOLOGY AND PATHOPHYSIOLOGY

- Reduced energy availability, or an imbalance between intake and output of calories, is the ultimate cause of REDs.
- Restriction of calories may be inadvertent (not taking in enough calories for the demand of the sport) or intentional (trying to lose weight).
- In many athletes, the emphasis on leanness in sport, along with the perceived benefits of low body weight (e.g., better fitness, agility, speed), causes increased focus on weight-control measures (2).
- Purging of calories may manifest as vomiting, laxative use, or excess exercise/training with little or no recovery time.
- The energy deficit leads to disruption of normal estrogen production through the hypothalamic–pituitary axis. The pituitary gland does not secrete pulses of luteinizing hormone (LH) at the correct frequency, which decreases bone formation and bone production and, in women, results in a change in menstrual function. Men may demonstrate reduced energy availability and thus a decrease in bone density, also owing to the preceding risk factors (5).

RISK FACTORS

- Sports emphasizing leanness or endurance, such as gymnastics, figure skating, cross-country running, or skiing, and diving
- Individual sports as opposed to team sports
- Early sport-specific training
- A sudden increase in training volume
- Punitive measures imposed for weight gain
- Unreasonable performance expectations by self or others
- Poor body self-image
- Social isolation

COMMONLY ASSOCIATED CONDITIONS

Psychological disorders such as depression, anxiety, eating disorders, and body dysmorphic disorders (6)

DIAGNOSIS

High index of suspicion required

HISTORY

- A thorough history of the athlete's *training, diet, lifestyle habits*, possible *REDs symptoms/signs*, and a general *review of symptoms*, including mental health, is required to make a diagnosis (2).
- For *training*, all the physical activity the athlete is doing is needed. This includes the training the athlete does with their team/coaches and what is done on their own.
- For *diet*, the athlete's typical daily intake, supplements, dietary restrictions, and fueling habits before, during, and after training sessions and competitions.
- Possible *REDs symptoms/signs* include:
  - Amenorrhea (primary and secondary) and other menstrual irregularities
  - Stress fracture(s)
  - Nonosseous overuse injuries (e.g., muscle strain)
  - Weight-control behaviors and/or weight loss
  - Cold intolerance
  - Sore throat/gastroesophageal reflux
  - Constipation/GI motility problems
  - Light-headedness/presyncope/syncope
  - Orthostatic hypotension
  - Fatigue/sleep difficulties
  - Nausea
  - Depression/anxiety
  - Worsened athletic performance
  - Worsened cognitive performance/focus difficulties

PHYSICAL EXAM

- Height, changes in weight, body mass index (BMI) ($<$18.5 kg/m^2 is underweight for patients $\geq$18 years of age.)
- Vital signs for evidence of bradycardia, hypotension, and/or orthostatic hypotension
- Observe for fat depletion and muscle wasting
- Integumentary exam for dry skin, lanugo, brittle hair/nails
- Ocular exam to evaluate for pituitary and thyroid disorders
- Dental examination for evidence of lingual enamel erosion secondary to vomiting
- Parotid gland observation/palpation for hypertrophy secondary to vomiting
- Thyroid palpation
- Cardiac auscultation for evidence of dysrhythmia and murmurs
- Complete neurologic examination, including cranial nerves and reflexes
- If amenorrheic, consider gynecology referral to rule out uterine pathology, outflow tract obstruction, and disorders of sexual differentiation as causes of primary amenorrhea
- Careful examination of any musculoskeletal pain, especially looking for stress injuries (2)

DIFFERENTIAL DIAGNOSIS

- Pregnancy in menstruating athletes
- Pituitary disease
- Hyperthyroidism
- Hypogonadism
- Hyperparathyroidism
- Primary ovarian insufficiency
- Polycystic ovarian syndrome
- Adrenal dysfunction
- Autoimmune disease
- Anabolic steroid use/abuse
- Excess glucocorticoid administration
- Malabsorption syndromes
- Overtraining syndrome

DIAGNOSTIC TESTS & INTERPRETATION

Initial Tests (lab, imaging)

- Pregnancy test (when applicable)
- Urinalysis for specific gravity (normal unless dehydration is present)
- Complete blood count (CBC) (normal or possible anemia)
- Erythrocyte sedimentation rate (normal)
- Serum electrolytes, blood urea nitrogen, and creatinine (normal, except possibly in the case of bulimia, which may cause electrolyte abnormalities or dehydration with malnutrition or refeeding syndrome)
- Thyroid function tests (normal or low T3)
- LH and follicle-stimulating hormone levels (low or normal)
- Estradiol level (low or normal)
- Serum prolactin (normal)
- Serum cortisol (normal or mildly elevated)
- Serum testosterone (low or normal in male athletes)
- BMD testing with dual energy x-ray absorptiometry (DEXA) if patient has had stress fracture from mild trauma or two prior stress fractures, 6 months evidence of hypoestrogenism (oligomenorrhea or amenorrhea) and/or disordered eating
- DEXA of weight-bearing sites (posteroanterior spine, total hip, femoral neck) using lower Z-score to base diagnosis of low BMD
- A DEXA with Z-score <-2.0 should prompt reevaluation of BMD in 1 year (2).

Diagnostic Procedures/Other

Progesterone challenge test (e.g., medroxyprogesterone acetate 10 mg PO daily $\times$ 10 days): If a period occurs, there is sufficient estrogen to stimulate the endometrium.

TREATMENT

GENERAL MEASURES

- Main goal of treatment is to modify diet and exercise behaviors to increase energy availability, subsequent resumption of normal physiologic functions (1).
- Counsel athlete that achieving energy balance may require increasing caloric intake and/or decreasing caloric expenditure (through decreased exercise).
- Athletes often resist treatment if negative energy balance is intentional. Treatment discussion requires good patient rapport and work with the appropriate mental health specialists (6).
- Emphasize performance and injury issues related to negative energy balance (e.g., stress fractures are related to low BMD).
- The International Olympic Committee's Relative Energy Deficiency in Sports Clinical Assessment Tool-Version 2 (IOC REDs CAT2) provides guidance on activity restrictions depending on the severity of the athlete's presentation (2).
- May need to restrict patient from sport/training if not making progress or participating in treatment plan
- Requires team approach (i.e., physician, psychologist, athletic trainer, parents, nutritionist, coach) and open communication among all involved
- Monitor progress closely, as indicated by severity and response to treatment.
- Prevention is best accomplished through education of athletes, coaches, trainers, and parents (2).

MEDICATION

- There is no strong evidence to support either hormone replacement therapy or oral contraceptive use to increase or protect BMD in athletes with functional hypothalamic amenorrhea, even if they remain amenorrheic (2),(7).
- Although oral contraceptives may restore regular menses, they do not normalize the underlying metabolic factors impairing bone health and will therefore be unlikely to reverse low BMD or fracture risk (7).
- Bisphosphonates are not recommended for women of reproductive age due to teratogenicity (7).
- Treating comorbid psychiatric conditions is essential, and pharmacotherapy for the specific disorder may be useful (6).
- Multivitamin supplements are commonly recommended.
- Supplement calcium between 1,000 and 1,300 mg/d and vitamin D 600 IU daily for adolescents and children, with higher doses for vitamin D deficiency (8).

ISSUES FOR REFERRAL

- Psychology referrals are recommended for cognitive-behavioral therapy; consider family therapy to help identify and cope with stressors (6).
- Nutrition consultant with disordered-eating experience recommended (2)

ADMISSION, INPATIENT, AND NURSING CONSIDERATIONS

- Electrolyte disturbances
- Severe bradycardia or dysrhythmia
- Severe dehydration
- Severe hypotension or orthostatic hypotension
- Significant psychiatric pathology

ONGOING CARE

FOLLOW-UP RECOMMENDATIONS

- Frequent follow-up to gauge compliance with treatment plan
- Athletes may be resistant to treatment, especially if their symptoms are severe.
- Monitor weight; address nutritional concerns and goals at each visit.
- Coordinate care with psychology and nutrition consultants.
- Assess physiologic and psychological functioning, sport performance (if participating).
- Menstruation usually occurs (may take a year or more) with improved nutrition and decreased exercise intensity (2).

PATIENT EDUCATION

- Education about low energy availability and its effects is generally lacking in populations at risk; effort to routinely discuss this condition is needed (9).
- Body weight and caloric intake below what is necessary for normal physiologic function are detrimental to athletic performance.
- BMD may be *permanently* lowered in adolescents. By 18 years of age, females have typically accumulated 90–95% of their peak BMD. Failure to achieve peak bone mass during this period predisposes to clinically low BMD throughout adulthood (8).
- Fertility is decreased with amenorrhea but is not totally impaired; it is possible to conceive without having a period. Fertility issues are not thought to be permanent and may normalize with resumption of menses.

PROGNOSIS

- Appropriate increase in energy availability has the potential to restore normal physiologic and psychological function (2).
- Athletes with both REDs and eating disorders (e.g., anorexia nervosa and bulimia nervosa) can be more difficult to treat and prognosis is guarded.
- Athletes who have perfectionist-driven tendencies are less likely to comply with treatment and have difficulty recovering.

COMPLICATIONS

Injury forcing the athlete to take time off from exercising can exacerbate disordered eating practices (e.g., caloric restriction or purging) or other mental health disorders.

REFERENCES

1. Mountjoy M, Sundgot-Borgen JK, Burke LM, et al. IOC consensus statement on relative energy deficiency in sport (RED-S): 2018 update. *Br J Sports Med*. 2018; 52(11):687–697.
2. Mountjoy M, Ackerman KE, Bailey D, et al. 2023 International Olympic Committee's (IOC) consensus statement on relative energy deficiency in sports (REDs). *Br J Sports Med*. 2024; 57(17):1073–1097.
3. Gallant TL, Ong LF, Wong L, et al. Low energy availability and relative energy deficiency in sport: a systematic review and meta-analysis. *Sports Med*. 2025;55(2):325–339.
4. Stellingwerff T, Mountjoy M, McCluskey WT, et al. Review of the scientific rationale, development and validation of the International Olympic Committee relative energy deficiency in sports clinical assessment tool: V.2 (IOC REDs CAT2)—by a subgroup of the IOC consensus on REDs. *Br J Sports Med*. 2023;57(17):1109–1118.
5. Burke LM, Ackerman KE, Heikura IA, et al. Mapping the complexities of relative energy deficiency in sports (REDs): development of a physiological model by a subgroup of the International Olympic Committee (IOC) consensus on REDs. *Br J Sports Med*. 2024; 57(17):1098–1108.
6. Pensgaard AM, Sundgot-Borgen J, Edwards C, et al. Intersection of mental health issues and relative energy deficiency in sport (REDs): a narrative by a subgroup of the IOC consensus on REDs. *Br J Sports Med*. 2023;57(17):1127–1135.
7. Aalberg K, Stavem K, Norheim F, et al. Effect of oral and transdermal oestrogen therapy on bone mineral density in functional hypothalamic amenorrhea: a systemic review and meta-analysis. *BMJ Open Sport Exerc Med*. 2021;7(3):e001112.
8. De Souza MJ, Nattiv A, Joy E, et al. 2014 Female athlete triad coalition consensus statement on treatment and return to play of the female athlete triad: 1st international conference held in San Francisco, California, May 2012 and 2nd international conference held in Indianapolis, Indiana, May 2013. *Br J Sports Med*. 2014;48(4):289.
9. Lodge MT, Ackerman KE, Garay J. Knowledge of the female athlete triad and relative energy deficiency in sport among female cross-country athletes and support staff. *J Athl Train*. 2022;57(4):385–392.

SEE ALSO

Menstrual Disorders in the Athlete

CLINICAL PEARLS

- REDs is a syndrome that consists of a spectrum of physiologic and psychological dysfunction due to low energy availability (1).
- When one aspect of REDs is found, the others should be investigated.
- Treatment requires a multidisciplinary approach, and should emphasize positive energy balance (with increased nutritional intake and decreased physical activity), resulting in resumption of normal menses. The use of hormones to augment bone density is not recommended.
- The IOC REDs CAT2 is a clinically validated tool clinicians may use to stratify risk and determine return to play for affected athletes (2).

RENAL TRAUMA

Angelina R. Edwards, MD, FASN • David S. Edwards, MD, CAQSM

BASICS

Genitourinary (GU) trauma comprises approximately 10% of all trauma but is relatively infrequent in sport-related injury. The most commonly injured organ is the kidney (1),(2).

EPIDEMIOLOGY

- Renal trauma occurs in 5% of all trauma cases and in 8–10% of patients with abdominal trauma. Up to 11% of blunt trauma in adults is sports related (3).
- Over the last two decades, incidence is rising due to motor vehicle collisions (MVC), particularly in young men (mean age 30.8 years) (2).
- Approximately 10% of blunt trauma in children includes renal involvement (2).
- Registry data indicate that 80–90% of renal injuries occur in children due to blunt trauma with 6.6% of cases secondary to sports (62% of these occur in football, 51% due to bicycling or falls, and 6% due to other team sports).
- Renal injuries are divided into renal laceration, renal contusion, and renal vascular injury (4),(5).

ETIOLOGY AND PATHOPHYSIOLOGY

- The major mechanisms that generate renal injury are blunt, iatrogenic during an interventional procedure, or intraoperative (4).
- The most common causes of renal injury are blunt trauma to the abdomen or back/flanks, especially with rapid deceleration as occurs in MVC, contact/collision sports, or fall from a height. Deceleration may avulse the renal pedicle and ureteropelvic junction (3).
- Penetrating injuries can cause up to 20% of renal injuries in urban areas (1).

RISK FACTORS

- Pediatric consideration: Children and adolescents are at increased risk due to greater kidney size relative to body size, less protection from ribs and perinephric fat, and weaker abdominal muscles (2),(6).
- Risk factors are heavily dependent on patient population and location and are seen in a variety of sports from cycling and equestrian events to snow sports or use of all-terrain vehicles (2),(6).

COMMONLY ASSOCIATED CONDITIONS

- Lower rib fractures
- Thoracolumbar vertebral fractures
- Intra-abdominal visceral injury

DIAGNOSIS

HISTORY

- Typical mechanisms include direct impact to the abdomen or flank, blow to the back, fall from a height, and rapid deceleration (1).
- In cases of penetrating trauma, the type or caliber of weapon or blade size can be helpful.
- A history of underlying renal abnormality can increase the risk of injury (5).
- In the absence of trauma: Painful hematuria suggests nephrolithiasis or infection, whereas painless hematuria in an adult could indicate bladder cancer or exercise-induced hematuria (5).

PHYSICAL EXAM

- Determine the stability of the patient with attention to primary survey, secondary survey, and vital signs, particularly blood pressure (BP):
  - Pediatric consideration: Hypotension may not correlate with degree of hypovolemia in children, so serial physical exams, BP measurements, and labs are essential (2),(6).
- Inspect for ecchymosis or hematoma to the abdomen and/or flanks.
- Inspect for penetrating injury to the abdomen, flanks, or lower chest.
- Evaluate for tenderness in the right or left upper quadrant, or flank pain.
- Palpate ribs and thoracolumbar spine for tenderness, crepitance, or step-offs.
- Auscultate and then palpate the abdomen for signs of visceral injury or peritonitis.
- Up to 50% of athletes with significant intra-abdominal injury do not have red flags on the initial exam (6).

DIFFERENTIAL DIAGNOSIS

Hematuria: renal contusion; renal infarction; renal laceration; nephrolithiasis; exercise-induced trauma to the bladder, urethra, or prostate; urinary tract infection; malignancy

DIAGNOSTIC TESTS & INTERPRETATION

Initial Tests (lab, imaging)

- Obtain basic labs with emphasis on hemoglobin/hematocrit, prothrombin time (PT)/international normalized ratio (INR), partial thromboplastin time (PTT), creatinine, and urinalysis with microscopy.

ALERT

- Order blood type and cross-match if suspicion for active bleeding.
- Gross hematuria is present in 95% of renal trauma.

- Increased creatinine suggests baseline renal impairment.
- Microscopic hematuria:
  - Three or more red blood cells (RBCs) per high-power field (HPF) in adults
  - Five or more RBCs per HPF in children (>50 RBCs per HPF in children per some sources)
- Neither degree nor absence of hematuria predicts severity of injury.
- The focused assessment with sonography in trauma (FAST) exam is a screening tool, developed for evaluation of blunt abdominal trauma (sensitivity 85–96%, specificity 98%) for free intraperitoneal fluid (6).
  - Accuracy is operator dependent.
  - If used on sideline, should not replace emergency room (ER) evaluation if suspicion for intra-abdominal trauma is high
  - If clinical suspicion is high, but negative FAST exam, further evaluation required as FAST may not reveal intra-abdominal organ injury if no hemoperitoneum.
- The preferred imaging modality is computed tomography (CT) of abdomen and pelvis with intravenous (IV) contrast and with immediate and delayed images (5)[C],(6)[C]:
  - Renal imaging during the FAST is limited by inability to detect depth of laceration and inability to differentiate extravasated blood from urinoma.
- Indications for CT abdomen and pelvis with IV contrast include:
  - Gross/microscopic hematuria (may be absent in 25–50% of ureteropelvic junction injuries) (5)[B]
  - Hypotension (systolic BP <90 mm Hg) (5)[B]
  - History or physical exam consistent with renal injury (even in the absence of hematuria) (5)[C]
  - Suspicion of renal injury or multiorgan trauma
- Indications for delayed contrast-enhanced CT (excretory phase imaging 5 to 10 minutes after contrast):
  - Evaluate the collecting system:
    - Parenchymal laceration (superficial <1 cm vs. deep >1 cm, can be poorly enhancing due to clotted blood and may mask a urine leak)
    - Perirenal hematoma (crescentic if small, lens-shaped/biconvex if large, enters perinephric space if capsule is lacerated) versus urinoma
- If too unstable for CT, consider intraoperative "single-shot" IV pyelogram (5)[C]:
  - Identifies a functional contralateral kidney
  - Provides staging information on the renal pelvis and ureter

ALERT

Repeat imaging in a stable patient is not warranted unless there is an acute change in their status.

- The American Association for the Surgery of Trauma (AAST) grading system correlates well with CT findings and need for surgery and should be used to grade severity. Grade 2 or higher is considered a "major" injury (3):
  - Grade 1: contusion or subscapular hematoma (75–85% of renal trauma) (3)
  - Grade 2: cortical renal laceration <1 cm and lack of urinary extravasation on excretory phase CT imaging or perirenal hematoma that is nonexpanding
  - Grade 3: deep renal laceration extending to the medulla, without urinary extravasation
  - Grade 4: laceration extending through the collecting system with extravasation, vascular injury or segmental infarction, hilum preserved, contained hematoma
  - Grade 5: shattered or fractured kidney or hilar avulsion and devascularization

TREATMENT

- The approach to renal injuries has changed over time, from aggressive surgical interventions to more conservative, nonoperative observational, or endovascular management (1).
- Typically, conservative in 95% of cases:
  - Prehospital/sidelines evaluation: primary survey, secondary survey if feasible, urgent transport via ambulance
  - Emergency department: primary and secondary survey if not already done, close hemodynamic monitoring, labs, imaging, IV resuscitation, and consultation with trauma and/or urology colleagues
  - Inpatient ward versus intensive care unit: depending on clinical status:
    - Noninvasive if hemodynamically stable (5)[B]
    - Hemodynamic monitoring
    - Bed rest until macroscopic hematuria clears.

- Serial examination and hemoglobin/hematocrit measurement
- Broad-spectrum IV antibiotics can be used if there is damage to the collecting system/urine leak, perinephric abscess, and/or concern for infected retroperitoneal hematoma in the setting of devitalized tissue, bowel or pancreatic injury, comorbidities, or immunosuppression (3).

– Conservative care for:
- Grades 1 to 2: differentiate contusion from segmental infarction on CT (5)[B]
- Grade 3: if hemodynamically stable (5)[B]
- Pediatric patients with grades 3 to 5: if hemodynamically stable (4)[A]

SURGERY/OTHER PROCEDURES

- There is a 64% rate of nephrectomy when renal injuries are explored surgically, regardless of the indication for exploration (3):
  - Goal of surgery is to control hemorrhage and salvage kidney function (5)[C].
  - Indications for surgery:
    - Hemodynamic instability, brief or no response to volume resuscitation (5)[C]
    - Hemodynamic instability, evidence of active bleeding (5)[C]:
      - Large perirenal hematoma (increased size is associated with higher rates of surgery or angioembolization)
      - Contrast leak from vasculature
      - Expanding, uncontained retroperitoneal hematoma
    - Renal pedicle avulsion
    - Persistent urinary leak
    - Worsening abdominal exam in children
- Endovascular management (5)[C]:
  - Transcatheter arterial angioembolization (TAE), with or without placement of stents/grafts, is becoming the preferred management of traumatic arterial injuries in those who are hemodynamically stable, without other indication for exploratory laparotomy.
  - Indication for endovascular management:
    - Diagnostic angiography and selective embolization of parenchymal injuries
    - Strongly recommended for high-grade injuries in hemodynamically stable children with continued or delayed bleeding (4)[B]
    - Stenting of renal arterial thrombosis
    - Segmental arterial injuries
  - May prevent nephrectomy in 78% of grade 4 and 83% of grade 5 renal injuries
  - Grades 4 and 5 lesions may require a second endovascular intervention to treat recurrent bleeding.
  - Postembolization syndrome:
    - Common side effect following TAE
    - Constellation of fever, abdominal pain, paralytic ileus with nausea and vomiting, leukocytosis
    - Severity of symptoms is dependent on the volume of infarcted tissue.
    - Moderate hematuria can occur depending on degree of infarction.
    - Treatment is supportive and duration is self-limited, resolving in a few days.
- Urinary drainage performed only in the presence of complications such as fever, increased pain, ileus, fistula, or infection (5)[C].

ONGOING CARE

FOLLOW-UP RECOMMENDATIONS

- Follow-up CT scan if any clinical signs of complications (5)[C]
- Follow-up CT scan after 48 hours indicated if deep injury or grades 4 to 5 injury (5)[C]
- Complications occur in 3–33% of renal trauma, especially with higher grade injuries, and include:
  - The leading complication is extravasation of urine and infection of this urinoma:
    - Small urinomas often reabsorb spontaneously.
    - Perinephric abscess is best treated by percutaneous drainage.
  - Early (acute, <1 month): worsening flank pain, uncontrolled bleeding, abdominal distention
  - Late:
    - Page kidney phenomenon/arterial hypertension (up to 40% of cases): extrinsic compression of renal parenchyma leading to intrarenal ischemia and activation of the renin-angiotensin system
    - Hypertension and renal impairment develop and can occur in native kidneys and renal allografts.
    - Hydronephrosis, stones, chronic pyelonephritis
- Outpatient follow-up:
  - Low-grade injury: 3 months for physical exam, urinalysis, measurement of electrolytes and creatinine, serial BP (5)[C]
  - Pediatric patients: Serial BP are strongly recommended; more research is needed on interval of checks and length of follow-up (4)[B].
- Return to play:
  - There is no evidenced-based statement or guideline.
  - Resolution of pain, healing of any procedural wound (if present), resolution of hematuria (including microscopic), and return to previous cardiovascular fitness
  - Hematuria usually resolves in 4 to 6 weeks.
  - Most sports-related renal injuries heal in 2 to 8 weeks, with high-grade injuries typically requiring more healing time.
- Considerations in renal transplant patients:
  - Kidney transplant remains an ideal treatment for end-stage renal disease, and although transplant patients make up a small percentage of trauma patients, large outcome data is lacking.
  - Retrospective reviews have challenged the common presumption among physicians that trauma patients with organ transplants do worse than nontransplanted patients.
  - Trauma registries show rare direct renal allograft injuries, few acute kidney injury events, and no greater infection risk from traumatic injuries.
  - An increased risk of posttrauma rejection was observed, perhaps due to trauma-related activation of the immune system, triggering a proinflammatory state.
  - Transplant trauma patients should be assessed by a transplant surgeon as soon as possible, and graft function should be closely followed, with input by the transplant nephrologist, during the hospitalization and after discharge.

REFERENCES

1. da Costa IA, Amend B, Stenzl A, et al. Contemporary management of acute kidney trauma. *J Acute Dis*. 2016;5:29–36.
2. Bernard JJ. Renal trauma: evaluation, management, and return to play. *Curr Sports Med Rep*. 2009;8(2):98–103.
3. Erlich T, Kitrey ND. Renal trauma: the current best practice. *Ther Adv Urol*. 2018;10(10):295–303.
4. Hagedorn JC, Fox N, Ellison JS, et al. Pediatric blunt renal trauma practice management guidelines: collaboration between the Eastern Association for the Surgery of Trauma and the Pediatric Trauma Society. *J Trauma Acute Care Surg*. 2019;86(5):916–925.
5. Morey AF, Broghammer JA, Hollowell CMP, et al. Urotrauma guideline 2020: American Urological Association guideline. *J Urol*. 2021;205(1):30–35.
6. Mathiasen RE, Hogrefe CP. Emergency abdominopelvic injuries. *Clin Sports Med*. 2023;42(3):409–425.

ADDITIONAL READING

- Bryk DJ, Zhao LC. Guideline of guidelines: a review of urological trauma guidelines. *BJU Int*. 2016;117(2):226–234.
- Coghlan K, McDermott J, Molloy M, et al. A narrative review of contact sports participation in children and young athletes with a solitary (functioning) kidney. *Am J Sports Med*. 2024;52(11):2939–2947.
- Freeman CM, Kelly ME, Nason GJ, et al. Renal trauma: the rugby factor. *Curr Urol*. 2015;8(3):133–137.
- Nicola R, Menias CO, Mellnick V, et al. Sports-related genitourinary trauma in the male athlete. *Emerg Radiol*. 2015;22(2):157–168.
- Rice SG; American Academy of Pediatrics Council on Sports Medicine and Fitness. Medical conditions affecting sports participation. *Pediatrics*. 2008;121(4):841–848.

CLINICAL PEARLS

- AAST grades 1 to 3 injuries have a low risk of complications with no need for follow-up CT scan in the setting of ongoing clinical improvement.
- The leading vascular injury due to blunt trauma is renal artery occlusion, manifesting as a well-defined segmental or global absence of parenchymal enhancement on CT scan. Collateral perfusion can create the "cortical rim sign" within 8 hours of trauma.
- Regardless of the grade of injury, nonoperative management, including observation, supportive therapy, and endovascular interventions, in hemodynamically stable patients, is favored over surgical intervention.
- Participation in contact or collision sport in the athlete with a single kidney is controversial. Please see the "Additional Reading" section for details (see Coghlan et al.).
- Although no consensus statement exists for return to play, athletes should not return to play until hematuria has resolved. For those in contact sports with grades 1 to 3 injuries, 2- to 6-week recovery time is reasonable. For those with more extensive injuries, more prolonged recovery on the order of 6 to 12 months may be required before returning to contact sports.

RETINAL DETACHMENTS AND TEARS

Brandon Schabacker, MD ▪ Catherine Carragee, MD ▪ Kenneth S. Taylor, MD, FAAFP, CAQSM

BASICS

DESCRIPTION

- Retinal detachment occurs when the neurosensory layer of the retina separates from the underlying retinal pigment epithelium and choroid.
- Three distinct classifications of retinal detachments:
  - Rhegmatogenous retinal detachment (RRD)
  - Tractional retinal detachment (TRD)
  - Exudative retinal detachment (ERD)
- RRD:
  - Occurs when a break in the sensory retina allows fluid from the vitreous to enter the subretinal space
  - Often preceded by posterior vitreous detachment (PVD)
- TRD:
  - Occurs because of contraction of fibrovascular or fibrotic tissue pulling the sensory retina off of the pigment epithelium
- ERD:
  - Abnormal collections of fluid are produced below the retina, separating the layer of the retina.

EPIDEMIOLOGY

- RRD is the most common type.
- Incidence increases with age.
- Average age of atraumatic onset ~55 years old.
- Male > female
- Occurs in 5–25% of patients with Marfan syndrome

ETIOLOGY AND PATHOPHYSIOLOGY

- RRD occurs as a result of either structural or developmental abnormalities of the eye or trauma:
  - High myopia
  - Lattice degeneration
  - PVD
  - Trauma is less common etiology however produces more retinal dialysis and giant tears.
- TRD:
  - Diabetic retinopathy
  - Proliferative vitreoretinopathy
  - Retinopathy of prematurity
  - Sickle cell retinopathy
  - Toxocariasis
  - Trauma
- ERD arises from transudative fluid:
  - Tumors of the choroid or retina
  - Inflammatory disorders such as Coats or Harada disease
  - Central serous retinopathy
  - Hypertensive retinopathy
  - Toxemia of pregnancy (preeclampsia)

RISK FACTORS

- Extreme myopia
- Cataract surgery
- Aphakia
- Trauma
- Retinal detachment in contralateral eye
- Glaucoma
- Vitreoretinal tufts: caused by focal areas of vitreous traction
- Meridional folds: redundant retina
- Family history of retinal detachment

GENERAL PREVENTION

- Early identification of retinal tears and treatment may prevent progression to retinal detachment and significant vision loss.
- Protective eyewear may prevent traumatic RRD.

DIAGNOSIS

HISTORY

- Sudden painless loss of visual acuity (filmy, cloudy or curtain like)
- Floaters
- Flashes of light (photopsias)
- Expanding shadow
- Progressive peripheral visual field defect
- May be asymptomatic

PHYSICAL EXAM

- Visual acuity and visual field testing:
  - May be decreased depending on location of tear/detachment
  - Important to differentiate macula on versus macula off
  - Macula on involves only peripheral vision.
  - Macula off involves central vision/acuity.
- Pupil exam:
  - May have relative afferent pupillary defect
- Dilated funduscopic exam:
  - RRD:
    - Mobile, convex retina
    - Retinal tears
    - Subretinal fluid does not shift with changes in head position.
    - Pigmented cells within the vitreous ("tobacco dust")
    - Vitreous hemorrhage
    - Chronic RRD: pigmented demarcation lines, intraretinal cysts, static retinal folds
  - TRD:
    - Smooth elevated retina
    - Fibrovascular proliferation
  - ERD:
    - Smooth elevated retina
    - Subretinal fluid shifts with changes in head position.
- Depressed peripheral retinal exam:
  - Indirect ophthalmoscopy using pressure to depress sclera in order to examine the peripheral retina for tears

DIFFERENTIAL DIAGNOSIS

- Senile retinoschisis
- Juvenile retinoschisis
- Choroidal detachment
- Vitreous hemorrhage
- Vitreous inflammation (e.g., *Toxoplasma* chorioretinitis)
- Central retinal artery occlusion (CRAO)
- Central retinal vein occlusion (CRVO)
- Occipital lobe stroke
- Ocular lymphoma
- Intraocular foreign body

DIAGNOSTIC TESTS & INTERPRETATION
B-scan ultrasound:
- Smooth, convex, mobile retina visualized as hyperechoic lesion in vitreous cavity
- In ERD, hyperechoic areas will shift with head movement.
- In TRD, will have tented appearance with vitreous adhesions

TREATMENT

ISSUES FOR REFERRAL
- Urgent ophthalmologic consultation (ideally within 24 hours)
- A retina specialist ultimately will need to care for the patient if retinal detachment is present.

SURGERY/OTHER PROCEDURES
- PVD management:
  - Most patients who present with PVD and do not have any retinal breaks or tears require only reassurance and education.
  - Full dilated exam with indirect ophthalmoscopy at least twice during the 6 weeks following onset of symptoms
- RRD:
  - Vitrectomy preferred for most RRDs
  - Vitrectomy and scleral buckling have similar outcomes (1)[A].
  - Pneumatic retinopexy can be performed in the office and is a cost-effective treatment for uncomplicated RRD (2)[B],(3)[A].
  - RRDs that do not yet involve the macula ("macula on") require repair within **24 to 48 hours**.
  - RRDs involving the macula ("macula off") may be repaired within **2 to 4 days**. There is no evidence that more urgent repair affects the outcome (4)[C].
- TRD:
  - Vitreoretinal surgery (vitrectomy with or without scleral buckling) to release traction if necessary
  - Observation unless macula is threatened or combined traction-rhegmatogenous detachment develops
- ERD:
  - Identify and treat etiology; surgical repair is not recommended in most cases.

ADMISSION, INPATIENT, AND NURSING CONSIDERATIONS
- Bed rest and minimal reading prior to surgery.
- Postoperatively, if intraocular gas has been used, the patient may need specific head positioning and may need to avoid all air travel or high altitudes.

ONGOING CARE

PROGNOSIS
RRD:
- Pneumatic retinopexy leads to successful retinal attachment 70–80% of the time after one procedure (5)[A]:
  - Offers better visual acuity outcomes in subset of patients (3)[A],(6)[C]
  - In cases of failure, treat with scleral buckle placement and/or vitrectomy.
- Scleral buckle placement is successful 80–90% of the time after one procedure (5)[A]:
  - Failed cases usually are treated with vitrectomy.
- Vitrectomy has an 80–90% success rate after one surgery (5)[A]:
  - In failed cases, more extensive vitreoretinal procedures are required.
- Virtually, all patients aged >50 years will develop progressive cataract following vitrectomy.

REFERENCES

1. Sun Q, Sun T, Xu Y, et al. Primary vitrectomy versus scleral buckling for the treatment of rhegmatogenous retinal detachment: a meta-analysis of randomized controlled clinical trials. *Curr Eye Res.* 2012;37(6):492–499.
2. Dhami A, Shah KK, Ratra D. Pneumatic retinopexy outcomes as primary or secondary surgical option for treating rhegmatogenous retinal detachment. *Indian J Ophthalmol.* 2018;66(3):420–425.
3. Roshanshad A, Shirzadi S, Binder S, et al. Pneumatic retinopexy versus pars plana vitrectomy for the management of retinal detachment: a systematic review and meta-analysis. *Ophthalmol Ther.* 2023;12(2):705–719.
4. Wykoff CC, Flynn HW Jr, Scott IU. What is the optimal timing for rhegmatogenous retinal detachment repair? *JAMA Ophthalmol.* 2013;131(11):1399–1400.
5. Sena DF, Kilian R, Liu SH, et al. Pneumatic retinopexy versus scleral buckle for repairing simple rhegmatogenous retinal detachments. *Cochrane Database Syst Rev.* 2021;11(11):CD008350.
6. Shah S, Chou B, Patel M, et al. Review and analysis of history and utilization of pneumatic retinopexy after pneumatic retinopexy versus vitrectomy for the management of primary rhegmatogenous retinal detachment outcomes randomized trial (PIVOT). *Curr Opin Ophthalmol.* 2024;35(3):217–222.

ADDITIONAL READING

- Lee TH, Chen YH, Kuo HK, et al. Retinal detachment associated with basketball-related eye trauma. *Am J Ophthalmol.* 2017;180:97–101.
- Read SP, Young RC, Flynn HW Jr. Outcomes in bullous retinal detachment. *Am J Ophthalmol Case Rep.* 2016;6:18–20.
- Yokoyama S, Kojima T, Mori T, et al. Clinical outcomes of endoscope-assisted vitrectomy for treatment of rhegmatogenous retinal detachment. *Clin Ophthalmol.* 2017;11:2003–2010.

CLINICAL PEARLS
- Concern for retinal tear or detachment should prompt urgent ophthalmology consultation.
- Although trauma is an uncommon etiology, protective eyewear may help to prevent traumatic causes of retinal detachment.
- Return to play:
  - The injured eye should feel comfortable and have adequate return of vision.
  - Eye protectors must be worn.

RHABDOMYOLYSIS

Vijay Jotwani, MD • Haris Vakil, MD

BASICS

DESCRIPTION

- The breakdown and necrosis of skeletal muscle with subsequent release of intracellular contents, such as myoglobin and creatine phosphokinase (CK)
- A combination of myoglobinuria, hypovolemia, and aciduria may lead to acute renal disease.
- Can be a result of trauma/crush injury or as a result of a training error where exertion persists beyond the point of fatigue (exertional rhabdomyolysis [ER]), often due to novel activity

EPIDEMIOLOGY

- Occurs in up to 85% of trauma patients
- 10–50% of patients with rhabdomyolysis will develop acute renal failure (ARF)
- ~26,000 people are affected in the United States each year.
- Exact incidence of ER is unknown but is likely comparable to military reports of 0.5–4% (1).

ETIOLOGY AND PATHOPHYSIOLOGY

- Muscle damage and/or necrosis that results in elevation in CK levels, electrolyte disturbances, and renal compromise as a result of:
  - Trauma/crush injuries (motor vehicle accidents, fall from seizure or stroke, struggle against restraints, abuse, prolonged tourniquet)
  - ER occurs due to exercise past the point of fatigue.
- Skeletal muscle necrosis occurs due to an increase in intracellular calcium resulting in rupture of the cellular membrane.
- Cell damage results in the release of intracellular contents including myoglobin, which is nephrotoxic. Myoglobin can be detected in the urine and causes darkening of urine color.
- Skeletal muscle damage also results in release of potassium, which can trigger arrhythmia and sudden death.

Genetics

Metabolic myopathies (1):

- Considered in recurrent cases or persistent CK elevation or kidney injury >2 weeks
- Inherited disorders:
  - McArdle disease
  - Carnitine palmitoyl transferase deficiency
  - Fatty acid oxidation deficiency
  - Aconitase deficiency
  - Myoadenylate dehydrogenase deficiency
  - Mitochondrial myopathies
  - Muscular dystrophy

RISK FACTORS

- Sudden increase in exercise intensity and repetitive muscular loading
- Inadequate conditioning
- Poor hydration
- Exercise in high heat or humidity
- Stimulant and supplement use (phentermine, creatine)
- High body mass
- High-risk medication or drug use (cocaine, amphetamines, alcohol, nonsteroidal anti-inflammatory drugs [NSAIDs], antihistamines, statins, etc.)
- Ongoing infection/exercise while febrile
- Sickle cell trait
- Heritable muscle enzyme deficiencies
- The majority of U.S. military cases occurred between June and August in black, non-Hispanic males <20 years of age (1).

DIAGNOSIS

- Symptoms of muscle injury along with an increase in CK levels are used to make the diagnosis. Typical threshold is a CK level 5 to 10 times the upper limit of normal (~1,000 IU/L) (1)[B].
- Symptoms include muscle pain, swelling, and weakness. Other general symptoms may include malaise, fever, tachycardia, and nausea.
- History and physical are insensitive in making the diagnosis and a high level of suspicion is needed for athletes with risk factors above.
- Serum CK level must be checked if any clinical suspicion exists (1)[B].
- Serum electrolytes, BUN, creatinine, calcium, and liver enzyme levels should be obtained:
  - Urine dipstick that is positive for heme, but absent for RBCs suggests rhabdomyolysis(myoglobinuria):
    - Because of rapid urinary excretion of myoglobin, up to 26% of patients with rhabdomyolysis have a negative urine dipstick.

HISTORY

- Wide range of severity of symptoms
- Classic triad of symptoms: muscle pain, weakness, and dark urine (seen in <10% of patients)
- General symptoms may include malaise, fever, tachycardia, nausea/emesis.
- ER typically due to error in training and will occur soon after exertion of increased intensity (i.e., early season training sessions, "two a days," new, intense, and group-based exercise programs, punishment-based workouts)

PHYSICAL EXAM

- Muscle tenderness, swelling, or weakness (proximal upper and lower extremities, calves, and lower back are most involved) (2)[B]
- Change in urine color; orange to cola-colored to black (not a reliable finding occurring in as few as 25% of cases)
- Visible crush injury in traumatic rhabdomyolysis
- Patient may be either alert or obtunded.
- Hypovolemic state, dry mucous membrane, poor skin turgor, tachycardia, hypotension
- Hypothermia/hyperthermia
- Decreased urine output

DIFFERENTIAL DIAGNOSIS

The following conditions can also cause muscle pain or swelling:

- Muscle strain
- Delayed onset muscle soreness
- Muscle infection
- Sickle cell crisis
- Nontraumatic myopathies
- Hypercalcemia/hyperparathyroidism
- Hypo/hyperthyroidism
- Renal failure
- Tumor

DIAGNOSTIC TESTS & INTERPRETATION

Initial Tests (lab, imaging)

- CK levels are the most sensitive; CK-MM isoenzyme is most elevated.
- CK rise of 5 to 10 times normal upper limit (~1,000 IU/L) is concerning for rhabdomyolysis (2)[B].
- CK levels rise within 12 hours, typically peak in 1 to 4 days, and gradually return to normal over days to weeks.

ALERT

CK levels can rise well above levels of 100,000 IU/L, but the severity of CK rise does not necessarily correlate to presence of myoglobinuria or severity of renal failure.

- Physical exertion can increase CK levels without rhabdomyolysis as well:
  - Black military recruits had a mean rise in CK to 1,226 IU/L at day 7 of basic training (but range as high as 35,000) without rhabdomyolysis (2).
  - Study of ultramarathoners found a mean CK increase to 2,400 IU/L also without symptoms of rhabdomyolysis.
- Urine dipstick will show blood, but no RBCs due to myoglobinuria.
- Serum and urine myoglobin levels are useful in acute phase but have short half-life and may return to normal within 6 to 8 hours.
- Metabolic profile to check for hyperkalemia, hypocalcemia, hyperphosphatemia, hyperuricemia
- Toxicology screen in absence of physical injury
- Prothrombin time/partial thromboplastin time, platelet count, fibrinogen, fibrin-split products if disseminated intravascular coagulopathy is suspected.
- Magnetic resonance imaging (MRI) is sensitive in visualizing muscle injury but is not typically obtained because it does not affect treatment.

Diagnostic Procedures/Other

Forearm ischemic test:

- To differentiate genetic causes of rhabdomyolysis
- Performed after rhabdomyolysis is resolved
- Obtain baseline ammonia and lactic acid levels.
- Inflate sphygmomanometer to >200 mm Hg.
- Patient performs hand-grip exercises to fatigue.
- Cuff is removed and serial blood tests are drawn.

- Minimal or no rise in lactic acid suggests carbohydrate metabolism disorder or McArdle disease.
- Delayed rise or no rise in the ammonia level suggests myoadenylate deaminase deficiency.
- Normal rise in ammonia and lactic acid levels suggests the presence of a disorder of lipid metabolism.

TREATMENT

- Aggressive fluid resuscitation is paramount to limiting renal compromise.
- Prehospital:
  - Need for rapid extrication in case of crush injury
  - Early intravenous (IV) fluids to prevent complications (hypovolemia, ARF, hyperkalemia, etc.)
- Emergency department (ED) treatment:
  - Directed toward treating or reversing the underlying cause of rhabdomyolysis
  - Prevent ARF (3)[B]:
    - Immediate IV isotonic saline
    - Bicarbonate administration can be considered for alkalization of urine to decrease myoglobin toxicity to renal tubules.
    - Mannitol following IV saline promotes diuresis, acts as renal vasodilator, and may act as free-radical scavenger, but clinical effects are unproven.
    - Furosemide administration is controversial.
  - Hyperkalemia: IV fluid, sodium bicarbonate, dextrose, insulin, telemetry monitor/electrocardiogram
  - Drug overdose: activated charcoal, lavage, antidote
  - Infection: broad-spectrum antibiotics
  - Compartment syndrome: fasciotomy (compartment pressure >35 mm Hg)
  - Neuroleptic malignant syndrome: dantrolene, bromocriptine
  - Need for hemodialysis: refractory to treatment, hyperkalemia, hyperphosphatemia, hyperuricemia, volume overload, overdose

MEDICATION

Medication guidelines (2),(3):

- Administer IV isotonic saline at 400 to 2,000 mL/h initially followed by maintenance at 120 to 400 mL/h (3).
- Goal: to achieve urine output of 200 to 300 mL/h until myoglobinuria resolves

First Line

IV fluids: isotonic saline

Second Line

- Addition of potassium chloride, bicarbonate, and mannitol has been recommended but has unproven benefit.
- Furosemide administration is controversial.

ADMISSION, INPATIENT, AND NURSING CONSIDERATIONS

- Initial stabilization:
  - Airway, breathing, and circulation (ABCs)
  - Immobilization of trauma/crush injuries
  - IV fluids for hypotension and hypovolemia
- Admission criteria:
  - Because it is impossible to predict which patients will develop complications, all patients with significant elevated CK or suspicion for rhabdomyolysis should be admitted.
  - Admit to telemetry-monitored bed for patients with electrolyte abnormalities.
  - Admit to intensive care unit bed for patients who might require hemodialysis or closer fluid and electrolyte monitoring.
  - Consider nephrology consultation if significant or persisting renal injury is noted.
  - CK levels should be reevaluated at least once daily (3)[B].
- IV fluids:
  - Plasma volume resuscitation with isotonic saline is first-line treatment.
- Nursing:
  - Monitor input/output closely with attention to urinary output.
- Discharge criteria:
  - No specific CK level is necessary for discharge, but level should be decreasing before considering discharge.
  - Myoglobinuria, when present, should be resolved.
  - Stable electrolytes and adequate renal function required before discharge from hospital.
  - Patient should demonstrate tolerance for PO hydration. Patient should follow up within 1 week after discharge.

ONGOING CARE

- Underlying cause of rhabdomyolysis should be determined if etiology was not discovered during hospital stay.
- Genetic testing and muscle biopsy should be considered when there is a suspicion for underlying genetic conditions.
- Medications, if implicated, should be stopped.
- Metabolic-modifying supplements and enhancing agents should be stopped.
- Activity modification if presumed exercise-induced

FOLLOW-UP RECOMMENDATIONS

- No evidence-based guidelines exist for return to exercise after ER, but graded return is encouraged (3).
- Return-to-play considerations:
  - Symptoms should be completely resolved.
  - Blood work should be trending toward normal limits.
  - Myoglobinuria should be resolved.
  - Infection and fever should be resolved.
  - Examination should demonstrate normal muscle strength and resolution of muscle pain.
  - Gradual return to exercise should first begin in cool, controlled environments to allow acclimatization before moving outdoors (4).
  - Return to exercise should begin with low-impact aerobic activities involving concentric muscle contractions and gradually advance toward higher impact resistance and eccentric exercise (4).

Patient Monitoring

Initially, patient should be monitored clinically at regular short intervals with close physician follow-up.

DIET

- Education should be provided about hydration.
- Specific diet recommendations may be considered for specific myopathies.

PATIENT EDUCATION

Prevention strategies for return to sports after rhabdomyolysis:

- Appropriate hydration counseling should be provided.
- Gradual return to exercise may include acclimatization.
- Return to exercise should begin with mild to moderate intensity.
- Athlete should be advised to stop activity if he or she experiences similar symptoms and physician should be contacted immediately.

COMPLICATIONS

- Early complications:
  - Hyperkalemia
  - Hypocalcemia
  - Cardiac arrhythmia
  - Cardiac arrest
  - Compartment syndrome
- Late complications (past 12 hours):
  - ARF with oliguria
  - Hypercalcemia
  - Disseminated intravascular coagulation
  - Compartment syndrome

REFERENCES

1. Nye NS, Kasper K, Madsen CM, et al. Clinical practice guidelines for exertional rhabdomyolysis: a military medicine perspective. *Curr Sports Med Rep.* 2021;20(3):169–178.
2. Gupta A, Thorson P, Penmatsa KR, et al. Rhabdomyolysis: revisited. *Ulster Med J.* 2021;90(2):61–69.
3. Fernandes PM, Davenport RJ. How to do it: investigate exertional rhabdomyolysis (or not). *Pract Neurol.* 2019;19(1):43–48.
4. Schleich K, Slayman T, West D, et al. Return to play after exertional rhabdomyolysis. *J Athl Train.* 2016;51(5):406–409.

CLINICAL PEARLS

- Consider rhabdomyolysis in any athlete with muscle pain, swelling, or weakness or following significant trauma.
- ER is a preventable condition that occurs secondary to training error when exertion persists beyond fatigue.
- CK elevation >5 times the upper limit and symptoms of muscle injury are required for diagnosis, but CK levels can vary significantly amongst cases and can also be elevated in cases of asymptomatic physical exertion.
- Inpatient monitoring of kidney function and IV fluid administration is required for treatment.
- Discharge from hospital can be made when CK and creatinine values are trending toward normal and return to sport must be gradual and individualized.

RHEUMATOID ARTHRITIS IN SPORTS

Shane Hudnall, MD, CAQSM • Hunter Rafoth, MD •
Kenneth P. Barnes, MD, MSc, CAQSM, FACP, FACSM, FAMSSM

BASICS

Chronic systemic inflammatory autoimmune disorder that primarily affects the small joints of the body causing a symmetric polyarthritis

DESCRIPTION

- Polyarthritis most commonly affects the joints of the wrist, the proximal interphalangeal (PIP) and metacarpophalangeal (MCP) joints of the hands, and the metatarsophalangeal (MTP) joints of the feet.
- Less commonly affects cervical spine (although higher risk of atlantoaxial instability than general population), ankles, knees, hips, elbows, and shoulders
- Extra-articular manifestations: anemia, rheumatoid nodules (20–30%), pleuritis, pericarditis, entrapment neuropathies (carpal tunnel syndrome), episcleritis and scleritis (<1%), splenomegaly, renal disease, interstitial lung fibrosis, pericarditis, interstitial lung disease, vasculitis, Sjögren syndrome, Felty syndrome (rheumatoid arthritis [RA], splenomegaly, neutropenia)

EPIDEMIOLOGY

Incidence

- Annual incidence 3/10,000
- Prevalence and disease burden higher in industrialized countries
- Prevalence overall 1%; varies from 0.1% to 5% based on ethnic background
- Predominant gender: female > male (2 to 5:1; ratio increases in patients >60 years old)
- Onset most common between 30 and 50 years of age, although mean age of onset is 52 years

ETIOLOGY AND PATHOPHYSIOLOGY

- Characterized by the presence of pannus (a proliferative mass of inflammatory vascularized tissue that may erode bone or cartilage)
- Macrophages produce cytokines (e.g., tissue necrosis factor α [TNF-α]), which produce many of the systemic features (e.g., fatigue, weight loss, elevated C-reactive protein [CRP] and erythrocyte sedimentation rate [ESR], and joint damage).

RISK FACTORS

- Female gender (Pregnancy and oral contraceptive use may be protective.)
- Nulliparity
- Family history (identical twins 3 to 4 times more likely to share disease than fraternal twins)
- Certain human leukocyte antigen (HLA)-DRB1 alleles that code the same epitope
- Cigarette smoking (Risk is amplified when present along with specific HLA-DRB1 alleles.)
- Obesity
- Silica or asbestos exposure
- Electrical workers
- Wood workers

DIAGNOSIS

HISTORY

- Clinical diagnosis: usually symmetric synovitis (warmth, swelling, tenderness) of small joints (MCPs, PIPs, MTPs, wrists) with morning stiffness >1 hour that improves with activity
- Progression to joint destruction and deformities (ulnar deviation at MCPs, volar subluxation at MCPs and wrists, swan-neck, and/or boutonnière deformities of fingers)
- Constitutional symptoms are quite common (e.g., low-grade fever, fatigue, myalgia, weight loss).
- American College of Rheumatology/European League Against Rheumatism (ACR/EULAR) classification criteria (6+ points needed to classify as definite RA) (1):
  - Joint involvement (only one of the below):
    - 2 to 10 large joints—1 point
    - 1 to 3 small joints—2 points
    - 4 to 10 small joints—3 points
    - >10 joints including 1 small joint—5 points
  - Serology
    - Low positive rheumatoid factor (RF) or anti-citrullinated protein antibody (ACPA)—2 points
    - High positive RF or ACPA—3 points
  - Acute-phase reactants
    - Abnormal CRP and/or ESR—1 point
  - Duration of symptoms
    - 6+ weeks—1 point
- Note that ~25% of patients have monoarticular involvement at initial presentation.
- Extra-articular manifestations (e.g., chest pain, shortness of breath, skin changes, nodules, dry eyes, or mouth)

PHYSICAL EXAM

- Examine joints thoroughly for synovitis (warmth, swelling, tenderness, erythema).
- Look for deformities (swan-neck, boutonnières, ulnar deviation of digits/wrists, volar subluxation at MCP or wrist, subcutaneous [SC] nodules).
- Nail fold infarcts
- Splinter hemorrhages
- Rheumatoid nodules
- Splenomegaly
- Pericardial rub
- Pleural effusions
- Rales (interstitial lung disease)
- Eye exam for scleritis/episcleritis

DIFFERENTIAL DIAGNOSIS

- Osteoarthritis (typically involves distal interphalangeal joints, knees, hips)
- Systemic lupus erythematosus (SLE)
- Gout
- Pseudogout
- Polymyalgia rheumatica
- Reactive arthritis
- Psoriatic arthritis
- Lyme disease
- Septic arthritis

DIAGNOSTIC TESTS & INTERPRETATION

- Joint fluid exam most helpful: >10,000 white blood cells (WBCs) with neutrophilic predominance characteristic but nondiagnostic (should also consider infection)
- RF positive >80% of the time but is not sufficient for diagnosis or to rule out diagnosis; if positive, more likely to have severe disease and extra-articular involvement
- Antinuclear antibodies (ANA) also not diagnostic
- ESR and CRP are not specific but may be elevated and part of diagnostic criteria.
- Complete blood count (CBC): leukocytosis, thrombocytosis, anemia: hemoglobin >9; level correlates with disease severity
- Abnormal liver function tests: low albumin directly linked to disease severity; elevated alkaline phosphatase
- Anticyclic citrullinated peptide (anti-CCP) antibodies: sensitivity of 67%, specificity of 95% for diagnosis of RA; associated with erosive disease
- X-rays: erosions or bony decalcification in wrist or posteroanterior hand radiographs
- Early: Obtain posteroanterior view of hands and wrists, anteroposterior view of both feet for future comparison of bony destruction.
- Magnetic resonance imaging (MRI) and ultrasound much more sensitive for detecting early signs of damage and revealing erosions or edematous bony lesions that were not demonstrated on plain radiography

TREATMENT

- Achieving the benefits of early intervention depends on making the diagnosis as early as possible before irreversible damage has occurred.
- Nonpharmacologic treatment:
  - Patient education, relative rest, routine exercise, physical and occupational therapy, cognitive-behavioral therapy, dietary therapy
  - Cognitive-behavioral therapy and self-management educational interventions have been shown to reduce pain and disability.
  - Counseling-based physical activity promotion changes physical activity behavior in those with RA (2)[A].
  - Exercise in the appropriate intensity and frequency improves fitness and muscle strength in patients with RA (2)[A].
  - Aerobic exercise has been shown to improve pain scores and quality of life.
  - Occupational therapy hand exercise programs in RA improve hand function.
  - Limit and treat cardiovascular risk factors (smoking, hyperlipidemia, hypertension, diabetes) given RA increases risk of atherosclerotic disease.
- Pharmacologic treatment:
  - Disease-modifying antirheumatic drugs (DMARDs) monotherapy preferred in patients who have never taken one before regardless of disease activity
  - Review specific side-effect profiles and monitoring parameters for medications.

MEDICATION

- Analgesia: nonsteroidal anti-inflammatory drugs (NSAIDs) helpful in controlling pain and inflammation, improving daily function, but they do not alter natural course of disease:
  - High-dose aspirin (12 to 16 tablets/d) or ibuprofen (2,400 mg/d) (rarely used because of gastrointestinal [GI] risks)
- DMARDs: These drugs have the potential to reduce or prevent joint damage and to preserve joint integrity and function. These should be offered to all patients as early as possible in disease course; divided into nonbiologic and biologic agents (3)[A],(4)[A]

- Nonbiologic agents:
  - Methotrexate is the most used nonbiologic agent and is first-line monotherapy for a DMARD-naive patient. Takes effect as early as 4 weeks; not to take in pregnancy; monitor for hematologic, hepatic, or pulmonary side effects (use folic acid supplementation 1 mg daily with methotrexate):
    - If fails, combine therapy with other DMARDs (methotrexate + sulfasalazine + hydroxychloroquine) or use a biologic agent with or without methotrexate
  - Sulfasalazine
  - Hydroxychloroquine
  - Leflunomide
- Biologic agents:
  - Effective at modifying disease and preventing erosions but increased risk of infection
  - Tuberculosis skin test prior to initiation because it can reactivate mycobacterial infections
  - As general rule, do not combine biologic agents with one another.
  - TNF inhibitors
    - Etanercept: inhibits action of TNF-α; SC injection 50 mg every week or 25 mg twice weekly.
    - Infliximab: antibody to TNF-α; periodic intravenous (IV) infusion
    - Adalimumab: anti-TNF monoclonal antibody; SC injection 40 mg every other week
    - Golimumab: anti-TNF monoclonal antibody; SC injection 50 mg once per month
    - Certolizumab: anti-TNF monoclonal antibody; initial: 400-mg SC injection, repeat dose 2 and 4 weeks after initial dose; maintenance: 200 mg SC every other week
  - Other biologic agents include rituximab, tocilizumab, sarilumab, and abatacept.
- Corticosteroids:
  - Mostly used as an adjunct for temporary control of disease in patients starting/switching DMARD therapy or those with acute disease flare; on their own, they do not provide long-term benefit for disease control or joint injury prevention.
  - For isolated joint involvement, intra-articular glucocorticoid injections may be effective and avoid the need for systemic steroid treatment.
  - Widespread flares can be treated by initiating oral glucocorticoids.
  - Pulse IV methylprednisolone is reserved for severe flares with systematic manifestations.
  - Prednisolone <7.5 mg/d is safe; greater doses should be considered only for short periods of time(4)[A].

ADDITIONAL THERAPIES

Consider total joint replacement for severe disability or pain that is unresponsive to medical therapy.

ONGOING CARE

PATIENT EDUCATION

- Exercise and increase in activity are associated with decreased level of pain, increased function, and better outcomes in patients with RA (best data shown for whole-body low-intensity group and individual exercise) (5).
- Start exercising slowly; over time, increase the length and intensity of workouts.
- Adjust workouts depending on symptoms.
- Athletes with a history of cervical spine involvement and high-risk sports need flexion/extension radiographs of C1 and C2 to assess risk of motion (atlantoaxial instability) and subsequent spinal cord injury.
- Generally, can play most sports, although contact sports and sports with a trampoline confer much greater risk and may be discouraged
- Athletes with ocular involvement should be screened by an ophthalmologist before being allowed to play; may need eye protection
- The presence of systemic idiopathic (juvenile) RA or HLA-B27–associated RA requires a cardiovascular assessment.

PROGNOSIS

- Clinical course and severity highly variable, ranging from insidious onset, slowly progressive disease with little destruction of joint spaces and few deformities (majority of cases), to a rapidly progressive disease leading to severe bony destruction and deformities (10–15%)
- Poor prognostic factors:
  - Functional limitation
  - Extra-articular disease
  - RF positivity or anti-CCP antibody positive
  - Bony erosions by x-ray
  - Cigarette smoking
- Disease remission occurs when there is little or no evidence of clinical disease activity.
- ACR Remission Criteria (must have minimum of 5 for >2 months) (6):
  - Morning stiffness not to exceed 15 minutes
  - No fatigue
  - No joint pain
  - No joint tenderness to palpation
  - No soft tissue swelling in joints or tendons
  - ESR <30 mm/h (women) or <20 mm/h (men)
- Achieving remission does not entirely preclude the development of further erosive changes.

COMPLICATIONS

- 50% increased risk of cardiovascular disease death in those with RA
- Increased risk of stroke (especially ischemic) with RA
- 70% higher risk for developing infection (related to immune dysfunction)
- Increased likelihood to develop lymphoma correlates directly with RA disease severity.

REFERENCES

1. Kay J, Upchurch KS. ACR/EULAR 2010 rheumatoid arthritis classification criteria. *Rheumatology (Oxford)*. 2012;51(Suppl 6):vi5–vi9.
2. Osthoff AKR, Juhl CB, Knittle K, et al. Effects of exercise and physical activity promotion: meta-analysis informing the 2018 EULAR recommendations for physical activity in people with rheumatoid arthritis, spondyloarthritis and hip/knee osteoarthritis. *RMD Open*. 2018;4(2):e000713.
3. Fraenkel L, Bathon JM, England BR, et al. 2021 American College of Rheumatology guideline for the treatment of rheumatoid arthritis. *Arthritis Care Res (Hoboken)*. 2021;73(7):924–939.
4. Smolen JS, Landewé RBM, Bergstra SA, et al. EULAR recommendations for the management of rheumatoid arthritis with synthetic and biological disease-modifying antirheumatic drugs: 2022 update. *Ann Rheum Dis*. 2023;82(1):3–18.
5. England BR, Smith BJ, Baker NA, et al. 2022 American College of Rheumatology guideline for exercise, rehabilitation, diet, and additional integrative interventions for rheumatoid arthritis. *Arthritis Rheumatol*. 2023;75(8):1299–1311.
6. van Tuyl LHD, Vlad SC, Felson DT, et al. Defining remission in rheumatoid arthritis: results of an initial American College of Rheumatology/European League Against Rheumatism consensus conference. *Arthritis Rheum*. 2009;61(5):704–710.

ADDITIONAL READING

- Aviña-Zubieta JA, Choi HK, Sadatsafavi M, et al. Risk of cardiovascular mortality in patients with rheumatoid arthritis: a meta-analysis of observational studies. *Arthritis Rheum*. 2008;59(12):1690–1697.
- Baillet A, Zeboulon N, Gossec L, et al. Efficacy of cardiorespiratory aerobic exercise in rheumatoid arthritis: meta-analysis of randomized controlled trials. *Arthritis Care Res (Hoboken)*. 2010;62(7):984–992.
- Bradley LA, Young LD, Anderson KO, et al. Effects of psychological therapy on pain behavior of rheumatoid arthritis patients. Treatment outcome and six-month follow-up. *Arthritis Rheum*. 1987;30(10):1105–1114.
- Doran MF, Crowson CS, Pond GR, et al. Frequency of infection in patients with rheumatoid arthritis compared with controls: a population-based study. *Arthritis Rheum*. 2002;46(9):2287–2293.
- Finckh A, Gilbert B, Hodkinson B, et al. Global epidemiology of rheumatoid arthritis. *Nat Rev Rheumatol*. 2022;18(10):591–602.
- Goekoop-Ruiterman YPM, de Vries-Bouwstra JK, Allaart CF, et al. Clinical and radiographic outcomes for four different treatment strategies in patients with early rheumatoid arthritis (the BeSt study): a randomized, controlled trial. *Arthritis Rheum*. 2005;52(11):3381–3390.
- Häkkinen A, Sokka T, Kotaniemi A, et al. A randomized two-year study of the effects of dynamic strength training on muscle strength, disease activity, functional capacity, and bone mineral density in early rheumatoid arthritis. *Arthritis Rheum*. 2001;44(3):515–522.
- Lamb SE, Williamson EM, Heine PJ, et al. Exercises to improve function of the rheumatoid hand (SARAH): a randomized controlled trial. *Lancet*. 2015;385(9966):421–429.
- Nishimura K, Sugiyama D, Kogata Y, et al. Meta-analysis: diagnostic accuracy of anti-cyclic citrullinated peptide antibody and rheumatoid factor for rheumatoid arthritis. *Ann Intern Med*. 2007;146(11):797–808.
- Rantalaiho V, Korpela M, Hannonen P, et al. The good initial response to therapy with a combination of traditional disease-modifying antirheumatic drugs is sustained over time: the eleven-year results of the Finnish rheumatoid arthritis combination therapy trial. *Arthritis Rheum*. 2009;60(5):1222–1231.
- Solomon DH, Goodson NJ, Katz JN, et al. Patterns of cardiovascular risk in rheumatoid arthritis. *Ann Rheum Dis*. 2006;65(12):1608–1612.
- van Drongelen V, Holoshitz J. Human leukocyte antigen—disease associations in rheumatoid arthritis. *Rheum Dis Clin North Am*. 2017;43(3):363–376.
- Warsi A, LaValley MP, Wang PS, et al. Arthritis self-management education programs: a meta-analysis of the effect on pain and disability. *Arthritis Rheum*. 2003;48(8):2207–2213.

CLINICAL PEARLS

- Treatment of patients with RA should be aimed for the best care and must be based on shared decision making between the patient and their rheumatologist.
- Exercise is helpful and should be encouraged as part of every patient's treatment.
- Treatment decisions are based on disease activity, safety issues, and other patient factors, such as comorbidities and progression of structural damage.
- Rheumatologists are the specialists who should primarily care for patients with RA.
- Patients require access to multiple drugs with different modes of action to address the heterogeneity of RA; they may require multiple successive therapies throughout life.
- RA incurs high individual, medical, and societal costs, all of which should be considered in its management by the treating rheumatologist.

ROTATOR CUFF TEARS

Weng Leong Choy, MD • Kenneth M. Bielak, MD, MBA, FAAFP, FACSM

BASICS

DESCRIPTION

- Partial or complete tears or disruption of any one or combination of the four rotator cuff muscles of the glenohumeral joint
- Supraspinatus and infraspinatus muscle-tendon complexes are the most common tears.
- Rotator cuff muscles are the supraspinatus, infraspinatus, teres minor, and subscapularis muscles.

EPIDEMIOLOGY

- Rare in young athletes
- More common in athletes >40 years of age, especially those with a history of many years of repetitive overhead sports
- More common than osteoarthritis (Shoulder is the only joint where soft tissue often wears out before joint.)

RISK FACTORS

- Older-than-40-years "weekend warrior" with years of repetitive overhead use (e.g., swimming, tennis, volleyball, gymnastics, weight lifting, and throwing sports)
- Previous trauma
- Sports with potential fall risk, such as equestrian, skiing, and body surfing

ETIOLOGY AND PATHOPHYSIOLOGY

- Can present following specific trauma (acute traumatic tear)
- Usually degenerative (chronic impingement syndrome), especially in older athlete with overhead sports
- Asymptomatic tears are more prevalent with age >40 years.

DIAGNOSIS

HISTORY

Mechanism of injury:

- Acute traumatic events such as a fall, direct blow, or forceful boxing punch
- Traumatic hyperextension of abducted arm
- Traumatic external or internal rotation of abducted arm
- Anterior dislocation

ALERT
Chronic overhead arm use may develop insidiously.

ALERT
Nocturnal pain and pain on sleeping on the affected side are common.

- Pain location can be variable (anterior, lateral, or posterior shoulder).
- Pain may radiate to elbow.
- Pain typically is aggravated with reaching motions: laterally (abduction), toward the back (internal rotation) and/or overhead.

PHYSICAL EXAM

- Diminished active range of motion (ROM)
- Pain with arm abduction, especially at 80 to 120 degrees of arc (1)[B]
- Atrophy of cuff muscles, especially if chronic
- Crepitus of supraspinatus muscle during abduction
- Rotator cuff muscle weakness
- Drop-arm test is positive for partial-thickness tear (14.3% sensitive, 88.4% specific) and full-thickness tear (34.9% sensitive, 87.5% specific) (1)[B]:
  - Arm is passively abducted to 90 degrees.
  - Patient is instructed to slowly return the arm to the side.
  - Severe pain or inability to do so is positive test for a torn rotator cuff complex.
- Empty can test is positive for large or full-thickness tears of supraspinatus (88% sensitive, 70% specific) (2)[B]:
  - Resistance applied to arm abducted 90 degrees, angled 30 degrees anteriorly with a medially rotated forearm (thumbs down, "empty can")
  - Test is positive for inability to do so or severe pain.
- Test external rotation (infraspinatus/teres minor) strength (partial tear 19.4% sensitive, 68.9% specific; full tear 50.5% sensitive, 84% specific) (1)[B]:
  - Perform test with elbow flexed 90 degrees at the side.
- Lift-off lag test (subscapularis): inability to lift the dorsum of the hand off the back hip
- Internal rotation lag test (modified lift-off test): Inability to maintain lift-off position and springs back (toward the back) is more accurate (3)[B], with 97% sensitivity and 83% specificity (4)[A].
- External rotation lag test (inability to maintain position of full external rotation) has sensitivity of 47% and specificity of 94% (4)[A].
- Significant pain with internal rotation can preclude an accurate test.
- Poor scapular stability is often present.
- Anterior glenoid-humeral laxity may be noted.
- Comprehensive testing of active and passive ROM, strength testing, and adequate neurovascular testing are recommended.

ALERT
In a multicenter review, the authors found that anatomic features defining the severity of atraumatic rotator cuff tears are not associated with the pain level. Factors associated with pain are comorbidities, lower education level, and race (4)[C].

DIFFERENTIAL DIAGNOSIS

- Rotator cuff strains
- Glenoid labrum tear
- Subluxation or unstable shoulder
- Subacromial impingement
- Isolated bicipital tendinitis
- Acromioclavicular joint disorders
- Glenohumeral arthritis
- Rare subacromial abscess or tumors
- Adhesive capsulitis
- Cervical radiculopathy can radiate to the shoulder.

DIAGNOSTIC TESTS & INTERPRETATION

Initial Tests (lab, imaging)

- Plain radiographs, although not specific for rotator cuff tears, may show some findings that are suggestive:
  - Calcifications along the tendons of the rotator cuff muscle (repetitive/chronic injury)
  - Subacromial osteophytes (may predispose to tears)
  - Superior or anterior migration of the humeral head (indicates full-thickness tear) (5)[B]
- Magnetic resonance imaging (MRI) demonstrates an 80–97% sensitivity in detecting full-thickness rotator cuff tears. Partial tears are more difficult to detect, with a sensitivity of 67–89%. This improves if fat suppression is used (6)[B].
- One caution is the use of MRI evaluation in patients with severe osteoarthritis of the glenohumeral joint as one study suggests that although MRI is highly sensitive, it has a low positive predictive value and moderately low specificity and accuracy in detecting full-thickness rotator cuff tears in patients with severe glenohumeral osteoarthritis (7)[C].
- 40% asymptomatic >50 years old have full rotator cuff tear (8),(9)[B].
- 60% asymptomatic >60 years old have partial or full rotator cuff tear (8)[B].
- One other study differs slightly on asymptomatic tears: 26–56% asymptomatic tears age: 63.1 ± 9 years
- Double-contrast arthrotomography (DCAT) is 100% sensitive and 94% specific in diagnosing complete rotator cuff tears but is much less sensitive for partial tears; probably more appropriate when concern for instability rather than pain alone
- Ultrasound (US) advantages are inexpensive and can localize areas of tenderness and dysfunction with patient present and in dynamic examination (technician dependent) (10)[B]. One study found no statistically significant difference between US and MRI in detection of rotator cuff tears of any type (11)[C].

ALERT
Diagnostic accuracy of shoulder US when evaluating rotator cuff tears can reach 91–100% for partial- and full-thickness tears detection, respectively, having been reported to be as accurate as MRI in experienced hands (12)[C].

Diagnostic Procedures/Other

Diagnostic injection: Subacromial bursa injection (10 mL of 1% lidocaine) may distinguish minor impingement and tendinosis from distinct tears of the rotator cuff (no pain relief or strength improvement from the injection).

TREATMENT

GENERAL MEASURES

- Acute treatment
- Analgesia:
  - Nonsteroidal anti-inflammatory drugs (NSAIDs) are the drugs of choice initially, but long-term use prior to operative repair can result in inferior long-term outcomes (13)[C].
  - More potent analgesics should rarely be necessary temporarily to relieve nocturnal symptoms.
- Immobilization: Sling may provide some relief for the acutely injured shoulder, but limit to initial 2 to 3 weeks as needed.
- Subacromial corticosteroid injection may provide short term (<8 weeks) limited pain benefit (14)[C].

ADDITIONAL THERAPIES

- Prolonged rehabilitation emphasizing increased ROM and strengthening is indicated for a partial tear.
- Normalizing scapulothoracic stabilization and posterior capsular flexibility with a 1:1 strength ratio for rotator cuff to anterior/middle cuff deltoid muscle
- *Future considerations as more research is published*:
  - A small study found that prolotherapy using dextrose solution reported excellent or good outcomes in 53 patients (92.9%) compared to 56.8% in the control group of 25 patients with partial tears (15)[C].
  - One author's review suggests of the myriad options being currently trialed that the platelet-rich plasma (PRP) fibrin matrix version holds the greatest promise for improving clinical success after rotator cuff tendon repair (16)[C].
  - A recent meta-analysis published in 2021 reveals that clinical evidence for the efficacy of PRP in rotator cuff tendinopathy remains equivocal at this time. Current studies suggest that corticosteroids are possibly superior in improving shoulder function in the short term. However, PRP treatments are more likely to produce favorable long-term improvements in rotator cuff recovery (15)[A],(17)[A].
  - PRP has not yielded statistically significant improvements in functional outcomes or range of movements thus far. Further studies for the ideal formulation of PRP in muscle healing is indicated (17)[A].
  - Steroid injections are indicated for bursitis and/or tendinitis to reduce inflammation and have been used successfully and without compromise to tendon repairs 6 weeks out from repair (18)[C].
  - Perioperative steroid injections within 1 month can increase risk of surgical site infections (19)[B].

SURGERY/OTHER PROCEDURES

- For complete tears, surgery may be warranted in the young patient or active athlete.
- Early operative repair provides the best chance for functional recovery. Severely retracted tendons/muscles create additional challenges to the surgeon for optimal recovery (20)[C].

ONGOING CARE

FOLLOW-UP RECOMMENDATIONS

Orthopedic surgeon referral encouraged for acute full-thickness tears early and partial tears after failed conservative therapy

PATIENT EDUCATION

Overhead athletes undergoing surgical repair may require 6 months or longer before being able to return to full active sports participation.

REFERENCES

1. Park HB, Yokota A, Gill HS, et al. Diagnostic accuracy of clinical tests for the different degrees of subacromial impingement syndrome. *J Bone Joint Surg Am*. 2005;87(7):1446–1455.
2. Holtby R, Razmjou H. Validity of the supraspinatus test as a single clinical test in diagnosing patients with rotator cuff pathology. *J Orthop Sports Phys Ther*. 2004;34(4):194–200.
3. Hertel R, Ballmer FT, Lombert SM, et al. Lag signs in the diagnosis of rotator cuff rupture. *J Shoulder Elbow Surg*. 1996;5(4):307–313.
4. Hermans J, Luime JJ, Meuffels DE, et al. Does this patient with shoulder pain have rotator cuff disease?: the rational clinical examination systematic review. *JAMA*. 2013;310(8):837–847.
5. Dunn WR, Kuhn JE, Sanders R, et al. Symptoms of pain do not correlate with rotator cuff tear severity: a cross-sectional study of 393 patients with a symptomatic atraumatic full-thickness rotator cuff tear. *J Bone Joint Surg Am*. 2014;96(10):793–800.
6. Weiner DS, Macnab I. Superior migration of the humeral head. A radiological aid in the diagnosis of tears of the rotator cuff. *J Bone Joint Surg Br*. 1970;52(3):524–527.
7. Burks RT, Crim J, Brown N, et al. A prospective randomized clinical trial comparing arthroscopic single- and double-row rotator cuff repair: magnetic resonance imaging and early clinical evaluation. *Am J Sports Med*. 2009;37(4):674–682.
8. Sershon RA, Mather RC, Sherman SL, et al. Low accuracy of interpretation of rotator cuff MRI in patients with osteoarthritis. *Acta Orthop*. 2013;84(5):479–482.
9. Moosikasuwan JB, Miller TT, Burke BJ. Rotator cuff tears: clinical, radiographic, and US findings. *Radiographics*. 2005;25(6):1591–1607.
10. Mall NA, Kim HM, Keener JD, et al. Symptomatic progression of asymptomatic rotator cuff tears: a prospective study of clinical and sonographic variables. *J Bone Joint Surg Am*. 2010;92(16):2623–2633.
11. Teefey SA, Middleton WD, Yamaguchi K. Shoulder sonography. State of the art. *Radiol Clin North Am*. 1999;37(4):767–785.
12. Elmorsy A, Keightley A, Flannery M. Accuracy of ultrasonography (US) and magnetic resonance imaging (MRI) in detection of rotator cuff tears in district general hospital. *Pol J Radiol*. 2017;82:634–637.
13. Corazza A, Orlandi D, Fabbro E. Dynamic high-resolution ultrasound of the shoulder: how we do it. *Eur J Radiol*. 2015;84(2):266–277.
14. Inderhaug E, Kollevold KH, Kalsvik M, et al. Preoperative NSAIDS, non-acute onset and long-standing symptoms predict inferior outcome at long-term follow-up after rotator cuff repair. *Knee Surg Sports Traumatol Arthrosc*. 2017;25(7):2067–2072.
15. Peng Y, Li F, Ding Y, et al. Comparison of the effects of platelet-rich plasma and corticosteroid injection in rotator cuff disease treatment: a systematic review and meta-analysis. *J shoulder elbow surg*. 2023;32(6):1303–1313.
16. Seven MM, Ersen O, Akpancar S, et al. Effectiveness of prolotherapy in the treatment of chronic rotator cuff lesions. *Orthop Traumatol Surg Res*. 2017;103(3):427–433.
17. Hamid MSA, Sazlina SG. Platelet-rich plasma for rotator cuff tendinopathy: a systematic review and meta-analysis. *PLoS One*. 2021;16(5):e0251111.
18. Barber FA. Platelet-rich plasma for rotator cuff repair. *Sports Med Arthrosc Rev*. 2013;21(4):199–205.
19. Forsythe B, Agarwalla A, Puzzitiello RN, et al. The timing of injections prior to arthroscopic rotator cuff repair impacts the risk of surgical site infection. *J Bone Joint Surg Am*. 2019;101(8):682–687.
20. Kim IB, Jung DW. An intra-articular steroid injection at 6 weeks postoperatively for shoulder stiffness after arthroscopic rotator cuff repair does not affect repair integrity. *Am J Sports Med*. 2018;46(9):2192–2202.

ADDITIONAL READING

Rashid MS, Cooper C, Cook J, et al. Increasing age and tear size reduce rotator cuff repair healing rate at 1 year. *Acta Orthop*. 2017;88(6):606–611.

CLINICAL PEARLS

- Diagnostic accuracy of shoulder US when evaluating rotator cuff tears can reach 91–100% for partial- and full-thickness tears detection, respectively, having been reported to be as accurate as MRI in experienced hands.
- Surgery is an option, especially for the young and/or active athlete, and should be considered early on for diagnosis of complete tears of the rotator cuff.
- Rehabilitation of a partial tear of the rotator cuff is a prolonged process that may take months to return to preinjury status.

SAGITTAL BAND RUPTURE/BOXER'S KNUCKLE

Laika M. Nur, MD ▪ Bryan Leek, MD ▪ Kenneth S. Taylor, MD, FAAFP, CAQSM

BASICS

DESCRIPTION

- Boxer's knuckle describes injuries to the sagittal band of the extensor hood at the metacarpal phalangeal (MCP) joint.
- Injury may result in instability of the extensor tendon, subluxation or dislocation of the extensor tendon over the MCP joint.
- Type 1 injury: sagittal band injury without instability of the extensor tendon
- Type 2 injury: sagittal band injury with subluxation of the extensor tendon
- Type 3 injury: sagittal band injury with dislocation of extensor tendons

EPIDEMIOLOGY

- Most commonly seen after traumatic injury with hand in a closed fist position
- This injury represents 16% of all hand and wrist injuries in boxers.
- Injury may occur spontaneously or a low energy mechanism; seen more commonly in patient with preexisting inflammatory conditions
- Middle finger is most frequently involved. This is likely due to greater prominence of 3rd metacarpal head.
- Ulnar displacement of the extensor tendon is almost always seen, because the MCP joints are slightly ulnar deviated and the juncture tendinae acts as a tether against radial deviation of the extensor tendon.
- Instability may be a normal atraumatic, asymptomatic variant.

ETIOLOGY AND PATHOPHYSIOLOGY

- The extensor hood at the MCP joint is a transverse fibrous complex made of two bands of tissue (sagittal bands).
- The sagittal bands envelope the extensor tendon with thin superficial band and thicker deep band that provide stability to the extensor tendon during finger flexion.
- The centrally located extensor tendons pass longitudinally through these bands.
- Longitudinal or oblique tear of either the superficial or deep band can lead to instability of the extensor tendon due to unopposed force from the remaining intact sagittal band.

GENERAL PREVENTION

None

COMMONLY ASSOCIATED CONDITIONS

None known

DIAGNOSIS

HISTORY

- Direct blow to hand in a closed fist position
- Spontaneous/atraumatic injuries can occur with activities of daily living and are more prevalent in patients with preexisting inflammatory arthropathy.
- Sudden onset of pain and swelling at the MCP joint
- Pain with flexion and limited flexion at MCP joint
- Mechanical popping felt at MCP joint

PHYSICAL EXAM

- Swelling and fullness over MCP joint
- Decreased active flexion at MCP joint
- Instability of the extensor tendon with flexion at MCP confirms diagnosis but can be difficult to appreciate in the presence of swelling.
- It is important to evaluate the contralateral hand, as instability may be a normal variant in some people.

DIFFERENTIAL DIAGNOSIS

- Metacarpal neck fracture
- Proximal phalanx fracture
- Extensor tendon rupture
- MCP joint injury (subluxation, osteochondral fracture, capsular injury)
- MCP arthritis
- MCP collateral ligament injury
- Trigger digit

DIAGNOSTIC TESTS & INTERPRETATION

ALERT

- X-rays may be negative but should be obtained to rule out associated fracture, dislocation, or arthritis (1)[C].
- MRI findings of extensor hood injuries in T2 weighted imaging correlate well with operative findings (1)[C].
- Ultrasound (US) may demonstrate soft tissue swelling with normal echogenicity of extensor tendons.
- Dynamic US can also be very useful in evaluating dynamic instability of the extensor tendon with flexion of MCP joint compared to static MRI (2)[C].

TREATMENT

GENERAL MEASURES

- Good functional outcome can be achieved with appropriate treatment.
- Nonoperative management with splinting in extension at the MCP for at least 6 to 8 weeks (1)[C],(3)[C]
- Nonoperative treatment has been suggested for patients evaluated within the first 3 to 6 weeks of injury who do not require high levels of physical performance or meticulous dexterity (3)[C].

ISSUES FOR REFERRAL

- There is no defined optimal treatment and no randomized controlled trials comparing surgical repair to nonsurgical management.
- Boxers knuckle may warrant a surgical referral for complete discussion of treatment options.
- Retrospective reviews have suggested up to a 50% failure rate in nonsurgical treatment of traumatic ruptures especially when associated with higher level soft tissue injuries (types 2 and 3) or an associated joint capsule injury. These cases should have a surgical consultation.
- Successful nonsurgical treatment has been demonstrated in case series, one series demonstrated only 1 in 11 patients electing for surgery after splinting. However, 30% of patients did have some residual subluxation.
- High demand patients should have surgical evaluation (1)[C],(3)[C],(4)[C].
- Late presentation (>4 weeks) are less likely to have success with nonsurgical management and warrant surgical evaluation (3)[C].

PROGNOSIS

- Prognosis is generally good in sagittal band ruptures with return to pain-free function using both nonsurgical and surgical treatment.
- Nonoperative management can be very effective with early treatment.
- Repair and reconstruction of sagittal band is effective in improving symptomatic MCP joint with recurrent extensor tendon instability or in high demand patients (4)[C].
- Recurrent swelling and subluxation may occur with surgical and nonsurgical management with acceptable patient satisfaction.

REFERENCES

1. Kleinhenz BP, Adams BD. Closed sagittal band injury of the metacarpophalangeal joint. *J Am Acad Orthop Surg.* 2015;23(7):415–23.
2. Watté N, Walschot L, Vanhoenacker F. Boxer's knuckle. *J Belg Soc Radiol.* 2021;105(1):79.
3. Grandizio LC, Klena JC. Sagittal band, boutonniere, and pulley injuries in the athlete. *Curr Rev Musculoskelet Med.* 2017;10(1):17–22.
4. Matharu GS, Gatt IT, Delaney R, et al. Extensor hood injuries in elite boxers: injury characteristics, surgical technique and outcomes. *J Hand Surg Eur Vol.* 2022;47(11):1162–1167.

ADDITIONAL READING

- Arai K, Toh S, Nakahara K, et al. Treatment of soft tissue injuries to the dorsum of the metacarpophalangeal joint (boxers knuckle). *J Hand Surg Br.* 2002;27(1) 90–95.
- Bueno BT, Smith TA, Lotito MJ, et al. Successful non-operative management of metacarpophalangeal collateral ligament and sagittal band rupture of the long finger: a case report. *Cureus.* 2022;14(6):e26231.
- Catalano LW III, Gupta S, Ragland R III, et al. Closed treatment of nonrheumatoid extensor tendon dislocations at the metacarpophalangeal joint. *J Hand Surg Am.* 2006;31(2):242–245.
- Hame SL, Melone CP Jr. Boxer's knuckle in the professional athlete. *Am J Sports Med.* 2000;28(6):879–82.
- Loosemore M, Lightfoot J, Gatt I, et al. Hand and wrist injuries in elite boxing: a longitudinal prospective study (2005–2012) of the Great Britain Olympic Boxing Squad. *Hand (N Y).* 2017;12(2):181–187.
- Mok KL. Boxer's knuckle of non-boxer patients. *Hong Kong J Emerg Med.* 2006;13(3)161–167.

CLINICAL PEARLS

- Sagittal band rupture, both traumatic and spontaneous, is a clinical diagnosis most commonly seen at the 3rd MCP joint.
- If diagnosed early, it can be managed nonoperatively with splinting in extension for 6 to 8 weeks.
- Counsel patients on the option for surgical management with delayed presentation and in patients with a need for more reliable treatment expectations such as high-level athletes or patients with high dexterity demands.

SCAPHOLUNATE DISSOCIATION

David E. Price, MD, FAMSSM • Alexandra M. Frank, MD

BASICS

DESCRIPTION

Scapholunate (SL) dissociation may be more accurately characterized as a spectrum of SL instability resulting from a tear of the SL interosseous ligament (SLIL). Concomitant or subsequent injury to secondary ligamentous restraints alters the biomechanics of the wrist, resulting in progressive carpal instability and leading to a predictable pattern of debilitating, degenerative changes of the wrist (1),(2).

EPIDEMIOLOGY

- Most common ligamentous instability of the wrist
- Frequently associated with a distal radius fracture
- Precise epidemiologic data is lacking.

ETIOLOGY AND PATHOPHYSIOLOGY

- Often a fall on an outstretched hand with impact on the base of the wrist and hypothenar region in extension, ulnar deviation, and supination (1),(2)
- Axial compression can drive the capitate between the scaphoid and lunate (1).
- Repetitive motion after an isolated SLIL injury may produce attritional changes in the secondary stabilizers leading to their eventual failure, thus completing the SL dissociation (1).
- May also result from repetitive minor trauma

RISK FACTORS

Active individuals who have ulnar-negative variance; shorter distal ulna compared with the radius on a neutral anteroposterior (AP) radiograph of the wrist.

DIAGNOSIS

- Early diagnosis and surgery offer the best chance for a successful outcome (1),(3).
- There are different levels of injury, which can be classified by increasing severity of wrist instability (1),(3),(4):
  - Occult instability: isolated tear or attenuation of a portion of the SLIL. There is no radiologic evidence of SL widening, and wrist pain is usually only with mechanical loading.
  - Dynamic instability: subtotal or complete tear of the SLIL, including the dorsal portion, with a partial secondary ligament injury; may have normal static radiographs, but instability will be apparent on stress radiographs
  - SL dissociation: involves a complete tear of the SLIL with additional tear of one or more secondary ligaments. SL widening is apparent on static radiographs (>3 mm).
  - Dorsal intercalated segment instability (DISI) and volar intercalated segment instability (VISI): terms used to describe the shifted positions of the bones of the carpus, as viewed on lateral radiograph, due to lack of association between the lunate and scaphoid (1).
  - SL advanced collapse (SLAC): end stage of the spectrum of instability (1). There is predictable and progressive degeneration and arthritis of the carpus due to the irreversible postural changes of the scaphoid, capitate, and lunate.

HISTORY

- Patient may report a fall or sudden load applied to the wrist but may not recall any specific fall or injury.
- Painful and/or decreased wrist motion
- Pain and/or swelling over the dorsal wrist (1)
- Decreased grip strength
- May not seek immediate care

PHYSICAL EXAM

- In the acute setting, pain may be poorly localized about the periscaphoid area. Swelling may be diffuse or localized to the SL region.
- In the subacute setting, there is usually well-localized tenderness about the scaphoid and dorsal SL interval.
- The patient may have weakness of grip and pinch strength.
- Test for paradoxical scaphoid motion:
  - Physician places their thumb over anatomic snuff box.
  - Ask patient to flex the thumb.
  - If SL ligaments not intact, body of the scaphoid should move dorsally against the examiner's thumb.
- Watson scaphoid shift test should be performed:
  - Place patient's wrist in ulnar deviation.
  - The physician puts dorsal pressure on the palmar scaphoid with the thumb. The physician then radially deviates the patient's wrist. Relief of thumb pressure will allow the scaphoid to reduce, often with an audible or palpable clunk. Pain or a clunk represents a positive test.
  - Compare to contralateral side as false positives are common.
- The shift and motion tests may become negative in chronic cases as arthritis stabilizes the scaphoid.

DIFFERENTIAL DIAGNOSIS

- Scaphoid or other carpal fracture
- Lunotriquetral instability
- Radial styloid or distal radius fracture
- Synovitis
- Radioscaphoid impingement
- Occult ganglion cyst
- Triangular fibrocartilage complex tear
- Osteoarthritis or rheumatoid arthritis
- Kienböck disease

DIAGNOSTIC TESTS & INTERPRETATION

- Imaging should be obtained in individuals with appropriate history and/or positive shift test.
- Initial plain films should include AP, lateral, and stress views.
- Radiographs of the opposite wrist can be obtained for comparison.
- Normal static and stress films in the acute setting do not always rule out serious injury because it may take time for instability to develop (4)[C].
- By the time frank dissociation is present on static films, significant damage is already present (1).
- Key findings on the lateral film (wrist in neutral):
  - SL angle >70 degrees is considered highly suggestive of diagnosis (normal 30 to 60 degrees) (1),(3).
  - Radiolunate angle exceeding 15 degrees indicates DISI (1).
- Key findings on the AP film:
  - Scaphoid ring sign: Distal scaphoid tubercle is superimposed on the scaphoid waist when scaphoid is flexed >70 degrees (1).
  - Gap >3 mm (3),(4) between scaphoid and lunate on AP is indicative of SL dissociation with 97% specificity (4).
- "Pencil grip posteroanterior (PA)" is the most useful stress view (3)[C]. It profiles the SL joint and demonstrates pathologic SL widening (>3 mm) under axial-loaded conditions. Additional stress view could include AP in ulnar deviation (3).
- Radiography has a sensitivity of 57–81% and specificity of 73–98% (4).
- Cineradiography (functional fluoroscopy) has a sensitivity of 86–96% and specificity of 80–97% (4).

- CT arthrography has been reported as having a sensitivity of 80–100%, whereas magnetic resonance (MR) arthrography has a sensitivity of 85–100%; both have a specificity of 80–100% (4). Traction MR arthrography has been proposed to have greater sensitivity and specificity (3).
- Traditional arthrography is limited by its static nature and the high prevalence of degenerative tears, which are often asymptomatic and bilateral (1).
- Static imaging modalities often miss early cases of instability when intervention may be most effective.
- The dorsal SL ligament can be assessed with ultrasound.
- Wrist arthroscopy remains the gold standard for diagnosis (1),(3),(4).

TREATMENT

- Treatment must be predicated by the patient's symptoms and clinical exam, not imaging.
- Management of injuries may depend on age, sport, position, level of competition, and schedule (3)[C].
- The treatment is often surgical, so do not delay referral.
- The goal of surgery is to restore or stabilize carpal kinematics to arrest the degenerative process (3).

MEDICATION

Nonsteroidal anti-inflammatory drugs (NSAIDs) or acetaminophen for pain

ADDITIONAL THERAPIES

- Occult instability may be successfully treated with immobilization for 4 to 6 weeks followed by therapy (3)[C].
- There has been some success with casting, splinting, NSAIDs, and therapy without surgical intervention for dynamic instability. This would include a short arm cast for 4 to 6 weeks, followed by removable splint for active range of motion (ROM) exercises and gentle strengthening across the wrist.
- All treatment courses should be followed by rehabilitation consisting of strengthening and proprioceptive training (3)[C].

SURGERY/OTHER PROCEDURES

- In general, unstable wrists should undergo surgical repair as soon as possible if the athlete desires to return to play. The procedures performed are dictated based on the timing and severity of the wrist instability.
- Occult instability:
  - There has been some success with arthroscopic débridement with or without pinning, but usually, this is treated with conservative measures (3)[C]. There is also some evidence for Kirschner wire (K-wire) fixation and/or electrocautery for electrothermal collagen shrinkage following arthroscopic débridement (1),(3),(5)[C]. However, the mechanism for pain reduction is felt to be a result of denervation rather than mechanical stabilization.
  - Electrocautery to denature type 1 collagen, leading to tightening of the stretched ligaments is currently being studied (5)[C].
- Acute, dynamic instability:
  - Usually require early surgical intervention
  - Some will use closed reduction and K-wire fixation, attempting to allow the torn ligaments to heal (1)[C]. Otherwise, attempt is made to repair the damaged ligaments before they degenerate (3),(5)[C],(6). Arthroscopic repair has been proposed as a less invasive technique (6)[C].
- Subacute or chronic injuries:
  - Typically require ligament reconstruction (3)[C]
- Chronically injured wrists with fixed deformity such as DISI, VISI, or SLAC:
  - Salvage procedures are sometimes needed to alleviate pain (1)[C].
  - A salvage procedure is performed to restore alignment, improve load distribution, and attempt to slow degenerative changes. Unfortunately, salvage procedures are likely to indicate the end of an athletic career (3)[C].
  - Salvage procedures may include scaphoid excision, carpal fusion, or proximal row carpectomy (1)[C].

ONGOING CARE

FOLLOW-UP RECOMMENDATIONS

- Following repair, immobilize the wrist for 8 weeks and then slowly rehab.
- Decisions about return to play must be individualized based on sport-specific demands and competition level.
- In general, an athlete may return after demonstrating progression in strength and ROM in a supervised rehabilitation program.
- Physical therapy should be performed within pain tolerance.
- Avoid power gripping and weight-bearing exercises of the upper extremity.

COMPLICATIONS

- Injury has the potential to be career ending (3).
- Arthritis of the wrist, which can be severe and debilitating

REFERENCES

1. Manuel J, Moran SL. The diagnosis and treatment of scapholunate instability. *Orthop Clin North Am.* 2007;38(2):261–277.
2. Wessel LE, Wolfe SW. Scapholunate instability: diagnosis and management—anatomy, kinematics, and clinical assessment—part I. *J Hand Surg Am.* 2023;48(11):1139–1149.
3. Morrell NT, Moyer A, Quinlan N, et al. Scapholunate and perilunate injuries in the athlete. *Curr Rev Musculoskelet Med.* 2017;10(1):45–52.
4. Cheriex KCAL, Sulkers GSI, Terra MP, et al. Scapholunate dissociation; diagnostics made easy. *Eur J Radiol.* 2017;92:45–50.
5. Dréant N. Treatment of chronic scapholunate instability according to the functional demand of the wrist. *Hand Surg Rehabil.* 2023;42(3):175–183.
6. Mathoulin C, Merlini L, Taleb C. Scapholunate injuries: challenging existing dogmas in anatomy and surgical techniques. *J Hand Surg Eur Vol.* 2021;46(1):5–13.

CLINICAL PEARLS

- Most common ligamentous injury of the wrist
- Normal static and stress films do not always rule out serious injury.
- Radiographs of the contralateral side should be obtained.
- Early diagnosis and treatment is essential.

SCHEUERMANN'S KYPHOSIS

David McClaskey, MD, ATC

BASICS

DESCRIPTION
- Juvenile osteochondrosis of the spine
- Scheuermann kyphosis is rigid and most commonly affects the thoracic spine.
- Vertebrae grow unevenly with regard to the sagittal plane (posterior angle is greater than the anterior), resulting in the signature "wedging" shape of the vertebrae, causing kyphosis.
- Defined radiographically by anterior wedging ≥5 degrees in three or more adjacent vertebral bodies
- Type I (typical)—thoracic spine only, apex of curve T7–T9
- Type II (atypical)—lower thoracic and lumbar spine involvement

EPIDEMIOLOGY

Prevalence
- 0.4–8% in the United States (1)
- Most common age of diagnosis is 12 to 17 years.
- Male-to-female ratio ranges between 2:1 and 7:1 (1).

ETIOLOGY AND PATHOPHYSIOLOGY
- Results from mechanical stress on a weakened vertebral endplate
- The vertebral endplate is weakened due to defective growth, likely from predisposing genetic defects. Hormonal abnormalities are postulated to contribute as well.
- Defective endplate may also affect the health of the adjacent intervertebral disk, resulting in early disk disease.

Genetics
- Suspected autosomal dominant inheritance (1)
- Seen more commonly in monozygotic twins
- Heritability (percentage of all cases that can be attributed to genetics) is 74% (2),(3).

RISK FACTORS
Altered biomechanics (such as poor posture or repetitive strain from sports or manual labor) may increase or accelerate the severity of the kyphosis. Contribution of elevated body mass index (BMI) to this condition is not well defined.

COMMONLY ASSOCIATED CONDITIONS
- Scoliosis
- Cervical or lumbar hyperlordosis (compensatory curvature due to the thoracic kyphosis)
- Spondylolysis
- The above conditions occur in up to 1/3 of patients with Scheuermann kyphosis.

DIAGNOSIS

HISTORY
- Affected patient will present with cosmetic deformity, back pain, and hamstring tightness.
- Thoracic kyphosis may produce pain at the thoracic spine and/or result in strain on the cervical or lumbar spine.
- Pain is typically insidious with no traumatic event.
- The pain worsens with activity and improves with rest.
- Cosmetic deformity may be noticed by parents or during school-based screenings, preparticipation examinations, or routine wellness exams.
- A family history of Scheuermann kyphosis may be present in most cases.

PHYSICAL EXAM
- Spinal range of motion should be carefully evaluated and documented in all planes of motion.
- Physical exam shows a rigid, hyperkyphotic curve that is accentuated with forward protrusion of the head and compensatory cervical and lumbar lordosis.
- The kyphosis does not resolve with postural maneuvers (extension, lying supine, prone, etc.). The kyphosis cannot be consciously corrected.
- Loss of vertebral height, thus appearing shorter
- May result in kyphoscoliosis, scoliosis, or cervical/lumbar hyperlordosis
- Patients typically have tight hamstrings to compensate for excessive lumbar curvature.
- Excessive curvature (>100 degrees) may cause restrictive lung disease, which can be confirmed with pulmonary function tests.
- Rarely, may cause neurologic deficits, therefore, a complete neurologic exam is warranted
- Look for findings that may suggest other causes of kyphosis, such as marfanoid body habitus, hypermobile joints (Marfan or Ehlers-Danlos syndrome), cafe-au-lait spots (neurofibromatosis), etc.

DIFFERENTIAL DIAGNOSIS
- Postural kyphosis (improves with postural maneuvers)
- Ankylosing spondylitis
- Scoliosis
- Neuromuscular disorders
- Ehlers-Danlos syndrome
- Marfan syndrome
- Rickets
- Congenital kyphosis (Klippel-Feil syndrome, vertebral anomalies [V], anal atresia [A], cardiac malformations [C], tracheoesophageal fistula [TE], renal dysplasia [R], and limb abnormalities [L] syndrome)

DIAGNOSTIC TESTS & INTERPRETATION

Initial Tests (lab, imaging)
- X-rays:
  - Anteroposterior (AP)/lateral radiographs confirm the diagnosis, demonstrating kyphosis >40 degrees, or anterior wedging ≥5 degrees in three or more adjacent vertebral bodies (3)[B].
  - Cobb angle is used to measure angle of kyphotic deformity; this angle is the intersection of the lines drawn from the endplates of the terminal vertebrae, which are most tilted toward each other.
  - Sagittal balance can also quantify spinal deformity by measuring the horizontal distance between the center of C7 and the superior endplate of S1 on a lateral radiograph. An abnormal balance (plumb line passing >2 cm in front of, or behind, the posterosuperior S1 body) is predictive of dysfunction.
  - May show signs of an irregular vertebral endplate, including Schmorl nodes, loss of disk space height, spondylolysis, or spondylolisthesis (3)[B]
  - Schmorl nodes are the herniation of the nucleus pulposus through the vertebral endplate into the body of the adjacent vertebra.
- Magnetic resonance imaging (MRI):
  - Useful for evaluating disk and spinal cord abnormalities in the presence of neurologic deficits
  - Can be used for preoperative planning
  - May show disk herniations, disk degeneration, or Schmorl nodes

TREATMENT

GENERAL MEASURES
- Treatment is determined primarily by symptoms and the severity of deformity.
- The goals of treatment are to optimize alignment and cosmetic appearance while reducing symptoms and neurologic deficits (1)[B].
- Majority of cases are treated with nonoperative management.
- Thoracic kyphosis of 50 to 80 degrees is an indication for nonsurgical treatment (1)[B].
- Physical therapy:
  - Focuses on stretching and strengthening of the paraspinal and hamstring musculature as well as postural control
  - Manual medicine may have a role in treatment among providers who are familiar with treating this condition.
- Lifestyle modification:
  - Avoidance of sports or exercises that place excessive pressure on the spine, such as weight lifting or rugby
  - OK to participate in athletics if kyphosis is nonpainful and being treated nonoperatively.

- Bracing:
  - Painful, mild to moderate kyphosis can be treated with bracing for 12 to 24 months.
  - Most effective in the skeletally immature patient due to vertebral remodeling
  - Bracing may effectively slow progression but may not resolve the kyphosis (1)[B].
  - Types of braces: Milwaukee brace, kyphologic brace, thoracolumbosacral orthosis-style Boston brace
  - Efficacy of braces is limited by compliance; requires the patient to wear up to 18 to 20 hours/d
- Emotional support:
  - Spinal deformity may negatively impact self-esteem and body image, particularly because this condition occurs during adolescence.
  - Treatment is time-consuming and may significantly impact daily activities.
  - Options for support groups and therapy should be explored and offered.

MEDICATION

First Line

Nonsteroidal anti-inflammatory drugs (NSAIDs) or acetaminophen is typically used for pain control.

ISSUES FOR REFERRAL

Referral for surgical correction should be considered for the following cases (4)[B]:

- Persistent or worsening symptoms despite nonsurgical management
- Progressive kyphosis >70 degrees despite nonsurgical management
- Neurologic deficits
- Unacceptable cosmetic deformity
- Pulmonary compromise (restrictive lung defect) secondary to kyphosis
- Patient/parent preference

SURGERY/OTHER PROCEDURES

- Significant variability among threshold to treat surgically
- Curve magnitude typically exceeds 70 to 80 degrees among surgical candidates, but decision to operate is individualized and influenced by patient age and maturity, level of pain, response to nonsurgical measures, and patient/parent preference (5)[B].
- Surgery involves release of spine structures, correction of the kyphosis, and arthrodesis.
- Surgery should be customized to the patient's biomechanics and spinal balance (5)[B].
- Arthrodesis may occur through combined anterior-posterior or posterior-only approach.
- Recent trends have favored the posterior-only approach due to its similar efficacy and slightly reduced complication profile when compared to the combined anterior-posterior approach (5)[B].
- Even with surgery, the kyphosis may progress over time, both in the fusion as well as at the levels above or below the fusion (junctional kyphosis) (6)[B].
- Risks of surgery include postoperative infection, neurologic injury, and reoperation. Risks are increased when more levels are fused.

ONGOING CARE

FOLLOW-UP RECOMMENDATIONS

- A sports medicine or spine specialist should follow patients every 4 to 6 months to monitor progression, particularly during skeletal maturation.
- Serial imaging should be performed at 6 to 12 months intervals until skeletally mature; can perform in shorter intervals if the kyphosis is progressive and the patient is skeletally immature

PATIENT EDUCATION

- Athletic activity is allowed for patients with non-painful kyphosis in nonoperative treatment. Given the potential for progression, high-impact or sports that strain the spine should be avoided.
- An extension-based stretching program incorporating hamstring stretches and postural exercises should be used.

PROGNOSIS

- The majority of patients maintain high functional scores with nonsurgical treatments.
- A high incidence of back pain is reported among patients long term with nonsurgical and surgical treatments (6).
- Kyphosis <60 degrees generally has few long-term complications.

COMPLICATIONS

- Untreated Scheuermann kyphosis may result in a higher risk of back pain and lower quality of life in the later adult years.
- Restrictive lung disease may occur with severe kyphosis (>100 degrees).
- Surgical complications include junctional kyphosis, neurologic complications, hardware failure, infection, and lung or kidney injury (5).

REFERENCES

1. O'Donnell JM, Wu W, Youn A, et al. Scheuermann kyphosis: current concepts and management. *Curr Rev Musculoskelet Med*. 2023;16(11):521–530.
2. Damborg F, Engell V, Nielsen J, et al. Genetic epidemiology of Scheuermann's disease. *Acta Orthop*. 2011;82(5):602–605.
3. Gokce E, Beyhan M. Radiological imaging findings of Scheuermann disease. *World J Radiol*. 2016;8(11):895–901.
4. Haselhuhn JJ, Odland K, Soriano PBO, et al. A novel surgical indication for Scheuermann's kyphosis. *J Am Acad Orthop Surg Glob Res Rev*. 2024;8(3):e23.00187.
5. Huq S, Ehresman J, Cottrill E, et al. Treatment approaches for Scheuermann kyphosis: a systematic review of historic and current management. *J Neurosurg Spine*. 2019;32(2):235–247.
6. Graat HCA, Schimmel JJP, Hoogendoorn RJW, et al. Poor radiological and good functional long-term outcome of surgically treated Scheuermann patients. *Spine (Phila Pa 1976)*. 2016;41(14):E869–E878.

ADDITIONAL READING

- Kaur S, Lalam R. Scheuermann's disease. *Semin Musculoskelet Radiol*. 2023;27(5):522–528.
- Ragborg L, Dragsted C, Dahl B, et al. Scheuermann's kyphosis: a 39-year follow-up from diagnosis in non-operated patients. *Eur Spine J*. 2020;29(8):2091–2099.

CLINICAL PEARLS

- Scheuermann kyphosis is distinguished as a rigid kyphosis that does not resolve with postural maneuvers and most commonly affects the thoracic spine.
- The diagnosis is confirmed with AP/lateral radiographs that demonstrate kyphosis >40 degrees or anterior wedging ≥5 degrees in three or more adjacent vertebral bodies.
- The majority of cases are treated successfully with nonsurgical management. Surgical considerations are influenced not only by the degree of kyphosis (typically >70 degrees) but also by individual patient considerations, including age, maturity, pain, response to nonsurgical measures, and patient or parent preference.
- The kyphosis may progress despite bracing and surgical management.
- Mild to moderate kyphosis <60 degrees has fewer long-term complications than more severe kyphosis.

S

SCIATICA

Dhiren J. Naidu, MD, FRCPC, Dip. Sport Med.

BASICS

- Sciatica is referred in the medical literature as lumbosacral radicular syndrome, radiculopathy, or nerve root pain.
- The classic description of sciatica or radiculopathy is a compromised spinal nerve with resultant pain, weakness, and/or sensory impairment in the distribution of the affected nerve root (1).
- Sciatica pain radiates from the lower back into the leg with typical radiation below the knee into the foot.
- Sciatica should not be confused with mechanical lower back pain because sciatic pain is typically worse in the leg than the back.

DESCRIPTION

- Radicular pain in the distribution of a lumbosacral nerve root (L4, L5, S1, S2, or S3), usually producing symptoms along the posterior or lateral aspect of the lower extremity and extending to the ankle or foot (1).
- Typically described as a burning-type pain with numbness and tingling
- Weakness can occur in the myotomal distribution depending on severity of nerve root compression (1).

EPIDEMIOLOGY

- Lower back pain is extremely common in the general population and the athletic population (e.g., football, gymnastics, tennis).
- General population: 5% annual occurrence; 60–90% lifetime incidence (2):
  - Men and women equally affected
  - Common reason to visit primary care physician
  - Leading cause of job-related disability in the United States
- Sciatica:
  - Sciatica is a common cause of pain and disability but less common than lower back pain.
  - Occurs in approximately 5% of the population (2)
  - 10–25% have >6 weeks of symptoms.
  - Up to 30% continue to have pain for a year or longer (3)
  - In males, typically occurs in 40s
  - In females, typically occurs in 50s to 60s
  - L5 and S1 are the most common nerve roots involved (90%).
  - Characterized by motor, reflex, and/or sensory changes (3)

ETIOLOGY AND PATHOPHYSIOLOGY

The usual etiology of sciatica or radicular pain is direct mechanical compression to the affected nerve root by a disk herniation and/or from irritation of the nerve root by chemical substances, commonly referred to as radiculitis (1).

RISK FACTORS

Occupations or activities that require repetitive lifting, flexion, or rotation movements; these may occur in laborers or dancers and golfers.

COMMONLY ASSOCIATED CONDITIONS

- Cauda equina syndrome
- Urinary retention
- Motor loss
- Neuropathic pain

DIAGNOSIS

HISTORY

- Determine mechanism of injury.
- Onset of pain can be variable from immediate (acute) or over days (subacute).
- Pain is described as sharp, "electrical," burning, or as a numbness or tingling.
- Pain is in the leg more than the lower back.
- Usually unilateral pain
- Pain is worse in the morning.
- Pain is aggravated by flexion-based activities, rotation, prolonged sitting, Valsalva maneuvers (coughing, sneezing, straining with bowel movement), and occasionally with prolonged standing.
- Alleviating factors include extension-based postures or lying in prone position.
- Radiation of pain is into the buttock and leg in a posterolateral distribution to the foot.
- Rule out any identified red flags that warrant further investigations.
- The red flags for lower back pain include:
  - Age <20 years or >50 years
  - Pain persists >6 weeks.
  - History or signs and symptoms of infection
  - History of cancer or immunosuppression
  - Unexplained weight loss
  - Severe worsening or atypical pain
  - Significant trauma
  - Intravenous (IV) drug use
  - Abdominal pain
  - Significant neurologic deficit
  - Neurologic bowel/bladder dysfunction
  - Saddle anesthesia
- Evaluate and manage any positive red flags.
- Determine if any constitutional symptoms are present.
- Psychosocial issues that may add to symptoms and prolong pain.

PHYSICAL EXAM

- Inspection may reveal fasciculations or muscle atrophy in long standing conditions.
- Lumbar flexion and rotation range of motion is restricted; usually extension is comfortable and may relieve pain.
- Sensation is decreased or lost in a dermatomal pattern:
  - Sensory loss:
    - L4: anteromedial leg, medial malleolus
    - L5: lateral lower leg, web space on dorsum of foot between the great and 2nd toes
    - S1: back of lower leg, lateral aspect of heel
- Strength is decreased in a myotomal pattern:
  - Motor weakness:
    - L4: ankle dorsiflexion
    - L5: big toe extension
    - S1: ankle plantar flexion
- Reflexes are absent or decreased:
  - Reflexes:
    - L4: patellar tendon (knee jerk)
    - L5: none
    - S1: Achilles tendon (ankle jerk)
- Straight-leg raise (SLR): Patient is in supine position and examiner passively raises fully extended leg. A positive test is reproduction of leg pain at approximately 30 degrees of hip flexion.
- Crossed SLR: Passive raising the contralateral leg results in reproduction of leg pain on the affected (opposite) side.
- Seated SLR: Performed while patient is sitting with knees flexed to 90 degrees; passive extension of the knee reproduces radicular leg pain (modification of SLR).
- Slump test: Performed with patient sitting with hands behind back, then patient flexes spine (slumps), followed by neck flexion. The examiner places hand on top of head, and patient extends knee. A positive test is if radicular leg pain occurs in the slumped position and decreases when patient moves out of neck flexion. This test has limited sensitivity and specificity in patients with a disk herniation.
- Examination of rectal tone and anal sensation in setting of suspected cauda equina syndrome or spinal cord injury
- Vascular examination to include peripheral pulses

DIFFERENTIAL DIAGNOSIS

- Ankylosing spondylitis
- Cauda equina syndrome
- Extrinsic nerve compression (wallet or prolonged cycling)
- Facet arthropathy
- Pathologic, traumatic, or osteoporotic compression fracture
- Herniation of the nucleus pulposus
- Infection (osteomyelitis, epidural abscess)
- Neoplasm, primary or metastatic
- Osteoarthritis of hip or spine
- Trochanteric bursitis
- Tarsal tunnel syndrome

- Paget disease
- Piriformis syndrome
- Sacroiliitis
- Spinal stenosis
- Spondylolisthesis
- Synovial cyst
- Trauma (hematoma, musculoligamentous strain, fracture)
- Nonspinal causes (abdominal aortic aneurysm, herpes zoster, hip arthritis or bursitis, iliotibial band syndrome, psychogenic, vascular claudication)

DIAGNOSTIC TESTS & INTERPRETATION

- X-rays: Anteroposterior and lateral radiographs of lumbar sacral spine usually are not indicated unless red flags are present (see "History").
- Magnetic resonance imaging (MRI): imaging of choice with excellent sensitivity. Consider ordering if red flags are present, especially in the setting of:
  - Suspected cauda equina syndrome
  - Neurologic deficits
  - Suspected malignancy or history of malignancy
  - Suspected infection or abscess
  - 6 weeks of failed conservative therapy for sciatica
- Computed tomography (CT) scan is the study of choice for identifying vertebral bone injuries. It should also be used if an MRI is contraindicated (hardware or pacemaker present).
- Ultrasound or a CT scan of the abdomen can evaluate for pathologies such as an abdominal aortic aneurysm.
- Electrodiagnostic studies: Nerve conduction velocity (NCV) studies and electromyography (EMG) can localize a specific level of injury. It is helpful to differentiate between a peripheral nerve and nerve root injury. It can also differentiate between acute or chronic injury (denervation vs. reinnervation).

TREATMENT

GENERAL MEASURES

- 6 weeks of nonoperative management should be tried before obtaining imaging or invasive procedures unless red flags are present or develop (4).
- Acute low back pain: Avoid inactivity.
- Sciatica: activity level not found to make a difference (5)
- Nonsteroidal anti-inflammatory drugs (NSAIDs) show global improvement compared to placebo, however, have increased side effects (6).
- Oral steroids: 5-day course seems to improve function but not pain (7).
- Physical therapy to teach core stability; core stability is adversely affected in patients with lumbosacral radiculopathy (8).
- Physical therapy directed toward restoring motor or strength deficits (8)
- For the best physical therapy outcomes, both aerobic conditioning and core strengthening are essential.
- The McKenzie method (extension-based exercises) is better for enhancing function in the long term versus manual therapy (9).
- Epidural steroid injections provide short-term improvement in pain but do not affect long-term outcomes. They may also serve as a preoperative assessment tool (10).
- Surgery should be considered for failure of response to nonoperative management for 6 weeks. Surgery more reliably alleviates leg pain than back pain (4).
- Patients with lumbar disk herniations not responding to conservative management should be considered for lumbar decompression and discectomy (4).
- In the absence of severe intractable radicular pain, neurologic deficits, and/or severe disease, surgery should be avoided.

COMPLEMENTARY & ALTERNATIVE MEDICINE

- Yoga-based education and exercises are beneficial for patients with lower back pain (8).
- Manual spine treatment is helpful in acute nonradicular lower back pain (8).
- Acupuncture is supported as an adjuvant treatment in the management of lower back pain (8).

ONGOING CARE

PATIENT EDUCATION

- Weight loss is beneficial.
- Aerobic exercise and core stability are the mainstays of an exercise-based treatment approach.
- Emphasis should be on staying active (5).
- Avoid long-term pain medication.
- Stop smoking.

PROGNOSIS

- Acute pain is almost always self-limited.
- Estimated recovery time: 75–90% by 6 weeks (2)

REFERENCES

1. Kennedy DJ, Noh MY. The role of core stabilization in lumbosacral radiculopathy. *Phys Med Rehabil Clin N Am.* 2011;22(1):91–103.
2. Konstantinou K, Dunn KM. Sciatica: review of epidemiological studies and prevalence estimates. *Spine (Phila Pa 1976).* 2008;33(22):2464–2472.
3. Thoomes E, Falla D, Cleland JA, et al. Conservative management for lumbar radiculopathy based on the stage of disorder: a Delphi study. *Disabil Rehabil.* 2023;45(21):3539–3548.
4. Bruggeman AJ, Decker RC. Surgical treatment and outcomes of lumbar radiculopathy. *Phys Med Rehabil Clin N Am.* 2011;22(1):161–177.
5. Dahm KT, Brurberg KG, Jamtvedt G, et al. Advice to rest in bed versus to advice to stay active for acute low-back pain and sciatica. *Cochrane Database Syst Rev.* 2010;(6):CD007612.
6. Rasmussen-Barr E, Held U, Grooten WJ, et al. Non-steroidal anti-inflammatory drugs for sciatica. *Cochrane Database Syst Rev.* 2016;10(10):CD012382.
7. Goldberg H, Firtch W, Tyburski M, et al. Oral steroids for acute radiculopathy due to a herniated lumbar disk: a randomized clinical trial. *JAMA.* 2015;313(19):1915–1923.
8. Carneiro KA, Rittenberg JD. The role of exercise and alternative treatments for low back pain. *Phys Med Rehabil Clin N Am.* 2010;21(4):777–792.
9. Namnaqani FI, Mashabi AS, Yaseen KM, et al. The effectiveness of McKenzie method compared to manual therapy for treating chronic low back pain: a systematic review. *J Musculoskelet Neuronal Interact.* 2019;19(4):492–499.
10. Leung SM, Chau WW, Law SW, et al. Clinical value of transforaminal epidural steroid injection in lumbar radiculopathy. *Hong Kong Med J.* 2015;21(5):394–400.

ADDITIONAL READING

- Berry JA, Elia C, Saini HS, et al. A review of lumbar radiculopathy, diagnosis, and treatment. *Cureus.* 2019;11(10):e5934.
- Kreiner DS, Hwang SW, Easa JE, et al. An evidence-based clinical guideline for the diagnosis and treatment of lumbar disc herniation with radiculopathy. *Spine J.* 2014;14(1):180–191.

CLINICAL PEARLS

- Sciatica is referred to as a lumbar radiculopathy and occurs from impingement on a nerve root usually from a disk herniation.
- Obtaining a history focusing on the red flags is of prime importance to rule out more emergent conditions that require urgent imaging and medical attention.
- Nonsurgical management is the mainstay of early treatment.
- Surgical referral is warranted if symptoms persist for >6 weeks despite nonsurgical management.
- Most radiculopathies improve by 6 weeks.

SCOLIOSIS (ADOLESCENT IDIOPATHIC SCOLIOSIS [AIS])

Erin S. Barnes, MD • Mark E. Lavallee, MD, CSCS, FACSM, FAMSSM

BASICS

A group of conditions characterized by structural deformities of the spine

DESCRIPTION

- Three-dimensional (3D) deformity of the spine
- Identified by lateral curvature of the spine with a Cobb angle measuring >10 degrees, accompanied by rotation
- Spine curvature measuring <10 degrees is considered within normal limits of skeletal asymmetry and is often called spinal asymmetry.
- Four main categories:
  - *Neuromuscular scoliosis*—caused by insufficient active spine stabilizers secondary to neurologic or musculoskeletal conditions. These include cerebral palsy, myelomeningocele, and muscular dystrophy, which cause muscular imbalance and impairments in truncal control. Most patients will have other findings related to an underlying disorder.
  - *Syndromic scoliosis*—develops as part of genetic syndrome disorders including Marfan, Ehlers-Danlos, Loueys-Deitz, and Down syndrome; osteogenesis imperfecta; and neurofibromatosis.
  - *Congenital scoliosis*—results from vertebral asymmetry secondary to congenital abnormalities including hemivertebrae, wedge vertebrae, and failure of segmentation. This may not be evident at birth but usually manifests before adolescence.
  - *Idiopathic scoliosis*—The most common type, with an unknown cause. It is a diagnosis of exclusion and is sub-categorized by age: infantile (0–3), juvenile (3–9), and adolescent (≥10). Any scoliosis diagnosed before age 10 is considered early-onset.
- Early-onset scoliosis is a heterogenous diagnosis involving all scoliosis diagnosed in children <10 years of age. This includes congenital, neuromuscular, syndromic, and infantile/juvenile idiopathic cases.

EPIDEMIOLOGY

- **Adolescent (AIS)**: The most common type, (80–90% of idiopathic cases).
  - Affects 2–3% of the population (curves >10°).
  - Females are affected 2:1 over males; this ratio increases with curve severity.
  - Only 10% of AIS patients (0.3% of the population) require treatment.
- **Infantile**: Rare (<1% of idiopathic cases); 80% of these regress.
- **Juvenile**: 10–12% of idiopathic cases.
- **Curve location**: Thoracic and thoracolumbar/lumbar curves are the most frequent (80% of all curves).

ETIOLOGY AND PATHOPHYSIOLOGY

- The specific cause of AIS is unknown but considered multifactorial.
- Proposed contributing factors include:
  - **Genetic**: AIS frequently runs in families.
  - **Neurologic**: The most supported theory involves abnormal balance and proprioception.
  - **Connective tissue**: Certain markers might help predict curve progression.
  - **Hormonal**: Lower melatonin levels have been observed in AIS patients.

RISK FACTORS

- Positive family history
- Joint hypermobility
- Low body mass index (BMI)
- Females with delayed puberty and/or menarche
- Increased height and growth velocity

GENERAL PREVENTION

- None
- Benefit of preclinical detection not proven at this time
- U.S. Preventive Services Task Force recommends against the routine screening of asymptomatic adolescents for idiopathic scoliosis.

DIAGNOSIS

- AIS is a diagnosis of exclusion for patients **10 years or older** who have a spinal curve with a **Cobb angle of at least 10 degrees**.
- The initial evaluation aims to rule out other causes, clinically assess the curve, determine the need for X-rays, and evaluate the risk of progression.

HISTORY

- Developmental history: Rule out other causes of scoliosis.
- Age on onset: determine subtype
- Skeletal maturity
  - Age of menarche: Pubertal growth starts just before menarche.
  - Important for determining remaining linear growth and need for intervention
- Rate of progression: faster rate of progression concerning for nonidiopathic cause
- Family history: if positive, may suggest AIS
  - Inquire about biologic parental heights to estimate growth potential.
- History of lower limb injury: Fracture, joint infection or arthritis may result in limb length discrepancy.
- Neurologic dysfunction: Weakness, sensory deficits, bowel or bladder dysfunction, gait abnormalities, these signs would be concerning for nonidiopathic causes, should rule out intraspinal pathology.
- Difficulty breathing: Severe thoracic scoliosis may compromise respiratory function.
- Nocturnal pain: Rule out tumor.
- Pain: not a common complaint of AIS, although 25% present with nonspecific pain, often localized to back or chest wall

PHYSICAL EXAM

- Growth and puberty assessment:
  - Plot height and weight on growth curve to monitor peak growth velocity.
  - Assess Tanner stage, as risk for progression is greatest during the pubertal spurt. Tanner stage 2 precedes the onset of pubertal growth spurt in boys. Tanner stage 2 follows the onset of pubertal growth spurt in girls. 90% of females reach terminal height within 24 months of menarche.
- Skeletal inspection:
  - Spine symmetry (coronal and sagittal planes)
  - Shoulder height difference
  - Scapular positioning
  - Trunk shift
  - Chest cage deviation
  - Iliac crest symmetry
    - Adam forward bend test: Instruct patient to bend forward at the waist with straight knees. Asymmetry is observed by rib or paraspinous elevations, demonstrating rotational component.
    - Scoliometer: tool (physical or phone application) used to measure trunk rotation; used to measure angle of trunk rotation (ATR) with Adam forward bend test
      - An angle of 7 degrees corresponds to Cobb angle of 20 degrees.
      - Important consideration: Not all patients with radiographic scoliosis have trunk rotation and may be missed by Adam forward bend test.
- Rule out other causes:
  - Skin changes such as café au lait spots, hair tufts, sacral dimple to rule out other related causes such as neurofibromatosis or spinal dysraphism
  - Foot deformities such as cavo varus suggest neuromuscular disorder such as Friedreich ataxia.
  - Evaluate for congenital anomalies.
  - Assess for contracture or excessive laxity that can be associated with Ehlers-Danlos syndromes and Marfan syndrome.
  - Leg length discrepancy can be evaluated by block testing or tape measure from ASIS to medial malleolus, as small as 10 mm may result in scoliosis.
  - Perform neurologic exam; abnormalities may suggest neuromuscular or intraspinal causes.

DIFFERENTIAL DIAGNOSIS

- Scoliosis: neuromuscular, congenital, syndromic
- Postural abnormalities
- Leg length discrepancy

DIAGNOSTIC TESTS & INTERPRETATION

- Lab work is unnecessary unless used to rule out associated metabolic conditions.
- Initial radiographs are plain standing full-length posteroanterior (PA) and lateral views of the entire spine, C7 to sacrum.
- Direction of curve labeled by convexity:
  - Right-sided curve—dextroscoliosis
  - Left-sided curve—levoscoliosis
- Location is identified by apical vertebra that is most deviated and rotated from midline (cervical, thoracic, lumbar, lumbosacral).
- Curve magnitude is calculated using the Cobb method. Lines are drawn parallel to the superior endplate of the most cephalad vertebrae with the greatest tilt and to the inferior endplate of the most caudal vertebrae of the curve. The angle at which these lines intersect is the Cobb angle.
- Assessing skeletal maturity guides treatment timing and predicts progression risk. Radiographic methods include the Risser sign and Sanders Staging System.
- *Risser sign*: visual grading of the degree of ossification and fusion of the iliac apophysis on PA spinal radiographs.
- Risser grades:
  - 0—no ossification
  - 1—up to 25% ossification
  - 2—26–50% ossification
  - 3—51–75% ossification
  - 4—>76% ossification
  - 5—complete apophyseal fusion
- A lower Risser grade indicates there is more growth remaining and therefore more risk of progression.
- Sanders Skeletal Maturity Staging System: a measure using hand and wrist PA radiograph to classify skeletal maturity in eight stages
- Magnetic resonance imaging (MRI) is not routinely necessary but is indicated in certain cases including:
  - Neurologic abnormalities
  - Children <10 years old with a curve >20 degrees
  - Other findings suggestive of a neuromuscular disorder
- Pulmonary function tests (PFTs) are indicated for severe cases with restrictive lung disease.
- EOS slot-scanning technology is full-body imaging showing two-dimensional (2D) x-ray images and 3D rendering of the spine that is a low-dose radiation

alternative to serial radiographs, an important consideration in this population in which there is a concern for increased cancer risk due to repeated radiation exposure (1)[A].

TREATMENT

- Options for treatment include serial observation, physical therapy, bracing, and surgery. Concepts for treatment are based on the severity of the deformity and on the likelihood of progression.
- Guidelines for management:
  - Cobb angles <25 degrees are monitored with serial XR, usually at 3-, 6-, or 12-month intervals, with younger patients and those with curves nearing 20 degrees followed more frequently.
    - Physiotherapeutic scoliosis-specific exercises (PSSEs) indicated if Cobb angle >15 degrees
    - Skeletally immature patients (Risser grade 0 to 2) with Cobb angle 20 to 29 degrees should be followed closely and braced if angle increases by ≥5 degrees over 3 to 6 months.
  - Cobb angles of 25 to 45 degrees in skeletally immature patients are candidates for bracing until skeletal maturity.
  - Cobb angles >45 degrees in skeletally immature patients or >50 degrees in skeletally mature patients should be referred for surgical evaluation.
  - Skeletally mature with Cobb angles <40 degrees can be reassured and discharged.
  - Skeletally mature with Cobb angles 40 to 50 degrees are managed on an individual basis.

GENERAL MEASURES

- Rehabilitation
  - Limited data suggest **Physiotherapeutic Scoliosis Specific Exercises (PSSE)** maybe potentially useful to promote 3D self-correction in skeletally immature patients with curves over 15°. In high-risk patients (curves 25–40°), combining PSSE with bracing has shown potential effectiveness, with one study noting that 89% of patients avoided significant curve progression (2)[B].
- Bracing
  - Only indicated for skeletally immature patients
  - Criteria are currently based on low-sensitivity Risser classifications.
  - Sanders Maturity Staging System correlates with rapid growth phase and curve progression and has greater reliability, but no treatment criteria have been defined (3)[A].
  - Indicated if patient is Risser grade 0 to 3 and Cobb angle of 30 to 60 degrees at time of diagnosis
  - Indicated if patient is Risser grade 0 to 2 and has progression of 5 degrees or more over 6- to 8-month period of observation
  - Bracing recommended to be worn 21 to 23 hours/d. Effectiveness of bracing diminishes if worn <18 hours daily.
  - Types of braces:
    - Thoracolumbosacral orthosis (TLSO), or Boston brace, historically most common rigid brace, capable of one-dimensional correction
    - Rigo Chêneau orthosis (RCO) is a derotational type of brace that provides corrective forces in multiple planes. Unique compared to the traditional TLSO in that it is capable of curve derotation and treats scoliosis in three dimensions and has been shown to be superior to TLSO in reducing apical vertebral rotation (4)[A].
    - Night-wear brace options are available and may be considered for skeletally immature patients with a single major curve of 25 to 35 degrees and an apex below T8.
    - SpineCor nonrigid or flexible brace may improve compliance; however, conflicting studies on success when compared to rigid bracing
    - Cervical TLSO (Milwaukee brace) is less well tolerated and no longer used commonly in modern scoliosis care.
  - Bracing cessation is indicated once peak growth has stopped (Risser grade 4 or 2 years after menarche in girls or Risser grade 5 in boys).

SURGERY/OTHER PROCEDURES

- Indications
  - Skeletally immature patients with curves >45 degrees or those that show progression
  - Skeletally mature patients with curves >50 degrees
  - Signs of pulmonary compromise
  - Certain syndromic or congenital type scoliosis curves, especially in presence of pain
- Procedures
  - Posterior spinal fusion (PSF) with instrumentation using segmental rods and bone grafting is the mainstay of treatment.
  - Anterior spinal fusion (ASF) is also used but has a higher risk of pulmonary complications.
  - ASF in conjunction with PSF is required at times to prevent the anterior spine from continuing to grow after the PSF (crankshaft phenomenon).
  - Bony fusion is paramount; pseudoarthrosis or failure to fuse is a complication of surgery. Sports restriction for 9 to 12 months following surgery, and the surgeon must clear for contact sports.
  - Vertebral body tethering is a new surgical technique using an anterior approach, spinal instrumentation with vertebral body screws, and a cable compressing the convexity of the curve to correct scoliotic curves. Data on long-term outcomes are lacking (5)[A].

ONGOING CARE

FOLLOW-UP RECOMMENDATIONS

- Follow-up recommended for 12 to 24 months after reaching skeletal maturity
- Skeletally mature patients do not need routine follow-up if Cobb angle <40 degrees; care for curves beyond 40 degrees should be individualized.

PROGNOSIS

- Skeletal maturity and curve size are the strongest predictors of progression in AIS.
  - **Juvenile scoliosis**: Curves progress slowly until age 10, then accelerate with growth. They are more likely to become severe and resist conservative treatment.
  - **Factors for increased progression risk**:
    - **Curve size**: Cobb angles ≥20°. Curves >30° are at greatest risk to progress, even after skeletal maturity.
    - **Skeletal immaturity**: More remaining growth (e.g., Risser 0–1, Sanders ≤3) equals higher risk.
    - **Age**: Diagnosis before age 12.
    - **Gender**: Females have a 3- to 10-fold increased risk.
    - **Curve type**: Double and thoracic curves progress more often than nonthoracic curves.
- Overall, prognosis is good in the majority of cases, with only 10% of all diagnosed cases requiring treatment.
- Slightly greater rates of nulliparity, infertility treatment, and prepartum back pain are noted in women with AIS; however, there does not appear to be an increased risk of pregnancy-related complications in the AIS population (6)[A].
- Mortality rate is increased in those with severe thoracic curves (90 to 100 degrees) that result in cor pulmonale or right heart failure. Otherwise, mortality rates in those with AIS is the same as the general population.

COMPLICATIONS

- An association with AIS (treated or untreated) and mild to moderate back pain has been noted in multiple studies.
- Progression of lumbar curves >50 degrees in adult life is associated with degenerative disk disease and pain.
- Reduced pulmonary function in patients with thoracic curves >60 degrees
- Psychosocial complications have been reported.

REFERENCES

1. Lau LCM, Hung ALH, Chau WW, et al. Sequential spine-hand radiography for assessing skeletal maturity with low radiation EOS imaging system for bracing treatment recommendation in adolescent idiopathic scoliosis: a feasibility and validity study. *J Child Orthop*. 2019;13(4):385–392.
2. Karavidas N, Tzatzaliaris D. Brace and physiotherapeutic scoliosis specific exercises (PSSE) for adolescent idiopathic scoliosis (AIS) treatment: a prospective study following Scoliosis Research Society (SRS) criteria. *Arch Physiother*. 2022;12(1):22.
3. Vira S, Husain Q, Jalai C, et al. The interobserver and intraobserver reliability of the Sanders classification versus the Risser stage. *J Pediatr Orthop*. 2017;37(4):e246–e249.
4. Minsk MK, Venuti KD, Daumit GL, et al. Effectiveness of the Rigo Chêneau versus Boston-style orthoses for adolescent idiopathic scoliosis: a retrospective study. *Scoliosis Spinal Disord*. 2017;12:7.
5. Raitio A, Syvänen J, Helenius I. Vertebral body tethering: indications, surgical technique, and a systematic review of published results. *J Clin Med*. 2022;11(9):2576.
6. Dewan MC, Mummareddy N, Bonfield C. The influence of pregnancy on women with adolescent idiopathic scoliosis. *Eur Spine J*. 2018;27(2):253–263.

CLINICAL PEARLS

- If any of the signs mentioned are seen in conjunction with significant back pain, an x-ray or referral is indicated. The scoliometer is also a useful tool in screening patients.
- Scoliosis associated with osteoid osteoma is the suggested diagnosis for children who present with scoliosis and back pain that occurs especially at night and is relieved with aspirin.
- Scoliosis is not preventable. Wearing heavy backpacks, calcium deficiency, or poor posture is not related to deformity development.

SCUBA DIVING INJURIES: DECOMPRESSION SICKNESS AND ARTERIAL GAS EMBOLISM

Edgar M. VanHorne, MD ▪ Terrance L. Leighton III, BS, DO

BASICS

DESCRIPTION

- Decompression sickness (DCS) and arterial gas embolism (AGE) are adverse medical conditions which may manifest in the self-contained underwater breathing apparatus (SCUBA) environment due to sudden changes in ambient pressure.
- When diving, ambient gases (predominately nitrogen) present in the atmosphere are diffused throughout the human body and distributed via the circulatory system into tissues and organs.
- In the diver, ambient pressure increases with increasing underwater depth, compressing gases, resulting in gas diffusion into the blood and bodily tissues.
- As a diver ascends from depth, the reverse process occurs, and ambient gases diffuse back into circulation, expand, and eventually are breathed away through routine respiration.
- Rapid ascent or decompression can result in trapping/coalition/expansion of nitrogen bubbles in the tissues, joints, and vasculature causing pathologic illness (DCS).
- In severe cases (AGE), nitrogenous bubble expansion can cause harm pending the anatomical location of the bubble. It can obstruct vasculature, inhibiting circulatory flow directly causing cerebral, spinal cord, or cardiac ischemia with associated inflammatory vascular response, rupture of pulmonary alveoli or pulmonary embolism (PE), and other associated pathologic end-organ damage.
- DCS may be subdivided into two categories:
  - *Type I* DCS: manifest by milder symptoms of musculoskeletal pain, dermatologic rash, and vague constitutional symptoms. Extreme fatigue may be a prelude to a more severe decompression illness (DCI).
  - *Type II* DCS: characterized by moderate to severe neurologic impairment, cardiorespiratory dysfunction, and vestibular symptoms (1)
- AGE: a central nervous system (CNS) or cardiac injury occurring due to pulmonary barotrauma/pulmonary overinflation syndrome (POIS), whereby air released from over-pressurized alveoli enters the pleural space (pneumothorax), mediastinum (pneumomediastinum), interstitium, and pulmonary capillary circulation, with subsequent access to systemic circulation
- Nitrogen gas bubbles returning to the heart may also reach the arterial circulation paradoxically via patent foramen ovale (PFO) or a right-to-left shunt, which can then embolize and obstruct cardiac or cerebral circulation (1).
- Type II DCS and AGE present similar symptoms and are best differentiated by time of onset.
- AGE symptoms typically present *immediately* or within minutes after resurfacing (<10 minutes), whereas DCS symptoms usually develop *hours to days* after diving.
- Synonym(s): the bends; air embolism; caisson disease; DCI

EPIDEMIOLOGY

- The incidence rate of DCI is estimated between 0.01% and 0.09% per dive in recreational divers (2). Divers Alert Network (DAN) estimates 3 cases per 10,000 person-dives in the recreational community (1). Based on international dive surveys, minor incidents occur at a rate of 1.3% of all dives (3).
- Predominant age is young adulthood 20 to 29 years, and predominant sex is male.

RISK FACTORS

- Inexperience
- Fatigue
- Hypovolemia/dehydration
- Poor physical conditioning
- Obesity
- Acute illnesses (ear, nose, and throat [ENT]; pulmonary; or gastrointestinal [GI])
- Chronic obstructive pulmonary disease (COPD) or poorly controlled asthma (increases risk for pulmonary barotrauma) (2),(4)
- Previous history of cerebral, spinal, inner ear, or cutaneous DCI
- Migraine with aura (MWA)
- PFO
- Atrial septal defect (ASD)
- History of anxiety, panic attacks, or claustrophobia
- Panic or anxiety while diving
- Rapid ascent from depth
- Holding breath during ascent
- Omitted decompression stops
- Prolonged dive at depth of >33 feet sea water (>10 m sea water or 2 ATA)
- Multiple/repetitive dives
- Cold water, rough sea, or strong current dives
- Free diving (breath-hold diving)—high frequency within short time period
- Inadequate rest/recovery between dives
- Strenuous physical activity while diving (commercial diving), tunnel, bridge, or oil platform work (caisson disease)
- Elevated body temperature
- Strenuous exertion after diving
- Flying <24 hours after SCUBA diving
- Inadequate aircraft cabin pressurization when flying

GENERAL PREVENTION

- Maintain adequate hydration.
- Do not dive under the influence of alcohol, drugs, or sedative medication.
- Ensure dive equipment is in good condition and proper working order.
- Ensure adequate wetsuit protection for projected water immersion temperatures.
- Always dive with a partner (dive buddy).
- Do not dive with sinus or ear infection, eustachian tube dysfunction, or inability to effectively perform Valsalva maneuver.
- Do not dive with poorly controlled asthma or other upper respiratory illness.
- Do not dive with any ongoing or active GI disturbance.
- Have a plan and know the current diving conditions.
- Use a dive computer to control exposure and ensure performance of adequate safety stops.
- Review dive tables prior in case dive computer malfunctions.
- Avoid holding breath during ascent.
- High-oxygen/low-nitrogen dive breathing gas mixture, or nitrox, may decrease tissue uptake of nitrogen but may also increase potential for oxygen toxicity at shallower depth. Specific training is recommended for heliox and nitrox.
- Wait 24 hours after diving before flying or traveling to higher altitudes.

DIAGNOSIS

HISTORY

- Determine time of onset of symptoms and any change in type or severity of symptoms.
- Obtain an independent account from a dive buddy or dive instructor, particularly if altered consciousness or mental status was impaired.
- Information from a dive computer (if the patient was equipped with one) may help to determine recent dive history, dive profile, and rate of ascent.
- Determine history of diving followed by exposure to altitude or past history of DCI.
- Note any significant past medical history of asthma, COPD, seizures, cardiac abnormality, prescription medications, recreational drug, or alcohol use.

PHYSICAL EXAM

- General manifestations of gas deposition in the CNS may mimic a transient ischemic attack (TIA), cerebrovascular accident (CVA), or seizure (epilepsy): manifest by confusion, personality changes, altered level of consciousness, delirium, numbness, weakness, aphasia, paresthesias, rapidly ascending paraplegia, or paralysis.
- Bubble formation in the inner ear can cause tinnitus, sensorineural hearing loss, and disequilibrium, with associated nausea, vomiting, ataxia, and nystagmus.
- Cardiac findings include tachyarrhythmia or bradyarrhythmia, signs of myocardial infarction, or congestive heart failure.
- Pulmonary examination may detect decreased breath sounds or pneumothorax, tachypnea, cough, wheeze, rales (the chokes), and decreased oxygen saturation with pulse oximetry.
- Joints may exhibit erythema and edema of periarticular surfaces, vague soreness, muscle weakness or fatigue, and pain with movement.
- Gas deposition in soft tissues may manifest as urticaria, mottled skin rash (cutis marmorata), or subcutaneous emphysema.

DIFFERENTIAL DIAGNOSIS

- Near drowning and hypoxic brain injury
- CVA
- Migraine
- Middle ear or sinus barotrauma with cranial nerve compression

- Inner ear barotrauma
- Seizure (hypoglycemia, epilepsy) and postictal state
- Spinal cord compression (disk herniation, hematoma, or tumor)
- Guillain-Barré syndrome
- Multiple sclerosis
- Transverse myelitis
- Acute myocardial infarction
- Cold water immersion pulmonary edema
- Swimming-induced pulmonary edema (SIPE)
- Contaminated breathing gas (carbon monoxide)
- Urticaria/anaphylaxis
- Seafood toxin poisoning (ciguatera, puffer fish, paralytic shellfish, sea snake envenomation)
- Malingering

DIAGNOSTIC TESTS & INTERPRETATION

- Chest radiography to assess for pneumothorax, mediastinal emphysema, and heart enlargement
- Chest computed tomography (CT) to screen PE
- CT scan or magnetic resonance imaging (MRI) to diagnose cerebral or spinal cord abnormalities
- Transesophageal bubble contrast echocardiogram to detect PFO
- Nonacute plain radiography, scintigraphy, MRI, and ultrasound of long bones and joints if dysbaric osteonecrosis is suspected
- If a high index of suspicion, recommend treating immediately with nonrebreather 100% oxygen and contacting hyperbaric oxygen chamber.

TREATMENT

- Hyperbaric oxygen therapy (HBOT), which is performed in a hyperbaric chamber where the patient is placed in the chamber and pressure is increased simulating descending to a depth of 60 feet underwater (2.8 ATA; 1 ATA is the atmospheric pressure at sea level). Once at the depth, the patient is placed on 100% oxygen for prescribed time periods with scheduled breaks off of oxygen to prevent oxygen toxicity. HBOT involves compression of nitrogen gas bubbles causing the symptoms of DCS, whereas the oxygen administered replaces nitrogen in the circulatory system improving tissue oxygenation while the nitrogen gas diffuses out of affected tissues over time, alleviating the symptoms of DCS.
- To locate the nearest HBOT chamber resources, access the DAN emergency hotline (+1-919-684-9111).
- DCS type I: Mild cases of DCS type I may be treated without HBOT by breathing 100% oxygen via a nonrebreather mask. Consider HBOT if conservative measures fail to alleviate symptoms (1)[C].
- DCS type II: recompression therapy in a hyperbaric oxygen chamber as soon as possible
- Treatment is typically administered based on the U.S. Navy Treatment Table 6 (TT6), which lasts approximately 4 hours and 45 minutes.
- Significant improvement of symptoms soon after arrival to a depth of 60 ft (2.8 ATA) supports the diagnosis of DCS.
- Treatment tables may be modified to extend protocol or repeated until symptoms completely resolve.
- AGE: Check for spontaneous breathing and circulation. If necessary, call 911 and initiate cardiopulmonary resuscitation (CPR). Administer 100% oxygen via a nonrebreather mask if available. Access the nearest emergency room facility via emergency medical services (EMS).
- Once stabilized, assess for hypoglycemia, CVA, spinal cord trauma, and PE/pneumothorax. Initiate correction of any volume deficit with isotonic intravenous (IV) fluid resuscitation. Once stable, prepare for transfer to a hyperbaric oxygen chamber facility.
- Initiate HBOT using U.S. Navy TT6 protocol.
- If symptoms do not improve significantly at the standard 2.8 ATA, TT6 may be modified by an extended initial 30-minute period of 50% oxygen at 6 ATA. Treatment is continued until symptoms resolve or plateau (5)[C].

ADDITIONAL THERAPIES

- Diazepam 5 to 15 mg IV may be considered for inner ear bends to alleviate symptoms of nausea and vomiting associated with severe vertigo.
- Deep venous thrombosis (DVT) prophylaxis may be indicated for patients immobilized by severe CNS bends.
- Avoid nonsteroidal anti-inflammatory drugs (NSAIDs) administration to patients with pain symptoms of DCS until hyperbaric treatment has been initiated.
- Fever in a patient with DCS should be worked up to rule out source of infection because hyperthermia may adversely affect prognosis.
- Additional resources:
  – International DAN (iDAN +1-919-684-9111)

ONGOING CARE

FOLLOW-UP RECOMMENDATIONS

- Patients may be discharged home if minor cutaneous symptoms are present and the patient responded to conservative therapy administered in the emergency department.
- Follow-up should be made with a physician knowledgeable in dive medicine.
- Wait 24 hours before flying after SCUBA diving.
- Exposure to altitude can precipitate relapse of DCS symptoms post-HBOT. If possible, postpone travel for 3 days at sea level after reaching a clinical plateau.
- In-flight oxygen supplementation may prevent DCS relapse.
- Type I DCS: 2 weeks is recommended before returning to diving.
- Type II DCS with minor neurologic symptoms: 6 weeks is recommended before return to diving.
- Type II DCS with severe neurologic symptoms: Diving is no longer recommended (1),(5)[C].

PROGNOSIS

- The prognosis is excellent for early symptomatic recognition and timely treatment.
- Delay in treatment of severe symptoms negatively affects outcome due to the ischemic effects of the occlusive nitrogen bubble.
- Rehabilitation of the injured diver may continue to improve residual sequelae by continuing hyperbaric treatment for up to 2 years.

COMPLICATIONS

- Oxygen toxicity
- Transient myopia due to ocular lens oxygen toxicity (older patients), which may resolve in 4 to 6 weeks
- Sensorineural hearing loss
- Dysbaric osteonecrosis
- Residual neurologic deficits in CNS bend (46–75%), despite comprehensive treatment
- Permanent paralysis may occur if recompression is not initiated promptly.
- Residual paralysis may occur even in adequately treated patients if initial presentation is severe.

REFERENCES

1. Pollock NW, Buteau D. Updates in decompression illness. *Emerg Med Clin North Am*. 2017;35(2):301–319.
2. Cooper JS, Hanson KC. *Decompression Sickness*. StatPearls; 2023. Updated December 13, 2023. Accessed September 10, 2025. https://www.ncbi.nlm.nih.gov/books/NBK537264/
3. Klapa S, Meyne J, Kähler W, et al. Decompression illness with hypovolemic shock and neurological failure symptoms after two risky dives: a case report. *Physiol Rep*. 2017;5(6):e13094.
4. Eichhorn L, Leyk D. Diving medicine in clinical practice. *Dtsch Arztebl Int*. 2015;112(9):147–157.
5. U.S. Navy. *U.S. Navy Diving Manual, Volume 1: Diving Principles and Policies, Revision 7*. Naval Sea Systems Command; 2016.

ADDITIONAL READING

- Divernet: http://www.divernet.com/medical-health/
- Wingelaar TT, van Ooij PAM, van Hulst RA. Oxygen toxicity and special operations forces diving: hidden and dangerous. *Front Psychol*. 2017;8:1263.

CLINICAL PEARLS

- DCS and AGE occur when compressed dissolved nitrogen gas reexpands into tissues and circulation as a result of rapid ascent from underwater depth.
- DCS should lead the differential diagnosis in any individual with recent history (hours to days) of SCUBA diving who presents with associated clinical symptomatology.
- AGE should be suspected in divers who surface with immediate (<10 minutes from time of surfacing) signs of severe neurologic or cardiopulmonary pathology.
- AGE is associated with PFO and/or persistent cardiac septal defects.
- HBOT is the definitive treatment for DCS and AGE.
- HBOT is contraindicated with an unresolved pneumothorax; recommended to place a chest tube and then treat with HBOT
- Proper diagnosis of DCS is supported if the patient's symptoms improve within a relatively short period of time after recompression.
- U.S. Navy TT6 is the preferred protocol for HBOT treatment.

SEIZURES AND EPILEPSY IN SPORTS

Nilesh Shah, MD, FAAFP, CAQSM • Jessica C. Tomazic, MD, CAQSM

BASICS

DESCRIPTION
- A seizure is an abnormal paroxysmal electrical discharge in the brain, usually with mental status changes.
- Individuals who have two unprovoked seizures that occur >24 hours apart are deemed to have epilepsy.
- Status epilepticus: one continuous seizure lasting >5 minutes or two or more seizures between which there is no full return of consciousness
- Seizure types:
  - Generalized: sudden onset involving an altered level of consciousness, usually bilateral and symmetrical
  - Partial: either simple (no alteration of consciousness) or complex (alteration/loss of consciousness often with semi-purposeful inappropriate movements)
- Synonym(s): convulsions; fits; attacks; spells

EPIDEMIOLOGY
- Incidence of seizure disorders is approximately 49 per 100,000 persons/y (1).
- Prevalence of active epilepsy is 6.4 per 1,000 persons internationally (1).
- Up to 10% of people will have at least one seizure during their lifetime (2).
- 21 to 30 per 100,000 new cases/y in 10- to 59-year-olds (1)
- 70% of people with epilepsy can go into remission if diagnosed and treated properly (3).

RISK FACTORS
- Family history
- Cerebrovascular disease
- Brain tumors
- Alcohol or drug abuse
- Previous head injury
- Malformations of cortical development
- Infections
- Abnormal early neurologic development

GENERAL PREVENTION
- Exercise may decrease seizure frequency (4).
- Sufficient and regular sleep (4)
- Practice proper nutrition and hydration (4).
- Adhering to antiepileptic drug (AED) therapy (4)

COMMONLY ASSOCIATED CONDITIONS
- Behavioral problems (personality disorders)
- Hematologic disorders (sickle cell disease, porphyria, and antiphospholipid syndrome)
- Learning disabilities
- Migraine headaches
- Mood disorders (anxiety/depression)
- Psychiatric conditions
- Systemic autoimmune conditions (systemic lupus erythematosus [SLE])

DIAGNOSIS

HISTORY
- Convulsions (focal or generalized)
- Change in muscle tone
- Decreased level of consciousness
- Staring spells
- Loss of control of bowel or bladder
- Postictal confusion
- Postictal psychosis
- Todd paralysis (temporary weakness or paralysis in a part or all of their body immediately following an epileptic seizure)
- Actual account by first-hand observer is extremely helpful or smartphone video.
- Previous history of seizure
- Previous history of head trauma
- Medications
- Social/family history

PHYSICAL EXAM
- Fever: suggests infectious etiology
- Focal neurologic deficit: possible localized trauma or tumor
- Meningismus: may be present in meningitis
- Papilledema: secondary to increased intracranial pressure
- Tongue biting (low sensitivity, high specificity)
- Look for injuries that may have occurred during the seizure.
- Look for evidence of acutely increased intracranial pressure, such as pupillary dilatation or posturing, indicating an emergency.
- Expect postictal confusion that gradually clears after a seizure.

DIFFERENTIAL DIAGNOSIS
- Alcohol withdrawal
- Arteriovenous malformation
- Electrolyte abnormalities (hypoglycemia, hyponatremia)
- Fever
- Hepatic failure
- Illicit drug use/abuse/withdrawal
- Infection
- Intracranial swelling/second-impact syndrome
- Primary/secondary brain tumor
- Posttraumatic (impact) seizure
- Stroke
- Syncope
- Uremia
- Vascular disease

DIAGNOSTIC TESTS & INTERPRETATION

Initial Tests (lab, imaging)
- Electrolytes, including glucose, calcium, magnesium, and phosphorus
- Renal/liver function tests, including ammonia level
- Complete blood count (CBC), urinalysis
- Blood/urine toxicology
- Anticonvulsant level(s): Inadequate levels are a significant cause of recurrent seizures.
- Computed tomography (CT) or magnetic resonance imaging (MRI) indicated for individuals with first-time seizure to evaluate for structural brain abnormality
- CT scan: rules out acute bleeding or intracranial masses
- MRI: may better define posterior fossa tumors, vascular abnormalities, and temporal lobes
- Electroencephalography (EEG): may define true seizure activity and focus, although a negative EEG result does not rule out seizure disorder. Sometimes, a sleep-deprived EEG may be required.

Diagnostic Procedures/Other
- Electrocardiogram (ECG): evaluates for cardiogenic causes of hypoxia-related seizure
- Spinal tap to rule out infectious etiology, elevated intracranial pressure, some congenital etiologies

TREATMENT

GENERAL MEASURES
- Supportive: airway, breathing, and circulation (ABCs)
- Roll patients with active tonic-clonic seizures on their side in the "recovery position."
- Do *not* use bite block or tongue depressor.
- Keep area clear: Ensure that the patient does not injure self or others.
- If in the setting of trauma, stabilize C-spine.
- Transfer to emergency department (ED) if the patient has no known seizure disorder:
  - ED treatment:
    - Immediate ED treatment includes benzodiazepines or other AEDs if patient is in status epilepticus.
    - Workup as above for etiology
    - Consider neurology consultation.

MEDICATION
- If no reversible cause is found, place patient on AEDs.
- A number of drugs are available.
- Use depends on etiology of seizures.
- Most AEDs are approved by the National Collegiate Athletic Association (NCAA) and International Olympic Committee (IOC).

First Line
- Benzodiazepines for status epilepticus
- Common AEDs: levetiracetam, fosphenytoin/phenytoin, and valproic acid

Second Line
Depends on etiology of seizure

ISSUES FOR REFERRAL
Neurology:
- First-time unprovoked seizure
- Initiation of AEDs
- Outpatient EEG

ADMISSION, INPATIENT, AND NURSING CONSIDERATIONS

- Hospitalization recommended for immediate care of uncontrolled seizures
- Abnormal mental status associated with seizures
- Ongoing studies (i.e., sleep study or 24-hour EEG monitoring)
- Need for intravenous (IV) access:
  - Ongoing IV drug administration
  - Correction of electrolyte abnormalities
  - Correction of dehydration

ONGOING CARE

FOLLOW-UP RECOMMENDATIONS

Patient Monitoring

Monitor levels of AEDs, especially in first couple months of training.

PATIENT EDUCATION

- People with chronic diseases, including epilepsy, should be encouraged to exercise, as should the general population. The mental and physical advantages of regular exercise are regarded as highly beneficial to a group that is normally sedentary, overweight, and with higher rates of depression (3)[A].
- Recommendations with respect to fitness to participate in a specific sport should consider the probability of a seizure occurring, the seizure type, the usual timing of seizure occurrence, and other factors (4)[C].
- International League Against Epilepsy (ILAE) proposed sports be classified into three categories based on potential risk of injury/death should a seizure occur (4)[C]:
  - Group 1 sports (no significant additional risk to person with epilepsy or bystanders):
    - Athletics
    - Bowling
    - Most collective contact sports (judo, wrestling, etc.)
    - Collective sports on the ground (baseball, basketball, cricket, field hockey, football, soccer, rugby, volleyball, etc.)
    - Cross-country skiing
    - Curling
    - Dancing
    - Golf
    - Racquet sports (squash, table tennis, tennis, etc.)
  - Group 2 sports (moderate risk to persons with epilepsy but no risk for bystanders):
    - Alpine skiing
    - Archery
    - Athletics (pole vault)
    - Biathlon, triathlon, modern pentathlon
    - Canoeing
    - Collective contact sports involving potentially serious injury (e.g., boxing, karate)
    - Cycling
    - Fencing
    - Gymnastics
    - Horse riding (e.g., Olympic equestrian events—dressage, eventing, show jumping)
    - Ice hockey
    - Shooting
    - Skateboarding
    - Skating
    - Snowboarding
    - Swimming
    - Water skiing
    - Weight lifting
  - Group 3 sports (high risk to persons with epilepsy and, for some sports, also risks for bystanders):
    - Aviation
    - Climbing
    - Diving (platform, springboard)
    - Horse racing (competitive)
    - Motor sports
    - Parachuting (and similar sports)
    - Rodeo
    - Scuba diving
    - Ski jumping
    - Solitary sailing
    - Surfing, windsurfing
- One or more acute symptomatic seizures:
  - Group 1 sports permitted
  - Group 2 and 3 sports at neurologist discretion
- Single unprovoked seizure:
  - Group 1 sports permitted after medical/neurologic assessment
  - Group 2 and 3 sports after seizure free for 12 months
- Sleep-related seizures only:
  - Group 1 sports permitted
  - Group 2 sports at neurologist discretion or after 12 months follow-up if seizures confirmed to be exclusively associated with sleep and sports does not involve alterations in the sleep-wake cycle
  - Group 3 sports generally barred
- Seizures without impaired awareness:
  - Group 1 sports permitted
  - Group 2 sports at neurologist discretion or after 12 months follow-up if seizure occurs exclusively without impairment of awareness
  - Group 3 sports generally barred
- Seizures with impaired awareness:
  - Group 1 sports permitted
  - Group 2 sports at neurologist discretion
  - Group 3 sports generally barred
- Resolved epilepsy (age-dependent epilepsy syndrome past applicable age, seizure free for 10 years, and off antiseizure medications for at least 5 years):
  - Group 1, 2, and 3 sports permitted
- Medication withdrawal:
  - Group 2 or 3 sports are not permitted for 6 months.
  - If seizure reoccurs, group 2 and 3 sports are not permitted for a period of 3 months after previously effective treatment is reinstated and no further seizures.

PROGNOSIS

Prognosis is generally excellent with well-controlled seizures.

COMPLICATIONS

- Exercise at high altitudes (>2,000 m) can predispose to hypoxia and induce seizures.
- Hyperhydration (consumption that outpaces demand) in combination with sodium loss can result in hyponatremic seizures.
- AED side effects may include impaired concentration or coordination.
- Certain AEDs can predispose athletes to heat-related illness and hyperthermia which is a known seizure trigger.

REFERENCES

1. Carter JM, McGrew C. Seizure disorders and exercise/sports participation. *Curr Sports Med Rep*. 2021;20(1):26–30.
2. Falco-Walter J. Epilepsy—definition, classification, pathophysiology, and epidemiology. *Semin Neurol*. 2020;40(6):617–623.
3. Duñabeitia I, Bidaurrazaga-Letona I, Diz JC, et al. Effects of physical exercise in people with epilepsy: a systematic review and meta-analysis. *Epilepsy Behav*. 2022;137(Pt A):108959.
4. Guidry A, Crutchfield K. Athletes with neurologic disease. *Handb Clin Neurol*. 2018;158:445–462.
5. Carrizosa-Moog J, Ladino LD, Benjumea-Cuartas V, et al. Epilepsy, physical activity and sports: a narrative review. *Can J Neurol Sci*. 2018;45(6):624–632.

ADDITIONAL READING

- Almeida MRG, Bell GS, Sander JW. Epilepsy and recreational scuba diving: an absolute contraindication or can there be exceptions? A call for discussion. *Epilepsia*. 2007;48(5):851–858.
- Arida RM. Physical exercise and seizure activity. *Biochim Biophys Acta Mol Basis Dis*. 2021;1867(1):165979.
- Dimitri P, Joshi K, Jones N, et al. Moving more: physical activity and its positive effects on long term conditions in children and young people. *Arch Dis Child*. 2020;105(11):1035–1040.
- Kiriakopoulos E. Summer safety for people with seizures. Published June 12, 2023. Accessed August 26, 2025. https://www.epilepsy.com/stories/summer-safety-people-seizures
- Sırtbaş G, Yalnızoğlu D, Livanelioğlu A. Comparison of physical fitness, activity, and quality of life of the children with epilepsy and their healthy peers. *Epilepsy Res*. 2021;178:106795.

CLINICAL PEARLS

- In general, individuals with epilepsy or new-onset seizure disorder should avoid high-risk activities such as scuba diving, skydiving, and group 3 sports (4)[C].
- There is no definitive evidence of any relationship between repetitive minor head injury and deterioration of the epileptic patient (1)[C]; therefore, most collision/contact sports are acceptable (but no boxing).
- Swimming is acceptable with a certified lifeguard who should be made aware of the situation. Motor sports should be undertaken only by individuals with well-controlled seizures. Sports in which falling is a potential (e.g., gymnastics, rock climbing, hang gliding) should be judged on an individual basis based on the type and frequency of seizure.
- Sports need not be avoided for children, or adults (3)[A], who experience seizures. Improving overall health may reduce the number of seizures experienced by a child (1)[C].
- Data suggests exercise can improve quality of life, cognitive, emotional well-being, and overall fitness in people with epilepsy (3)[A].
- On rare occasions, exercise may induce seizure occurrence (5)[C]. Therefore, clinicians should be aware of:
  - Seizure types (as temporal reflex epilepsy may be more prone to exercise-induced seizures than other forms) (5)[C]
  - Seizure triggers (5)[C]
  - Side effects of AEDs on athlete perception and alertness (4)[C]

S

SEPTIC ARTHRITIS AND BURSITIS

Matthew Rachwalski, DO • Kevin B. Gebke, MD

BASICS

DESCRIPTION

- Infection of articular joint(s) or bursae with a bacterial, mycobacterial, spirochetal, fungal, viral, or parasitic source
- Usually acute, but bursitis can be chronic
- May be an indication of systemic infection
- Synonym(s): infectious arthritis; purulent synovitis; infectious bursitis

EPIDEMIOLOGY

- Incidence 29 cases per 100,000 person-years (1)
- Monoarticular or oligoarticular pattern for acute bacterial infection, chronic mycobacterial infection, or fungal infection
- Acute polyarticular involvement usually signifies disseminated neisserial infection or acute hepatitis B.
- Septic arthritis from gonorrhea now very rare
- Olecranon and prepatellar bursae most common

RISK FACTORS

- Soft tissue/joint penetration or recent surgery
- Trauma, including repetitive microtrauma (bursitis)
- Abnormal joint architecture (rheumatoid arthritis [RA], osteoarthritis [OA], joint replacement) (1)
- Intravenous drug abuse (IVDA), alcoholism, tobacco use (1)
- Intravascular devices, urinary catheters
- Sexually active person at risk for sexually transmitted infections (STIs) (rare etiology)
- Significant comorbid diseases (diabetes, malignancy, hepatic failure, sickle cell disease, immunocompromised states)
- Elderly (age >80 years)

DIAGNOSIS

HISTORY

- Rapid onset (1 to 2 weeks) in septic arthritis; may have rapid or insidious onset with septic bursitis
- Single joint involvement in >85% of patients
- Most commonly involves knee (50%) > hip > shoulder, ankle, wrist, or elbow joints (2)
- Hematologic spread: presence of infection leading to bacterial seeding of joint (Skin infection, pneumonia, and pyelonephritis are commonly the source.)

PHYSICAL EXAM

- Usually, severe pain in region of joint or bursa with motion
- Swelling (bursitis) or joint effusion (arthritis)
- Decreased range of joint motion (especially with septic arthritis may not have with bursitis)
- Localized or systemic fever
- Concomitant urethral discharge (gonorrhea)
- Erythema and tenderness to palpation of affected joint or bursa
- IV drug abuse often develops bacterial arthritis in axial joints, such as the sternoclavicular and sternomanubrial joint; may develop bacterial arthritis as a consequence of infective endocarditis
- Rare cutaneous lesions (infective endocarditis, Lyme disease, meningococcal infection, gonorrhea)

DIFFERENTIAL DIAGNOSIS

- Cellulitis
- Osteomyelitis
- Gout, pseudogout (calcium pyrophosphate deposition disease)
- RA, juvenile inflammatory arthritis (JIA), rheumatic fever
- Lyme disease
- Spondyloarthropathy (reactive arthritis, psoriatic arthritis, ankylosing spondylitis, irritable bowel disease)
- Sarcoidosis, amyloidosis
- Synovitis, synovial papilloma
- HIV/AIDS, bacterial endocarditis

DIAGNOSTIC TESTS & INTERPRETATION

- Laboratory evaluation of joint or bursal aspirate is gold standard for diagnosis. Collect prior to starting antibiotics (1)[C],(2)[C],(3)[A].
- Complete blood count (CBC); blood cultures; erythrocyte sedimentation rate (ESR) ≥10 mm/h (98% sensitive); C-reactive protein (CRP) ≥15 mm/h (94% sensitive); blood cultures × 2, procalcitonin >0.5 ng/mL (higher specificity than CRP); ESR/CRP helpful but not diagnostic (1)[C],(2)[C]
- Contaminated overlying tissue (i.e., cellulitis) should be avoided during arthrocentesis or bursal aspiration.
- Cloudy indicates high likelihood of infection synovial or bursal fluid aspirate should be sent for white blood cell (WBC) count and differential, Gram stain and examination for crystals, and culture (aerobic/anaerobic bacteria, mycobacteria, and fungi). Order serum testing and confirmatory polymerase chain reaction (PCR) testing for Lyme disease if high suspicion (1)[C],(2)[C].
- In acute septic arthritis, synovial WBC counts typically average 50,000 WBC/mL with >90% neutrophils (>100,00 WBC/mL more specific) (1)[C],(3)[A],(4)[B]

- In prosthetic joint infections, synovial WBC counts may be as low as 1,100 WBC/mL with >64% neutrophils.
- Plain radiographs initially may be normal—help rule out fracture, osteopenia first radiologic sign, and then diffuse joint space narrowing.
- Ultrasound (US) is useful for identifying joint effusions and to aid in aspiration of bursa or joint.
- Computed tomography (CT) visualizes bone edema, bone erosions, and sclerosis.
- Magnetic resonance imaging (MRI) preferably with and without contrast better for detection joint effusion and differentiate between bone and soft tissue infections
- Bone scan is indicated for identification of region affected by inflammatory process.

TREATMENT

- Septic bursitis:
  - Systematic review suggests nonsurgical management is superior to surgical débridement/bursectomy.
  - Most common organisms include *Staphylococcus aureus* (80%), β-hemolytic *Streptococcus*, and *S. epidermidis* (1)[A].
  - With repetitive microtrauma and hematogenous seeding may broaden coverage
  - Primary therapy includes penicillinase-resistant penicillins (nafcillin or dicloxacillin) or 1st-generation cephalosporins (cefazolin). If allergic, then use Bactrim or clindamycin (1)[C],(2)[C]. If concern for methicillin-resistant *S. aureus* (MRSA) then use IV vancomycin.
  - No consensus on duration but generally 10 to 14 days
  - Hospitalization for parenteral therapy is required when signs of systemic or bony extension of infection are observed.
  - Surgical intervention includes endoscopic versus open bursectomy; reserved for persistent infection despite antibiotic treatment, presence of foreign body, or underlying osteomyelitis (5)[B]
- Septic arthritis:
  - Septic arthritis is considered an emergency, and prompt drainage and administration of IV antibiotics can prevent joint damage.
  - Empiric IV broad-spectrum antibiotic should be initiated based on Gram stain result (2)[C],(6)[B].
  - If Gram stain shows gram-positive cocci (likely staph/strep species), treat with vancomycin plus cephalosporin, carbapenem, or fluoroquinolone; may start PO clindamycin and fluroquinolone if started within 1 week of surgery/arthrocentesis with similar outcome to IV therapy (2)[B]
  - If Gram stain shows gram-negative cocci or bacilli, treat with a 3rd-generation cephalosporin such as ceftriaxone. If *pseudomonas* is suspected, then start 4th-generation cephalosporin such as cefepime. If β-lactam allergy, then use aztreonam or ciprofloxacin (2)[C].
  - If Gram stain negative, start vancomycin in immunocompetent and add 3rd-generation cephalosporin in immunocompromised and at risk for STIs (2)[C].
  - Infection eradication is complicated by the presence of joint prostheses, and removal of the prosthesis may be necessary (5)[B],(6)[B].
  - No indication for intra-articular antibiotics (2)[C]
  - No consensus on duration of antibiotic therapy, Infectious Diseases Society of America (IDSA) recommends 4-week course of parenteral therapy in *S. aureus* and gram-negative bacilli infections (3)[C].
  - Patients treated for gonorrhea also should receive doxycycline 100 mg PO BID × 7 days to cover possible concurrent *Chlamydia* infection.
  - Longer treatment is required for joints affected by arthritis.
  - Surgical intervention via arthroscopic lavage or arthrotomy is indicated only if needle drainage is ineffective (fluid loculation or inaccessible joint).
  - After initial joint drainage, therapeutic response monitored with serial synovial fluid analysis

ONGOING CARE

- Complete resolution and restoration of joint function is the goal.
- Possible adverse outcomes include death, impaired joint function (e.g., decreased motion, fusion, dislocation), septic necrosis, sinus formation, ankylosis, osteomyelitis, synovitis, and limb length changes.

FOLLOW-UP RECOMMENDATIONS

- Recurrent arthrocentesis is recommended as joint fluid reaccumulates to rule out persistent/recurrent infection.
- Regular office visits are recommended after hospital discharge for reevaluation and early recognition of persistent or new problems.
- Prosthesis replacement is possible in the future after clearance of infection.

REFERENCES

1. Khodaee M. Common superficial bursitis. *Am Fam Physician*. 2017;95(4):224–231.
2. Earwood JS, Walker TR, Sue GJC. Septic arthritis: diagnosis and treatment. *Am Fam Physician*. 2021;104(6):589–597.
3. McBride S, Mowbray J, Caughey W, et al. Epidemiology, management, and outcomes of large and small native joint septic arthritis in adults. *Clin Infect Dis*. 2020;70(2):271–279.
4. Miller JM, Binnicker MJ, Campbell S, et al. A guide to utilization of the microbiology laboratory for diagnosis of infectious diseases: 2018 update by the Infectious Diseases Society of America and the American Society for Microbiology. *Clin Infect Dis*. 2018;67(6):813–816.
5. Cho HJ, Burke LA, Lee M. Septic arthritis. *Hosp Med Clin*. 2014;3(4):494–503.
6. Lieber SB, Fowler ML, Zhu C, et al. Clinical characteristics and outcomes of septic bursitis. *Infection*. 2017;45(6):781–786.

CLINICAL PEARLS

- Nonsurgical management of septic bursitis is preferred.
- Septic arthritis is considered an emergency, and prompt drainage and administration of IV antibiotics can prevent joint damage.
- Knee joint is most common, although axial joints are more common in IVDA.
- Complete restoration of joint function is expected if early diagnosis and treatment occur before articular damage is seen.
- Sign of hip infection, more common in children, is hip held in flexed and externally rotated position.

SESAMOID DYSFUNCTION AND FRACTURE

William C. Nace, DO • James R. Borchers, MD, MPH

BASICS

Anatomy:

- Two sesamoid bones: the larger tibial (medial) sesamoid and fibular (lateral) sesamoid
- Located on the plantar side of the 1st metatarsophalangeal (MTP) joint, just proximal to the metatarsal head, embedded within the flexor hallucis brevis tendon and connected by the intersesamoid ligament
- The sesamoids' articular surfaces are located dorsally and articulate with the plantar facets on the 1st metatarsal head.
- Blood supply is usually from a single artery, with a lack of significant secondary blood supply (which increases risk for nonunion of fractures) (1).
- Can have multiple ossification centers that may lead to a bipartite sesamoid, which can be difficult to distinguish from an acute fracture (1)
- Vitally important in the biomechanics of the foot
  - When the 1st MTP joint dorsiflexes, the sesamoids are pulled distally, covering and protecting the plantar surface of the 1st metatarsal head and absorbing up to 3 times body weight during normal gait.
  - Flexor hallucis brevis provides the active plantarflexion force at the 1st MTP joint, and the sesamoid complex provides an increased mechanical advantage in plantarflexion.

DESCRIPTION

- Stress fractures:
  - Most common sesamoid pathology (1)
  - More common in athletes than in general population (2)
- Sesamoiditis:
  - General term that encompasses multiple conditions including osteonecrosis, chondromalacia, or inflammatory changes (1)
  - Usually involves the medial (tibial) sesamoid (1)
- Acute fracture:
  - Typically caused by forced dorsiflexion (1)
  - Often, a transverse fracture line is seen on imaging with sharp edges (3).

EPIDEMIOLOGY

- Sesamoiditis is seen more commonly in young, active adults.
- Stress fractures are more common in athletes.
- The sesamoid complex is involved in 9% of foot and ankle injuries and 1.2% of running injuries (1),(4).

RISK FACTORS

- Repetitive, forceful dorsiflexion, or loading (pushing off) of the MTP joint
- At-risk sports include dancing (especially ballet), running, gymnastics, volleyball, basketball, high-impact aerobics, football, and soccer (1),(5).
- Asymmetrical sesamoids
- Overpronation (3)
- Playing on artificial turf (1)
- Wearing shoes without adequate forefoot support (i.e., high heels)

GENERAL PREVENTION

- Wearing shoes with adequate forefoot support
- Use of orthotics to offload the 1st MTP joint
- An aperture (donut) padding can also off-load the sesamoids in at-risk athletes.

DIAGNOSIS

HISTORY

- Gradual onset of pain on the plantar surface of the 1st hallux
- Pain with dorsiflexion or weight-bearing (1)
- Pain with "pushing off" while walking or running
- Unilateral symptoms are typical.
- Pain typically is located at the medial sesamoid.
- Acute fracture usually occurs with a history of hyperextension injury of the big toe (1).

PHYSICAL EXAM

- Tenderness with direct palpation of the sesamoids ± swelling or ecchymosis
- Pain with resisted plantarflexion of the 1st hallux
- Pain with passive dorsiflexion of the 1st MTP
- Erythema or swelling may be present.
- Decreased range of motion at 1st MTP and/or decreased plantarflexion strength
- An enlarged bursa on the plantar surface may be present.
- Presence of significant pes cavus, pes planus, or cock-up deformity of the hallux

DIFFERENTIAL DIAGNOSIS

- Turf toe
- Flexor hallucis longus tendonitis
- Hallux rigidus
- Hallux valgus
- Neuroma
- Metatarsalgia
- Osteochondritis (more common in young women)
- Osteoarthritis or inflammatory arthritis
- Osteonecrosis
- Avascular necrosis of the sesamoids
- Neoplasm
- Nerve impingement (less common)
- Nonunion of a sesamoid fracture

DIAGNOSTIC TESTS & INTERPRETATION

- X-ray examination of the foot should include weight-bearing anteroposterior, lateral, medial and lateral oblique views. Comparison views of the contralateral foot may be helpful (2)[A].
- If possible, an axial view of the 1st MTP joint in dorsiflexion, known as the "sesamoid view" (2)[A]:
  - Bipartite sesamoids are more common in the tibial sesamoid, are bilateral in 85% of cases, and are present in 7.8–35.5% of the normal population.
  - An acutely fractured sesamoid is characterized by sharp, irregular edges, comminution, or widely spaced fragments in contrast to the sclerotic edges of a nonunion or the smooth edges of a bipartite sesamoid (1),(3).
  - Magnetic resonance imaging (MRI) or bone scan are helpful in differentiating sesamoid injuries from normal bipartite variant because they can detect soft tissue or bony edema before radiographically evident (1).
- Computed tomography (CT) or single-photon emission computed tomography (SPECT) are more specific for sesamoid fractures (3)[C].

TREATMENT

- Sesamoiditis or stress fracture/nonunion:
  - Initially, conservative therapy is recommended for at least 4 to 6 weeks (1)[A]:
    - Relative rest with immobilization by off-loading the 1st MTP complex with orthotics or rocker sole shoes (forefoot unloader shoe), a dancer's pad, or metatarsal bar; taping the great toe in plantarflexion may be considered for severe symptoms(5)[A],(6)[A].
    - Ice
    - Oral nonsteroidal anti-inflammatory drugs (NSAIDs) or other analgesics (6)[C]
    - Avoid offending movements such as the demi relevé position in dancing (6).
    - 86% of patients who underwent conservative therapy returned to sport on average at 13.9 weeks (6).
    - Rarely, injections with corticosteroids can be considered (6).
    - There is increasing evidence for use of platelet-rich plasma (PRP) and other orthobiologics (4).
  - Long-term treatment includes:
    - Correction of any mechanical abnormalities with the use of taping, orthotics, or a stiff-soled shoe to limit dorsiflexion of the 1st MTP joint
    - Eliminating or minimizing the stressing activity (1)[C]
    - Surgery, usually to excise the sesamoid, to treat prolonged symptoms despite several months of conservative management (see below)
- Acute fractures:
  - Non–weight-bearing immobilization with a short leg cast/ankle foot orthosis (AFO) for 6 to 8 weeks, followed by protected weight-bearing in cast/AFO for 4 to 6 additional weeks (2)[A],(5)[A]
  - Surgical options include internal fixation, percutaneous screw fixation, or sesamoidectomy (2)[A],(3)[A],(5)[A].

SURGERY/OTHER PROCEDURES

Surgical options are available for prolonged symptoms if nonoperative treatment fails, but mechanical defects can lead to long-term problems:

- Sesamoidectomy (surgical excision) (1),(5)[A]:
  - Most common procedure for sesamoid pathology
  - Can be partial or complete
  - Can result in overload of the metatarsal head or flexor hallucis longus tendon
  - Excision of both sesamoids generally is not recommended owing to development of cock-up deformity and biomechanical morbidity (1).
  - Sesamoidectomy resulted in fastest return to sport, but internal fixation resulted in best chance of returning to previous level of sport (5).
  - 80% of athletes had a mean return to play of 4.6 months postoperatively (6).
- Curettage and bone grafting (1)
- Shaving of the sesamoid (1)

ONGOING CARE

- Custom orthotics ± cutouts for the sesamoid bones (3)
- Short-leg walking cast can be considered for recalcitrant cases (1).
- Corticosteroid injection into the sesamoid area can be considered with caution.

FOLLOW-UP RECOMMENDATIONS

- Periodic follow-up every 4 to 8 weeks until the patient is asymptomatic
- Continued modification of activities and use of orthotics
- Referral to orthopedic surgeon or podiatrist if symptoms persist >6 months

PROGNOSIS

- Conservative management is generally successful in treating most sesamoid pathology.
- More severe cases that require surgical intervention are at risk for iatrogenic complications.

COMPLICATIONS

- Nonunion of fractures
- Development of stress fractures or avascular necrosis in untreated sesamoiditis

REFERENCES

1. Dedmond BT, Cory JW, McBryde A Jr. The hallucal sesamoid complex. *J Am Acad Orthop Surg.* 2006;14(13):745–753.
2. Mittlmeier T, Haar P. Sesamoid and toe fractures. *Injury.* 2004;35(Suppl 2):SB87–SB97.
3. Ribbans WJ, Hintermann B. Hallucal sesamoid fractures in athletes: diagnosis and treatment. *Sports Orthop Traumatol.* 2016;32(3):295–303.
4. Le HM, Stracciolini A, Stein CJ, et al. Platelet rich plasma for hallux sesamoid injuries: a case series. *Phys Sportsmed.* 2022;50(2):181–184.
5. Stein CJ, Sugimoto D, Slick NR, et al. Hallux sesamoid fractures in young athletes. *Phys Sportsmed.* 2019;47(4):441–447.
6. Ivanova V, Todd NW, Yurgelon J. Dance-related foot and ankle injuries and pathologies. *Clin Podiatr Med Surg.* 2023;40(1):193–207.

CLINICAL PEARLS

- Medial sesamoid is injured most commonly.
- Acute fractures are almost exclusively unilateral.
- Bilateral bipartite sesamoids are usually benign.
- Tenderness over the sesamoids or pain with dorsiflexion that improves with non–weight-bearing should arise suspicion for sesamoid pathology.
- Nonoperative treatment, especially immobilization, is the mainstay of therapy.
- Sesamoidectomy is the most common surgical procedure to treat chronic symptoms.

SEVER DISEASE/CALCANEAL APOPHYSITIS

Christopher Jordan, MD, ATC, CAQSM • Marcus Farrand, DO

BASICS

DESCRIPTION

- Sever disease, also known as *calcaneal apophysitis*, is an overuse syndrome and one of the most common causes of late childhood and adolescent heel pain.
- This traction apophysitis is the foot equivalent to Osgood-Schlatter disease.
- Synonym(s): calcaneal apophysitis

EPIDEMIOLOGY

Incidence

- Typically occurs during an adolescent growth spurt
- Most common activities are ones requiring repetitive running or jumping (track, basketball, soccer, gymnastics).
- Occurrence in general population: 3.7/1,000 individuals age 6 to 17 years old
- Predominant age: described most often between the ages of 9 and 12 years; most frequent at age 11 years in girls and at age 12 years in boys
- Predominant gender: male > female
- Occurs bilaterally in just over 60% of cases
- Makes up 2–16% of all youth musculoskeletal injuries (1)

ETIOLOGY AND PATHOPHYSIOLOGY

- The posterior calcaneus develops as a secondary ossification center.
- This secondary ossification center provides attachment for the Achilles tendon.
- During a growth spurt, bone growth greater than the ability of the muscle-tendon unit to sufficiently stretch creating increased tension
- The apophysitis is the weakest point of the chain.
- Repetitive stress results in microtrauma and chronic irritation leading to thickening and pain.
- Ongoing stress may lead to stress fracture of the body of the calcaneus.
- The calcaneal physis typically closes between the ages of 12 and 15 years.
- There are six stages of calcaneal ossification during peak height velocity—Sever typically occurs during stage 1, 2, or 3 (2).

RISK FACTORS

- Adolescent growth spurt
- Increased or excessive sport and play activity without period of rest
- Tight gastrocsoleus complex
- Weak ankle dorsiflexors
- Biomechanical factors such as genu varum and forefoot varus
- Poor-quality or worn-out athletic shoes
- Poorly cushioned or low-heeled shoes such as soccer, baseball, track, or cycling cleats
- Running on hard surfaces
- High-impact sports
- Obesity (3)

DIAGNOSIS

HISTORY

- An 8- to 13-year-old child presents with heel pain worsened with increased activity (2)[C],(3)[B]
- Sports requiring a lot of running and jumping activities are particularly prone to cause this overuse syndrome.
- Pain is typically unilateral but may be bilateral and is often relieved with rest (4)[C].
- May have significant impact on health-related quality of life (1),(4)[C]

PHYSICAL EXAM

- Signs and symptoms include:
  - Intermittent or continuous posterior heel pain (1)[C]
  - No swelling
  - No ecchymoses or skin changes
- Physical examination includes the following:
  - Pain with single-heel rise test (Sever sign) (3)[C]
  - Tenderness with medial and lateral compression of the calcaneus (heel squeeze test) (4)[C]
  - Tenderness at Achilles insertion on heel (4)[C]
  - Heel cord inflexibility with sometimes <10 degrees of dorsiflexion
  - Biomechanical contributors such as forefoot varus, hallux valgus, pes cavus, and pes planus (4)[C]

DIFFERENTIAL DIAGNOSIS

- Nerve entrapment (plantar)
- Neuroma (plantar)
- Plantar fasciitis (plantar)
- Heel pad syndrome (plantar)
- Calcaneal stress fracture (plantar)
- Peroneal tendinopathy (midfoot/lateral)
- Sinus tarsi syndrome (midfoot/lateral)
- Tarsal tunnel syndrome (midfoot/medial)
- Achilles tendinopathy (posterior)
- Haglund deformity (posterior)
- Osteomyelitis
- Retrocalcaneal bursitis

DIAGNOSTIC TESTS & INTERPRETATION

- Radiographs may show fragmentation, sclerosis, and increased density of the apophysis, but these radiographic changes can be normal (4)[C].
- Imaging is not necessary to make this clinical diagnosis but may be helpful to rule out other causes of heel pain (3)[B],(4)[C].
- Consider imaging when considering alternative diagnoses (3)[B].
- If radiograph demonstrates ossification at stage 4 or later, consider alternative diagnosis (2)[C].

TREATMENT

- Rest or reduce activity to a pain tolerance level (4)[C].
- Ice (4)[C]
- Nonsteroidal anti-inflammatory drugs (NSAIDs) for pain control (1),(2),(4)[C]
- Taping may provide immediate pain relief (3)[B].
- Heel lifts (1)[C]
- Shock-absorbing heel inserts (1)[C]
- Custom orthosis (5)[C]
- Gastrocsoleus stretching exercises: knee straight and knee flexed stretch with the heel maintained on the floor or ground (4)[C]
- Eccentric calf strengthening exercises (4)[C]
- If not responsive to conservative treatment, then a short leg cast or boot walker or even immobilization may be necessary (4)[C].

ADDITIONAL THERAPIES

- Strengthening of the quadriceps and gastrocsoleus to better equip these muscle groups to act as shock absorbers (4)[C]
- Strengthening of the foot dorsiflexors
- Good-quality shoe with adequate shock absorption and firm heel counter (4)[C]
- The use of heel raises over prefabricated orthoses may have a relative advantage in the first 2 months of treatment, but there is no difference in pain or impact at 12 months (5)[C].
- Custom orthosis may demonstrate greater improvement than heel lifts (5)[C].
- Off-the-shelf orthoses are much more cost-effective and can be tried first before custom orthoses are considered. Time to symptom resolution varies, but symptoms abate totally with skeletal maturity (2)[C].
- No reports of long-term sequelae from Sever disease (4)[C]

SURGERY/OTHER PROCEDURES

Not indicated

ONGOING CARE

FOLLOW-UP RECOMMENDATIONS

Referral/disposition necessary only when clinician is uncertain of diagnosis.

COMPLICATIONS

Persistent pain that does not respond to conservative measures may indicate there is a calcaneal stress fracture.

REFERENCES

1. Sweeney EA, Little CC, Wilson JC, et al. Comparison of braces for treatment of Sever's disease (Calcaneal Apophysitis) in barefoot athletes: a randomized clinical trial. *J Athl Train*. 2023;58(5):437–444.
2. Duong MM, Nicholson AD, Li SQ, et al. Relationship between Sever disease and skeletal maturity. *J Pediatr Orthop*. 2020;40(2):93–96.
3. Fares MY, Salhab HA, Khachfe HH, et al. Sever's disease of the pediatric population: clinical, pathologic, and therapeutic considerations. *Clin Med Res*. 2021;19(3):132–137.
4. Belikan P, Färber LC, Abel F, et al. Incidence of calcaneal apophysitis (Sever's disease) and return-to-play in adolescent athletes of a German youth soccer academy: a retrospective study of 10 years. *J Orthop Surg Res*. 2022;17(1):83.
5. Alfaro-Santafé J, Gómez-Bernal A, Lanuza-Cerzócimo C, et al. Effectiveness of custom-made foot orthoses vs. heel-lifts in children with calcaneal apophysitis (Sever's disease): a CONSORT-compliant randomized trial. *Children (Basel)*. 2021;8(11):963.

ADDITIONAL READING

- Hendrix CL. Calcaneal apophysitis (Sever disease). *Clin Podiatr Med Surg*. 2005;22(1):55–62.
- Tu P. Heel pain: diagnosis and management. *Am Fam Physician*. 2018;97(2):86–93.

CLINICAL PEARLS

- Conservative therapy remains the mainstay of treatment.
- Diagnosis should be made clinically without radiography unless signs and symptoms are atypical.
- Total rest may hasten the recovery from this heel pain but may not be necessary.
- Reducing the amount of activity may allow sports participation without worsening the heel pain and increase patient buy-in.
- Current evidence does not suggest any long-term sequelae.

SHOULDER ADHESIVE CAPSULITIS

Lyndsey N. Booker, MD, CAQSM • Amanda T. Wise, DO, CAQSM

BASICS

DESCRIPTION

- Commonly known as "frozen shoulder"
- Progressively painful loss of both passive and active glenohumeral joint range of motion (ROM) with arm dysfunction
- Adhesive capsulitis (AC) is classified into two categories:
  - Primary: idiopathic without a preceding event
  - Secondary: due to trauma, intrinsic shoulder disease such as rotator cuff tendinopathy, prolonged immobilization, or underlying systemic illness (e.g., diabetes mellitus, thyroid disease, autoimmune conditions)

EPIDEMIOLOGY

- 2–5% of the general population
- Slight predominance in females, 1.4:1
- Mean age of onset is ~56.4 ± 13.1 years (1).
- 15% experience bilateral disease.
- 13.4% of patients with diabetes mellitus develop AC.
- 30% of patients with AC have diabetes mellitus (2),(3).

ETIOLOGY AND PATHOPHYSIOLOGY

- Exact pathophysiology of AC is poorly understood.
- Current evidence suggests immunologic and inflammatory etiology leading to thickening of the coracohumeral ligament, fibrosis, and contraction of the glenohumeral joint capsule.
- Inflammation, fibrosis, contracture, and hypervascularity leads to pain, restricted ROM, and disability (2)
- Rarely, also arises from clinically significant trauma to shoulder, cervical radiculopathy, brachial plexus pathology, or rotator cuff tendonitis
- Autoimmune theory of disease: Microvascular disease causes abnormal collagen repair, leading to capsular fibrosis.
- Diabetes theory of disease: High serum glucose increases collagen glycosylation of joint capsule tissue leading to inflammation → fibrosis → contracture. Current evidence suggests a dose dependence with cumulative HbA1C > 7.0 over time increasing risk of AC by 2.77% (4).

RISK FACTORS

- Shoulder immobilization—increases risk by 5 to 9 times over the general population (2)
- Class 1 obesity (body mass index [BMI] 30 to 34.9 kg/m^2) (1)
- Diabetes mellitus—5 times more likely to develop AC (2)
- Thyroid disease—particularly hypothyroidism or subclinical hypothyroidism, and not hyperthyroidism (2),(3)
- Stroke
- Female sex
- Hispanic/Latino (odds ratio [OR] 4.85) and African American (OR 1.71) (1)
- Parkinson disease in the elderly

GENERAL PREVENTION

Avoidance of prolonged shoulder immobilization or severe restriction of movement

DIAGNOSIS

HISTORY

- Insidious onset of pain over several weeks to months
- Pain is worse with any shoulder movement, both active and passive.
- Pain is worse at night and may interfere with sleep.
- Pain usually is not only present in the region of the deltoid but also may radiate into the upper or arm and neck.
- Common functional impairments include difficulty bathing, dressing, combing one's hair, and reaching into one's back pocket.
- A careful medical history to exclude associated conditions should be conducted.
- Four clinical phases (2),(3):
  - Phase 1: pre-adhesive phase—insidious onset of nocturnal pain, progresses to pain at rest, ROM is preserved
  - Phase 2: freezing phase—progressive limitation of ROM in all directions
  - Phase 3: frozen phase—stiffness is present, although pain may be improved.
  - Phase 4: thawing phase—ROM gradually improving, although stiffness may persist; pain is typically resolved.
  - The time course of each phase varies, but each may last several months.
  - Total duration of symptoms ranges from 15 to 30 months.

PHYSICAL EXAM

- The hallmark of AC is decreased glenohumeral ROM (both active and passive) that is associated with pain.
- Observation may reveal limited use of the limb and lack of arm swing with walking.
- Often occurs in nondominant arm first
- Pain at end ROM may be the only finding in the early phase with the greatest limitation commonly being seen in external rotation (2).
- In later stages, all ROM usually are limited.
- Focal tenderness is not common, but vague pain of the anterior and posterior shoulder may be present.
- Impingement (Neer, Hawkins) and biceps tendinopathy (Speed) maneuvers may be positive.
- Shoulder girdle muscle atrophy is possible later in the process due to disuse.

DIFFERENTIAL DIAGNOSIS

- Rotator cuff tendinopathy
- Subacromial-subdeltoid bursitis
- Biceps tendinopathy
- Osteoarthritis of the glenohumeral joint
- Cervical radiculopathy
- Autoimmune disease
- Infection
- Fracture of the humerus or glenoid
- Calcific tendonitis
- Thoracic outlet syndrome (TOS)
- Neoplasm

DIAGNOSTIC TESTS & INTERPRETATION

- Radiographs are useful to assess the presence of osteoarthritis, calcific tendonitis, or other diagnoses but are often normal in appearance.
- Magnetic resonance imaging (MRI) is not required for diagnosis but can support the clinical exam and investigate for other diagnoses.
- Ultrasound findings (i.e., coracohumeral ligament and axillary pouch thickening) have been shown to be as reliable as MRI for diagnosis.

TREATMENT

- Treatment should be focused on relief of symptoms and optimization of ROM (2)[C],(3)[C].
- Topical and potentially a short course of oral non-steroidal anti-inflammatory drugs (NSAIDs) can be used, if tolerated, to aid with pain control in the initial phase (2)[C],(3)[C].
- Oral steroids also can provide short-term benefit in pain relief and improved ROM and function; however, oral steroids are not clinically indicated because they have side effects (3)[C].
- Hydrodilatation with corticosteroid can reduce pain and improve ROM and function in the short term (3)[C],(5)[A],(6)[A].
- A program of therapeutic exercise comprising gentle ROM exercises, stretching, and graded resistance training has been associated with increased ROM and decreased pain. The program should be guided by the patient within the limits of his or her pain, and vigorous programs that increase symptoms should be avoided (5)[A].
- Dynamic splinting (e.g., using a continuous passive motion device or specialized adjustable splints) may be considered as an adjunct, particularly in the later stages of AC or postoperatively, to facilitate gradual and sustained increases in ROM. These devices apply a constant, gentle stretch to the joint, helping to lengthen tightened soft tissues and improve flexibility over time without constant therapist presence.
- Manipulation under anesthesia (MUA) and arthroscopic capsular release are considered if symptoms persist despite nonoperative treatment. >80% of nondiabetic patients have successful outcomes with arthroscopic capsular release (2)[C].
- Diabetic patients may have an increased risk of recurrent pain, decreased ROM, and a need for revision surgery (2)[C].

REFERENCES

1. Kingston K, Curry EJ, Galvin JW, et al. Shoulder adhesive capsulitis: epidemiology and predictors of surgery. *J Shoulder Elbow Surg*. 2018;27(8):1437–1443.
2. Leafblad N, Mizels J, Tashjian R, et al. Adhesive capsulitis. *Phys Med Rehabil Clin N Am*. 2023;34(2):453–468.
3. Ramirez J. Adhesive capsulitis: diagnosis and management. *Am Fam Physician*. 2019;99(5):297–300.
4. Chan JH, Ho BS, Alvi HM, et al. The relationship between the incidence of adhesive capsulitis and hemoglobin A1c. *J Shoulder Elbow Surg*. 2017;26(10):1834–1837.
5. Challoumas D, Biddle M, McLean M, et al. Comparison of treatments for frozen shoulder: a systematic review and meta-analysis. *JAMA Netw Open*. 2020;3(12):e2029581.
6. Catapano M, Mittal N, Adamich J, et al. Hydrodilatation with corticosteroid for the treatment of adhesive capsulitis: a systematic review. *PM R*. 2018;10(6):623–635.

ADDITIONAL READING

- Al Khayyat SG, Falsetti P, Conticini E, et al. Adhesive capsulitis and ultrasound diagnosis, an inseparable pair: a novel review. *J Ultrasound*. 2023;26(2):369–384.
- Latzka E, Cali M, Ishii H, et al. Hydrodilatation versus corticosteroid injection in treatment for adhesive capsulitis. *PM R*. 2023;15(12):1580–1587.

CLINICAL PEARLS

- Frozen shoulder typically presents with insidious shoulder stiffness and decreased active and passive ROM of the shoulder, often starting with limited external rotation.
- Shoulder X-ray, ultrasound, and MRI can help distinguish between AC and shoulder osteoarthritis, as they present similarly with both pain and loss of active and passive ROM.
- Prolonged shoulder immobilization, thyroid disease, and diabetes are risk factors for developing AC.
- The four clinical phases include the pre-adhesive phase, freezing phase, frozen phase, and thawing phase.
- There are high rates of spontaneous recovery after 15 to 30 months.
- Conservative treatment options include a home exercise program and physical therapy but may also include NSAIDs and intra-articular corticosteroids, with or without hydrodilatation.

SHOULDER INSTABILITY, ANTERIOR

Kristy Smith, MD ▪ Sravya Kamarajugadda, BS

BASICS

DESCRIPTION

- A symptomatic anteroinferior subluxation or dislocation of the glenohumeral (GH) joint
- Synonym(s): GH dislocation; GH subluxation; dead-arm syndrome

EPIDEMIOLOGY

- One of the most commonly dislocated joints in the body due to its significant mobility. In a study of 8,056 dislocations, 45% involved the GH joint.
- Anterior traumatic dislocation accounts for 96% of all GH dislocations.

ALERT

Recurrence rate for athletes aged <25 years is >85% in those who have suffered an initial traumatic event.

RISK FACTORS

- History of previous dislocation
- Younger patients
- Athletes participating in repetitive overhead sports (i.e., throwing/volleyball) or contact sports (i.e., football, wrestling, ice hockey)

DIAGNOSIS

HISTORY

- Patients usually describe a history of prior dislocation/subluxation event(s). The symptoms will be reported to occur when the arm is placed in the provocative position of abduction and external rotation.
- Patients also may complain of a "dead arm," which typically occurs with subluxation.

PHYSICAL EXAM

- Patients note the feeling of impending dislocation with the arm in a provocative position. Pain itself is generally not a sign of pure instability.
- A thorough exam of the cervical spine, proximal humerus, and scapula should be performed when evaluating anyone with shoulder pain. If multidirectional instability is suspected, an assessment of ligamentous laxity should be addressed. A complete neurologic exam should be performed to identify any central or peripheral neuropathy.
- Apprehension test: Arm is placed at 90 degrees of abduction and gently externally rotated. A sense of "impending" dislocation is regarded as a positive test.
- Relocation test: During the apprehension test, a posteriorly directed force is applied to the proximal humerus with the scapula stabilized by the examiner's opposite hand. If symptoms abate, the test result is positive.
- Load and shift test: The patient is seated while the examiner stabilizes the scapula with one hand and with the thumb and forefinger of the free hand on the proximal humerus attempts to sublux the head anteriorly and posteriorly. In general, this test works better with thinner patients and requires a fair amount of patient relaxation.

DIFFERENTIAL DIAGNOSIS

- Diagnoses that can mimic anterior instability include multidirectional instability, acromioclavicular instability, superior labrum anterior and posterior (SLAP) lesions, biceps tendon subluxation, and subscapularis tear.
- One should always rule out referred pain from the cervical spine.

DIAGNOSTIC TESTS & INTERPRETATION

- Imaging studies should include orthogonal views to evaluate for associated bony injuries and to ensure that the humeral head is located within glenoid.
- Radiography: The initial series includes an anteroposterior (AP), true shoulder AP, axillary lateral, and scapular Y. Additional views, if necessary, may include the West Point view (good for identifying a bony Bankart/anteroinferior glenoid rim fracture) and Stryker notch view (good for identifying a Hill-Sachs lesion/posterolateral humeral head compression fracture).
- Velpeau view if initial radiographs are inconclusive, or patient is unable to be appropriately positioned for axillary radiograph (if required to stay in sling).
- Postreduction views are necessary for the acute treatment of shoulder dislocation to ensure relocation and assess for possibility of a fracture.
- Magnetic resonance imaging (MRI) can identify rotator cuff tears, biceps abnormalities, and occasionally lesions associated with humeral avulsion of the GH ligament. Because of the normal variation of the labrum and GH ligaments, most studies overestimate the frequency of labral tears. Use of arthrogram with MRI increases sensitivity and specificity in evaluation of labral tears.

TREATMENT

GENERAL MEASURES

- Nonoperative management in young, active patients is associated with a high incidence of recurrent instability but can be considered in older/low-demand patients or in-season athletes waiting for surgical evaluation after completion of their season. Motion control braces can limit abduction and external rotation and decrease the position of vulnerability for instability events (1)[C],(2)[C],(3)[C].
- Early treatment consists of brief immobilization, followed by early protected range of motion (ROM) and strengthening. The anterior capsular structures must be protected throughout rehabilitation, and therefore, all stressors to the anterior structures should be limited.
- Rotator cuff strengthening: Initial strengthening should begin in the plane of the scapula. Internal and limited-range external rotation exercises can start with light free weights or resistance bands.
- Scapular stabilization: Exercises include rowing, modified push-ups with maximal protraction, scaption (elevation of the humerus in external rotation in the scapular plane), modified flies, and press-ups (later stage).

SURGERY/OTHER PROCEDURES

- Indications for surgery: rotator cuff tear >50%, Hill-Sachs lesion >25%, glenoid defect >20%, failure to return to activities after nonoperative therapy (2)[C],(3)[C]
- Relative indications for surgery: first-time dislocations in young (<30 years) athletes or laborers, >2 dislocations in one season, participation in overhead or contact sports, bony Bankart lesion, significant glenoid bone loss (2)[C],(3)[C]
- Surgical techniques for the management of anterior shoulder instability are evolving. Both soft tissue (arthroscopic or open Bankart repair) and bone augmentation (Latarjet) procedures exist. Multiple factors will be considered when deciding on which surgical procedure to perform: possible pathology of labrum or rotator cuff, extent of bony Bankart of the glenoid or Hill-Sachs injury of the humeral head, and desired postsurgical activities (1)[C],(2)[C],(3)[C].
- Decreasing risk of recurrent instability while maximizing ROM is the ultimate goal of surgical stabilization (1)[C],(2)[C],(3)[C].

ONGOING CARE

FOLLOW-UP RECOMMENDATIONS

- Any patient with recurrent anterior dislocations or a young, athletic, first-time dislocator should discuss surgical options with a qualified sports medicine physician.
- Any patient failing nonoperative modalities also should be referred for surgical evaluation.

REFERENCES

1. Carpinteiro EP, Barros AA. Natural history of anterior shoulder instability. *Open Orthop J*. 2017;11:909–918.
2. Elsenbeck MJ, Dickens JF. Return to sports after shoulder stabilization surgery for anterior shoulder instability. *Curr Rev Musculoskelet Med*. 2017;10(4):491–498.
3. Pickett A, Svoboda S. Anterior glenohumeral instability. *Sports Med Arthrosc Rev*. 2017;25(3):156–162.

ADDITIONAL READING

- Bankart AS. Recurrent or habitual dislocation of the shoulder-joint. *Br Med J*. 1923;2(3285):1132–1133.
- Bedi A, Ryu RK. The treatment of primary anterior shoulder dislocations. *Instr Course Lect*. 2009;58:293–304.
- Cave EF, Burke JF, Boyd RJ. *Trauma Management*. Year Book Medical; 1974.
- Iannotti JP, Williams GR. *Disorders of the Shoulder: Diagnosis and Management*. Lippincott Williams & Wilkins; 1999.
- Jobe FW, Pink MM. *Operative Techniques in Upper Extremity Sports Injury*. Mosby; 1996.
- Kazár B, Relovszky E. Prognosis of primary dislocation of the shoulder. *Acta Orthop Scand*. 1969;40(2):216–224.
- Ludewig PM, Reynolds JF. The association of scapular kinematics and glenohumeral joint pathologies. *J Orthop Sports Phys Ther*. 2009;39(2):90–104.
- Neviaser RJ, Neviaser TJ, Neviaser JS. Anterior dislocation of the shoulder and rotator cuff rupture. *Clin Orthop Relat Res*. 1993;(291):103–106.
- Ochoa E Jr, Burkhart SS. Glenohumeral bone defects in the treatment of anterior shoulder instability. *Instr Course Lect*. 2009;58:323–336.
- Rowe CR, Patel D, Southmayd WW. The Bankart procedure: a long-term end-result study. *J Bone Joint Surg Am*. 1978;60(1):1–16.

CLINICAL PEARLS

- Young athletes, particularly those participating in overhead or contact sports, continue to be at increased risk of anterior shoulder instability.
- Recurrent instability is common after the initial episode.
- Primary surgical stabilization should be considered after the first dislocation in the young athlete in a high-risk activity/sport.

S

SHOULDER INSTABILITY, MULTIDIRECTIONAL

Kevin C. Jillson, MD, CAQSM • Hans A. Erickson, MD

BASICS

DESCRIPTION

- Multidirectional instability (MDI) is a symptomatic increase in glenohumeral translation in more than one direction (inferior, anterior, or posterior; rarely superior) causing either subluxation or dislocation.
- The extent of laxity is not always correlated with the degree of symptoms. Some individuals may be symptomatic with minimal millimeters of laxity, whereas others may have minimal symptoms with significant (3+) laxity.

EPIDEMIOLOGY

- MDI is more common than previously realized but still represents <5% of all shoulder instability.
- Most patients are in their 3rd decade of life but range in age from teenagers to middle age.

ETIOLOGY AND PATHOPHYSIOLOGY

Etiology is likely multifactorial. MDI may occur as a result of repetitive microtrauma, acute injury, or underlying connective tissue disorder and often involves anatomic, biochemical, and neuromuscular abnormalities:

- Anatomic:
  - Often associated with a large, patulous inferior pouch and wide rotator interval
  - Pathologic changes in labral height and Bankart lesions have also been observed in patients with MDI (1).
- Biochemical:
  - Patients with MDI have been shown to have alterations in the type and quantity of collagen, specifically types III and IV collagen, as seen in Ehlers-Danlos syndrome (1).
- Neuromuscular:
  - Loss of strength or neuromotor coordination of the rotator cuff and scapular stabilizers may also contribute to MDI.
  - Impaired proprioception has also been seen in MDI; however, further investigation is needed to determine whether impaired proprioception is a cause or effect of shoulder instability.

RISK FACTORS

- Repetitive microtrauma (especially overhead motion): butterfly and backstroke swimmers, gymnasts, baseball pitchers, weightlifters, and racquet sports
- Generalized ligamentous hyperlaxity (e.g., connective tissue disorders)

DIAGNOSIS

HISTORY

- MDI is often associated with recurrent or "low-energy" trauma.
- Most common complaint is vague pain radiating to the deltoid insertion, initially occurring after activity and progressing to pain at rest; may also be associated with pain at night
- Transient neurologic symptoms, such as numbness ("dead arm") or tingling may also occur following subluxation, usually affecting ulnar > median nerve distribution.
- 30–70% of patients with MDI have symptoms in the opposite shoulder.
- Previously unsuccessful shoulder reconstruction for presumed unidirectional instability may indicate MDI.
- Inferior instability: pain, numbness, tingling while carrying a briefcase or heavy suitcase; this is caused by traction on the brachial plexus.
- Posterior instability: pain while arm in forward-flexed, internally rotated position (e.g., pushing open a heavy door, performing push-ups or bench press, blocking in football, or during pull-through phase of rowing stroke)
- Anterior instability: pain with arm in overhead, abducted, externally rotated position (e.g., during windup or early acceleration of a throw)

PHYSICAL EXAM

- General ligamentous laxity is often present (e.g., thumb to forearm, elbow hyperextension, metacarpophalangeal joint hyperextension, genu recurvatum, patellofemoral subluxation).
- Sulcus test involves inferior traction on the arm while at the side. Inferior translation of at least 1 to 2 cm causing concavity of skin inferior to acromion (positive sulcus sign) indicates inferior instability.
- Anterior and posterior load and shift test and/or drawer test usually result in anterior and posterior displacement (graded trace to III). Always remember to stabilize the scapula with one hand while the patient remains in either a seated or supine position.
- Apprehension test involves placing the shoulder in the position of instability (throwing position: abduction and external rotation for anterior instability; adduction, flexion, and internal rotation for posterior instability). A positive test is seen when the patient senses pending subluxation or has involuntary guarding. It is apprehension, not pain, which is most reliable in confirming shoulder instability.
- Relocation test involves relief of apprehension and symptoms when applying a stabilizing counterforce (posterior force on humeral head for anterior instability; anterior force on humeral head for posterior instability) to the arm in the provocative position with the scapula stabilized.
- Cervical range of motion, upper extremity strength, sensory function (including axillary nerve), and reflexes should also be evaluated.
- Muscle guarding may make the examination difficult, repeat exams may be necessary for confirmation of diagnosis.

DIFFERENTIAL DIAGNOSIS

- Unilateral instability (anterior, posterior, inferior)
- Acute dislocation or subluxation
- Voluntary dislocator
- Primary impingement
- Rotator cuff tear
- Thoracic outlet syndrome
- Cervical disc disease
- Brachial plexitis
- Connective tissue disorder (i.e., Ehlers-Danlos syndrome)

DIAGNOSTIC TESTS & INTERPRETATION

- MDI is a clinical diagnosis based on the history and physical exam.
- Orthogonal plain radiographs should be obtained to evaluate for bony defects such as Bankart and Hill-Sachs lesions as well as glenoid dysplasia.
- Specialty views include Stryker notch and West Point view.
- Magnetic resonance imaging (MRI) is often performed to rule out underlying ligamentous, capsule, or labral pathology. Magnetic resonance (MR) arthrogram may also be used to evaluate for capsular redundancy.

TREATMENT

GENERAL MEASURES

- Analgesia: Nonsteroidal anti-inflammatory drugs (NSAIDs) can decrease pain acutely, but long-term analgesic usage is typically not necessary.
- Reduction: often reduce spontaneously or self-reduce
- Immobilization:
  - May consider short-term sling for up to 3 weeks in younger patients (<30 years of age) with an acute, initial dislocation
  - Immobilization for recurrent dislocators is of less value.
  - Use caution in immobilizing older patients who are more likely to develop adhesive capsulitis.

ADDITIONAL THERAPIES

- First-line treatment is a prolonged course of physical therapy/independent exercise program (at least 6 months) focused on strengthening anterior deltoid, rotator cuff muscles, and scapular stabilizers while improving proprioceptive control (2)[B].
- Watson program is a six-stage rehabilitation program lasting 3 to 6 months; targets scapula and humeral head biomechanics prior to progressing to range of motion and functional, sports-specific exercises (3),(4)[B]
- It is important to continue a maintenance exercise program indefinitely.
- If patient is pain free with normal strength after 6 months, prior activity may be resumed.
- May need to adjust prior activity (i.e., a butterfly stroke swimmer may need to choose a different stroke, or a pitcher may need to change his or her delivery or position)

SURGERY/OTHER PROCEDURES

- Surgery is indicated only for symptomatic, painful shoulders after the patient fails aggressive, prolonged physical therapy (usually minimum 6 months) (5)[C].
- MDI is managed differently than unilateral anterior shoulder dislocation, as the etiology is often multifactorial and may be related to an underlying connective tissue disorder.
- ~10–13% of patients require bilateral surgical repair.
- Laxity alone is not a typical indication for surgery.
- Surgical techniques include open capsular shift (first described "Dr. CS Neer in 1974"), although arthroscopic repair is now considered more common.
- Studies have shown that arthroscopic plication with suture anchors results in relatively good functional outcomes (around 8–31% of patients report postoperative instability) (6)[B].
- Thermal capsulorrhaphy (capsular shrinkage through laser or radiofrequency energy) was previously used; however, this technique is no longer recommended due to a high failure rate and complications such as glenohumeral chondrolysis and axillary nerve injury (5).
- Note: Probably the earliest "sports surgery" was thermal capsulorrhaphy for anterior instability in ancient Egypt, where warriors with instability were treated with a hot poker to thermally shrink anterior structures to try to allow them to throw a spear.

ONGOING CARE

FOLLOW-UP RECOMMENDATIONS

- Most patients with MDI should be referred for physical therapy. Patients who fail physical therapy can be referred to an orthopedist for consideration of surgical treatment.
- Resumption of full sports is generally 6 months. If surgery is required, then postoperative immobilization with a sling is typically for 3 to 6 weeks, with early supervised range of motion exercises. Light sports and throwing can start at ~4 months postoperatively if strength is at least 90% and full range of motion is achieved.

REFERENCES

1. Bahu MJ, Trentacosta N, Vorys GC, et al. Multidirectional instability: evaluation and treatment options. *Clin Sports Med*. 2008;27(4):671–689.
2. Stokes DJ, McCarthy TP, Frank RM. Physical therapy for the treatment of shoulder instability. *Phys Med Rehabil Clin N Am*. 2023;34(2):393–408.
3. Watson L, Warby S, Balster S, et al. The treatment of multidirectional instability of the shoulder with a rehabilitation program: part 1. *Shoulder Elbow*. 2016;8(4):271–278.
4. Watson L, Warby S, Balster S, et al. The treatment of multidirectional instability of the shoulder with a rehabilitation program: part 2. *Shoulder Elbow*. 2017;9(1):46–53.
5. Hippensteel KJ, Uppstrom TJ, Rodeo SA, et al. Comprehensive review of multidirectional instability of the shoulder. *J Am Acad Orthop Surg*. 2023;31(16):871–880.
6. Mitchell BC, Siow MY, Carroll AN, et al. Clinical outcomes, survivorship, and return to sport after arthroscopic capsular repair with suture anchors for adolescent multidirectional shoulder instability: results at 6-year follow-up. *Orthop J Sports Med*. 2021;9(2):2325967121993879.

ADDITIONAL READING

- Caprise PA Jr, Sekiya JK. Open and arthroscopic treatment of multidirectional instability of the shoulder. *Arthroscopy*. 2006;22(10):1126–1131.
- Foster CR. Multidirectional instability of the shoulder in the athlete. *Clin Sports Med*. 1983;2(2):355–368.
- Neer CS II, Foster CR. Inferior capsular shift for involuntary inferior and multidirectional instability of the shoulder. A preliminary report. *J Bone Joint Surg Am*. 1980;62(6):897–908.
- Schenk TJ, Brems JJ. Multidirectional instability of the shoulder: pathophysiology, diagnosis, and management. *J Am Acad Orthop Surg*. 1998;6(1):65–72.

CLINICAL PEARLS

- MDI is symptomatic laxity of the shoulder in more than one direction (often including inferior).
- Diagnosis is clinical; imaging is not required although x-rays and MRI are often performed to evaluate for underlying pathology.
- First-line treatment is prolonged course of physical therapy with emphasis on glenohumeral and scapula positioning, strength, and proprioceptive control.
- Surgery is indicated only for symptomatic, painful shoulders after the patient fails aggressive, prolonged physical therapy (usually minimum 6 months).

SINDING-LARSEN-JOHANSSON SYNDROME (PATELLAR APOPHYSITIS)

Ian D. McKeag, MD, MS, CAQSM

BASICS

DESCRIPTION

- Sinding-Larsen-Johansson (SLJ) syndrome is a condition considered to be a chronic overuse injury caused by excessive and repetitive traction applied to the patella by the patellar tendon (i.e., jumping). Forces exerted gradually avulse the inferior pole of the patella at the apophysis:
  - Pain and swelling at the lower pole of the patella
  - Ossicle formation or fragmentation of inferior patellar pole on radiographs
- System: musculoskeletal
- Synonym: patellar apophysitis

EPIDEMIOLOGY

Incidence

Child and adolescent boys and girls with increased rate with those participating in organized sports

Prevalence

- A relatively common cause of anterior knee pain in adolescents
- Typically unilateral
- Cause of nearly 10% of all anterior knee pain in high school–aged females; only 3% in middle school

ETIOLOGY AND PATHOPHYSIOLOGY

- Traction apophysitis with reactive calcification of the partially avulsed proximal patellar tendon
- Noninflammatory traction injury due to repetitive microtrauma (1)[C]
- 4-fold increased risk in athletes with early sports specialization (2)[B]

Genetics

None

RISK FACTORS

- Early sports specialization (2)[B].
- Participation in running, jumping, and kneeling sports
- Shortened/tight hamstring tendons; increased posterior tibial slope (3)[C]

GENERAL PREVENTION

- Avoid sports specialization (2)[B].
- Avoid high intensity and repetitive quadriceps loading.
- Preseason muscular and flexibility training to help avoid sudden increases in training load

COMMONLY ASSOCIATED CONDITIONS

- Osgood-Schlatter disease and other overuse injuries (4)[B]
- Spastic lower extremities (cerebral palsy)

DIAGNOSIS

HISTORY

- Gradual and progressive anterior knee pain at the inferior pole of the patella
- Pain exacerbated with kneeling and exercise, especially with jumping activities

PHYSICAL EXAM

- Tenderness to palpation at the inferior pole of the patella
- Swelling at inferior patellar pole and the absence of a knee effusion
- Worsening pain with knee loading and/or prolonged knee flexion of the effected knee
- Erythema may be present at inferior patellar pole.
- Functional testing: Single-leg squat and knee extension against resistance may reproduce pain.

DIFFERENTIAL DIAGNOSIS

- Patellofemoral pain syndrome
- Patellar tendinitis/tendinosis
- Chondromalacia patellae
- Patellar sleeve fracture
- Osgood-Schlatter disease
- Infrapatellar bursitis
- Superficial patellar bursitis
- Osteochondroma
- Tibial fracture
- Patellar tendon lipoma

DIAGNOSTIC TESTS & INTERPRETATION

Initial Tests (lab, imaging)

- Diagnosis can be made clinically and imaging is not always necessary.
- Plain radiographs: widening, fragmentation, and/or irregular calcification of the ossification centers of the inferior pole of the patella (1)[C]
- Ultrasound: fragmentation of the inferior patellar pole, insertional patellar tendon thickening, and infrapatellar bursitis
- Magnetic resonance imaging (MRI): can be useful in severe cases to rule out more sinister etiologies (e.g., patellar sleeve avulsion) (5)[C]

Follow-Up Tests & Special Considerations

- Ultrasound can be considered for monitoring.
- Follow-up x-rays are typically unnecessary.

TREATMENT

GENERAL MEASURES

- Nearly all cases can be treated with nonoperative management and rest (1)[C].
- Avoidance of aggravating activities, such as running, kneeling, squatting, jumping, and stair climbing

MEDICATION

First Line

- Relative rest and activity modification
- Compressive knee sleeve or patellar counterforce strap
- Stretches (hamstring, quadriceps, heel cord) (3)[C]
- Ice
- Nonsteroidal anti-inflammatory drugs (NSAIDs)

ISSUES FOR REFERRAL

- Chronic pain
- Acute muscle weakness or atrophy
- Acute knee pain with inability to extend knee

ADDITIONAL THERAPIES

- Physical therapy for core strengthening, specifically with the quadriceps and hip flexors
- Cross training

SURGERY/OTHER PROCEDURES

- For chronic pain and recurrence despite nonoperative measures, surgical intervention can be considered (6)[C].
- Necrotic area may be present in portion of patellar tendon, in which excision has been reported to be clinically successful in treatment (6)[C].

COMPLEMENTARY & ALTERNATIVE MEDICINE

- Very brief knee immobilization for the most severe cases (rare)
- Patellar banding with activity

ADMISSION, INPATIENT, AND NURSING CONSIDERATIONS

No urgent admission and inpatient treatment is needed for this condition.

ONGOING CARE

FOLLOW-UP RECOMMENDATIONS

- Continue with core strengthening exercises.
- Proper quadriceps and hamstring stretching and warm up prior to activity or competition

Patient Monitoring

Monitor for any recurrent signs of anterior knee pain after resuming activity.

PATIENT EDUCATION

Sports specialization in one sport has been found to be associated with increased risk of developing this condition, especially in adolescent females, compared to multisport athletes.

PROGNOSIS

- Resolution typically occurs within 12 to 24 months from treatment onset (1)[C].
- Complete resolution closely associated with skeletal maturity, patellar ossification, and apophyseal closure (1)[C]

COMPLICATIONS

In some instances, surgery is required if the skeletally mature ossicles become painful.

REFERENCES

1. Kraus E, Rizzone K, Walker M, et al. Stress injuries of the knee. *Clin Sports Med*. 2022;41(4):707–727.
2. Hall R, Foss KB, Hewett TE, et al. Sports specialization's association with an increased risk of developing anterior knee pain in adolescent female athletes. *J Sport Rehabil*. 2015;24(1):31–35.
3. Patel DR, Villalobos A. Evaluation and management of knee pain in young athletes: overuse injuries of the knee. *Transl Pediatr*. 2017;6(3):190–198.
4. McCormick KL, Tedesco LJ, Bixby EC, et al. Sinding-Larsen-Johansson disease: analysis of the associated factors in the largest cohort to date. *Orthop J Sports Med*. 2022;(5 Suppl2):2325967121S00503.
5. Schmidt-Hebbel A, Eggers F, Schütte V, et al. Patellar sleeve avulsion fracture in a patient with Sinding-Larsen-Johansson syndrome: a case report. *BMC Musculoskelet Disord*. 2020;21:267.
6. Kajetanek C, Thaunat T, Guimaraes T, et al. Arthroscopic treatment of painful Sinding-Larsen-Johansson syndrome in a professional handball player. *Orthop Traumatol Surg Res*. 2016;102(5):677–680.

ADDITIONAL READING

- Draghi F, Danesino GM, Coscia D, et al. Overload syndromes of the knee in adolescents: sonographic findings. *J Ultrasound*. 2008;11(4):151–157.
- Duri ZAA, Patel DV, Aichroth PM. The immature athlete. *Clin Sports Med*. 2002;21(3):461–482.
- Foss KDB, Myer GD, Hewett TE. Epidemiology of basketball, soccer, and volleyball injuries in middle-school female athletes. *Phys Sportsmed*. 2014;42(2):146–153.
- Valentino M, Quiligotti C, Ruggirello M. Sinding-Larsen-Johansson syndrome: a case report. *J Ultrasound*. 2012;15(2):127–129.

CLINICAL PEARLS

- Common cause of anterior knee pain without effusion in children/adolescents
- Diagnosis is typically made clinically, and imaging is not always necessary.
- Nonoperative measures, including relative rest, NSAIDs, physical therapy, and stretching, tend to resolve most cases of this condition.

SINUS TARSI SYNDROME

C. Trent Davis, MD • LaRae L. Seemann, MD • George G. A. Pujalte, MD, FACSM, FAMSSM, FAAFP

BASICS

Sinus tarsi syndrome is a persistent, anterolateral ankle pain often associated with previous ankle injury (1).

DESCRIPTION

- Sinus tarsi is the lateral extension of the tarsal canal formed by the sulcus of the talus and calcaneus (2).
- Within the sinus tarsi are the talocalcaneal interosseous ligament; cervical ligament; the subtalar joint capsule; synovium; and the medial, intermediate, and lateral roots of the inferior extensor retinaculum (2):
  - Talocalcaneal interosseous ligament is involved in movements of the subtalar joint (2). It functions to maintain apposition of the talus and calcaneus in all positions (2). Its rich innervation suggests that the sinus tarsi may be susceptible to neurogenic inflammation and may be a center of articular nociception (2).

EPIDEMIOLOGY

- Patients with sinus tarsi syndrome are usually between their 3rd and 4th decades of life (3).
- Often associated with dancers, volleyball players, basketball players, overweight individuals, and patients with foot deformities, usually flexible flat feet (4)

ETIOLOGY AND PATHOPHYSIOLOGY

- Soft tissue inversion injuries of the ankle most commonly involve the ligamentous structures of the lateral aspect of the ankle and sinus tarsi (5).
- Chronic inflammation may lead to fibrotic changes in the wall and surrounding tissue of veins, causing disturbance of venous outflow and increased intrasinusal pressure, and may be a factor in the pathogenesis of sinus tarsi syndrome (6).
- Sinus tarsi is not only a talocalcaneal joint space with interosseous ligaments but also a source of nociceptive and proprioceptive information on the movements of the foot and ankle (2).
- Sinus tarsi syndrome may result from disorders of nociception and proprioception of the foot (2).

RISK FACTORS

Forefoot and calcaneal valgus, mechanical factors predisposing to supination ankle injuries, may lead to sinus tarsi syndrome after such injuries (7). In the majority of cases, the lateral ankle pain follows a history of an inversion ankle sprain (6).

COMMONLY ASSOCIATED CONDITIONS

- 70% of cases are posttraumatic.
- 30% can be attributed to causes including systemic disease, structural abnormalities, and soft tissue masses, such as ganglions (8).

DIAGNOSIS

Four clinical characteristics have been used to describe and diagnose the syndrome (3)[A]:

- Pain at the lateral opening of the sinus tarsi, increasing with pressure, usually ceasing at rest
- Perception of instability of the rear foot on uneven ground
- Marked reduction of pain and discomfort following an injection of local anesthetic into the sinus tarsi
- Clinical and stress radiographic examination showing no or minimal instability

HISTORY

- Deep aching, throbbing, or sharp pain within the sinus tarsi may be associated with a sense of rear foot instability. Pain over the lateral part of the ankle and hindfoot, over the sinus tarsi, is often the primary complaint, but because the synovitis and the associated fibrotic tissues take time to develop, athletes with injuries to the subtalar joint may not initially have symptoms that are localized to the sinus tarsi (1). A previous sprain or other injury is often the inciting event:
  - Initial injury may have responded to conservative therapies, but recurrent pain or pain settling into the sinus tarsi may be experienced with activities of daily living.
- Can result in severe pain and instability of the ankle and the subtalar joints, particularly in athletes (5)
- Pain and paresthesia may also be felt over the dorsolateral aspect of the foot (9). Intermittent pain often radiates into the leg, with resulting paresthesia over the distal aspect of the foot (9). Swelling may and may not be present.
- Patients most often complain of "ankle" pain, when the pain is emanating from the subtalar area. When asked to identify the site of maximal tenderness, patients often point directly to the sinus tarsi region.
- Pain may involve the anterior and lateral ankle, although this pain is less intense.
- The perception of ankle symptoms may be secondary to previous trauma, referred pain, or an altered gait in an attempt to reduce pain.

PHYSICAL EXAM

- Diagnosis is often clinical; tenderness over the sinus tarsi often leads to the diagnosis of sinus tarsi syndrome.
- Pain over the sinus tarsi at the end range of ankle plantarflexion with foot supination is typical (1).
- Discomfort usually worsens with pressure over the lateral opening of the sinus tarsi, becoming more severe with the foot in varus position (6).
- Symptoms are usually alleviated when the foot is immobilized in a valgus position (6).
- Injury to the ligaments may result in laxity of the joints of the ankle complex; neuromuscular deficits are also likely to occur due to the injury to the nervous and musculotendinous tissue (10).
- Neuromuscular deficits may be manifested as impaired balance, reduced joint position sense, slower firing of the peroneal muscles on inversion, slowed nerve conduction velocity, impaired cutaneous sensation, strength deficits, and decreased dorsiflexion range of motion (10).
- Assessment of patients with lateral ankle sprain not only must address joint laxity and swelling but also should include examination for neuromuscular deficits (2).

DIFFERENTIAL DIAGNOSIS

- Peripheral mononeuropathies
- Radiculopathy
- Lateral ankle sprain
- Anterolateral soft tissue impingement
- Bifurcate ligament injury
- Stress fractures of the cuboid, talus, or calcaneus (11)

DIAGNOSTIC TESTS & INTERPRETATION

Initial Tests (lab, imaging)

- Radiologic examination usually will not reveal a bone lesion or any insufficiency of the ankle ligaments, and dynamically, there is usually no restriction of talocalcaneonavicular joint range of motion (6).
- Magnetic resonance imaging (MRI), with or without arthrography, may better reveal abnormalities and show enhanced signal on T2 imaging, representative of inflammation and fibrotic changes at the sinus tarsi and tarsi canal (1).
- Single photon emission computed tomography/computed tomography (SPECT/CT) can be used in those with contraindication to MRI. It is found to have sensitivity and specificity of 95% and 83%, respectively (12).

Diagnostic Procedures/Other

- Pain and functional instability in the region have been found to be reduced for a few hours after the injection of a local anesthetic into the opening of the sinus tarsi (7).
- A reduction in electrical activity or complete electrical silence of both the peroneus brevis and longus muscles have been noted on electromyographic studies (2).

TREATMENT

- Relative rest, avoidance of aggravating activities, and use of nonsteroidal anti-inflammatory drugs (NSAIDs) as needed for pain may give temporary relief.
- Orthotics may be used to address forefoot valgus and calcaneal valgus, mechanical factors predisposing to supination ankle sprains (7)[B].
- Conservative treatment includes physical therapy, corticosteroid injections, immobilization in a cast or walking boot, application of local anti-inflammatory gels or local irritants such as capsaicin, and short-term use of systemic drugs aimed at reducing neuralgic pain.
- When there is ankle instability or feeling of giving way, physical therapy should be tried first. Physical therapy should be focused on balance, progressive stability, and proprioceptive training (13)[B].
- Other methods such as mobilization, ice massage, friction massage, and deep massage using ultrasound, soft laser, transcutaneous electrical stimulation, or any other method of deep massage
- Athletic training footwear is also a consideration, and recommendation includes those with a straight last, a firm heel counter, and rigid material through the midsole (13)[B].
- Corticosteroid injections mixed with local anesthetics have been shown to be effective (12)[A].
- Conservative treatment has been shown to be effective in up to 2/3 of patients (3)[A]. There seem to be no clear studies that delineate the length of time conservative measures should be tried, and the determination appears to be on a case-to-case basis for the most part, although, in our practice, a time frame of 4 to 6 weeks is the most commonly used length of time for any conservative treatment chosen and applied to sinus tarsi syndrome.

MEDICATION

- A local anesthetic injection may be given as initial treatment for the pain of sinus tarsi syndrome; may also be diagnostic (5)[B]
- A mixed local anesthetic and corticosteroid injection may also be given as treatment for the pain of sinus tarsi syndrome, with 5 to 6 injections at weekly intervals usually sufficient (3)[B],(5)[B].

ISSUES FOR REFERRAL

Referral to orthopedic surgery may be appropriate after failure of conservative measures (5)[B].

SURGERY/OTHER PROCEDURES

Surgical treatment of sinus tarsi syndrome may involve excision of the lateral half of the sinus tarsi contents, followed by below-knee casting for 3 weeks and physical therapy (5)[B].

ONGOING CARE

FOLLOW-UP RECOMMENDATIONS

Postoperatively, patients may be immobilized with a walking boot for around 4 weeks and then made to undergo physical therapy, usually for another 4 to 6 weeks (3)[A].

PROGNOSIS

- 2/3 of sinus tarsi syndrome cases respond to conservative treatment.
- In the remaining 1/3 of cases, surgical intervention has been shown to cure or improve 90% of patients (3).

COMPLICATIONS

- Sinus tarsi syndrome responds well to therapeutic interventions, often mixed local anesthetic and corticosteroid injections (12).
- Should surgery be required, there are usually few postoperative complications (1),(14).
- The most common reported complication from surgical intervention is a transient neurapraxia involving branches of the superficial peroneal nerve (15).

REFERENCES

1. Helgeson K. Examination and intervention for sinus tarsi syndrome. *N Am J Sports Phys Ther*. 2009;4(1):29–37.
2. Akiyama K, Takakura Y, Tomita Y, et al. Neurohistology of the sinus tarsi and sinus tarsi syndrome. *J Orthop Sci*. 1999;4(4):299–303.
3. Taillard W, Meyer JM, Garcia J, et al. The sinus tarsi syndrome. *Int Orthop*. 1981;5(2):117–130.
4. Herrmann M, Pieper KS. Sinus tarsi syndrome: what hurts? Article in German. *Unfallchirurg*. 2008;111(2):132–136.
5. Mabit C, Boncoeur-Martel MP, Chaudruc JM, et al. Anatomic and MRI study of the subtalar ligamentous support. *Surg Radiol Anat*. 1997;19(2):111–117.
6. Schwarzenbach B, Dora C, Lang A, et al. Blood vessels of the sinus tarsi and the sinus tarsi syndrome. *Clin Anat*. 1997;10(3):173–182.
7. Duddy RK, Duggan RJ, Visser HJ, et al. Diagnosis, treatment, and rehabilitation of injuries to the lower leg and foot. *Clin Sports Med*. 1989;8(4):861–876.
8. Dozier TJ, Figueroa RT, Kalmar J. Sinus tarsi syndrome. *J La State Med Soc*. 2001;153(9):458–461.
9. Giorgini RJ, Bernard RL. Sinus tarsi syndrome in a patient with talipes equinovarus. *J Am Podiatr Med Assoc*. 1990;80(4):218–222.
10. Rab M, Ebmer J, Dellon AL. Innervation of the sinus tarsi and implications for treating anterolateral ankle pain. *Ann Plast Surg*. 2001;47(5):500–504.
11. Shear MS, Baitch SP, Shear DB. Sinus tarsi syndrome: the importance of biomechanically-based evaluation and treatment. *Arch Phys Med Rehabil*. 1993;74(7):777–781.
12. Mahato A, Mukherjee PB, Jha DK, et al. Sinus tarsi syndrome: diagnosed on ^{99m}Tc-MDP bone SPECT/CT. *Asia Ocean J Nucl Med Biol*. 2020;8(2):153–156.
13. Yamashita MH. Evaluation and selection of shoe wear and orthoses for the runner. *Phys Med Rehabil Clin N Am*. 2005;16(3):801–829.
14. Oloff LM, Schulhofer SD, Bocko AP. Subtalar joint arthroscopy for sinus tarsi syndrome: a review of 29 cases. *J Foot Ankle Surg*. 2001;40(3):152–157.
15. Frey C, Feder KS, DiGiovanni C. Arthroscopic evaluation of the subtalar joint: does sinus tarsi syndrome exist? *Foot Ankle Int*. 1999;20(3):185–191.

CLINICAL PEARLS

- Sinus tarsi syndrome is a persistent, anterolateral ankle pain often associated with previous ankle injury and most common in individuals aged 20 to 40 years, previous ankle inversion injury, and forefoot deformities making them more prone to pronation.
- Diagnostic requirements include pain at the lateral opening of the sinus tarsi, perception of instability, relief following an injection of local anesthetic into the sinus tarsi, and clinical and stress radiographic examination showing no or minimal instability.
- Imaging does not usually reveal an injury to the bone or soft tissue of the sinus tarsi but may help show abnormalities in the anatomy of the sinus tarsi leading them to have sinus tarsi syndrome.
- Conservative therapy is the first-line treatment and includes relative rest, orthotics, NSAIDs, and corticosteroid injections, followed by physical therapy to improve instability.
- Referral to an orthopedic surgeon is reasonable if conservative therapy fails, which occurs in up to 1/3 of patients.

S

SLAP TEARS

Marjorie Delo, MD, CAQSM, RMSK

BASICS

DESCRIPTION

- Superior labrum anterior-to-posterior (SLAP) tears are a type of tear of the glenoid labrum of the shoulder.
- The glenoid labrum is a fibrocartilaginous ring that deepens the bony socket to provide stability to the glenohumeral joint, as well as serving as an attachment site for the glenohumeral ligaments and the long head of the biceps tendon (LHBT).
- The LHBT attaches to the superior aspect of the labrum and the bony supraglenoid tubercle.
- SLAP tears involve the superior labrum/biceps tendon junction.
- The most common cause of SLAP tears is sports injury.

ETIOLOGY AND PATHOPHYSIOLOGY

The majority of SLAP tears are likely multifactorial. Etiologies include:

- Torsional forces through the "peel-back" mechanism of the biceps insertion on the superior labrum during the cocking phase of throwing
- Traction forces on the biceps tendon during the deceleration phase of throwing
- Posteroinferior capsular contractures increasing shear forces on the LHBT
- Labral degeneration from compressive grinding forces within the joint due to altered shoulder mechanics
- Acute traumatic events such as falls, traction injuries, or forceful heavy lifting

RISK FACTORS

- Athletes engaging in repetitive throwing or overhead sports
- Acute injury such as a fall on an outstretched hand (FOOSH), traction injury to the arm, or shoulder dislocation
- Degenerative tearing or fraying from general aging >40 years
- Careers involving heavy repetitive overhead motion

COMMONLY ASSOCIATED CONDITIONS

- Rotator cuff pathology
- Glenohumeral instability

DIAGNOSIS

HISTORY

- Typical complaint is anterior or deep shoulder pain with a decrease in sports performance.
- Symptoms intensify with lifting overhead or in the cocking position.
- Mechanical symptoms may be present like catching, clicking, or grinding.
- A sense of instability may be present.
- Symptoms may be vague or similar to those associated with other shoulder pathology; it is important to maintain a degree of clinical suspicion for labral injury.

PHYSICAL EXAM

- Comprehensive evaluation of glenohumeral and scapulothoracic range of motion (ROM) compared to the uninvolved shoulder
- Glenohumeral joint stability evaluation
- The literature has found that single exam tests for SLAP tears have poor diagnostic accuracy. A combination of tests increases sensitivity and specificity.
- A recent meta-analysis found that all combinations of three or more of the following tests had a specificity of >94% (1)[A].
  - O'Brien active compression test: The shoulder is positioned in 90 degrees of flexion, 10 to 15 degrees adduction, full internal rotation with a pronated forearm. Manual resistance is then applied in a downward direction. The shoulder is then repositioned into neutral rotation with forearm supination, and manual resistance again applied. A positive test occurs when there is pain or clicking with the first position which reduces or resolves in the second.
  - Yergason test: The patient is seated with the shoulder at rest, elbow in flexion, and the forearm neutral. Active elbow flexion and forearm supination is resisted by the examiner. The test is positive if it reproduces pain along the proximal biceps.
  - Speed test: The patient shoulder is positioned in forward flexion and external rotation, with full elbow extension and forearm supination. Manual resistance is then applied in a downward direction. The test is positive if pain is reproduced along the proximal biceps.
  - Crank test: The shoulder is elevated to 160 degrees in the scapular plane and compression is applied to the joint, with passive internal/external rotation. The test is positive if there is pain, clicking, or catching.
  - Anterior slide: The patient is positioned standing with their hand on their ipsilateral hip with the thumb pointing posteriorly. The examiner then applies an axial load in an anterosuperior direction from the elbow to the shoulder. The test is positive if it reproduces pain.
  - Jobe relocation test: Patient is positioned supine with the elbow flexed to 90 degrees and the shoulder abducted to 90 degrees. The first part of the test is the apprehension test, where the shoulder is passively externally rotated. Subsequently, the examiner applies a posterior force to the humeral head. If pain or apprehension is reduced, then the relocation test is positive.

DIFFERENTIAL DIAGNOSIS

- Rotator cuff tear or tendinopathy
- Rotator cuff impingement syndrome
- Refractory bicipital tendinosis
- Symptomatic glenohumeral instability
- Glenohumeral osteoarthritis

DIAGNOSTIC TESTS & INTERPRETATION

Initial Tests (lab, imaging)

- Plain radiographs are usually normal.
- Nonenhanced magnetic resonance imaging (MRI) can show the anatomy of the labral biceps complex but is not as sensitive for superior labral detachments.
- Gadolinium-enhanced MRI (magnetic resonance [MR] arthrogram) increases the accuracy of identifying superior labral pathology.
- 3T magnets improve diagnostic accuracy of superior labral tears (2)[A].
- Musculoskeletal ultrasound may be helpful identifying associated shoulder pathology; however, it is not useful for examining SLAP tears.
- Arthroscopy is the gold standard for diagnosis.

Test Interpretation

The majority of SLAP tears can be classified by the original Snyder classification:

- Type I: fraying of the superior labrum with an intact biceps tendon origin

- Type II (most common type): labral fraying with detachment of the biceps tendon from the supraglenoid tubercle
- Type III: bucket handle tear of the superior labrum with an intact biceps attachment to bone
- Type IV: bucket handle tear of the superior labrum that extends into the biceps tendon
- There are several variations that could be subcategorized within these types.

TREATMENT

GENERAL MEASURES

- Stable labral tears without mechanical symptoms may be successfully treated nonoperatively with nonsteroidal anti-inflammatory drugs (NSAIDs) or acetaminophen (Tylenol) and physical therapy.
- Therapy should involve ROM including specifically addressing posterior capsule contractures, along with rotator cuff and scapular stabilizer strengthening.
- Shoulder exercises should be supplemented with core and lower extremity strengthening in the throwing or overhead athlete.
- Return to play can be graduated as tolerated.

ISSUES FOR REFERRAL

- Overhead athletes or patients with high-demand occupations should be considered for shoulder specialist referral.
- Unstable tears should be referred.
- If an athlete or patient cannot progress after 3 to 6 months of conservative management, operative intervention should be considered.

SURGERY/OTHER PROCEDURES

- Unstable SLAP tears require arthroscopic surgery.
- Young active patients, often with type II SLAP tears, can undergo primary SLAP repair.
- Older patients with chronic symptoms or degenerative labral tissue, often type I SLAP tears, may undergo débridement or biceps tenodesis (3)[C].
- Regenerative medicine may have a role in stable labral tears; however, more research is needed.

ONGOING CARE

FOLLOW-UP RECOMMENDATIONS

- After surgical repair, time is needed for healing and recovery prior to the reinitiation of physical therapy, usually about 6 weeks.
- A throwing program can usually start within 3 to 4 months of surgery.
- Return to full throwing may take 9 to 12 months.
- Prognosis/return to play
  - Nonsurgical treatment is normally recommended first; a recent systematic review found a return-to-play rate of only 53.7%; however, with formal rehabilitation, this increased to 78% (4)[B].
  - Studies of surgical repair reveal a similar return-to-play rate as formal rehabilitation (5)[B].
  - Statistically, overhead athletes undergoing surgical or nonsurgical treatment both can have difficulty returning to prior level of performance.
  - Return-to-play rates are affected by concomitant rotator cuff pathology.
  - Biceps tenodesis has demonstrated positive results in the general population.

COMPLICATIONS

- Breakage or dislodgment of nonabsorbable anchors
- Foreign body reaction to surgical materials
- Healing complications

REFERENCES

1. Dean RS, Onsen L, Lima I, et al. Physical examination maneuvers for SLAP lesions: a systematic review and meta-analysis of individual and combinations of maneuvers. *Am J Sports Med.* 2023;51(11):3042–3052.
2. Ajuied A, McGarvey CP, Harb Z, et al. Diagnosis of glenoid labral tears using 3-tesla MRI vs. 3-tesla MRA: a systematic review and meta-analysis. *Arch Orthop Trauma Surg.* 2018;138(5):699–709.
3. Calcei JG, Boddapati V, Altchek DW, et al. Diagnosis and treatment of injuries to the biceps and superior labral complex in overhead athletes. *Curr Rev Musculoskelet Med.* 2018;11(1):63–71.
4. Steinmetz RG, Guth JJ, Matava MJ, et al. Return to play following nonsurgical management of superior labrum anterior-posterior tears: a systematic review. *J Shoulder Elbow Surg.* 2022;31(6):1323–1333.
5. Smith R, Lombardo DJ, Petersen-Fitts GR, et al. Return to play and prior performance in Major League Baseball pitchers after repair of superior labral anterior-posterior tears. *Orthop J Sports Med.* 2016;4(12):2325967116675822.

ADDITIONAL READING

- Gismervik SØ, Drogset JO, Granviken F, et al. Physical examination tests of the shoulder: a systematic review and meta-analysis of diagnostic test performance. *BMC Musculoskelet Disord.* 2017;18(1):41.
- Ireland ML, Hatzenbuehler JR. Superior labrum anterior to posterior (SLAP) tears. Updated December 6, 2024. Accessed August 20, 2025. https://www.uptodate.com/contents/superior-labrum-anterior-to-posterior-slap-tears#:~:text=Superior%20labrum%20anterior%20to%20posterior%20(SLAP)%20tear%20refers%20to%20a,laborers%20involved%20in%20overhead%20activities

CLINICAL PEARLS

- SLAP tears are injuries to the superior labrum/biceps tendon complex.
- Type II tears are the most common and are seen in overhead or throwing athletes.
- Physical exam techniques have low sensitivity and sensitivity; thus, multiple tests should be performed in series to determine the need for imaging.
- MR arthrogram is the diagnostic study of choice to evaluate for a SLAP lesion.
- Many athletes will do well with conservative rehabilitation; however, if symptoms persist after 3 to 6 months, surgical consultation should be obtained.

S

SLIPPED CAPITAL FEMORAL EPIPHYSIS

Jarrod Yamanaka, MD, CAQSM

BASICS

DESCRIPTION

- A disorder of unknown cause in which the proximal femoral epiphysis (head of the femur) begins to "fall off or slip off" the femoral neck
- The slippage occurs at the epiphyseal plate, which begins to weaken as it matures.
- There are four presentation patterns for slipped capital femoral epiphysis (SCFE):
  - Early SCFE (previously named "preslip")
  - Acute
  - Acute on chronic
  - Chronic
- SCFEs are classified based on the intensity and duration of symptoms present as well as the radiographic findings.

EPIDEMIOLOGY

- The disorder affects 0.2 to 10/100,000 children (1).
- Predominant age: The mean age at which it occurs is 12 years in girls and 13.5 years in boys. Age decreases with increasing obesity.
- The disorder is bilateral in 18–63% of affected children.
- The disorder frequently occurs in two distinct body types: (i) slender, tall, rapidly growing and (ii) large, obese adolescents.
- Pacific Islanders have the highest incidence, followed by African Americans, Hispanics, Native Americans, Americans, and children of Indonesian/Malay descent.

ETIOLOGY AND PATHOPHYSIOLOGY

- Biomechanical and biochemical factors play a role in SCFE.
- Biomechanical factors include obesity, femoral retroversion, and increased physeal obliquity.
- Biochemical factors include increased growth hormone during puberty, which increases the height of the zone of hypertrophy, and increased testosterone, which decreases physeal strength.

RISK FACTORS

- Rapid growth spurt
- Obesity
- Endocrine disorders that weaken the physis, particularly in preadolescent children
- Radiation therapy and renal failure
- Obesity

COMMONLY ASSOCIATED CONDITIONS

- Obesity
- Hypothyroidism
- Multiple endocrine neoplasia syndrome type 2
- Panhypopituitarism
- Renal failure
- Radiation therapy

DIAGNOSIS

- Determined by history, physical examination, and pelvis anteroposterior (AP) and frog-leg lateral view radiographs.
- It is important to always examine both sides owing to possibility of bilateral disease (1),(2).
- Acute SCFE: sudden-onset severe pain usually of <3-week duration that prevents weight-bearing; usually associated with trauma; joint effusion and no metaphyseal remodeling. Examination reveals external rotational deformity, shortening of the affected limb, decreased range of motion at the hip, and severe pain with attempted manipulation.
- Acute on chronic SCFE: history of at least 3 weeks of hip pain and/or limp with a sudden increase in pain and inability to bear full weight. Patients usually have a joint effusion and metaphyseal widening.
- Chronic SCFE: Vague intermittent symptoms of hip, thigh, or knee pain, worsened by activity and relieved by rest. Exam reveals antalgic gait and even a Trendelenburg or waddling depending on whether unilateral or bilateral. Often the affected foot is turned outward. Often there is pain with internal rotation, abduction, and flexion of the hip with reduced movement in these planes. Metaphyseal modeling is present but no effusion.

PHYSICAL EXAM

- A common presenting complaint is hip pain and a limp (antalgic gait). Trendelenburg test is positive when the patient stands on the affected leg and a downward pelvic tilt occurs due to hip weakness on the affected side (3). Pain is localized to groin, lateral or posterolateral hip, and thigh with pain commonly radiating to the knee (4).
- Pain can be gradual in onset, and symptoms occur even when minimal displacement is present or can be acute and dramatic with sudden severe hip or knee pain and inability to bear weight.
- The physical exam reveals tenderness over the hip joint capsule, and an external rotation deformity of the lower extremity may be present.
- There is restricted hip motion, especially internal rotation, abduction, and forward flexion.
- The hip tends to rotate externally and abduct as it is flexed (Whitman sign).
- In chronic late presenting cases, the affected leg may be 1 to 3 cm shorter than the normal leg, and the thigh muscles may be atrophied.

DIFFERENTIAL DIAGNOSIS

- Septic arthritis
- Transient synovitis
- Iliac apophysitis or apophyseal avulsion fracture at avulsion anterior inferior iliac spine (AIIS) and avulsion anterior superior iliac spine (ASIS)
- Femoral cutaneous nerve entrapment (more common in muscular girls)
- Proximal femur fracture
- Avascular necrosis
- Juvenile rheumatoid arthritis
- Legg-Calvé-Perthes disease (in younger age range)

DIAGNOSTIC TESTS & INTERPRETATION

- AP pelvis and frog-leg lateral radiograph views confirm the diagnosis. The affected side always should be compared with the unaffected leg. Up to 10% of SCFE patients have normal radiographs initially:
  - AP pelvis can be useful to measure "Klein" line which is an imaginary line parallel to superior border of femoral neck and should intersect with ~1/3 of the epiphysis.
  - The sensitivity and reliability are improved by measuring the epiphyseal width lateral to Klein line, which if differing by 2 mm (0.079 inch) or more between hips suggests the diagnosis of SCFE.
- Magnetic resonance imaging (MRI) is useful for detecting early SCFE that may be symptomatic but have normal radiographs.
- Computed tomography (CT) is occasionally useful for grading chronic slips.
- The capital epiphysis is seen to displace posteriorly and downward, whereas the femoral neck displaces upward and anteriorly. In some patients, displacement is not obvious, but the physeal plate is widened (early SCFE).
- Classification is based on the severity of the slip. Type 1 slips involve <33% of the width of the femoral epiphysis. Type 2 involves a 33–50% slip, and a type 3 involves >50% of the width of the femoral epiphysis.
- Consider endocrinology workup with atypical SCFE presentations including thyroid and renal studies (4).

TREATMENT

GENERAL MEASURES

- Orthopedic referral should be made immediately on diagnosis (4).
- Patients should immediately be made non–weight-bearing.

SURGERY/OTHER PROCEDURES

- Surgical stabilization is the mainstay of treatment for all types of slippages (1),(4).
- Current controversy exists surrounding the need for prophylactic surgical stabilization of the unaffected contralateral side. This is due to the prevalence of bilateral SCFE and inability to predict who will develop bilateral disease (2).

ADMISSION, INPATIENT, AND NURSING CONSIDERATIONS

- Acute treatment involves cessation of weight-bearing and surgical stabilization (5),(6).
- A displaced epiphysis may require reduction before fixation.
- In the early SCFE phase, with widening of the physeal plate evident on radiographs, in situ operative fixation is recommended.
- Weight-bearing begun at 6 weeks postoperatively.

ONGOING CARE

FOLLOW-UP RECOMMENDATIONS

- Orthopedic referral should be made immediately on diagnosis.
- Patients should be made non–weight-bearing if the diagnosis is suspected.

PROGNOSIS

- Prognosis is usually good, except in patients with acute traumatic separation.
- Slight shortening of the leg of <1.25 cm may result, along with a mild external rotation deformity.
- The internal fixation devices are removed after the physeal plate closes in 1 to 2 years.
- In acute traumatic separations, avascular necrosis of the femoral head is a common complication, and this usually results in severe arthritis of the hip.
- Another complication is acute cartilage necrosis or lysis of the articular cartilage of the hip joint. A painful fibrous ankylosis of the hip joint is frequently the result.

REFERENCES

1. Peck DM, Voss LM, Voss TT. Slipped capital femoral epiphysis: diagnosis and management. *Am Fam Physician*. 2017;95(12):779–784.
2. Swarup I, Goodbody C, Goto R, et al. Risk factors for contralateral slipped capital femoral epiphysis: a meta-analysis of cohort and case-control studies. *J Pediatr Orthop*. 2020;40(6):e446–e453.
3. Frank JS, Gambacorta PL, Eisner EA. Hip pathology in the adolescent athlete. *J Am Acad Orthop Surg*. 2013;21(11):665–674.
4. Haider S, Podeszwa DA, Morris WZ. The etiology and management of slipped capital femoral epiphysis: current concept review. *J Pediatr Orthop Soc N Am*. 2022;4(4):589.
5. Rosenbaum DG, Cooper AP. Slipped capital femoral epiphysis: emphasis on early recognition and potential pitfalls. *Skeletal Radiol*. 2025;54(4):807–818.
6. Gorgolini G, Caterini A, Efremov K, et al. Surgical treatment of slipped capital femoral epiphysis (SCFE) by Dunn procedure modified by Ganz: a systematic review. *BMC Musculoskelet Disord*. 2022;22(Suppl 2):1064.

ADDITIONAL READING

Armstrong AD, Hubbard MC. *Essentials of Musculoskeletal Care*. 5th ed. American Academy of Orthopedic Surgeons; 2016.

CLINICAL PEARLS

- SCFE can present unilaterally or bilaterally with only knee or thigh pain; not all cases have hip pain.
- All adolescent patients with thigh or hip pain should get x-rays. The recommended radiographs are AP and frog-leg lateral pelvis views, not individual hip radiographs.
- Treatment includes non–weight-bearing status and immediate referral for surgical stabilization.

S

SNAPPING SCAPULA AND WINGING OF THE SCAPULA

Brandon W. Barsky, MD, FAAP, CAQSM

BASICS

DESCRIPTION

Snapping scapula syndrome (SSS) is a disorder of the scapulothoracic articulation resulting in crepitation with overhead arm motion that may or may not be painful. It can be the result of anatomic impediment to normal scapular motion from weakness, inflexibility, postural imbalances, or inadequate proprioception of 1 or more of the 17 muscles that insert on the scapula, which cause excessive friction between the scapula and thorax. Winged scapula (WS) results from a nerve injury, usually of the long thoracic nerves (LTN) or spinal accessory nerves (SAN). This results in profound weakness of the serratus anterior or trapezius muscles, respectively, producing functional shoulder pain and dysfunction.

EPIDEMIOLOGY

Incidence

- SSS is relatively common but likely underdiagnosed.
- Altered scapular position and motion has been reported in 68–100% of patients with shoulder injuries.

Prevalence

- SSS:
  - Relatively common
  - Altered scapular position and motion has been reported in 31% of asymptomatic individuals.
- WS:
  - Rare
  - LTN palsy has been reported 15/7,000 electromyography (EMG) patients, 1/38,500 orthopedic patients, 3/12,000 neurologic evaluations.
  - SAN palsy prevalence is difficult to assess.

ETIOLOGY AND PATHOPHYSIOLOGY

- SSS:
  - Anatomic (1):
    - Thoracic rib disorders (fracture with prominent callus or displacement)
    - Thoracic spine disorder (costovertebral dysfunction, scoliosis, Scheuermann kyphosis, postural kyphosis)
    - Scapular disorders (fracture with prominent callus or displacement, hooked superior medial edge [Luschka tubercle], osteochondroma)
    - Soft tissue tumor (elastofibroma)
  - Inadequate strength, flexibility, and proprioception:
    - Weakness (mostly in serratus anterior, middle and lower trapezius)
    - Inflexibility (mostly in pectoralis minor, levator scapulae, and upper trapezius)
    - Abnormal firing patterns associated with repetitive motion (asymmetric strength training, throwing mechanics, swimming technique, etc.) may lead to bursitis in 1 of the 6 bursae.
- WS:
  - Blunt trauma:
    - LTN: sudden depression of the shoulder
    - SAN: blow over the posterior cervical triangle
  - Sports related: archery, ballet, baseball, basketball, bowling, football, golf, gymnastics, hockey, soccer, tennis, weight lifting, wrestling
  - Iatrogenic:
    - LTN: chiropractic manipulation, crutches, surgery
    - SAN: surgery to the neck area
  - Other: postviral neuritis, exposure to toxin or drugs, muscular dystrophy

DIAGNOSIS

HISTORY

- SSS:
  - Palpable crepitus and audible snapping with shoulder motion, with or without pain, usually along the medial scapular border (superior > inferior > middle)
  - Classic anterior impingement complaints (pain with overhead activities)
  - Involved in higher incident, overhead sports (baseball, swimming, tennis)
- WS:
  - LTN: shoulder pain that usually is more toward the upper medial scapula. It may occur a few weeks after onset of palsy when the trapezius starts to stretch from the unopposing serratus anterior. Severe pain may occur with postviral neuritis. Burning neuralgic pain at the inferior scapular pole may occur with acute trauma.
  - SAN: stiffness, heaviness, pain, and weakness, especially with overhead activities or prolonged exertion

PHYSICAL EXAM

- Cervical spine evaluation, including range of motion of the cervical spine, strength, sensation, deep tendon reflexes in the upper extremity, Spurling maneuver
- Spine and shoulder inspection: standing and forward flexed, analyzing for asymmetry and posture
- Scapular position:
  - SSS (may be normal scapular position with classic "teenager posture" with rounded shoulders, dynamic thoracic kyphosis, forward flexed head, and suboccipital extension)
  - LTN (scapula is superior and adducted medially)
  - SAN (drooping shoulder with scapula abducted laterally)
- Scapular winging tests:
  - LTN (entire medial scapula will protrude with shoulder forward flexion [FF] or wall push-up)
  - SAN (superior medial scapula will laterally displace causing downward rotation with shoulder abduction or resisted external rotation; no winging with shoulder FF)
- Range-of-motion deficit:
  - LTN (<120 degrees of FF and 110 degrees of abduction)
  - SAN (normal FF and <90 degrees of abduction)
- Scapular motion with shoulder movement, assessing for any asymmetry or abnormality

DIFFERENTIAL DIAGNOSIS

- Cervical discogenic neuropathy
- Thoracic outlet syndrome
- Rotator cuff tear
- Glenohumeral instability
- Glenohumeral arthritis
- Acromioclavicular joint pathology
- Suprascapular nerve entrapment
- Primary neuromuscular disease
- Neurofibromatosis
- Primary pulmonary pathology

DIAGNOSTIC TESTS & INTERPRETATION

Initial Tests (lab, imaging)

- Radiographs of the cervical spine, shoulder, chest, and ribs will usually be normal.
- Computed tomography (CT) scans and magnetic resonance imaging (MRI) are rarely necessary unless concern about bone or soft tissue masses. Isolated left thoracic scoliosis should be evaluated with cervical spine MRI secondary to its association with congenital anomalies (syringomyelia, Arnold-Chiari malformations).

Diagnostic Procedures/Other

EMG is the only definitive diagnostic test for nerve dysfunction and muscle paralysis associated with WS. Abnormalities found on the EMG include resting denervation potentials, decreased motor unit recruitment, and polyphasic motor unit potential with volitional activities. EMG does not correlate with clinical improvement and cannot be used to predict the extent of recovery (2)[C].

TREATMENT

GENERAL MEASURES

Emergency department (ED) treatment (3)[C]:

- Acute injury may result in WS, but the symptoms of pain and nerve dysfunction may not present for a few weeks.
- Avoiding painful activities, especially overhead activities, is important.
- Brief sling immobilization may be necessary for pain control.

MEDICATION

- Analgesic medications may be necessary for acute injuries and severe pain, like with postviral neuritis.
- Subacromial bursa steroid injection and oral anti-inflammatories may be used with SSS in order to decrease pain while physical therapy is retraining normal muscle firing patterns.
- Ultrasound-guided anesthetic and corticosteroid at the medial scapular border have also been proven effective for pain relief (4).

ADDITIONAL THERAPIES

- SSS (treat the etiology) (1)[C]:
  - Anatomic lesions (fracture callus, fracture displacement, mass lesion): assessment for surgical consultation, depending on their contribution to the pain and dysfunction
  - Thoracic dysfunction: Thoracic scoliosis and Scheuermann kyphosis may require bracing and surgery. Segmental thoracic dysfunction (resulting in malalignment) may benefit from manual manipulation followed by stabilization rehabilitation.
  - Scapular dyskinesis: requires an astute clinician to direct the subtle relationships that need to be restored (2)[C]. Outlined below are the most common components of most scapular dyskinesis:
    - Release the muscular and capsular restrictions:
      - Glenohumeral posterior capsule tightness
      - Pectoralis minor tightness
    - Improve muscular strength and scapular force focusing on scapular stabilization and balance.
- WS (3)[C]:
  - LTN: 75% will respond to conservative management but will take anywhere from 6 to 24 months. There are some that do not improve serratus anterior firing but improve their function by muscular compensation with other scapulothoracic stabilizers (usually trapezius):
    - In the early phase of rehabilitation, avoid further injury by limiting any overhead or painful activities.
    - As pain decreases, progress to gentle range of motion to avoid adhesive capsulitis. Avoid stretching the serratus anterior muscle by limiting passive scapular retraction.
    - As the serratus strength improves, shoulder girdle strengthening exercises can be started. Reducing the amount of winging during rehab and activities of daily living (ADLs) is important.
    - Doing rehab while lying supine will stabilize the WS.
  - SAN: Conservative management is not as effective. A trial of protection, bracing, and progression as above is advised for 6 to 12 months.

SURGERY/OTHER PROCEDURES

- WS: If symptoms continue despite compliant conservative management for 12 (SAN) to 24 months (LTN), surgical intervention must be considered. Dynamic muscle transfer procedures show improved function, fewer symptoms of pain and winging, and are replacing many of the older procedures (5)[C].
- SSS: Surgical management is reserved for patients with impinging anatomic structures and recalcitrant bursitis that are not responding to conservative management.
- Previous surgical intervention had been an open approach, but arthroscopic intervention has become the standard of treatment as it is minimally invasive, allows for faster recovery, and produces good outcomes (4)[C].

REFERENCES

1. Martin RM, Fish DE. Scapular winging: anatomical review, diagnosis, and treatments. *Curr Rev Musculoskelet Med*. 2008;1(1):1–11.
2. Osias W, Matcuk GR Jr, Skalski MR, et al. Scapulothoracic pathology: review of anatomy, pathophysiology, imaging findings, and an approach to management. *Skeletal Radiol*. 2018;47(2):161–171.
3. Didesch JT, Tang P. Anatomy, etiology, and management of scapular winging. *J Hand Surg Am*. 2018;44(4):321–330.
4. Milton AH, Arefin S, Khan KJ, et al. Scapulothoracic bursitis or the snapping scapula syndrome may mimic with shoulder pain. *JORAPAIN*. 2021;7(1):12–15.
5. Hanson JA, Liles JL, Dey Hazra RO, et al. Arthroscopic treatment of snapping scapula syndrome with scapulothoracic bursectomy and partial scapulectomy. *Arthrosc Tech*. 2022;11(7):e1175–e1180.

ADDITIONAL READING

- Baldawi H, Gouveia K, Gohal C, et al. Diagnosis and treatment of snapping scapula syndrome: a scoping review. *Sports Health*. 2022;14(3):389–396.
- Seror P, Lenglet T, Nguyen C, et al. Unilateral winged scapula: clinical and electrodiagnostic experience with 128 cases, with special attention to long thoracic nerve palsy. *Muscle Nerve*. 2018;57(6):913–920.

CLINICAL PEARLS

- Scapular dyskinesis should be considered in patients with shoulder pain. Whether it is a primary cause or a secondary problem, it is an important component of restoring shoulder function.
- LTN: 75% will respond to conservative management but will take anywhere from 6 to 24 months. There are some that do not improve serratus anterior firing but improve their function by muscular compensation with other scapulothoracic stabilizers (usually trapezius).
- CT scans and MRI are rarely necessary unless concern about bone or soft tissue masses. Only definitive test is EMG.

SPINAL STENOSIS

Salvador Portugal, DO, MBA, FAAPMR, CAQSM • Jina Libby, DO, FAAPMR •
Maria Janakos, MD, FAAPMR, CAQSM

BASICS

DESCRIPTION

- Stenosis of the spinal canal is defined as narrowing of the available space within the spinal canal causing impingement on the neural and/or vascular elements of the spine (1).
- A general consensus defines lumbar spinal stenosis as a lumbar canal diameter of <12 mm (relative stenosis) and <10 mm (absolute stenosis) (1).
- A general consensus defines cervical spinal stenosis as an anteroposterior diameter of <13 mm from C3–C7.
- Stenosis can lead to pain in the leg or buttock with or without associated back pain.
- Spinal stenosis classification is divided into congenital (primary) and acquired (secondary) forms (1).

EPIDEMIOLOGY

- Most often occurs in the lumbar spine but can occur in the cervical (C)-spine
- Rarely occurs in the thoracic spine

Prevalence

- Symptoms of lumbar spinal stenosis are estimated to be 11% in the general public but 25–39% in the clinical setting (1).
- Estimated to be 47% in those > 60 years old (1)

ETIOLOGY AND PATHOPHYSIOLOGY

- Degenerative pathology/arthritis affecting the spine is the most common cause of lumbar spinal stenosis and can affect the lateral recess, central canal or neuroforamen, or any combination of these locations (1).
- Clinical manifestations differ based on the anatomical structures involved (1).
  - The spinal cord and nerve roots are safeguarded within the central canal, surrounded by bony, ligamentous, and intervertebral disk structures (1).
  - These structures can undergo hypertrophy and degeneration, leading to encroachment of the canal and subsequent compression of neurovascular tissue (1).
  - This compression may result in mechanical and/or chemical irritation (1).

Genetics

Genetics play a role in some cases of spinal stenosis in conditions such as spondyloarthropathies, dwarfism, and spina bifida.

RISK FACTORS

- Degenerative changes in the intervertebral disks, ligaments, and facet joints as well as osteophyte formation surrounding the canal
- Older age (>50 years)
- Spondylitic disease of the spine may contribute to stenosis.

GENERAL PREVENTION

- Degenerative changes may not be able to be prevented, but symptom severity may be limited by maintaining a healthy back.
- Core strengthening, appropriate flexibility and posture, and maintaining a healthy body weight may slow the progression of symptoms.

COMMONLY ASSOCIATED CONDITIONS

- Degenerative arthritis
- Disk bulging
- Facet osteophytes
- Ligamentum flavum hypertrophy
- Spondylolisthesis (1)

DIAGNOSIS

HISTORY

- Typically, the earliest complaint is back pain.
- The most common symptom is claudication. Claudication, which is bilateral leg pain, numbness and/or tingling often involving the buttocks and thighs and spreading toward the feet that worsens with ambulation and standing.
- Symptoms are relieved by sitting and forward bending (shopping cart sign).
- The pain may be described as burning, cramping, or a dull fatigue.
- In severe late-stage cases where the sacral roots are impinged, visceral disturbance may manifest with urinary incontinence.
- The history for cervical spinal stenosis may include transient quadriplegia after a tackle or just bilateral "stingers" (numbness and pain down both arms).
- Red flag symptoms such as fever, chills, night sweats, unexplained weight loss and pain that worsens with lying supine/at rest may suggest neoplasm or infection.

PHYSICAL EXAM

- A slow, broad-based gait is often present.
- Abnormal Romberg test
- The spine must be examined for abnormal curvature or limitation in range of motion (ROM).
- Commonly, flexion relieves symptoms, and extension is painful.
- The spine should be examined for tenderness, which may suggest a fracture, neoplasm, or infection.
- A full neurologic exam must be done including manual muscle testing, deep tendon reflexes, sensory exam, and gait analysis.
- The straight-leg test should be done to rule out disk herniation. Generally, patients with lumbar spinal stenosis do not have a positive straight-leg test.
- The physical examination also should include an examination of the skin, nails, and distal pulses of the feet to evaluate for possible vascular claudication. Patients with vascular claudication often will have pallor, nail dystrophy, absence of hair, and diminished distal pulses in their feet.

DIFFERENTIAL DIAGNOSIS

- Vascular claudication
- Space-occupying lesion such as a neoplasm
- Herniated disk
- Trauma, for example, compression fracture
- Degenerative subluxation of the vertebrae (spondylolisthesis)
- Infectious process, for example, discitis or epidural abscess

DIAGNOSTIC TESTS & INTERPRETATION

- Imaging can be used to confirm the clinical diagnosis, but spinal stenosis can be seen in asymptomatic individuals.
- Plain films are not diagnostic or specific but may demonstrate degenerative spinal disease.
- In the C-spine, a vertebral canal–vertebral body ratio <0.8 was defined by Torg as spinal stenosis. The Torg ratio, however, is not used exclusively to evaluate cervical spinal stenosis. Even though it carries about a 93% sensitivity, it leads to many false-positive results and has a poor positive predictive value for predicting cervical cord neurapraxia (2)[C].
- Computed tomography (CT) scans ± intrathecal contrast material injection (CT myelogram) may demonstrate encroachment of the canal by osteophytes, hypertrophied lamina, or other degenerative changes.
- Magnetic resonance imaging (MRI) is the preferred method to establish a diagnosis and exclude other conditions. MRI is both noninvasive and visualizes the soft tissue structures that may be obstructing the canal (3)[B].
- There are multiple imaging grading classifications for stenosis with no clear consensus on diagnosis.

TREATMENT

GENERAL MEASURES

- First-line therapy is activity modification, analgesia, and physical therapy (4).
- Nonsurgical management of lumbar stenosis may be attempted initially in patients who do not have severe pain or significant weakness.
- Patients on warfarin, chronic anticoagulants, or those who have severe risks for complications with decompressive surgery may not be candidates for invasive procedures.
- Nonsteroidal anti-inflammatory drugs (NSAIDs) and exercises may provide some relief for patients with lumbar spinal stenosis. Flexion exercises that reduce lumbar lordosis are especially useful.
- Morbidly obese patients should be encouraged to lose weight.
- Research is limited to suggest support for or against specific nonsurgical approaches, but studies are currently ongoing.
- Prehospital:
  - Management of acute symptomatic cervical spinal stenosis after trauma includes stabilization of the spine with a cervical collar and transport to an emergency setting.

MEDICATION

There is little evidence that pharmacologic therapy provides long-term relief in spinal stenosis (3)[B].

ADDITIONAL THERAPIES

- Epidural steroid injections may provide short-term relief (2 to 3 weeks), but long-term efficacy results are conflicting (3),(4)[B].
- 6 weeks of physical therapy is as effective as initially undergoing decompression surgery (5).

SURGERY/OTHER PROCEDURES

- Typically, multilevel decompressive laminectomies are needed if surgery is required because the canal stenosis often occurs at multiple levels.
- Multilevel laminotomies, foraminotomies, and even decompression of the lateral recesses may be alternative methods of treatment.
- Most patients with radiographic and clinical evidence of spinal stenosis get significant long-term relief from decompressive surgery.

COMPLEMENTARY & ALTERNATIVE MEDICINE

- Lumbosacral corset bracing may provide symptomatic relief *without the complications of surgery* (5).
- Acupuncture may provide pain relief, but further research is needed to validate the efficacy.

ONGOING CARE

PROGNOSIS

- According to the North American Spine Society, patients followed for 2 to 10 years with mild to moderate stenosis have a 20–40% chance of requiring surgical intervention.
- Of those who do not have surgery, 50–70% will have improvement in their pain (3)[C].

REFERENCES

1. Deer TR, Grider JS, Pope JE, et al. Best practices for minimally invasive lumbar spinal stenosis treatment 2.0 (MIST): consensus guidance from the American Society of Pain and Neuroscience (ASPN). *J Pain Res*. 2022;15:1325–1354.
2. Torg JS, Guille JT, Jaffe S. Injuries to the cervical spine in American football players. *J Bone Joint Surg Am*. 2002;84(1):112–122.
3. Snyder DL, Doggett D, Turkelson C. Treatment of degenerative lumbar spinal stenosis. *Am Fam Physician*. 2004;70(3):517–520.
4. Katz JN, Zimmerman ZE, Mass H, et al. Diagnosis and management of lumbar spinal stenosis: a review. *JAMA*. 2022;327(17):1688–1699.
5. Zania F, Tomkins-Lane C, Carragee E, et al. Surgical versus nonsurgical treatment for lumbar spinal stenosis. *Spine (Phila Pa 1976)*. 2016;41(14):E857–E868.

ADDITIONAL READING

- Atlas SJ, Delitto A. Spinal stenosis: surgical versus nonsurgical treatment. *Clin Orthop Relat Res*. 2006;443:198–207.
- Bronfort G, Nilsson N, Haas M, et al. Non-invasive physical treatments for chronic/recurrent headache. *Cochrane Database Syst Rev*. 2004;(3):CD001878.
- Gross AR, Hoving JL, Haines TA, et al. A Cochrane review of manipulation and mobilization for mechanical neck disorders. *Spine (Phila Pa 1976)*. 2004;29(14):1541–1548.
- Lurie J, Tomkins-Lane C. Management of lumbar spinal stenosis. *BMJ*. 2016;352:h6234.
- Matz PG, Meagher RJ, Lamer T, et al. *Clinical Guidelines for Multidisciplinary Spine Care: Diagnosis and Treatment of Degenerative Lumbar Spondylolisthesis*. 2nd ed. North American Spine Society; 2014.

CLINICAL PEARLS

- Experience with the National Center for Catastrophic Sports Injury Research suggests that athletes with significant cervical spinal stenosis are at increased risk for quadriplegia and should not participate in contact or collision sports. Referral to a spine specialist is indicated for competitive athletes wishing to return to play.
- To evaluate a patient with surgical hardware for spinal stenosis, CT myelogram is the preferred imaging modality.

S

SPLENIC CONTUSION AND RUPTURE

Tyler D. Ingersoll, DO, CAQSM, ABOFP ▪ Austin Patterson, DO ▪ David S. Edwards, MD, CAQSM

BASICS

DESCRIPTION

- The spleen is an encapsulated hematopoietic organ that lies within the posterior aspect of the left upper quadrant (LUQ) in the peritoneal cavity with proximity to the 9th, 10th, and 11th ribs (1).
- The spectrum of splenic trauma consists of contusion, hematoma, laceration, and rupture.
- Splenic rupture is divided into two major categories: traumatic and nontraumatic rupture.

EPIDEMIOLOGY

- The spleen is the most injured intra-abdominal organ in blunt abdominal trauma. (1)
- Sequela from splenic injury is the leading cause of preventable mortality in sports-related abdominal blunt force trauma (2).

ETIOLOGY AND PATHOPHYSIOLOGY

- The most prevalent mechanism is the result of motor vehicle injury. Direct abdominal blows and falls are leading causes of traumatic rupture (3).
- The spleen is highly vascularized; thus, significant blood loss can occur.

RISK FACTORS

- Participation in collision and contact sports.
- Children have a smaller and more compliant rib cage that offers less protection.
- Underlying hepatic disease, neoplasm, or infection

COMMONLY ASSOCIATED CONDITIONS

- Rib fractures
- Thoracolumbar vertebral fractures
- Other intra-abdominal visceral injury

DIAGNOSIS

HISTORY

- Blunt, splenic injury can occur through a variety of mechanisms.
- Ask focused questions regarding surgical history, recent infections, hepatic diseases, medications such as Nonsteroidal anti-inflammatory drugs (NSAIDs), and bleeding disorders.
- LUQ pain is often accompanied by referred left shoulder pain (Kehr sign) because intra-abdominal bleeding causes irritation of the diaphragm.

PHYSICAL EXAM

- Determine the stability of the patient with attention to primary survey, secondary survey, and vital signs, particularly hypotension (systolic <90 mm Hg), orthostatic hypotension, tachycardia, and tachypnea:
  - Pediatric considerations: Hypotension may not correlate with degree of hypovolemia in children. Serial physical exams, blood pressure (BP) measurements, and labs are essential.
  - Neurologic status: altered mentation
  - Poor perfusion to extremities
- Inspect for ecchymoses or hematoma of the abdomen with close attention to discoloration of the periumbilical area (Cullen sign) or flank (Turner sign) that are consistent with intra-abdominal bleeding; may take up to 24 hours to develop
- Cannot rule out splenic injury with visual findings alone as up to 20% of patients may not display them on initial exam (1)
- Inspect for penetrating injury to the abdomen, flanks, or lower chest.
- Palpate ribs and thoracolumbar spine for tenderness, crepitus, or step-offs.
- Auscultate and then palpate the abdomen for signs of visceral injury or peritonitis.
- Spleen exam in the stable, cooperative patient with no neck or spine injury:
  - Place the patient in the right lateral decubitus position, permitting gravity to anteriorly displace the spleen.
  - Ensure that the patient's hips and knees are flexed to relax the abdominal muscles.
  - Proceed with gentle palpation during deep inspiration.
- Palpation of the spleen >2 cm below the left costal margin is an abnormal finding in adults.

DIFFERENTIAL DIAGNOSIS

- Rib fracture
- Diaphragmatic injury
- Thoracic aorta rupture
- Peritonitis due to liver injury or ruptured hollow viscus
- Pelvic fracture
- Genitourinary trauma
- Rectus sheath hematoma
- Splenomegaly with rupture secondary to:
  - Congestion: liver disease
  - Infiltration: amyloidosis; hematologic malignancies such as leukemia, lymphoma, myeloproliferative disorder
  - Inflammation: acute or chronic such as HIV, tuberculosis, parasitic diseases
  - Extramedullary hematopoiesis

DIAGNOSTIC TESTS & INTERPRETATION

- Complete blood count (CBC)
- Serum electrolytes
- Type and screen or type and crossmatch (hemodynamically unstable patient in preparation for transfusion).
- Serial hemoglobin and hematocrit (suspected evolving bleed; 48 to 72 hours postinsult)
- Urinalysis for evaluation of renal injury
- For the hemodynamically stable patient with blunt splenic injury and no peritonitis, the preferred imaging modality is computed tomography (CT) of abdomen and pelvis with intravenous (IV) contrast (4)[B]:
  - Contrast extravasation ("blush") alone is not an absolute indication for surgery or angiography (4)[C].
  - Focal accumulation of contrast in the parenchyma suggests a contained vascular injury.
- For the hypotensive patient (systolic BP <90 mm Hg), splenic imaging during the focused assessment with sonography in trauma (FAST) is warranted.
- Ultrasound can be helpful and accurate in diagnosis of splenic injury with ability to visualize as little as 100 mL of free fluid in the abdomen with 90% sensitivity (2).
- The American Association for the Surgery of Trauma (AAST) spleen injury scale:
  - 1994: widely used to grade severity
    - Location of hematoma or laceration
    - Percent of spleen damaged
    - Involvement of hilar vessels
  - Advance grade I for multiple injuries up to grade III
  - Some patients will require emergent surgery without preoperative grading.
  - Grade I:
    - Hematoma–subcapsular, <10% surface area (SA)
    - Laceration–capsular tear, extension into parenchyma <1 cm
  - Grade II:
    - Hematoma–subcapsular (10–50% SA) and/or intraparenchymal, <5 cm diameter
    - Laceration–capsular tear, extension into parenchyma 1 to 3 cm, spares trabecular vessels
  - Grade III:
    - Hematoma–subcapsular (>50% SA or expanding), ruptured hematoma in subcapsular or intraparenchymal location, intraparenchymal hematoma ≥5 cm or expanding
    - Laceration–extension into parenchyma >3 cm or involving trabecular vessels
  - Grade IV:
    - Laceration–extension into segmental or hilar vessels, major devascularization >25% of spleen
  - Grade V:
    - Laceration–shattered spleen
    - Vascular–extension into hilar vessels, devascularized spleen
- The World Society of Emergency Surgery (WSES) classification system (3):
  - Defines spleen injuries associated with blunt or penetrating trauma as minor, moderate, or severe
  - Advantages:
    - Incorporates the AAST grading system
    - Accounts for hemodynamic status
    - Applicable to pediatric and adult populations
  - Minor spleen injury: WSES class I:
    - Correlates with AAST I and II in a hemodynamically stable patient
    - CT scan advised
  - Moderate spleen injury: WSES II:
    - Correlates with AAST III in a hemodynamically stable patient
    - CT scan advised
  - Moderate spleen injury: WSES III:
    - Correlates with AAST IV and V in hemodynamically stable patient
    - CT scan advised
  - Severe spleen injury: WSES IV:
    - Correlates with AAST I to V in any hemodynamically unstable patient
    - CT scan is not recommended.

TREATMENT

- The approach to blunt splenic injuries has changed over time from aggressive surgical interventions to more conservative, nonoperative management (NOM) or endovascular management.
- NOM has become the standard management technique in hemodynamically stable patients with spleen injuries (3)[C].
- In hemodynamically unstable patients, the first-line intervention is splenic artery embolization (SAE) based on WSES Census 2022 (3)[C]
- Regarding age stratification for current treatment guidelines, pediatric patients are identified as <15 years of age and adults >15 years of age (5).
- Typically conservative in 75–93% of children and 35–65% of adults (4):
  - Prehospital/sidelines evaluation: primary survey, secondary survey if feasible, urgent transport via ambulance
  - Emergency department: primary and secondary survey if not already done, close hemodynamic monitoring, labs, imaging, IV resuscitation, consultation with trauma surgery, and perhaps interventional radiology colleagues
  - Arrange for urgent transport to a higher level of care if unable to provide close monitoring, serial assessment, and an operative room in the event of laparotomy (4)[B].
  - Inpatient ward versus intensive care unit (ICU): depending on clinical status:
    - Hemodynamic monitoring
    - Serial physical examination and three hemoglobin measurements every 8 hours
    - In the absence of specific complications, deep venous thrombosis (DVT) and venous thromboembolism (VTE) prophylaxis with low-molecular-weight heparin (LMWH) within 48 to 72 hours from hospital admission (3)
    - Consider ICU admission and critical care consultation for:
      - Transfusion requirement
      - Arterial "blush" on CT, grade IV and V injuries
  - Exam significant for hemodynamic instability or diffuse peritonitis warrants urgent laparotomy (2)[A].
- Angiography/angioembolization:
  - Indications:
    - Consider for all blunt or penetrating spleen injury in the hemodynamically stable patient without peritonitis (6).
    - AAST grade ≥3, "blush," moderate hemoperitoneum, clinical evidence of ongoing bleeding (3)
    - Stable patient with high-grade injury (WSES classes II to III, AAST grade >III) as effective adjunct to NOM (6)
  - Complications: 20% of patients (4):
    - Failure to control bleed
    - Missed injuries
    - Splenic abscess
    - Postembolization syndrome (PES) presenting in 90% of pediatric cases. Symptoms consist of abdominal pain, nausea, ileus, and fever; self-limited with spontaneous resolution in 6 to 9 days

ADDITIONAL THERAPIES

- Immunizations in asplenic patients as per Centers for Disease Control (CDC) guidelines are:
  - Seasonal influenza vaccine yearly
  - Tdap vaccine
  - Hib vaccine
  - Pneumococcal vaccines (PCV13 and PPSV23)
  - Meningococcal vaccines against all three serogroups (B, C, and Y)
  - Zoster vaccine in adults >60 years of age
  - Human papillomavirus (HPV) vaccine series in men until 21 years of age and women until 26 years of age
  - Measles, mumps, rubella (MMR) vaccine
  - Varicella vaccine
- Consider tailored antibiotic prophylaxis regimens in high-risk asplenic patients:
  - <6 years of age
  - >50 years of age
  - Inadequate response to pneumococcal vaccine
  - History of previous invasive pneumococcal disease
  - Malignancy or ongoing immunosuppression

ONGOING CARE

FOLLOW-UP RECOMMENDATIONS

- There are no high-quality evidence-based guidelines for return to sport. For adults treated with NOM:
  - WSES class I/AAST grade I to II: no vigorous activities for 3 to 5 weeks.
  - WSES classes II to III/AAST grade III to V: 2 to 4 months
  - Consider contrast-enhanced CT or contrast-enhanced ultrasound before return to vigorous activities.
  - Pediatric consideration: Regardless of injury grade on CT scan, children treated with NOM should avoid vigorous activities for 4 weeks (3)[C].
- Some elite athletes with splenectomy have returned to full sport in as little as 3 weeks. Most injuries take 2.0 to 2.5 months to heal. Return to sport decisions should be individualized (6).
- Reimaging need/frequency determined by response to resuscitation, persistent abdominal pain, persistent evidence of systemic inflammatory response syndrome (SIRS), drop in hemoglobin (5)[C]
- Repeat CT scan in 48 to 72 hours postadmission for WSES class II (AAST grade III) and at 5 to 7 days of trauma (only if remarkable changes are noted at 72 hours) (6)[C].
- Complications:
  - Delayed rupture (within 4 to 8 days) in 1–8% of adults and 0.5–7.5% of children (6)
  - Splenic pseudocyst
  - Overwhelming postsplenectomy infection (OPSI)—50% mortality:
    - Encapsulated organisms: *Streptococcus pneumoniae*, *Neisseria meningitidis*, *Haemophilus influenzae* type B (Hib)
    - Parasites: malaria, babesia
    - Others: *Capnocytophaga canimorsus* from dog/human bites
- Outpatient follow-up: Immunizations are administered at 14 days postsurgery but should be given prior to hospital discharge if follow-up reliability is questioned.

REFERENCES

1. Akoury T, Whetstone DR. *Splenic Rupture*. StatPearls Publishing; 2023. Accessed date August 20, 2025. https://www.ncbi.nlm.nih.gov/books/NBK525951/
2. Gannon EH, Howard T. Splenic injuries in athletes: a review. *Curr Sports Med Rep*. 2010;9(2):111–114.
3. Podd M, De Simone B, Ceresoli M, et al. Follow-up strategies for patients with splenic trauma managed non-operatively: the 2022 World Society of Emergency Surgery consensus document. *World J Emerg Surg*. 2022;17(1):52.
4. Stassen NA, Buhllar I, Cheng JD, et al. Selective nonoperative management of blunt splenic injury: an Eastern Association for the Surgery of Trauma practice management guideline. *J Trauma Acute Care Surg*. 2012;73(5 Suppl 4):S294–S300.
5. Larsen JW, Thorsen K, Soreide K. Splenic injury from blunt trauma. *Br J Surg*. 2023;110(9):1035–1038.
6. Juyia RF, Kerr HA. Return to play after liver and spleen trauma. *Sports Health*. 2014;6(3):239–245.

ADDITIONAL READING

- Crichton JCI, Naidoo K, Yet B, et al. The role of splenic angioembolization as an adjunct to nonoperative management of blunt splenic injuries: a systematic review and meta-analysis. *J Trauma Acute Care Surg*. 2017;83(5):934–943.
- El-Matbouly M, Jabbour G, El-Menyar A, et al. Blunt splenic trauma: assessment, management and outcomes. *Surgeon*. 2016;14(1):52–58.
- Putukian M, McGrew CA, Benjamin HJ, et al. American Medical Society of Sports Medicine position statement: mononucleosis and athletic participation. *Clin J Sport Med*. 2023;33(4):359–367.

CLINICAL PEARLS

- Splenic contusion and rupture occur in a variety of sports and can be subtle initially. Consider spleen injury in the differential of patients with abdominal pain.
- "Delayed rupture" of the spleen can occur several days after initial injury. A high index of suspicion is essential.
- Evidence-based guidelines regarding return to play are lacking. Patients with infectious mononucleosis require of minimum of 3 weeks before reevaluation. Most patient require 8 to 10 weeks for full recovery. Return to play is an individualized decision that varies based on sport and training level. It is ultimately determined by the managing physician. Most patients require 8 to 10 weeks for full recovery.

S

SPONDYLOARTHROPATHIES (SERONEGATIVE RA)

Brent H. Messick, MD, MS, FAAFP, FASCM, CAQSM • Kevin E. Burroughs, MD, CAQSM, FAMSSM

BASICS

DESCRIPTION

- Spectrum of chronic inflammatory disorders that impair spinal function and mobility over time
- Spondyloarthropathy (SpA) is a term applied to the clinical, radiologic, and immunogenetic features shared by a group of diseases that include:
  - Ankylosing spondylitis (AS)
  - Reactive arthritis (ReA)
  - Psoriatic arthritis (PsA)
  - Arthritis associated with inflammatory bowel disease (IBD)
  - Juvenile onset spondyloarthritis
  - Undifferentiated spondyloarthropathy (USpA):
    - These conditions are variably associated with the human leukocyte antigen B27 (HLA-B27). Individuals with these conditions frequently exhibit overlapping clinical and radiologic features.
- Synonym(s): seronegative spondyloarthropathies; HLA-B27–related SpA

EPIDEMIOLOGY

- AS and USpA are the most common types of SpA.
- AS and ReA are more common in males.
- SpA is seen in all age groups, but most cases present at 20 to 50 years of age.

Incidence

ReA incidence: 3–8% (1)

Prevalence

- SpA: 0.5–2% of the Caucasian population
- AS: 1 to 2/1,000
- ReA: 1/1,000
- PsA develops in 5% of patients with psoriasis.

ETIOLOGY AND PATHOPHYSIOLOGY

- Most cases of SpA are associated with HLA-B27.
- ReA is triggered by an infectious agent (*Yersinia, Escherichia coli, Shigella, Salmonella, Campylobacter, Chlamydia*, and others) (1),(2).
- Inflammation and immune system activation at the entheses and subchondral bone leads to bone destruction.

Genetics

- HLA-B27 positivity:
  - AS 90–95%
  - ReA 80%
  - USpA 70%, PsA 40%
  - IBD associated 30%
- 8% of Caucasians and 4% of African Americans are HLA-B27 positive.
- <20% of HLA-B27–positive individuals will develop SpA.

RISK FACTORS

- Male
- Caucasian
- Unprotected sex
- Positive family history
- Populations with high HLA-B27 prevalence, such as Northern European
- ReA is significantly increased in persons with HIV.
- More common in patients who were not breast fed

DIAGNOSIS

- There are several sets of criteria used for research purposes, including the European Spondyloarthropathy Study Group (ESSG) criteria. More recently, the Assessment of Spondyloarthritis International Society (ASAS) criteria have been shown to be the most specific (3).
- ASAS criteria:
  - Sacroiliitis on imaging plus one of the following or HLA-B27 and two of the following:
    - Sausage digit
    - Psoriasis—family history of SpA
    - Inflammatory back pain
    - Nonsteroidal anti-inflammatory drugs (NSAIDs) good response
    - Enthesitis
    - Arthritis
    - Crohn/colitis—elevated C-reactive protein (CRP)
    - Uveitis

HISTORY

- Inflammatory back pain:
  - Insidious onset of low back pain before the age of 40 years
  - Morning stiffness (>30 minutes)
  - Often associated with night pain
  - Persists for >3 months
  - Improved with exercise and NSAIDs (inflammatory vs. mechanical back pain)
- Low back pain at night with prominent early morning stiffness (sacroiliitis, spondylitis)
- Peripheral joint pain and swelling (often lower limb and asymmetric)
- Pain and inflammation at the insertion of tendons or ligaments (enthesitis), sausage digits (dactylitis)
- Other joint or enthesis involvement; eye, bowel, skin, mucous membrane, gut, genitourinary symptoms

PHYSICAL EXAM

- Ocular: conjunctivitis, iritis
- Gastrointestinal (GI): oral ulcerations, gut inflammation
- Skin and nails: psoriasis, keratoderma blennorrhagica, psoriatic nail dystrophy
- Genitourinary: urethritis, cervicitis, circinate balanitis
- Constitutional: fever and weight loss (ReA)
- Lumbar spine: restricted range of motion:
  - Schober test: Mark the spinous process of L5 and make a mark 10 cm above that point. Ask the patient to bend forward. The distance between the two points should increase by >5 cm in a normal subject.
- Peripheral joints: tender and/or warm
- Enthesitis: tenderness around the heel (Achilles or plantar fascia)

DIFFERENTIAL DIAGNOSIS

- Rheumatoid arthritis
- Osteoarthritis
- PsA
- Seronegative arthritis
- Gout
- Septic (gonococcal) arthritis
- Sarcoidosis

DIAGNOSTIC TESTS & INTERPRETATION

- Elevated erythrocyte sedimentation rate (ESR) or CRP
- Elevated white blood cells (WBCs) in peripheral and synovial fluid:
  - These studies have poor sensitivity and specificity.
- Joint space narrowing, signs of inflammation, multiple joint involvement, and distal involvement in the hands and feet with added features of bone proliferation suggest seronegative SpA:
  - Differentiation of these relies on the distribution of radiographic abnormalities and clinical information.
- Peripheral arthritis with soft tissue swelling, juxta-articular osteopenia, joint space narrowing, and erosions
- Areas of periostitis or osteitis are not uncommon (PsA, ReA).
- PsA:
  - Typically involves the hands, wrists, and feet; bilateral or unilateral, symmetric or asymmetric
  - Involvement of several joints in a single digit produces the classic "sausage digit."

  - Irregular and indistinct appearance of marginal bone about the joint, characterized as "fuzzy" or "whiskering"; may also see one side of joint thinned, the other broad ("pencil in cup")
  - In foot sclerosis, enthesitis, periostitis, and soft tissue swelling can give an "ivory phalanx" appearance.
  - At the sacroiliac (SI) joint, advanced changes are usually bilateral and show bone erosions and narrowing to the point of fusion.
- ReA:
  - Similar features to PsA
  - Lower extremity involvement more common than upper. Sausage digit and pencil-in-cup deformities can also occur.
  - In the spine, large, comma-shaped, paravertebral ossification may also be seen.
- AS:
  - More commonly involves the axial skeleton, although peripheral joints can be affected
  - The spine findings are characterized by osteitis, syndesmophyte formation, facet inflammation, and eventual facet joint and vertebral body fusion (bamboo spine of AS).
  - SI joint disease is often bilateral and symmetric and typically precedes spine involvement.
  - Magnetic resonance imaging (MRI) may detect up to 75% of early sacroiliitis not seen on plain radiography.
  - Spine involvement is centered at the thoracolumbar or lumbosacral junction. Focal areas of osteitis become sclerotic and are termed *the shiny corner sign*.
  - Ultrasound may show areas of abnormal vascularization of the entheses.

TREATMENT

- The goal of treatment is to reduce pain and stiffness and maintain posture and function.
- Eye, skin, genitourinary, and bowel involvement should be treated accordingly.
- Patients with spondylitis should engage in a lifelong program of exercise to preserve posture and mobility.
- Antibiotic therapy is indicated for proven acute bacterial infections but does not reduce arthritis.

MEDICATION

First Line

NSAIDs and topical/intra-articular steroids for acute pain

Second Line

- Disease-modifying antirheumatic drugs: Adalimumab, certolizumab, etanercept, golimumab or infliximab, and methotrexate are used for chronic pain and inflammation (4).
- Sulfasalazine is not recommended for purely axial disease but can be useful for patients with peripheral disease (4).
- Pamidronate for refractory cases (4)[C]

ISSUES FOR REFERRAL

Referral to an ophthalmologist for ocular symptoms because these may require additional treatments

ADDITIONAL THERAPIES

- Joint splinting and rest may be indicated for acute flares.
- Physical therapy and home exercise plans

SURGERY/OTHER PROCEDURES

Joint arthroplasty may be required for those with severe peripheral joint disease.

REFERENCES

1. Denison HJ, Curtis EM, Clynes MA, et al. The incidence of sexually acquired reactive arthritis: a systematic literature review. *Clin Rheumatol.* 2016;35(11):2639–2648.
2. Townes JM, Deodhar AA, Laine ES, et al. Reactive arthritis following culture-confirmed infections with bacterial enteric pathogens in Minnesota and Oregon: a population-based study. *Ann Rheum Dis.* 2008;67(12):1689–1696.
3. Chung HY, Lau CS, Wu KP, et al. Comparison of performance of the Assessment of SpondyloArthritis International Society, the European Spondyloarthropathy Study Group and the modified New York criteria in a cohort of Chinese patients with spondyloarthritis. *Clin Rheumatol.* 2011;30(7):947–953.
4. Navarro-Compán V, Sepriano A, El-Zorkany B, et al. Axial spondyloarthritis. *Ann Rheum Dis.* 2021;80(12):1511–1521.

ADDITIONAL READING

- Akgul O, Ozgocmen S. Classification criteria for spondyloarthropathies. *World J Orthop.* 2011;2(12):107–115.
- Buckton KE, Jacobs PA, Court Brown WM, et al. A study of the chromosome damage persisting after x-ray therapy for ankylosing spondylitis. *Lancet.* 1962;2(7258):676–682.
- Callhoff J, Sieper J, Weiß A, et al. Efficacy of TNFα blockers in patients with ankylosing spondylitis and non-radiographic axial spondyloarthritis: a meta-analysis. *Ann Rheum Dis.* 2015;74(6):1241–1248.
- Kataria RK, Brent LH. Spondyloarthropathies. *Am Fam Physician.* 2004;69(12):2853–2860.
- López-Medina C, Ramiro S, van der Heijde D, et al. Characteristics and burden of disease in patients with radiographic and non-radiographic axial spondyloarthritis: a comparison by systematic literature review and meta-analysis. *RMD Open.* 2019;5(2):e001108.
- Mandl P, Navarro-Compán V, Terslev L, et al. EULAR recommendations for the use of imaging in the diagnosis and management of spondyloarthritis in clinical practice. *Ann Rheum Dis.* 2015;74(7):1327–1339.
- Montoya J, Matta NB, Suchon P, et al. Patients with ankylosing spondylitis have been breast fed less often than healthy controls: a case-control retrospective study. *Ann Rheum Dis.* 2016;75(5):879–882.
- Olivieri I, Salvarani C, Cantini F, et al. Ankylosing spondylitis and undifferentiated spondyloarthropathies: a clinical review and description of a disease subset with older age at onset. *Curr Opin Rheumatol.* 2001;13(4):280–284.
- Oostveen J, Prevo R, den Boer J, et al. Early detection of sacroiliitis on magnetic resonance imaging and subsequent development of sacroiliitis on plain radiography. A prospective, longitudinal study. *J Rheumatol.* 1999;26(9):1953–1958.
- Ramiro S, Stolwijk C, van Tubergen A, et al. Evolution of radiographic damage in ankylosing spondylitis: a 12 year prospective follow-up of the OASIS study. *Ann Rheum Dis.* 2015;74(1):52–59.
- Walsh JA, Magrey M. Clinical manifestations and diagnosis of axial spondyloarthritis. *J Clin Rheumatol.* 2021;27(8):e547–e560.

CLINICAL PEARLS

- SpA is a term applied to the clinical, radiologic, and immunogenetic features shared by a group of diseases including AS, ReA, PsA, IBD, and USpA.
- Most patients will exhibit sacroiliitis on imaging, HLA-B27, and some or all of the following: sausage digit, inflammatory back pain, relief with NSAIDs, psoriasis, enthesitis, arthritis, Crohn/colitis, and uveitis.
- Treatment should address pain relief, joint preservation, maintenance of activity, and management of eye, skin, GI, or GU involvement.

SPONDYLOLYSIS AND SPONDYLOLISTHESIS

Timothy Tiu, MD, FAAPMR, CAQSM • Edwin Amirianfar, DO

BASICS

DESCRIPTION

- From Greek, spondylo (vertebra) + lysis (loosening), or listhesis (slippage)
- Spondylolysis:
  - Involves a defect in the pars interarticularis of the vertebral complex
  - Usually an acquired stress fracture or stress reaction of the lower lumbar spine (L-spine)
  - Can be unilateral or bilateral; if bilateral, can lead to spondylolisthesis (1)
- Spondylolisthesis:
  - Results from displacement of a vertebral body on the subjacent vertebra; defect may be secondary to fracture, arthrosis, or systemic disease.
  - Vertebral translation can be a source of pain, radiculopathy (spinal nerve injury), or spinal cord injury.

EPIDEMIOLOGY

- Spondylolysis and spondylolisthesis are the most common causes of back pain in children and adolescents >10 years old (2).
- Spondylolysis:
  - Most common cause of significant back pain in young athletes
  - Prevalence: 23–63% in young athletes (3)
  - Frequently develops between 7 and 10 years of age; very rare in patients <5 or >20 years of age (3)
  - Highest incidence in sports emphasizing extension activities
  - Seen most commonly in adolescent male athletes
  - Most commonly involves L5 (95% of cases) (1)
- Spondylolisthesis:
  - Most common segment involved is the L5–S1 level, followed by L4–L5 (4).
  - 75% of cases are grade I (4).
  - Incidence of isthmic spondylolisthesis: 6–7% by the age of 18 years (4)

ETIOLOGY AND PATHOPHYSIOLOGY

- Spondylolysis:
  - May be either an overuse injury (continued microtrauma to pars interarticularis from repetitive spinal flexion, extension and rotation, and shear forces to the L-spine) or a traumatic fracture
  - Shear forces on the normal lumbar lordosis are increased in extension and accentuated by combined extension and lateral side bending.
- Spondylolisthesis:
  - Isthmic (spondylolytic) spondylolisthesis:
    - Listhesis caused by breakdown/fracture of bilateral pars interarticularis
    - Most common cause of listhesis in patients <50 years old, representing up to 50% in some series
    - Most common cause of listhesis in athletes
    - Usually occurs at L5–S1
  - Dysplastic (congenital) spondylolisthesis:
    - Caused by failure of development of the superior facets
    - Represents 20% of all cases of listhesis
    - Major slippage can occur
    - Usually occurs at L5–S1
  - Degenerative spondylolisthesis:
    - Caused by facet joint osteoarthritis, degenerative disk disease, and ligamentum flavum hypertrophy
    - Most common cause of listhesis in patients >50 years old
    - Typically occurs at L4–L5
    - Major cause of spinal stenosis
    - Has higher incidence of cauda equina or nerve root compression
  - Traumatic spondylolisthesis:
    - Disruption of the posterior elements of the neural arch other than pars (pedicles or lamina)
    - Requires large force (also likely to have other fractures)
  - Pathologic spondylolisthesis:
    - Due to osteoporosis, rheumatoid arthritis, tumor, or infection (5)

RISK FACTORS

- Genetics: Up to 70% of patients with spondylolysis have a first-degree relative with spondylolysis (3).
- Sports involving extreme spinal motion, especially repetitive hyperextension and rotational movements (e.g., football linemen, diving, Olympic weight lifting, wrestling, rowing, gymnastics, throwing sports, and high jump in track and field)
- Adolescent growth spurts (fatigue fractures)
- Anatomic variations: spina bifida occulta, transitional vertebrae, elongated pars interarticularis, scoliosis
- Biomechanics: increased lumbar lordosis and/or increased pelvic inclination (contributed to by tight hip flexors and weak abdominal muscles), increased hamstring tightness (3)

DIAGNOSIS

- Classification of spondylolisthesis by direction:
  - Anterolisthesis (most common): forward slippage of superior vertebra over inferior vertebra
  - Retrolisthesis: backward slippage of superior vertebra over inferior vertebra
- Grading of spondylolisthesis (Meyerding classification)
  - Displacement of cranial vertebral body relative to caudal as visualized on lateral x-ray:
    - Grade I: <25%
    - Grade II: 25–50%
    - Grade III: 50–75%
    - Grade IV: 75–100%
    - Grade V: >100%; also termed spondyloptosis (5)

HISTORY

- Spondylolysis:
  - May be found incidentally on radiographic examination (1)
  - If symptomatic, most commonly complain of insidious onset of low back pain
  - Pain is usually worse with activity, especially spine flexion and extension/lateral side bending and better with rest (1).
  - Pain may radiate into the buttocks or posterior thigh, but patients rarely experience neurologic signs or symptoms (1).
  - May note increase in symptoms with an increase in intensity or volume of training; uncommon reports of numbness, paresthesias, weakness, bowel or bladder changes, gait disturbance, or constitutional symptoms (fever, weight loss, night pain, or rashes)
- Spondylolisthesis:
  - Majority are asymptomatic (5). If symptomatic, typically derive from mechanical etiology or spinal stenosis. Over half of symptomatic individuals report sciatica or radicular symptoms (usually after long-standing back pain).
  - May have cauda equina or claudication symptoms

PHYSICAL EXAM

- Symptomatic patient may be tender to palpation of the spinous process or paraspinal musculature.
- Can exhibit hamstring tightness (crouch gait) and hyperlordosis (5)
- May exhibit limited range of motion and pain with extension
- Some suggest performing the "stork" test or single leg lumbar hyperextension test:
  - Ipsilateral back pain when a patient stands on one leg and hyperextends the back may indicate active spondylolysis (not sensitive or specific for spondylolysis)
- If significant listhesis is present (≥ grade III), may appreciate a step-off when palpating the spinous processes (5).
- Gait abnormality if severe pain
- Neurologic findings are rare.

DIFFERENTIAL DIAGNOSIS

- Infection
- Tumor
- Herniated nucleus pulposus
- Mechanical low back pain
- Spinal stenosis
- Muscle strain
- Fibromyalgia

DIAGNOSTIC TESTS & INTERPRETATION

- Plain films:
  - Anteroposterior (AP) and lateral views (for spondylolisthesis), and oblique views (for spondylolysis)
  - Fracture is not appreciated on lateral views; oblique views may be helpful but not ideal as iliac wings may obscure L5 and S1 vertebra (1)[C].
  - May be normal in the acute or subacute stage
  - Standing lateral x-ray can help with grading of listhesis.
  - Weight-bearing x-rays may worsen the apparent slip by up to 25%.
  - Oblique films may allow visualization of the "Scottie dog"; a radiolucent line through the "dog's neck" may represent a defect through the pars interarticularis (2)[C]. Because of radiation exposure, most centers are not including oblique views.
  - Indirect sign of spondylolysis on AP view include lateral deviation of the spinous process and sclerosis of the contralateral pedicle (2)[C]
  - On standing AP view, an "inverted Napoleon hat sign" can be seen with large (grade IV/V) slips, representing the radiographic appearance of spondyloptosis. This increases risk of cauda equina syndrome.
- Triple-phase bone scan: used to evaluate the acuity of the injury
  - Can demonstrate defects unseen on plain x-ray
  - Can be positive as soon as 48 to 72 hours after injury
  - High false-positive rate in older patients, especially those with significant osteoarthritis of the L-spine
  - Not recommended in asymptomatic patients or in patients with symptoms >1 year
- Single-photon emission computed tomography (SPECT) scan:
  - If normal radiographs in setting of high clinical suspicion of spondylolysis, SPECT of the lumbosacral spine is useful for further workup (5)[C].
  - Improves resolution of planar bone scans (allows for precise localization)

- Most sensitive tool in diagnosing spondylolysis (2)[C]
- May be more helpful in demonstrating stress reactions at the pars and provides excellent resolution of the bony anatomy to characterize cortical defects, incomplete fractures, and sclerotic changes associated with pars injury (2)[C]
- Advantage: may help delineate the acute "hot" lesion with potential to heal versus more chronic "cold" lesion that may not heal or progress to a fibrous union:
  - Pars defect on imaging with normal SPECT scan indicates inactive healed lesion or nonunion (3)[B].
- Disadvantage: may not be widely available, much greater radiation exposure than computed tomography (CT) scans (3), and cannot distinguish spondylolysis from facet spondylosis, infection, or osteoid osteoma

- CT scan:
  - Best to visualize spondylolysis with pars fracture
  - Can delineate neural compression and assess fracture healing (2)[C]
  - Useful after SPECT to help stage and determine treatment stratification
  - Reverse gantry thin-cut CT used at the level seen on SPECT scan to define morphology of defect
  - Advantage: visualization of bony anatomy, assessment of healing at later interval (6 months)
  - Disadvantage: radiation exposure (50 times plain films), not reliable to identify early stress fracture and to distinguish acute from chronic fractures (2)[C]
- Magnetic resonance imaging (MRI):
  - MRI has recently emerged as a potential initial diagnostic imaging rather than CT or SPECT for suspected lumbosacral spondylolysis (2)[C].
  - Addition of tau or short-tau inversion recovery sequence improves the sensitivity for bone marrow edema to detect early pars stress reactions (2),(3)[B].
  - Compared to bone SPECT, MRI has demonstrated a high sensitivity and specificity for distinguishing normal pars from grade 1 or higher injury (2)[C].
  - Advantages: lack of radiation, ability to detect other pathology (discitis, disk pathology, tumor), good to evaluate nerve root compression, able to detect early pars stress reactions that cannot be seen on x-ray or CT
  - Needed if cauda equina symptoms present
  - Disadvantages: unable to determine if lesion is improving or worsening, can miss spondylolysis, and may see false positives in younger patients secondary to normal bone marrow edema
  - If negative results when MRI used as initial diagnostic test, further radiographic follow-up should be performed (2).

TREATMENT

GENERAL MEASURES

- Goal is to return the athlete to pain-free participation in sports along with the prevention of further slippage and spondylolisthesis.
- Spondylolysis:
  - Rest from activity is indicated at least until pain is alleviated. Some suggest a minimum 3 months of restriction from sport.
  - Physical therapy is generally recommended with exercises directed at core strengthening (i.e., deep abdominal musculature) and back extensors (e.g., lumbar multifidi).
  - Timing of physical therapy is controversial. Some advocate early therapy, whereas other recommend initiating therapy after period of restriction.
  - Bracing:
    - Controversial
    - Biomechanical studies have shown that the bracing poorly stabilizes lower lumbar vertebral segments which are most commonly affected.
    - Satisfactory outcomes can be achieved with or without bracing.
    - Most suggest using the brace if initial conservative management fails.
    - Reported duration is variable (6 weeks to 6 months).
    - If used, should continue until patient is asymptomatic with all activities
    - Positive x-ray and negative bone scan demonstrate a chronic injury that usually does not need bracing (2)[C].
  - For lesions with chronic features on CT, healing is unlikely; however, rest should continue until full resolution of symptoms (6)[C].
  - Surgical intervention is indicated only for individuals who have failed >12 months conservative management or for advanced cases causing neural compromise.
  - Surgical intervention can include direct repair of the pars interarticularis (Buck screw, Scott wiring technique, and Morscher hook screw) or posterolateral fusion (2)[C].
  - Fusion has high efficacy (>70%) in providing pain relief (1)[C].
  - One study showed that Buck procedure resulted in 18/19 patients returning to sport within 7 months (2)[C].
- Spondylolisthesis:
  - Low-grade slips (grades I and II) treated similarly to spondylolysis (2)[C]
  - 70–90% of athletes can expect to return to activities with 3 to 6 months of conservative treatment (5)[C].
  - If low-grade and failed conservative treatment for 6 to 12 months, consider surgery (2)[C].
  - Higher grade listhesis (>50%), high slip angle (>55 degrees), slip progression, or any neurologic findings should be evaluated by a surgeon (5)[C].

ADDITIONAL THERAPIES

Physical therapy:

- Initial treatment will include modalities followed by strengthening activity.
- Typical rehabilitation includes hamstring/hip stretching and core strengthening (low back, hip, and abdominal musculature) (2)[C]
- Water therapy, including water running, is very helpful when available.
- Aerobic conditioning with progression to sport-specific drills

ONGOING CARE

FOLLOW-UP RECOMMENDATIONS

- Monitor symptoms and gait abnormalities, and radiographic progression of spondylolisthesis
- In the skeletally immature, monitoring is more important because changes are common during growth (3).
- X-rays: Data on the timing and frequency of follow-up x-rays are not clear; may consider plain x-ray every 6 to 12 months if skeletally immature; monitoring radiographic progression is no longer recommended if patient is responding well to treatment (6).
- Risk factors to consider when assessing for slip progression of listhesis:
  - Female, obesity, facet sagittalization, baseline slip, decreased intervertebral disc space, increased laxity on flexion/extension x-rays, high pelvic incidence, high L4 or L5 vertebral angle, high lumbar lordotic angle (7)

PROGNOSIS

- Most young athletes with symptomatic spondylolysis are successfully managed nonoperatively (1).
- Most patients with acute spondylolysis eventually will have mild to no symptoms with conservative treatment.
- 92% of athletes are able to return to sport with little to no pain within 6 months of conservative treatment (6).
- Progression of listhesis uncommon after age 20 years due to ossification of growth plate (1)
- Following fusion for spondylolysis/spondylolisthesis, varying opinions based on surgeon's preference with some being against return to contact sports altogether (8)

REFERENCES

1. Li N, Amarasinghe S, Boudreaux K, et al. Spondylolysis. *Orthop Rev (Pavia).* 2022;14(3):37470.
2. Chung CC, Shimer AL. Lumbosacral spondylolysis and spondylolisthesis. *Clin Sports Med.* 2021;40(3):471–490.
3. Choi JH, Ochoa JK, Lubinus A, et al. Management of lumbar spondylolysis in the adolescent athlete: a review of over 200 cases. *Spine J.* 2022;22(10):1628–1633.
4. Tenny S, Gillis CC. *Spondylolisthesis.* StatPearls Publishing; 2023. Updated May 22, 2023. Accessed August 8, 2025. https://www.ncbi.nlm.nih.gov/books/NBK430767/
5. Li N, Scofield J, Mangham P, et al. Spondylolisthesis. *Orthop Rev (Pavia).* 2022;14(4):36917.
6. Selhorst M, Allen M, McHugh R, et al. Rehabilitation considerations for spondylolysis in the youth athlete. *Int J Phys Ther.* 2020;15(2):287–300.
7. Atalay B, Gadjradj PS, Sommer FS, et al. Natural history of degenerative spondylolisthesis. A systematic review and meta-analysis. *World Neurosurg.* 2023;176:e634–e643.
8. Prakash AA. Return to play after spondylolysis: an overview. *Med J Armed Forces India.* 2021;77(1):6–14.

ADDITIONAL READING

Achar S, Hwang D, Finkenstaedt T, et al. Deep-learning-aided evaluation of spondylolysis imaged with ultrashort echo time magnetic resonance imaging. *Sensors (Basel).* 2023;23(18):8001.

CLINICAL PEARLS

- Initial imaging for suspected spondylolysis or spondylolisthesis, in the absence of neurologic abnormalities, should be x-ray with AP and lateral views.
- SPECT scan is the most sensitive imaging modality in diagnosing spondylolysis; however, radiation exposure from SPECT surpasses that of CT (3).
- Bilateral spondylolysis can potentially progress to isthmic spondylolisthesis.
- Pars defect on x-ray with normal SPECT scan indicates inactive healed lesion or nonunion (3).
- Use of bracing for conservative management of spondylolysis is controversial. Most recommend using brace if initial conservative management fails.
- Important to assess for neurologic deficits in athletes with spondylolysis and spondylolisthesis

SPORTS HERNIAS

Warren Young, MD, FAAP

BASICS

DESCRIPTION

- The sports hernia is a syndrome of chronic pain owing to weakness or injury to the posterior inguinal canal, conjoined tendon, common adductor origin, external oblique aponeurosis, and/or rectus abdominis.
- Typically described as an activity-related pain of either insidious or acute onset, predominantly in the lower abdominal or groin area with no other obvious pathology, such as a hernia, to explain the symptoms.
- Historically considered to be an early direct inguinal hernia, but recent evidence shows that no true hernia exists. Therefore, the term sports hernia is a misnomer.
- Per the Doha agreement, injuries should be named and classified as one of three distinct groin pain groups: defined groin pain, hip-related groin pain, or other groin pain.
- Synonym(s): core muscle injury, athletic pubalgia; sportsman's hernia; Gilmore groin; inguinal disruption; inguinal-related groin pain; footballer's groin; hockey groin syndrome

EPIDEMIOLOGY

Incidence

- Unknown
- Male predominance: accounts for >90% of cases
- Most common in soccer players but also described in football, hockey, baseball, rugby, skiing, wrestling, and tennis players among others
- Mostly diagnosed in professional or high-level athletes, but increasing in recreational athletes

ETIOLOGY AND PATHOPHYSIOLOGY

Pathogenesis is unclear:

- May be related to overuse and excessive inguinal wall stress due to underlying muscle strength, balance, stability, or endurance inequality between a weaker abdominal musculature and a stronger hip adductor muscle group
- Posterior inguinal canal weakness seen in 85% of surgical cases
- Multiple injured structures are often seen operatively, including:
  - Distal rectus abdominis
  - Conjoint tendon
  - External oblique aponeurosis
  - Inguinal ligament
  - Adductor longus muscle/tendon

RISK FACTORS

Activities with sudden acceleration and deceleration, kicking, cutting, twisting, and turning

GENERAL PREVENTION

Strength and conditioning programs that stress flexibility and core strength, decrease muscle imbalances (such as between abdominal oblique and rectus abdominus), and emphasize sport-specific movements may play a preventative role

COMMONLY ASSOCIATED CONDITIONS

- Groin pain is often multifactorial.
- High rate of coexisting adductor longus tendinosis and femoroacetabular impingement (FAI)

DIAGNOSIS

HISTORY

- Activity-related lower abdominal and proximal adductor-related pain with quick acceleration, deceleration, kicking, twisting, or lateral movement
- Often occurs in soccer players from hard or long kicks
- Relieved with rest but returns with resumption of sports
- Often gradual in onset but may occur after sudden tearing sensation
- Early in course, pain is felt after activity or toward the end of activity.
- As condition progresses, pain is more severe and occurs earlier in activity. Decreased ability to twist, turn, or stride out is observed.
- Later in course, pain occurs with running and may progress to affect daily activities.
- Usually unilateral but may radiate to uninvolved side or scrotum or be bilateral in etiology
- Exacerbated by sudden movements, sit-ups, coughing/sneezing, Valsalva maneuver (i.e., mimics hernia pain)
- Ask about hip joint–related mechanical symptoms including catching, locking, and giving way.

PHYSICAL EXAM

- Diagnosis of sports hernia may be made if at least three of the following five signs exist (1)[C]:
  - Pinpoint tenderness to the pubic tubercle at conjoint tendon insertion
  - Tenderness over deep inguinal ring
  - Pain and/or dilation of the external ring with no palpable hernia
  - Pain at origin of adductor longus tendon
  - Dull diffuse groin pain often radiating to perineum and inner thigh or across the midline
- Classification of defined groin pain entities by exam (2)[C]:
  - Hip adductor origin tenderness *and* pain with resisted adduction suggest adductor-related groin pain.
  - Tenderness at pubic symphysis suggests pubic-related groin pain.
  - Pain with resisted hip flexion *and/or* stretching of hip flexors suggests iliopsoas-related groin pain.
    - Pain in the inguinal canal region *and* pain on palpation along the canal is suggestive of inguinal-related groin pain. Likelihood for this increases with pain after cough/Valsalva *or* resistance testing of abdominal muscles.
- Physical exam for hip-related groin pain may elicit pain with passive range of motion (ROM); flexion, adduction, and internal rotation (FADIR); and flexion, abduction, external rotation (FABER) tests.
  - Adductor-related, pubic-related, iliopsoas-related, inguinal-related, hip joint–related, other groin pain.
- Thorough hip/genitourinary exam should be performed to assess for nonorthopedic causes of groin pain. These causes are classified as other groin pain.

DIFFERENTIAL DIAGNOSIS

- Inguinal or femoral hernia
- Hip adductor strain
- Rectus abdominis strain
- FAI
- Osteitis pubis
- Bursitis
- Snapping hip syndrome
- Femoral neck stress fracture
- Pubic ramus fracture
- Hip apophysitis or avulsion fracture
- Nerve entrapment:
  - Obturator
  - Ilioinguinal
  - Genitofemoral
  - Iliohypogastric
- Referred pain from lumbar spine or sacroiliac joint
- Intra-articular hip pathology
- Testicular/ovarian pathology
- Spondyloarthropathy
- Lymphadenopathy

DIAGNOSTIC TESTS & INTERPRETATION

- No diagnostic imaging test is specific for sports hernia. Many patients will have no pathologic findings at all on any imaging study.
- Magnetic resonance imaging (MRI) is the advanced imaging modality most commonly performed.
- To identify associated muscle, tendon, cartilage, bony intra-articular pathology, or occult stress fractures as well as nerve entrapment
- Plain radiographs can evaluate for fractures, degenerative disease, FAI, dysplasia, pubic symphysis disruption.
- Bone scan/computed tomography (CT) scan may identify stress fractures, osteitis pubis.
- Dynamic ultrasound may visualize posterior inguinal wall insufficiency, but it is highly operator dependent.
- Herniography is not recommended due to invasive nature and complication risk.
- Electromyography, nerve conduction studies, and ultrasound may demonstrate nerve entrapment or injury.

TREATMENT

GENERAL MEASURES

- Nonoperative treatment should be attempted for at least 3 months prior to surgical consideration.
- Nonsurgical rehabilitation treatment:
  - Initial 6- to 8-week period of rest with supportive care (nonsteroidal anti-inflammatory drugs [NSAIDs], ice, heat) followed by a 6- to 8-week rehabilitation program with gradual return to sports activity
  - Initial focus on hip adductor stretching, with progression to hip and abdominal strengthening, core stabilization and balance exercises, followed by sports-specific functional exercise (3)[B]
- Ultrasound-guided injection to rectus abdominis insertion, conjoint tendon, or adductor tendon may be considered, but there is limited evidence for its efficacy.
- Nerve ablation has been described for nerve entrapment or surgical release.

SURGERY/OTHER PROCEDURES

- Surgery should be considered if nonoperative treatment fails after 3 or more months.
- Herniorrhaphy is the definitive treatment.
- Surgical techniques vary, but general principles are the repair of injured structures and decreasing tension.
- Open or laparoscopic surgical techniques appear equally effective with similar success rates.
- Laparoscopic technique theoretically allows for quicker recovery.
- Time to full return to sports ranges from 4 to 12 weeks depending on type of surgery.
- Postsurgery: 80–95% rate of return to prior level of activity

REFERENCES

1. Sheen AJ, Stephenson BM, Lloyd DM, et al. "Treatment of the sportsman's groin": British Hernia Society's 2014 position statement based on the Manchester Consensus Conference. *Br J Sports Med*. 2014;48(14):1079–1087.
2. Weir A, Brukner P, Delahunt E, et al. Doha agreement meeting on terminology and definitions in groin pain in athletes. *Br J Sports Med*. 2015;49(12):768–774.
3. Abouelnaga WA, Aboelnour NH. Effectiveness of active rehabilitation program on sports hernia: randomized control trial. *Ann Rehabil Med*. 2019;43(3):305–313.

ADDITIONAL READING

- Forlizzi JM, Ward MB, Whalen J, et al. Core muscle injury: evaluation and treatment in the athlete. *Am J Sports Med*. 2023;51(4):1087–1095.
- Kopscik M, Crisman JL, Lomasney L, et al. Sports hernias: a comprehensive review for clinicians. *Cureus*. 2023;15(8):e43283.
- Lee SC, Endo Y, Potter HG. Imaging of groin pain: magnetic resonance and ultrasound imaging features. *Sports Health*. 2017;9(5):428–435.
- Padaki AS, Lynch TS, Larson CM, et al. Femoroacetabular impingement and core muscle injury in athletes: diagnosis and algorithms for success. *Sports Med Arthrosc Rev*. 2021;29(1):9–14.

CLINICAL PEARLS

- A sports hernia is a misnomer and should be classified into defined, hip-related, or other groin injury.
- There is no palpable or true hernia on exam.
- Symptoms can resolve with prolonged rest and appropriate therapy; however, there is a high recurrence rate of symptoms on resumption of activity.
- Imaging for sports hernia is nonspecific and is primarily to rule out other causes of chronic groin pain and diagnose coexisting conditions.
- Negative imaging studies does not rule out sports hernia; rather, it is a diagnosis of exclusion.
- Surgery is indicated for failed nonoperative treatment.
- Groin pain is often multifactorial. Coexisting causes such as adductor-related groin pain and hip- related groin pain should be concurrently addressed for best outcomes.

STERNOCLAVICULAR JOINT INJURY

Douglas Comeau, DO, FAAFP, FAMSSM • Justin Lockrem, MD, CAQSM

BASICS

- The sternoclavicular joint (SCJ) is a saddle-type joint that participates in all movements of the upper extremity. It is one of five joints that contains a meniscus.
- The SCJ provides free movement of the clavicle in nearly all planes.
- The joint is weakest inferiorly and reinforced superiorly, anteriorly, and posteriorly by the interclavicular, anterior, and posterior sternoclavicular and costoclavicular ligaments.

DESCRIPTION

- SCJ injuries are graded into three types:
  - Grade I: incomplete tear or stretching of the sternoclavicular and costoclavicular ligaments; joint stability and minimal pain
  - Grade II: complete tear of the sternoclavicular ligament and a partial tear of the costoclavicular ligament secondary to an anterior or posterior subluxation of the clavicle from the manubrium; pain and swelling of joint with mild deformity
  - Grade III: complete rupture of the sternoclavicular and costoclavicular ligaments; massive pain, swelling, and deformity
- The ligaments and capsule of the SCJ contribute to its stability, making it one of the least dislocated joints in the body.
- Dislocations are primarily due to trauma from vehicular or athletic injuries (>80%); congenital dislocations are extremely rare.

EPIDEMIOLOGY

Incidence

- 1% of all dislocations; 3% of all shoulder injuries in contact sport athletes (1)
- Overall incidence is higher in males than in females.
- Incidence is increased in young adult males.

ETIOLOGY AND PATHOPHYSIOLOGY

- *Anterior dislocation* is much more common than posterior dislocation (9:1 ratio):
  - Caused by an anterolateral force compressing the shoulder that rotates the shoulder backward and transmits stress to the joint
- *Posterior dislocation* is caused either from a direct anterior-to-posterior blow to the medial clavicle or from a posterolateral force compressing the shoulder followed by forward rolling.
- *Posterior dislocation is a surgical emergency and has an estimated 25% complication rate:*
  - Compression of trachea, esophagus, and great vessels in the mediastinum demand immediate reduction.

DIAGNOSIS

- Mechanism of injury, time from injury, and initial symptoms
- Immediate respiratory, neurologic, and vascular assessments
- Appropriate analgesia for patient comfort

HISTORY

- Mechanism of injury: Direct trauma (motor vehicle accident, athletic injury), falls, and dislocations can also be secondary to congenital, degenerative, and inflammatory processes.
- Symptoms: chest and/or shoulder pain exacerbated by arm movement or by lying down, dyspnea, dysphagia, or paresthesia

PHYSICAL EXAM

- Patient presents with the affected arm foreshortened and supported across the chest by opposite hand.
- Inability to abduct or externally rotate the affected arm because of severe pain over sternoclavicular junction
- In *anterior dislocation*, medial end of the clavicle is visibly prominent, palpable, and may be fixed or mobile.
- In *posterior dislocation*, loss of normal inner prominence of the clavicular head may be masked by significant local swelling:
  - Head tilted toward injured side because of spasm of the sternocleidomastoid muscle
  - Venous congestion in the neck or upper extremities, diminished pulses on affected extremity, shortness of breath, hoarseness, dysphagia, or signs of shock may suggest life-threatening impingement of the posteriorly displaced clavicle on vascular structures in the mediastinum.
- Check vital signs and perform a complete neurovascular examination of the affected extremity.
- Due to rare injury type, SCJ is often not completely examined in the setting of shoulder injury.

Pediatric Considerations

- True dislocations of the SCJ are extremely rare in children because of the strong ligamentous attachments about the medial physis.
- The medial physeal growth plates of the clavicles may not be radiographically apparent until age 18 years and generally fuse between ages 22 and 25 years. It is the last physis to close.
- Presumed SCJ dislocations are often actually fractures through the medial physis.
- In patients <25 years of age, SCJ dislocations are classified as Salter-Harris type I or type II fractures.
- In skeletally immature patients, 23% of SCJ/physeal clavicle injuries have been missed on initial emergency department (ED) evaluation (2).

DIFFERENTIAL DIAGNOSIS

- Sternoclavicular sprain/subluxation
- Sternal contusion
- Medial clavicle fracture
- Rib fracture
- Septic joint
- Osteoarthritis

DIAGNOSTIC TESTS & INTERPRETATION

- Routine radiographs can be difficult to interpret and may appear normal.
- In patients with posterior dislocations, a plain chest radiograph is needed to rule out possible associated pneumothorax.
- Rockwood view (serendipity view): a specialized view that allows for better visualization of the position of the medial clavicle:
  - X-ray beam aimed at manubrium in a 40 degrees caudal tilt
- Point of care ultrasound can be useful, especially for prompt diagnosis in posterior dislocations (3).
- Computed tomography (CT) scan is the best study to evaluate the SCJ:
  - Useful in the ED when plain films are inconclusive
  - Accurately differentiates fractures from dislocations
  - Demonstrates the position of the medial end of the clavicle in relation to the structures in the mediastinum
  - Shows detailed anatomy of the structures of the thoracic outlet and mediastinum
- Magnetic resonance imaging (MRI) can be used to distinguish a dislocation from a physeal injury in children and young adults.

TREATMENT

Pediatric Considerations

- During childhood, the medial physeal growth plate of the clavicle provides 80% of longitudinal bone growth.
- Fractures in the medial clavicle have tremendous capability for healing and remodeling.
- Nonunion and significant malunion rarely occur.
- Anteriorly displaced fractures of the medial clavicle that mimic SCJ dislocation can be placed in a figure-8 splint without reduction.
- Posteriorly displaced fractures uniformly require reduction and should be considered a surgical and orthopedic emergency.
- Prehospital:
  - The close proximity of the sternum and clavicle to vital structures of the neck and chest predispose patients with SCJ injuries to additional severe and life-threatening injuries.

- Airway, breathing, and circulation (ABCs) must first be addressed in these patients.
- Vital signs and an initial neurovascular examination should be completed.
- For patients with isolated SCJ injuries, the affected extremity should be splinted and immobilized to stabilize the joint and minimize pain prior to transport to the hospital.

- ED treatment:
  - Grade I and II usually with conservative treatment (immobilization or early functional therapy) (4)
  - Grade III usually closed reduction and immobilization versus open reduction and internal fixation (ORIF) (4)
  - *Anterior dislocations* may be reduced in the ED.
  - Conscious sedation is often necessary for pain control and muscle relaxation.
  - A rolled towel is placed between the shoulder blades in the supine position:
    - Longitudinal traction is applied to the ipsilateral arm in the extended position with the shoulder abducted at 90 degrees.
    - An assistant can maintain gentle inward pressure over the displaced medial end of the clavicle.
    - After reduction, immobilization is achieved using a well-padded figure-8 dressing.
    - Many anterior dislocations remain unstable after reduction; however, ORIF is rarely indicated, as the deformity is mainly cosmetic without functional loss.
  - *Posterior dislocations* require prompt reduction, best achieved in the operating room (OR) under general anesthesia:
    - If surgical intervention is not immediately available to reduce a posterior dislocation, reduction may be attempted in the ED to relieve serious airway, neurologic, or vascular compromise.
    - Surgical interventions may include ligament reconstruction in a figure-8 orientation using an autograft or allograft tendon, local soft tissue repair +/− augmentation, medial clavicular resection +/− ligament transfer, or ORIF (5).

MEDICATION

Anti-inflammatory agents and analgesics are the drugs of choice to decrease inflammation and reduce pain:

- Acetaminophen: 500 to 1,000 mg q6–8h PRN
- Ibuprofen: 400 to 800 mg q4–8h PRN with meals
- Careful consideration of narcotics based on weight, prior history, and level of discomfort

ADMISSION, INPATIENT, AND NURSING CONSIDERATIONS

- Initial stabilization:
  - Patients in respiratory distress require endotracheal intubation and immediate reduction.
  - Emergent reduction is also needed in patients with hoarseness, dysphagia, or neurovascular compromise (upper extremity weakness, paresthesia, diminished pulses, signs of shock).
  - *Patients with posterior dislocations represent true orthopedic and surgical emergencies*, and appropriate consults should be obtained promptly.
  - Appropriate analgesia (e.g., narcotics or nonsteroidal anti-inflammatory drugs [NSAIDs]) necessary for pain control
- Admission criteria:
  - All posterior dislocations of the SCJ require admission for prompt reduction in the OR and evaluation for potential intrathoracic complications.
- Discharge criteria:
  - Anterior dislocations of the SCJ that can be reduced and splinted, in the absence of neurovascular compromise, may be discharged with appropriate orthopedic follow-up.

ONGOING CARE

FOLLOW-UP RECOMMENDATIONS

Patient Monitoring

- Patients with sprains should initially restrict activity, and depending on the amount of pain or discomfort, a sling can be used for immobilization.
- Reductions performed in the ED require stabilization of the affected shoulder with a soft figure 8 or sling; immobilization for 4 weeks
- Anterior dislocations should restrict activity and follow up with their physician as directed.
- Patients with posterior dislocations who are discharged home should return for medical care if they exhibit symptoms of mediastinal injury.

PROGNOSIS

Prognosis depends on extent and type of joint damage, but most patients have adequate upper extremity function following SCJ injuries. In a 2018 review study of 108 surgical cases, a majority of surgeries, regardless of technique had favorable outcomes, with return to work, normal function, or sport in 54–100% of cases. Surgical complication rates were 15.6% and only 4% had recurrent instability (5).

COMPLICATIONS

- Tracheal rupture
- Pneumothorax
- Laceration of superior vena cava
- Occlusion of the subclavian artery
- Recurrent dislocation
- Deformity

REFERENCES

1. Hellwinkel JE, McCarty EC, Khodaee M. Sports-related sternoclavicular joint injuries. *Phys Sportsmed*. 2019;47(3):253–261.
2. Lee JT, Nasreddine AY, Black EM, et al. Posterior sternoclavicular joint injuries in skeletally immature patients. *J Pediatr Orthop*. 2014;34(4):369–375.
3. Bengtzen RR, Petering RC. Point-of-care ultrasound diagnosis of posterior sternoclavicular joint dislocation. *J Emerg Med*. 2017;52(4):513–515.
4. Garcia JA, Arguello AM, Momaya AM, et al. Sternoclavicular joint instability: symptoms, diagnosis and management. *Orthop Res Rev*. 2020;12:75–87.
5. Kendal JK, Thomas K, Lo IKY, et al. Clinical outcomes and complications following surgical management of traumatic posterior sternoclavicular joint dislocations: a systematic review. *JBJS Rev*. 2018;6(11):e2.

ADDITIONAL READING

- Gobet R, Meuli M, Altermatt S, et al. Medial clavicular epiphysiolysis in children: the so-called sterno-clavicular dislocation. *Emerg Radiol*. 2004;10(5):252–255.
- Jang ES, Park CN, Levine WN, et al. A current concepts review of clavicle injuries in ice hockey from sternoclavicular to acromioclavicular joint. *Orthop J Sports Med*. 2020;8(9):2325967120951413.
- Sernandez H, Riehl J. Sternoclavicular joint dislocation: a systematic review and meta-analysis. *J Orthop Trauma*. 2019;33(7):e251–e255.

CLINICAL PEARLS

- SCJ injuries are graded (I, II, III) based on severity of tearing of associated ligaments.
- Dislocations are usually from trauma (direct blows/falls), especially in contact sports. Anterior dislocation is most common. Posterior dislocations are less common but require prompt reduction and is a surgical emergency.
- Physical exam may show swelling and deformity of SCJ, and athlete may have restricted shoulder motion in abduction and external rotation.
- Treatment for grade I and II is usually conservative. Grade III injuries may require surgery.

STRESS FRACTURES

Bridget Doyle, DO, MPH • Daniel C. Herman, MD, PhD, FAAPMR, FACSM, FISBS, CAQSM • Sara N. Raiser, MD, FAAPMR, CAQSM

BASICS

- A stress fracture (SF) is the damage to bone caused by repetitive loading that exceeds healing capacity. SF injury can range from a mild periosteal reaction to a displaced fracture.
- SFs are grouped as low or high risk. Examples of low-risk stress fractures (LRSFs) include the pelvis, femoral shaft, posteromedial tibia, fibula, metatarsal shafts, cuboid, calcaneus, and cuneiform. These can be treated nonoperatively.
- Examples of high-risk stress fractures (HRSFs) include the femoral neck, anterior tibial shaft, patella, medial malleolus, proximal 2nd metatarsal, proximal 5th metatarsal, sesamoids, tarsal navicular, and talus.
- HRSFs have a greater risk of complications; thus, early advanced imaging and specialty referral is recommended. Operative treatment is indicated in some HRSF cases.
- SFs occur in the pelvis and lower extremities in military recruits, endurance athletes, dancers, and soccer and basketball players.
- SFs may also occur in the spine and upper extremities in certain sports (e.g., gymnastics, baseball, tennis, rowing). SFs are particularly common in females, occurring in up to 40% of athletes at some point in their career. Female athletes with one component of the female athlete triad (low energy availability, menstrual dysfunction, and low bone mineral density) have a 15–20% risk, which increases to 30–50% with multiple components. The female athlete triad has an expanded focus and now has been incorporated in the relative energy deficiency in sport (REDs) terminology.
- A prolonged state of low energy availability (REDs) substantially increases the risk of SFs in all athletes.
- Overall, 90% of athletes return to sport after an SF.

EPIDEMIOLOGY

Incidence

- The incidence among female athletes is as high as 13%, with lower extremity SFs representing 80–95% of all cases.
- High incidence in female military recruits (21%)
- Incidence varies with activity/sport.

Prevalence

- SFs account for >10% of all orthopedic injuries and up to 20% of injuries seen in sports medicine clinics.
- 80–95% of SFs involve the lower extremity.
- Tibia, tarsals, and metatarsals are the most common sites with 49% prevalence in the tibia, 25% in tarsal bones, and 9% in metatarsals.

ETIOLOGY AND PATHOPHYSIOLOGY

- Repetitive load plus inadequate rest
- Bone resorption is faster than bone formation.
- Microfractures lead to cortical break.
- Anatomical sites of HRSFs have reduced vascularity and bear high tensile load.

Genetics

Genes that regulate bone remodeling have shown an association with SFs in recent studies. More research is needed to establish a clear genetic link.

RISK FACTORS

- Female gender
- Female body mass index (BMI) <19 kg/m^2
- Late menarche ≥15 years old
- Prior SF
- Pes cavus or planus
- >5 degrees knee valgus/external rotation (ER)
- Inadequate caloric intake
- Excessive caffeine, alcohol, or tobacco use
- Osteopenia
- Chronic corticosteroid use
- Rapid increase in training loads (e.g., volume, intensity)
- Recreational runners >20 miles/wk
- Poor footwear
- Running on hard surfaces
- Low 25-hydroxy vitamin D
- Amenorrhea/oligomenorrhea (females)
- Low testosterone (males)
- Activities that increase the risk of SF in different locations of the body:
  - **Tibia**: military recruits, runners, and children participating in rigorous activity; sports that involve jumping and sudden deceleration
  - **Fibula**: children taking part in sports or ballet and adults participating in running or jumping activities
  - **Metatarsal**: ballet dancers (specifically the 2nd metatarsal); endurance athletes
  - **Navicular**: sprinting or jumping activities; runners, dancers, military recruits, and adolescent boys and girls playing on artificial turf
  - **Cuneiform**: sprinters
  - **Shoulder girdle**: throwers
  - **Forearm**: weight lifting, cycling, gymnastics, crutch walking, and racket sports
  - **Wrist and hand**: softball, tennis, rowing, and military activity
  - **Ribs**: swinging sports (i.e., golf, tennis); rowing
  - **Femoral neck**: long-distance runners, ballet dancers, military recruits

GENERAL PREVENTION

- Adequate calories and nutrition
- 1,000 to 1,300 mg calcium and 400 to 800 IU vitamin D per day
- Screen for female athlete triad, REDs
- Padded insoles and orthotics (military recruits)
- Replace footwear every 3 months or 300 miles.
- Limit training increase (intensity, duration, frequency) to 10% per week.

COMMONLY ASSOCIATED CONDITIONS

- REDs
- Chronic corticosteroid use
- Osteopenia/osteoporosis
- Amenorrhea/oligomenorrhea

DIAGNOSIS

HISTORY

- Insidious local pain from repetitive activity
- Worse with continued activity
- Pain at rest (e.g., night pain)
- Assess risk factors and training history (miles per week, intensity, frequency).
- Assess for prior history of SF.
- Detailed nutrition history, including total caloric intake, calcium and vitamin D intake, dietary restrictions/changes, and any recent weight changes
- Menstrual irregularity or amenorrhea, age of menarche
- Corticosteroid use
- Osteopenia/osteoporosis

PHYSICAL EXAM

- Direct bony tenderness ± edema
- Palpate for callus or bony step-off.
- Limping/pain on weight-bearing
- Pain with axial compression
- Tender "N" spot (dorsal central third of the navicular bone between the anterior tibial and hallucis longus tendons) suggestive of SF.
- Hop test: pain with single leg hop suggestive of SF
- Calcaneal squeeze test: simultaneous pressure on the medial and lateral aspects of calcaneus, pain suggestive of SF
- Fulcrum test: pain at the site with bending the long bone over a table edge or examiner's leg or forearm; useful for tibial and femoral shaft SFs
- Log roll test: Passive internal rotation (IR)/ER of the thigh may elicit groin pain in a femoral neck SF.
- Sacroiliac joint pain tests, Flamingo test: useful for sacral SF
- Assess lower extremity alignment and foot type that would predispose to SF.
- Assess for poor lower quarter mechanics, especially core and pelvic stability.

DIFFERENTIAL DIAGNOSIS

- Muscle strain/tendinopathy
- Fasciitis/periostitis
- Exertional compartment syndrome
- Nerve/artery entrapment
- Bone tumor
- Femoral neck SF may mimic adductor or hip flexor strain.
- Anterior and posteromedial tibial SF can be confused with shin splints.
- Proximal posteromedial tibial SF can mimic pes anserine bursitis.

DIAGNOSTIC TESTS & INTERPRETATION

Initial Tests (lab, imaging)

- X-rays:
  - Initial low-cost, widely available test but has low sensitivity (10–56%) in early stages (1)[C]
  - Repeat x-rays after 2 to 3 weeks show improved sensitivity (30–70%) with possible lucency or callus formation (1)[C].
- Bone scan:
  - Highly sensitive (74–100%) but less specific, can be falsely positive with infection or tumor, involves radiation exposure (2)[C]
- Computed tomography (CT) scan:
  - Useful for detailed assessment of high-risk fractures, although less sensitive than magnetic resonance imaging (MRI) and involves significant radiation (1)[C]
  - Bone scan combined with single photon emission CT may be more accurate than MRI for pars interarticularis SF (1)[C].
- Diagnostic ultrasound:
  - Useful for superficial structures like metatarsals with a sensitivity of 83% and specificity of 75% in small studies (1)[C]
- MRI:
  - The gold standard, with a sensitivity of 86–100% and specificity of 100%, preferred for early and accurate diagnosis, showing bone marrow edema and fractures lines (1)[C]
  - Excludes other diagnoses and can grade severity which can aid in prognosis

- Obtain labs based on clinical suspicion of nutritional, endocrine, and metabolic factors.
- Complete blood count (CBC), comprehensive metabolic panel (CMP), magnesium, phosphorous, 25-OH vitamin D_3 and parathyroid hormone, thyroid function tests (thyroid-stimulating hormone [TSH], free T4, total and free T3), iron studies (iron, ferritin, transferrin, total iron-binding capacity)
- Females with menstrual dysfunction: follicle-stimulating hormone (FSH), luteinizing hormone (LH), estradiol, testosterone, human chorionic gonadotropin (hCG)
- Testosterone if low testosterone suspected in males
- Dexamethasone suppression test if excess cortisol suspected

Follow-Up Tests & Special Considerations

- X-rays: useful in follow-up to demonstrate callus formation and union
- CT: provides greater detail to assess healing in follow-up
- Bone scan: not useful for follow-up as it remains positive for over a year
- MRI: may show positive findings after the patient is asymptomatic, useful for ongoing assessment

Diagnostic Procedures/Other

Bone biopsy may sometimes be necessary to differentiate a tumor from an SF.

TREATMENT

GENERAL MEASURES

- Stop the offending activity: Cessation of all activities that contribute to the SF for a period of 6 to 8 weeks is generally recommended for most SFs (2)[C].
- Use a cast, pneumatic boot, rigid sole shoe, or crutches to help off-load stress from the affected area and to ensure pain-free relative rest.
- A compression boot for tibial SFs may lead to earlier return to play (1)[C].
- Allow progressive weight-bearing based on symptomatic improvement.
- Select site-specific treatments (2)[C]:
  - **Medial malleolus**: Nondisplaced fractures in nonelite athletes are managed conservatively with limited weight-bearing, although elite athletes may require surgical fixation.
  - **Talus**: treated with non–weight-bearing for at least 6 weeks, followed by assisted weight-bearing in a cast or CAM boot
  - **Navicular**: Nondisplaced fractures are treated conservatively with a non–weight-bearing short leg cast for 6 to 8 weeks.
  - **Femoral neck**: Nondisplaced compression-sided fractures affecting <50% diameter may be treated with prolonged non–weight-bearing (typically at least 6 weeks). Tension-sided fractures of any amount should be treated surgically.
  - **Tibia**: medial managed conservatively with pain-free protected weight-bearing. Anterior requires 6 weeks non–weight-bearing, and those that fail to heal may require surgery.
  - **Sesamoid**: initially treated conservatively with limited weight-bearing with off-loading sesamoid pad or non–weight-bearing. Surgery may be necessary if conservative treatment fails.

MEDICATION

- Acetaminophen for pain; off-loading should be first line of action.
- Avoid nonsteroidal anti-inflammatory drugs (NSAIDs) due to potential for inhibition of bone healing.
- Although bisphosphonates like pamidronate have shown some efficacy in reducing pain and aiding in sports-specific participation, their use is controversial and not recommended for prevention (2)[C].
- Teriparatide may be considered to facilitate bone healing in select patients.

ISSUES FOR REFERRAL

- Urgent orthopedic/sports medicine consultation for HRSFs
- Early advanced imaging of HRSFs is crucial for the early detection and management of HRSFs to prevent complications and determine the need for surgical intervention.

ADDITIONAL THERAPIES

- Electromagnetic or ultrasonic bone stimulation may be considered for recalcitrant cases, but evidence is lacking for efficacy (1)[C].
- A retrospective chart review study demonstrated that extracorporeal shockwave therapy is a safe and effective treatment for managing bone stress injuries in runners, with most patients (97.5%) returning to pain-free running after an average of 5 ± 2 treatments (3)[B].
- Run gait retraining may help runners reduce impact and abnormal bone loading patterns which may help prevent SFs.

SURGERY/OTHER PROCEDURES

- Superolateral femoral neck SF (tension side) requires emergent surgical fixation (4)[C].
- Anterior tibial SF has a high rate of nonunion, and surgery is recommended if 3 to 6 months of conservative treatment has failed.
- Navicular SF is often treated surgically in elite athletes, but outcomes are comparable with nonoperative treatment (4)[C].
- Proximal 5th metatarsal SF involving zones 2 or 3 (distal to the tuberosity) benefit from surgical fixation with reduced complications and earlier return to sport (4)[C].

ONGOING CARE

FOLLOW-UP RECOMMENDATIONS

- Athletes are typically followed every 2 to 4 weeks to assess for symptomatic improvement and allow a gradual increase in weight-bearing. A progressive protocol can be used for return to running.
- Follow-up imaging is often used in HRSFs and complicated cases. Athletes with LRSFs may be followed on the basis of clinical signs and symptoms without repeat imaging.

DIET

- Adequate calories, protein, and carbohydrates for age, body type, and sport
- Daily calcium 1,000 to 1,300 mg and vitamin D 400 to 800 IU

PATIENT EDUCATION

- Athletes should understand their individual intrinsic and extrinsic risk factors and modify when possible. Individualize training to reduce injury and optimize performance.
- Advise athletes not to ignore pain symptoms and to avoid overtraining and underfueling.

PROGNOSIS

- Excellent for most if treated early with adequate rest
- Poor for anterior tibial SF with evidence of cortical disruption (dreaded black line on x-ray)
- Completed femoral neck SF can be associated with long-term morbidity and disability.

COMPLICATIONS

Delayed union, nonunion, refracture, completed fracture, avascular necrosis, and failure to (timely) return to sport.

REFERENCES

1. Patel DS, Roth M, Kapil N. Stress fractures: diagnosis, treatment, and prevention. *Am Fam Physician.* 2011;83(1):39–46.
2. Abbott A, Bird M, Brown SM, et al. Part II: presentation, diagnosis, classification, treatment, and prevention of stress fractures in female athletes. *Phys Sportsmed.* 2020;48(1):2532.
3. Beling A, Tenforde A. Outcomes using focused shockwave for the treatment of stress fractures in runners: 2602. *Med Sci Sports Exerc.* 2023;55(9 Suppl):863.
4. McInnis KC, Ramey LN. High-risk stress fractures: diagnosis and management. *PM R.* 2016;8(Suppl 3):S113–S124.

ADDITIONAL READING

- Abbott A, Bird ML, Wild E, et al. Part I: epidemiology and risk factors for stress fractures in female athletes. *Phys Sportsmed.* 2020;48(1):17–24.
- Hoenig T, Ackerman KE, Beck BR, et al. Bone stress injuries. *Nat Rev Dis Primers.* 2022;8(1):26.
- Hoenig T, Eissele J, Strahl A, et al. Return to sport following low-risk and high-risk bone stress injuries: a systematic review and meta-analysis. *Br J Sports Med.* 2023;57(7):427–432.
- Mountjoy M, Ackerman KE, Bailey DM, et al. 2023 International Olympic Committee's (IOC) consensus statement on relative energy deficiency in sport (REDs). *Br J Sports Med.* 2023;57(17):1073–1097.

CLINICAL PEARLS

- Diagnosis is based on index of suspicion, risk factors, and clinical findings. Negative x-rays do not exclude SFs.
- Obtain urgent advanced imaging in patients with clinical findings consistent with an HRSF.
- MRI is the advanced imaging study of choice.
- HRSFs warrant orthopedic or sports medicine specialty evaluation.
- High-demand athletes may elect for early surgery for a more rapid return to play.

SUBCONJUNCTIVAL HEMORRHAGE

Holly Beach, MD, CAQSM

BASICS

DESCRIPTION

- Benign condition of the eye characterized by the rupture of small vessels leading to an accumulation of blood in the subconjunctival space, the potential space between the conjunctiva and the sclera (1)
- Synonym(s): conjunctival hemorrhage

EPIDEMIOLOGY

- One of the most frequently encountered eye problems in primary care offices accounted for 2.9% of visits to outpatient eye clinics in one study
- Uncommon in children, especially infants, and when encountered abuse should be considered (2)

RISK FACTORS

- Sudden increase in ocular pressure, which may result from coughing, sneezing, vomiting, or straining.
- Uncontrolled hypertension (HTN)
- Acute conjunctivitis
- Vigorous eye rubbing
- Aspirin or other anticoagulant use
- Underlying hematologic or systemic disease
- Contact sports and activities involving projectiles

DIAGNOSIS

HISTORY

- No visual changes
- Eye trauma, including rubbing
- Use of aspirin or other anticoagulant
- Medical conditions leading to increased intraocular pressure or straining, including uncontrolled HTN, constipation, prostatic hypertrophy, cough, sneezing, and vomiting (3)[C]
- Exercise or activities involving exertional straining (i.e., weightlifting)
- Diagnosis of or symptoms suggestive of bleeding disorders, such as easy bruising, menorrhagia, and so forth

PHYSICAL EXAM

- Asymptomatic
- Extreme redness of eye without changes in vision
- Extensive subconjunctival hemorrhage may cause a protruding sac of blood, beyond the lid margin.
- Bright red area of blood, either focally or diffusely in potential space under conjunctiva
- Blood pressure (BP) measurement to evaluate for uncontrolled HTN.
- Stigmata of bleeding or other hematologic disorders (petechiae, bruising, etc.)
- Associated signs suggestive of acute hemorrhagic conjunctivitis

DIFFERENTIAL DIAGNOSIS

- Acute hemorrhagic conjunctivitis: a highly contagious disease caused by enterovirus 70 and coxsackievirus A24; pain, photophobia, blurred vision, and epiphora develop acutely, with 80% developing bilateral disease within 24 hours. Ocular signs may include subconjunctival hemorrhage as well as discharge, punctate corneal epithelial keratitis, and lid edema. Patients also may complain of fever, headache, upper respiratory infection symptoms, myalgia, and may have tender preauricular lymphadenopathy. Symptoms usually resolve without treatment over 5 to 7 days, with persistent subconjunctival hemorrhages resolving over an additional few weeks.
- Scleral rupture should be suspected in a post-traumatic patient with a bullous subconjunctival hemorrhage, especially in the presence of blood in the vitreous, decreased intraocular pressure, or a shallow anterior chamber.
- Orbital hemorrhage may present with massive subconjunctival hemorrhage as well as proptosis and limitation of extraocular movements, usually after trauma.
- Infrequently, adenoviral conjunctivitis, bacterial conjunctivitis, and even allergic conjunctivitis may present with an associated subconjunctival hemorrhage.

TREATMENT

GENERAL MEASURES

- Reassurance; no analgesia; condition is self-limited.
- Condition is nonpainful; the presence of pain should alert the examiner to a more serious condition (4)[C].
- Large subconjunctival hemorrhages that cover most of the sclera should be evaluated by an ophthalmologist as they may mask an underlying occult rupture or perforation/penetration of the globe (5).
- Topical steroids are contraindicated, especially with suspicion of acute hemorrhagic conjunctivitis, due to risk of clinical deterioration and permanent side effects.

ADDITIONAL THERAPIES

- Again, reassurance: Hemorrhages usually resolve spontaneously in 1 to 3 weeks.
- Further treatment should be directed at reduction of risk factors and treatment of any identified underlying etiology (bleeding problems, HTN).
- Treat secondary bacterial conjunctivitis and allergic conjunctivitis, as indicated.

ONGOING CARE

FOLLOW-UP RECOMMENDATIONS

- Prognosis is good with no long-term complications.
- Consider ophthalmology consultation if history of ocular trauma is present or in the presence of associated ocular injury (6)[C].
- Consider hematology consultation if hemorrhages are idiopathic and recurrent.

REFERENCES

1. Joshi RS, Bandgar RR. Incidence of non-traumatic subconjunctival hemorrhage in an Indian rural population. *Clin Ophthalmol.* 2021;15:183–188.
2. Wolford JE, Berger RP, Eichman AL, et al. Injuries suggestive of physical abuse in young children with subconjunctival hemorrhages. *Pediatr Emerg Care.* 2022;38(2):e468–e471.
3. Sahinoglu-Keskek N, Cevher S, Ergin A. Analysis of subconjunctival hemorrhage. *Pak J Med Sci.* 2013;29(1):132–134.
4. Micieli JA, Easterbrook M. Eye and orbital injuries in sports. *Clin Sports Med.* 2017;36(2):299–314.
5. Ohana O, Alabiad C. Ocular related sports injuries. *J Craniofac Surg.* 2021;32(4):1606–1611.
6. Tarlan B, Kiratli H. Subconjunctival hemorrhage: risk factors and potential indicators. *Clin Ophthalmol.* 2013;7:1163–1170.

ADDITIONAL READING

- Cronau H, Kankanala RR, Mauger T. Diagnosis and management of red eye in primary care. *Am Fam Physician.* 2010;81(2):137–144.
- Fukuyama J, Hayasaka S, Yamada K, et al. Causes of subconjunctival hemorrhage. *Ophthalmologica.* 1990;200(2):63–67.
- Goroll AH, May LA, Mulley AG, eds. *Primary Care Medicine: Office Evaluation and Management of the Adult Patient.* Lippincott Williams and Wilkins; 1995.
- Kaimbo D, Kaimbo W. Epidemiology of traumatic and spontaneous subconjunctival haemorrhages in Congo. *Bull Soc Belge Ophthalmol.* 2009;(311):31–36.
- Mimura T, Usui T, Yamagami S, et al. Subconjunctival hemorrhage and conjunctivochalasis. *Ophthalmology.* 2009;116(10):1880–1886.
- Pavan-Langston D, ed. *Manual of Ocular Diagnosis and Therapy.* 4th ed. Little Brown; 1996.
- Wright PW, Strauss GH, Langford MP. Acute hemorrhagic conjunctivitis. *Am Fam Physician.* 1992;45(1):173–178.

CLINICAL PEARLS

- Benign condition with most cases resolving completely without intervention over the course of 1 to 3 weeks.
- Presence of pain suggests alternative diagnosis.
- Only recurrent or persistent cases require evaluation by an ophthalmologist.

SUBCORACOID IMPINGEMENT

Sarah Kennedy, DO, CAQSM • Joshua Schulte, MD

BASICS

DESCRIPTION

Subcoracoid impingement is the pathologic narrowing of the subcoracoid space, defined by the lateral coracoid process and the lesser tuberosity of the humerus. Typically, the subscapularis and biceps tendons traverse this space, and narrowing can therefore lead to inflammation of these tendons. Persistent impingement and tendonitis then leads to anterior shoulder pain, especially with forward flexion, adduction, and internal rotation of the shoulder (1),(2).

- Etiology can be categorized into bony and soft-tissue stenosis, indicated by the initial cause of subcoracoid space narrowing (1), whereas others have categorized the etiology as idiopathic, iatrogenic, or traumatic (3),(4).

EPIDEMIOLOGY

The epidemiology of subcoracoid impingement has not been reported in the literature.

ETIOLOGY AND PATHOPHYSIOLOGY

- The subcoracoid canal (sometimes referred to as the coracohumeral canal) is the space created by the coracoid process and anterior scapular neck medially and the coracohumeral ligament, biceps tendon, and lesser tuberosity laterally (1).
- Narrowing of this space or increased tissue mass within a normal space can lead to pain.
- Narrowing of the space is typically secondary to anatomic variants or restructuring/trauma of the coracoid or lesser tuberosity (4). Via imaging and cadaver studies, narrowing of the space is typically <7 mm, whereas normal space may be as much as 11 mm (1),(4).
- Inflammation or thickening in the subscapularis tendon can cause narrowing of the space and increased tissue within the space (5).

RISK FACTORS

- Anatomic variations in the lateral coracoid or lesser tuberosity of the humerus
- Traumatic injury to the humerus, scapula, or clavicle (4)
- Subscapularis calcification/ossification/hypertrophy
- Ganglion cysts (4)

GENERAL PREVENTION

Early modification of scapular dyskinesis and avoidance of repetitive shoulder movements (1)

COMMONLY ASSOCIATED CONDITIONS

- Subacromial impingement
- Subscapularis tendinopathy (more common) and other rotator cuff tendinopathies (less common)
- Biceps tendinopathy (1),(2),(3)

DIAGNOSIS

HISTORY

- Most commonly, patients will complain of nonspecific, dull, anterior shoulder pain, aggravated by overhead activities especially with forward flexion, adduction, and internal rotation of the shoulder (McKernan).
- Commonly, patients will have pain with activities such as driving, writing on a whiteboard, or the follow-through motion of throwing.
- Asking about a history of trauma or surgery can aid in categorizing the impingement.

PHYSICAL EXAM

- Visual inspection for surgical scars or bony deformities (2)[C]
- Tenderness to palpation medial or lateral to coracoid process is common while pain radiating into the upper extremity (1)[C].
- If there is paresthesia, it will not be associated with a cervical territory (2)[C],(3)[C].
- Patients may have limited range of motion in horizontal adduction and internal rotation (1)[C],(2)[C],(3)[C].
- Positive modified Kennedy-Hawkins impingement sign (1)[C],(3)[C]
- Subscapularis—belly press and weakness in external rotation (typically pain occurs between 80 and 130 degrees of elevation) (1)[C]
- Biceps tendinopathy (concomitant vs. alternative)—Speed test and Yergason test (1)[C]

DIFFERENTIAL DIAGNOSIS

- Subacromial Impingement
- Superior labrum anterior-to-posterior (SLAP) lesion
- Biceps tendinopathy
- Rotator cuff tendinopathy
- Osteoarthritis
- Shoulder instability

DIAGNOSTIC TESTS & INTERPRETATION

Initial Tests (lab, imaging)

AP and axillary x-ray are used to rule out fractures and can demonstrate bony abnormalities (4)[C]. Chevron-shaped coracoid process is pathognomonic for subcoracoid impingement (3)[C].

Follow-Up Tests & Special Considerations

- Studies have shown ultrasound (with proper technique and training), which tends to be cheaper and more widely available, can aid in showing coracohumeral space narrowing with similar sensitivity and specificity to computed tomography (CT) and magnetic resonance imaging (MRI) (1)[C]. Ultrasound can also demonstrate subscapularis tendon abnormalities (1)[C].
- CT and MRI (especially dynamic if available) are also used to demonstrate coracohumeral interval, with low sensitivity and high specificity. MRI is especially useful in evaluating soft tissue lesions (1)[C],(4)[C].

Diagnostic Procedures/Other

Ultrasound-guided anesthetic injection and ultrasound-guided steroid injection are diagnostic if they relieve pain (1)[C],(2)[C].

TREATMENT

GENERAL MEASURES

Initial treatment includes activity modification, rest, and ice/heat.

MEDICATION

First Line

- The primary medications used are to help control pain and inflammation. These include, but are not limited to, nonsteroidal anti-inflammatory drugs (NSAIDs) (ibuprofen, meloxicam, etc.) and acetaminophen (Tylenol) (2)[C].
- NSAIDs are to be avoided in patients with kidney disease or history of peptic ulcer disease.

ISSUES FOR REFERRAL

Similar to many orthopedic shoulder pathologies, follow-up should be scheduled for weeks to months to allow a sufficient course of rest, activity modification, and/or steroid injection.

ADDITIONAL THERAPIES

Physical therapy (PT) is a mainstay in the initial treatment and can be done before, during, or after a steroid injection (1)[C],(2)[C],(4)[C].

SURGERY/OTHER PROCEDURES

- Typically reserved for patients who have failed conservative management. Follow-up typically starts with weeks, is stretched to months, and then can be extended to years or as needed (1)[C],(2)[C],(4)[C].
- Arthroscopic subcoracoid decompression (coracoplasty) with or without a subscapularis tendon repair (1)[C],(6)[B]
- Open coracoplasty—There has not been evidence to support one surgical technique over the other (1)[C].
- Current studies have not shown benefit in performing coracoplasty over subscapularis tendon repair alone (1)[C],(6)[B].

ONGOING CARE

FOLLOW-UP RECOMMENDATIONS

Following injection and PT, follow-up is typically 2 to 4 months. Following surgery, follow-up is typically tapered, starting with 1 to 2 weeks follow-up paired with PT which then extends to 2 to 3 months. If healing progresses appropriately, follow-up can be on an as-needed basis (2),(5).

PATIENT EDUCATION

- Early postsurgical PT is essential to recovery of mobility and strength without pain (5).
- Graded weight-bearing and activity tolerate is recommended after surgery. Full return to normal activities may take several months (5)[C].

PROGNOSIS

Most patients have improvements in range of motion, strength, and pain after PT, steroid injection, and/or surgical interventions. These outcomes are reported to continue for years (as most studies limited follow-up 1 to 2 years) (1).

COMPLICATIONS

- With any injection or surgical intervention, patients are at risk for infection, bleeding, and pain.
- Damage can be done to musculoskeletal and axillary nerves as well as the cephalic vein (2).
- Some patients may undergo surgery and not have resolution of pain or regain complete range of motion/strength (6).

REFERENCES

1. McKernan MJ, Schickendantz MS, Frangiamore SJ. Diagnosis and management of subcoracoid impingement. *J Am Acad Orthop Surg*. 2021;29(3):100–107.
2. Horowitz EH, Aibinder WR. Shoulder impingement syndrome. *Phys Med Rehabil Clin N Am*. 2023;34(2):311–334.
3. Osti L, Soldati F, Del Buono A, et al. Subcoracoid impingement and subscapularis tendon: is there any truth? *Muscles Ligaments Tendons J*. 2013;3(2):101–105.
4. Bolia IK, Collon K, Bogdanov J, et al. Management options for shoulder impingement syndrome in athletes: insights and future directions. *Open Access J Sports Med*. 2021;12:43–53.
5. Garofalo R, Conti M, Massazza G, et al. Subcoracoid impingement syndrome: a painful shoulder condition related to different pathologic factors. *Musculoskeletal Surg*. 2011;95(Suppl 1):S25–S29.
6. Karnaugh RD, Sperling JW, Warren RF. Arthroscopic treatment of coracoid impingement. *Arthroscopy*. 2001;17(7):784–787.

ADDITIONAL READING

Pearce SS, Ruzbarsky JJ, Ernat JJ, et al. Arthroscopic subcoracoid decompression, coracoplasty, and subscapularis repair for subscapularis tears in the setting of subcoracoid impingement. *Arthroscopy Tech*. 2022;11(3):e333–e338.

CLINICAL PEARLS

- Subcoracoid impingement is defined as an abnormal narrowing of the coracohumeral space and is categorized by bony and soft tissue stenosis.
- Subcoracoid impingement typically causes anterior shoulder pain especially with flexion, adduction, and interior rotation and is commonly accompanied by subscapularis tendinopathy.
- Diagnosis is mostly clinical but can be aided with ultrasound and MRI.
- Treatment is typically conservative, consisting of activity modification, PT, and steroid injection. However, surgical interventions are available.
- Early postsurgical rehabilitation has shown good long-term results in increased range of motion and decreased pain.

SUBUNGUAL EXOSTOSIS AND HEMATOMA

Nicole L. Leonard, MD ▪ Glenn H. Sapp II, MD ▪ Daniel C. Herman, MD, PhD, FAAPMR, FACSM, FISBS, CAQSM

BASICS

DESCRIPTION

- Subungual exostosis: a chronic, benign, and osteocartilaginous growth from the distal phalanx's terminal tuft that commonly causes pain and/or deformity of the nail
- Subungual hematoma: an acute, traumatic subungual collection of blood appearing as a red, blue, or black discoloration, usually caused by a direct, blunt impact or chronic, repetitive stresses to the distal phalanx
- Both cause pain not only due to mechanism of injury but also to the pressure resulting from growth or blood accumulation.
- Synonym(s) for subungual hematoma: tennis toe; jogger's toe; sportsman's toe

EPIDEMIOLOGY

Subungual exostosis:

- Relatively uncommon
- Average age of presentation is 26 years old; however, adolescents carry the majority of the diagnoses (1).
- About 55% of cases occur in patients aged <18 years. (1)
- 80% of cases target the great toe but may also occur at the lesser toes or fingers (1).
- Subungual exostosis growths account for about 17% of surgeries on the hallux (1).
- No gender preference (2)

ETIOLOGY AND PATHOPHYSIOLOGY

- Subungual hematomas are seen more commonly in sports that require frequent pivoting, abrupt stops, or repetitive kicking (e.g., basketball, handball, racquet sports, soccer, football, running).
- Repeated contact of the toes with the front of the shoebox causes toenail dyshesion and subsequent hemorrhage (3).
- If the activity continues, it may lead to chronic nail dystrophy, nail loss, and callus formation of the tip of the toe (3).
- Acute overt trauma is the most common cause of subungual hematomas (e.g., fingertip slammed in a car door, hammer blow, or blunt trauma), and although exact etiology is unknown, the current theory is that subungual exostosis is the result of metaplasia caused by chronic microtrauma (4).

RISK FACTORS

- Microtrauma
- Chronic infection
- Hereditary abnormality (i.e., hereditary multiple osteochondroma)

GENERAL PREVENTION

Subungual hematoma:

- Wearing well-fitted, task-appropriate footwear with a snug midfoot and a wide toe box (e.g., steel-toed shoes for construction workers)
- Using orthotic devices to prevent foot sliding
- Maintaining toenails trimmed straight across without curved edges

DIAGNOSIS

HISTORY

- Subungual exostosis: typically weeks to months with reports of toenail pain, a localized mass or swelling in the toenail, or shoe wear discomfort. Previous history may include trauma or infection (4).
- Subungual hematoma: an acute history of digital trauma with resultant nail discoloration and pain. Inquiry into participation in athletic activities and day-to-day activities involving use of hands or feet may help elucidate etiology.
- Other pertinent history includes whether the discoloration was present at birth or acquired.
- A medication history to identify drugs that may contribute to abnormal nail pigmentation or increased the risk of bleeding (3).

PHYSICAL EXAM

- Subungual exostosis:
  - Presence of a firm mass noted at the distal portion of the terminal phalanx
  - Pain is typically elicited through direct palpation.
  - Exam may demonstrate a lifted nail bed and even a detached nail (onycholysis) if exostosis is large enough.
  - Most common physical finding is a deformed nail bed (onychodystrophy).
  - Gait may be affected secondary to pain and swelling related to the exostosis.
- Subungual hematoma:
  - Collection of blood that appears as a reddish to blackish pigmentation, under the nail with or without edema/erythema
  - The pigment in a subungual hematoma is homogenous in distribution, whereas melanocytic lesions have cellular inclusions (3).
  - Observe for any extension of discoloration from under the nail plate into the proximal nail fold and nail matrix (Hutchinson melanotic whitlow sign); suspect subungual melanoma.
  - Variable pain presentation that can range from painless to extreme throbbing
  - Examine all 20 nail units, periungual skin, and oral mucosa for additional lesions (for signs of Peutz-Jeghers syndrome or Laugier-Hunziker syndrome) (3).
  - May note a callus on the skin distal to the affected nail
  - Toes most likely affected in a sport-specific pattern are:
    - "Tennis toe": more commonly lateral nail of the hallux or 2nd toe, depending on which is longer
    - "Jogger's toe": 2nd through 5th toes
    - Kicking sports: 2nd or 3rd toe

DIFFERENTIAL DIAGNOSIS

- Subungual exostosis (2):
  - Subungual osteochondroma: Histologically, exostosis has a fibrocartilage cap, and the osteochondroma has hyaline cartilage that is confluent with the underlying trabecular and cortical bone (2).
  - Fibroma
  - Subungual verruca vulgaris
  - Subungual squamous cell carcinoma
  - Glomus tumor
  - Enchondroma protuberans
  - Multiple exostosis: Consider an autosomal-dominant multiple exostosis syndrome.
- Subungual hematoma (3):
  - Subungual benign and malignant tumors (e.g., melanoma)
  - Onychomycosis
  - Glomus tumor
  - Subungual exostosis

DIAGNOSTIC TESTS & INTERPRETATION

Initial Tests (lab, imaging)

- Subungual exostosis:
  - Diagnosis primarily through radiographs, especially if hard subungual mass is noted on exam
  - Radiographs show overgrown pedunculated radiopaque mass located at the dorsal bone of the distal toe/finger composed of trabeculae (5).
  - Imaging will differentiate subungual exostosis, osteochondroma, and enchondroma (which can rarely affect the distal phalanx).
  - Radiographically, an exostosis lacks clear contiguity of the medullary cavity and cortex, unlike an osteochondroma.
- Subungual hematoma:
  - Three-view radiographs should be obtained when a hematoma involves ≥50% of the visible nail to assess for fracture.
  - Point-of-care ultrasound has been shown to be a promising tool for traumatic nail bed injuries with sensitivity of 93.4% and specificity of 100% (5).

Diagnostic Procedures/Other

A chronic nontraumatic lesion or a patient with a history of melanoma each may require a biopsy of the underlying nail matrix and/or nail bed to rule out a pigmented lesion (3).

TREATMENT

- Subungual exostosis:
  - Excision of the tumor
- Subungual hematoma:
  - Immediate elevation and application of ice or immersion in ice water may reduce pain and bleeding.
  - An acute subungual hematoma can be evacuated by trephination—puncturing the nail plate overlying the hematoma using thermal cautery, laser, or a drill (i.e., 18-gauge needle, scalpel blade, dental bur) (6).
  - Evacuation is performed by directing the preferred heated trephine perpendicular to the nail plate overlying the hematoma; slow and gentle pressure is applied until blood is expressed from the nail plate.
  - Nail removal if the normal architecture of the nail plate or its surrounding structures have been damaged (6)
  - Wound and laceration repair if needed. Prophylactic antibiotics are not recommended.

ISSUES FOR REFERRAL

Chronic nail lesions, patients with history of melanoma, and pigmented lesions involving the periungual should be referred for evaluation for the possibility of a subungual melanoma.

ONGOING CARE

FOLLOW-UP RECOMMENDATIONS

Further evaluation with radiographs (excluding exostosis) and possibly a biopsy is required when a suspected subungual hematoma does not grow out distally as the nail plate grows or if there is a recurrence of the hematoma (3).

PATIENT EDUCATION

Subungual hematoma:

- To prevent infection following a trephination of the hematoma, instruct the patient on proper wound care, including:
  - Observing and reporting any signs of infection
  - Keeping the area clean and dry
  - Avoidance of swimming, hot tub, and whirlpool use
- Inform the patient that they may eventually lose the affected nail and a new nail will grow out, typically within 2 to 6 months.
- Wear well-fitting footwear with a snug midfoot and a wide toe box.
- Keep nails trimmed.
- Orthotic devices if appropriate

PROGNOSIS

Prognosis for both subungual exostosis and hematoma is excellent.

COMPLICATIONS

- A recurrence of the exostosis secondary to an incomplete excision
- Onychodystrophy, the discoloration or malformation of a nail, may result from disruption of nail bed and matrix (2).
- Infection following excision of a subungual exostosis or an evacuation of a subungual hematoma
- Recurring subungual hematomas of the same nail bed secondary to repetitive trauma may predispose the nail bed to onychomycosis.

REFERENCES

1. Ardebol J, Mubarak A. Subungual exostosis recurrence in a 16-year-old athletic male. *Oxf Med Case Reports*. 2020;2020(4–5):omaa033.
2. DaCambra MP, Gupta SK, Ferri-de-Barros F. Subungual exostosis of the toes: a systematic review. *Clin Orthop Relat Res*. 2014;472(4):1251–1259.
3. Braun RP, Baran R, Le Gal FA, et al. Diagnosis and management of nail pigmentations. *J Am Acad Dermatol*. 2007;56(5):835–847.
4. Li H, Li H, Qi X, et al. Clinical diagnosis and treatment of subungual exostosis in children. *Front Pediatr*. 2022;10:1075089.
5. Gungor F, Akyol KC, Eken C, et al. The value of point-of-care ultrasound for detecting nail bed injury in ED. *Am J Emerg Med*. 2016;34(9):1850–1854.
6. Pingel C, McDowell C. *Subungual Hematoma Drainage*. StatPearls Publishing; 2023. Updated June 24, 2025. Accessed August 8, 2025. https://www.ncbi.nlm.nih.gov/books/NBK482508/

CLINICAL PEARLS

- Not all dark patches under the nail are subungual hematomas. Consider the diagnosis of melanoma and other tumors when the history of trauma and the physical examination are not consistent with a simple subungual hematoma.
- Chronic subungual hematomas can be a manifestation of child abuse. If history and exam are suspicious, please notify a member of social services if warranted.

SUDDEN CARDIAC ARREST: COMMOTIO CORDIS

Elizabeth A. Williams, DO

BASICS

ALERT
Early resuscitation with automated external defibrillator (AED)/defibrillation improves survival.

DESCRIPTION

Commotio cordis (CC), Latin for "agitation or disruption of the heart," is blunt, nonpenetrating trauma to the precordium, which results in an irregular heart rhythm such as ventricular tachycardia or ventricular fibrillation (VF). This is a rare event but must be considered secondary to its lethal nature.

EPIDEMIOLOGY

- This condition occurs primarily in young males, with the highest incidence in sports such as baseball and hockey, although it has been reported in nearly all sports. It may occur in any sport when the sports person (male/female) is struck in the precordial region with a firm object such as a ball, puck, other player, and so on.
- CC was first described in the 1700s.
- More than half of reported cases occurred during competitive sporting events.
- The mean age is 15 years (1).
- 95% of cases are male (2).
- Youth baseball accounts for most of the cases, 45% of sports-related cases (3).

Incidence

- 60–75% of reported CC events involve sports.
- Highest incidence of CC is seen in youth baseball with pitches of standard baseballs thrown at speeds between 30 and 50 mph.
- Velocities above and below this range did not seem to carry the same risk; faster speeds incurred risk of contusio cordis.

Prevalence

- The CC registry has >200 cases, and only 5 cases were reported prior to 1983 (2).
- Historically low prevalence (prior to 1983) possibly due to lack of recognition/underreporting
- 53% of cases occur during organized competitive sports, with total of 77% occurring with all sports participation.
- Estimated 10 to 20 per year

ETIOLOGY AND PATHOPHYSIOLOGY

- Several variables must combine for an impact to result in CC: type (size and hardness) of projectile, force of projectile, location of impact, and timing of impact in the cardiac cycle.
- Impact to the precordium during the vulnerable period of the repolarization upslope of the T wave (10 to 30 milliseconds before the T-wave peak) may lead to VF. VF is the most common initial rhythm in CC (4).
- Low-energy impact directly over the heart, specifically over the center of the left ventricle (LV), carries the highest risk. Blows at noncardiac sites does not carry the same risk.
- Causative theories on predisposition to VF/CC include rapid rises in LV pressures to forces between 250 and 450 mm Hg that may potentiate the associated arrhythmia. Stretch channels may be activated due to associated myocardial stretch with impact, and potassium adenosine triphosphate channel activation has been implicated (4).
- Sympathetic activation occurring during sports participation may increase the likelihood of CC, but this has not been substantiated in research studies.

Genetics

- No specific genes or genetic conditions have been attributed to the condition.
- It is unclear why there is a male predilection for this condition. One possibility is increased male relative to female participation in competitive youth baseball.

RISK FACTORS

- Participation in competitive sports
- Maron et al. found a significantly increased risk of death when CC occurred during recreational activities or normal daily activities as compared to occurrence in organized competitive sports (2).
- Lee et al. study also found that non–sport-related CC had a higher rate of morality than sport-related CC (88% vs. 66%, respectively) (3).
- Harder projectiles used in certain sports
- Smaller round objects (size of a golf ball) had greater risk of inducing VF than a larger object (size of a baseball), and the flat objects of equal weight did not induce VF.
- Velocity of projectile, distance from center of LV and peak LV pressure induced by impact (1)
- Younger age: postulated that younger people are at greater risk due to the increased compliance of their chest wall
- Prolonged corrected Q-T interval (QTc) may increase susceptibility.
- African Americans are 8 times less likely to survive when compared to white counterparts (2).

GENERAL PREVENTION

- The U.S. Consumer Product Safety Commission recommends use of softer "safety baseballs" to reduce the risk of soft tissue trauma. These "safety baseballs" reduced the risk of onset of VF after precordial impact in a swine model study, and there is a linear correlation between CC events and the relative hardness of a baseball. Safety balls may decrease the risk but do not eliminate it.
- Kumar et al. demonstrated that more effective chest protectors could be developed. In a swine model, they demonstrated reduced incidence of VF from 54% to 5% for certain chest protectors. The advancement of materials is believed to contribute to improved performance (5). The performance of the newer materials will need further evaluation once used in sport. Previously available barriers were shown to have little protective benefit.
- National Operating Committee on Standards for Athletic Equipment (NOCSAE) updated its criteria for testing chest guards in February of 2018 in attempts to produce more effective chest protectors.
- Changes in coaching techniques to eliminate chest blocking are theorized to potentially reduce CC events.
- Public health measures, such as youth, parents, and coaches learning cardiopulmonary resuscitation (CPR), and the increased availability and use of AED may provide the biggest impact on improving CC outcomes, recognizing this does not prevent CC.

COMMONLY ASSOCIATED CONDITIONS

- Contusio cordis (myocardial contusion with tissue damage)
- Rule out other causes of sudden cardiac death (SCD) causing arrhythmia such as hypertrophic cardiomyopathy (HCM).

DIAGNOSIS

HISTORY

Witnessed trauma to the precordium followed by collapse should elicit suspicion of CC:

- There may be a delay from impact to collapse.

PHYSICAL EXAM

- In the setting of collapse, any physical exam should be focused on brief assessment of pulse and, if absent, initiating CPR with use of AED as soon as possible. CC is a diagnosis made based on witnessed precordial blow and confirmed by AED recognition of subsequent arrhythmia. There are no specific labs/imaging tests to aid in diagnosis.
- Note: There may be a brief period of consciousness after impact and before collapse; must maintain a high level of suspicion
- Pathologic findings:
  - Autopsy is notable for absence of any significant cardiac or thoracic injury.

DIFFERENTIAL DIAGNOSIS

- HCM
- Anomalous coronary artery
- Long QT syndrome
- Wolff-Parkinson-White syndrome
- Arrhythmogenic right ventricle dysplasia
- Brugada syndrome
- Dilated cardiomyopathy
- Ruptured/dissected aorta
- Severe aortic valve stenosis
- Mitral valve prolapse
- Coronary artery disease
- Asthma
- Heat stroke
- Drug abuse

TREATMENT

Treatment consists of immediate institution of basic life support (BLS)/advanced cardiac life support (ACLS) protocols, including implementation of an AED. Early defibrillation is critical to survival with CC. Increased survival if defibrillated within 3 minutes of collapse. Survival has been reported up to 58% most likely due to increased availability of AEDs (2)[C].

ADDITIONAL THERAPIES

All CC survivors should be referred to a cardiologist for a complete cardiac evaluation to investigate for structural heart disease (i.e., electrocardiogram [ECG], echocardiogram, cardiac magnetic resonance imaging [MRI], ambulatory ECG monitoring, stress testing). Additional testing to investigate for Brugada and long QT syndromes with pharmacologic testing is case dependent (6)[C].

ONGOING CARE

FOLLOW-UP RECOMMENDATIONS

Patient Monitoring

- All patients should be admitted to the hospital for observation and monitoring after the event.
- Patients should be followed after discharge to assess for potential cardiac or neurologic deficit.

PATIENT EDUCATION

- An individual athlete's susceptibility to CC should be considered in any return to play decisions regarding contact sports.
- Decisions are made on a case-by-case basis, with consideration given to residual cardiac deficit, neurologic deficit, or other morbidity. Cardiology consultation should be involved in these decisions (6)[C].

PROGNOSIS

- CC is a condition that carries a grave prognosis. Despite use of BLS/ACLS protocols, the condition is often lethal.
- Lee et al. reported a 66% mortality rate (3).
- Use of an AED has been found to be an independent predictor of survival (2).
- Improved survival if AED used within 3 minutes of event (3)
- Sustaining blunt cardiac trauma while participating during organized competitive sporting activity was found to be an independent predictor of survival (2).
- Maron et al. demonstrated that 71% of CC survivors achieved complete physical recovery (2).

COMPLICATIONS

- Neurologic impairment may occur secondary to cerebral hypoperfusion.
- Cardiac sequela resulting in decreased left ventricular ejection fraction

REFERENCES

1. Madias C, Maron BJ, Dau N, et al. Size as an important determinant of chest blow-induced commotio cordis. *Med Sci Sports Exerc*. 2018;50(9):1767–1771.
2. Maron BJ, Haas TS, Ahluwalia A, et al. Increasing survival rate from commotio cordis. *Heart Rhythm*. 2013;10(2):219–223.
3. Lee RN, Rodrigues TS, Gan JT, et al. Commotio cordis in non-sport-related events: a systematic review. *JACC Clin Electrophysiol*. 2023;9(8 Pt 1):1321–1329.
4. Krexi L, Sheppard MN. Blow/trauma to the chest and sudden cardiac death: commotio cordis and contusio cordis are leading causes. *Med Sci Law*. 2018;58(2):93–96.
5. Kumar K, Mandleywala SN, Gannon MP, et al. Development of a chest wall protector effective in preventing sudden cardiac death by chest wall impact (commotio cordis). *Clin J Sport Med*. 2017;27(1):26–30.
6. Link MS, Estes NAM III, Maron BJ, et al. Eligibility and disqualification recommendations for competitive athletes with cardiovascular abnormalities: task force 13: commotio cordis: a scientific statement from the American Heart Association and American College of Cardiology. *Circulation*. 2015;132(22):e339–e342.

ADDITIONAL READING

- Alsheikh-Ali AA, Madias C, Supran S, et al. Marked variability in susceptibility to ventricular fibrillation in an experimental commotio cordis model. *Circulation*. 2010;122(24):2499–2504.
- Doerer JJ, Haas TS, Estes NAM III, et al. Evaluation of chest barriers for protection against sudden death due to commotio cordis. *Am J Cardiol*. 2007;99(6):857–859.
- Huis In 't Veld MA, Craft CA, Hood RE. Blunt cardiac trauma review. *Cardiol Clin*. 2018;36(1):183–191.
- Kalin J, Madias C, Alsheikh-Ali AA, et al. Reduced diameter spheres increases the risk of chest blow-induced ventricular fibrillation (commotio cordis). *Heart Rhythm*. 2011;8(10):1578–1581.
- Link MS. Commotio cordis: ventricular fibrillation triggered by chest impact-induced abnormalities in repolarization. *Circ Arrhythm Electrophysiol*. 2012;5(2):425–432.
- Link MS, Maron BJ, Wang PJ, et al. Upper and lower limits of vulnerability to sudden arrhythmic death with chest-wall impact (commotio cordis). *J Am Coll Cardiol*. 2003;41(1):99–104.
- Palacio LE, Link MS. Commotio cordis. *Sports Health*. 2009;1(2):174–179.
- The National Registry of Sudden Death in Young Athletes: https://cihlab.com/

CLINICAL PEARLS

- Witnessed precordial impact to a young athlete with resultant distress/collapse should elicit consideration of CC. Immediate institution of BLS/ACLS protocols with use of AED provides the best chance of survival.
- Use of age-appropriate safety baseballs has been shown to reduce CC events.
- Chest wall protective devices should be used in high-risk positions (catchers/goalies) but have not been proven to prevent CC. Newer materials show promise of being more effective in prevention of CC based on animal models.
- Thorough evaluation of all CC survivors should be undertaken, with return-to-play considerations made on a case-by-case basis.
- Awareness and availability of AED has increased survival rate; nevertheless, there is still a high mortality rate.

SUPERFICIAL RADIAL NERVE (WARTENBERG DISEASE)

Bailey J. Meccariello, DO, CAQSM • Karl B. Fields, MD, CAQSM, FAMSSM

BASICS

DESCRIPTION

- Compression mononeuropathy of the superficial branch of radial nerve in the distal forearm
- Radial nerve, arises from C5–C8, provides motor function to the extensors of the forearm, wrist, and fingers and motor function for supinators of forearm. Superficial radial nerve (SRN) provides sensory function to extensor surface of the forearm via posterior cutaneous nerve and the web of skin between the thumb and index finger.
- SRN becomes susceptible to injury as it passes beneath the tendon of the brachioradialis and pierces the deep fascia.
- Synonym(s): Wartenberg syndrome entrapment; cheiralgia paresthetica; prisoner's palsy; handcuff disease; radial sensory nerve entrapment

EPIDEMIOLOGY

- The incidence is not known but estimated to be rare at 0.003% of the population (1).
- It is rare, although often is not recognized.
- More common in women

RISK FACTORS

- Wrist compression (i.e., tight bands, tape, watches, archery guards, gloves, or straps of a racquetball racquet, cast, soft tissue mass, ganglion cyst)
- Anomalous or two bellied brachioradialis muscle or split brachioradialis tendon (1)
- Has been documented after carpal tunnel syndrome splinting (1)[C]
- Direct trauma in contact sports
- Laceration and postsurgical injury
- Sports involving repetitive pronation and supination at the wrist (e.g., batting, throwing, and rowing)

COMMONLY ASSOCIATED CONDITIONS

de Quervain syndrome

DIAGNOSIS

HISTORY

- Determine whether pain or sensory deficit is the primary symptom. If pain is the main complaint, then de Quervain syndrome seems a more likely diagnosis.
- Duration of symptoms
- Location of symptoms
- Characteristics of symptoms to suggest sensory involvement

PHYSICAL EXAM

- Symptoms primarily limited to the dorsoradial aspect of the distal forearm and hand (wrist, hand, dorsal thumb, and index finger)
- Paresthesias (numbness and tingling)
- Hyperesthesia
- Less commonly, pain or burning
- Positive Tinel sign along the radial aspect of the midforearm
- Wrist flexion, ulnar deviation, and pronation place traction on the nerve and increase symptoms.
- Sensation deficit on the dorsoradial aspect of the forearm and/or hand
- Finkelstein test typically negative, as opposed to de Quervain syndrome, which usually has positive Finkelstein test
- Pain at rest more typical of Wartenberg Syndrome and not de Quervain syndrome
- With SRN injury, pain can be present with thumb abduction and adduction, differentiating this from de Quervain syndrome in which extension and flexion create more symptoms.
- Diagnostic nerve block to the cutaneous nerve in the proximal forearm just distal to the cubital crease and adjacent to the cephalic vein may help define its contribution to any pathology.
- Ultrasound evaluation can be useful to assess for areas of nerve compression and evidence of mononeuropathy (i.e., enlargement, hypoechogenicity, enlarged nerve fascicles, neovascularization) (2)[C].
- Lidocaine test: This test is effective because the terminal branch of the lateral antebrachial cutaneous nerve (LABCN) often shares distribution with the SRN, its compression can mimic that involving the SRN.
- Nerve conduction study (NCS) may be useful for diagnosis (3)[C].
- The most common technique records the sensory nerve action potentials from the web space between the thumb and index finger with stimulation originating in the distal forearm.
- Ideally, it is preferable to perform NCS on both the SRN and the LABCN (4)[C].
- Sensory action potential, conduction velocity, and amplitude are decreased.
- Motor testing of radial nerve is normal.

DIFFERENTIAL DIAGNOSIS

- de Quervain syndrome
- Intersection syndrome
- Lateral antebrachial cutaneous neuropathy
- Thumb carpometacarpal arthritis
- C6 radiculopathy

TREATMENT

GENERAL MEASURES

- Almost all patients do well with conservative treatment.
- Remove the offending compressive agent (5)[C].
- Avoid repetitive trauma to the area. Consider padding the area if unable to avoid trauma during the athletic season.
- Avoid repetitive pronation, wrist flexion, and ulnar deviation.
- Thumb spica splint for brief period of immobilization may be needed.
- Nonsteroidal anti-inflammatory drugs (NSAIDs)
- Hydrodissection of the nerve at the area of compression and maximal pain can be helpful.
- Desensitization
- No information exists about neuropathic pain agents, and use of vitamin B_6 is anecdotal.

SURGERY/OTHER PROCEDURES

If conservative treatment fails, then surgical decompression should be considered (6)[C].

COMPLEMENTARY & ALTERNATIVE MEDICINE

No studies of acupuncture or other alternative products reported

REFERENCES

1. Węgiel A, Karauda P, Zielinska N, et al. Radial nerve compression: anatomical perspective and clinical consequences. *Neurosurg Rev*. 2023;46(1):53.
2. Serçe A, Karaca Umay E, Karaahmet ÖZ, et al. An unexpected side effect: Wartenberg syndrome related to the use of splint during carpal tunnel syndrome treatment. *Turk J Phys Med Rehabil*. 2017;64(1):83–86.
3. Xiao TG, Cartwright MS. Ultrasound in the evaluation of radial neuropathies at the elbow. *Front Neurol*. 2019;10:216.
4. Cho NS, Kim KH, Park BK, et al. Superficial radial sensory neuropathy: medial and lateral branch injury. *Muscle Nerve*. 2016;53(5):690–693.
5. Kon T, Suzuki C, Hotta R, et al. Utility of nerve conduction studies for diagnosis of injury to the medial branch of the superficial radial nerve. *eNeurologicalSci*. 2017;8:38–39.
6. Doughty CT, Bowley MP. Entrapment neuropathies of the upper extremity. *Med Clin North Am*. 2019;103(2):357–370.

ADDITIONAL READING

- Anto C, Aradhya P. Clinical diagnosis of peripheral nerve compression in the upper extremity. *Orthop Clin North Am*. 1996;27(2):227–236.
- Dang AC, Rodner CM. Unusual compression neuropathies of the forearm, part I: radial nerve. *J Hand Surg Am*. 2009;34(10):1906–1914.
- Nuber GW, Assenmacher J, Bowen MK. Neurovascular problems in the forearm, wrist, and hand. *Clin Sports Med*. 1998;17(3):585–610.
- Plancher KD, Peterson RK, Steichen JB. Compressive neuropathies and tendinopathies in the athletic elbow and wrist. *Clin Sports Med*. 1996;15(2):331–371.
- Spies CK, Unglaub F, Müller LP, et al. Endoscopically assisted release of the superficial radial nerve. *Arch Orthop Trauma Surg*. 2015;135(5):737–741.
- Terrono AL, Millender LH. Management of work-related upper-extremity nerve entrapments. *Orthop Clin North Am*. 1996;27(4):783–793.

CLINICAL PEARLS

- If the symptoms are present >3 days, the neurapraxic injury may require up to 3 months to reach maximum improvement.
- The splint usually needs to be worn 2 to 4 weeks or until symptoms resolve.
- The protective padding needs to be worn until symptoms resolve or if engaging in sports with repetitive forearm trauma.

SUPRASCAPULAR NERVE PALSY

Tony Olmert, MD, MPhil · Brianna Martinez, MD · Kenneth S. Taylor, MD, FAAFP, CAQSM

BASICS

DESCRIPTION

Injury of the suprascapular nerve causing pain or weakness with or without functional limitation of supraspinatus and/or infraspinatus muscles

EPIDEMIOLOGY

- True incidence unknown; thought to be relatively uncommon; however, recognition and diagnosis are increasing and could be responsible for 1–2% of all cases of shoulder pain (1).
- Diagnosis skews young (<40 years old), more common in overhead athletes (1)

ETIOLOGY AND PATHOPHYSIOLOGY

- The suprascapular nerve is a mixed motor and sensory nerve, arising from the upper trunk of the brachial plexus, carrying fibers from the C5 and C6 nerve roots with variable contributions from C4.
- It crosses the posterior triangle of the neck and passes under the superior transverse scapular ligament via suprascapular notch.
- Crossing the supraspinous fossa, it sends motor branches to supraspinatus and receives sensory branches, including from the posterior shoulder capsule and glenohumeral joint.
- The nerve turns around the spinoglenoid notch (passing under the spinoglenoid ligament, also known as the inferior transverse scapular ligament, when present) and passes into the infraspinous fossa, where its branches terminate into infraspinatus.
- This anatomy explains the propensity for nerve injury, most commonly at the suprascapular and spinoglenoid notches; injury at the former affects both supraspinatus and infraspinatus, whereas the latter only affects infraspinatus (1),(2).
- Chronic or acute suprascapular nerve injuries can occur via mechanisms including compression, traction, and vascular compromise.
- Chronic injuries are attributed to repetitive movements causing traction and/or compression, extrinsic compression from paralabral or ganglion cysts, or secondary to systemic conditions (1),(2).
- Acute injuries can arise secondary to massive, retracted rotator cuff tears or other trauma, or, in rare reports, iatrogenic injury (1),(2).

RISK FACTORS

- Anatomic factors such as the morphology of the suprascapular notch, superior transverse scapular ligament, and associated vascular structures can contribute to risk of nerve injury.
- Suprascapular notch morphology has been described as six different subtypes, with the "deep V-shaped" notch at risk for nerve injury (2).
- The variably present anterior coracoscapular ligament, which runs inferior to the superior transverse scapular ligament, can also contribute to injury, depending on its morphology (2).
- Repetitive overhead motions, such as those incurred by volleyball, baseball, and tennis players is a risk factor for chronic injury, as evidenced by the high rate of suprascapular neuropathy documented in these athletes (1),(2).
- Nerve compression against the scapular spine is thought to occur with supraspinatus and/or infraspinatus contraction with extreme abduction and external rotation for example during the volleyball serve motion (1),(2).
- This compression can be exacerbated by either compression or traction injury from cross-body adduction incurred in a pitching, throwing, or serving motion (1),(2).
- Either direct (scapular fracture) or indirect (retracted rotator cuff tear) trauma is also a risk factor for development of nerve injury by compression (paralabral cysts) or traction.

DIAGNOSIS

HISTORY

- Most common symptom is shoulder pain, localized to the posterior or lateral shoulder; however, radiation to the neck or arm can occur.
- Symptoms help identify the site of injury—pain suggests proximal (suprascapular notch), whereas painless weakness or atrophy suggests a distal (spinoglenoid notch) lesion.
- Fewer than half of patients recall a traumatic event (2).
- Younger patients more often overhead athletes, older patients more often associated with rotator cuff injury

PHYSICAL EXAM

- Inspect for supraspinatus and/or (especially) infraspinatus atrophy, comparing side by side.
- If proximal lesion, may have posterior/lateral shoulder pain along with weakness and atrophy of supraspinatus and infraspinatus
- If lesion is distal to sensory branches, painless, isolated infraspinatus atrophy with or without weakness of external rotation may be seen.
- Tenderness to palpation can often be elicited at the site of the lesion.
- External rotation testing against resistance to evaluate infraspinatus strength, but deficits may be compensated by teres minor and posterior deltoid.
- Jobe test to evaluate supraspinatus strength
- Evocative tests include cross-body adduction with internal rotation and the suprascapular stretch (1).
- The above should be accompanied by full shoulder examination to evaluate for associated injury.
- Investigate for cervical radiculopathy and other cervical spine pathology (complete neck exam, including the Spurling maneuver).
- Complete neurologic examination should be performed as well; deep tendon reflexes should not be affected in isolated suprascapular neuropathy.
- Ultrasound-guided injection of local anesthetic into the suprascapular or spinoglenoid notch may help to determine source of pain but is rarely necessary.

DIFFERENTIAL DIAGNOSIS

- Rotator cuff tendonitis/tear
- Labral pathology
- Cervical radiculopathy
- Parsonage-Turner syndrome/brachial neuritis
- Brachial plexopathy (stinger)

DIAGNOSTIC TESTS & INTERPRETATION

Initial Tests (lab, imaging)

- Plain films of the neck and shoulder evaluate for bony abnormalities; Stryker notch view can be particularly effective for evaluating suprascapular notch (1),(2).
- Computed tomography (CT) may be considered following plain films if nerve injury due to osseous compression is suspected.
- Radiographs are typically followed by magnetic resonance imaging (MRI) to identify contributory lesions such as paralabral cysts or rotator cuff tears.
- Magnetic resonance neurography, performed with 3.0-T MRI, is advantageous for its ability to image the nerve directly, identify the etiology of injury, and evaluate for other conditions on the differential (3)[B].
- Ultrasound can also be used to detect compressive lesions affecting the suprascapular nerve (1),(2),(3).

Diagnostic Procedures/Other

- Electromyography and nerve conduction velocity are considered the gold standard diagnostic tests for suprascapular nerve injury (1).
- Shortcomings of these studies include possible false-negative results, inability to identify etiology of injury, and operator dependence.

TREATMENT

MEDICATION

In the absence of a well-defined lesion causing suprascapular nerve compression, initial nonoperative therapy, including a course of nonsteroidal anti-inflammatory drugs is recommended (2)[C],(4)[A].

ADDITIONAL THERAPIES

- Initial nonoperative therapy also includes physical therapy.
- Peripheral nerve stimulation, pulsed radiofrequency, and transcutaneous electrical nerve stimulation can also be considered for minimally invasive pain management (4).

SURGERY/OTHER PROCEDURES

- Surgery (either open or arthroscopic) should be considered for patients with suprascapular nerve entrapment leading to nerve compression (4)[A],(5)[A]; it may also be of benefit in patients who fail nonsurgical management (4)[A],(5)[A].
- Surgery has a high rate of patient-reported improvement in symptoms and return to activity; the most common adverse outcome is ongoing pain (5).
- Ultrasound-guided cyst aspiration has been reported as well however can result in recurrent symptoms (2).
- Ultrasound-guided suprascapular nerve block has been shown in a meta-analysis to be superior to physical therapy and comparable to intra-articular injection for chronic shoulder pain (6); suprascapular nerve hydrodissection may provide superior results as well.

ONGOING CARE

COMPLICATIONS

Two areas which have shown mixed results include (i) ganglion cyst aspiration performed concomitantly with repairs of superior labral tears from anterior to posterior and (ii) suprascapular nerve release performed alongside rotator cuff repair (2),(4),(5).

REFERENCES

1. Bozzi F, Alabau-Rodriguez S, Barrera-Ochoa S, et al. Suprascapular neuropathy around the shoulder: a current concept review. *J Clin Med*. 2020;9(8):2331.
2. Strauss EJ, Kingery MT, Klein D, et al. The evaluation and management of suprascapular neuropathy. *J Am Acad Orthop Surg*. 2020;28(15):617–627.
3. Chalian M, Faridian-Aragh N, Soldatos T, et al. High-resolution 3T MR neurography of suprascapular neuropathy. *Acad Radiol*. 2011;18(8):1049–1059.
4. Vij N, Fabian I, Hansen C, et al. Outcomes after minimally invasive and surgical management of suprascapular nerve entrapment: a systematic review. *Orthop Rev (Pavia)*. 2022;14(3):37157.
5. Sandler AB, Wells ME, Tran C, et al. High rates of return to sport after suprascapular nerve decompression: an updated systematic review. *JSES Rev Rep Tech*. 2024;4(4):654–661.
6. Chang KV, Hung CY, Wu WT, et al. Comparison of the effectiveness of suprascapular nerve block with physical therapy, placebo, and intra-articular injection in management of chronic shoulder pain: a meta-analysis of randomized controlled trials. *Arch Phys Med Rehabil*. 2016;97(8):1366–1380.

CLINICAL PEARLS

- Diagnosis of suprascapular neuropathy requires a high index of suspicion, which may be aided by history of overhead athletics.
- Nonoperative management is the first-line treatment unless a discrete compressive lesion can be identified as the target of surgery.
- Return of muscle strength usually occurs over time once the cause of the injury has been treated, however, especially with long-standing, severe lesions, muscle atrophy may not fully resolve.

S

SURFER'S EAR

Matthew J. Jepson, MD, MS, CAQSM ▪ Tenley Murphy, MD, FAAFP, CAQSM ▪ Jason J. Stacy, MD

BASICS

- Surfer's ear, or external auditory exostosis, is a benign overgrowth of the temporal bone in the external auditory meatus that occurs after prolonged exposure to cold water.
- Patients are usually asymptomatic but may present with recurrent ear infections, conductive hearing loss, and/or pain.

DESCRIPTION

- Benign overgrowth of temporal bone into external auditory meatus
- Usually bilateral
- May have multiple exostoses in a canal
- Occurs after prolonged exposure to cold water

EPIDEMIOLOGY

Rates are highly correlated with time spent in the associated activities. Typically, condition becomes symptomatic after 5 to 7 years of surfing or other cold-water activities with development of exostoses in 90% of cold-water surfers at 10 years (1).

Prevalence

In the general population, the prevalence of external auditory exostoses is 6.3 per 1,000 people (2). Prevalence increases with time spent in the associated activities. Surfers have higher rates of exostoses with increasing years of surfing experience (3).

ETIOLOGY AND PATHOPHYSIOLOGY

Regular irritation of the auditory meatus by exposure to cold water was implicated in the causation of exostoses. Increasing size of exostoses can lead to recurrent infections, conductive hearing loss, and/or pain.

RISK FACTORS

- Occurs after prolonged and/or repetitive exposure to cold water (1),(3)
- Most common in surfing; also seen in kayaking, white water rafting, and diving (breath holding and scuba) (3),(4)

GENERAL PREVENTION

- Screening susceptible individuals in order to recommend appropriate prevention (5)
- Best method of prevention is molded earplugs worn during activity.
- Special headbands that cover ears are also preventive.
- Earplugs and headbands may be used in combination.

COMMONLY ASSOCIATED CONDITIONS

- Otitis externa
- Furunculosis
- Acute cellulitis
- Rare: perichondritis, chondritis, bullous myringitis

DIAGNOSIS

- Visual diagnosis during otoscopic exam
- Weber and Rinne test to evaluate for conductive hearing loss
- Computed tomography (CT) demonstrates broad-based or more focal circumferential bony overgrowth of the osseous external auditory canal (6).

HISTORY

Key points:

- Amount of cold-water exposure
- Use of preventive aids
- Previous surgeries
- Presence of recurrent infections or progressive hearing loss

DIFFERENTIAL DIAGNOSIS

- Fibrous dysplasia
- Otitis externa
- Acute otitis media
- Cholesteatoma
- Osteoma
- Mastoiditis
- Referred pain
- Temporomandibular joint syndrome

TREATMENT

MEDICATION

Medications typically are not needed, unless to treat related bacterial infection or cerumen impaction.

ISSUES FOR REFERRAL

- Referral to audiology to establish degree of hearing loss
- Referral to ear, nose, and throat (ENT) specialist indicated for recurrent infections, pain, or hearing loss (7)[B]

SURGERY/OTHER PROCEDURES

- Surgery is definitive care for exostoses.
- Reserved for severe, symptomatic cases; presence of exostoses without symptoms would not necessitate surgical intervention.
- Several approaches are used; postauricular is the most common and seems to minimize complications (7)[B].
- Transcanal approaches are being revisited because the use of an endoscope allows for this lower morbidity approach while lowering risk of damage to the tympanic membrane or facial nerve (8)[C].
- If hearing loss is present, generally, there is a good response to surgery with restored hearing.
- Some patients require repeated surgeries if cold-water exposure continues (usually after ≥5 years of additional exposure).

ONGOING CARE

PROGNOSIS

Correctable with surgery but may recur with continued exposure

REFERENCES

1. Alexander V, Lau A, Beaumont E, et al. The effects of surfing behaviour on the development of external auditory canal exostosis. *Eur Arch Otorhinolaryngol*. 2015;272(7):1643–1649.
2. Bart RM, Lau H, Cooper JS. *Surfer's Ear*. StatPearls Publishing; 2023. Updated April 30, 2023. Accessed August 27, 2025. https://www.ncbi.nlm.nih.gov/books/NBK534874/
3. Lennon P, Murphy C, Fennessy B, et al. Auditory canal exostoses in Irish surfers. *Ir J Med Sci*. 2016;185(1):183–187.
4. Sheard PW, Doherty M. Prevalence and severity of external auditory exostoses in breath-hold divers. *J Laryngol Otol*. 2008;122(11):1162–1167.
5. Simas V, Hing W, Pope R, et al. Australian surfers' awareness of 'surfer's ear.' *BMJ Open Sport Exerc Med*. 2020;6(1):e000641.
6. Fallshaw A, Walizai T, Knipe H, et al. External auditory canal exostoses. Radiopaedia. Updated October 5, 2024. Accessed August 27, 2025. https://doi.org/10.53347/rID-4054
7. House JW, Wilkinson EP. External auditory exostoses: evaluation and treatment. *Otolaryngol Head Neck Surg*. 2008;138(5):672–678.
8. Kozin ED, Remenschneider AK, Shah PV, et al. Endoscopic transcanal removal of symptomatic external auditory canal exostoses. *Am J Otolaryngol*. 2015;36(2):283–286.

ADDITIONAL READING

Cooper A, Tong R, Neil R, et al. External auditory canal exostoses in white water kayakers. *Br J Sports Med*. 2010;44(2):144–147.

CLINICAL PEARLS

- Benign bony overgrowth of the temporal bone into the external auditory meatus
- Causes repeated ear infections, hearing loss, or pain in surfers (or other cold-water athletes)
- Preventable with earplugs and/or headbands
- Surgery is definitive treatment when hearing loss is present.

S

SWIMMING-INDUCED PULMONARY EDEMA (SIPE)

James Suchy, MD, CAQSM • Caitlyn C. Mooney, MD, FAAP, CAQSM

BASICS

DESCRIPTION

- Acute, noncardiogenic pulmonary edema that occurs during swimming or other water-based exercise, often in cold water and high-exertion conditions.
- Presents with sudden onset of dyspnea, cough (often producing frothy or blood-tinged sputum), and hypoxemia during or shortly after a swim, without evidence of water aspiration or underlying cardiac failure
- Caused by the leakage of fluid from the pulmonary capillaries into the alveoli during physical activity in water
- Can range in severity from mild symptoms that quickly resolve to potentially life-threatening respiratory failure
- Synonym: immersion pulmonary edema (IPE)

EPIDEMIOLOGY

Incidence

- First described in healthy scuba divers in the 1980s
- Since then, hundreds of cases have been reported among triathletes, swimmers, snorkelers, free divers, and scuba divers. A surge in triathlon and open-water swimming events has coincided with increased swimming-induced pulmonary edema (SIPE) case reports.
- SIPE is considered uncommon overall, and true incidence is hard to determine due to misattribution to drowning events and underreporting of mild cases.
- Estimates of SIPE incidence vary considerably across populations with reported rates ranging from ~0.01% in triathlon races up to 26% in small studies of military trainee swims (1).
- In a large 4-year prospective study at a mass open-water swim event (47,573 individual swims), SIPE incidence was 0.44% of swims (2).
- In this same study, women and older athletes were at significantly higher risk; SIPE incidence was 0.75% in women versus 0.09% in men (8.59 times higher odds), and increased from 0.08% in young adults to ~1.1% in swimmers >60 years old (12.74 times higher odds) (2).
- Precise mortality rates are unknown, because fatal SIPE episodes are often misclassified as drowning (autopsy findings can be similar).
- Some experts suspect SIPE to be a leading cause of sudden death in triathlon swimming segments and an underrecognized contributor to dive fatalities. In one analysis of United States triathlon deaths from 2008 to 2015, 72.4% occurred during the swim. Many of those victims had unexpected left ventricular hypertrophy (LVH) on autopsy—a marker of SIPE susceptibility–suggesting SIPE as a possible cause (3).

ETIOLOGY AND PATHOPHYSIOLOGY

- The exact pathophysiology of SIPE is not fully understood, and ongoing research is needed.
- SIPE appears to result from a combination of hemodynamic and environmental factors that overwhelm the body's compensatory mechanisms, leading to pulmonary edema.
- SIPE is multifactorial, with both environmental conditions and individual anatomic/physiologic factors contributing to an excessive fluid transudation from pulmonary capillaries into alveoli.
- Pulmonary edema occurs when fluid accumulates in the lung interstitium and alveoli secondary to extravasation from pulmonary vasculature.
- Pulmonary edema occurs due to an imbalance in (Starling) forces across the alveolar membrane resulting in a net influx of fluid into the alveoli; thus, capillary hydrostatic pressure overcomes the plasma oncotic pressure.
- Factors that increase the hydrostatic pressure include increased external pressures, increased central blood volume, changes in pulmonary resistance, and increased cardiac output.
- Factors increasing central blood volume:
  - Water immersion at depth increases hydrostatic pressure on the extremities.
  - Cold water causing peripheral vasoconstriction to maintain core body temperature
  - Tight wet suits compressing the extremities
  - Excessive prehydration increasing overall blood volume (particularly in triathletes concerned about dehydration during competition and scuba divers believing it will protect them from decompression illness)
- Factors increasing pulmonary resistance:
  - Cold water causing peripheral vasoconstriction and thus increased afterload on the ventricle
  - Reduced diastolic relaxation (often from long-standing hypertension) causing increased pulmonary resistance in the lungs
  - Exercise causing increased cardiac-filling pressures
  - Breathing against a negative pressure relative to the pressure at the lung centroid (snorkels and scuba diving breathing equipment)
- Additionally, damage to the capillary membrane may also create a leaky membrane that may also contribute.
- Together, these factors, which increase central blood volume and pulmonary resistance, result in increased hydrostatic pressure and subsequent alveolar edema.

RISK FACTORS

- Hypertension
- Preexisting cardiopulmonary disease
- Pulmonary hypertension
- LVH
- Cold water immersion
- Intense exercise/exertion
- Long-duration swims or race distance
- Age >50 years
- Female sex
- Depth of immersion
- Elevated negative inspiratory pressure
- Stressors such as emotional stress or sleep deprivation
- Overhydration
- Tight-fitting wet suit
- *Note:* SIPE occurs even among otherwise healthy and well-conditioned athletes (3),(4).

GENERAL PREVENTION

- **Awareness:** Educate swimming event organizers, dive instructors, medical staff, and participants about SIPE. They should recognize that even healthy and experienced athletes can develop SIPE, and be vigilant for its signs (unexplained breathlessness, cough, etc., in the water). Early recognition is key to preventing severe outcomes.
- **Manage medical risk factors:** Optimize control of hypertension and treat any cardiovascular disease in individuals who plan to engage in strenuous aquatic activities. Evaluating and addressing conditions like LVH, arrhythmias, or pulmonary hypertension may reduce risk.
- **Modifiable behavior for athletes:**
  - Avoid overhydrating before immersion. Start well-hydrated but not excessively so to prevent unnecessary volume load.
  - Ensure wet suits are properly fitted—not overly tight, especially around the chest and limbs. A well-fitted wet suit limits excessive peripheral compression.
  - Mitigate race anxiety and avoid all-out exertion at the very start. Calming techniques and pacing strategies can help reduce surges in blood pressure.
  - Perform a warm-up swim before competition to acclimate to the water temperature and exertion.
  - This may help the body adjust and potentially reduce sympathetic spikes upon race start.
- **Pharmacologic prophylaxis:** In athletes with a prior history of SIPE, small studies have reported fewer recurrences with off-label use of pulmonary vasodilators such as sildenafil or nifedipine, presumably by lowering pulmonary artery pressures. Although evidence is inconclusive and not yet incorporated into guidelines, prophylactic sildenafil has been used empirically in SIPE-susceptible Navy swimmers with some reported success (4)[C].

DIAGNOSIS

HISTORY

- Acute onset of symptoms either during or immediately following exertion in water activities, swimming, or diving
- Symptoms may include dyspnea, cough, chest pain/tightness, and hemoptysis.
- No history of water aspiration (Near-drowning presents with similar symptoms, signs, and radiographic findings.)
- Returned to surface at a safe rate (divers); thus, symptoms are not explained by decompression sickness or lung barotrauma.
- Swimmers and triathletes may report dyspnea above normal exertion levels.
- Divers may report malfunctioning breathing equipment, when it is in fact perfectly fine.
- Other early indicators in divers are using their own or a companion's secondary air supply or flushing a closed-circuit system.

PHYSICAL EXAM

- Tachypnea
- Hypoxemia (ranging from mild to severe)
- Abnormal airway sounds to auscultation, such as crackles, rales, and wheezing, but lung exam can be normal.

DIFFERENTIAL DIAGNOSIS

- Near/fatal drowning
- Pulmonary decompression sickness
- Pulmonary overinflation syndrome
- Respiratory tract infection
- Exercise-induced bronchospasm or asthma exacerbation
- Exercise-induced pulmonary edema
- Congestive heart failure
- Noncardiogenic pulmonary edema
- Cardiopulmonary arrest

DIAGNOSTIC TESTS & INTERPRETATION

- Chest x-ray is usually sufficient for diagnosis in the appropriate clinical context.
- Chest x-ray findings are consistent with pulmonary edema (diffuse interstitial infiltrates or patchy alveolar infiltrates) and sometimes pleural effusions (bilateral or unilateral).
- Point-of-care ultrasound can help distinguish SIPE from other causes of dyspnea (like asthma or aspiration) in an acute setting.
- Ultrasound often shows diffuse B-lines (vertical comet-tail artifacts) in multiple lung fields, reflecting interstitial edema.
- Chest computed tomography (CT) scan is usually not necessary but can rule out other pathologies.
- Rule out other acute cardiopulmonary disease with chest x-ray, electrocardiogram (ECG), cardiac enzymes, and echocardiogram.

TREATMENT

GENERAL MEASURES

- Normalize the environment by stopping activity, removing the patient from the water, removing any constricting gear, and placing them upright in a warm environment (all of which reverse the common physiologic causes of SIPE).
- Do *not* provide additional fluids (which can worsen pulmonary edema).
- Provide supplemental oxygen. If available, administer prompt noninvasive positive-pressure ventilation (NPPV) as either continuous positive airway pressure (CPAP) mask or a portable positive expiratory pressure (PEP) device; this is highly effective for reversing SIPE and preventing hospitalization and intubation (5)[B].
- Race medical teams should be aware of the value of having a CPAP (or PEP device) for safely and effectively treating SIPE.
- Should be monitored by medical staff until complete resolution of symptoms and be prepared to transfer to a higher level of care that can provide advanced respiratory support if needed

MEDICATION

First Line

Traditional treatments such as diuretics or vasodilators have been reported anecdotally (e.g., case reports of using sublingual nitrates or furosemide alongside noninvasive ventilation), but there are no controlled trials supporting medication therapy.

ADMISSION, INPATIENT, AND NURSING CONSIDERATIONS

- Implementation of the above strategies may be able to avoid hospitalization.
- Patients who have severe or deteriorating respiratory symptoms should be transferred to a higher level of care.
- Cases of SIPE with severe respiratory failure may require admission to the intensive care unit (ICU) for intubation and mechanical ventilation to treat pulmonary edema.

ONGOING CARE

FOLLOW-UP RECOMMENDATIONS

- Although SIPE has traditionally been thought to resolve within 24 to 48 hours, newer data show symptoms often persist longer. In a 30-month longitudinal study, 38% of patients had symptoms beyond 2 days, 21% beyond 5 days, 15% at 10 days, and 4% still had symptoms after 1 year (1).
- Persistent cough, dyspnea, or exercise intolerance beyond 48 hours does not exclude SIPE and may reflect a slower recovery trajectory.
- Most patients recover fully, but clinical follow-up is recommended. Further evaluation (e.g., pulmonary function testing, imaging) may be warranted if symptoms are unusually prolonged to exclude other pathology.
- Evaluation for underlying cardiopulmonary conditions (e.g., ECG, echocardiogram, stress testing) should be considered after symptom resolution to identify and manage potential contributing factors.
- Asthma is a key modifiable risk factor—associated with both prolonged symptoms (odds ratio [OR] ~2.6) and recurrence (OR ~6.9)—and should be optimally managed in patients with a history of SIPE (1).

PATIENT EDUCATION

- Educate patients about the recurrence risk of SIPE, which occurred in approximately 28% of individuals who resumed open-water swimming (1).
- Many (58%) choose to avoid open-water swimming after an episode (5), but those wishing to return should be counseled on recurrence prevention strategies:
  - Proper conditioning and warm-up
  - Avoiding overexertion in cold water
  - Using a well-fitted wet suit to reduce chest squeeze
  - Consideration of prophylactic inhaler use in asthmatics
- Athletes resuming activity should be aware of early warning signs—such as unexplained shortness of breath or persistent cough—and should stop activity and exit the water if symptoms arise.

PROGNOSIS

- Although SIPE can be life-threatening in acute cases, particularly due to respiratory failure or drowning risk, most cases are self-limited and resolve over time.
- Long-term outcomes are generally favorable: 90% of patients in a follow-up study reported unchanged or improved health and fitness after 30 months postincident, and most maintained or increased their physical activity levels (5).
- With appropriate evaluation, management, and precautions, athletes can often safely return to training and competition following a SIPE episode.

REFERENCES

1. Kristiansson L, Seiler C, Lundeqvist D, et al. Symptom duration, recurrence, and long-term effects of swimming-induced pulmonary edema: a 30-month follow-up study. *Chest.* 2023;164(5):1257–1267.
2. Hårdstedt M, Kristiansson L, Seiler C, et al. Incidence of swimming-induced pulmonary edema: a cohort study based on 47,600 open-water swimming distances. *Chest.* 2021;160(5):1789–1798.
3. Moon RE, Martina SD, Peacher DF, et al. Deaths in triathletes: immersion pulmonary oedema as a possible cause. *BMJ Open Sport Exerc Med.* 2016;2(1):e000146.
4. Moon RE, Martina SD, Peacher DF, et al. Swimming-induced pulmonary edema: pathophysiology and risk reduction with sildenafil. *Circulation.* 2016;133(10):988–996.
5. Seiler C, Kristiansson L, Klingberg C, et al. Swimming-induced pulmonary edema: evaluation of prehospital treatment with CPAP or positive expiratory pressure device. *Chest.* 2022;162(2):410–420.

CLINICAL PEARLS

- Recent increases in the popularity of aquatic endurance events have raised awareness of SIPE as a cause of morbidity and mortality in water athletes.
- If identified early, there are steps that can be taken to decrease the severity of SIPE. SIPE is likely due to multiple factors but may occur in completely healthy individuals during exertional activities in water.
- Initial treatment of SIPE is to stop swimming, remove the individual from the water, and place them upright in a warm environment. Prompt NPPV is an effective and safe way to reverse SIPE.
- After an episode of SIPE, evaluate for underlying cardiopulmonary disease or other risk factors. There is a risk of SIPE recurrence and death due to acute respiratory failure in the water.

S

SYNCOPE IN SPORTS

Elizabeth A. Williams, DO

BASICS

ALERT

- Need to differentiate cardiac syncope (CS) from noncardiac syncope (NCS) due to increased risk of sudden cardiac death with CS
- Syncope may be the initial presentation of an underlying cardiac condition that increases the risk of sudden cardiac death.

DESCRIPTION

- Syncope: sudden loss of postural tone with loss of consciousness (LOC) due to global cerebral hypoperfusion and spontaneous recovery
- Exercise-related syncope (ERS): syncope occurring during exertion

EPIDEMIOLOGY

- Syncope is a common occurrence, especially in young females and is usually due to a benign etiology.
- Important to differentiate between syncope occurring *during* exertion, postexertional syncope (immediately after exertion), and nonexertional syncope as their underlying etiology and risk to the individual are drastically different.

ALERT

One study showed that 50% of syncope that occurred during exertion was due to underlying cardiac pathology, therefore with increased risk of sudden cardiac death (1).

Incidence

- Most syncopal events are not related to exertion:
  - Colivicchi et al. showed of ~7,500 athletes (mean age 16 years old), 6.2% self-reported syncope within the past 5 years. Of those with syncope, 87% were unrelated to exercise, 12% were postexertional, and ~1% occurred while exercising (2).
- Postexertional collapse: most common reason medical attention is sought after marathon/ultramarathon; 59–85% of all visits to medical tent after those races

Prevalence

To date, there is no major epidemiologic study investigating syncope in athletes.

ETIOLOGY AND PATHOPHYSIOLOGY

- Syncope is due to decreased cerebral perfusion (specifically to the reticular activating system in the brainstem).
- Causes of syncope vary with general categories, including CS and NCS, such as orthostatic hypotension and reflex (neutrally mediated) syncope (1),(3).
- Syncope in athletes is most commonly due to noncardiac etiologies (3).
- Postexertional collapse: collapse and occasionally syncope after a period of exercise, usually after endurance activities
- Postexercise syncope is due to hypotension and hypocapnia (3).
  - Impaired postexercise vasoconstriction is a key factor in predisposing athletes to postexercise hypotension and collapse/syncope.
  - Postexertional hypotension can be due to impaired vasoconstriction from obligatory etiologies (sympathoinhibition, histaminergic vasodilation, and downregulation of cardiovagal baroreflex) and situation etiologies (dehydration, hyperthermia, gravitational stress).
  - Additionally, when athlete stands still after exertion, they lose the muscle pump which contributes to venous pooling in their legs.
  - Postexercise hypocapnia from hyperventilation and orthostasis-induced hypocapnia when recovery takes place with athlete standing
  - Hypocapnia leads to cerebral vasoconstriction.
- Hyperthermic collapse: collapse with or without complete LOC due to prolonged exertion and decreased cardiac output due to dehydration (body temperature >104°F), part of the heat illness spectrum
- Orthostatic hypotension: decrease of systolic blood pressure (SBP) >20 mm Hg or diastolic blood pressure (DBP) >10 mm Hg within 3 minutes of position change:
  - Increased susceptibility in middle-aged and older athletes possibly due to volume depletion and decreased vasomotor tone (1)
- Cardiac etiologies can be divided into the following categories: bradyarrhythmia, tachyarrhythmia, and low cardiac output (4).

Genetics

Depends on the etiology for syncope, for example:

- Hypertrophic cardiomyopathy (HCM): autosomal dominant inheritance
- Long QT syndrome (LQTS): three main types (LQTS1, LQTS2, and LQTS3); predominantly inherited autosomal dominant, rarely autosomal recessive
- Clinical suggestion of inheritable susceptibility to vasovagal syncope, although a specific gene has not yet been identified

RISK FACTORS

- CS: underlying condition that increases risk
- NCS: dehydration, strong emotional response, inadequate fueling, environmental conditions
- Medications such as macrolide antibiotics, antihistamines/decongestants, recent illness (5)

GENERAL PREVENTION

- NCS:
  - Hydration
  - Proper fueling
  - Continued movement immediately after an endurance event and proper cool down
  - Dressing appropriately for climate and ideally time for climate acclimation
  - Adequate training
- CS: identifying those at risk and implementing treatment strategy

DIAGNOSIS

HISTORY

Detailed history is critical to determining etiology:

- Obtain details from witness if available about events surrounding the syncopal episode such as muscle activity, tongue biting, loss of bladder control, time duration of LOC (usually brief, a few seconds):
  - Myoclonus can occur independently of seizure.
- Determine if prodromal symptoms were present such as light-headedness, dizziness, tunnel vision, nausea, and so forth:
  - Syncope with prodrome more likely to be NCS
  - Syncope without prodromal state is more concerning for CS. Lack of prodrome increases risk of injury as individual is unable to place themselves into a more protective position.
- Determine circumstances surrounding syncope:
  - Was the athlete still exercising (suggestive of CS) or was syncopal event at rest/after exercise (suggestive of NCS)?
  - Was syncope triggered by loud noise or cold water (suggestive of CS, specifically LQTS)?
- Evaluate mentation status after regaining consciousness (i.e., groggy vs. mentally sharp):
  - NCS: tend to be very fatigued/groggy after event
  - CS: can be alert immediately following event
- Obtain details of family history (5)[B].
- Consider calculation of CS risk stratification schemes such as Evaluation of Guidelines in Syncope Study (EGSYS)—emergency room tool validated for adults (5)[B]. Környei et al. indicate it can identify arrhythmic syncope in children (6)[C].

PHYSICAL EXAM

- Sideline/field assessment:
  - Rapidly assess for consciousness and pulse. If no pulse, initiate Emergency Action Plan and start cardiopulmonary resuscitation (CPR) with rapid use of automated external defibrillator (AED).
  - If regains consciousness:
    - Check blood pressure on both arms.
    - Assess patient while he or she is supine with legs elevated.
    - Consider rectal temperature (if concern for hyperthermia, must have rectal temperature; oral/temporal temperature is not adequate).
    - Full neurologic evaluation
- In-office evaluation post syncope:
  - Obtain a detailed history specifically of events and family history of syncope, cardiac condition, or sudden death in family member (5)[B].
  - Vital signs, including orthostatic vital signs
  - Cardiac auscultation:
    - Standing, supine, and supine with Valsalva
    - Murmurs
    - Irregular pulse
  - Neurologic evaluation
  - Evaluate for Marfan stigmata.

DIFFERENTIAL DIAGNOSIS

- CS (usually occurs during exertion):
  - HCM
  - Anomalous coronary artery
  - Severe aortic valve stenosis
  - Coronary artery disease
  - Myocarditis
  - Arrhythmogenic right ventricular cardiomyopathy (ARVC)
  - Brugada syndrome
  - Catecholaminergic polymorphic ventricular tachycardia (CPVT)
  - LQTS
  - Right ventricular outflow tract ventricular tachycardia

- NCS (usually occurs after exertion or unrelated to exertion):
  - Heat stroke
  - Hypoglycemia
  - Hyponatremia
  - Orthostatic hypotension
  - Seizure
  - Vasovagal syncope
  - Drug abuse

DIAGNOSTIC TESTS & INTERPRETATION

Initial Tests (lab, imaging)

- Electrocardiogram (ECG) (5)[B]
- Lab work: comprehensive metabolic panel (CMP), complete blood count (CBC), thyroid-stimulating hormone (TSH), finger glucose test:
  - Additional labs based on differential (i.e., troponin if concerned for cardiac ischemia)
- Orthostatic vital signs

Follow-Up Tests & Special Considerations

- Cardiogenic syncope:
  - Echocardiogram—if concern for cardiac etiology (4)[C]
  - Holter monitor/event recorder—for unexplained syncope or high suspicion for arrhythmogenic etiology with normal initial testing (4)[C]
  - Consider the following in conjunction with sports cardiology consultation:
    - Cardiac magnetic resonance imaging (MRI) with gadolinium
    - Exercise treadmill testing
    - Electrophysiology (EP) testing
    - Genetic testing (LQTS, Brugada syndrome, HCM)
- Noncardiogenic syncope:
  - If history is consistent with noncardiac etiology, usually no additional testing required, although may obtain addition testing if portions of history and physical exam are concerning

TREATMENT

GENERAL MEASURES

- For safety, all athletes with syncope or near syncope should be restricted from sports until further evaluation is completed (7)[B].
- If immediate reversible etiologies are identified, proceed with treating identified condition (i.e., hypoglycemia, hyponatremia, heat stroke).
- Treatment of CS depends on etiology.
- All syncope occurring during exertion should be restricted from sports until evaluation is completed (7)[B]:
  - CS: Restriction from sport is dictated by underlying condition (7)[C].
  - NCS: Athlete is able to return to sports after risk factors are addressed to prevent recurrent syncope (7)[C].
  - Syncope of unknown etiology: advised to refrain from sporting events that may place themselves and others at risk should they syncopize. Water-based sports could be an example (7)[C].

MEDICATION

- Dictated by underlying etiology for cause of syncope
- Refractory cases of vasovagal syncope could consider midodrine or fludrocortisone (5)[B]. Be mindful of level of sport and prohibition for in-competition usage of these medications.

ISSUES FOR REFERRAL

- All syncopal events occurring during exercise should be evaluated by a sports medicine team.
- If doubt about etiology or concern for cardiac etiology, consider referral for further evaluation by sports cardiologist and possibly an electrophysiologist.
- If recurrent postexertional collapse, strongly consider cardiac evaluation.
- If concern for nutritional status, consider referral to dietitian to work with athlete about proper fueling and hydration.

ONGOING CARE

DIET

- Encourage proper fueling prior to exertion to ensure adequate fuel for activity. Nutrition plans will vary with the athlete, but allow for adequate time for athlete to adjust to the fueling plan.
- Encourage proper hydration techniques, which will vary depending on event, environmental climate, and athlete.

PATIENT EDUCATION

- Discuss with athlete the importance of hydration, prerace and postrace nutrition, and continued after races with a cooldown.
- Hydration strategies especially for endurance events
- Proper clothing for the climate—especially important for endurance athletes
- Education about syncopal warning signs and how to protect themselves if they develop:
  - Counter maneuvers in patients with prodrome can be helpful in preventing syncope (5)[B].
- AED operation and locations of AEDs
- Awareness of emergency action plans (EAPs) and practice of EAPs

PROGNOSIS

- NCS and postexertional collapse usually has excellent prognosis with implementation of activity modification (i.e., proper cooldown and continued movement immediately after event).
- CS return to play is debated; decisions regarding return to play need to be based on joint decision-making by all stakeholders involved.
- CS: Access to AED is imperative if returning to sport.

COMPLICATIONS

- Potential for trauma from syncope
- Neurologic impairment may occur secondary to cerebral hypoperfusion if prolonged decreased blood flow due to nonperfusing cardiac rhythm.
- Possible cardiac sequela depending on underling etiology

REFERENCES

1. Vettor G, Zorzi A, Basso C, et al. Syncope as a warning symptom of sudden cardiac death in athletes. *Cardiol Clin*. 2015;33(3):423–432.
2. Colivicchi F, Ammirati F, Santini M. Epidemiology and prognostic implications of syncope in young competing athletes. *Eur Heart J*. 2004;25(19):1749–1753.
3. Christou GA, Christou KA, Kiortsis DN. Pathophysiology of noncardiac syncope in athletes. *Sports Med*. 2018;48(7):1561–1573.
4. D'Ascenzi F, Zorzi A, Sciaccaluga C, et al. Syncope in the young adult and in the athlete: causes and clinical work-up to exclude a life-threatening cardiac disease. *J Cardiovasc Transl Res*. 2020;13(3):322–330.
5. Shen WK, Sheldon RS, Benditt DG, et al. 2017 ACC/AHA/HRS guideline for the evaluation and management of patients with syncope: a report of the American College of Cardiology/American Heart Association Task Force on Clinical Practice Guidelines and the Heart Rhythm Society. *Circulation*. 2017;136(5):e60–e122.
6. Környei L, Szabó A, Róth G, et al. Frequency of syncope as a presenting symptom in channelopathies diagnosed in childhood. Can the multivariable EGSYS score unmask these children? *Eur J Pediatr*. 2021;180(5):1553–1559.
7. Zipes DP, Link MS, Ackerman MJ, et al. Eligibility and disqualification recommendations for competitive athletes with cardiovascular abnormalities: Task Force 9: arrhythmias and conduction defects: a scientific statement from the American Heart Association and American College of Cardiology. *J Am Coll Cardiol*. 2015;66(21):2412–2423.

ADDITIONAL READING

- Ackerman MJ, Zipes DP, Kovacs RJ, et al. Eligibility and disqualification recommendations for competitive athletes with cardiovascular abnormalities: Task Force 10: the cardiac channelopathies: a scientific statement from the American Heart Association and American College of Cardiology. *J Am Coll Cardiol*. 2015;66(21):2424–2428.
- Asplund CA, O'Connor FG, Noakes TD. Exercise-associated collapse: an evidence-based review and primer for clinicians. *Br J Sports Med*. 2011;45(14):1157–1162.
- Bader YH, Link MS. Syncope in the athlete. *Cardiac Electrophysiol Clin*. 2013;5(1):85–96.
- Maron BJ, Levine BD, Washington RL, et al. Eligibility and disqualification recommendations for competitive athletes with cardiovascular abnormalities: Task Force 2: preparticipation screening for cardiovascular disease in competitive athletes: a scientific statement from the American Heart Association and American College of Cardiology. *Circulation*. 2015;132(22):e267–e272.
- Maron BJ, Udelson JE, Bonow RO, et al. Eligibility and disqualification recommendations for competitive athletes with cardiovascular abnormalities: Task Force 3: hypertrophic cardiomyopathy, arrhythmogenic right ventricular cardiomyopathy and other cardiomyopathies, and myocarditis: a scientific statement from the American Heart Association and American College of Cardiology. *Circulation*. 2015;132(22):e273–e280.

CLINICAL PEARLS

- Differentiating CS from NCS is key in determining next steps in evaluation and return-to-play decision-making.
- If concern for CS, consult with sports cardiology if available.
- Return-to-play decisions after a syncopal episode should be made using the joint decision model.
- Have EAP documented and practiced regularly with all responsible parties involved.

TALON NOIR

Chris Nelson, MD, CAQSM • Matthew Waldrop, MD • Jeremy Swisher, MD

BASICS

DESCRIPTION

- Asymptomatic, benign, self-limiting dermatologic condition also known as "black heel"
- Characterized by intraepidermal hemorrhage in areas of recurrent or sudden trauma due to shearing forces

EPIDEMIOLOGY

- Most often occurs in young athletes with a history of sport-related activities, repetitive trauma, mountain climbing, or patients taking anticoagulant therapy.
- A study of 596 healthy young athletes aged 12 to 24 years showed an incidence of 2.85%.
- No gender differences

ETIOLOGY AND PATHOPHYSIOLOGY

- Repetitive trauma to the area
- Leakage of blood from the deeper dermis to the more superficial epidermis, specifically the stratum corneum; this blood is not accessible for phagocytes to clear out.

RISK FACTORS

- New or ill-fitting shoes
- Walking long distances
- Peripheral vascular disease
- Type 2 diabetes mellitus
- Smoking

GENERAL PREVENTION

- Proper-fitting shoes
- Cushioned inserts and appropriate arch support

DIAGNOSIS

HISTORY

- Typically, an asymptomatic dark-colored spot noticed incidentally on the heel, sole, or toe of the foot
- History of repetitive trauma
- Often unilateral
- Does not cause pain, sensory deficits, or difficulty ambulating

PHYSICAL EXAM

- Asymmetric black, brown, or red-colored macules of varying size and shape
- Nontender to palpation
- No blanching or fluctuance

DIFFERENTIAL DIAGNOSIS

- Acral melanoma
- Acral nevi
- Plantar wart
- Corn
- Tinea nigra
- See Table.
- See Figure 1 in Appendix C.

DIAGNOSTIC TESTS & INTERPRETATION

- Not indicated (1)[C]
- Can consider hemoccult testing of skin shavings to support diagnosis (1)[C]
- Can consider benzidine staining of skin shavings for blood to support diagnosis

Initial Tests (lab, imaging)

- Dermoscopy can be performed if clinical diagnosis is in question (2)[C].
- There will be hyperkeratosis, epidermal acanthosis, and focal hemorrhages within the stratum corneum.

TREATMENT

GENERAL MEASURES

- Does not require treatment (1)[C],(3)[C]
- Spontaneously resolves within 4 to 6 weeks of cessation of the inciting activity (1)[C],(2)[C]
- Can be cosmetically treated by pairing of lesion with scalpel (2)[C]
- Eliminate inciting cause if possible

MEDICATION

Can consider vitamin C supplementation to assist with healing of capillary fragility (2)[C]

ISSUES FOR REFERRAL

If symptomatic or concerned for malignancy, refer to dermatology for further evaluation (3)[C].

Diagnosis	Distinguishing Factors	Testing
Talon noir	Asymptomatic, repetitive foot trauma, normal-appearing skin after removing hemorrhagic material	Pair with scalpel, dermoscopy, hemoccult card
Acral melanoma	Parallel ridge pattern with irregular pigmentation on dermoscopy, age >40 years, slow growing	Dermoscopy, biopsy
Acral nevi	No significant change over time, regular shape, any age, no risk factors needed	Dermoscopy
Plantar wart	Verrucous surface with disrupted skin lines, pinpoint bleeding from tips of papillae when paired with scalpel	Pair with scalpel, dermoscopy
Pyogenic granuloma	Painless red fleshy nodule, rapid growth over weeks due to trauma, proliferation of capillaries with keratin border	Dermoscopy
Angiokeratoma	Blue-red hyperkeratotic papule, dark lacunae from dilated capillaries in dermis with overlying white veil	Dermoscopy, biopsy
Corn	Painful, callus-like, epidermal hyperplasia with thick stratum corneum and stratum spinosum, dermal fibrosis	Dermoscopy
Tinea nigra	Fungal infection, brown macule, usually asymptomatic, can itch, more common in those who sweat excessively	Potassium hydroxide (KOH) scraping, dermoscopy, biopsy

SURGERY/OTHER PROCEDURES

- Can use a scalpel to pair the lesion for cosmetic purposes or for testing (2)[C]
- Punch biopsies are considered for unsure lesions (2)[C],(3)[C].

ONGOING CARE

FOLLOW-UP RECOMMENDATIONS

Follow-up in 4 to 6 weeks to monitor clinical resolution (1)[C],(2)[C]

Patient Monitoring

- It may recur if the inciting activity continues.
- To prevent recurrence, educate on properly fitted footwear with adequate cushion and arch support (2)[C].
- Consider using a heel gel cup or pad in shoes (3)[C].

PATIENT EDUCATION

Reassure the patient on the benign nature of talon noir.

PROGNOSIS

There is an excellent prognosis for talon noir as it resolves spontaneously with cessation of the inciting activity.

COMPLICATIONS

- Persistence of skin pigmentation with continuation of inciting activity
- Improper diagnosis may lead to unnecessarily invasive testing, psychological trauma of a potential cancer diagnosis, and time away from sport.

REFERENCES

1. Emer J, Sivek R, Marciniak B. Sports dermatology: part 1 of 2 traumatic or mechanical injuries, inflammatory conditions, and exacerbations of pre-existing conditions. *J Clin Aesthet Dermatol.* 2015;8(4):31–43.
2. Choudhury S, Mandal A. Talon noir: a case report and literature review. *Cureus.* 2023;15(3):e35905.
3. Carr PC, Cropley TG. Sports dermatology: skin disease in athletes. *Clin Sports Med.* 2019;38(4):597–618.

ADDITIONAL READING

- Burkhart CG, Nguyen N. Talon noire (black heel, calcaneal petechiae, runner's heel, basketball heel, tennis heel, hyperkeratosis hemorrhagica, pseudochromhidrosis plantaris, chromidrose plantaire, eccrine intracornee, post-traumatic punctuate hemorrhage of the skin, post-traumatic cutaneous intracorneal blood, disseminated punctuate intraepidermal hemorrhage, black palm, playstation thumb, tennis toe). Dermatology Advisor. Published March 13, 2019. https://www.dermatologyadvisor.com/home/decision-support-in-medicine/dermatology/talon-noire-black-heel-calcaneal-petechiae-runners-heel-basketball-heel-tennis-heel-hyperkeratosis-hemorrhagica-pseudochromhidrosis-plantaris-chromidrose-plantaire-eccrine-intracorne
- Cunliffe T. Talon noir. Primary Care Dermatology Society. Published November 19, 2021. https://www.pcds.org.uk/clinical-guidance/talon-noir
- Martin SB, Lucas JK, Posa M, et al. Talon noir in a young baseball player: a case report. *J Pediatr Health Care.* 2021;35(2):235–238.
- Seervai R, Wiggins CJ. Calcaneal petechiae. DermNet. Published 2020. https://dermnetnz.org/topics/calcaneal-petechiae
- Tallon B. Talon noir pathology. DermNet. Published 2011. https://dermnetnz.org/topics/talon-noir-pathology

CLINICAL PEARLS

- Talon noir is a clinical diagnosis suggested by a history of repetitive trauma in young athletes with the heel being the most common location affected.
- Pairing the lesion with a scalpel blade can be both diagnostic and therapeutic.
- Hyperpigmented lesions are not always worrisome for melanoma, and it is important to reassure the patient.

TARSAL TUNNEL SYNDROME/POSTERIOR TIBIAL NERVE ENTRAPMENT

Christopher Jordan, MD, ATC, CAQSM • Joshua F. Loiseau, MD

BASICS

DESCRIPTION

- A compression neuropathy which causes pain and/or paresthesia along the medial ankle and plantar foot secondary to entrapment of the posterior tibial nerve or one of its branches as it passes through the tarsal tunnel on the medial side of the ankle
- Synonym: posterior tibial nerve entrapment

EPIDEMIOLOGY

- Unknown
- Likely underdiagnosed or misdiagnosed due to low clinician suspicion
- Women > men
- More common in athletes and individuals with prolonged weight-bearing

ETIOLOGY AND PATHOPHYSIOLOGY

- Three etiologies: compressive, idiopathic, and venous dilatation (1)
- Tarsal tunnel is formed by the distal tibia anteriorly, talus and calcaneus laterally, and the flexor retinaculum (laciniate ligament) medially. The flexor retinaculum forms the roof of the tunnel. Contents of the tunnel include the posterior tibial nerve, tibial artery and vein, the flexor hallucis longus (FHL), flexor digitorum longus (FDL), and posterior tibial tendons (PTTs).
- The tibial nerve branches within the tarsal tunnel into medial and lateral plantar nerves and the medial calcaneal nerve.
- The medial plantar nerve provides sensation to the plantar medial foot and the medial 3.5 toes.
- The lateral plantar nerve provides sensation to the lateral plantar foot and the lateral 1.5 toes.
- The medial calcaneal nerve provides sensation to the posterior and medial aspects of the heel.
- Tarsal tunnel entrapment can be differentiated into distal and proximal syndromes based on whether the tibial nerve itself is compressed (proximal) or a terminal branch is compressed (distal).

RISK FACTORS

- Decreased volume or increased pressure within the tarsal tunnel
- Hypertrophy of or within the tarsal tunnel (e.g., flexor retinaculum, abductor hallucis muscle)
- Space-occupying lesions (e.g., ganglion or lipoma, bone spurs, osteophytes, varicose veins) (2)
- Tenosynovitis
- Local trauma
- Prior surgery in the area
- Scar tissue formation
- Abnormal foot/ankle mechanics (e.g., pes planus)
- Hindfoot deformities (e.g., heel valgus or varus)
- Repetitive activity
- Weight gain
- Lower extremity edema
- Accessory muscles (e.g., accessory soleus)
- Systemic diseases (e.g., diabetes)

DIAGNOSIS

HISTORY

- Tarsal tunnel syndrome (TTS) presents with a nonspecific, highly variable clinical picture.
- History of trauma or repetitive activity (e.g., running)
- Numbness, tingling, and burning to the medial aspect and plantar surface of the foot; can include calf symptoms and radiation to the toes
- Foot cramping in the medial longitudinal arch
- Typically, unilateral
- Symptoms typically worsen throughout the day.
- Prolonged standing or walking often exacerbates the symptoms.
- Rest may alleviate the symptoms.
- Habit of removing shoes to obtain relief
- Patients lack morning pain and often lack heel pain.
- Nocturnal pain may awaken the patient, especially after excessive activity.

PHYSICAL EXAM

- Numbness/tingling that progresses to a burning sensation at the plantar aspect of the foot; intermittent initially; can become constant
- Plantar foot pain accentuated by walking and foot dorsiflexion
- Nocturnal pain often relieved with walking
- Pain worse at the end of the day
- Occasional fusiform swelling over the nerve course
- Motor weakness or loss as late finding: poor prognostic indicator
- Muscle fasciculations
- Pain radiation proximally into the midcalf during percussion over the tunnel (Valleix phenomenon)
- Inspect for biomechanical abnormalities such as excessive heel varus or valgus positioning.
- Observe for swelling.
- Observe for toe contractures, which can occur late.
- Palpate for soft tissue thickening or lesions; light touch–induced paresthesias
- Diminished pinprick sensation to plantar foot
- Intrinsic muscle weakness, although possibly present, is difficult to assess.
- Atrophy of abductor hallucis or abductor digiti minimi as a late finding
- Tinel sign: paresthesia during percussion over the tunnel
- Cuff sign: pain with pneumatic pressure device around leg
- Dorsiflexion-eversion test: pain elicited when placing the foot in maximum dorsiflexion and eversion and then maximally dorsiflexing the metatarsophalangeal joints and holding this position for 5 to 10 seconds.
- Trepman test: maximal plantar flexion and inversion resulting in pain and numbness at the ankle or plantar surface of the foot.
- Triple compression stress test: combination of Tinel test and Trepman test for 30 seconds; the ankle is placed in full plantarflexion, and the foot in inversion, with even constant pressure applied to the posterior tibial nerve.

DIFFERENTIAL DIAGNOSIS

- Plantar fasciitis
- Calcaneal bursitis or spurs
- Tendinitis/tenosynovitis (FHL, PTT, FDL)
- Nerve root avulsions
- Osteomyelitis
- Morton metatarsalgia
- Heel pad atrophy
- Nerve entrapment at more proximal locations (e.g., beneath the piriformis muscle, posterior knee or fibula)
- Peripheral vascular disease, including popliteal artery entrapment
- Peripheral neuropathy
- Systemic disease (e.g., diabetes, vitamin B_{12} deficiency, Reiter disease, rheumatoid arthritis, gout)
- Bony abnormalities (e.g., degenerative changes, previous fractures, calcaneal stress fracture)
- L3–S1 radiculopathies

DIAGNOSTIC TESTS & INTERPRETATION

- Plain x-ray (weight-bearing) and computed tomography (CT) scan to rule out morphologic or structural abnormalities (2)[C].
- Magnetic resonance imaging (MRI) is gold standard for evaluating compression of the tunnel due to soft tissue structures such as anomalous or hypertrophied muscles, ganglion cysts, and/or tumors (3)[C].
- Electrodiagnostic studies to rule out proximal nerve pathology causing a double crush syndrome (4)[C]
- Electromyography (EMG) to evaluate for motor latencies; has a high false-positive rate when evaluating intrinsic foot muscles (4)[C]
- Nerve conduction studies (NCSs) evaluating for sensory action potentials may increase the sensitivity but are best for adjunctive assessment for confirmation of diagnosis as they often yield false-negative results (4)[C].
- Ultrasound (US) can evaluate enlarged tibial nerve cross-sectional area (CSA). Imaging was positive for TTS in patients with CSA >15 mm^2 within the tunnel (74% sensitivity, 100% specificity) and/or within-tunnel-to-proximal tunnel CSA ratio >5 mm^2 (81% sensitivity, 100% specificity) (3)[B].
- Improved distal response after lidocaine injection into the abductor hallucis muscle may aid in differentiating between distal and proximal TTS (5)[C].

TREATMENT

GENERAL MEASURES

Conservative treatments are recommended prior to NCSs or surgical interventions (4)[C]:

- Acute treatment:
  - Custom orthotics with arch support
  - Immobilizing braces
  - Muscular stretching and strengthening of the lower leg and foot musculature
  - Acupuncture
  - Transcutaneous electrical nerve stimulation (TENS)
  - Corticosteroid injections
- Long-term treatment:
  - Activity modification
  - Weight loss for obese patients
  - Optimize proper gait biomechanics.
  - Surgery

MEDICATION

- Nonsteroidal anti-inflammatory drugs (NSAIDs)
- Corticosteroid injection
- Tricyclic antidepressants (4)[C]
- Vitamin B complex supplementation
  - Gabapentin (2)[C]

ISSUES FOR REFERRAL

- Indicated for acute cases with space-occupying lesions, patients who present with obvious muscle atrophy, and cases which do not respond to conservative management
- Best surgical results in patients with tumor or tarsal coalition
- Surgical referral should be considered for patients recalcitrant to a high-quality nonoperative treatment program.

ADDITIONAL THERAPIES

- Ice
- Relative rest
- Discontinued use of any external compression (e.g., shoes, clothing)
- Rehabilitation:
  - May last up to 24 weeks (3)[C]
  - May aid tissue and nerve mobility (2)[C]
  - Optimize proper biomechanics.
  - Strengthen foot intrinsic and extrinsic muscles.

SURGERY/OTHER PROCEDURES

- Endoscopic tarsal tunnel decompression allows for earlier mobilization and may cause less soft tissue trauma and scarring (6)[A].
- Flexor retinaculum release
- Surgical decompression of the tibial nerves and its branches
- Fascial release of the abductor hallucis muscle
- Postoperative physical therapy is aimed at controlling pain, edema, and inflammation.
- Ultrasound-guided release of the flexor retinaculum may be considered in proximal tarsal tunnel cases (3)[C].

ONGOING CARE

COMPLICATIONS

- Poor nerve recovery outcomes are more likely when surgical intervention is delayed for >10 months (3).
- Untreated patients risk permanent nerve damage resulting in persistent pain, motor deficits, and potentially plantar ulcerations and complex regional pain syndrome.
- Recurrence of symptoms following surgical release is likely secondary to inadequate initial decompression (6)[A].

REFERENCES

1. Lalevée M, Coillard JY, Gauthé R, et al. Tarsal tunnel syndrome: outcome according to etiology. *J Foot Ankle Surg*. 2022;61(3):583–589.
2. Nelson SC. Tarsal tunnel syndrome. *Clin Podiatr Med Surg*. 2021;38(2):131–141.
3. Khodatars D, Gupta A, Welck M, et al. An update on imaging of tarsal tunnel syndrome. *Skeletal Radiol*. 2022;51(11):2075–2095.
4. Pomeroy G, Wilton J, Anthony S. Entrapment neuropathy about the foot and ankle: an update. *J Am Acad Orthop Surg*. 2015;23(1):58–66.
5. Nelson SC. Tarsal tunnel syndrome. *Clin Podiatr Med Surg*. 2021;38(2):131–141.
6. Gkotsoulias EN, Simonson DC, Roukis TS. Outcomes and safety of endoscopic tarsal tunnel decompression: a systematic review. *Foot Ankle Spec*. 2014;7(1):57–60.

ADDITIONAL READING

- Reichert P, Zimmer K, Wnukiewicz W, et al. Results of surgical treatment of tarsal tunnel syndrome. *Foot Ankle Surg*. 2015;21(1):26–29.
- Tu P. Heel pain: diagnosis and management. *Am Fam Physician*. 2018;97(2):86–93.

CLINICAL PEARLS

- TTS is often underdiagnosed due to low clinician suspicion.
- Many cases of TTS can be managed conservatively with relative rest from exercise, biomechanical control, and anti-inflammatory drugs.
- Identification of surgically treatable causes is necessary to avoid permanent nerve compression, sensory deficits, and motor weakness.
- Early surgical intervention of intrinsic causes such as space occupying lesions
- Surgical intervention for persistent syndromes despite conservative management improves outcomes.

TEMPOROMANDIBULAR JOINT INJURY

Tammy Ng, MD • Giorgio A. Negron, MD • Daniel C. Herman, MD, PhD, FAAPMR, FACSM, FISBS, CAQSM

BASICS

Temporomandibular joint (TMJ) injuries, although relatively uncommon, do occur in sport. Players in collision sports (e.g., football, field hockey, soccer, lacrosse, boxing, mixed martial arts) may be at particular risk, along with divers.

DESCRIPTION

- TMJ complex consists of the mandibular condyle inserting into the mandibular fossa of the temporal bone (1).
- Temporomandibular disorders (TMD) are a myriad of painful conditions involving the TMJ, muscles of mastication, and surrounding bony/soft tissue parts:
  - TMD are categorized as intra-articular or extra-articular.
  - Trauma, dentoskeletal malocclusion, and bruxism are important contributors.
- If pain persists >3 months, it is considered chronic.
- Up to 70% of sufferers may have a displacement of the articular disk (typically anteromedially), made up of fibrocartilage (2).
- Osteoarthrosis is another common cause of TMJ pain.
- May be related to whiplash injuries, hyperextension associated with cervical trauma, or related acceleration-deceleration injuries in sport (2)

EPIDEMIOLOGY

Incidence

- Clinical symptoms of TMD affect 10–15% of the adult population (~5% seeking treatment at some point in their lives) (1).
- Incidence depicted by bimodal peaks between 20 and 40 years of age (1).
- Predominant gender: female > male (2:1, although this ratio may be reversed in athletes)

RISK FACTORS

- ~1/3 of TMD sufferers report a previous history of macrotrauma.
- Psychosocial conditions such as fibromyalgia, depression, and anxiety are risk factors for the development of chronic temporomandibular dysfunction (1).
- Generalized joint hypermobility (3)

GENERAL PREVENTION

- Use of mouth guards in sports may protect against traumatic causes:
  - Omission of use carries 1.6 to 1.9 times risk of orofacial trauma (4).
  - Biomechanical stresses from impacts to the TMJ are decreased, regardless of the occlusion type of the mouth guard.
- Proper technique in sports-specific activities
- Avoidance of repetitive or unilateral chewing

COMMONLY ASSOCIATED CONDITIONS

In cases of trauma, other facial injuries may be related:

- Mandibular or other orofacial fractures
- Cervical neck injury may occur in whiplash-type injuries.
- Auditory canal injuries (5)

DIAGNOSIS

- Primarily based on history and physical exam findings
- Exclude other causes of unilateral facial or head pain.

HISTORY

- History of pain with jaw movement (particularly repetitive chewing), headache, and/or ear discomfort (1)
- Related history of oromaxillofacial trauma

PHYSICAL EXAM

- On inspection, assess for facial asymmetry, swelling, mastication muscle hypertrophy, and uncorrected deviation on maximum mouth opening (2).
- Limited range of motion of the mandible
- Tenderness over the muscles of mastication is most consistent with TMD.
- Tenderness over TMJ capsule, surrounding neck and shoulder muscles
- A "popping," "clicking," or "locking" sensation may be noted with jaw movement (1):
  - The first click upon jaw opening may be associated with anterior disk displacement; the second click when closing indicates recapture of displaced disk.
  - Crepitus may indicate osteoarthritis.
- Pain when clenching jaw
- Assess for dentoskeletal malocclusion:
  - TMJ dislocation and mandibular jaw fracture both present with malocclusion.
  - To determine fracture from TMJ injury, examiner's index finger may be pressed outward along the interior border of mandible (pain and movement of bone segment indicates jaw fracture) (4)[C].

DIFFERENTIAL DIAGNOSIS

- Mandibular fracture
- Myocardial ischemia
- Carotid or vertebral artery dissection
- Intracranial hemorrhage (subarachnoid hemorrhage)
- Temporal arteritis
- Multiple sclerosis (MS) may present with pain similar to trigeminal neuralgia.
- Trigeminal or glossopharyngeal neuralgia
- Postherpetic neuralgia (1)
- Vascular headache
- Dental abnormalities
- Salivary gland disorder, otitis media, external otitis, and sinusitis
- Elongated styloid process pain often is precipitated by swallowing or turning the head.
- Autoimmune conditions (systemic lupus erythematosus [SLE], Sjögren, rheumatoid arthritis) (1)

DIAGNOSTIC TESTS & INTERPRETATION

- No specific laboratory tests are indicated.
- Imaging is not necessary for diagnosis; may be helpful to evaluate for other disorders with similar symptoms
- Initial studies include transcranial and transmaxillary plain radiography and/or panoramic radiography.
- Magnetic resonance imaging (MRI) to further evaluate joint pathology and disk position (ultrasound if MRI not available) (1),(2)

TREATMENT

- Typically treated as outpatients with pain medication, muscle relaxants, and warm compresses
- In general, symptoms from acute injury resolve within 7 to 10 days, although a significant percentage of patients may have long-term sequelae.
- Prehospital:
  - Evaluate the patient to rule out other more serious injuries:
    - Cervical spine injuries
    - Orofacial fractures
    - Dental abscess (1)
  - In acute injuries, conservative measures are applied:
    - Protection from further injury
    - Icing
    - Nonsteroidal anti-inflammatory drugs (NSAIDs) for pain relief if indicated
    - Decreased stimulation (i.e., chewing) on affected side
- Emergency department (ED) treatment:
  - Pain control
  - Radiographs to rule out other injuries as clinically indicated (plain film, computed tomography [CT])
  - For TMJ dislocation, you may perform digital intraoral reduction (bimanual traction) (3)[C]:
    - May use local anesthesia for auriculotemporal nerve block
  - For severe bruxism, refer to dentist or oral and maxillofacial surgeon for occlusal splints (1)[C].

MEDICATION

- Topical NSAIDs or short-term oral NSAIDs (preferably naproxen) as first line (1)[A]
- Muscle relaxants to improve muscle spasms
- Additional adjunct therapies:
  - Tricyclic antidepressants (mainstay management for chronic conditions) (1)[C]
  - Intra-articular and local injections of anesthetics or steroids for severe cases (1)[A]
  - Inconclusive evidence for hyaluronic acid injection (1)[A]

ISSUES FOR REFERRAL

- Pain or loss of function uncontrolled by the preceding may benefit from referral to maxillofacial or orofacial surgeons (1)[C].
- Surgery is rarely required but may consist of:
  - Arthrocentesis and arthroscopy
  - Hemiarthroplasty
  - Osteotomy
  - Total joint replacement is considered a salvage procedure.
- Treatment of recurrent TMJ dislocation may involve intermaxillary fixation combined with autologous blood injection (6)[C].

ADDITIONAL THERAPIES

- Warm/cold compresses
- Biofeedback (1)[C]
- Acupuncture to treat myofascial pain
- Physical therapy exercises to strengthen muscles of mastication, and maintain range of motion (1)[C]
- Although not studied extensively, a mouthpiece or mouth guard may help to relieve some postinjury pain.

ONGOING CARE

DIET

- A soft diet may be effective in reducing pain severity during episodes.
- Chewing gum also may make symptoms worse.

PROGNOSIS

Typically self-limited but can progress to a chronic state of inflammation and pain

REFERENCES

1. Gauer RL, Semidey MJ. Diagnosis and treatment of temporomandibular disorders. *Am Fam Physician*. 2015;91(6):378–386.
2. De Rossi SS, Greenberg MS, Liu F, et al. Temporomandibular disorders: evaluation and management. *Med Clin North Am*. 2014;98(6):1353–1384.
3. Cohen A, Sela MC, Ran LZ, et al. Increased prevalence of generalized joint hypermobility observed in patients with recurrent temporomandibular joint dislocation. *J Oral Maxillofac Surg*. 2023;81(8):950–955.
4. Fillingim RB, Ohrbach R, Greenspan JD, et al. Potential psychosocial risk factors for chronic TMD: descriptive data and empirically identified domains from the OPPERA case-control study. *J Pain*. 2011;12(11 Suppl):T46–T60.
5. Reghunadhan P, Upasi AP, Rai KK, et al. A spectrum of auditory canal injuries ensuing from direct or indirect trauma to the temporomandibular joint: a 2-year prospective study. *J Craniomaxillofac Surg*. 2022;50(10):765–770.
6. Abrahamsson H, Ericksson L, Abrahamsson P, et al. Treatment of temporomandibular joint luxation: a systematic literature review. *Clin Oral Investig*. 2020;24(1):61–70.

ADDITIONAL READING

Tanaka E, Detamore MS, Mercuri LG. Degenerative disorders of the temporomandibular joint: etiology, diagnosis, and treatment. *J Dent Res*. 2008;87(4):296–307.

CLINICAL PEARLS

- Consideration of possible underlying psychosocial factors may significantly aid in the treatment of TMD.
- The practitioner should take care at the time of presentation to evaluate for more serious masquerading conditions.
- Although acute cases typically resolve within 1 to 2 weeks, close follow-up should be scheduled for consideration of additional treatment options to prevent progression to chronic pain states.

TENOSYNOVIAL GIANT CELL TUMOR (TGCT)

Fouad Sayde, MD, ABIM, ABEM, FACP

BASICS

DESCRIPTION

- A proliferative disorder of the synovial membrane; locally aggressive but almost always benign (1)
- Histologically, a tenosynovial giant cell tumor (TGCT) with proliferation of two types of cells, small, histiocyte-like cells and larger cells with lobulated nucleus, with surrounding multinucleated giant cells and hemosiderin-laden macrophages (1)
- There are two types: nodular (localized) and diffuse.
- Both types can be intra-articular or extra-articular.
- Can affect the synovium of bursae and the tenosynovial sheaths of tendons
- Typically affects large joints (diffuse type) with the knee being the most common but can also affect the hands/fingers (nodular type) (1)

EPIDEMIOLOGY

- Epidemiologic data is scarce and heterogenous.
- Typically presents in the 3rd, 4th, and 5th decades (2)
- More common in females
- Mean age at diagnosis is 35 to 50 years but may reflect a delay in diagnosis of up to 10 years.
- Reported incidence rates for nodular (localized) type varies from 30 to 34/1,000,000 (1).
- Reported incidence rates for diffuse type range from 5 to 8.4/1,000,000.
- One study reported the prevalence of nodular and diffuse type as 44/100,000 and 11/100,00, respectively (2).
- Hospital-based studies report higher rates of diffuse type (70–90%) compared to nodular, possibly due to complexity of cases referred to hospitals.
- Lower incidence in pediatric age group

ETIOLOGY AND PATHOPHYSIOLOGY

- Characterized by aberrations in the expression of CSF-1 gene and subsequent synovial cell hyperplasia (1)
- History of trauma and recurrent local hemorrhage of the affected joint is another proposed etiology.
- Nodular type (formerly localized pigmented villonodular synovitis [PVNS]):
  - Lesions are pedunculated/lobular and localized to one area of synovium (3).
  - Most commonly affects the flexor tendons and interphalangeal joint in the hands (1)
  - Nodular type rarely affects the large joints.
- Diffuse type:
  - Histologically similar to nodular type; however, involvement is noted throughout most or all of the involved joint, bursa, or tendon sheath (3).
  - Knee is the most commonly affected joint; however, can involve the hip, ankle, shoulder, and elbow.
  - Higher recurrence rate following treatment than local form (2)
  - More destructive course and typically leads to more end-stage joint disease than nodular type
  - Disease progression leads to recurrent hemarthrosis, worsening stiffness, and joint destruction.

Genetics

- Abnormal expression of CSF-1 gene (1)
- 1p13 chromosomal translocation is present in the majority of PVNS cases.

RISK FACTORS

Risk factors are unknown.

DIAGNOSIS

HISTORY

- Insidious onset
- Symptoms are often vague, may be intermittent, and are typically slowly progressive.
- Patients can present with painless swelling.
- Monoarticular involvement is the norm, with the knee the most commonly involved joint in the diffuse type (2).
- Rarely presents as a polyarthropathy
- Localized type can lead to locking, catching, and instability.
- Diffuse type typically presents as a slow insidious onset of pain, swelling, and stiffness.
- Symptoms often mistaken for early arthritis, meniscal, or ligamentous injuries.

PHYSICAL EXAM

- Localized type:
  - May have a palpable synovial mass
  - Most common in hand flexor tendon and anterior compartment of the knee (anterior horn of medial meniscus) (1)
  - Other common locations include infrapatellar fat pad, suprapatellar pouch, intercondylar notch, anterior horn of lateral meniscus.
  - Tenderness to palpation
  - Decreased range of motion
- Diffuse type:
  - Global effusion of joint
  - Decreased and often painful range of motion
  - Tenderness to palpation

DIFFERENTIAL DIAGNOSIS

- Osteoarthritis: similar exam/radiographs, but TGCT does not have osteophytes
- Hemophilia: similar exam/radiographs but without history of hemophilia
- Synovial hemangioma: similar exam/radiograph but age of presentation different (TGCT 3rd to 4th decades, synovial hemangioma 1st to 3rd decades)
- Rheumatoid arthritis: similar exam/radiographs but TGCT monoarticular
- Tuberculous arthritis: similar exam but without periarticular osteoporosis/abscesses on radiographs/magnetic resonance imaging (MRI)
- Lipoma arborescens: similar exam and MRI findings, but lesions show low signal enhancement with contrast versus no enhancement

DIAGNOSTIC TESTS & INTERPRETATION

Initial Tests (lab, imaging)

- Inflammatory blood markers like erythrocyte sedimentation rate (ESR) and C-reactive protein (CRP) are often normal.
- Joint aspiration that yields blood is suggestive, especially in patients with no history of trauma (2).
- Plain radiographs:
  - Often are normal
  - May see periarticular erosions/subchondral cysts
  - Reciprocal erosions on opposite sides of the joint, with a preserved joint space, are highly suggestive (1)[C].

- CT scan:
  - Appears as a high-density soft tissue mass compared with skeletal muscle
  - Bone erosion and cysts may be seen.
  - CT scan with contrast material displays the synovial changes.
- MRI:
  - Most sensitive imaging modality (1)[A]
  - Helps to determine extent of disease
  - Local type: MRI reveals synovial nodular mass with bone erosion; T1/T2-weighted images show low signal owing to hemosiderin (1).
  - Diffuse type:
    - T1/T2-weighted images show diffuse mass/synovial thickening with periarticular "dark on dark" erosions (3).
    - Fat-suppressed images show high-signal synovial mass (hemosiderin deposits not seen).
    - Fast field echo shows hemosiderin deposits.
    - Thallium-201 uptake also useful

Diagnostic Procedures/Other

- Biopsy and pathologic evaluation is the diagnostic standard (1)[A].
- Aspiration/joint fluid evaluation may reveal blood-tinged aspirate, but aspirate may be clear.

ALERT

Blood-tinged aspirate without a history of trauma is highly suggestive of TGCT.

- Aspirate may show hemosiderin pigment and macrophages.

TREATMENT

- Should be managed by multidisciplinary team with experience in sarcoma (1)
- Active surveillance is an option for asymptomatic patients.
- Surgical synovectomy is traditionally the treatment of choice for diffuse type (1)[A].
- Preferred treatment for nodular type is marginal excision.
  - Open versus arthroscopic surgery is still debated and depends on location of lesions.
  - Recurrence rate is low in patients with nodular type.
  - Extent of disease, location of lesions, and patient preference/comorbidities determine if arthroscopy or open surgery is selected.
- Surgery is the gold standard treatment when it can be done without significant morbidity.
  - Some studies report positive outcomes with radiotherapy, but data is insufficient for making reliable recommendations (1)[A].
  - Cryotherapy is investigational with little available data.
- Systemic treatment:
  - Consider for symptomatic patients who are poor surgical candidates.
  - Pexidartinib (1)[A]
    - The only approved treatment
    - An oral CSF1 receptor inhibitor
    - Risk of hepatotoxicity
    - Available in very few countries
  - Imatinib
    - Inhibits CSF1 receptor
    - Generic is widely available.
    - Favorable safety profile

ONGOING CARE

FOLLOW-UP RECOMMENDATIONS

Patient Monitoring

- No clear-cut guidelines
- Frequency of follow-up should be individualized.
- Recurrence is common especially with diffuse type.
- For diffuse type, experts recommend MRI every 6 to 12 months.
- More frequent follow-up (every 3 to 4 months) is appropriate for patients receiving system therapy.
- Pain management should be involved for very symptomatic patient.

COMPLICATIONS

- Recurrence
- Joint erosion
- End-stage joint disease as result of erosion
- Pexidartinib-induced hepatotoxicity
- Surgical complications
- Malignancy and metastasis (extremely rare)

REFERENCES

1. Stacchioti S, Dürr HR, Schaefer IM, et al. Best clinical management of tenosynovial giant cell tumor (TGCT): a consensus paper from the community of experts. *Cancer Treat Rev*. 2023;112:102491.
2. Fecek C, Carter KR. *Pigmented Villonodular Synovitis*. StatPearls Publishing; 2023. Updated August 7, 2023. Accessed August 8, 2025. https://www.ncbi.nlm.nih.gov/books/NBK549850/
3. Falek A, Niemunis-Sawicka J, Wrona K, et al. Pigmented villonodular synovitis. *Folia Med Cracov*. 2018;58(4):93–104.

CLINICAL PEARLS

- Insidious onset
- Symptoms can be vague with swelling and stiffness out of proportion to pain.
- Aspirate may be blood-tinged and show hemosiderin pigment and macrophages.
- MRI is the most sensitive imaging modality.
- Surgical excision/synovectomy is treatment of choice when it can be done safely.

T

TFCC (TRIANGULAR FIBROCARTILAGE COMPLEX) TEARS

Jordan W. Lyons, MD, MBA, FAAFP

BASICS

- The TFCC acts as a primary stabilizer to the distal radioulnar joint (DRUJ) and a cushion to the ulnar-sided carpal bones, transmitting up to 18–21% of the load on the wrist.
- TFCC tears are part of the spectrum of ulnar-sided wrist pain with associated clicking, instability, or grip weakness.
- TFCC injury can be disabling to the athlete.
- TFCC tears are either traumatic or degenerative or combination of both.
- Traumatic tears may be acute or acute on chronic, repetitive events.
- Traumatic tears are either from acute collision (axial load with rotation, hyperpronation-supination, or traction) or repetitive injury (chronic loading of ulnar wrist).

DESCRIPTION

- The TFCC has five major components:
  - Triangular fibrocartilage disc distal to the ulna
  - Meniscus homologue (ulnocarpal meniscus)
  - Radioulnar ligaments (dorsal and volar)
  - Subsheath of the extensor carpi ulnaris (ECU)
  - Ulnotriquetral and ulnolunate ligaments
- Fibers of the TFCC originate on the distal radius, inserting on the distal ulna, base of the ulnar stylus, and extending to lunate (ulnolunate ligament), triquetrum (lunotriquetral ligament), and base of the 5th metacarpal.
- TFCC acts as a stabilizer of the DRUJ (pronation, supination, volar and dorsal movement) and a cushion for the ulnocarpal forces.
- The periphery of the TFCC is vascular, and the central aspect is avascular; therefore, peripheral lesions often do well with repair.

EPIDEMIOLOGY

- Degenerative tears are seen with advancing age. A systematic review noted the prevalence of TFCC abnormalities ranged from 27% in the youngest group (<30 years old) to 49% in patients >70 years old regardless of symptoms (1).
- Magnetic resonance imaging (MRI) scans revealed TFCC abnormalities with a similar prevalence in asymptomatic participants: 34% in <30-year-olds and 100% in those >60 years old (2).
- Degenerative tears often are seen in an older population.
- Traumatic tears are seen frequently in the athletic population.

ETIOLOGY AND PATHOPHYSIOLOGY

- The thickness of the TFCC is inversely related to the ulnar variance (the more ulnar plus, the thinner the TFCC).
- In neutral mechanics, with axial load on, the load on the forearm is 82% at the distal radius and 18% at the TFCC; with removal of the TFCC, the radius takes 95% of the load (3).
- Palmer classified TFCC tears in to two types: traumatic and degenerative (3):
  - Traumatic:
    - 1A: central perforation
    - 1B: ulnar avulsion ± distal ulnar fracture
    - 1C: avulsion from lunate or triquetrum
    - 1D: avulsion from sigmoid notch of radius
  - Degenerative:
    - 2A: TFCC wear
    - 2B: TFCC wear + lunate and/or ulnar chondromalacia
    - 2C: TFCC perforation + lunate and/or ulnar chondromalacia
    - 2D: TFCC perforation + lunate and/or ulnar chondromalacia + ligament tear
    - 2E: TFCC perforation + lunate and/or ulnar chondromalacia + ligament tear + ulnocarpal arthritis
- Several mechanisms have been described to cause TFCC tears.
- Axial loading the ulnar side of the wrist with a rotational force (often a fall on an outstretched hand)
- Hyperrotation with hyperpronation or hypersupination
- Traction to the ulnar side of the wrist
- Chronic repetitive loading the ulnar carpus

RISK FACTORS

- Type of sport can lead to tears from collision, falling on outstretched hand, and hyperrotation or traction.
- Racquet sports (tennis, racquetball), pole vault, gymnastics, golf, weight training (bench press), hockey (collision and hyperrotation with a slapshot), and water skiing (traction)
- Positive ulnar variance is associated with TFCC tears.
- Distal radius fractures are associated with tears of the TFCC. Symptomatic nonunion of the ulnar styloid is also associated with tear of the TFCC (often with distal radius fractures).

COMMONLY ASSOCIATED CONDITIONS

- Positive ulnar variance (result of distal radius fracture or congenital) can cause increased load of ulnar carpus on TFCC.
- Distal radius fractures can result in disruption of radial-ulnar aspect of TFCC (DRUJ instability) or increased ulnar variance.
- Nonunion of base of the ulnar styloid fracture may result in symptomatic TFCC tears.
- Instability (subluxation or dislocation) of the DRUJ, midcarpus, or triquetrum-lunate
- Ulnar impaction syndrome (abutment syndrome, impingement syndrome) with positive ulnar variance and risk factors (sport, repetitive trauma): There is central tear to TFCC, and chondromalacia develops in the lunate, triquetrum, and ulnar head.

DIAGNOSIS

HISTORY

- In athletes, there is a history of:
  - Acute trauma such as a fall on an outstretched hand, especially with ulnar load or ulnar deviation
  - Traction or hyperrotation
  - Previous Colles fracture
  - Previous dislocated/subluxed DRUJ
  - "Insignificant" wrist injury
- Overuse and repetitive trauma to the ulnar side of the wrist as seen in club and racquet sports
- Patients often report ulnar-sided pain ± clicking.
- Weak hand grip
- Subjective sense of wrist instability
- Pain with pronation, supination, or extension with axial load

PHYSICAL EXAM

- TFCC impaction/load/compression test: Axially load the wrist and ulnar deviate; a positive test reproduces pain ± click.
- May have pain/weakness with isometric resisted wrist flexion (patient tries to lift table in supination); this is seen with dorsal-sided peripheral tears.
- Pain/weakness pushing out of a chair (wrist extension with axial load)
- The fovea sign describes point tenderness at the recess of the TFCC with a sensitivity of 95.2% and specificity of 86.5% correctly identifying TFCC injury. The fovea lies between the ulnar styloid process and the flexor carpi ulnaris (FCU) tendon. Distally, it is bounded by the pisiform bone and proximally by the volar surface of the ulnar head.
- Tests to evaluate for associated instability:
  - Shuck test (excessive anteroposterior [AP] glide with either fixed ulna in relation to radius or vice-versa in pronation, supination, and neutral)
  - AP translation of triquetrum to fixed lunate
  - AP translation of lunate to fixed triquetrum
  - Ulnar compression test: Squeeze ulnar head against sigmoid notch of distal radius.
- Diagnostic injection with lidocaine to either the ECU, FCU tendons, the TFCC interval, or the DRUJ—sigmoid notch may be useful to differentiate the source of pain

DIFFERENTIAL DIAGNOSIS

- Tendinopathy (ECU, FCU)
- DRUJ instability (dislocation, subluxation) and arthritis
- Carpal instability (lunotriquetral, midcarpal)
- Fracture (distal radius, ulnar styloid nonunion, triquetrum, hamate, pisiform)
- Ulnar carpal impingement (ulnar abutment syndrome)
- Kienböck disease

DIAGNOSTIC TESTS & INTERPRETATION

Initial Tests (lab, imaging)

- Radiographs: Lateral and posteroanterior [PA] in neutral, zero rotation to rule out associated fractures and determine ulnar variance. Presurgical assessment could include PA in full pronation with hand grip view to accentuate the ulnar variance.
- MRI, especially high-resolution scanners with experienced radiologists, is useful to detect TFCC pathology, with sensitivity and specificity reported as high as 99% and 90%, respectively (4)[C].
- MR arthrography with traction reduces vacuum effect and improves visualization of the TFC and ligament tears and is a good option for elite athletes, presurgical study or if there are unexplained clinical symptoms in lieu of a prior nonarthrographic MRI. Note: MRI arthrography can better delineate intrinsic ligament tears and the articular surface cartilage.
- Peripheral lesions of the TFCC are difficult to image with MRI, and arthroscopy remains the gold standard for diagnosing TFCC pathology in addition to being therapeutic. The trampoline sign is when a surgical probe fails to spring back when peripheral tears exist (4)[C].
- MR arthrogram and high-resolution dedicated MRI are nearly perfect in accuracy to diagnose traumatic TFCC tears.
- Peripheral lesions are difficult to diagnose with imaging (4)[C].

Diagnostic Procedures/Other

Diagnostic injection with lidocaine into ECU, FCU, TFCC space, DRUJ, midcarpus, or lunotriquetral may help to differentiate pain.

TREATMENT

- Initial treatment for traumatic and symptomatic degenerative tears is conservative, for up to 8 to 12 weeks and includes:
  - Nonsteroidal anti-inflammatory drugs (NSAIDs), relative rest (avoid painful activities):
    - Immobilization (ulnar deviation, slight volar flexion) in a short arm cast for 4 to 6 weeks, if traumatic
    - Followed by physical therapy and use of a removable splint (5)[C]
- A more aggressive approach has been recommended for high-level athletes (6)[C]:
  - A trial of immobilization of the wrist for 2 to 3 weeks if distal DRUJ is stable
  - Arthroscopic surgery if that fails or there is any associated instability
- Care to not load the ulnar wrist or load in pronosupination is important.
- Peripheral lesions often will heal owing to the improved vascularity.
- Injections with corticosteroids or PRP can be used in recalcitrant cases, but there is no evidence for efficacy to support this approach (5).
- If there is instability of the DRUJ (distal ulna is dorsal), immobilization in 30 degrees of supination for 4 weeks followed by gradual return to neutral for the next 2 weeks (5)[C]
- Surgery is indicated if symptoms persist or there is failure to improve after a short course of immobilization, any instability of the DRUJ or lunotriquetral, and positive ulnar variance (5)[C].

MEDICATION

Trial of NSAIDs for pain

ISSUES FOR REFERRAL

- If any instability to the DRUJ or lunotriquetral is noted, refer for arthroscopy (6)[C].
- If the wrist is stable and not responding to initial immobilization, refer for arthroscopy (6)[C].

ADDITIONAL THERAPIES

For competitive, elite athletes, a more aggressive approach has been recommended (6)[C].

SURGERY/OTHER PROCEDURES

- No significant clinical outcomes for TFCC repair with either open or arthroscopic technique in 75 patients over 10 years. But, although not significant, there were more complaints of superficial ulnar nerve pain in the open repair group. Also, female gender was associated with a higher rate of reoperation (5)[C].
- For Palmer type 1A lesions, arthroscopic débridement/repair is recommended (5)[C].
- For Palmer type 1B/C/D, arthroscopy with mini-open repairs is performed (5)[C].
- Palmer 2A/B arthroscopic débridement (Consider osteotomy if + ulnar variance.) (5)[C]
- Palmer 2C/D with neutral ulna variance, no lunotriquetral instability—arthroscopic débridement (5)[C]
- Palmer 2C/D if ulna variance <2 mm, arthroscopy and:
  - Without lunotriquetral instability—wafer procedure indicated
  - With lunotriquetral instability—osteotomy indicated
- Palmer 2C/D with ulna variance >2 mm arthroscopy and osteotomy (5)[C]
- Palmer 2E arthroscopy has mixed results, often a salvage surgery is performed (5)[C].
- For degenerative Palmer type 2 lesions, ulnar variance is assessed as well as midcarpal stability and wear:
  - If ulnar variance is 3 mm or less, wafer procedure is recommended.
  - If ulnar variance is >3 mm, wafer + ulnar shortening is recommended (6)[C].
  - Wafer procedure is arthroscopic decompression of the ulnocarpal joint with débridement of the TFCC.
  - Atzei and Luchetti offer an alternative classification and treatment algorithm based on tear size, location and associated DRUJ instability to direct intervention (7)[C].

ONGOING CARE

FOLLOW-UP RECOMMENDATIONS

After initial injury, follow-up should be at 2 to 3 weeks to gauge response to immobilization.

PROGNOSIS

- Return to play:
  - A conservative approach postoperatively to avoid ulnar synovitis: 6 weeks of immobilization in a short arm or Muenster cast followed by 6 weeks of progressive range of motion and strength, with full return to sport at 3 to 6 months postoperatively with circumferential compression during activity (7)[C].
  - Return to restricted sport (golf and tennis) 4 to 6 weeks after débridement of central TFCC tear (type 1A) and 3 to 4 months after repair (6)[C].
- Prognosis:
  - If no associated instability of DRUJ or lunotriquetral and no positive ulnar variance, long-term results are good.
  - Excellent results for return to play with improvement in pain relief after arthroscopic surgery in high-level athletes. Those who did not return to play at 3 months had DRUJ instability and ulnar-carpal abutment but returned to play after an additional period postoperatively, 5 to 7 months (5)[C].

COMPLICATIONS

Previously undiagnosed carpal or DRUJ instability or ulnar-carpal abutment syndrome

REFERENCES

1. Chan JJ, Teunis T, Ring D. Prevalence of triangular fibrocartilage complex abnormalities regardless of symptoms rise with age: systematic review and pooled analysis. *Clin Orthop Relat Res.* 2014;472(12):3987–3994.
2. Iordache SD, Rowan R, Garvin GJ, et al. Prevalence of triangular fibrocartilage complex abnormalities on MRI scans of asymptomatic wrists. *J Hand Surg Am.* 2012;37(1):98–103.
3. Palmer AK. Triangular fibrocartilage complex lesions: a classification. *J Hand Surg Am.* 1989;14(4):594–606.
4. Zhao X, Yu A, Zhao H, et al. Diagnostic value of MRI in traumatic triangular fibrocartilage complex injuries: a retrospective study. *BMC Musculoskelet Disord.* 2024;25(1):63.
5. Jawed A, Ansari MT, Gupta V. TFCC injuries: how we treat? *J Clin Orthop Trauma.* 2020;11(4):570–579.
6. Rettig AC. Athletic injuries of the wrist and hand: part II: overuse injuries of the wrist and traumatic injuries to the hand. *Am J Sports Med.* 2004;32(1):262–273.
7. Dineen HA, Greenberg JA. Ulnar-sided wrist pain in the athlete. *Clinics in Sports Medicine.* 2020;39(2):373–400.

ADDITIONAL READING

- Ahn AK, Chang D, Plate AM. Triangular fibrocartilage complex tears: a review. *Bull NYU Hosp Jt Dis.* 2006;64(3–4):114–118.
- Coggins CA. Imaging of ulnar-sided wrist pain. *Clin Sports Med.* 2006;25(3):505–526.
- Dumontier C. Physical examination of wrist instabilities. Accessed March 7, 2018. https://mo-journal.com/posts/physical-examination-of-wrist-instabilities-247
- Nagle DJ. Triangular fibrocartilage complex tears in the athlete. *Clin Sports Med.* 2001;20(1):155–166.
- Palmer AK, Werner FW. Biomechanics of the distal radioulnar joint. *Clin Orthop Relat Res.* 1984;(187):26–35.
- Smith TO, Drew B, Toms A, et al. Diagnostic accuracy of magnetic resonance imaging and magnetic resonance arthrography for triangular fibrocartilaginous complex injury: a systematic review and meta-analysis. *J Bone Joint Surg Am.* 2012;94(9):824–832.
- Steinberg B. Acute wrist injuries in the athlete. *Orthop Clin North Am.* 2002;33(3):535–545.
- Tse YL, Chau WW, Wong CW. A structured non-operative treatment program for traumatic triangular fibrocartilage complex tear: a quasi-experimental study. *Hand Surg Rehabil.* 2023;42(6):492–498.

CLINICAL PEARLS

- Ulnar-sided wrist pain has been described as the "low back pain" of the wrist due to the complexity of the functional anatomy, of which the TFCC contributes.
- A detailed history and careful examination can demystify this condition and lead to diagnosis of TFCC tears with or without resultant instability of the DRUJ, lunotriquetral intervals. This is also important rather than relying only on obtaining radiographs.
- Conservative therapy is recommended as first-line treatment with bracing/splinting, NSAIDS and physical therapy.
- Early referral for MRI or arthroscopy is indicated when suspecting TFCC tears in the athlete, with any instability of the DRUJ or lunotriquetral intervals or when the TFCC fails to improve with conservative management after a short period of immobilization.
- The key to long-term treatment success in large part depends on positive ulnar variance—if present, consider referral to evaluate for ulnar shortening procedure.

THORACIC OUTLET SYNDROME

Brent Pickett, DO ▪ Jeffrey R. Bytomski, DO, FAOASM, FAMSSM

BASICS

DESCRIPTION

- Neurogenic or vascular symptoms in the upper extremity due to compression of the neurovascular bundle (brachial plexus and subclavian vessels) by skeletal and/or muscular structures above the 1st rib and behind the clavicle
- Symptoms are variable and based on the structure that is compressed or irritated.

ALERT

Three subtypes (1):
- Neurogenic: >95% of cases
- Venous: 4% of cases
- Arterial: <1% of cases

ETIOLOGY AND PATHOPHYSIOLOGY

- Brachial plexus nerve roots, subclavian artery, and subclavian vein pass through the scalene triangle formed by the 1st rib, anterior scalene muscles, and middle scalene muscles.
- Increased risk of positional compression of the neurovascular bundle at the thoracic outlet due to:
  - Congenital anatomic predisposition (cervical rib, abnormally long transverse process of C7, anomalous fibromuscular band)
  - Acquired extrinsic factors (anterior scalene hypertrophy, pectoralis minor tightness, poor posture causing decreased diameter of the costoaxillary canal, trauma, shortening of the scalene muscles due to active trigger points)
- Upper extremity venous thrombosis or Paget-Schroetter syndrome:
  - Overhead athletes may develop "effort thrombosis" due to repetitive shoulder hyperabduction and external rotation, which can compress the axillary-subclavian veins, damage the intimal lining, and transiently restrict venous flow. Over time, this creates a favorable environment for thrombus formation.

RISK FACTORS

Overhead athletes: swimmers, pitchers, weight lifters, volleyball, and tennis players
- Poor posture
- Poor overhead/movement mechanics
- Middle-aged female
- Congenital abnormalities:
  - Cervical rib
  - Abnormally long transverse process of C7
  - Anomalous fibromuscular band in the thoracic outlet
- Trauma
- Obesity

DIAGNOSIS

Thoracic outlet syndrome is largely a clinical diagnosis.

HISTORY

- Neurogenic and vascular symptoms related to certain positions
- Worse with lifting heavy objects, overhead activities, shoulder abduction, and external rotation
- Neurogenic:
  - Arm, shoulder, and neck pain
  - Paresthesia and numbness:
    - Frequently seen in the ulnar distribution
  - Headaches
  - Cramping of forearm muscles
  - Difficulty with fine motor skills of the hand
  - Sensory loss, motor weakness, atrophy (late findings)
  - Gilliatt-Sumner hand: severe wasting of the abductor pollicis brevis and, to a lesser extent, the interossei and hypothenar muscles (<1% of patients)
- Venous:
  - Pain
  - Edema
  - Cyanosis
  - Feeling of heaviness in the arm or hand
  - Venous distension of the arm and hand
- Arterial (often asymptomatic until embolization occurs):
  - Ischemic pain
  - Paresthesia and numbness
  - Claudication
  - Cool extremity
  - Pallor
  - Decreased distal pulse
  - Pulsating lump above the clavicle

PHYSICAL EXAM

- Swelling or discoloration of the affected extremity
- Muscle atrophy
- Decreased or absent distal pulse with activity or position changes
- Bruit auscultated in the supraclavicular space
- Provocative testing (low overall sensitivity and specificity) (1):
  - Elevated arm stress test (EAST):
    - Arms abducted above the head in a "stick-em-up" position
    - Patient opens and closes fists at moderate speed for 3 minutes.
    - Positive test if position reproduces pain or paresthesias
  - Upper limb tension tests:
    - Position 1: Abduct arms to 90 degrees.
    - Position 2: Extend wrists.
    - Position 3: Tilt head to one side—ear to shoulder—and then, tilt head to other side.
    - Positions 1 and 2 should cause ipsilateral pain, and position 3 should cause contralateral pain.
    - Strongest response is an onset of symptoms with position 1 and an increase in severity with positions 2 and 3.
  - Adson maneuver:
    - Neck extended and turned to the affected side while the shoulder is slightly abducted and extended
    - Feel for radial pulse while patient takes a deep breath.
    - Positive test if pulse lost and symptoms reproduced (only useful if this position causes arterial compression)
    - False positives/false negatives are common.
  - Wright test:
    - Affected arm is progressively hyperabducted and externally rotated.
    - Positive test if radial pulse lost
    - Just like the Adson maneuver, the thoracic outlet anatomy can vary significantly. Some individuals might have enough space in their thoracic outlet to avoid compression even with the hyperabduction and external rotation of the Wright test.
    - Subjectivity to determine with pulse is lost.
  - Allen test:
    - Flex elbow to 90 degrees; abduct and externally rotate the shoulder.
    - Patient rotates head away from the test arm.
    - Positive test if radial pulse lost.
    - Same limitations as Wright and Adson tests

DIFFERENTIAL DIAGNOSIS

- Cervical disc disorders
- Rotator cuff tear/impingement syndrome
- Brachial plexus neuritis
- Carpal tunnel syndrome
- Ulnar nerve entrapment
- Complex regional pain syndrome
- Polymyalgia rheumatica
- Fibromyalgia
- Subclavian steal
- Vasculitis
- Raynaud disease
- Multiple sclerosis
- Tumors of the spinal cord
- Pancoast tumor
- Neurofibroma
- Adhesive capsulitis
- Glenohumeral/acromioclavicular osteoarthritis

DIAGNOSTIC TESTS & INTERPRETATION

Initial Tests (lab, imaging)

- X-rays of the cervical spine, shoulder, and/or chest: useful to evaluate for a cervical rib or other thoracic pathology (1),(2),(3),(4),(5)[C]
- Magnetic resonance imaging (MRI): helpful to evaluate for rotator cuff derangement, cervical contribution to symptoms, or soft tissue mass (1),(2),(4)[C]
- Duplex ultrasound (US): to document degree of stenosis, presence of an aneurysm, or confirm thrombosis (2)[C]

Diagnostic Procedures/Other

- Electromyogram/nerve conduction studies (1),(4),(5),(6)[C]
- Diagnostic US with or without dynamic maneuvers (5)
- Diagnostic anesthetic injection to scalene or pectoralis minor musculature (4),(6).
- Can consider MRI brachial plexus (1),(6)
- Computed tomography (CT)/MRI arteriography/venography: reserved for cases of suspected arterial or venous thoracic outlet syndrome (vTOS) and for surgical planning (1),(2),(4),(5),(6)[C]

TREATMENT

- Conservative therapy is the initial approach, except in cases of thromboembolic phenomena with acute vascular occlusion, stenosis, arterial dilatation, or progressive neurologic deficits (1).
- Medications (2),(4)[C]: (under 2 weeks)
  - Nonsteroidal anti-inflammatory drugs (NSAIDs)
  - Muscle relaxants
- Activity modification (2)[C]
- Weight loss (2),(6)
- Physical therapy (1),(2),(5),(6)[C]:
  - Postural retraining
  - Pectoral and scalene stretching/strengthening
    - Caution with aggressive strengthening/stretching of pectoralis muscles in neurogenic thoracic outlet syndrome (nTOS) as it can worsen symptoms (4)
  - Scapulothoracic stability/mobility
  - Trigger point treatment
  - Soft tissue mobilization
- US-guided steroid, onabotulinumtoxinA, or anesthetic injections (1),(4),(5),(6)[C]:
  - Consider as a short-term adjunct to nonoperative therapy with physical therapy or as a bridge to surgery.
  - US-guided scalene block with local anesthetic to relax the anterior scalene muscle and lower the 1st rib to relieve the tension on the brachial plexus. If the injection provides symptomatic relief, it indicates likely benefit of a 1st rib resection/anterior scalenectomy (1),(2),(4)[C].
  - US-guided injection to pectoralis minor insertion on coracoid process with or without diagnostic block of the suprascapular nerve (1)
- vTOS with thrombus present (4)[C]:
  - Catheter-directed thrombolysis versus thrombolytics and anticoagulation (2)

SURGERY/OTHER PROCEDURES

- Surgery is an option for nTOS that has not responded to aggressive nonoperative treatments. Treatments can include 1st rib resection, pectoralis minor release, with consideration for suprascapular nerve release, subclavius release, or brachial plexus neurolysis (1),(2),(4)[C].
- For vTOS subtypes, can consider possible thoracic outlet decompression following thrombolysis or systemic anticoagulation (2)
- For arterial thoracic outlet syndrome (aTOS), can consider scalenectomy, 1st rib resection, and/or arterial reconstruction or bypass (2)

ONGOING CARE

FOLLOW-UP RECOMMENDATIONS

- Surgical referral if signs of vascular compromise or severe neurogenic symptoms are present
- Surgical referral when a cervical rib or extra-long transverse process of C7 is associated with loss of sensation, muscle atrophy, or weakness
- Surgical referral if symptoms persist despite an adequate course of aggressive, nonoperative therapy

COMPLICATIONS

- Poststenotic dilatation of the subclavian artery resulting in aneurysm formation and the potential for thromboembolism to the affected upper extremity (aTOS)
- Pulmonary embolism, residual symptoms, and high recurrence rate (vTOS)
- Progressive motor deficits (nTOS)

REFERENCES

1. Ahmed AS, Lafosse T, Graf A R, et al. Modern treatment of neurogenic thoracic outlet syndrome: pathoanatomy, diagnosis, and arthroscopic surgical technique. *J Hand Surg Glob Online*. 2023;5(4):561–576.
2. Panther EJ, Reintgen CD, Cueto RJ, et al. Thoracic outlet syndrome: a review. *J Shoulder Elbow Surg*. 2022;31(11):e545–e561.
3. Foley JM, Finlayson H, Travlos A. A review of thoracic outlet syndrome and the possible role of botulinum toxin in the treatment of this syndrome. *Toxins (Basel)*. 2012;4(11):1223–1235.
4. Troyer W, Gardner JE, Bowers RL. Neurogenic thoracic outlet syndrome in the overhead and throwing athlete: a narrative review. *PM R*. 2023;15(5):629–639.
5. Stewman C, Vitanzo PC Jr, Harwood MI. Neurologic thoracic outlet syndrome: summarizing a complex history and evolution. *Curr Sports Med Rep*. 2014;13(2):100–106.
6. Jones MR, Prabhakar A, Viswanath O, et al. Thoracic outlet syndrome: a comprehensive review of pathophysiology, diagnosis, and treatment. *Pain Ther*. 2019;8(1):5–18.

ADDITIONAL READING

Illig KA, Thompson RW, Freischlag JA. *Thoracic Outlet Syndrome*. Springer International Publishing; 2013.

CLINICAL PEARLS

- Thoracic outlet syndrome is a largely clinical diagnosis, although radiographic studies can be helpful if diagnosis is unclear.
- Treatment is often conservative, consisting of activity modification, physical therapy, and medication for pain.
- If diagnosis is equivocal, refer for US-guided diagnostic/therapeutic procedures prior to surgical referral.
- Surgical referral is reserved for patients with severe neurologic/vascular compromise (emergent) or refractory symptoms despite adequate treatment (subacute).

THORACIC SPINE INJURY

Kenneth Vitale, MD, FACSM, FAAPMR ▪ David Bakal, MD

BASICS

DESCRIPTION

- Thoracic spine injuries occur to bone, ligament, muscle, disk, and nerve
- Thoracic spine fractures:
  - Range from minor, stable fractures to serious, unstable or catastrophic fractures
  - Higher risk in collision sports (e.g., hockey, football, wrestling)
  - Catastrophic injuries are rarely seen in sports.
  - The spinal column is divided into three distinct columns (anterior, middle, and posterior). If two of three are disrupted, the spinal column traditionally is considered unstable and requires emergent surgical referral. The posterior ligamentous complex (PLC) is part of the posterior column and consists of the supraspinous and interspinous ligaments, ligamentum flavum, and facet capsule. It is now considered the most critical predictor of stability (three-column theory only moderately reliable in determining stability)
  - Typically, **stable** fractures:
    - Transverse process, spinous process, or isolated articular fracture
    - Pars interarticularis fracture (more common in lumbar spine)
    - Compression fracture (axial, flexion, or lateral compression force); although if anterior compression >40–50%, likely PLC disrupted and unstable
    - Extension injury: facet, lamina, spinous process fracture, or disruption of *all* three

ALERT

Typical **unstable** fractures:

- Burst fracture (higher energy axial compression with centripedal displacement)
- Flexion-rotation injury (slice fracture): PLC typically fails and is unstable.
- Fracture-dislocation injury: bilateral facet dislocation (jumped facets) typically unstable as all three columns disrupted
- Flexion-distraction (Chance fracture): most common at thoracolumbar junction and posterior and middle column fractures. It happens when the spine bends forward with significant force, often while the body is restrained by a lap belt. This is why it's sometimes called a "seatbelt fracture"; may occur with **abdominal pain**: due to the mechanism of injury, there is a high chance of associated abdominal injuries.

- Thoracic discogenic pain and disk herniation:
  - The three basic structures of normal vertebral disks:
    - Nucleus pulposus: gelatinous core, composed mostly of water and proteoglycans
    - Annulus fibrosus: concentric collagen lamellae surrounding nucleus; outer third innervated and may be clinically painful if tear present
    - Vertebral endplates: aid in the diffusion of nutrients into the disks, absorb hydrostatic pressure of axial loading, prevent nucleus from herniating into vertebral body
  - Thoracic disk herniations rare (~1% of all herniated nucleus pulposus):
    - **Central**: higher potential for spinal cord injury; monitor for weakness, spasticity, hyperreflexia, abnormal gait, bowel/bladder incontinence
    - **Centrolateral**: Often in younger patients with history of trauma, may have contralateral pain and sensory changes resembling Brown-Séquard syndrome (rare neurological condition caused by damage to one half of the spinal cord)
    - **Lateral**: may cause radicular pain to rib area and visceral sites
- Muscular contusions: caused by a direct blow with intramuscular bleeding, often contact sports or falls. Check for potential rib fracture, pneumothorax, hemothorax, and pulmonary contusion.
- Musculoligamentous strain/sprain:
  - Stretch/tear of thoracic muscles and/or ligaments
  - Seen most frequently in twisting/turning sports
- Facet syndrome:
  - Facet dysfunction/irritation and capsule microtears can lead to mild subluxation, synovitis, and fibrosis.
  - May have localized pain and rib asymmetry
- Scheuermann (juvenile) kyphosis:
  - Osteochondrosis of thoracic vertebral ossification centers with at least 5% anterior wedging of at least three consecutive thoracic vertebrae
  - Often asymptomatic (~20% adolescents report pain)
  - Progressive, degenerative condition

ALERT

Spinal tumors:

- Pediatric Considerations: Maintain high index of suspicion in younger patients with night pain, fevers, systemic symptoms; persistent back pain in adolescents is never considered "normal."
- Vertebral tumors:
  - Primary: rare, usually younger adults, grow slowly; osteosarcoma most common malignant tumor
  - Metastatic: more common, seen in 30–70% of cancer patients; painful with constitutional symptoms; primary malignancies include breast, lung, thyroid, kidney, prostate, colon, lymphoma, melanoma, sarcoma, myeloma
- Extramedullary tumors: usually benign, grow slowly and therefore are found in middle age and older individuals (meningioma, schwannoma, neurofibroma)
- Intramedullary tumors: also usually benign and found later in life but surgical excision difficult (intramedullary lipoma most common in thoracic; astrocytoma, ependymoma common in cervical)

EPIDEMIOLOGY

- Thoracic spine fractures:
  - 19–50% thoracolumbar fractures result in neurologic damage and spinal cord compression.
  - 15% of spinal fractures occur in sports; third most common etiology after motor vehicle accident (45%) and falls (20%):
    - In sports-related injuries, the most common cause of fracture is water sports (65%).
    - Of water sports, diving is most common (60%).
  - Male-to-female ratio of spinal fractures 4:1
  - Mean age: 24 ± 12 years
- Scheuermann kyphosis: 5% of general population; typically seen at 10 to 15 years, slight male predominance
- Facet syndrome: 15% (up to 40%) of back pain (including lumbar) thought to be facet-mediated pain
- Disk disease: evidence of degenerative disk disease and disk herniation in up to 58% of athletes (vs. 38% control population); may be sport specific

ETIOLOGY AND PATHOPHYSIOLOGY

- The thoracic spine is very rigid owing to the rib cage and the costovertebral articulations.
- T2–T10 better protected from ribs and facet orientation in coronal plane (limits motion, allows rotation)
- Cervicothoracic and thoracolumbar junctions susceptible to shear and flexion-extension forces
- Extreme flexion-extension plus axial loads are not well tolerated and may lead to injury.
- Thoracic spine fracture:
  - Most thoracic spine fractures (>50%) occur at thoracolumbar junction region (T11–L2) due to fulcrum effect.
  - Rotational or extension forces may fracture the pars interarticularis and damage facets.
- Thoracic discogenic pain:
  - Up to 90% of herniated disks are due to degenerative processes. With aging, disk water content decreases, leading to decreased disk height and loss of axial absorption capacity.
  - Trauma may be implicated in up to 10–20%, typically a twisting/torsional movement.
- Facet syndrome:
  - Acute excessive motion that traumatizes joint versus chronic overuse

Genetics

Scheuermann kyphosis:

- 74% heritability pattern (autosomal dominant)
- Histology shows disorganized endochondral ossification, collagen reduction, increased endplate mucopolysaccharides

RISK FACTORS

- Scheuermann kyphosis:
  - Possible additional risk factor from repetitive flexion sports at young age (e.g., water skiing has a higher prevalence)
  - Scheuermann may predispose to subsequent thoracic disk herniations.
- Facet syndrome:
  - Often in sports with powerful hyperextension or extremes of spinal range of motion (ROM) (e.g., gymnasts and figure skaters)
  - Facet syndrome can lead to facet osteoarthritis.
- Sport-specific risk factors:
  - Football players have increased risk of degenerative disk disease, facet degeneration, and chronic back pain proportional to years of involvement in sport.
  - Weightlifting is associated with degenerative disk disease and musculoligamentous sprains/strains.
  - Endurance athletes also may be at risk (e.g., butterfly swimmers and rowers are at risk for rib subluxation from the transverse processes [often 6th or 7th rib]).
  - Disk herniation risk is higher in athletes participating in axial rotation sports, such as golf.

DIAGNOSIS

- Rapid evaluation of airway, breathing, and circulation (ABCs), primary and secondary trauma survey
- Detailed spine and neurologic exam, with specific attention to bony deformity or tenderness, and lower extremity neurologic deficits

HISTORY

- Thoracic spine fracture:
  - Significant force is required for thoracic vertebral fractures, so associated injuries may obscure symptoms directly related to thoracic fractures.
  - Common symptoms:
    - Pain or tenderness:
      - Localized—usually midline
      - Referred—paraspinals, ribs, anterior chest wall, and/or visceral pain
    - Paresthesia or dysesthesia

ALERT

Bowel or bladder incontinence, saddle anesthesia, leg weakness, and/or gait instability indicates probable spinal cord injury and is a medical emergency that requires immediate consultation with a surgeon.

- Thoracic discogenic pain and disk herniation:
  - Most commonly insidious onset without history of trauma
  - Pain is the most common symptom (60% of patients), may be band-like, dull, localized to the thoracic spine or referred to visceral, sternal, or inguinal regions.
  - Paresthesia and dysesthesia are present in 25% of patients, typically dermatomal.
  - Abdominal and intercostal weakness present in 17% of patients; suspect myelopathy if lower extremities is affected.
  - Bladder abnormalities present in only 2% of patients, suspect cord compression (1),(2)[B].
- Muscular strains: typically, mild pain following a sporting activity
- Scheuermann kyphosis:
  - Symptoms are typically insidious onset with no history of major trauma.
  - Often seen with history of repetitive microtrauma, osteoporosis, osteochondrosis, necrosis of the ring apophysis, and/or tight hamstrings

PHYSICAL EXAM

Thoracic spine fracture: localized soft tissue deformity

ALERT
- Neurologic deficits
  - Assess for leg or saddle paresthesia, weakness or paraplegia, spasticity, and hyperreflexia, all are signs of critical spinal cord injury.
  - Reflexes: Hyperactive reflexes signify upper motor neuron lesions; hypoactive reflexes signify lower motor neuron lesions (spinal cord ends ~L1–L2).
- Spinal shock
  - Assess for hypotension, bradycardia, hyporeflexia, which can happen acutely after spinal cord injury.

- Thoracic discogenic pain and disk herniation:
  - Musculoskeletal findings are often nonspecific but may reveal local myofascial pain and stiffness.
  - Sensory deficits to light touch or pinprick along a thoracic dermatomal pattern
  - Motor examination should include testing muscle strength, flexibility, and tone:
    - Include abdominal muscles; T9 and T10 lesions can affect lower abdominal muscles but spare upper abdominal muscles.
    - Lower extremity weakness, spasticity, or hyperreflexia is serious, indicating myelopathy.
  - In isolated thoracic discogenic pain, upper extremity reflexes are normal (otherwise, suspect cervical injury) and lower extremity reflexes are normal (otherwise, suspect lumbosacral pathology or spinal cord injury) (1)[B],(2)[B].
- Scheuermann kyphosis:
  - Thoracic hyperkyphosis deformity that does not correct with passive extension
  - Compensatory lumbar hyperlordosis common
  - Tight hip flexors, hamstrings, lumbar fascia

DIFFERENTIAL DIAGNOSIS
- Arthritis (degenerative and rheumatoid)
- Spondyloarthropathy (e.g., ankylosing spondylitis)
- Congenital malformation (e.g., spina bifida)
- Pathologic fracture
- Spinal infection
- Paget disease

DIAGNOSTIC TESTS & INTERPRETATION
- Pain or tenderness, MVA, or falls from height are indications for anteroposterior (AP) and lateral plain-film views of the spine.
- Thoracic spine fracture:
  - CT scan is more sensitive and specific than plain radiographs for the detection of thoracic spine fractures and should be used in any patient with a traumatic injury suspicious for fracture based on history, exam, or initial plain films.
  - If suspicion is high and initial radiographs unremarkable, CT is still indicated.
  - Urgent MRI is ideal for evaluating spinal cord and ligamentous injuries.
- Thoracic discogenic pain and disk herniation:
  - Plain radiographs can be used in the initial evaluation of fracture, cancer, or infection.
  - X-ray findings that suggest disk herniation:
    - Disk calcification is present in up to 70% of patients with thoracic disk herniation versus only 4–6% of patients without herniation.
    - Other signs of disk degeneration: osteophyte formation, disk space narrowing, kyphosis
  - MRI: best visualization of the disk, spinal cord, and nerve roots; should be urgently ordered if symptoms suggest spinal cord injury
  - Can consider CT myelography in patients with contraindications to MRI (3)[C]
- Scheuermann kyphosis: Plain radiographs are usually diagnostic:
  - Irregular appearing vertebral endplates
  - Anterior disk space narrowing
  - Wedging of >5 degrees of three adjacent vertebrae (4)[C]
  - Kyphosis of >40 degrees with apex typically T7–T9 (4)[C]
- Spinal tumors:
  - Must rule out tumor when a patient has nocturnal back pain or significant constitutional symptoms
  - If concern for malignancy, lab workup should include complete blood count with differential, ESR, CRP, chemistries.
  - Imaging should start with plain x-ray; however, may not show abnormality until there is 30–50% loss of cancellous bone
  - Technetium-99m bone scan is sensitive but not specific; can find smaller metastases than x-rays
  - 18F positron emission tomography shows improved specificity; good for evaluating metastatic spread
  - MRI, especially with gadolinium, demonstrates soft tissue and osseous changes well.

TREATMENT
- Thoracic spine fracture:
  - Stable fractures often treated with brace immobilization for ~6 to 12 weeks (e.g., a thoracolumbosacral orthosis [TLSO] for a stable thoracic compression fracture)
  - Unstable fractures or neurologic deficits often require surgical intervention.
- Thoracic discogenic pain:
  - Conservative; largely involves activity modification, passive interventions such as soft tissue mobilization, and gradual reintroduction of activity including strengthening and postural training (5)[B]
  - Can consider epidural corticosteroid injections for refractory discogenic pain though high-level evidence is lacking (3)[C]
  - Early surgical consult indicated for lower extremity neurologic symptoms
- Muscular contusions/strains:
  - Conservative treatment: ice to reduce pain, limit bleeding and swelling
  - Moist heating pad after 72 hours.
  - Gentle massage after initial pain has resolved
  - Analgesics as needed for pain
  - Restrict activity until pain-free ROM, full strength.
  - Physical therapy (PT) for ROM, strengthening, core stabilization exercises, teach biomechanics (5)[B]

- Facet syndrome:
  - Conservative: rest, avoid triggering activity.
  - PT with manual therapy techniques (5)[B]
  - Teach postural correction to prevent recurrence (5)[B].
  - If no response, can consider a diagnostic/therapeutic intra-articular facet injection or medial branch block
- Scheuermann kyphosis:
  - PT to stretch tight hamstring muscles, core strengthening, and thoracic extensor muscle strengthening (4)[C]
  - Consider a brace in skeletally immature patients with fixed thoracic kyphosis between 50 and 80 degrees (4)[C].
  - Milwaukee brace for high thoracic curves; Boston brace for lower thoracic curves (apex below T7) (4)[C]
  - Surgical indications are ill-defined; decision should be individualized based on pain, neurologic deficits, worsening deformity despite bracing (4)[C].

MEDICATION

- Acute traumatic thoracic spinal cord injury:
  - May consider a 24-hour infusion of high-dose methylprednisolone if benefits outweigh risks, although conflicting clinical evidence (6)[C]
- Other causes of back pain: analgesics/Nonsteroidal anti-inflammatory drugs (NSAIDs) PRN

ADDITIONAL THERAPIES

- Soft tissue mobilization, massage, PT and other manual therapy services can be helpful ancillary treatments for chronic thoracic pain (5)[B].
- Posture classes and methods (e.g., yoga, Pilates, Feldenkrais, many others) also can be considered for chronic symptoms.
- Emergency department (ED) treatment:
  - Perform all needed resuscitation and diagnostic tests with the patient in full spinal immobilization.
  - If spinal cord injury is suspected, consult a neurosurgeon or orthopedic spine surgeon urgently.
  - If spinal fracture or instability is suspected without neurologic impairment, order stat CT scan/MRI and consult neurosurgery or orthopedic spine surgery.
  - Pain control should be administered if needed. NSAIDs, opiates, are the mainstays of treatment.

ADMISSION, INPATIENT, AND NURSING CONSIDERATIONS

- Follow the ABCs of trauma resuscitation.
- Airway intervention should be done with inline cervical immobilization (always stabilize the spine to prevent further injury and preserve residual function).
- Admission criteria:
  - Unstable spinal column injury
  - Spinal cord injury
  - Ileus
  - Severe intractable pain
  - Concomitant other injury/polytrauma
  - Patients with significant fracture or spinal cord injury should be treated in a regional trauma center.
- Discharge criteria: stable minor fractures after orthopedic or neurosurgical evaluation

ONGOING CARE

PATIENT EDUCATION

Keys to prevent recurrence include postural correction, core strengthening, and teaching proper biomechanics.

PROGNOSIS

Most thoracic injuries respond well to relative rest, activity modification, PT, and gradual reintroduction of activities.

REFERENCES

1. Cornips EMJ. Crippling upper back pain after whiplash and other motor vehicle collisions caused by thoracic disc herniations: report of 10 cases. *Spine (Phila Pa 1976)*. 2014;39(12):988–995.
2. Brown CW, Deffer PA, Akmakjian J, et al. The natural history of thoracic disc herniation. *Spine (Phila Pa 1976)*. 1992;17(Suppl 6):S97–S102.
3. Manchikanti L, Knezevic NN, Navani A, et al. Epidural interventions in the management of chronic spinal pain: American Society of Interventional Pain Physicians (ASIPP) comprehensive evidence-based guidelines. *Pain Physician*. 2021;24(S1):S27–S208.
4. O'Donnell JM, Wu W, Youn A, et al. Scheuermann Kyphosis: current concepts and management. *Curr Rev Musculoskelet Med*. 2023;16(11):521–530.
5. Heneghan NR, Gormley S, Hallam C, et al. Management of thoracic spine pain and dysfunction: a survey of clinical practice in the UK. *Musculoskelet Sci Pract*. 2019;39:58–66.
6. Karsy M, Hawryluk G. Modern medical management of spinal cord injury. *Curr Neurol Neurosci Rep*. 2019;19(9):65.

ADDITIONAL READING

- Diaz JJ Jr, Cullinane DC, Altman DT, et al. Practice management guidelines for the screening of thoracolumbar spine fracture. *J Trauma*. 2007;63(3):709–718.
- Nannapaneni R, Marks SM. Posterolateral thoracic disc disease: clinical presentation and surgical experience with a modified approach. *Br J Neurosurg*. 2004;18(5):467–470.
- Papagelopoulos P, Mavrogenis A, Savvidou O, et al. Current concepts in Scheuermann's kyphosis. *Orthopedics*. 2008;31(1):52–60.
- Ye C, Sun T, Li J, et al. Patterns of sports- and recreation-related spinal cord injuries in Beijing. *Spinal Cord*. 2009;47(12):857–860.

CLINICAL PEARLS

- 73% of thoracic herniations are asymptomatic; therefore, consider avoiding thoracic MRI during workup unless there is a concern for spinal cord injury.
- Return to play only when the athlete is pain free, neurologically intact, with normal ROM, and normal strength.
- If suspicious for a spine fracture or spinal cord injury, immobilize the patient on a spine board immediately and consult surgery urgently.
- Patients with neurologic deficit, weakness, bowel/bladder symptoms, or significant gait instability should be transported directly to a trauma center.

TIBIAL BONE STRESS INJURIES

Andrew J.M. Gregory, MD, FAAP, FACSM

BASICS

Bone stress injury of the tibia refers to an overuse injury of the bone as a result of repetitive loading that overwhelms its capacity to heal. It must be differentiated from medial tibial stress syndrome, which is not a stress fracture. In general, bone stress injury of the tibia can be classified into low risk or high risk. The more common low-risk bone stress injury of the tibia occurs on the posterior medial aspect of the bone (compression side) and heals well if treated appropriately. The less common high-risk bone stress injury of the tibia occurs on the anterior aspect of the bone (tension side) and often does not heal well even when treated appropriately.

EPIDEMIOLOGY

- True incidence and prevalence is unknown.
- 19–64% of all stress fractures
- Predominantly younger athletes (<20 years old)
- Predominantly female athletes

Incidence

Incidence of tibial bone stress injuries is not known and varies greatly among sports and studies.

Prevalence

Prevalence of tibial bone stress injuries is not known and varies between sports and studies.

ETIOLOGY AND PATHOPHYSIOLOGY

Repetitive impact activities causes these injuries.

Genetics

Little is known about the genetic predisposition for bone stress injury.

RISK FACTORS

- Previous history of bone stress injury
- Track and field athletes
- Female gender
- Younger age
- Increase in training volume or intensity
- Multisport athletes
- Chronic steroid use
- Relative energy deficiency syndrome (RED-s) patients with:
  - Osteopenia/osteoporosis, disordered eating
  - Oligomenorrhea/amenorrhea

GENERAL PREVENTION

Most bone stress injuries can be prevented by:

- Gradual increases in activity such as the 10% rule: no more than a 10% increase in load—intensity, duration, and/or frequency per week.
- Appropriate footwear such as properly fitted running shoes and orthotics if indicated (particularly in the military population(1)[B])
- Running on softer surfaces is probably justified to lower risk.
- Appropriate nutrition to match energy intake with expenditure; nutrition consult may be appropriate.

COMMONLY ASSOCIATED CONDITIONS

RED-s or any of the following signs:

- Osteopenia/osteoporosis from chronic steroid use
- Amenorrhea/oligomenorrhea: either primary or secondary
- Low energy availability from disordered eating or excess exercise

DIAGNOSIS

- Primarily based on history and physical examination and a high index of suspicion based on risk factors
- X-rays can be helpful if positive but are often unremarkable in the first 6 weeks of stress injury.
- Hallmark is point tenderness on physical examination. A wide area of tenderness may be more suggestive of medial tibial stress syndrome.
- It is important to distinguish high-grade anterior bone stress injuries (the dreaded black line) from posteromedial ones because the prognosis for anterior injuries can be catastrophic.

HISTORY

- Pain in the shin area:
  - Severe enough to limit activity
  - Worse with activity and better with rest
  - Worsens over time if the activity is continued
  - Often associated with an increase in training duration, frequency, or intensity
  - Usually no associated injury
- Assess for risk factors:
  - Training history should include days per week, hours per day and intensity, and footwear (how often changed and what type).
  - Dietary history (calories, foods avoided, and vitamin D and calcium intake; weight changes)
  - Menstrual history (number of missed periods, use of hormonal birth control, history prior to birth control use)
  - Family or personal history of bone stress injuries or osteoporosis/osteopenia
  - Medications known to decrease bone density (contraceptives, glucocorticoids, antiseizure medications)
  - Supplements (sex hormones or precursors, vitamin D, calcium)

PHYSICAL EXAM

- Focal tenderness to palpation on examination is the primary method for diagnosis of a stress fracture.
- Palpate for fracture callus, step-off, or crepitus.
- Hop test: pain at the site with hopping on one leg—be cautious with this because high index of suspicion can worsen fracture.
- Fulcrum test: pain at the site with bending the long bone over a fulcrum (table edge or examiner's leg)
- Examine foot type and function for biomechanical factors that predispose to bone stress injury (pes planus, pes cavus, heavy heel strike).
- X-rays can be helpful in diagnosing stress fractures but is often negative initially.
- History and clinical examination are often all that is necessary.
- Magnetic resonance imaging (MRI) is the gold standard for diagnosis.
- Bone scan or computed tomography (CT) scan can be useful adjuncts.

DIFFERENTIAL DIAGNOSIS

- Medial tibial stress syndrome (shin splints)
- Chronic exertional compartment syndrome
- Popliteal artery entrapment syndrome
- Pes anserine bursitis
- Osgood-Schlatter disease
- Posterior/anterior tibialis tendonitis
- Osteoarthritis of the knee
- Superficial nerve entrapment
- Other bony processes: bone cysts, osteoid osteoma, tumor, infection

DIAGNOSTIC TESTS & INTERPRETATION

Initial Tests (lab, imaging)

Initial approach:

ALERT

- X-rays:
  - May be negative through course; often negative for 3+ weeks; shows a lucency or fracture callus
  - For anterior cortical fractures, shows the "dreaded black line"
  - Sensitivity ranged from 12% (0–29%) to 56% (39–72%) (2).
  - Specificity ranged from 88% (55–100%) to 96% (87–100%) (2).
- Bone scan:
  - Sensitivity ranged from 50% (23–77%) to 97% (90–100%) (2).
  - Specificity ranged from 33% (12–53%) to 98% (93–100%) (2).
  - Poor accuracy (52%)
  - Helpful in multiple areas of concern, such as bilateral tibia or if MRI is not possible
- MRI:
  - Gold standard (2)[B]
  - Sensitivity ranged from 68% (45–90%) to 99% (95–100%) (2).
  - Specificity from 4% (0–11%) to 97% (88–100%) (2)
  - Best at demonstrating the exact location and extent of injury; accuracy (90%) (3)[B]
  - Shows fracture line on T1 and edema on T2
  - MRI grading may offer prognostic value for time to return to play after conservative treatment (3)[A].
- CT scan:
  - Not useful in the acute setting
  - Sensitivity ranged from 32% (8–57%) to 38% (16–59%) (2).
  - Specificity from 88% (55–100%) to 98% (91–100%) (2)
  - Useful in assessing healing of fractures
- Musculoskeletal ultrasound (MSK US):
  - Sensitivity ranged from 43% (26–61%) to 99% (95–100%) (2).
  - Specificity ranged from 13% (0–45%) to 79% (61–96%) (2).
- Follow-up and special considerations:
  - X-rays will show healing of an existing injury in most cases; look for callus formation or nonunion.
  - Bone scan can remain positive for over a year; therefore, not useful to determine healing
  - MRI may continue to show edema after the fracture is asymptomatic.
  - CT is useful for assessing fracture healing for fractures that are difficult to see on plain film.
  - Bone density scan (dual energy x-ray absorptiometry [DEXA]) may be considered if risk factors for RED-s are found.

Diagnostic Procedures/Other

Occasionally, bone stress injuries can be confused with tumor on imaging. A biopsy of the anterior tibia should be avoided if possible because it may increase the risk of nonunion.

TREATMENT

- Treatment of most bone stress injuries of the tibia is the same as other bone stress injuries, which is to remove the offending activity (usually impact activity).
- However, the treatment of anterior versus posterior tibial bone stress injuries is quite different:
  - Posterior medial tibial bone stress injuries can be allowed to continue to participate in limited activity as pain allows. Decrease practice to allow more participation in games.
  - Anterior tibial bone stress injuries or fracture (the "dreaded black line") should not continue to participate because of the risk of fracture completion and/or nonunion; requires prolonged non–weight-bearing or often surgery for internal fixation and/or bone grafting to heal
- Prehospital:
  - PRICE:
    - Protection: bracing
    - Rest
    - Ice
    - Compression
    - Elevation
  - Acetaminophen
  - Walking boot or long Aircast, crutches if necessary based on the amount of pain with weight-bearing
- Emergency department (ED) treatment:
  - Continued PRICE
  - Acetaminophen
  - Avoidance of scheduled nonsteroidal anti-inflammatory drugs (NSAIDs)
  - Walking boot
  - Crutches as needed
  - Consider non–weight-bearing or surgery for anterior tibial bone stress injuries or nonunion of tibial bone stress injuries.
  - Addressing other risk factors: nutritional, menstrual, osteopenia

MEDICATION

- No medications currently available to help stress fracture healing but can treat with pain medications
- Pain medications with anti-inflammatory drugs may be contraindicated because they may delay the healing of fractures.

ISSUES FOR REFERRAL

- Most athletes with anterior tibial stress injuries should be referred for surgical treatment (4)[B].
- Conservative treatment with casting and strict non–weight-bearing for 2 to 3 months can be considered but still may result in nonunion.

ADDITIONAL THERAPIES

- Measures to alleviate the pain associated with bone stress injuries include ice, acetaminophen, a controlled ankle movement (CAM) walker boot, and crutches.
- Some evidence that use of a pneumatic or stirrup brace may shorten the time to return to activity.
- Physical therapists and coaches can check and possibly correct poor biomechanics. Foot orthoses were found to be effective for prevention of tibial bone stress injuries in the military population (1)[B].

SURGERY/OTHER PROCEDURES

Surgical treatment of anterior tibial bone stress injuries consists of intermedullary nailing, with or without bone graft (3).

COMPLEMENTARY & ALTERNATIVE MEDICINE

Bone stimulators: Current evidence is insufficient to conclude a benefit in improving the rate of union in patients with a fresh fracture, osteotomy, delayed union, or nonunion or on time to healing in tibial bone stress injuries or a reduction in pain (1)[A].

ADMISSION, INPATIENT, AND NURSING CONSIDERATIONS

Not applicable in most cases

ONGOING CARE

- Low-risk bone stress injuries of the tibia: Ongoing activity modification and pain management is usually sufficient.
- High-risk bone stress injuries of the tibia require intermedullary nailing and grafting or non–weight-bearing and casting for 8 to 12 weeks, after which intermedullary nailing and grafting still may be necessary (approximately 70% require surgery) (4).
- Return to play
  - Suggested criteria include resolution of bony tenderness, pain-free walking, evidence of radiographic healing, strength/function/loading tests as well as identification of risk factors (5)[B].

DIET

- Nutritional evaluation is important not only for healing of the current fracture but also for prevention of recurrence.
- Current recommendations from the National Osteoporosis Foundation are 1,000 mg of calcium and 400 to 800 IU of vitamin D daily for adults aged <50 years.

PATIENT EDUCATION

- Athletes should understand that training, nutrition, biomechanical, and footwear errors must be remedied.
- Athletes with a prior bone stress injury are at increased risk for a future bone stress injury.

PROGNOSIS

- Good for low-risk bone stress injuries of the tibia
- Poor for high-risk bone stress injuries of the tibia

COMPLICATIONS

- Posteromedial bone stress injuries of the tibia: potential for slower healing if continued participation is allowed
- Anterior bone stress injuries of the tibia: Risk of nonunion and delayed or partial union is high, requiring surgery (6).

REFERENCES

1. Lavigne A, Chicoine D, Esculier JF, et al. The role of footwear, foot orthoses and training-related strategies in the prevention of bone stress injury. a systematic review and meta-analysis. *Int J Exerc Sci.* 2023;16(3):721–743.
2. Wright AA, Hegedus EJ, Lenchik L, et al. Diagnostic accuracy of various imaging modalities for suspected lower extremity stress fractures: a systematic review with evidence-based recommendations for clinical practice. *Am J Sports Med.* 2016;44(1):255–263.
3. Hoenig T, Tenforde AS, Strahl A, et al. Does magnetic resonance imaging grading correlate with return to sports after bone stress injuries? A systematic review and meta-analysis. *Am J Sports Med.* 2022;50(3):834–844.
4. Robertson GAJ, Wood AM. Return to sports after stress fractures of the tibial diaphysis: a systematic review. *Br Med Bull.* 2015;114(1):95–111.
5. George ERM, Sheerin KR, Reid D. Criteria and guidelines for return to running following tibial bone stress injury: a scoping review. *Sports Med.* 2024;54(9):2247–2265.
6. Mallee WH, Weel H, van Dijk CN, et al. Surgical versus conservative treatment for high-risk stress fractures of the lower leg (anterior tibial cortex, navicular and fifth metatarsal base): a systematic review. *Br J Sports Med.* 2015;49(6):370–376.

ADDITIONAL READING

- Busse JW, Kaur J, Mollon B, et al. Low intensity pulsed ultrasonography for fractures: systematic review of randomised controlled trials. *BMJ.* 2009;338:b351.
- Fredericson M, Bergman AG, Hoffman KL, et al. Tibial stress reaction in runners. Correlation of clinical symptoms and scintigraphy with a new magnetic resonance imaging grading system. *Am J Sports Med.* 1995;23(4):472–481.
- Kaeding CC, Yu JR, Wright R, et al. Management and return to play of stress fractures. *Clin J Sport Med.* 2005;15(6):442–447.
- Mitchell C, McDonnel S, Oganezova K, et al. The effect of surface compliance on overground running biomechanics: a systematic review and meta-analysis. *Sports Biomech.* 2025;24(5):1143–1167.
- Mollon B, da Silva V, Busse JW, et al. Electrical stimulation for long-bone fracture-healing: a meta-analysis of randomized controlled trials. *J Bone Joint Surg Am.* 2008;90(11):2322–2330.
- Snyder RA, Koester MC, Dunn WR. Epidemiology of stress fractures. *Clin Sports Med.* 2006;25(1):37–52.
- Whitelaw GP, Wetzler MJ, Levy AS, et al. A pneumatic leg brace for the treatment of tibial stress fractures. *Clin Orthop Relat Res.* 1991;(270):301–305.

SEE ALSO

Other bone stress injury chapters

CLINICAL PEARLS

- Distinguish low-risk from high-risk bone stress injury based on imaging and exam.
- Tenderness to palpation is the main physical examination finding.
- MRI is the imaging study of choice.
- Evaluate for training errors.
- Evaluate for additional risk factors (RED-s).

TIBIALIS POSTERIOR TENDINOPATHY

Matthew W. Wise, DO, CAQSM

BASICS

DESCRIPTION

- Overuse or underuse injury of a nonruptured tendon presenting as medial ankle pain
- Stage 1: mild swelling and pain, single leg heel raise (SLHR) is normal but painful
- Stage 2: progressive pain with flattening of the arch, inability to perform SLHR, flexible hindfoot
- Stage 3: All signs of stage 2 except the hindfoot deformity is fixed.
- Synonyms: posterior tibial tendon dysfunction; posterior tibial tendinopathy

EPIDEMIOLOGY

- Incidence of 2.3–3.6% in runners presenting to sports medicine clinics in earlier studies (1)
- Tibialis posterior tendon (TPT) dysfunction is the major cause of acquired flatfoot deformity in adults.

ETIOLOGY AND PATHOPHYSIOLOGY

- Caused by muscular imbalance resulting in overloading the tendon
- Tendon experiences structural and inflammatory changes resulting in reduced energy-storing capacity, dysfunction, and pain.

RISK FACTORS

- Change in activity or exercise
- Severe pronation of the foot
- Recent steroid exposure
- History of trauma or surgery to foot or ankle

COMMONLY ASSOCIATED CONDITIONS

- Pes planus and plantar fasciopathy
- Associated with hypertension, diabetes, and obesity in patients >50 years of age
- Associated with rheumatologic disease when present bilaterally

DIAGNOSIS

HISTORY

- Pain along the course of the posterior tibialis tendon, particularly around the medial malleolus
- Pain can radiate into medial foot arch.
- Recent change in type, frequency, or intensity of activity or exercise
- Worsened by prolonged strenuous activity requiring forceful plantarflexion (e.g., running or jumping)
- Alleviated by relative rest

PHYSICAL EXAM

- Always compare to contralateral side.
- Medial ankle swelling
- Flattened foot arch
- Increased hindfoot valgus
- "Too many toes sign:" More toes are seen laterally when observing the patient posteriorly.
- Tenderness along posterior tibialis tendon
- Pain and weakness with resisted ankle inversion and plantarflexion
- SLHR: Depending on the degree of pathology, any of the following may be present—pain, decreased hindfoot pronation, inability to elevate fully or at all.

DIFFERENTIAL DIAGNOSIS

- Subluxation of the posterior tibialis tendon
- Tendinopathy of flexor hallucis longus or flexor digitorum longus
- Osteoarthritis of tibiotalar, subtalar, midfoot joints
- Os naviculare syndrome
- Tarsal tunnel syndrome
- Lumbosacral radiculopathy: L4–S2 nerve roots
- Medial ankle sprain
- Stress injury or fracture of the medial malleolus, talus, or navicular bone

DIAGNOSTIC TESTS & INTERPRETATION

- Imaging is not required for diagnosis.
- Radiographs are helpful to evaluate differential diagnoses. Recommend weight-bearing x-rays of the ankle (anteroposterior, lateral, mortise views) and foot (anteroposterior, lateral views). Hindfoot valgus and flattened arch may be appreciated depending on severity of tendinopathy.
- Ultrasound evaluation by an experienced ultrasonographer can more accurately diagnose than 3T magnetic resonance imaging (1)[B]. Consider a referral to primary care sports medicine or musculoskeletal radiology for ultrasound.

TREATMENT

- Early treatment is essential to prevent progression between stages.
- Use the Education, Unloading, Reloading, and Prevention (EdUReP) model for nonsurgical management of tendinopathy (2)[A]:
  - Education: 5 As construct for behavioral counseling—assess, advise, agree, assist, and arrange
  - Unloading: over-the-counter or custom orthotics for medial arch support; relative rest (cross-training—pool running or swimming as tolerated) (3)[B]
  - Reloading: Refer to physical therapy for controlled reloading with focused concentric or eccentric exercises, transition to weight-support training (treadmill in pool) and weaning from unloading braces or orthotics.
  - Prevention: prevention of disease progression and disease recurrence through gradual resumption of activity

MEDICATION

Focus on control of pain and inflammation particularly during the initial phase of symptoms where the latter is more prevalent.

ISSUES FOR REFERRAL

Stage 1 or 2 should be treated conservatively for at least 3 months. If symptoms are unimproving, consider referral for additional therapies.

ADDITIONAL THERAPIES

- A systematic review of prospective, noncontrolled studies of corticosteroid injections into tendon sheaths including TPT showed short-term improvement in pain and function but increased the risk of posterior tibialis tendon rupture (4)[A].
- An umbrella review of randomized controlled trials found that extracorporeal shockwave therapy (ESWT) offered moderate improvement in pain and function.
- In the same umbrella review, platelet-rich plasma (PRP) had mixed results. Leukocyte-rich PRP offered the best results in function relative to other injections (5)[A].
- Although there is a lack of research on percutaneous ultrasound-guided needle tenotomy (PUNT) specifically for TPT, it has been shown to be effective in the short and long term for other tendinopathies and fasciopathy with minimal complications (6)[A].

ALERT

Steroid injections into the synovial sheath and especially into the tendon itself carry a risk of tendon rupture. Clinical practice guidelines recommend against injecting the PTT tendon sheath because risks of rupture outweigh short term benefits (7)[C],(8)[C].

SURGERY/OTHER PROCEDURES

- Consider surgical intervention for stage 1 or 2 if unimproving after conservative and additional therapies:
  - Endoscopic tendon sheath release, scar tissue excision, and/or partial synovectomy
- Because stage 3 disease has a fixed deformity, tendon reconstruction will not correct the problem. Subtalar or triple arthrodesis may be needed.

ONGOING CARE

PATIENT EDUCATION

Consider printing and reviewing the "Foot and Ankle Conditioning Program" from the American Academy of Orthopedic Surgeons with the patient (https://orthoinfo.aaos.org/globalassets/pdfs/2017-rehab_foot-and-ankle.pdf).

REFERENCES

1. Arnoldner MA, Gruber M, Syrè S, et al. Imaging of posterior tibial tendon dysfunction—comparison of high-resolution ultrasound and 3T MRI. *Eur J Radiol*. 2015;84(9):1777–1781.
2. Davenport TE, Kulig K, Matharu Y, et al. The EdUReP model for nonsurgical management of tendinopathy. *Phys Ther*. 2005;85(10):1093–1103.
3. Houck J, Neville C, Tome J, et al. Randomized controlled trial comparing orthosis augmented by either stretching or stretching and strengthening for stage II tibialis posterior tendon dysfunction. *Foot Ankle Int*. 2015;36(9):1006–1016.
4. Cushman DM, Carefoot A, Lisenby S, et al. A systematic review of the efficacy of corticosteroid injections of tendon sheaths, excluding stenosing tenosynovitis of the wrist and hand. *Am J Phys Med Rehabil*. 2021;100(7):683–688.
5. Irby A, Gutierrez J, Chamberlin C, et al. Clinical management of tendinopathy: a systematic review of systematic reviews evaluating the effectiveness of tendinopathy treatments. *Scand J Med Sci Sports*. 2020;30(10):1810–1826.
6. Shomal Zadeh F, Shafiei M, Shomalzadeh M, et al. Percutaneous ultrasound-guided needle tenotomy for treatment of chronic tendinopathy and fasciopathy: a meta-analysis. *Eur Radiol*. 2023;33(10):7303–7320.
7. Rouzier P, Ehrlich A, Shaughnessy A. Posterior Tibialis Tendon Dysfunction. Updated July 12, 2024. Accessed October 4, 2025. https://www.dynamedex.com/condition/posterior-tibialis-tendon-dysfunction
8. Kohls-Gatzoulis J, Angel JC, Singh D, et al. Tibialis posterior dysfunction: a common and treatable cause of adult acquired flatfoot. *BMJ*. 2004;329(7478):1328–1333.

ADDITIONAL READING

- Alvarez RG, Marini A, Schmitt C, et al. Stage I and II posterior tibial tendon dysfunction treated by a structured nonoperative management protocol: an orthosis and exercise program. *Foot Ankle Int*. 2006;27(1):2–8.
- Andres BM, Murrell GA. Treatment of tendinopathy: what works, what does not, and what is on the horizon. *Clin Orthop Relat Res*. 2008;466(7):1539–1554.
- Augustin JF, Lin SS, Berberian WS, et al. Nonoperative treatment of adult acquired flat foot with the Arizona brace. *Foot Ankle Clin*. 2003;8(3):491–502.
- Bernasconi A, Sadile F, Welck M, et al. Role of tendoscopy in treating stage II posterior tibial tendon dysfunction. *Foot Ankle Int*. 2018;39(4):433–442.
- Chao W, Wapner KL, Lee TH, et al. Nonoperative management of posterior tibial tendon dysfunction. *Foot Ankle Int*. 1996;17(12):736–741.
- Geideman WM, Johnson JE. Posterior tibial tendon dysfunction. *J Orthop Sports Phys Ther*. 2000;30(2):68–77.
- Krause F, Bosshard A, Lehmann O, et al. Shell brace for stage II posterior tibial tendon insufficiency. *Foot Ankle Int*. 2008;29(11):1095–1100.
- Premkumar A, Perry MB, Dwyer AJ, et al. Sonography and MR imaging of posterior tibial tendinopathy. *AJR Am J Roentgenol*. 2002;178(1):223–232.
- Richie DH Jr. Biomechanics and clinical analysis of the adult acquired flatfoot. *Clin Podiatr Med Surg*. 2007;24(4):617–644.
- Scott A, Backman LJ, Speed C. Tendinopathy: update on pathophysiology. *J Orthop Sports Phys Ther*. 2015;45(11):833–841.
- Wadehra A, Fallat LM, Jarski R. Surgical management of stage 2 adult and pediatric acquired flatfoot without tendon transfer or arthrodesis: a retrospective study. *J Foot Ankle Surg*. 2018;57(4):658–663.

CLINICAL PEARLS

- Tibialis posterior tendinopathy is caused by overuse and needs relative rest with orthotics, bracing, or a cam walker boot followed by gradual return to activity via home exercise program and cross-training.
- If patients are not improving after 3 months, nonsurgical interventions should be considered including but not limited to steroid injections into the tendon sheath, PRP injections, ESWT, and PUNT. Shared decision-making should be used to determine the optimal intervention for each patient.
- If patients are still not improving after conservative and additional therapies or if they have a fixed hindfoot, consider surgical referral.

TILLAUX FRACTURES, PEDIATRIC

Suraj A. Achar, MD, FAAFP, CAQSM ▪ Jivan Achar, BA ▪ Andrew Pennock, MD

BASICS

DESCRIPTION

- Salter-Harris (SH) type III avulsion fracture of the anterolateral distal tibial epiphysis
- Mechanism of injury: traumatic external rotatory force pulling through the anterior inferior talofibular ligament
- Classically seen in adolescent girls aged 11 to 14 years and boys aged 13 to 16 years
- Described by Paul Jules Tillaux in 1892 (1)

EPIDEMIOLOGY

- Relatively uncommon—15–18% of fractures of the long bones involve the epiphyseal growth plate, and 2.9% of these represent pediatric Tillaux fractures (2).
- Fractures typically occur within 1 year of physeal closure involving the anterolateral portion of the growth plate which is the last to close.

RISK FACTORS

- Participation in activities that involve rotational force through the ankle
- Traumatic, forceful external rotation of the foot when the distal tibial physis is fusing centrally but not yet laterally in girls 13 to 15 years old and in boys 15 to 17 years old (3)

DIAGNOSIS

HISTORY

- Acute ankle pain after forceful supination and external rotation of the joint
- Also seen with internal rotation of the lower leg on a firmly planted foot
- Difficulty with bearing weight

PHYSICAL EXAM

- Swelling and/or ecchymosis particularly anterolaterally
- Tenderness over the anterolateral ankle and syndesmosis
- Limited active ankle range of motion (ROM)
- Pain with passive ankle motion
- Weight-bearing—limited
- Examine for concurrent fibular injury or medial malleolus fracture.
- Extremity neurovascular examination

DIFFERENTIAL DIAGNOSIS

- Ankle or syndesmosis injury/sprain
- Triplane fracture: more severe transitional fracture (SH IV) with extension of the fracture into the posterior tibial metaphysis
- Talar dome injury/osteochondritis dissecans
- Distal fibular physeal injury

DIAGNOSTIC TESTS & INTERPRETATION

- Radiography: ankle anteroposterior (AP), lateral, and mortise views
- Consider comparison of uninjured ankle to assess physeal closure.
- Computed tomography (CT): Patients with transitional distal tibial fractures may benefit from CT to better determine fracture pattern, amount of displacement, and need for surgery (4)[C].

TREATMENT

- Initial: immobilization, non–weight-bearing, ice, elevation, acetaminophen, and nonsteroidal anti-inflammatory drugs (NSAIDs)
- Nondisplaced or minimally displaced fractures (<2.5 mm) can be treated nonoperatively (5),(6)[B].
- For more displaced fractures >2.5 mm, may attempt a closed reduction by positioning foot in neutral or slight internal rotation/inversion
- If postreduction gap is <2.5 mm, may proceed with nonoperative treatment (6),(7)[B]
- *Postreduction evaluation*: neurovascular exam and repeat radiographs: ankle AP, lateral, and mortise views. Postreduction is the optimal time to perform a CT if indicated.

- *Immobilization*:
  - 4 to 6 weeks non–weight-bearing in a short leg or long leg cast. Recent data suggests that a long-leg cast may not be necessary to control rotational stability of the fracture (5)[B].
  - After period of immobilization, may transition to a cam walker or rigid shell boot for several weeks
  - Weight-bearing is started based on radiographic healing and clinical exam but typically 4 to 6 weeks postinjury.
- *Complications*: rare, but include late displacement of the fracture, ankle stiffness, residual pain, posttraumatic arthritis, complex regional pain syndrome, and premature physeal closure (6)

SURGERY/OTHER PROCEDURES

- Indicated if ≥2.5 mm of displacement (6)
- Surgeon preference: typically, open reduction with internal fixation, but some fractures are amenable to closed reduction with percutaneous fixation or arthroscopically assisted reduction and fixation (3)[B],(7)[B]
- Overall good reported surgical outcomes if residual displacement is <2.5 mm (6),(7)[C]
- *Complications*: similar to nonoperative complications, but also includes soft tissue issues (wound dehiscence, infection, and keloid formation), symptomatic implants requiring implant removal, and rare iatrogenic neurovascular and tendinous injuries (6)

ADDITIONAL THERAPIES

Rehabilitation:

- Sport-specific drills
- Strengthening of dynamic stabilizers
- Proprioception training
- Proper shoe wear
- Consideration of a lace-up ankle brace

ONGOING CARE

FOLLOW-UP RECOMMENDATIONS

For nonsurgically treated:

- Follow up with x-rays at 7 to 10 days to confirm no fracture displacement.
- After 4 to 6 weeks of immobilization, repeat radiographs to confirm healing. Patient can then be transitioned to a walking cast or cam walker for an additional 2 weeks.

PROGNOSIS

- Generally good outcomes if residual displacement is <2.5 mm at the time of healing
- Early arthritis: risk based on displacement and residual displacement
- Physeal arrest extremely rare and typically of low concern given patients are near physeal closure
- Many patients can return to full activity after 3 months postinjury.

REFERENCES

1. Cassas KJ, Jamison JP. Juvenile Tillaux fracture in an adolescent basketball player. *Phys Sportsmed*. 2005;33(2):30–33.
2. Spiegel PG, Cooperman DR, Laros GS. Epiphyseal fractures of the distal ends of the tibia and fibula. A retrospective study of two hundred and thirty-seven cases in children. *J Bone Joint Surg Am*. 1978;60(8):1046–1050.
3. Tak S, Qureshi MK, Ackland JA, et al. Adolescent Tillaux fractures: a systematic review of the literature. *Cureus*. 2021;13(1):e12860.
4. Nenopoulos A, Beslikas T, Gigis I, et al. The role of CT in diagnosis and treatment of distal tibial fractures with intra-articular involvement in children. *Injury*. 2015;46(11):2177–2180.
5. Tiefenboeck TM, Binder H, Joestl J, et al. Displaced juvenile Tillaux fractures: surgical treatment and outcome. *Wien Klin Wochenschr*. 2017;129(5–6):169–175.
6. Lurie B, Van Rysselberghe N, Pennock AT, et al. Functional outcomes of Tillaux and triplane fractures with 2 to 5 millimeters of intra-articular gap. *J Bone Joint Surg Am*. 2020;102(8):679–686.
7. Choudhry IK, Wall EJ, Eismann EA, et al. Functional outcome analysis of triplane and Tillaux fractures after closed reduction and percutaneous fixation. *J Pediatr Orthop*. 2014;34(2):139–143.

ADDITIONAL READING

Feng SM, Sun QQ, Wang AG, et al. "All-inside" arthroscopic treatment of Tillaux-Chaput fractures: clinical experience and outcomes analysis. *J Foot Ankle Surg*. 2018;57(1):56–59.

CLINICAL PEARLS

- Possible complications include posttraumatic arthritis and asymmetric physeal growth.
- Nonoperative options are optimal for fractures with minimal displacement (<2.5 mm).
- If treated nonoperatively, 4 week non–weight-bearing in a short leg cast followed by 2 to 4 weeks in a walking cast or cam walker. If stabilized with internal fixation, patients are kept non–weight-bearing for 4 to 6 weeks. A cam boot or cast is typically used for 4 to 6 week post-op (5)[C].
- Return to sports after >12 weeks if well-healed on x-ray, pain-free with activity, and have full ROM and strength.
- Peroneal strengthening and proprioception training are essential rehab components.
- Proper mechanics and proper shoe wear

TINEA GLADIATORUM (CAPITIS, CORPORIS, CRURIS, PEDIS)

Philipp J. Underwood, MD, FAAEM, FACEP, FAAFP, CAQSM, RDMS • Clarence Kong, MD

BASICS

DESCRIPTION

- This group of topical fungal infections commonly affects athletes, particularly wrestlers, judo, or other contact sports due to close contact and potentially mat contamination. They are classified by site of infection: Tinea capitis involves the scalp and hairline; tinea corporis involves the trunk, face, or extremities; tinea cruris involves inguinal folds; tinea pedis involves the feet. Infection is caused by a dermatophyte, most commonly from the *Trichophyton, Epidermophyton,* and *Microsporum* species.
- This is typically an infection of the stratum corneum that results in thickening of the epidermis and scale formation. Majocchi granuloma is an infection of the dermis, usually due to fungal entry through hair follicles.
- Synonym(s): ring worm (tinea corporis); jock itch (tinea cruris); athlete's foot (tinea pedis); tinea gladiatorum (most commonly *Trichophyton tonsurans* 92% and *Trichophyton rubrum* ~3%)

EPIDEMIOLOGY

ALERT

In the United States, dermatophytic infections present in 4.3–100% of all wrestlers during any given season (1).

- Carrier rates of up to 84% in United States wrestlers (1)
- 10–20% lifetime risk for nonathletes
- More common in African Americans and Asians
- 2 to 20 days from inoculation to subsequent development of identifiable skin lesions

RISK FACTORS

- Spread by direct contact with a pet or human carrier
- Fomite transmission may occur from wrestling mats, pieces of athletic equipment, shower floor, and so forth.

GENERAL PREVENTION

- Good personal hygiene
- Do not share towels, razors, or clothing.
- Wipe down surfaces before and after use (wrestling mats).
- Shower immediately after practice.
- Wash clothing and bedding regularly in hot water (60°C) (at least once a week).

DIAGNOSIS

Scraping of the leading edge of the skin plaque and preparation with potassium hydroxide (KOH) 10–20% can be examined under the microscope. This will reveal hyphae and pseudohyphae, which are diagnostic of tinea infection. For *tinea capitis*, spores are visualized by KOH preparation of the hair shaft. *Microsporum canis* may fluoresce bright green under a Wood lamp. Fungal culture using Sabouraud dextrose agar also can be used, but in athletes, use is limited by time and expense involved. Most tinea infections do not fluoresce under Wood light examination.

HISTORY

- Determine when and where lesions appeared and exposure history.
- Are other wrestlers and wrestling partners on the team infected?

PHYSICAL EXAM

- Lesions typically noted on surface of trunk, head/neck, or upper extremities, unusual on lower extremities.
- Lesions present with erythema, pruritus, and scaling.
- Tinea capitis: two distinct types:
  - Black dot: most common form seen in United States and most caused by *T. tonsurans*. Usually children and elderly. Erythematous, scaling patch that enlarges slowly. Hairs then break off flush with scalp leaving residual hair giving black dot appearance; can cause alopecia, which may be permanent
  - Gray patch: uncommon in United States and caused by *M. canis* contracted usually from dogs and cats. Erythematous, scaling patch that enlarges slowly. Hairs break off 1 to 2 mm above the scalp.
- Tinea corporis: circular, erythematous, scaling plaques with central clearing on trunk, face, and extremities
- Tinea cruris: pruritic, scaling, erythematous patches in inguinal folds and/or medial thighs. If lesions present on penis or scrotum, consider candida infection rather than tinea.
- Tinea pedis: pruritic, erythematous scaly skin along the sole of foot. Cracking and maceration of the web spaces also may be present. Bullous form will have bullae or vesicles filled with clear fluid.

DIFFERENTIAL DIAGNOSIS

- Tinea capitis: alopecia areata, impetigo, psoriasis, seborrhea, trichotillomania
- Tinea corporis: impetigo, eczema, psoriasis, contact or atopic dermatitis, drug eruption, cutaneous herpes, lupus, pityriasis rosea
- Tinea cruris: contact dermatitis, candida intertrigo, erythrasma, psoriasis, seborrhea
- Tinea pedis: eczema, contact or atopic dermatitis, dyshidrosis, pitted keratolysis, psoriasis

TREATMENT

MEDICATION

- Primary treatment for tinea corporis, cruris, and pedis is with topical antifungal agents. Primary treatment for tinea capitis is oral antifungal agents.
- Initial treatment also may include a topical corticosteroid. This may help reduce the associated pruritus and erythema; however, this may exacerbate tinea infections and can lead to treatment failure or recurrent infections (1).
- Azoles were slightly less effective in clinical cure compared to azoles + steroid combination.
- Tinea capitis and diffuse, multiple lesions in other areas should be treated with oral antifungal agents.
- When using oral agents, give consideration to drug interactions, potential for toxicity, and cost of medication.
- Prevention is key: Emphasize proper personal hygiene; use dry, cotton clothing; and keep athletic equipment disinfected properly.
- Naftifine is both fungicidal and fungistatic.
- Shampooing hair and body with selenium (Selsun Blue) may be useful prophylaxis.
- Failure to treat all areas simultaneously may result in treatment failure.

- *Tinea capitis* requires oral treatment:
  - Griseofulvin: Treat for 6 weeks. Monitor complete blood count (CBC), liver function tests (LFTs). Side effects: photosensitivity, headache, neutropenia, elevated LFTs, paresthesia, rash; pregnancy category C:
    - Adults: 500 mg microsize or 330 to 375 mg ultramicrosize daily for 6 weeks
    - Children: 11 mg microsize/kg/d or 7.3 mg ultramicrosize/kg/d for 6 weeks
  - Terbinafine: Treat for 4 weeks. Monitor CBC, LFTs; pregnancy category B:
    - 10 to 20 kg: 62.5 mg daily
    - 20 to 40 kg: 125 mg daily
    - >40 kg: 250 mg daily
    - Recent studies have shown cases of resistance to terbinafine treatment (2).
  - Itraconazole: Treat for 2 to 6 weeks. Monitor LFTs. Caution: hypoglycemia with sulfonylureas, rhabdomyolysis with HMG-CoA reductase inhibitors; pregnancy category C:
    - Adults: 100 mg daily, up to 200 mg BID (3)[B]
    - Children: 3 to 5 mg/kg daily
  - Fluconazole: Treat for 2 to 4 weeks; increased international normalized ratio (INR) on warfarin; pregnancy category C:
    - Adults: 200 mg daily
    - Children: 6 mg/kg/d
- *Tinea corporis, cruris*, and *pedis*: Topical antifungals are first-line treatment. Topical nystatin is ineffective; oral therapy for failed topical, extensive lesions or immunocompromised:
  - Topical therapy: Treat for 2 to 6 weeks (continue treatment additional week after resolution of rash):
    - Naftifine: gel, apply twice daily; cream, apply once daily.
    - Terbinafine: Apply once to twice daily.
    - Ciclopirox: Apply twice daily.
    - Clotrimazole: Apply twice daily.
    - Econazole: Apply once daily.
    - Ketoconazole: Apply once daily.
    - Miconazole: Apply twice daily.
    - Oxiconazole: Apply once to twice daily.
    - Sertaconazole: Apply twice daily.
    - Sulconazole: Apply once to twice daily.
    - Tolnaftate: Apply twice daily.
  - Oral therapy: Treat for 2 to 6 weeks:
    - Griseofulvin: 500 mg daily *or* 500 mg BID *or* 250 mg TID
    - Fluconazole: 150 to 200 mg once weekly for 2 to 4 weeks or 400 mg one-time dose
    - Itraconazole: 100 to 200 mg daily
    - Terbinafine: 250 mg daily
- If an outbreak occurs on a team, particularly in a contact or collision sport, all team members should be screened.

ADDITIONAL THERAPIES

Prophylaxis for tinea gladiatorum:

- Recommended for recurrent episodes (exclude immunocompromised state)
- Used by some prior to wrestling tournaments or during season:
  - Fluconazole: 200 mg once weekly
  - Itraconazole: 400 mg once every 2 months

ONGOING CARE

ALERT

Wrestling return to play:

- National Collegiate Athletic Association (NCAA): A minimum of 2 weeks of systemic antifungal therapy is required for scalp lesions. A minimum of 72 hours of topical therapy is required for skin lesions. Wrestlers with extensive and active lesions will be disqualified. Activity of treated lesions can be judged either by use of KOH preparation or a review of therapeutic regimen. Wrestlers with solitary or closely clustered, localized lesions will be disqualified if lesions are in a body location that cannot be "properly covered" (a gas-permeable dressing, e.g., Opsite, Tegaderm, Bioclusive, Duoderm, and then covered by elastic/stretch tape). The disposition of tinea cases will be decided onsite and on an individual basis as determined by the examining physician and/or athletic trainer (NCAA Sports Medicine Handbook 2013–2014).
- National Federation of State High School Associations (NFHS): tinea lesions (ringworm scalp, skin): oral or topical treatment for 72 hours on skin and 14 days on scalp (NFHS revised/approved April 2024)

FOLLOW-UP RECOMMENDATIONS

Most infections are easily treated with topical or oral antifungal agents; therefore, referral is rare. However, for cases that do not respond as expected, further evaluation to rule out an immunocompromised state or other systemic illness should be considered.

REFERENCES

1. Zalewski A, Goldust M, Szepietowski JC. Tinea gladiatorum: epidemiology, clinical aspect, and management. *J Clin Med*. 2022;11(14):4066.
2. Leung AKC, Lam JM, Leong KF, et al. Tinea corporis: an updated review. *Drugs Context*. 2020;9:5–6.
3. Dellière S, Joannard B, Benderdouche M, et al. Emergence of difficult-to-treat tinea corporis caused by trichophyton mentagrophytes complex isolates, Paris, France. *Emerg Infect Dis*. 2022;28(1):224–228.

ADDITIONAL READING

Khurana A, Agarwal A, Agrawal D, et al. Effect of different itraconazole dosing regimens on cure rates, treatment duration, safety, and relapse rates in adult patients with tinea corporis/cruris: a randomized clinical trial. *JAMA Dermatol*. 2022;158(11):1269–1278.

CLINICAL PEARLS

- All areas of tinea infection need to be treated simultaneously to reduce risk of reinfection.
- Prevention strategies can reduce the risk to the participant and others.
- First-line treatment for simple infections includes topical medications.
- Consider oral fluconazole for extensive and resistant lesions as well as prophylaxis.

TRACHEAL AND LARYNGEAL INJURIES

Jeffrey P. Feden, MD, FACEP, CAQSM • Razib Khaund, MD

BASICS

DESCRIPTION

- Injuries to the larynx and trachea may result from either blunt or penetrating trauma involving the head, neck, or upper chest.
- Although they are relatively uncommon and sometimes subtle, these potentially life-threatening injuries must not be overlooked.

EPIDEMIOLOGY

- Laryngotracheal (LT) trauma occurs at an estimated frequency from 1/5,000 to 1/30,000 emergency department (ED) visits.
- Laryngeal injuries comprise <1% of blunt and 7% of penetrating trauma cases; only 10% result from athletic trauma (1).
- Mortality is as high as 20% and 40% for penetrating and blunt injuries, respectively (2).

ETIOLOGY AND PATHOPHYSIOLOGY

- LT trauma may cause obstructive edema, submucosal hematomas, cartilage fractures, mucosal tears, or complete LT separation.
- Low-velocity trauma may cause soft tissue swelling, lacerations, contusions, and abrasions.
- High-velocity trauma may injure laryngeal muscles and nerves.
- Forceful compression to the chest against a closed glottis may cause laryngeal fractures and mucosal disruption.

RISK FACTORS

- Contact and collision sports
- Sports with high-velocity projectiles (i.e., baseball, hockey, lacrosse)
- Motor sports

COMMONLY ASSOCIATED CONDITIONS

- Penetrating trauma is associated with additional injury to the chest, esophagus, vasculature, or nerves in 86% of cases; esophageal injury occurs 50% of the time.
- Blunt trauma is associated with intracranial injury (17%), cervical spine injury (13%), chest injury (13%), and esophageal injury (13%) (2).
- Pneumothorax may accompany distal tracheal injuries.

DIAGNOSIS

HISTORY

- Index of suspicion should exist when there is trauma to the anterior neck.
- Hoarse voice, dysphagia, odynophagia, cough, hemoptysis, anterior neck pain
- Signs or symptoms may be absent initially in up to 1/3 of those with LT trauma.

PHYSICAL EXAM

- Dysphonia (e.g., hoarseness) and neck/throat pain are most common (3)[C].
- Respiratory distress, stridor
- Loss of anatomic landmarks, anterior cervical tenderness, sternoclavicular (SC) crepitus, cervical ecchymosis, or hematoma

DIAGNOSTIC TESTS & INTERPRETATION

Initial Tests (lab, imaging)

- Chest radiograph to evaluate for associated trauma
- Cervical spine radiographs to evaluate for cervical spine injury
- Plain radiographs may show hyoid bone elevation or prevertebral air.
- Computed tomography (CT) imaging of the cervical region is recommended if the airway is stable because it provides additional anatomic detail useful for management decisions; however, CT may lack sensitivity for laryngeal cartilage fractures and hyoid bone fractures (4)[C].

Diagnostic Procedures/Other

Flexible bedside laryngoscopy is the preferred initial method for evaluating the stable airway and can provide detail about laryngeal anatomy and vocal cord function.

TREATMENT

- Prehospital:
  - Initial treatment focuses on the primary survey and airway, breathing, and circulation (ABCs) in accordance with Advanced Trauma Life Support guidelines.
  - Control the airway and immobilize the cervical spine.
  - Rapidly transport to the nearest ED while continuing to manage the airway.
  - Oral airways, combitubes, and laryngeal mask airways fail to provide a definitive airway by virtue of their supraglottic position.
  - Orotracheal intubation and cricothyroidotomy may be contraindicated in cases of significant trauma or complete LT separation; either must be undertaken with extreme caution to avoid losing the airway or causing greater injury.
- ED treatment:
  - Airway management is the priority (3)[C].
  - Prompt assessment of the stable airway includes fiberoptic laryngoscopy in consultation with ear, nose, throat (ENT) specialist, followed by close observation, further imaging with CT scan, or surgical management in the operating room (3)[C].
  - Preferred management of an unstable airway includes awake tracheostomy under local anesthesia in the operating room (2)[C].

ADDITIONAL THERAPIES

- Conservative management is appropriate for patients with mild edema or small hematomas.
- Observation in an intensive care unit (ICU) for at least 24 hours may be indicated for significant LT trauma that does not require emergent surgical intervention.
- Some patients may develop signs or symptoms up to 48 hours after injury.
- Monitor for signs of progressive airway compromise, and prepare for the possibility of urgent tracheotomy.
- Humidified air and head of the bed elevation
- Serial endoscopic examinations
- Vocal rest
- Minimize laryngeal irritation from gastric acid with H_2 blockers or proton pump inhibitors.
- Antibiotics and systemic corticosteroids are controversial (steroids may reduce laryngeal edema).
- Use narcotic pain medications and sedatives with caution to avoid their effects of respiratory depression.
- Following initial treatment, prompt phoniatric evaluation is mandatory for all patients.
- Speech therapy may be required to restore vocal quality or to avoid permanent restrictions of phonation.

SURGERY/OTHER PROCEDURES

- Indications for surgery include initial airway instability, progressive airway decline despite conservative treatment, and complex LT injuries.
- Operative interventions range from tracheotomy to open reduction and internal fixation (ORIF) of the injured cartilaginous structures.
- 25–80% of patients with LT trauma will require surgery.

ONGOING CARE

- Long-term treatment goals involve restoring the anatomy, airway patency, and vocal quality.
- All athletes should be sent for phonic and speech therapy evaluations; speech therapy may be necessary to restore vocal quality.

PATIENT EDUCATION

- Dysphonia is the most common and problematic complication after LT trauma.
- Phoniatric evaluation is essential, and speech therapy may be important even after minor injuries.

PROGNOSIS

- Prognosis depends on injury severity, but complications may be avoided by early diagnosis and proper initial management.
- Voice disorders typically are associated with the most severe injuries, but even minor injuries can cause permanent problems with phonation.
- Most patients can expect excellent airway patency and good voice quality following LT trauma that has been recognized and treated appropriately.
- Prognosis is worse for those with late presentations (who already may have laryngeal stenosis).

COMPLICATIONS

- Dysphonia, hoarseness, voice fatigue, and poor vocal control are most common.
- Vocal cord paralysis owing to recurrent laryngeal nerve injury
- Permanent phonic disorders owing to laryngeal scarring or infection

REFERENCES

1. Paluska SA, Lansford CD. Laryngeal trauma in sport. *Curr Sports Med Rep*. 2008;7(1):16–21.
2. Atkins BZ, Abbate S, Fisher SR, et al. Current management of laryngotracheal trauma: case report and literature review. *J Trauma*. 2004;56(1):185–190.
3. Mendis D, Anderson JA. Blunt laryngeal trauma secondary to sporting injuries. *J Laryngol Otol*. 2017;131(8):728–735.
4. Nganzeu C, Esce A, Abu-Ghanem S, et al. Laryngeal trauma. *Otolaryngol Clin North Am*. 2023;56(6):1039–1053.

ADDITIONAL READING

- Becker M, Duboé PO, Platon A, et al. MDCT in the assessment of laryngeal trauma: value of 2D multiplanar and 3D reconstructions. *AJR Am J Roentgenol*. 2013;201(4):W639–W647.
- Bhojani RA, Rosenbaum DH, Dikmen E, et al. Contemporary assessment of laryngotracheal trauma. *J Thorac Cardiovasc Surg*. 2005;130(2):426–432.
- Kim JD, Shuler FD, Mo B, et al. Traumatic laryngeal fracture in a collegiate basketball player. *Sports Health*. 2013;5(3):273–275.

CLINICAL PEARLS

- LT trauma may be immediately life-threatening.
- Diagnosis often requires a high index of suspicion.
- Prompt recognition and airway management are essential.
- Complications and airway compromise may not develop until 24 to 48 hours following injury.
- Consideration of associated traumatic injuries is also important.

TRANSIENT OSTEOPOROSIS OF THE HIP

Uziel Sauceda, MD, CAQSM

BASICS

DESCRIPTION

- Transient osteoporosis of the hip (TOH) is a clinical presentation of acute hip pain, characterized by bone marrow edema of the femoral head, bone resorption, and subsequent resolution.
- Also known as primary bone marrow edema of proximal femur
- Similar bone marrow edema syndromes happen in the knee, ankle, and foot.

EPIDEMIOLOGY

- Condition is rare and of unknown incidence or prevalence; most information derived from case series
- Common in middle-aged men, average age of 40 years with wide age of distribution
- Also common in females in 3rd trimester of pregnancy
- Rare in children

ETIOLOGY AND PATHOPHYSIOLOGY

- Etiology largely unknown, often indistinguishable from early avascular necrosis (AVN)
- Other authors propose it is a subset of complex regional pain syndrome type 1 (1).
- Proposed pathophysiology involves an initial insult, followed by edema leading to separation of bone trabeculae, and then increased bone resorption. Resorption is self-limited, and last stage involves resolution of edema, pain, and return of bone formation.
- Another proposed etiology involves femoral head vein dysfunction causing increased intraosseous pressure and venous hypertension, leading to transient osteoporosis (2).
- Inferred from histologic findings
- Initial insult: trauma, microfracture, infection, ischemic injury, venous hypertension, surgery, drugs, alcohol, or neurovascular dysfunction

RISK FACTORS

- Pregnancy in 3rd trimester, alcohol, abnormal vascularity, inflammatory state, mechanical injury, osteogenesis imperfecta, hypothyroid, neurologic, and metabolic derangements
- A case series of pregnant patients also revealed risk factors of smoking, family history of osteoporosis, relative advanced maternal age (age 34 +/− 4), IVF conception, and low body mass index pre pregnancy (average 22) and at term (average of 27) (3).
- Viral illness such as covid has a recent case report, unclear if a significant precipitant.
- Drugs: thiazolidinediones, serotonin reuptake inhibitors, nonsteroidal anti-inflammatory drugs (NSAIDs), steroids, and HIV protease inhibitors (4)
- Many risk factors are the same as initial insult proposed in pathophysiology.

COMMONLY ASSOCIATED CONDITIONS

- Pregnancy
- Osteogenesis imperfecta
- Migratory osteoporosis
- Generalized low bone mass

DIAGNOSIS

Note that TOH is diagnosis of exclusion; therefore, a thorough evaluation for more common etiologies is warranted.

HISTORY

- Often spontaneous onset of acute unilateral or bilateral hip pain without obvious causal factor or trauma
- 3rd trimester of pregnancy
- Often unable to bear weight
- Ask about recent new medicine, illicit substances, alcohol, smoking, or new activity. Presentation can vary from vague pain to severe pain and immobility.

PHYSICAL EXAM

- Pain may be out of proportion to exam findings.
- Antalgic gait
- Decrease in full range of motion (ROM), along with pain, specifically on internal/external rotation.
- Percussion of hip bone causes pain on the affected side.
- Various exam maneuvers may cause pain in the hip and are unlikely to be specific.

DIFFERENTIAL DIAGNOSIS

- Osteoarthritis
- AVN of femoral head
- Infection: septic hip joint, osteomyelitis
- Tumor: metastasis versus primary versus benign (osteoid osteoma)
- Fracture: acute, compression, or stress type
- Femoroacetabular impingement
- Chondral defect: labral tear, osteochondritis dissecans
- Inflammatory joint disease
- Radicular pain

DIAGNOSTIC TESTS & INTERPRETATION

- There are no lab tests specific to TOH.
- To evaluate for systemic disease: complete blood count with differential, blood urea nitrogen (BUN)/creatinine and electrolytes, liver enzymes, and coagulation panel. Erythrocyte sedimentation rate (ESR) and C-reactive protein (CRP) help in determining if there is underlying inflammatory component.
- *X-ray*: may be normal, but evaluate for osteopenia (compared to contralateral) and obvious tumors or fractures
- *Bone scan*: increased uptake at femoral head; seen in all phases of condition and persists for weeks after clinical improvement
- *Dual energy x-ray absorptiometry (DEXA)*: may show osteoporosis
- *Magnetic resonance imaging (MRI) is the* best confirmation test (2)[C],(5)[C].
- Differentiate AVN versus TOH.
- High signal intensity on T2 sequences, homogenous, without distinct border or focal defect, located on femoral head; edema may extend to the neck or intertrochanteric region.
- Joint effusion is often seen.
- Subchondral changes favors AVN diagnosis (subchondral radiolucency crescent sign).

TREATMENT

GENERAL MEASURES

- The majority have self-limited course and complete resolution with conservative management within 6 months (ranges from 4 to 12 months).
- Analgesia should be tailored to individual; minimize weight-bearing/rest, analgesics, and ultrasound therapy (4)[C],(5)[C].
- Suppression of bone resorption or induction of bone formation may shorten recovery time (4)[C],(5)[C].
- Surgical treatment usually not required, unless symptoms refractory or femoral head fracture present

MEDICATION

- *Bisphosphonate therapy*:
  - Alendronate PO: 70 mg/wk:
    - Average recovery of 6 months in eight cases (5)[C]
  - Pamidronate intravenous (IV): Dosing varies in separate case reports: 45 mg every 3 days for 3 doses or 60 mg every 7 days for 4 doses (5)[C]:
    - Clinical recovery of 2 months in 15 cases
- *Other bone-remodeling agents*:
  - Calcitonin nasal: 200 IU daily for 4 to 6 weeks (5)[C]:
    - Recovery in 4.7 months in six cases
  - Teriparatide: 20 μg daily:
    - Recovery in 4 weeks in one case (5)[C]
  - Iloprost: a prostacyclin analogue; thought to increase vessel dilation and reduce permeability; can improve symptom of pain (5)[C]

Pregnancy Considerations

- Exposure to bisphosphonates before conception or during pregnancy may affect fetal skeletal mineralization, shorten gestational age, or cause birth defects/abortion.
- Calcitonin preferred because it does not cross placenta and safe to use during pregnancy (5)[C]

ISSUES FOR REFERRAL

- Refer to orthopedics if there is any suspicion of AVN or underlying femoral fracture.
- If considering medical therapy, consult endocrinology for recommendation on dosage and duration due to no formal guidelines.

ADDITIONAL THERAPIES

- *Hyperbaric oxygen therapy* (6)[C]
- In 41 total patients, half underwent combination analgesics and hyperbaric oxygen (O_2), whereas the control was treated with only analgesics.
- It showed improvement in Western Ontario and McMaster Universities Osteoarthritis Index (WOMAC) scores as well as MRI findings at 3 months.

SURGERY/OTHER PROCEDURES

- Core decompression therapy (4)[C]: usually used for AVN treatment of femoral head
- Has not been shown to improve outcomes more than medical therapy; data is limited to case reports.
- This approach is best left for patients that pain is unable to be controlled with conservative treatment.

ONGOING CARE

FOLLOW-UP RECOMMENDATIONS

- Follow-up MRI usually done; timing of repeat study uncertain; not unreasonable to repeat at 6 months, often hyperintense signal resolved or markedly improved.
- Weight-bearing activity as tolerated; unclear when high-impact activity can resume but likely when minimal imaging findings and patient clinically improved.

PATIENT EDUCATION

- Emphasize the importance of limited weight-bearing while symptomatic.
- Smoking cessation, alcohol moderation, and optimization of diet rich in calcium/vitamin D may help (2)[C],(4)[C].
- Medication to alter bone resorption is off-label and needs full informed consent.
- Diagnosis is self-limited and will resolve with time.

PROGNOSIS

- Limited data to suggest long-term abnormalities after TOH resolves
- Recurrence months to years afterward at a separate skeletal site (contralateral hip) is known to happen and suggests a diagnosis of regional migratory osteoporosis (4).
- TOH has not been shown to recur in subsequent pregnancies (3).

COMPLICATIONS

- Fracture is rare: subchondral, femoral neck, or subcapital; more frequently seen in females
- Progression to AVN or osteonecrosis is rare.

REFERENCES

1. Vaishya R, Agarwal AK, Kumar V, et al. Transient osteoporosis of the hip: a mysterious cause of hip pain in adults. *Indian J Orthop*. 2017;51(4):455–460.
2. Maisi N, Patoulias D, Tsagkaris C, et al. Transient hip osteoporosis: etiopathogenetic, clinical, and imaging approach. *Mediterr J Rheumatol*. 2022;33(2):196–200.
3. Toussia-Cohen S, Eshed I, Segal O, et al. Transient osteoporosis of the hip in pregnancy—a case series. *J Matern Fetal Neonatal Med*. 2023;36(1):2175659.
4. Patel S. Primary bone marrow oedema syndromes. *Rheumatology (Oxford)*. 2014;53(5):785–792.
5. Asadipooya K, Graves L, Greene LW. Transient osteoporosis of the hip: review of the literature. *Osteoporos Int*. 2017;28(6):1805–1816.
6. Capone A, Podda D, Ennas F, et al. Hyperbaric oxygen therapy for transient bone marrow oedema syndrome of the hip. *Hip Int*. 2011;21(2):211–216.

ADDITIONAL READING

- Ciaffi J, Vanni E, Facchini G, et al. Transient osteoporosis of the hip: a novel vascular manifestation of COVID-19? *Rheumatology (Oxford)*. 2023;62(4):e127–e128.
- Diwanji SR, Cho YJ, Xin ZF, et al. Conservative treatment for transient osteoporosis of the hip in middle-aged women. *Singapore Med J*. 2008;49(1):e17–e21.
- Fessel J. There are many potential medical therapies for atraumatic osteonecrosis. *Rheumatology (Oxford)*. 2013;52(2):235–241.
- Mirza R, Ishaq S, Amjad H. Transient osteoporosis of the hip. *J Pak Med Assoc*. 2012;62(2):196–198.
- Thiryayi WA, Thiryayi SA, Freemont AJ. Histopathological perspective on bone marrow oedema, reactive bone change and haemorrhage. *Eur J Radiol*. 2008;67(1):62–67.

CLINICAL PEARLS

- TOH is a diagnosis of exclusion; evaluate for common causes of hip pain before diagnosing.
- MRI is an imaging modality of choice and can distinguish between AVN and TOH.
- Most patients will recover with conservative treatment of rest, analgesia, and maintenance of ROM within 6 months.
- Follow-up at least every 3 months recommended after proper pain control
- Consider endocrine consult if considering using medications to alter bone resorption.
- Data on surgical management is limited.

TRICEPS TENDINITIS

Adam Culver, MD, CAQSM ▪ Anthony Martin, MD, CAQSM

BASICS

DESCRIPTION

- Inflammation of the triceps tendon at or proximal to the insertion onto the olecranon
- Classically an overuse injury due to repetitive extension of the elbow or extreme force placed on the tendon
- May result from direct trauma

EPIDEMIOLOGY

- Uncommon but higher prevalence observed in certain groups (see "Risk Factors")
- Male predominance (1)
- Has been described through a wide range of ages (1)

ETIOLOGY AND PATHOPHYSIOLOGY

Inflammation or swelling of the triceps tendon due to excessive force or repetitive use

RISK FACTORS

- Certain sports such as professional weight lifting, professional football (American), softball players (1)
- Use of anabolic steroids and history of local corticosteroid injections may also predispose to injury (2).
- Systemic disorders, including renal osteodystrophy, hyperparathyroidism, and diabetes mellitus (2)
- Commonly associated with posterior impingement, presence of loose bodies, classic tennis elbow, history of elbow arthroplasty, high-intensity interval training (2)

GENERAL PREVENTION

- Proper form when lifting weights
- Avoid excessive weight or force when using triceps.
- Dynamic warm-up prior to repetitive use of triceps or weight lifting

COMMONLY ASSOCIATED CONDITIONS

- Olecranon bursitis
- Triceps tendon rupture (1)
- Lateral epicondylitis (1)

DIAGNOSIS

HISTORY

- Increasing pain in the posterior elbow over several weeks that worsens over course of the day and associated with occasional morning stiffness
- Improvement can be seen with periods of inactivity.

PHYSICAL EXAM

- Pain in the posterior elbow
- Pain on full extension/flexion of the elbow
- Tenderness/swelling at or above the triceps insertion onto the olecranon
- Increased pain with resisted extension of the elbow
- Possible weakness with elbow extension (may be indicative of tendon rupture)

DIFFERENTIAL DIAGNOSIS

- Olecranon fracture/stress fracture
- Olecranon bursitis
- Triceps rupture
- Subtendinous bursitis
- Cervical radiculopathy
- Posterior interosseous neuropathy

DIAGNOSTIC TESTS & INTERPRETATION

- Anterior/posterior and lateral plain films may be helpful if concerned for tendon avulsion (3)[B].
- Ultrasound may be useful in distinguishing between triceps tendonitis and olecranon bursitis if the physical exam is unclear (4)[B].
- Ultrasound may distinguish acute versus chronic pathology with increased tendon thickness, hypoechogenicity of tendon fibers, and calcific deposits within the tendon being found in chronic pathology (often called tendinopathy) (3)[B].
- Magnetic resonance imaging (MRI) is rarely needed.

TREATMENT

- Acute treatment:
  - RICE: rest, ice, compression, elevation:
    - Rest: Avoid any that may exacerbate symptoms.
    - Ice: Use ice packs in the painful area for 5 to 10 minutes 3 to 4 times/d; may also perform ice massage

    - Compression: wrapping the affected area with an elastic bandage, strap, or brace
    - Elevation: If swelling is present, elevation will help alleviate the swelling.
  - Short-term use of nonsteroidal anti-inflammatory drugs (NSAIDs) is also a mainstay of therapy.
- Long-term treatment:
  - Prevention is vital in high-risk populations such as weight lifters, carpenters/construction workers, or guitar players; the key to prevention is dynamic warm-up, avoiding excessive force, and taking frequent breaks within activity.
  - Injection of platelet-rich plasma (PRP) is likely effective for improving function and decreasing pain intensity in the long term (5)[A].

MEDICATION

- Anti-inflammatories: NSAIDs (e.g., ibuprofen, etodolac)
- Acetaminophen

ISSUES FOR REFERRAL

- If history, physical exam, or other imaging studies suggest signs of tendon rupture, including profound weakness with elbow extension, referral to orthopedic surgery is necessary for potential surgical intervention.
- For high-risk patients, physical therapy may be beneficial to ensure proper form and stretching.

ADDITIONAL THERAPIES

- Special considerations:
  - Limit ice to 10 minutes 3 or 4 times daily to avoid cubital tunnel damage of the ulnar nerve.
- Rehabilitation:
  - Graduated eccentric strengthening following period of rest
  - French stretch: (i) Clasp fingers together with hands above head; (ii) keep elbows close to head; (iii) reach down behind head attempting to touch back; (iv) hold, and then repeat.
  - French press: as with stretch, except holding a dumbbell
  - Towel stretch: (i) injured arm overhead with uninjured reaching behind back; (ii) one end of towel in each hand; (iii) pull, hold, and repeat

SURGERY/OTHER PROCEDURES

- Surgical intervention should be considered after a minimum of 1 year of conservative management (3)[C],(6)[C].
- Rare, but operative treatment described with elliptical resection of diseased tissue

ONGOING CARE

FOLLOW-UP RECOMMENDATIONS

Return to sport/activity when no longer tender at or above tendon insertion, strength regained, and full range of motion.

REFERENCES

1. Taylor SA, Hannafin JA. Evaluation and management of elbow tendinopathy. *Sports Health*. 2012;4(5):384–393.
2. Keener JD, Sethi PM. Distal triceps tendon injuries. *Hand Clin*. 2015;31(4):641–650.
3. Donaldson O, Vannet N, Gosens T, et al. Tendinopathies around the elbow part 2: medial elbow, distal biceps, and triceps tendinopathies. *Shoulder Elbow*. 2014;6(1):47–56.
4. Blankstein A, Ganel A, Givon U, et al. Ultrasonographic findings in patients with olecranon bursitis. *Ultraschall Med*. 2006;27(6):568–571.
5. Fitzpatrick J, Bulsara M, Zheng MH. The effectiveness of platelet-rich plasma in the treatment of tendinopathy: a meta-analysis of randomized controlled clinical trials. *Am J Sports Med*. 2017;45(1):226–233.
6. Sibley PA, Harman TW, Bamberger HB. Triceps tendinopathy. *J Hand Surg Am*. 2015;40(7):1446–1448.

CLINICAL PEARLS

- Evidence suggests that the increased risk of rupture with injection serves as a contraindication to direct tendon injection with corticosteroid.
- Emerging evidence for PRP and its ability to promote faster healing and decrease pain may be beneficial in these types of injuries.

TRICEPS TENDON RUPTURE

Christopher Miles, MD, CAQSM • Zachary Sitton, MD

BASICS

DESCRIPTION

Triceps rupture occurs when the triceps tendon becomes detached from its insertion on the olecranon after an elbow injury (1).

EPIDEMIOLOGY

Incidence

- Least common of all tendon injuries (0.78%) (1),(2)
- Average age: 30 to 50 years (2)
- Predominant sex: male (2)
- Most common sports: football, soccer, weightlifting, and bodybuilding (especially with concomitant anabolic steroid use) (1),(2)

Pediatric Considerations

- Insertion of triceps tendon ossifies at age of 9 years, so it is not visible on radiographs before this age (3).
- In children with open growth plates, triceps tendon rupture injury typically causes avulsion of epiphysis with subsequent Salter-Harris type I or II injury (3).

ETIOLOGY AND PATHOPHYSIOLOGY

- Triceps muscle composed of long, lateral, and medial heads (4):
  - Long head originates from the infraglenoid tuberosity on the scapula.
  - Lateral head originates from the posterior-lateral portion of the humerus and the lateral intermuscular septum.
  - Medial head extends from distal to spiral groove to trochlea.
  - All three heads insert on the olecranon.
- Overloading an extended elbow (1)
- Abrupt eccentric contraction of triceps muscles (1)
- Direct posterior elbow trauma (4)

RISK FACTORS

- Extrinsic factors (1),(2):
  - Local steroid injection
  - Degenerative arthritic changes
  - Olecranon bursitis
  - Recent elbow arthroplasty
  - Anabolic steroid use
  - Fluoroquinolone use
- Intrinsic factors (1),(2):
  - Chronic renal failure
  - Secondary hyperparathyroidism
  - Hypocalcemic tetany
  - Rheumatoid arthritis
  - Marfan syndrome
  - Osteogenesis imperfecta
  - Systemic lupus erythematosus
  - Insulin-dependent diabetes

GENERAL PREVENTION

- Properly warm up and stretch prior to physical activity.
- Ensure accurate weight-lifting techniques.
- Avoid local steroid injections and anabolic steroid use.
- Ensure proper rehabilitation from elbow arthroplasty (1).

COMMONLY ASSOCIATED CONDITIONS

- Olecranon fracture (intra-articular)
- Triceps tendinosis
- Triceps contusion
- Avulsion fracture of the olecranon
- Radial head fracture
- Olecranon bursitis (1),(2)

DIAGNOSIS

HISTORY

- Fall on outstretched hand (4)[C]
- Direct elbow trauma (4)[C]
- Patients may feel a pop with resisted elbow extension such as with weightlifting or daily activities (1)[C].

PHYSICAL EXAM

- Swelling and ecchymosis at posterior elbow near triceps insertion site (2)[C]
- Elbow tender to palpation (4)[C]
- Palpable gap at, or proximal, to olecranon tip (1)[C]
- Decreased range of motion (ROM) with elbow extension (4)[C]
- Pain with active elbow extension (4)[C]
- Positive Viegas test (modified Thompson test), with this technique, lack of elbow extension after proximal compression of muscle mass can suggest a diagnosis of complete rupture (1)[C].

DIFFERENTIAL DIAGNOSIS

- Elbow strain
- Olecranon bursitis
- Radial head fracture
- Distal humerus fracture (1)[C]

DIAGNOSTIC TESTS & INTERPRETATION

- Anteroposterior (AP) and lateral elbow radiographs: "flake sign" (Dunn-Kusnezov sign) seen on lateral radiograph (1)[C],(2)[A],(4)[C]
- Ultrasound can help determine severity of tear (2)[C], (5)[C].
- Magnetic resonance imaging (MRI) elbow: gold standard if above inconclusive despite clinical suspicion (1)[C]; also necessary for guiding management and preoperative planning (2)[C]
- Partial versus complete triceps tendon tears:
  - MRI or ultrasound can be used to distinguish between partial and complete tendon tears (2)[C],(5)[C].

ALERT

It is important to note that with partial tears and even some complete central tendon tears, active elbow extension may be preserved due to an intact lateral triceps expansion and compensation from the anconeus muscle (2)[C],(5)[C]. As a result, up to 50% of acute triceps tendon ruptures have been misdiagnosed after initial evaluation (5)[C].

TREATMENT

GENERAL MEASURES

- Ice and acetaminophen or nonsteroidal anti-inflammatory drugs (NSAIDs) initially are appropriate.
- Arm should be placed in sling with 90 degrees or less of flexion initially after the injury. A posterior splint may be applied if necessary but should be in 90 degrees or less of flexion.

ISSUES FOR REFERRAL

Refer all patients with complete or partial triceps rupture >50% to orthopedics for surgical consultation.

ADDITIONAL THERAPIES

- Conservative (1)[C]:
  - Weeks 1 to 6: immobilization:
    - Immediate immobilization with 30 degrees elbow flexion by splint or brace
  - Weeks 6 to 12: ROM:
    - Gradually increase ROM with adjustable angle elbow brace after 6 weeks.
    - Full ROM targeted by 12 weeks postinjury
  - Weeks 12 and on: strengthening:
    - Goal of full extension strength by 6 to 9 months posttreatment
  - Shoulder, wrist, and hand ROM exercises may be started immediately.
  - After immobilization, physical therapy is important.
- Physical therapy
- Current studies are investigating the use of platelet-rich plasma (PRP) for partial ruptures.

SURGERY/OTHER PROCEDURES

Complete triceps rupture or partial triceps tendon rupture >50% and decreased strength with elbow extension (1)[C],(2)[C]:

- Primary repair of tendon within 3 weeks of initial rupture
- Transosseous cruciate and suture anchor repair are the most common techniques (6)[C]. Rerupture rate may be lower when the suture anchor technique is used (6)[B].
- ~90% return rate to preinjury activity level after surgery (2)[A]
- Postoperative physical therapy:
  - Weeks 0 to 6: postoperative adjustable elbow splint at 20 degrees flexion, increasing flexion by 10 degrees every week with passive elbow extension
  - Weeks 6 to 12: active elbow extension
  - Weeks 12 and on: active elbow extension against resistance
- Complete triceps rupture untreated within the first 6 weeks following rupture (4)[C]:
  - Triceps reconstruction
  - Achilles tendon allograft with a calcaneal bony attachment considered in some cases (4)[C]

ONGOING CARE

FOLLOW-UP RECOMMENDATIONS

Routine follow-up at 4 to 6 weeks (transition from immobilization to ROM), 12 weeks (transition from ROM to strengthening), and 6 months (medical clearance) (1)

PATIENT EDUCATION

Triceps extension ROM and strengthening exercises to begin after immobilization

PROGNOSIS

- Nonoperative treatment of partial tears generally resulted in full ROM and subjective strength within 3 to 9 months (4).
- Primary repair of partial tears typically resulted in full ROM and subjective strength by 3 to 6 months (4)
- Primary repair of complete tears generally resulted in full ROM by 3 months and baseline subjective strength by 6 months (4)
- Total triceps reconstruction typically resulted in some loss of ROM and full subjective strength by 2 to 3 years (4)

COMPLICATIONS

- Complete rupture untreated within the first 6 weeks will likely require triceps reconstruction.
- Partial rupture that progresses into complete rupture during conservative therapy
- Postoperative rerupture
- Postoperative wounds given thin subcutaneous tissue at posterior elbow
- Complex regional pain syndrome
- Compartment syndrome
- Heterotopic ossification
- Residual flexion contractures between 5 and 20 degrees (1)

REFERENCES

1. Demirhan M, Ersen A. Distal triceps ruptures. *EFORT Open Rev*. 2017;1(6):255–259.
2. Gaviria M, Ren B, Brown SM, et al. Triceps tendon ruptures: risk factors, treatment, and rehabilitation. *JBJS Rev*. 2020;8(4):e0172.
3. Paramanathan V, Brookfield S, Menon D. Paediatric triceps avulsion fracture identified with ultrasound. *Int J Surg Case Rep*. 2013;4(10):923–925.
4. Tom JA, Kumar NS, Cerynik DL, et al. Diagnosis and treatment of triceps tendon injuries: a review of the literature. *Clin J Sport Med*. 2014;24(3):197–204.
5. Walker CM, Noonan TJ. Distal triceps tendon injuries. *Clin Sports Med*. 2020;39(3):673–685.
6. Tran DV, Yetter TR, Somerson JS. Surgical repair of distal triceps rupture: a systematic review of outcomes and complications. *JSES Rev Rep Tech*. 2022;2(3):332–339.

ADDITIONAL READING

- Aunon-Martin I, Prada-Canizares A, Jimenez-Diaz V, et al. Treatment of a complex distal triceps tendon rupture with a new technique: a case report. *Arch Trauma Res*. 2016;5(1):e32221.
- Dunn JC, Kusnezov N, Fares A, et al. Triceps tendon ruptures: a systematic review. *Hand (N Y)*. 2017;12(5):431–438.
- Foulk DM, Galloway MT. Partial triceps disruption: a case report. *Sports Health*. 2011;3(2):175–178.
- Mair SD, Isbell WM, Gill TJ, et al. Triceps tendon ruptures in professional football players. *Am J Sports Med*. 2004;32(2):431–434.
- Mancini F, Bernardi G, De Luna V, et al. Surgical repair of isolated triceps tendon rupture using a suture anchor technique: a case report. *Joints*. 2017;4(4):250–252.

CLINICAL PEARLS

- Clinicians should maintain a high index of suspicion for triceps tendon tear when evaluating patients with an acute elbow injury (2)
- Significant swelling increases risk of missing diagnosis initially because it hinders ability to localize pain and gap at insertion site of triceps tendon on the olecranon (2).
- It is important to categorize triceps ruptures as partial or complete because this guides treatment (2),(5).
- It is important to note that active elbow extension may be preserved in even high-grade tears due to compensatory mechanisms and can lead to frequent misdiagnosis (5).
- Consider point-of-care (POC) ultrasound if rupture not visualized on radiographs, especially in children (3).
- MRI is most useful for determining the percentage of tears and hence is of paramount help in preoperative management (2).
- Delay in surgical repair past 3 weeks from injury increases risk of requiring triceps reconstruction and worse functional outcomes postoperatively (1).

TRIGGER FINGER

Amy B. Jones, MD ▪ Haris Vakil, MD

BASICS

DESCRIPTION
- Also called flexor tenosynovitis
- Type of stenosing tenosynovitis
- Nodule on flexor tendon catching on first annular (A1) pulley
- Can affect any digit; occasionally, multiple digits
- Ring and middle digit involvement most common in adults
- Almost exclusively thumb in children
- Diffuse versus nodular versus "congenital" (pediatric trigger thumb)

EPIDEMIOLOGY
- Predominant gender: female > male (3 to 6 times more common in females)
- Predominant age: bimodal: age <8 years old and 55 to 60 years old
- Seen more commonly in dominant hand
- Lifetime risk 2.6% in general population but 10% in diabetics
- In children, 25% will have bilateral involvement.

Incidence
28 cases/100,000 population

ETIOLOGY AND PATHOPHYSIOLOGY
- Inflammation of flexor digitorum superficialis (FDS) tendon leading to nodule formation
- A1 pulley spans from volar plate of distal metacarpal to base of proximal phalanx.
- Nodule catches on A1 pulley during finger flexion, leading to pain.
- Pain often greatest at metacarpophalangeal (MCP) joint
- Generally idiopathic
- Activity or occupation that involves repetitive use of the fingers
- Results from repetitive trauma but also occasionally sepsis from secondary infection (e.g., tuberculosis)

RISK FACTORS
- Diabetes, rheumatoid arthritis (RA), connective tissue disorders
- Repetitive trauma with compressive force against MCP area (e.g., arc welding)

GENERAL PREVENTION
Activity modification

COMMONLY ASSOCIATED CONDITIONS
- Diabetes
- RA
- Hypothyroidism
- Amyloidosis
- Mucopolysaccharidosis
- Connective tissue disorders

DIAGNOSIS

HISTORY
- Painful catching/clicking with finger flexion or extension
- Pain over MCP; may refer to palm or proximal interphalangeal (PIP) joint
- Digit may be locked, usually in flexion.
- Stiffness develops with prolonged symptoms.

PHYSICAL EXAM
- Tender, palpable nodule on flexor tendon, just proximal to MCP
- Active fist closing reproduces lock/snap.

DIFFERENTIAL DIAGNOSIS
- Dupuytren contracture
- Carpal tunnel syndrome
- Gamekeeper's thumb
- RA
- Tendon sheath ganglion
- Suppurative tenosynovitis

DIAGNOSTIC TESTS & INTERPRETATION

Initial Tests (lab, imaging)
- Lab not indicated, except to evaluate associated systemic disease
- Imaging not indicated; x-rays may be considered to rule out differentials.

Diagnostic Procedures/Other
None; steroid injection is both therapeutic and diagnostic.

TREATMENT

GENERAL MEASURES

- Activity modification
- Splinting options
  - Splinting of PIP with the best results if there is one joint involved × 8 weeks
  - Splinting of MCP joint at 10 to 15 degrees of flexion 6 to 10 weeks:
    - Reduces tendon motion in sheath
    - Allows resolution of surrounding synovitis
    - 47–93% with partial or full symptom resolution after 10 weeks (1)[A]
    - Distal interphalangeal (DIP) immobilization showed a negative effect (1)[A].

MEDICATION

First Line

Injected corticosteroids (see "Surgery/Other Procedures" below)

Second Line

Nonsteroidal anti-inflammatory drugs (NSAIDs) may help with pain relief; no specific evidence but commonly recommended

SURGERY/OTHER PROCEDURES

- Corticosteroid injection into tendon sheath:
  - Palmar or dorsolateral approach to avoid neurovascular bundle.
  - Subcutaneous (SC) infiltration equal or superior to intrasheath injection (2)[B]
  - May require repeat injection in 1 month
  - Up to 90% complete or partial reduction of symptoms (2)[B]
  - Only 50% response in diffuse type or diabetes
- Surgical release of A1 pulley:
  - Open or percutaneous procedure
  - First-line treatment for locked digit or pediatric trigger thumb, although there is increasing argument toward conservative management for the latter
  - Indicated if repeat injections ineffective
  - 81.7–100% complete resolution of symptoms (3)[A]

ONGOING CARE

FOLLOW-UP RECOMMENDATIONS

Patient Monitoring

May see increased glucose level following steroid injection in diabetes

PROGNOSIS

- Excellent; >90% symptom resolution with steroid or surgical therapy
- 23–63% of pediatric trigger digits may resolve spontaneously.

COMPLICATIONS

- If untreated:
  - PIP joint flexion contracture
  - Distal triggering from FDS tendon degeneration
- Of injection:
  - Fat atrophy and necrosis
  - Local skin depigmentation
  - Theoretical risk of tendon rupture
- Of surgical release:
  - Bowstringing of flexor tendon
  - Second annular (A2) pulley injury
  - Digital nerve injury
  - Infection
  - Long-term scar tenderness

REFERENCES

1. Lunsford D, Valdes K, Hengy S. Conservative management of trigger finger: a systematic review. *J Hand Ther*. 2019;32(2):212–221.
2. Tunçez M, Turan K, Aydın ÖD, et al. Ultrasound guided versus blinded injection in trigger finger treatment: a prospective controlled study. *J Orthop Surg Res*. 2023;18(1):459.
3. Garcia HRP, Mund E, Romeiro P. Ultrasound-guided vs. non-guided trigger finger release: a systematic review and meta-analysis. *Int Orthop*. 2024;48(9):2429–2437.

ADDITIONAL READING

- Akhtar S, Bradley MJ, Quinton DN, et al. Management and referral for trigger finger/thumb. *BMJ*. 2005;331(7507):30–33.
- Giugale J, Fowler JR. Trigger finger: adult and pediatric treatment strategies. *Orthop Clin North Am*. 2015;46(4):561–569.
- Ryzewicz M, Wolf JM. Trigger digits: principles, management, and complications. *J Hand Surg Am*. 2006;31(1):135–146.
- Teo SH, Ng DCL, Wong YKY. Effectiveness of proximal interphalangeal joint–blocking orthosis vs metacarpophalangeal joint–blocking orthosis in trigger digit management: a randomized clinical trial. *J Hand Ther*. 2019;32(4):444–451.

CLINICAL PEARLS

- Clinical diagnosis by painful catching at MCP joint
- Corticosteroid injection is safe and highly effective first-line treatment.
- Surgical release provides excellent results when conservative measures fail.
- Trigger finger in diabetics is less likely to respond to steroid therapy.

TURF TOE

Holly J. Benjamin, MD, FAMSSM, FACSM ▪ Abdullah Hasan Pratt, MD

BASICS

1st metatarsophalangeal (MTP) joint sprain

DESCRIPTION

- 1st MTP forced hyperextension injury to the plantar plate and sesamoid complex, resulting in sprain of the plantar capsuloligamentous complex (PLC)
- Chondral and osseous injuries can be associated.
- The common factors resulting in turf toe injury are hard playing surfaces, light flexible footwear, and axial loading.

EPIDEMIOLOGY

- The overall incidence and prevalence remain unknown, with most available data emanating from smaller studies.
- The incidence of this injury has increased secondary to athletic fields being covered by artificial turf as well as increased flexibility of the toe box in athletic shoes.
- Within college football, the overall incidence of turf toe injuries obtained over 5 years via the National Collegiate Athletic Association's (NCAA's) Injury Surveillance System (ISS) was 0.062 per 1,000 athlete exposures (1).

ALERT

In NCAA football players, there was an 85% higher risk of turf toe injury on third-generation "artificial fill turf" (0.087 per 1,000) as compared to natural grass (0.047 per 1,000), where artificial nonfill surfaces (Astroturf) had a rate of 0.057 per 1,000 (not significantly different than grass 0.017, 0.36) (2).

- The proposed theory for this discrepancy in injuries seen on different playing surfaces is that MTP hyperextension is increased with increased traction (i.e., less give as compared to grass and Astroturf).
- Although turf toe is seen more often in football, it also occurs in basketball, dancing, soccer, tennis, volleyball, and wrestling.
- There seem to be no differentiating ethnocultural, sex-related, or age-related determinants connected to turf toe (2).

ETIOLOGY AND PATHOPHYSIOLOGY

- The MTP joint bears most of the body weight (40–60%) during walking, increasing up to 2- to 3-fold during running, and up to an 8-fold increase during jumping.
- In the acute setting, 80% of turf toe typically occurs during an applied downward force, where the great toe is dorsiflexed beyond its biomechanical limits, resulting in tear of the capsule about the neck of the 1st MTP (1).
- In a minority of cases, forced plantarflexion ("sand toe") and valgus/varus mechanisms can also lead to symptoms consistent with turf toe.

RISK FACTORS

- Artificial turf and playing surfaces
- Athlete's experience and years of sports participation
- Athlete's position while playing sport
- Athlete's weight, where higher forces are transmitted with increased weight
- Flattening of the 1st MTP
- Football players (defensive and offensive running backs, wide receivers, linemen)
- Foot pronation
- Hallux degenerative joint disease
- Increased ankle dorsiflexion
- Increased friction between athletic shoe and turf
- Increased toe box flexibility and decreased number of cleats in the shoe
- Prior 1st MTP joint injury
- Pes planus

GENERAL PREVENTION

- Early identification of athletes with prior MTP injuries or existing ankle injuries requiring range of motion (ROM)-limiting support or braces is key toward preventative measures.
- Limited ROM at the MTP, specifically limited dorsiflexion <60 degrees, can predispose athletes to injuries secondary to hyperextension.
- Through vigilant screening during preparticipation physicals, as well as at early signs of MTP injury, the use of orthotic and rigid insoles can reduce the progression of injury and minimize inactive time secondary to injury.

COMMONLY ASSOCIATED CONDITIONS

In addition to plantar plate rupture, excessive forefoot hyperextension may also injure the articular cartilage, sesamoids, subchondral bone, resulting in stress fracture and hallux rigidus (late sequelae).

DIAGNOSIS

HISTORY

- Acute forced hyperextension of MTP joint resulting in painful weight-bearing, pain with ROM, and especially pain with applied pressure to MTP during running or jumping (toeing off)
- Swelling, tenderness, and possibly ecchymosis/bruising may also be reported.

PHYSICAL EXAM

- Swelling of 1st MTP, with or without ecchymosis
- Tenderness to palpation of MTP joint
- Decreased active ROM
- Pain with dorsiflexion and passive ROM
- Laxity within the ligamentous capsule and instability of the MTP joint may be seen in severe injury, resulting in a positive Lachman test (dorsal plantar drawer test to access the plantar plate of the toe).
- Grading system:
  - Grade 1 injuries are a capsular sprain without loss of its functional integrity. Clinically, there is mild edema and pain but no bruising, and ROM is preserved.
  - Grade 2 injuries represent partial-thickness tearing of the plantar plate and capsular structures. Clinically, there is both edema and ecchymosis of the 1st MTP, loss of ROM, moderate pain, and often have an antalgic gait.
  - Grade 3 injuries are acute injuries with complete disruption of the PLC. The plantar plate may be completely avulsed from the metatarsal neck, and impaction of the metatarsal head may occur during full extension of the joint. Clinically, there is marked edema and ecchymosis, severe pain to palpation, and they rarely can bear weight or ambulate during the immediate post injury period (3).

DIFFERENTIAL DIAGNOSIS

- Gout
- Plantar plate rupture
- 1st distal metatarsal or proximal phalangeal fracture
- Osteoarthritis of 1st MTP (hallux rigidus)
- Sesamoiditis
- Sesamoid stress fracture
- Flexor or extensor hallucis tendonitis

DIAGNOSTIC TESTS & INTERPRETATION

- Initial imaging should include anteroposterior, lateral, and oblique radiographs.
- If plantar tenderness, sesamoid views should also be obtained.
- Dynamic maneuvers with musculoskeletal (MSK) ultrasound can demonstrate discontinuity of the normal plantar plate.
- Magnetic resonance imaging (MRI) can be obtained to evaluate soft tissue edema or the true extent of the plantar plate injury but is often not required (4).
- The resulting earlier, more accurate diagnosis with MRI has changed the course of conservative treatment, provided a road map for potential surgery when indicated, and decreased overall morbidity (3).
- Grade 1 sprain:
  - X-ray: normal appearance
  - MRI: edema of any portion of the PLC, no tear
- Grade 2 sprain:
  - X-ray: normal appearance
  - MRI: partial tear of any portion of the PLC, edema if acute
- Grade 3 sprain:
  - X-ray: possible fracture, sesamoid retraction, or diastasis of bipartite sesamoid
  - MRI: full-thickness tear of any portion of the PLC, bony edema, sesamoid retraction, or diastasis of bipartite sesamoid

TREATMENT

GENERAL MEASURES

- Grade 1 sprain (3)[B]:
  - Ice, elevation, and nonsteroidal anti-inflammatory drugs (NSAIDs)
  - Toe spica taping with activity, which restricts excessive dorsiflexion
  - Gentle ROM exercises can be initiated typically 3 to 5 days post injury. Initial exercise consists of passive plantarflexion to prevent sesamoid adhesions while protecting the healing soft tissues.
- Grade 2 sprain (3)[B]:
  - Ice, elevation, and NSAIDs
  - Toe spica taping with activity as well as orthotics such as stiff sole/turf toe plate or walking boot
  - Gentle passive ROM exercises as tolerated, but explosive, push off activities should be restricted until low-impact exercise is tolerated without pain or limitation; usually up to 2 weeks
- Grade 3 sprain (3)[B]:
  - Treatment similar to grade 2 sprains
  - Weight-bearing as tolerated, with use of crutches if pain with ambulation
  - Prolonged progression typical due to severity of symptoms; clearance optimal when has progressed with weight-bearing and has returned to preinjury performance level; often up to 8 weeks

MEDICATION

- NSAIDs are used primarily to reduce pain.
- Steroid injections are not recommended.

ADDITIONAL THERAPIES

- Treatment of turf toe depends largely on the grade of injury. Once identified, some grade 1 and many grade 2 and grade 3 injuries should be referred to a sports medicine or orthopedic foot and ankle specialist for definitive treatment.
- Physical therapy can aid greatly in both acute management with gentle ROM techniques as well as in chronic cases where repeated injuries have resulted in restricted ROM at 1st MTP (4).

SURGERY/OTHER PROCEDURES

- In the acute setting, surgery is only indicated in plantar plate rupture, sesamoid fracture, severe chondral injury, new bunion/deformity, or significant fracture dislocation at MTP (2)[B],(3)
- In chronic turf toe, surgery may become a viable option if ROM is significantly limited affecting return to preinjury performance level, osteonecrosis of sesamoid, or persistent pain/instability despite conservative therapy (5).

ONGOING CARE

More severe or recurrent cases may require a rigid-soled shoe or rigid forefoot orthotic when participating in sports.

PROGNOSIS

The prognosis for full return to preinjury performance level is usually good unless repeated injury without fully healing or chronic injuries resulting in instability or limited ROM. Typical timeframe for return to play is weeks to months.

COMPLICATIONS

Chronic or severe cases can lead to significantly limited ROM, which can predispose to recurrent injury, so early controlled ROM is recommended after injury to minimize the risk of this complication.

REFERENCES

1. George E, Harris AHS, Dragoo JL, et al. Incidence and risk factors for turf toe injuries in intercollegiate football: data from the National Collegiate Athletic Association Injury Surveillance System. *Foot Ankle Int*. 2014;35(2):108–115.
2. Tran A, Kappa J, Smith E, et al. The effect of turf toe injuries on player performance in the National Football League. *Iowa Orthop J*. 2019;39(2):35–39.
3. Vopat ML, Hassan M, Poppe T, et al. Return to sport after turf toe injuries: a systematic review and meta-analysis. *Orthop J Sports Med*. 2019;7(10):2325967119875133.
4. Crain JM, Phancao JP. Imaging of turf toe. *Radiol Clin North Am*. 2016;54(5):969–978.
5. McCormick JJ, Anderson RB. Rehabilitation following turf toe injury and plantar plate repair. *Clin Sports Med*. 2010;29(2):313–323.

CLINICAL PEARLS

- Common injury; clinical diagnosis with adjunctive radiographs typical; MRI is not often needed.
- Return to play and progression of all three grades of sprains depending on severity of symptoms, and all must complete a gradual, functional progression over a period of 1 to 8 weeks typically.
- Early return to play is associated with chronic pain and a higher complication rate, particularly for grade 3 injuries.
- Corticosteroid injections have no role in the acute treatment of this condition.

ULNAR COLLATERAL LIGAMENT INJURIES OF THE ELBOW

Caroline M. Fryar, MD • Daniel C. Herman, MD, PhD, FAAPMR, FACSM, FISBS, CAQSM • Jason L. Zaremski, MD, CAQSM, FAAPMR, FACSM, FAMSSM

BASICS

DESCRIPTION

- Sprain or tearing of the ulnar collateral ligament (UCL) of the elbow secondary to acute or chronic valgus stress leading to pain, instability, and dysfunction
- Two main mechanisms: chronic deterioration of the UCL owing to repetitive valgus overload or, less commonly, an acute traumatic rupture

EPIDEMIOLOGY

- Most UCL injuries are seen in baseball players, but they also can be seen in wrestlers, javelin throwers, tennis players, football players, volleyball players, and in acute trauma victims.
- UCL injuries are more common in skeletally mature athletes, but the incidence in skeletally immature athletes is rising because of the improved detection with ultrasound (US) and magnetic resonance imaging (MRI).
- Predominant gender: male > female
- Although the exact prevalence of UCL injury is unknown, there has been a definite increase in the number of surgical reconstructions performed in professional, collegiate, and high school athletes in recent years (1).

ETIOLOGY AND PATHOPHYSIOLOGY

- The UCL is the primary restraint to valgus stress of the elbow in flexion.
- The UCL is composed of three ligaments: the anterior bundle, posterior bundle, and transverse ligament.
- The anterior bundle, which is composed of an anterior and posterior band with reciprocal functions, is the most important medial stabilizer of the elbow. Rupture of the anterior bundle is considered a complete tear of the UCL.
- The posterior bundle provides secondary restraint beyond 90 degrees of flexion.
- The transverse ligament is an extension of the joint capsule and does not contribute to valgus stability.
- Repetitive valgus load to the elbow is absorbed primarily by the UCL and the forearm flexor muscles.
- Over time, the UCL becomes overloaded, and microtraumatic tears occur, potentially leading to altered throwing kinematics.
- Cumulative microtrauma can lead to rupture of the UCL.
- Altered mechanics lead to decreased throwing accuracy and velocity.
- Acute rupture can occur in a previously attenuated ligament or in a normal ligament subjected to extreme valgus stress, such as an elbow dislocation.

RISK FACTORS

- Participation in sport that demands repetitive excessive valgus stress to the elbow, such as high-velocity throwing or overhead activity, is a risk factor for chronic injury.
- Contact sports or sports with significant fall risk are a factor in acute injury.
- Sport specialization, excessive throwing, poor pitching mechanics, and weak links in the kinetic chain

GENERAL PREVENTION

- Athletes who participate in throwing or overhead sports should be on a conditioning program that includes core stabilization, rotator cuff and forearm muscle strengthening, and posterior capsule stretching.
- Athletic technique should be reviewed to minimize valgus stress to the elbow.
- Throwing athletes should have a 3- to 4-month rest from throwing per 12 months as per MLB pitch smart guidelines

COMMONLY ASSOCIATED CONDITIONS

- Valgus extension overload syndrome: radiocapitellar and posteromedial olecranon impingement
- Ulnar neuritis or subluxation
- Osteochondral loose bodies

DIAGNOSIS

HISTORY

- In acute rupture, the athlete may experience sudden pain, sometimes with an audible pop, and cannot resume play.
- Chronic injuries present as persistent, insidious medial elbow pain, often accompanied by decreased command and velocity of throwing.

PHYSICAL EXAM

- Tenderness along the sublime tubercle
- Joint effusion and ulnar nerve tenderness may be present.
- Flexion contracture with pain at terminal extension is common.
- Valgus stress test: The examiner stabilizes the arm and flexes the elbow to 30 degrees; valgus stress is applied. The test is positive if the athlete has pain, apprehension, or instability.
- Milking maneuver: The forearm is supinated and the elbow flexed to 90 degrees; the examiner applies a valgus stress by pulling on the thumb while palpating along the UCL. Pain, apprehension, or instability indicates MCL injury, but this test can give a high number of false-positive results.
- Moving valgus stress test: This test is highly sensitive and specific for UCL injury. A constant valgus stress is placed on the elbow as the joint is moved through the arc of flexion and extension. The test is positive if the athlete's pain is reproduced between 70 and 120 degrees of flexion.

DIFFERENTIAL DIAGNOSIS

- Flexor/pronator tendonitis or rupture
- Ulnar neuritis or subluxation
- Medial triceps subluxation
- Loose bodies
- Olecranon osteophytosis
- Medial epicondyle avulsion
- Pronator syndrome

DIAGNOSTIC TESTS & INTERPRETATION

- X-rays: Three-view (anterior-posterior, lateral, and medial oblique) series of the elbow should be performed to evaluate for osteophytes, calcifications within the ligament or soft tissues, osteochondral damage, and loose bodies.
- Stress x-rays may show joint widening compared with the contralateral elbow; a difference in joint opening of >1 mm suggests UCL injury (2)[B].
- US also can reveal disruption of the UCL in the hands of an experienced user (stress US compared to the uninjured side may be particularly helpful).

- MRI arthrography is superior to MRI alone to diagnose UCL tears (2).
- MRI can visualize attenuation, partial tearing, or complete tearing of the UCL as well as evaluate the articular surface and surrounding soft tissue structures. Image enhancement is possible with saline or gadolinium.
- Arthroscopy can evaluate and treat associated articular injuries but cannot visualize the UCL well. Stress testing under arthroscopy, however, can be diagnostic of UCL tear (3)[C].

TREATMENT

GENERAL MEASURES

- Acute treatment: Acute injuries should be treated with rest from sport, ice, nonsteroidal anti-inflammatory drugs (NSAIDs), and sling immobilization or long arm casting if pain is substantial with movement. Caution should be used to avoid direct ice application over the ulnar nerve.
- Long-term treatment:
  - Sprain consisting of edema seen on imaging but no definitive tear should be treated with rehabilitation, including sports-specific training.
  - Low-grade partial tear injuries are treated with removal from sport followed by prolonged rehabilitation and sports-specific training.
  - High-grade partial tears, particularly distally, as well as complete ruptures are treated with surgical intervention in the high-demand throwing or overhead athlete.
- Orthobiologic treatment (4)[B]:
  - Evidence is inconclusive that platelet-rich plasma can successfully improve outcomes versus rest and rehabilitation alone in partial tears.
- Rehabilitation (5):
  - Range-of-motion (ROM) exercises begin after pain decreases.
  - Once pain free, strengthening begins with wrist flexor and extensor groups followed by scapular stabilizers.
  - Throwing and valgus stresses are restricted for at least 6 weeks.
  - Long toss in practice and pitching should be avoided in skeletally immature for up to 9 to 12 months.
  - A structured sports-specific program, such as an interval throwing program, is begun when the athlete has full strength and painless valgus testing.
  - Athletes are rested at any period when they experience pain.

SURGERY/OTHER PROCEDURES

- Surgery is indicated for complete rupture or failure of 6 to 12 months of nonsurgical management in a high-demand competitive athlete with a partial tear.
- In some cases, with partial-thickness tears, UCL repair with internal bracing rather than reconstruction may be a viable option (6).
- Surgical reconstruction of the UCL is performed using the palmaris longus, toe extensor, or other tendon graft through a muscle-splitting approach in the flexor-pronator bundle.
- Surgical reconstruction is followed by lengthy postoperative rehabilitation:
  - After 10 to 14 days of immobilization, ROM exercises are initiated.
  - Hinged bracing is usually recommended until 6 weeks.
  - At that time, strengthening exercises begin.
  - Valgus stress is avoided until 4 months postoperatively.
  - An interval throwing program is initiated at approximately 4 months with soft tosses.
  - This is advanced in intervals, with return to competitive throwing allowed at 9 to 12 months if the athlete is pain free with full strength and ROM.
  - Athletes are rested at any step if pain recurs.
- The timeline for return to play after reconstruction is typically at least 12 months, longer if the athlete is an overhead throwing athlete, a pitcher, or is a javelin thrower.
- Return to play is typically shorter with surgical repair and internal bracing (6)
- Most modern techniques allow >90% of athletes to return to sport, although there is a slight decrease of returning to sport at previous level of competition (67–92%) (4)[A].

REFERENCES

1. Idowu OA, Boyajian HH, Lindsay-Rivera K, et al. Trends of ulnar collateral ligament reconstruction in the United States from 2003 to 2014: analysis of 3,133 patients. *Arthrosc Sports Med Rehabil*. 2020;2(6):e705–e710.
2. Roedl JB, Gonzalez FM, Zoga AC, et al. Potential utility of a combined approach with US and MR arthrography to image medial elbow pain in baseball players. *Radiology*. 2016;279(3):827–837.
3. Peters SD, Bullock GS, Goode AP, et al. The success of return to sport after ulnar collateral ligament injury in baseball: a systematic review and meta-analysis. *J Shoulder Elbow Surg*. 2018;27(3):561–571.
4. Bowers RL, Fryar CM, Cipriano K, et al. Orthobiologic treatment of throwing related injuries in sport: a focused review of the published literature. *Curr Sports Med Rep*. 2023;22(6):199–203.
5. Bogdanov JM, Bolia IK, Benvegnu N, et al. Rehabilitation following ulnar collateral ligament reconstruction in overhead-throwing athletes. *JBJS Rev*. 2021;9(4).
6. Wilk KE, Arrigo CA, Bagwell MS, et al. Repair of the ulnar collateral ligament of the elbow: rehabilitation following internal brace surgery. *J Orthop Sports Phys Ther*. 2019;49(4):253–261.

CLINICAL PEARLS

- UCL injuries are predominantly seen in high-velocity throwing or overhead athletes.
- Pain, apprehension, or laxity appreciated on valgus testing of the elbow should lead to MRI arthrography and/or US imaging to evaluate the integrity of the UCL.
- Most UCL sprains and low-grade tears injuries respond to rehabilitation and sports-specific training, but surgical reconstruction should be considered in high-level athletes that have high-grade partial tears and rupture.

ULNAR COLLATERAL LIGAMENT INJURY OF THUMB (SKIER'S THUMB/GAMEKEEPER'S THUMB)

Haruki Ishii, MD, CAQSM

BASICS

DESCRIPTION

- Synonym(s): skier's thumb; gamekeeper's thumb
- Injury of the ulnar collateral ligament (UCL) of the 1st metacarpophalangeal (MCP) joint with or without a bony avulsion from the insertion on the phalanx
- Acute tears have been described as a "skier's thumb."
- Chronic or attritional ruptures of the ligament have been described as a "gamekeeper's thumb" as a reference to chronic UCL injuries suffered by gamekeepers while twisting the necks of small game like rabbits while hunting.
- Stener lesion:
  - With a complete rupture, the adductor pollicis aponeurosis can become interposed between the ligament ends.
  - Occurs in 60–90% of cases of a complete rupture, preventing effective recovery without surgical intervention (1)

EPIDEMIOLOGY

- As high as 50 per 100,000 and 4 to 10 times more likely than radial collateral ligament injuries (2)
- Represents 6.6% of all skiing injuries and the third most common injury (3)

RISK FACTORS

Ski poles likely increase the risk of UCL injury:

- Wrist straps on the ski poles do not likely increase the risk of UCL injury further.

DIAGNOSIS

Avulsion of bony fragment at the insertion of UCL on the phalanx may be associated with this condition.

HISTORY

- A valgus force to the thumb in extended and/or abducted position
- Injuries can range from mild sprains to partial/complete tears.
- Commonly seen in skiing but often occurs in other sports, such as football, basketball, baseball, or cycling

PHYSICAL EXAM

- Localized tenderness, swelling, and ecchymosis may be present around the thumb MCP joint.
- When a Stener lesion is present, a palpable mass over the MCP joint may be felt.
- If patients have guarding due to pain, local anesthetic can improve clinical assessment (2)[C].
- Tenderness along the UCL and possibly the dorsal capsule or volar plate
- Valgus stress test to evaluate for complete UCL tears:
  - Tested at 0 and 30 degrees of MCP joint flexion
  - There is side-to-side variability even in the absence of injury (2)[C].
- The degree of laxity and presence of a firm end point is used to guide clinical decision-making:
  - Grade 1 (mild sprain): painful without laxity
  - Grade 2 (partial-thickness tear): laxity with a firm end point
  - Grade 3 (complete tear): laxity without a firm end point

DIFFERENTIAL DIAGNOSIS

- Radial collateral ligament sprain/rupture
- Fracture (i.e., metacarpal fracture, proximal phalanx fracture)
- MCP joint dislocation

DIAGNOSTIC TESTS & INTERPRETATION

- X-rays (posteroanterior [PA]/lateral) (2),(3):
  - Rule out bony avulsion or other fractures.
  - Stress x-rays to determine the degree of radial deviation
  - Stress views are used less frequently given a theoretical concern of worsening UCL injuries (3).
  - "Sag sign": volar subluxation of the proximal phalanx in relation to the metacarpal at the MCP joint due to the dorsal capsular injury (3)
  - "Two fleck sign": an avulsion of the adductor pollicis attachment and a distal UCL avulsion, describing a Stener lesion (3)
- Ultrasound (US) (3):
  - Although user dependent, it has been shown to be highly sensitive and specific comparable to those seen with magnetic resonance imaging (MRI) (4)[A].
    - A normal UCL has a homogeneous fibrillar structure.
    - Full-thickness tears are characterized by a focal hypoechoic/anechoic defect or cleft, typically associated with proximally retracted ligament.
- MRI:
  - Sensitivity 96% and specificity 100% (4)[A]
  - Stener lesions may have a "yo-yo on a string" appearance (3).

TREATMENT

- Ice, elevation, and immobilization should be used immediately after the injury for protection and pain control.
- Nonoperative treatment (grade 1 or 2 injuries):
  - Immobilization with a thumb spica for a minimum of 4 weeks (1)[C]
  - Start range of motion exercises after 4 to 6 weeks of immobilization.
  - Progress to strengthening exercises as tolerated.

- Operative treatment (3):
  - Complete UCL tears
  - Large avulsion fragments with intra-articular extension
  - Presence of Stener lesions
- Primary repair is preferred for acute tears. Reconstruction is usually reserved for chronic, irreparable tears, or cases of railed primary repair. (3)[C]:
  - Even after failure of nonoperative treatment up to >6 years, almost all patients achieve complete pain relief and normal strength, stability, and range of motion after surgical reconstruction (5)[A].
- Controversial:
  - Grade 3 UCL injuries without Stener lesion or joint subluxation
    - Potential for healing with conservative management with nondisplaced ligament disruption (1)[C]
  - Avulsion fractures at UCL origin
    - Results are promising with conservative management if there is stability with valgus stress on physical exam (1)[C].

MEDICATION

Acetaminophen or nonsteroidal anti-inflammatory drugs (NSAIDs) are generally adequate for pain control.

ADDITIONAL THERAPIES

Protected range of motion exercises recommended between 4 to 6 weeks for acute UCL tears and 6 to 8 weeks for chronic UCL tears postoperatively (1)[C].

SURGERY/OTHER PROCEDURES

- Acute operative treatment (2),(3):
  - Several different surgical techniques for repair are used and will depend on the exact nature of the injury and surgeon's preference.
- Postoperative protocol (1)[C]:
  - Thumb spica splint/cast for 4 weeks
  - Removable thumb spica splint with initiation of protected range of motion exercises at 4 to 6 weeks
  - Strengthening exercises are initiated at 6 to 12 weeks.
  - Full unrestricted activity is generally allowed at 10 to 12 weeks.
- Chronic operative treatment generally requires surgical reconstruction of the UCL (5)[A].
- Postoperative protocol (1)[C]:
  - Casting for 6 weeks
  - Removable thumb spica splint with initiation of protected range-of-motion exercises at 6 to 8 weeks
  - Strengthening exercises are initiated at 8 to 12 weeks.
  - Full unrestricted activity is generally allowed at 12 to 16 weeks.

ONGOING CARE

PROGNOSIS

- Prognosis is excellent for grade 1 or 2 injuries with nonoperative management with immobilization (1)[C],(3)[C].
- Prognosis is excellent for complete tears treated surgically (5)[A].
- Postoperative return-to-play rates are high with few complications (6)[A].

COMPLICATIONS

- Most common complication of UCL repair is stiffness.
- Other complications include implant or graft failure, the MCP joint arthritis, and persistent instability.

REFERENCES

1. Daley D, Geary M, Gaston RG. Thumb metacarpophalangeal ulnar and radial collateral ligament injuries. *Clin Sports Med*. 2020;39(2):443–455.
2. Chang AL, Merkow DB, Bookman JS, et al. Thumb metacarpophalangeal joint ulnar collateral ligament injuries: management and biomechanical evaluation. *J Am Acad Orthop Surg*. 2023;31(1):7–16.
3. Robinson DM, Kakar S, Jelsing E. Acute thumb metacarpophalangeal joint ulnar collateral ligament injury: diagnosis, management, and return to sports considerations. *Curr Sports Med Rep*. 2023;22(6):238–244.
4. Rashidi A, Haj-Mirzaian A, Dalili D, et al. Evidence-based use of clinical examination, ultrasonography, and MRI for diagnosing ulnar collateral ligament tears of the metacarpophalangeal joint of the thumb: systematic review and meta-analysis. *Eur Radiol*. 2021;31(8):5699–5712.
5. Samora JB, Harris JD, Griesser MJ, et al. Outcomes after injury to the thumb ulnar collateral ligament—a systematic review. *Clin J Sport Med*. 2013;23(4):247–254.
6. Allahabadi S, Kwong JW, Pandya NK, et al. Return to play after thumb ulnar collateral ligament injuries managed surgically in athletes—a systematic review. *J Hand Surg Glob Online*. 2023;5(3):349–357.

ADDITIONAL READING

- Avery DM III, Caggiano NM, Matullo KS. Ulnar collateral ligament injuries of the thumb: a comprehensive review. *Orthop Clin North Am*. 2015;46(2):281–292.
- Avery DM III, Inkellis ER, Carlson MG. Thumb collateral ligament injuries in the athlete. *Curr Rev Musculoskelet Med*. 2017;10(1):28–37.
- Knisely B, Noland SS, Melville DM. Ultrasound versus MRI in the evaluation of the thumb metacarpophalangeal joint. *J Ultrason*. 2023;23(95):e214–e222.

CLINICAL PEARLS

- UCL of the thumb injuries are common in athletes, ranging from mild sprains (grade 1) to complete rupture (grade 3). Grade 1 and 2 injuries are typically treated conservatively with immobilization for a minimum of 4 weeks followed by range of motion and strengthening exercises.
- A complete tear or presence of a Stener lesion or large avulsion fragments require surgical management. Protected range-of-motion exercises recommended between 4 to 6 weeks for acute UCL tears and 6 to 8 weeks for chronic UCL tears postoperatively. Both conservative and surgical treatment have a good prognosis if injuries are appropriately managed.

ULNAR IMPACTION SYNDROME

Jason L. Zaremski, MD, CAQSM, FAAPMR, FACSM, FAMSSM • Aimee Madsen, MD •
Daniel C. Herman, MD, PhD, FAAPMR, FACSM, FISBS, CAQSM

BASICS

DESCRIPTION

- Ulnar impaction syndrome (also referred to as ulnocarpal abutment or ulnocarpal impaction syndrome) is a degenerative condition of the ulnar-sided wrist due to excessive load across the ulnocarpal joint.
- It occurs most often with positive ulnar variance; in a normal wrist, approximately 20% of the load goes through the ulna and 80% through the radius. In positive ulnar variance, loads through the ulnocarpal joint approaching 40% (1).
- It can result in a myriad of pathology, including triangular fibrocartilage complex (TFCC) deterioration as well as degeneration of the ulnar head, lunate, triquetrum, and/or lunotriquetral interosseous ligament (LTIL).
- Ulnar impaction syndrome is also seen in neutral or negative variance due to dynamic impaction during high-impact activities.

EPIDEMIOLOGY

- Little is known about the demographics of ulnar impaction syndrome.
- Positive ulnar variance is more prevalent in people of Asian ancestry. Incidence may be higher in this population; however, further research is needed (1).

ETIOLOGY AND PATHOPHYSIOLOGY

- Ulnar impaction syndrome is a wrist condition caused by the ulna (the forearm bone on the pinky side) being too long in relation to the radius (the thumb-side forearm bone). This extra length, known as positive ulnar variance, causes the ulna to "jam" into the small bones and cartilage of the wrist.
- This seemingly small difference in bone length dramatically overloads the joint. A slightly longer ulna can more than double the force absorbed by the pinky side of the wrist (from a normal 18% to >40%) (2). This chronic impaction wears down the TFCC—the main cartilage cushion and the surfaces of the wrist bones, leading to degeneration and pain.
- This condition can occur for three main reasons:
  - Anatomy: A person is simply born with a longer ulna.
  - Previous injury: A poorly healed wrist fracture can shorten the radius, making the ulna relatively longer.
  - Repetitive stress: Activities with forceful gripping and twisting can functionally create the same jamming effect, even if the bones are of normal length, that is, repetitive forceful loading of the wrist in pronation and ulnar deviation, such as in gymnasts, boxers, and athletes of racquet sports (3).

GENERAL PREVENTION

Prevention in the repetitive loading population includes activity modification and functional bracing when needed. In patients with acquired ulnar impaction syndrome, most commonly secondary to traumatic shortening of the distal radius, open reduction and internal fixation of the radius is done to recreate a balanced wrist joint.

COMMONLY ASSOCIATED CONDITIONS

- Scapholunate dissociation
- TFCC tears
- Lunotriquetral ligament tears
- Radial shortening from Colles fracture

DIAGNOSIS

Ulnar impaction syndrome is a clinical diagnosis assisted by radiographic findings.

HISTORY

- Pain on the dorsal-ulnar side of distal radioulnar joint (DRUJ)
- Pain with pronation and ulnar deviation of wrist
- Pain with axial loading

PHYSICAL EXAM

- Painful range of motion (ROM) especially with rotation and ulnar deviation
- Positive ballottement test
- Positive ulnocarpal stress test
- Positive fovea test

DIFFERENTIAL DIAGNOSIS

- Pisotriquetral arthritis
- DRUJ arthrosis
- Neuritis of the dorsal cutaneous branch of the ulnar nerve
- Extensor carpi ulnaris (ECU) subluxation or tendinopathy
- Isolated TFCC tear

DIAGNOSTIC TESTS & INTERPRETATION

- Complete wrist radiograph series, including postero-anterior (PA) wrist to evaluate ulnar variance.
- A pronated grip PA radiograph to evaluate for dynamic ulnar variance
- Radiographic identification of subchondral sclerosis and cystic changes, particularly around the distal ulna and ulnar carpal bones, the lunate and the triquetrum
- Magnetic resonance imaging (MRI) of the wrist without contrast may assist in identifying bony edema and chondral lesions but is not required for diagnosis.

TREATMENT

GENERAL MEASURES

- Nonoperative treatment is first line and includes rest and/or immobilization for 6 to 12 weeks, nonsteroidal anti-inflammatory drugs (NSAIDs), and local corticosteroids (2).
- Female gender, length of symptoms, increased pain scores, and MRI enhancement are factors associated with a higher likelihood of splint immobilization treatment failure (2).

SURGERY/OTHER PROCEDURES

- If nonoperative treatment fails, surgical intervention may be indicated.
- Surgical intervention decreases loading across the ulnocarpal joint and may decompress the TFCC when there is a central lesion (4).
- Ulnar shortening osteotomy (USO) is the gold standard surgical option often paired with a wrist arthroscopy to evaluate TFCC, LTIL, and articular surfaces (5).
- A wafer procedure (WP) may be considered and consists of a partial distal ulnar resection of the dome of the ulnar head.
- USO results in better results in treating pronounced ulna positive variation, whereas WP results in improved grip strength (5).
- Wafer shortening of the ulnar head by 2 to 3 mm does not fix stylocarpal impaction or dorsal subluxation if present.
- If a positive ulnar variance is acquired due to a prior injury to the radius, operative intervention may focus on correcting the radius as opposed to the ulna.

ONGOING CARE

PROGNOSIS

- More studies are needed for prognosis of nonoperative treatment.
- A systematic review of operative treatment showed a 100% satisfaction rate for arthroscopic WP, 89% for open WP, and 84% for USO (6)[A].
- 88% of patients report being satisfied to very satisfied following USO at average of 10-year follow-up despite 30% of patients requiring hardware removal (5)[B].

COMPLICATIONS

Surgical complications include need for hardware removal in USO, nonunion, and need for revision procedures.

REFERENCES

1. Sammer DM, Rizzo M. Ulnar impaction. *Hand Clin.* 2010;26(4):549–557.
2. Shin EK. Impaction syndromes about the wrist. *Curr Rev Musculoskelet Med.* 2023;16(1):1–8.
3. Acott TR, Greenberg JA. Ulnar abutment syndrome in the athlete. *Orthop Clin North Am.* 2020;51(2):227–233.
4. Löw S, Herold A, Unglaub F, et al. Treatment of ulnar impaction syndrome with and without central TFC lesion. *J Wrist Surg.* 2018;7(2):133–140.
5. Yu H, Wang T, Wang Y, et al. Ulnar shortening osteotomy vs. wafer resection for ulnar impaction syndrome: a systematic review and meta-analysis. *Int J Surg.* 2022;104:106725.
6. Stockton DJ, Pelletier ME, Pike JM. Operative treatment of ulnar impaction syndrome: a systematic review. *J Hand Surg Eur Vol.* 2015;40(5):470–476.

CLINICAL PEARLS

- Ulnar impaction syndrome is a degenerative condition involving the abutment of the ulna onto the carpal bones.
- Occurs more frequently in those with positive ulnar variance
- Diagnosis is clinical, aided by radiographic findings.
- If patients do not improve with a course of nonoperative treatment, ulnar-sided osteotomy or WP maybe indicated.

ULNAR TUNNEL SYNDROME

Rachel Young, DO, ATC ▪ Richard A. Okragly, MD, FAMSSM

BASICS

DESCRIPTION

- Defined as compression of the ulnar nerve in Guyon canal at the level of the wrist
- Ulnar nerve is a terminal branch of the medial cord of the brachial plexus (C7–T1) (1),(2).
- Guyon canal is bordered by the volar carpal ligament, transverse retinacular ligament, and laterally by the hook of the hamate.
- The superficial sensory branch and/or the deep motor branch of the ulnar nerve can be involved.
- Synonyms: Handlebar palsy; Guyon canal syndrome
- Types (based on the Shea and McClain classification) (1),(2):
  - I—combined sensory and motor deficit (90%)
  - II—motor deficit only (19%)
  - III—sensory deficit only (61%)

ETIOLOGY AND PATHOPHYSIOLOGY

- Guyon canal is located at the base of the hand on the ulnar side:
  - The borders of Guyon canal are (2),(3),(4):
    - Pisiform (medially)
    - Hook of the hamate (laterally)
    - Volar carpal ligament/pisohamate ligament (volar, roof)
    - Transverse retinacular ligament (floor)
- Guyon canal contents (3):
  - Ulnar nerve
  - Ulnar artery
  - Associated vena comitans
- Traumatic injury to the nerve is caused by trauma to wrist and pressure over the hypothenar eminence (4).
- Nontraumatic ulnar nerve compression is typically caused by anatomic means/variation (4).
- A true motor, true sensory, or mixed injury pattern can be seen, depending on the location of compression.
- The mixed (motor and sensory) type is due to compression in the proximal aspect of Guyon canal before the division of the ulnar nerve into superficial and deep branches (type I).
- True motor type is due to compression of the ulnar nerve at the level of the lower wrist (type II).
- True sensory type is due to compression of the superficial branch of the ulnar nerve at the distal aspect of Guyon canal (type III).

RISK FACTORS

- Environmental trigger factors:
  - Repetitive occupational wrist trauma (occupational neuritis)
  - Baseball catchers, batters
  - Cyclists
  - Hockey goalies
  - Golf and racquet sports
  - Martial arts
  - Wheelchair athletes
  - Cross-country skiing
  - Weight lifters
- Anatomical
- Ganglion cyst
- Lipoma
- Palmaris brevis hypertrophy
- Inflammatory arthritis
- Congenital fibrous bands
- Hook of hamate/pisiform fracture
- Deviant hypothenar muscles
- Ulnar artery aneurysm/thrombosis

GENERAL PREVENTION

- Avoid excessive pressure to ulnovolar aspect of palm.
- Avoid repetitive wrist trauma.
- Ergonomic bicycle grips and/or gloves

COMMONLY ASSOCIATED CONDITIONS

- Cubital tunnel syndrome
- Carpal tunnel syndrome
- Radial nerve compression
- Hook of hamate fractures
- Martin-Gruber ulnar-median anastomosis (15% of population)
- Riche-Cannieu deep ulnar-median anastomosis
- Hypothenar hammer syndrome

DIAGNOSIS

HISTORY

- Ring (4th) and small (5th) finger paresthesias with variable weakness of grip
- Localized pain and tenderness over Guyon canal
- Paresthesias or vascular compromise (coldness and pallor of the 4th and 5th digits, cyanosis, and pain) if the ulnar artery is involved
- Coincidental involvement of the median nerve is common (tingling or numbness or weakness or pain in the 2nd and 3rd digits and the lateral aspect of the 4th digit) (1),(5)[C].

PHYSICAL EXAM

- Depending on the location of the lesion, motor, sensory, or mixed signs may be elicited.
- Sensory (1),(2),(3),(5)[C]:
  - Positive Tinel sign at the pisiform, affecting the medial aspect of the 4th digit and all of the 5th digit.
  - Sensory loss at tip of little finger
  - Hypoesthesia on volar sensory branch without involvement of dorsal sensory branch
- Motor (1),(2),(3),(5)[C]:
  - Weakness with resistance of adductor pollicis and all interossei muscles
  - Late atrophy of the first dorsal interosseous muscle
  - Positive Wartenberg sign: abduction of the small finger due to interosseous and lumbrical compromise
  - Positive Froment sign: activation of flexor pollicis longus to substitute for adductor pollicis
  - Decreased grip strength (40% due to ulnar-innervated muscles)
  - Ulnar claw hand with paralysis of the deep motor branch

DIFFERENTIAL DIAGNOSIS

- Proximal ulnar entrapment (elbow, cervicothoracic spine)
- Calcific tendonitis of flexor carpi ulnaris tendon
- Carpal instability
- Arthropathy of pisotriquetral joint
- Ligamentous wrist injury
- Ulnar artery thrombosis/hypothenar hammer syndrome
- Hypoesthesia on dorsal sensory branch does *not* involve compression in Guyon canal.

DIAGNOSTIC TESTS & INTERPRETATION

Initial Tests (lab, imaging)

Generally, imaging is not needed to make the diagnosis but can be used to establish the etiology or rule out other diagnoses (1),(2),(3),(4),(5)[C]:

- Radiographs to exclude carpal instability and fracture at hook of hamate or pisiform: carpal tunnel view
- Computed tomography (CT) scan to exclude hook of the hamate fractures
- Doppler ultrasound (US) to exclude thrombosis
- US/magnetic resonance imaging (MRI) to exclude ganglion cyst or lipoma as space-occupying lesions and evaluate areas of muscle denervation
- US imaging to assess ulnar nerve within the ulnar tunnel and assist in identifying underlying cause of ulnar tunnel syndrome, potentially guiding surgical planning (2),(3),(4)[C]

Diagnostic Procedures/Other

Electromyogram (EMG) studies to document ulnar nerve pathology (3),(5)[C] and localize area of compression

TREATMENT

Prehospital:

- Avoid aggravating activities, including but not limited to (1),(2),(3),(4),(5)[C]:
  - Repetitive hand motions and activities
  - Heavy grasping and gripping
  - Resting the palm against hard surfaces

MEDICATION

First Line

Nonsteroidal anti-inflammatory drugs (NSAIDs) (1),(2),(3),(4),(5)[C]

Second Line

Landmark or US-guided local injection of corticosteroids (3),(4),(5)[C]

ADDITIONAL THERAPIES

- Conservative treatment to include (1),(2),(3),(4),(5)[C]:
  - Splinting
  - Padding of gloves and handlebars
  - Physical therapy
  - Rest
- Adjust activity to avoid repetitive wrist trauma (4)[C].
- Adjusting bicycle fit and batting grip to reduce hand/wrist pressure

SURGERY/OTHER PROCEDURES

- Surgical exploration of Guyon canal with release of tendinous pisohamate arcade (3)[C],(5)[C]
- Surgery to remove compressive ganglion (3)[C],(5)[C]
- Hook of hamate excision in setting of fracture (3)[C]

ONGOING CARE

FOLLOW-UP RECOMMENDATIONS

Following surgery, proper wound care and pain control are essential.

REFERENCES

1. Węgiel A, Zielinska N, Tubbs RS, et al. Possible points of compression of the ulnar nerve: tricks and traps that await clinicians from an anatomical point of view. *Clin Anat*. 2022;35(2):155–173.
2. Kopcik K. Guyon canal syndrome and handlebar palsy —summary of available knowledge. *J Pre-Clin Clin Res*. 2023;17(1):23–26.
3. Scarborough A, MacFarlane RJ, Mehta N, et al. Ulnar tunnel syndrome: pathoanatomy, clinical features and management. *Br J Hosp Med (Lond)*. 2020;81(9):1–9.
4. Melson M, Tompary A, Karvelas K, et al. A review of current concepts in ultrasound evaluation and management of ulnar nerve pain. *Curr Phys Med Rehabil Rep*. 2022;10(4):265–272.
5. Plancher KD. The athletic elbow and wrist, part II: common overuse injuries. *Clin Sports Med*. 1996;15:347–353.

CLINICAL PEARLS

- Numbness and tingling in the hand are not always signs of carpal tunnel syndrome.
- A good history and physical examination are necessary to accurately diagnose this condition.
- US evaluation of ulnar nerve is a cost and time effective modality that allows for dynamic evaluation, possible identification of causative pathology, assistance in surgical planning and a tool for injection guidance in patients being managed conservatively.
- Nerve conduction velocity (NCV)/EMG can be normal if tested during first few weeks of symptoms.

U

ULTRAVIOLET KERATITIS

Carrie B. Zaslow, MD • Tracy L. Zaslow, MD, FAAP, CAQSM

BASICS

- Also known as photokeratitis or solar keratitis
- Acute syndrome occurs after exposure of the eyes to ultraviolet (UV) radiation.
- Painful but usually self-limited

DESCRIPTION

Exposure to various forms of UV radiation leads to acute onset of redness, pain, tearing, and photophobia in association with epithelial defects of the cornea and conjunctival injection.

ETIOLOGY AND PATHOPHYSIOLOGY

- Cornea transmits light in visible spectrum.
- Cornea absorbs light in UV spectrum:
  - 10–20% of light in UVA spectrum is absorbed.
  - Nearly 100% of UVC light is absorbed and a substantial amount of UVB (1).
- Damage to the cornea in UV keratitis:
  - Results from absorption of light at the transition point between UVB and UVC (290 nm)
  - Occurs from absorption in the corneal epithelium (the most anterior part of the cornea)
  - Causes surface epithelial cells to die and desquamate
  - The epithelial nociceptor terminal axons of the damaged cells are destroyed.
  - Axon destruction causes corneal pain secondary to stimulation of the subepithelial nerve plexus.
  - The eye's tear film is also disrupted by UV exposure.

Genetics

No genetic association

RISK FACTORS

- UV exposure to unprotected eyes associated with various recreational and occupational activities (2),(3)
- Sources of exposure:
  - Outdoor activities
  - Welder's arc burns
  - Snow blindness
  - High-voltage-line short circuits
  - Other solar exposure
  - Sunlamps
  - Damaged metal halide lamps
  - Aquaria disinfection lamps
  - Laboratory or germicidal UV lamps

GENERAL PREVENTION

The mode of prevention depends on the type of exposure:

- Recreational sun exposure: well-fitting sunglasses that meet the American National Standards Institute (ANSI) standards with protection against most UVA and UVB radiation
- Occupational exposure to solar and artificial-solar UV sources: ANSI-approved UV-blocking safety goggles
- Occupational exposure to metal halide or mercury vapor lamps: Adherence to the U.S. Food and Drug Administration (FDA) Radiological Health Program is recommended.

COMMONLY ASSOCIATED CONDITIONS

Facial/eyelid edema and erythema, resulting from the same UV exposure injury

DIAGNOSIS

- Accurate history, including:
  - Type of exposure
  - Timing and duration of exposure
  - Latency from exposure to symptom onset
  - Use of protective eyewear
- Visual acuity testing
- Complete bilateral ocular exam, including:
  - Extraocular movements
  - Slit-lamp exam with and without fluorescein stain of conjunctiva/sclera/cornea
  - Slit-lamp exam of anterior chambers (checking for cell and flare)
  - Intraocular pressure
  - Lenses
  - Eversion of the lids to check for foreign bodies
  - pH exam (to rule out chemical keratitis)

HISTORY

- Exposure without protective eyewear 20 minutes to 12 hours prior to onset of symptoms (4),(5)
- To assess amount of UV radiation with exposure, need to know time of day, season, hemisphere, clouds and haze, atmospheric scattering, and ground reflection
- Symptoms (usually bilateral):
  - Intense pain
  - Photophobia
  - Foreign body sensation
  - Mild to moderate decrease in visual acuity
  - Increased lacrimation

PHYSICAL EXAM

- Topical anesthetic generally is needed to obtain a good physical exam.
- Visual acuity normal or mildly reduced (6)
- Penlight exam:
  - Tearing, injection, chemosis of the bulbar conjunctiva, and corneal haze
  - No discharge present in the tarsal conjunctiva; lack of discharge distinguishes photokeratitis from infectious conjunctivitis.
  - Pupils are usually relatively miotic and react sluggishly.
- Fluorescein exam: confluent superficial punctuate staining between the lids
- Slit-lamp exam:
  - Eversion of the eyelids should not reveal a foreign body.
  - Superficial punctate staining of the cornea
  - Corneal edema and anterior chamber reaction (cell and flare) may be seen.
- A thorough eye exam including fluorescein staining and slit-lamp exam generally is sufficient for diagnosis.

DIFFERENTIAL DIAGNOSIS

- Foreign body of the cornea or eyelids
- Intraocular foreign body
- Corneal abrasion
- Thermal burns
- Toxic epithelial keratopathy (from exposure to chemicals or drugs)
- Exposure keratopathy
- Nocturnal lagophthalmos
- Conjunctivitis
- Stevens-Johnson syndrome
- Infectious keratitis
- Neurotrophic keratopathy
- Contact lens–related problems
- Trauma
- Dry eye syndrome
- Scleritis

DIAGNOSTIC TESTS & INTERPRETATION

Initial Tests (lab, imaging)

- Is typically a clinical diagnosis
- If intraocular foreign body suspected as comorbid condition: Orbit x-ray, computed tomography (CT), ultrasound, ultrasound biomicroscopy, or magnetic resonance imaging (MRI) can aid in diagnosis and localization; MRI and CT are best if globe injury is suspected (4)[B].

Diagnostic Procedures/Other

pH of tear lake: To distinguish from a chemical burn, check pH of tear lake in lower conjunctival fornix; pH should be normal in UV keratitis.

TREATMENT

GENERAL MEASURES

- Treatment is supportive.
- Severe pain from the syndrome should be treated with oral analgesics.
- Although they do have a role in the physical exam, topical anesthetics should *never* be prescribed.
- Emergency department (ED) treatment:
  - Oral analgesics:
    - Mild oral narcotics may be necessary.
    - Pain control is important to allow patient to sleep, thus creating an anatomic patch.
  - Ocular lubrication:
    - Over-the-counter (OTC) lubricant drops or ointment may provide comfort; may use up to 4 times per day. Preservative-free lubricants may be used more frequently without restriction.
  - Antibiotic ointment:
    - To provide prophylaxis against superinfection
    - Has secondary effect of providing lubrication and increasing comfort
  - Cycloplegic drops (optional):
    - May help to relieve photophobia
    - Will induce pupil dilation and inhibit accommodation (causing blurring of near vision)
      - This side effect may preclude use.
      - If used, short-acting agents (i.e., cyclopentolate) is preferable.
  - Pressure patch (optional):
    - Only to be used in very reliable patients who have scheduled follow-ups
    - On the worse eye for 24 hours
    - May provide some relief
    - Has not been proven to aid in expeditious healing

MEDICATION

- Antibiotic ointment (prescribed 3 to 4 times per day for 2 to 3 days):
  - Erythromycin
  - Bacitracin
  - Polymyxin-bacitracin
- Cycloplegics:
  - Cyclopentolate 1%

ADMISSION, INPATIENT, AND NURSING CONSIDERATIONS

- Initial stabilization:
  - Topical anesthesia helps to obtain:
    - More accurate documentation of visual acuity
    - More thorough eye exam and fluorescein staining
    - Do not prescribe on outpatient basis; interferes with healing and worsens keratitis
- Admission criteria:
  - Patients requiring bilateral patching with severely decreased visual acuity and whose social circumstances make it impossible for the patient to take care of his or her own needs
- Discharge criteria:
  - Nearly all patients may be discharged from the ED following treatment.
  - Lesions usually heal completely within 24 to 48 hours.
  - Ophthalmologist referral for patients who have other eye disorders, if vision is worse than 20/40, or for those who fail to improve significantly after 24 hours.

ONGOING CARE

- Corneal surface regenerates in 24 to 72 hours.
- Surface regeneration leads to symptom resolution.

FOLLOW-UP RECOMMENDATIONS

- Reexamination in 24 to 48 hours
- If symptoms improved: Patient can continue with topical antibiotics QID and discontinue cycloplegic.
- If symptoms not improved and superficial punctate staining is still present: Continue treatment with cycloplegics and antibiotics and refer to ophthalmologist.

Patient Monitoring

Long-term monitoring is generally unnecessary. Patients should be counseled on using protective eyewear.

PATIENT EDUCATION

Depending on their daily activities, patients should be referred to the appropriate resource to learn about protective eyewear:

- ANSI (https://www.ANSI.org)
- FDA Radiological Health Program (https://www.FDA.gov)

PROGNOSIS

Generally, acute, single episodes heal without long-term sequelae.

COMPLICATIONS

Chronic UV exposure can lead to other sequelae:

- Cutaneous melanoma
- Ocular melanoma
- Erythema
- Cataract
- Pinguecula/pterygium
- Nonmelanocytic skin cancer

REFERENCES

1. Young AR. Acute effects of UVR on human eyes and skin. *Prog Biophys Mol Biol*. 2006;92(1):80–85.
2. Izadi M, Jonaidi-Jafari N, Pourazizi M, et al. Photokeratitis induced by ultraviolet radiation in travelers: a major health problem. *J Postgrad Med*. 2018;64(1):40–46.
3. Kwon DH, Moon JD, Park WJ, et al. Case series of keratitis in poultry abattoir workers induced by exposure to the ultraviolet disinfection lamp. *Ann Occup Environ Med*. 2016;28:3.
4. Loporchio D, Mukkamala L, Gorukanti K, et al. Intraocular foreign bodies: a review. *Surv Ophthalmol*. 2016;61(5):582–596.
5. Leung KCP, Ko TCS. Improper use of germicidal range ultraviolet lamp for household disinfection leading to phototoxicity in COVID-19 suspects. *Cornea*. 2021;40(1):121–122.
6. Chan JYY, Chow VWS, Chan CKM, et al. Photokeratitis in outdoor event participants exposed to UV radiation display. *JAMA Ophthalmol*. 2024;142(6):568–571.

ADDITIONAL READING

- American National Standards Institute. Accessed September 20, 2025. https://www.ansi.org
- Bagheri N, Wajda B, eds. *The Wills Eye Manual: Office and Emergency Room Diagnosis and Treatment of Eye Disease*. 7th ed. Wolters Kluwer; 2016.
- U.S. Food and Drug Administration. Accessed September 20, 2025. https://www.fda.gov
- Verma AS, Dwarika D, Bhola RM, et al. Photokeratitis following the manipulation of aquaria disinfection lamps. *Emerg Med J*. 2007;24(3):232.

CLINICAL PEARLS

- A patient with eye pain should not be prescribed topical anesthetic eye drops.
- Abuse of these drops can lead to neurotrophic keratopathy, a loss of corneal sensation leading to epithelial defects.
- Patients must be counseled about use of protective eyewear.

URETERAL, BLADDER, AND URETHRAL TRAUMA

Scott Goodsell, DO • Alex Tomesch, MD, BCEM, CAQSM

BASICS

DESCRIPTION

- Sports-related trauma to the trunk and/or perineum can result in contusion, laceration, or complete transection of the ureter, bladder, or urethra.
- Injury to the genitourinary (GU) tract is overall uncommon. Lower GU tract injuries from blunt or penetrating mechanisms can involve the bladder, urethra, or the external genitalia.
- Ureteral, bladder, and urethral injuries may be associated with pelvic fractures.

EPIDEMIOLOGY

Injury to the GU tract is overall uncommon.

ALERT
Fractures of the pelvis can result in injuries to the urethra, bladder, and ureters.

- Ureteral injury is very rare compared with other GU organs, and traumatic ureteral injury rarely occurs in isolation from blunt trauma, but if present, it is highly associated with concomitant injuries.
- Ureteral injuries account for 1% of all GU injuries.
- Bladder injuries (contusion or rupture) occur in approximately 1.6% of blunt abdominal trauma:
  – Extraperitoneal in 60% and intraperitoneal in 30%
- Urethral injuries account for 4% of all GU trauma and are divided by the perineal membrane into the anterior and posterior urethra (1).
- With posterior urethral injuries, there is a concomitant bladder injury 15% of the time.
- Although males are susceptible to blunt injury of the urethra, this type of injury is uncommon in females due to shorter length, higher elasticity, and relative mobility. However, female urethral injuries are associated with up to 6% of pelvic fractures (1).
- Impingement of the bulbous urethra against the pubic symphysis results in urethral injuries from the straddle mechanism.
- Straddle injuries in females may result in labial hematoma and urinary retention. These injuries have been reported in in-line skating.
- Most posterior urethral injuries occur by a shearing mechanism.

ETIOLOGY AND PATHOPHYSIOLOGY

Bladder injuries are broadly classified as extraperitoneal (i.e., injury confined to extraperitoneal space) or intraperitoneal (i.e., injury communicating with the peritoneum).

Genetics

- No specific genetic predisposition for GU injuries
- Genetic malformations and solitary kidney are often diagnosed in young children after workup for GU trauma and must be considered for clearance to play.

RISK FACTORS

- In children with multiple injuries, GU injuries are common (2).
- Although rare, avulsion of the ureter secondary to blunt trauma is known to occur in children (3).
- Rupture of the bladder may occur following blunt or penetrating trauma. The bladder is especially at risk for injury when full (2),(4).
- Children have greater risk of bladder injury in trauma due to its position above the pelvic ring and less rectus muscle tone (2),(4),(5).
- Bladder injuries often occur in association with pelvic fractures (4),(5).

GENERAL PREVENTION

Appropriate protective equipment for contact sports is recommended.

COMMONLY ASSOCIATED CONDITIONS

- Urethral injuries in children may result from a straddle mechanism (i.e., direct trauma to the perineum commonly due to contact with the crossbar of a bicycle) (4).
- Patients admitted with multiple trauma injuries will have associated GU injuries 10% of the time (2).

DIAGNOSIS

HISTORY

- Ureter: trauma to the back or flank, hematuria, expanding flank mass (3)[C]:
  – Suspect traumatic ureteral injury if (i) an appropriate mechanism of injury; (ii) new symptoms of fever, flank pain, sepsis, and/or ileus occur following initial trauma stabilization; or (iii) following pelvic surgery (3)[C].
- Bladder: hematuria, urethrorrhagia, or inability to void following a traumatic injury to the abdomen (4)[C]
- Urethra: trauma to the pelvis possibly resulting in pelvic fracture, penile fracture, urethrorrhagia, hematuria, inability to void, and lower abdominal or perineum pain (1)[C]

PHYSICAL EXAM

- Clinical features that should increase suspicion for lower GU tract injury include suprapubic tenderness, hematuria, blood at the urethral meatus, and difficulty voiding, although these are nonspecific (3)[C].
- Ureter: flank pain, flank mass (urine or hematoma), lower abdominal pain, urinary urgency, hematuria, fever, chills, rarely shock (2),(3)[C]
- Bladder: hematuria, urethrorrhagia, or inability to void (3)[C]
- Urethra: urethrorrhagia and inability to void, especially if pelvic fracture is present or suspected, rectal exam reveals a floating or absent prostate; ecchymosis, hematoma, or swelling of the external genitalia or perineum, or blood at the urethral meatus (1),(3)[C]
- Urethral damage in females (usually with pelvic fractures) may show hematuria, labial swelling, or blood within the vaginal introitus (1)[C].
- Localized tenderness: ureter, flank pain; bladder, abdominal pain; urethra, perineum pain
- Peritoneal signs can occur with extravasation, especially of the bladder (3)[C].
- Look for ecchymosis in the pubic area or perineum (3)[C].
- Findings consistent with pelvic fracture (2),(5)[C]

DIFFERENTIAL DIAGNOSIS

- Hematuria: kidney contusion, kidney laceration, sports-induced hematuria, kidney failure, renal calculi, cystitis
- Inability to void: kidney failure, renal calculi, kidney laceration, prostatic hypertrophy, cauda equina

DIAGNOSTIC TESTS & INTERPRETATION

Initial Tests (lab, imaging)

ALERT
Hematuria on urinalysis, although nonspecific, can be an indication of lower collecting system injury (urethra, bladder, ureter) (2),(3)[C].

- The degree of hematuria is not necessarily correlated with the degree of injury. Small urethral injuries may present with significant gross blood. Large ureteral injuries may present with microscopic hematuria (1)[C].
- Hematuria is present in <1/2 of patients with a ureteral injury (3)[C].
- Pelvic fractures, lower rib fractures, and spinal vertebrae fractures, seen on either x-ray or CT, should raise suspicion of an associated GU injury (5)[C].
- Ureter: in hemodynamically stable patients, contrast-enhanced computed tomography (CT) scan of the abdomen/pelvis recommended to diagnosis of ureteral injury:
  – Identification of ureteral injuries requires a delay of 5 to 10 minutes after the administration of intravenous (IV) contrast to allow contrast to reach the ureters.
- Bladder: Retrograde cystography can establish presence of bladder rupture (3)[B].
- Urethra: Retrograde urethrography (RUG) is diagnostic (5),(6)[C].
- If urethral damage is suspected, one must perform an RUG prior to urethral catheterization, as to not worsen possible urethral injury (1)[C].
- Children should have CT scan if they have gross hematuria or significant microscopic hematuria >50 red blood cells (RBCs) per high-power field (5)[C].
- Isolated microscopic hematuria in children with blunt trauma are unlikely to have significant urologic injury. However, if there is associated injuries they are at much higher risk, and preexisting renal abnormalities are often diagnosed in the trauma setting for microscopic hematuria, so these should be worked up (5)[C].
- Ultrasound (US) is not reliable at differentiating urine and blood. Thus, US is not the imaging technique to use in patients with high risk of bladder injury (6)[B].

Follow-Up Tests & Special Considerations

- Direct inspection of the ureters in the operating room is the most sensitive method to assess for ureteral injury (3)[B].
- IV dyes (e.g., methylene blue, indigo carmine) can be used to aid the assessment looking for dye leakage along the course of the ureter (3),(4)[B].

Diagnostic Procedures/Other

When CT of the abdomen/pelvis and CT cystogram are both needed for the evaluation of pelvic trauma, the CT cystogram should be performed after the corticomedullary phase of the CT scan (to assess possible kidney injury) or the arterial phase (to assess other injuries).

- Waiting will prevent extravasated bladder contrast from obscuring vascular injuries that may benefit from urgent angioembolization (3),(6)[A].

Test Interpretation

- Pelvic fracture patterns associated with high risk of GU injury are pubic rami fractures of all four rami, ipsilateral rami fracture with massive posterior disruption of the sacrum, sacroiliac joint, or ilium (3)[B].
- Pelvic fracture patterns associated with low risk are single rami fractures, ipsilateral rami fractures without ring disruption (3)[B].
- Very little risk of ureteral injury with isolated fractures of acetabulum, ilium, and sacrum (6)[C]

TREATMENT

GENERAL MEASURES

ALERT
Because these injuries are often associated with trauma and multiple injuries, stabilization of the patient is the most important (3)[C].

- Signs of shock may be present and should be addressed immediately (3)[C].
- Other more life-threatening organ trauma, renal injuries, for example, likely will need to be addressed first (3)[C].
- Analgesia: Oral analgesia may be adequate; however, pain from associated trauma may require intramuscular (IM) or IV administration of narcotics (6)[C].
- Prognosis is good for full recovery if the injury is diagnosed early and treated appropriately (3)[A].
- Most patients will require urologic consultation and possible surgical intervention (6)[C].

ALERT
- Urinary drainage is an essential aspect of the acute management of a suspected lower GU tract injury. Blind catheter passage prior to lower GU tract imaging is discouraged (3),(6)[B].
- Co-management should address concerns regarding the placement of any suprapubic catheters in patients who are likely to need surgery to repair pelvic fractures (3)[C].
- Most pelvic fracture urethral injury (PFUI) cases should have suprapubic tube placement (open or percutaneous) for urinary drainage, preferably with Foley latex catheter 14 Fr or larger (6)[C].
- Bladder injuries are broadly classified anatomically as extraperitoneal (i.e., injury confined to extraperitoneal space) simple or complex or intraperitoneal (i.e., injury communicating with the peritoneum) (4)[C]:
  - Complex extraperitoneal bladder injuries include bladder neck injury, open pelvic fracture with impinging bone into the bladder, concomitant rectal and/or vaginal injury (3),(4),(6)[A].
- The management of bladder injuries is according to anatomic classification (4)[A]:
  - Simple extraperitoneal bladder injuries begin with conservative management with transurethral catheter drainage and prophylactic antibiotics, which are safe, having a high rate of spontaneous bladder healing within 2 to 3 weeks (4),(5),(6)[C].
  - Complex extraperitoneal bladder injuries are managed with early surgical repair rather than bladder catheter drainage alone. These injuries are not likely to heal with urethral catheter drainage alone (4)[C].
  - Early repair is also reasonable for patients with pelvic fracture who require open reduction/fixation or who have other indications for laparotomy (4)[C].
- Traumatic intraperitoneal bladder injuries should be repaired because they are typically large and will not heal with catheter drainage (4)[C].

ISSUES FOR REFERRAL

Referral to trauma and general surgery is emergent if a lower collecting system injury is suspected.

ADDITIONAL THERAPIES

- Special considerations:
  - Ureteral fistulas and strictures can occur as a result of missed injuries or from entrapment associated with fibrosis from healed dislocation of sacroiliac joints, which may require either stent placement or surgical intervention (3),(6)[C].
  - IV pyelogram should be performed prior to the cystogram (3)[C].
  - RUG should be performed prior to catheterization in the male athlete who has sustained a pelvic fracture and is unable to void following the trauma (4)[C].
- Rehabilitation:
  - No specific rehabilitation, but general reconditioning is usually required following the period of convalescence.
  - Following surgical procedures, rehabilitation exercises directed at the back or pelvic musculature may be necessary.

SURGERY/OTHER PROCEDURES

- Ureteral injuries generally require some form of treatment:
  - Minimal blunt ureteral injuries and partial penetrating injuries (<50% of circumference) may be amenable to ureteral stenting alone (5)[C].
  - Ureteral repair should be performed when injury is identified at the time of laparotomy, if possible.
  - For severe injuries, ligation of the ureter with urinary drainage and delayed reconstruction may be necessary.
  - Transection of the ureter requires prompt repair, ureteropyelostomy (2),(3)[C].
- Any bladder rupture associated with pelvic fracture where penetration of the bladder by a bony spicule is possible is best managed with surgical débridement (2),(3)[C].
- Intraperitoneal rupture of the bladder is appropriately treated with transperitoneal exploration, débridement, and repair (6)[C].
- Initial management of urethral injuries remains controversial. Although early exploration and realignment have been successful, lower complication rates have been found with conservative treatment and delayed realignment (4),(6)[C].

ONGOING CARE

FOLLOW-UP RECOMMENDATIONS

- Delayed diagnosis of ureteral injury can result in nephrectomy (6)[C].
- Small, uncomplicated extraperitoneal rupture of the bladder may be managed nonoperatively with a urethral catheter for 7 to 14 days (3)[C].
- Urethral Injuries can develop delayed stricture formation/recurrence, erectile dysfunction, and incontinence over at least the first year. Patient should follow up at 1-, 3-, 6-, and 12-month intervals and then yearly thereafter (1)[C].

Patient Monitoring

- After bladder injury, a repeat cystogram is usually recommended at 7 to 10 days to exclude persistent leakage (5)[C].
- Repeat imaging is recommended prior to catheter removal to ensure that bladder or urethral healing has occurred, regardless of whether the injury was managed conservatively or required surgery (3)[C].
- Bladder injuries requiring surgery are repaired with a two-layer closure with urethral catheter drainage for 2 to 3 weeks (3)[C].
- Dual catheter drainage (suprapubic tube, urethral catheter drainage) may be warranted in select circumstances (3)[C].
- Cystography is recommended prior to catheter removal to ensure complete healing has occurred regardless of whether the injury was managed conservatively or required surgery (3)[C].
- Avoidance of imaging for simple intraperitoneal repairs has also been advocated (3)[C].

PROGNOSIS

Full recovery and return to sports is expected but will be influenced by surgical procedure.

REFERENCES

1. Patel AB, Osterberg EC, Satarasinghe PN, et al. Urethral injuries: diagnostic and management strategies for critical care and trauma clinicians. *J Clin Med*. 2023;12(4):1495.
2. McGeady JB, Breyer BN. Current epidemiology of genitourinary trauma. *Urol Clin North Am*. 2013; 40(3):323–334.
3. Phillips B, Holzmer S, Turco L, et al. Trauma to the bladder and ureter: a review of diagnosis, management, and prognosis. *Eur J Trauma Emerg Surg*. 2017;43(6):763–773.
4. Gomez RG, Ceballos L, Coburn M, et al. Consensus statement on bladder injuries. *BJU Int*. 2004;94(1):27–32.
5. Singer G, Arneitz C, Tschauner S, et al. Trauma in pediatric urology. *Semin Pediatr Surg*. 2021;30(4): 151085.
6. Morey AF, Brandes S, Dugi DD III, et al. Urotrauma: AUA guideline. *J Urol*. 2014;192(2):327–335.

ADDITIONAL READING

- Asmundo L, Sgrazzutti C, Vanzulli A. Imaging of urologic trauma. *Urol Clin North Am*. 2025;52(1):61–73.
- Bryan ST, Coleman NJ, Blueitt D, et al. Bladder problems in athletes. *Curr Sports Med Rep*. 2008; 7(2):108–112.
- Chapple C, Barbagli G, Jordan G, et al. Consensus statement on urethral trauma. *BJU Int*. 2004;93(9):1195–1202.
- Johnsen NV, Dmochowski RR, Young JB, et al. Epidemiology of blunt lower urinary tract trauma with and without pelvic fracture. *Urology*. 2017; 102:234–239.
- Kong JP, Bultitude MF, Royce P, et al. Lower urinary tract injuries following blunt trauma: a review of contemporary management. *Rev Urol*. 2011;13(3):119–130.
- Lumen N, Kuehhas FE, Djakovic N, et al. Review of the current management of lower urinary tract injuries by the EAU Trauma Guidelines Panel. *Eur Urol*. 2015;67(5):925–929.
- Sahai A, Ali A, Barratt R, et al. British Association of Urological Surgeons (BAUS) consensus document: management of bladder and ureteric injury. *BJU Int*. 2021;128(5):539–547.
- Styn NR, Wan J. Urologic sports injuries in children. *Curr Urol Rep*. 2010;11(2):114–121.

CLINICAL PEARLS

- Suspect traumatic ureteral injury if (i) an appropriate mechanism of injury; (ii) new symptoms of fever, flank pain, sepsis, and/or ileus occur following initial trauma stabilization; or (iii) following pelvic surgery.
- Clinical features that should increase suspicion for lower GU tract injury include suprapubic tenderness, hematuria, blood at the urethral meatus, and difficulty voiding, although these are nonspecific.
- Repeat imaging is recommended prior to catheter removal to ensure that bladder or urethral healing has occurred, regardless of whether the injury was managed conservatively or required surgery.
- Retrograde cystography (fluoroscopic or CT imaging) is the only imaging study to establish a diagnosis of bladder injury.

U

VENOUS THROMBOEMBOLISM IN ATHLETES

Anant Shukla, MD • Caitlyn C. Mooney, MD, FAAP, CAQSM

BASICS

DESCRIPTION

- A deep vein thrombosis (DVT) is a blood clot in a deep vein (deep to the fascia). It is most common in the lower extremity but can occur elsewhere.
- A pulmonary embolism (PE) is a blockage of the pulmonary artery, most commonly from a DVT that has broken off and embolized to the lungs.
- PE and DVT are different ends of the clinical spectrum of the same disease process (venous thromboembolism [VTE]).
- Paget-Schroetter syndrome or "effort thrombosis" occurs most commonly in the dominant arm of overhead athletes due to repetitive arm activity. The location is typically in the axillary or subclavian veins.

EPIDEMIOLOGY

Incidence

- Estimated 900,000 affected in the United States yearly (1 to 2 per 1,000)
- Rates increase with age
- There is limited data on the incidence of VTE in athletes, with most data from case series.
- Untreated PE has a mortality rate as high as 30–50%.
- 15% of cases of sudden death are attributed to PE.
- Upper extremity DVTs are much less common than lower extremity and account for <10% of all DVTs.

ETIOLOGY AND PATHOPHYSIOLOGY

- Clot formation/dissolution is an intricately balanced system that can be influenced by many factors.
- When this balance is disrupted, a clot can form in the veins, forming a DVT. A PE occurs when part of that clot breaks off and travels to the pulmonary arteries disrupting blood flow to the lung.
- Virchow triad refers to three broad categories of factors contributing to thrombus formation: hypercoagulability, hemodynamic changes such as turbulence or stasis, and endothelial injury.

Genetics

Hereditary thrombophilia increase the risk of VTE and include factor V Leiden mutation, protein C or S deficiencies, prothrombin G20210 mutation, and antithrombin deficiency.

RISK FACTORS

- Regular exercise generally has a protective effect to VTE; however, athletes still may possess risk factors.
- It is postulated that athletes are at increased risk for VTE due to several reasons, including long travel distances, dehydration, hemoconcentration, direct trauma and microtrauma to tissues, stasis caused by bradycardia, venous compression from muscle hypertrophy, transient hypercoagulability after endurance events, and increased venous compliance. Case studies and expert opinion support these claims.
- Injured athletes may experience endothelial injury and stasis, both from injuries themselves and their management (immobilization or surgery).
- Some performance-enhancing drugs may increase the risk of VTE, including testosterone and erythropoietin.
- Additional risk factors:
  - Hypercoagulable states (often multiple concomitant):
    - Cancer (particularly lung, pancreas, colorectal, kidney and prostate)
    - Myeloproliferative disorders
    - Nephrotic syndrome
    - Sepsis
    - Infections such as COVID-19
    - Inflammatory conditions:
      - Ulcerative colitis, Crohn disease
    - Hormone alterations:
      - Pregnancy/postpartum
      - Exogenous hormones (oral contraceptive pills [OCPs], hormone replacement therapy [HRT])
      - Testosterone supplements
    - Antiphospholipid syndrome
    - Proteins S and C and antithrombin deficiencies, factor V Leiden, prothrombin gene mutations, lupus, others
  - Stasis:
    - Prolonged bed rest and immobility (from a cast)
    - Long plane, car, or train rides
    - Neurologic disorders with paralysis
    - Congestive heart failure (CHF)
  - Vascular concerns/damage:
    - Trauma
    - Surgery, particularly orthopedic surgeries
    - Intravenous drug abuse
    - Dialysis
    - Anatomic anomalies (May–Thurner syndrome, congenital heart disease, Paget–Schroetter)
    - Central lines/pacemaker placement
  - Multifactorial issues:
    - Advancing age
    - Obesity
    - Comorbid conditions (diabetes, hypercholesterolemia, hypertension)
    - Other medications (glucocorticoids, some antidepressants, and others)
    - Thoracic outlet syndrome
    - Tobacco use
    - Prior DVT or PE
  - Genetics:
    - Family hx of DVT/PE is an independent risk factor.

Pregnancy Considerations

Pregnancy is a risk factor for DVT up to 6 weeks postpartum. Treatment is multidisciplinary, including patient, ObGyn.

Geriatric Considerations

Age is a risk factor. Treatment considerations are complicated due to comorbid conditions, fall risk, etc.

GENERAL PREVENTION

- Avoid prolonged immobility.
- Hydrate adequately.
- Consider compression stockings when immobilized or for flights. (Cochrane Review demonstrated a decrease in asymptomatic DVT in flights >5 hours in high-risk/low-risk travelers with compression socks. Unable to show a reduction in symptomatic DVT/PE as no such events occurred (1)[A].
- Recommend use of low-estrogen pills or progestin-only contraceptives in high-risk groups (family hx of VTE for example).
- High-risk individuals can take a direct oral anticoagulant (DOAC), low-molecular-weight heparin (LMWH), or aspirin for prophylaxis for long flights.
- Move, hydrate, and avoid cramped seating for flights.
- Appropriate prophylaxis for hospitalized, injured, postop patients

DIAGNOSIS

- Despite being conditions with relatively high morbidity and mortality, athletes often have a delay in diagnosis of PE and DVT, which is likely multifactorial.
- Practitioners may be unfamiliar with recognizing VTE in young and active individuals.
- Many of the symptoms are common postexercise symptoms, such as muscle pain, cramping, leg discomfort, and even mild shortness of breath and thus may not be recognized as serious complaints.
- Athletes often have bradycardia and lung reserve and thus are less likely to present with tachycardia or shortness of breath at rest with a PE.
- In general, diagnosis is based on clinical suspicion followed by an evaluation of lab and imaging.
- The diagnosis of VTE in athletes requires a high index of suspicion as most clinical decision tools such as Wells DVT/PE or PE rule out criteria (PERC) have been shown to fail to pick up athletes with these conditions (2)[C].

HISTORY

- Classic symptoms of DVT are swelling, pain, and discoloration in the extremity; may be asymptomatic
- Classic symptoms of PE include sudden-onset pleuritic chest pain, shortness of breath, and cough. Patients can present with insidious onset of symptoms such as anxiety, light-headedness, palpitations, and fatigue. Additionally, patients can present with sudden cardiopulmonary collapse or cardiac arrest.

PHYSICAL EXAM

- Signs of DVT: Inspection of the extremity may reveal ipsilateral edema and erythema: >1- to 2-cm difference in leg circumference.
- Palpation of the extremity may reveal a palpable cord, increased warmth, and superficial venous dilation.
- Phlegmasia cerulea dolens: reddish purple lower extremity from venous engorgement and obstruction
- Homan sign is a test for DVT that involves abrupt passive dorsiflexion of the ankle with the knee in partial flexion. It has low sensitivity and specificity and minimal diagnostic value.
- Signs of pulmonary embolus: tachycardia (relative tachycardia for well-conditioned athletes); tachypnea; low-grade fever

DIFFERENTIAL DIAGNOSIS

- DVT
- Cellulitis
- Superficial thrombophlebitis
- Torn muscle and/or ligaments
- Ruptured Baker cyst (bilateral)
- Edema secondary to heart, liver, or kidney disease
- Delayed-onset muscle soreness
- Venous valvular insufficiency/varicose veins
- Leg edema from medical cause: drug induced, lymphedema
- Postthrombotic syndrome
- Stress fractures or other bony lesions
- PE
- Asthma
- Panic attack/anxiety
- Cardiogenic chest pain/pericarditis
- Costochondritis/musculoskeletal chest pain
- Acute chest syndrome
- Fat embolism
- Pneumothorax

DIAGNOSTIC TESTS & INTERPRETATION

- D-dimer: a protein product of blood clot breakdown
- D-dimer test: concentration of D-dimer in the blood; laboratory test for the evaluation of VTE
- D-dimer test is sensitive for VTE but not specific, meaning that a negative result essentially excludes VTE, but a positive result does not confirm.
- Compression ultrasound (US): imaging study for DVT
  - Standard first-line diagnostic test:
    - Proximal (common femoral/femoral/popliteal veins) or whole leg

- Normal veins compress; those with clots do not.
- Color Doppler can be useful for identifying the vein but does not substantially increase accuracy.
- Duplex scanning refers to the combination of compression B-mode US and color Doppler.
- Duplex US has a sensitivity in the high 90% range.
- Should be repeated in 48 to 72 hours in high-risk patients with negative US
- Current recommendations: Patients with low/moderate pretest probability should be screened using D-dimer first, followed by US only if positive. Patients with high pretest probability should be screened by the US only.
- Venography is the gold standard for the diagnosis of Paget-Schroetter syndrome.
- Chest x-ray (CXR) should be performed in upper extremity cases in addition to US.
- PE: computed tomography (CT) angiography (gold standard) (3)[A]:
  - High sensitivity (0.94) and specificity (0.98)
  - Contraindicated in kidney failure
- V/Q scan if CT angiography is not available
- In certain situations such as unprovoked VTE (one without an identifiable provoking cause), a lab workup should be considered for conditions that can cause thrombophilia, including factor V Leiden, prothrombin, serum homocysteine, factor VIII level, lupus anticoagulant, protein C and S levels, antithrombin activity, and anticardiolipin antibodies.
- Lab studies assist in determining the athlete's risk for recurrence and guide long-term anticoagulation tx.

TREATMENT

Outpatient treatment for proximal DVT and clinically significant PE:

- Anticoagulation (4)[A],(5)[A]
- Systemic anticoagulation:
  - Anticoagulation is recommended in the treatment of VTE in patients without contraindications due to morbidity and mortality associated with PE.
  - Options include unfractionated heparin, LMWH, warfarin, fondaparinux, or DOAC.
  - DOAC: factor Xa inhibitors or direct thrombin inhibitors (DTIs)
  - No specific medication has been proven to be superior. Still, due to ease of use, oral administration, short half-life, lack of required lab monitoring, and less major bleeding, DOACs, are currently the treatment of choice.
  - Dabigatran, rivaroxaban, and apixaban are typically first line except where contraindicated.
  - DOACs are not recommended in catheter-associated DVT, breastfeeding, and pregnant patients.
  - Absolute contraindications to anticoagulation include intracranial bleeding, severe active bleeding, recent brain, eye, and spinal cord surgery, pregnancy, and malignant hypertension.
  - Counseling on the risk of bleeding is important; can use VTE-BLEED scoring tool
  - Counsel athletes in sports with impact and contact to not participate while on anticoagulation.
- Treatment duration (5)[A]:
  - Provoked DVT/PE: Recommend 3 months of anticoagulation.
  - Unprovoked first time DVT/PE: Recommend 3 months of anticoagulation and nuanced discussion of risk-benefit of (extended-phase) anticoagulation for secondary prevention.
  - The use of lower dose DOACs is recommended when extended-phase treatment is offered.
- Inpatient management of PE varies based on disease severity and other patient factors. Management is currently rapidly evolving due to the emergence of less-invasive interventional treatment options. Anticoagulation medications remain the treatment of choice for most situations currently (5)[A].
- Cardiopulmonary life support may be required in severe cases.
- Vena cava filters (5)[A]
  - The main indication is for patients with contraindications to systemic anticoagulation and recurrent VTE with adequate anticoagulation.
    - Additional indications are controversial due to the lack of evidence of benefits and associated risks. Risk of complications include filter migration, embolization, breakage, and endothelial damage.
- Exercise/return to play:
  - Previously, bed rest was recommended during the acute phase. Recent studies suggest mobilization/walking is safe immediately after VTE and may reduce symptoms.
  - Strenuous exercise before 3 weeks is not recommended, as the clot stabilizes. After 3 weeks, a gradual progression in return to activity can be initiated, starting with activities with less load, such as swimming and stationary cycling. Contact sports should not be resumed until after the cessation of anticoagulation or with intermittent treatment.
  - For elite athletes who play a contact or impact sport and are on extended DOAC treatment, consideration of an intermittent DOAC may be applicable. In this setting, the short half-life of DOACs allows the athlete not to take the medications when active and restart a few hours later, in the absence of any major trauma (6)[C].

MEDICATION

- Rivaroxaban: 15 mg PO BID with food for 21 days and then 20 mg PO daily with food afterward; secondary prophylactic dosing 10 mg PO daily.
- Apixaban: 10 mg PO BID for 7 days and then 5 mg PO BID afterward; secondary prophylactic dosing 2.5 mg PO BID
- Dabigatran: 150 mg PO BID after 5 to 10 days of parenteral anticoagulation
- Enoxaparin: 1 mg/kg subcutaneous (SC) BID
- The risk of major bleeding events secondary to anticoagulation medication varies based on the patient population but is described as 1–4% per year.

ISSUES FOR REFERRAL

Cardiology, pulmonary, hematology, or anticoagulation referrals may be warranted based on physician comfort with VTE or for complex cases.

ONGOING CARE

FOLLOW-UP RECOMMENDATIONS

Patient Monitoring

Patients should be monitored for signs of VTE progression to PE, major bleeds, recurrence, and for possible complications such as signs and symptoms of postthrombotic syndrome and pulmonary hypertension.

PATIENT EDUCATION

When traveling, patients should sit in seats that allow leg extension, take hourly walking breaks, wear loose clothing, and avoid crossing their legs. Hydration is also important during travel. Patients should also be informed of the risks of blood clots prior to at-risk surgeries.

PROGNOSIS

- Both the primary disease process as well as treatment carry significant morbidity and mortality.
- Tx for DVT greatly reduces the risk of progression to PE; untreated risk as high as 50%
- In the setting of unmodifiable risk factors, risk of recurrence is high.
- Risk of recurrence is based on the patient risk factors; there are multiple calculators to assess the risk and thus guide ongoing management.
- Often, long-term anticoagulation tx is recommended for secondary prophylaxis in those who are at high risk for recurrence. Due to the risk of bleeding, long-term anticoagulation can be difficult for active athletes.
- Despite adequate treatment, 1/1,000 patients may develop chronic leg pain consistent with postthrombotic syndrome.
- Up to 50% of PE patients will experience complications, including dyspnea, pulmonary hypertension, cardiac dysfunction, and functional impairment.
- Anxiety, depression, and posttraumatic stress disorder have been recently recognized to affect many with PE, especially in young patients.
- Those on long-term anticoagulation risk bleeding, including life-threatening bleeding.

REFERENCES

1. Clarke MJ, Broderick C, Hopewell S, et al. Compression stockings for preventing deep vein thrombosis in airline passengers. *Cochrane Database Syst Rev*. 2021;4(4):CD004002.
2. Zaleski AL, Taylor BA, Pescatello LS, et al. Performance of wells score to predict deep vein thrombosis and pulmonary embolism in endurance athletes. *Phys Sportsmed*. 2017;45(4):358–364.
3. Patel P, Patel P, Bhatt M, et al. Systematic review and meta-analysis of test accuracy for the diagnosis of suspected pulmonary embolism. *Blood Adv*. 2020;4(18):4296–4311.
4. Wang X, Ma Y, Hui X, et al. Oral direct thrombin inhibitors or oral factor Xa inhibitors versus conventional anticoagulants for the treatment of deep vein thrombosis. *Cochrane Database Syst Rev*. 2023;4(4):CD010956.
5. Stevens SM, Woller SC, Kreuziger LB, et al. Antithrombotic therapy for VTE disease: second update of the CHEST guideline and expert panel report. *Chest*. 2021;160(6):e545–e608.
6. Moll S, Berkowitz JN, Miars CW. Elite athletes and anticoagulant therapy: an intermittent dosing strategy. *Hematology Am Soc Hematol Educ Program*. 2018;2018(1):412–417.

CLINICAL PEARLS

- Leg pain and swelling are common complaints, and DVT is a diagnosis one does not want to miss due to the high morbidity and mortality.
- Athletes have several risk factors that may favor hypercoagulability and VTE.
- VTE can be a clinical challenge, and there is often a delay in diagnosis. Diagnosis can be even more challenging in young, active patients who are less likely to present with classic signs and symptoms of VTE. A high index of suspicion and understanding of diagnosis is necessary.
- Athletes are generally not advised to participate in contact sports while on anticoagulation. Individualized anticoagulation plans for elite athletes may include intermittent dosing.
- Although athletes can still develop VTE, physical activity significantly decreases risk, and thus, encouraging physical activity and limiting sedentary behavior remains an important recommendation for prevention.

VOCAL CORD DYSFUNCTION

Sarah Merrill, MD, CAQSM

BASICS

DESCRIPTION

Vocal cord dysfunction (VCD) is not uncommon and often missed diagnosis in both athletes and nonathletes (1),(2). VCD—also known as paradoxical vocal fold motion or inducible laryngeal obstruction—occurs when inappropriate adduction of the vocal cords results in temporary partial airway obstruction (3),(4). The vocal cords close when they should open, impairing speech and breathing (3),(4). VCD can cause significant appearing symptoms of stridor, wheezing, and apparent upper airway obstruction during exercise (2),(3),(5). Due to these distinctive symptoms, patients or athletes with VCD are frequently misdiagnosed and subjected to unnecessary testing or invasive procedures, such as intubation or tracheostomy (4),(5). A high clinical suspicion and special testing can aid in the accurate diagnosis of VCD (3),(5). Although several interventions have been proposed, there is a lack of conclusive evidence on VCD treatment (5).

EPIDEMIOLOGY

Incidence

Due to widespread underdiagnosis, it is difficult to accurately assess incidence and prevalence (4).

Prevalence

- Prevalence estimates vary widely from 4% to 30% of adults (2),(4).
- 2/3 of those diagnosed with VCD are adults, and 1/3 are children (4).
- 2 to 3 times greater prevalence in females versus males (2),(3)

ETIOLOGY AND PATHOPHYSIOLOGY

- Normally, the true vocal cords open (abduct) on inspiration and close (adduct) on expiration (4),(5).
- Paradoxical vocal cord motion occurs when the true vocal cords inappropriately adduct on inspiration, causing a temporary and reversible partial airway obstruction and transient airway narrowing (5). The degree of the obstruction varies but can result in decreased air flow (5).
- Exercise, underlying asthma, inhaled irritants or allergens, rhinosinusitis, recent respiratory infections, or gastroesophageal reflux disease (GERD) can precipitate or exacerbate VCD (3),(4).
- VCD has also shown an association with social and emotional stressors; however, it is unclear if this correlation is causative or results from the stress of VCD exacerbations (4).
- Although precipitants have been identified, no reliable causative factor has been identified (3),(4).
- The higher female prevalence is thought to be related to female smaller larynx, which is more susceptible to laryngeal obstruction (4).

Genetics

There is no established genetic component to VCD (4).

RISK FACTORS

There is a higher rate of VCD in patients with GERD and chronic rhinitis (4). Exercise in cold air may be a unique trigger (4).

GENERAL PREVENTION

Avoidance of known triggers and treatment of comorbidities (3),(4),(5)

COMMONLY ASSOCIATED CONDITIONS

- Asthma
- Exercise-induced bronchoconstriction (EIB)
- Exercise-induced asthma (EIA)
- GERD
- Chronic rhinitis (2),(3),(5)

DIAGNOSIS

HISTORY

- Patients will typically report episodes of dyspnea on exertion, wheezing sometimes progressing to stridor, and cough (3). These episodes are typically brought on by increased activity, often leading to false or inaccurate diagnosis of EIA (3),(4); however, stress, environmental allergens, GERD, or chemical irritants can also trigger episodes (2),(4).
- Patients may complain of dyspnea, choking sensation, dysphonia, wheezing, and cough during these episodes (3),(4); however, symptoms are typically mild and intermittent (3),(4). They resolve with cessation of exercise (3),(4).
- VCD symptoms tend to occur during peak exercise or immediately following exercise and can last for hours to days (2). Symptoms typically stop and start precipitously (3),(4). EIA/EIB symptoms tend to occur 15 to 20 minutes after exercise and athletes have expiratory wheezing (2),(4). Laryngospasms tend to last a few seconds to minutes (6).
- Symptoms are not typically relieved with albuterol (4),(6).

PHYSICAL EXAM

- Physical exam outside of the acute episode may be normal (4),(5).
- During an acute episode, adventitious breath sounds and/or stridor can be heard on both inspiration and expiration, most prominently over the anterior neck (6).
- Unlike asthma, symptoms are more prominent with inspiration than expiration (3),(4).
- Although patients exhibit apparent air hunger, they often have a normal PaO_2 (>97% O_2 saturation). When there is a decrease in PaO_2, it is usually due to hypoventilation (3),(6).
- Dysphonia may be present as the vocal cords are partially closing on inspiration (3).

DIFFERENTIAL DIAGNOSIS

- Asthma
- EIA
- EIB
- Presence of foreign body
- Vocal cord tumor
- Laryngospasm
- Laryngeal angioedema
- Vocal fold paresis
- GERD
- Nerve injury after cervical or thyroid surgery
- Irritant exposure
- Rhinosinusitis
- Prolapse of supraglottic tissue
- Tracheomalacia
- Laryngomalacia
- Amyotrophic lateral sclerosis
- Psychogenic stridor

DIAGNOSTIC TESTS & INTERPRETATION

Initial Tests (lab, imaging)

- Flexible laryngoscopy is considered the gold standard for diagnosis (2). Laryngoscopy performed during or immediately following exercise (continuous laryngoscopy exercise [CLE] test) reveals inspiratory and early expiratory adduction of the anterior 2/3 of the true vocal cords (2),(3). This exam can be normal if not performed during an acute exacerbation (4).
- Spirometry is often used initially for patients with exertional dyspnea. A flattened inspiratory limb and forced expiratory flow (FEF) 50/forced inspiratory flow (FIF) 50 >1 suggests extrathoracic obstruction consistent with VCD but is not sensitive. Up to 70% of patients can also have a positive methacholine challenge (3).
- Chest x-ray can be used to evaluate for mass occupying lesions and/or infections (3).
- Recent studies found that CT larynx can show inappropriate vocal cord adduction (1).

Follow-Up Tests & Special Considerations

- Impulse oscillometry can be used in patients who cannot cooperate with spirometry, such as children (2).
- 4D computed tomography (CT) has been used experimentally in a small number of patients (2).

TREATMENT

- **Acute management:**
  - Because episodes are often self-limiting, reassurance and supportive measures can be effective (3),(4).
  - Encourage patient to pant, which forces abduction of the vocal cords. Breathing through a straw, pursed-lip breathing, or diaphragmatic breathing can produce similar results (2),(3),(4).
  - Inhalation of a combination of helium and oxygen (heliox) to reduce airway resistance (3),(4)
  - Coexisting asthma should be treated (3).
  - Continuous positive airway pressure (CPAP) (4)
- **Long-term management:**
  - There are no randomized control trials to support therapeutic decisions. Current recommendations are largely based on expert consensus and small studies (3).
  - Education of patient and family members regarding diagnosis (4)
  - Avoidance of known triggers (3)
  - Referral to speech language pathologist for behavioral speech and voice therapy (2),(3),(4),(5)
  - Speech therapy generally focuses on respiratory retraining and abortive techniques for acute episodes, laryngeal and whole-body relaxation techniques, vocal hygiene, and phonation retraining if appropriate (3). The number of recommended sessions has not been established (5).
  - Treat coexisting GERD, rhinitis/allergies, and asthma (3),(4).
  - Behavioral counseling for concurrent depression or anxiety (3),(4)
  - OnabotulinumtoxinA injections into laryngeal muscle spasms have been proposed for severe, recalcitrant cases (3),(4),(5).

MEDICATION

First Line

- A small subset of studies showed some benefit with use of low-dose amitriptyline (10 to 75 mg) (5)
- Case studies have shown some benefit with use of inhaled anticholinergics such as ipratropium prior to exercise (4).
- Generally, inhaled β_2-agonists (albuterol) do not ease symptoms of VCD unless there is a concomitant asthma component to symptoms (3),(5).

SURGERY/OTHER PROCEDURES

In severe, recalcitrant cases, long-term tracheostomy has been performed (3). This is not advocated by the current literature (3),(4),(5).

ONGOING CARE

Education of athletes, parents, and coaches regarding symptoms and treatments is essential for avoiding unnecessary hospitalizations and procedures.

REFERENCES

1. Koh J, Leong P, Bardin PG. A new paradigm for vocal cord dysfunction/inducible laryngeal obstruction: swift diagnosis and streamlined management pathways. *Respirology*. 2023;28(10):911–913.
2. Fretzayas A, Moustaki M, Loukou I, et al. Differentiating vocal cord dysfunction from asthma. *J Asthma Allergy*. 2017;10:277–283.
3. Malaty J, Wu V. Vocal cord dysfunction: rapid evidence review. *Am Fam Physician*. 2021;104(5):471–475.
4. Petrov AA. Vocal cord dysfunction: the spectrum across the ages. *Immunol Allergy Clin North Am*. 2019;39(4):547–560.
5. Mahoney J, Hew M, Vertigan A, et al. Treatment effectiveness for vocal cord dysfunction in adults and adolescents: a systematic review. *Clin Exp Allergy*. 2022;52(3):387–404.
6. Barnes KP. Exercise-induced bronchoconstriction and vocal cord dysfunction in athletes: a brief overview. *Athl Train Sports Health Care*. 2010;2(2):52–56.

CLINICAL PEARLS

- VCD results from the true vocal cords inappropriately adducting on inspiration, causing symptoms of shortness of breath, wheezing, and stridor.
- VCD can be accurately diagnosed by laryngoscopy examination done during or immediately following exercise.
- Treatment of coexisting medical conditions decreases VCD exacerbations.
- Speech therapy and breathing retraining exercises are the current mainstay of VCD therapy.

V

WARTS

Kathleen Weber, MD, MS

BASICS

DESCRIPTION

Warts (verrucas) are caused by a human papillomavirus (HPV) infection, resulting in a variety of lesions on the skin and mucous membranes. Several different HPV genotypes are associated with warts, as noted below.

EPIDEMIOLOGY

- >150 different genotypes of HPV have been identified (1)
- Cutaneous HPV infections, three types:
  - Common warts (verruca vulgaris): 70% of nongenital warts:
    - HPV types 1 to 5, 7, 27, 29 (2)
  - Plantar warts (verruca plantaris): 25–30%:
    - HPV types 1 to 4, 27, 29, 57 (2)
  - Flat warts (verruca plana): 3–4%:
    - HPV types 3, 10, 28, 29 (2)
- 10–30% of children will develop cutaneous warts, with the peak incidence occurring between 12 and 16 years old.
- Common in certain occupations: meat, poultry, and fish handlers
- Mucosal HPV infections:
  - Most common are genital warts (condyloma acuminatum). HPV types 6 and 11. In pediatrics, HPV 1 to 4, 16, and 18 were also detected.
  - Estimated prevalence rate of HPV genital infection in the U.S. adult population is 10–20% (3).

ETIOLOGY AND PATHOPHYSIOLOGY

- HPV infects epithelial tissues and mucous membranes.
- The virus infects the mucosa or the basal layer of the skin, causing cellular proliferation and vascular growth, resulting in a mucosal or skin lesion (3).
- Incubation period, once exposed, varies from weeks to more than a year.

RISK FACTORS

- Cutaneous HPV infections:
  - Transmission: direct or indirect contact; minor superficial abrasions of the skin promote infection (1)
  - Autoinoculation occurs especially in younger children.
  - Risk factors: atopic dermatitis, conditions with decreased cell-mediated immunity (immunocompromised), organ transplantation (1)
- Mucosal HPV infections:
  - Transmission: sexual contact; contact with contaminated objects; autoinoculation; vertical transmission during vaginal delivery (3)
  - Risk factors: unprotected sexual relations, multiple sex partners, immunocompromised

GENERAL PREVENTION

- Warts are infectious: Avoid touching; use footwear in public showers; do not reuse paring instruments such as nail files or pumice stone on normal skin/nails or share with others.
- Cutaneous lesions: no restrictions for participation; coverage recommended
- Mucosal lesions: condoms recommended but not completely effective
- Anogenital warts: The importance of Pap smears should be stressed; screen for other sexually transmitted diseases.
- HPV vaccination is indicated for use in patients who are between 9 and 26 years of age; not recommended for pregnant women (4)
- Ideally, should be vaccinated before first sexual intercourse
- Cervical screening continues to be important as the vaccination is not effective in clearing HPV infection, genital warts, or cervical intraepithelial neoplasia that is already present.
- Male circumcision may decrease male transmission rates (4).

COMMONLY ASSOCIATED CONDITIONS

- Cutaneous HPV infection: Warts may regress spontaneously, more commonly in children than adults (5); immunocompromised individuals may be refractory to all treatment.
- Condylomata recur commonly despite therapy.
- Condylomata are associated with cervical dysplasia and cervical squamous cell carcinoma, invasive carcinoma of genitalia, and anal squamous cell carcinoma.

DIAGNOSIS

- Warts are usually diagnosed based on their appearance (4),(5).
- Paring of the hyperkeratotic surface on common or plantar warts black dots, thrombosed capillaries can help with the diagnosis (5).
- Dermoscopy can help elucidate the difference between a plantar warts and a callus and can be used to monitor therapeutic effects of treatment (6).

HISTORY

- Cutaneous and anogenital warts are usually asymptomatic, but plantar warts can cause discomfort during activities.
- Without treatment, the wart can remain for months to years.

PHYSICAL EXAM

- Verruca vulgaris (common warts):
  - Skin-colored papule, hyperkeratotic with horny surface
  - Normal skin markings are disrupted.
  - Pathognomonic for warts are red-black dots seen on the surface.
  - Can be one or multiple lesions
  - Typically, asymptomatic but may be painful, especially if located over areas of pressure
  - Distribution: fingers, hands (most common), knees; may occur anywhere
- Verruca plantaris (plantar warts):
  - Skin-colored papule with coarse, keratotic surface; has characteristic red-black dots
  - Normal skin markings are disrupted.
  - Painful, especially if located over areas of pressure
  - Distribution: plantar surface of foot
- Verruca plana (flat warts):
  - Skin colored or lightly pigmented; well-defined, smooth, flat, or slightly elevated papules
  - Variety of shapes: round, oval, linear
  - Sizes vary from pinhead to a few millimeters.
  - Numbers range from a few to hundreds
  - Distribution: face; dorsum of the hands; extremities, especially shins
  - Commonly seen in children and less common in adolescents and adults
- Condylomata acuminata (anogenital warts):
  - Skin colored, slightly pigmented, or pink
  - Range from soft, tiny, isolated papules, filiform, and often pedunculated sessile papules to cauliflower masses (3)
  - Distribution: glans penis, prepuce, shaft, labia, vagina, cervix, perianal area, urethra, bladder, rectum, and oral cavity (3)
  - Most asymptomatic or subclinical; may go unrecognized

DIFFERENTIAL DIAGNOSIS

- Verruca vulgaris: callus, guttate psoriasis, molluscum contagiosum, seborrheic keratosis, cutaneous malignancies (squamous cell carcinoma and amelanotic melanoma)
- Verruca plantaris: callus, corn
- Verruca plana: lichen planus, molluscum contagiosum, seborrheic keratosis, moles, skin tags
- Condylomata acuminata: lichen planus, molluscum contagiosum, pearly penile papules, skin tags, squamous cell carcinoma, condyloma lata of secondary syphilis, seborrheic keratosis, vulvar intraepithelial neoplasia (4)

DIAGNOSTIC TESTS & INTERPRETATION

Diagnostic Procedures/Other

- Diagnosis is typically done via clinical examination.
- Lesions on the genital skin can be visualized as white patches by applying 5% acetic acid to the suspected area.
- Confirmed by biopsy if diagnosis unclear by exam

TREATMENT

Warts may eventually spontaneously resolve and may not require treatment (5).

- Reasons to treat: pain, functional impairment, cosmetic, persistent, immunosuppression, anogenital

MEDICATION

First Line

- Self-administered:
  - For cutaneous infections: salicylic acid preparations (10–40%) (2),(5)[A]. Apply directly to the wart, gel/solution apply once or twice daily or if a topical pad/strip apply every 48 hours for 6 to 12 weeks depending on preparation. Avoid facial, genital, mucous membrane, or to inflamed or infected skin.
  - For mucosal lesions: imiquimod 5% cream (4)[A]. Apply 3 times per week (alternating every other day) for up to 16 weeks.
- Clinician administered:
  - For cutaneous infections: cryosurgery (liquid nitrogen): Apply to wart and surrounding normal tissue (2 mm) until surrounding skin is visibly frozen ~15 to 30 seconds; repeat every 2 to 4 weeks for 3 months or six treatments (5); may be painful; if no response with six treatments, consider alternative treatment (2),(4)[B].
  - Combining cryotherapy and salicylic acid treatment has not been proven more effective.
  - For mucosal lesions: trichloroacetic acid 80% (3)[B]. Apply 1 to 3 times per week and repeat as needed.

ISSUES FOR REFERRAL

Referral to a dermatologist or gynecologist should be considered in recalcitrant warts or in immunocompromised patients.

ADDITIONAL THERAPIES

- There is some evidence supporting use of 5-fluorouracil for treatment of cutaneous infections and mucosal lesions (4),(5)[B].
- For mucosal lesions: podophyllotoxin and sinecatechins can be used as self-administered therapies. Podophyllin can be used as a clinician-administered therapy (4)[B].
- Podophyllotoxin and podophyllin are contraindicated during pregnancy (4)[C].
- Although used for cutaneous infections, there is limited evidence of effectiveness for use of duct tape; duct tape is sometimes used in conjunction to treatment with salicylic acid (2)[B].
- There is some evidence of effectiveness for use of pulsed dye laser (PDL) for treatment of cutaneous infections and mucosal lesions (2)[B].

SURGERY/OTHER PROCEDURES

- For cutaneous infections: excision, electrocautery, CO_2 laser surgery (5)[C], and intralesional injections (bleomycin, *Candida*, or mumps skin antigen) (2),(5)[B]
- For mucosal lesions: cryosurgery as described earlier (3)[B], electrocautery or excision (3)[A], CO_2 laser (4)[C]

ONGOING CARE

FOLLOW-UP RECOMMENDATIONS

Patient Monitoring

- Papanicolaou tests screening for cervical cancer at age 21 years old (exception: can consider screening earlier if HIV positive or immunocompromised)
- In cases of extensive or recalcitrant anogenital warts, consider diagnostic evaluation for immunodeficiency, especially HIV (5).

PATIENT EDUCATION

- Advise to observe for recurrence of infection.
- Counsel on associated risk of sexually transmitted infection (STI) transmission.
- Ensure eligible patients are up-to-date on HPV vaccine series (4).

COMPLICATIONS

- Skin irritation
- Infection
- Pain from procedure
- Damage to tendon or nerve

REFERENCES

1. Nunes EM, Talpe-Nunes V, Sichero L. Epidemiology and biology of cutaneous human papillomavirus. *Clinics (Sao Paulo)*. 2018;73(Suppl 1):e489s.
2. Mulhem E, Pinelis S. Treatment of nongenital cutaneous warts. *Am Fam Physician*. 2011;84(3):288–293.
3. Scheinfeld N, Lehman DS. An evidence-based review of medical and surgical treatments of genital warts. *Dermatol Online J*. 2006;12(3):5.
4. Karnes JB, Usatine RP. Management of external genital warts. *Am Fam Physician*. 2014;90(5):312–318.
5. Sterling JC, Gibbs S, Hussain SSH, et al. British Association of Dermatologists' guidelines for the management of cutaneous warts 2014. *Br J Dermatol*. 2014;171(4):696–712.
6. Bhatti A, Chowdhary S, Ferrise T, et al. Plantar verruca and dermoscopy: an update. *Clin Podiatr Med Surg*. 2021;38(4):513–520.

ADDITIONAL READING

- Cordoro KM, Ganz JE. Training room management of medical conditions: sports dermatology. *Clin Sports Med*. 2005;24(3):565–598.
- Curry SJ, Krist AH, Owens DK, et al. Screening for cervical cancer: U.S. Preventive Services Task Force recommendation statement. *JAMA*. 2018;320(7):674–686.
- Herman BE, Corneli HM. A practical approach to warts in the emergency department. *Pediatr Emerg Care*. 2008;24(4):246–251.
- Leerunyakul K, Thammarucha S, Suchonwanit P, et al. A comprehensive review of treatment options for recalcitrant nongenital cutaneous warts. *J Dermatolog Treat*. 2022;33(1):23–40.

CLINICAL PEARLS

- Warts are a result of HPV infection, which can result in common warts, plantar warts, flat warts, and anogenital warts.
- Warts are usually diagnosed based on history and clinical appearance.
- First-line therapy for cutaneous warts is salicylic acid or cryotherapy.
- First-line therapy for mucosal warts is imiquimod or trichloroacetic acid.
- Consider immune deficiency in cases of extensive or recalcitrant warts.

WOLFF-PARKINSON-WHITE (WPW) SYNDROME

Michael Troy, DO ▪ Catherine Carragee, MD ▪ Kenneth S. Taylor, MD, FAAFP, CAQSM

BASICS

DESCRIPTION
A disorder of cardiac conduction caused by accessory pathways between the atria and ventricles leading to ventricular preexcitation

EPIDEMIOLOGY
Incidence
New cases are diagnosed in the general population at a rate of 0.004% per year.

Prevalence
- Ranges from 0.1% to 0.3%
- No significant difference in prevalence is observed between athletic and nonathletic populations
- The syndrome is more commonly observed in males than in females.
- In pediatric cases, sudden cardiac death (SCD) may be the initial clinical manifestation in 10–48% of cases.
- The annual risk of SCD in patients with WPW is estimated to be 0.1–0.45%.
- WPW syndrome accounts for approximately 1% of cases of SCD in athletes (1).

ETIOLOGY AND PATHOPHYSIOLOGY
- The condition arises from the presence of at least one abnormal electrical pathway that bypasses the atrioventricular (AV) node, allowing for the premature delivery of electrical impulses to the ventricles, resulting in preexcitation of the ventricles. The accessory pathways may participate in reentrant tachyarrhythmias by engaging in electrical circuits involving both the accessory pathway and the AV node.
- Associated arrhythmias include:
  - **Orthodromic reentrant tachycardia (type A):** The most common arrhythmia associated with WPW syndrome, characterized by narrow complex supraventricular tachycardia (SVT). It is typically not associated with a significant risk of SCD.
  - **Antidromic reentrant tachycardia (type B):** a less common arrhythmia characterized by wide complex tachycardia
  - **Atrial fibrillation (AF):** Although not a direct result of WPW syndrome, AF in these patients may conduct through the accessory pathway, leading to degeneration into ventricular fibrillation (VF), which poses a significant risk for SCD (2).

Genetics
- Approximately 3–4% of WPW cases are familial.
- A mutation in the PRKAG2 gene has been associated with the syndrome, particularly in patients with left ventricular hypertrophy (3).
- The syndrome follows an autosomal dominant pattern of inheritance.

COMMONLY ASSOCIATED CONDITIONS
- Ebstein anomaly
- Hypertrophic cardiomyopathy
- Ventricular septal defect
- Atrial septal defect
- Corrected transposition of the great arteries

DIAGNOSIS

HISTORY
- Patients may present with symptoms such as palpitations, chest pain, dyspnea, dizziness, fatigue, nausea, or syncope. In some cases, SCD may be the first presenting event (1).
- Symptoms of WPW syndrome may include:
  - Palpitations
  - Chest pain
  - Dyspnea
  - Dizziness
  - Weakness
  - Fatigue
  - Nausea
  - Light-headedness
  - Syncope
- Initial presenting symptom may be SCD.

PHYSICAL EXAM
- Tachycardia:
  - Regular (reentrant SVT)
  - Irregular (AF)
- Signs of instability:
  - Hypotension
  - Chest pain
  - Change in mental status
  - Rales

DIFFERENTIAL DIAGNOSIS
- The differential diagnosis for WPW syndrome includes other causes of SVT, AF, VF, and ventricular tachycardia (VT).
- Electrocardiogram (ECG) finding:
  - The ECG may demonstrate a PR interval of <120 milliseconds in adults and <90 milliseconds in children.
  - A characteristic delta wave is present, representing a slurring of the QRS complex.
  - The QRS duration is typically >120 milliseconds in adults and >90 milliseconds in children.
  - Secondary ST- and T-wave abnormalities may also be noted.
  - Symptomatic patients may present with episodes of SVT, AF, VT, or VF (4).

DIAGNOSTIC TESTS & INTERPRETATION
Diagnostic Procedures/Other
- **Echocardiography** should be performed to assess for any underlying structural cardiac abnormalities.
- **Holter monitoring or event monitoring** may be used to detect paroxysmal arrhythmias.
- **Exercise stress testing** can provide additional information regarding the risk of arrhythmic events
- **Electrophysiologic studies (EPSs)** are performed to map and identify the accessory pathways and to assess the associated arrhythmic risk.
- Risk stratification:
  - Low-risk features:
    - Loss of preexcitation during exercise
    - Intermittent WPW pattern on the ECG
- High-risk features:
  - Short refractory period of the accessory pathway (<250 milliseconds)
  - Short preexcited RR interval during AF (<250 milliseconds)
  - Inducible atrioventricular reentrant tachycardia (AVRT)
  - Presence of multiple accessory pathways (5),(6)

TREATMENT

MEDICATION
Antiarrhythmic agents are generally less effective than catheter ablation and may adversely impact athletic performance.

ISSUES FOR REFERRAL
Patients with WPW on an ECG should be referred to cardiology for further evaluation. Risk stratification is essential to guide management decisions, including the choice of treatment and recommendations for sports participation. Symptomatic or high-risk asymptomatic patients should be considered for treatment interventions, including catheter ablation.

SURGERY/OTHER PROCEDURES
- **Radiofrequency catheter ablation (RFA)** is the treatment of choice for symptomatic patients and those at high risk of arrhythmic events.
- The success rate of RFA is approximately 95%, and recurrence rates range from 0% to 10% within the first year.
- Complications of RFA may include right bundle branch block (RBBB) in 0.5% of cases, left bundle branch block (LBBB) in 0.1%, valve regurgitation in 0.3%, hematoma in 1.4%, and atrioventricular block (AVB) in 0.9%.
- In patients with associated conditions, such as Ebstein anomaly, a repeat RFA may be necessary, with recurrence rates of 25% (7).

ADMISSION, INPATIENT, AND NURSING CONSIDERATIONS

- Stable narrow-complex tachycardia:
  - Vagal maneuvers (e.g., Valsalva or carotid massage, if no bruit is present) are first-line treatment.
  - Intravenous (IV) adenosine is the drug of choice, administered as a 6-mg bolus with a possible second dose of 12 mg if necessary. In pediatric patients, the dose is 0.1 mg/kg.
  - If hypotension or instability is present, fluid resuscitation and positioning (Trendelenburg) should be performed.
- Stable wide-complex tachycardia:
  - The use of procainamide (6 to 13 mg/kg IV bolus) may be effective in terminating the arrhythmia.
  - For cases refractory to pharmacologic therapy, synchronized cardioversion may be required.

ALERT

Never use calcium channel blockers, β-blockers, or digoxin. These medications block the AV node and lead to conduction occurring exclusively down the faster accessory pathway, resulting in fatal ventricular dysrhythmias.

- Unstable patients:
  - Synchronized cardioversion

ONGOING CARE

FOLLOW-UP RECOMMENDATIONS

- Following catheter ablation, patients can typically return to sports 2 to 4 weeks postprocedure.
- Routine follow-up is recommended to monitor for recurrence of arrhythmias, particularly in patients with persistent preexcitation.

PROGNOSIS

- Patients who undergo successful RFA have an excellent prognosis, with a very low risk of SCD.
- Nonablated patients, particularly those with symptomatic arrhythmias, have a higher long-term risk of SCD.
- The incidence of AF remains elevated in both ablated and nonablated patients, with long-term surveillance required for management (6),(8).

REFERENCES

1. Zipes DP, Link MS, Ackerman MJ, et al. Eligibility and disqualification recommendations for competitive athletes with cardiovascular abnormalities: task force 9: arrhythmias and conduction defects: a scientific statement from the American Heart Association and American College of Cardiology. *Circulation*. 2015;132(22):e315–e325.
2. Lampert R, Chung EH, Ackerman MJ, et al. 2024 HRS expert consensus statement on arrhythmias in the athlete: evaluation, treatment, and return to play. *Heart Rhythm*. 2024;21(10):e151–e252.
3. Lu C, Wu M, Chen H, et al. Epidemiological profile of Wolff-Parkinson-White syndrome in a general population younger than 50 years of age in an era of radiofrequency catheter ablation. *Int J Cardiol*. 2014;174(3):530–534.
4. Bunch TJ, May HT, Bair TL, et al. Long-term natural history of adult Wolff-Parkinson-White syndrome patients treated with and without catheter ablation. *Circ Arrhythm Electrophysiol*. 2015;8(6):1465–1471.
5. Di Mambro C, Russo MS, Righi D, et al. Ventricular pre-excitation: symptomatic and asymptomatic children have the same potential risk of sudden cardiac death. *Europace*. 2015;17(4):617–621.
6. Mah DY, Sherwin ED, Alexander ME, et al. The electrophysiological characteristics of accessory pathways in pediatric patients with intermittent preexcitation. *Pacing Clin Electrophysiol*. 2013;36(9):1117–1122.
7. Rao AL, Salerno JC, Asif IM, et al. Evaluation and management of Wolff-Parkinson-White in athletes. *Sports Health*. 2014;6(4):326–332.
8. Van Hare GF, Javitz H, Carmelli D, et al. Prospective assessment after pediatric cardiac ablation: recurrence at 1 year after initially successful ablation of supraventricular tachycardia. *Heart Rhythm*. 2004;1(2):188–196.

ADDITIONAL READING

- Baggish AL, Shah AB. MY APPROACH to the athlete with Wolff-Parkinson-White Syndrome (WPW). *Trends Cardiovasc Med*. 2018;28(2):154–155.
- Ceresnak SR, Dubin AM. Wolff-Parkinson-White syndrome (WPW) and athletes: Darwin at play? *J Electrocardiol*. 2015;48(3):356–361.
- Di Mambro C, Drago F, Milioni M, et al. Sports eligibility after risk assessment and treatment in children with asymptomatic ventricular pre-excitation. *Sports Med*. 2016;46(8):1183–1190.
- Mah DY, Sherwin ED, Alexander ME, et al. The electrophysiological characteristics of accessory pathways in pediatric patients with intermittent preexcitation. *Pacing Clin Electrophysiol*. 2013;36(9):1117–1122.
- Packer DL, Mark DB, Robb RA, et al. CABANA Trial Investigators. Catheter ablation versus antiarrhythmic drug therapy for atrial fibrillation: updated outcomes. *N Engl J Med*. 2023;388(9):816–827.
- Van Hare GF, Javitz H, Carmelli D, et al. Prospective assessment after pediatric cardiac ablation: demographics, medical profiles, and initial outcomes. *J Cardiovasc Electrophysiol*. 2004;15(7):759–770.

CLINICAL PEARLS

- Classic ECG findings are shortened PR interval and presence of delta wave.
- Asymptomatic athletes should be evaluated for the purpose of risk stratification for primary determination of the role of RFA.
- Symptomatic athletes presenting with symptoms clearly attributable to WPW-associated tachyarrhythmias should be considered for RFA prior to return to athlete participation.
- RFA is the first-line treatment for patients who are symptomatic or asymptomatic with high-risk pathways.
- AV nodal blocking agents should not be used in the management of acute tachyarrhythmias among patients with known or suspect WPW physiology.

Appendix A

MUSCULOSKELETAL RADIOGRAPHY

Karen Yik Ting Cheng, MD ▪ Tudor Hesketh Hughes, MD

It is important when ordering radiographic studies to know the most appropriate study to answer the questions at hand. To this end, it is necessary to know which images are obtained when a certain series is requested, and the advantages of each series and projection. Although all centers will have slightly different series, what follows is a general guideline.

As a general rule, computed tomography (CT) is a useful adjunct for intra-articular fracture preoperative planning in larger joints where the fractured bone is to be repaired rather than replaced, or complex areas such as the carpal or tarsal regions. Although CT scan does involve a significant dose of ionizing radiation, this is of most concern centrally rather than peripherally. A full x-ray series of the pelvis or lumbar spine can give a higher radiation dose and less useful information than coned-down CT scan of the area of interest.

Ultrasound (US) is an ideal inexpensive way of assessing superficial soft tissues for both trauma and masses. It has the distinct advantage of being dynamic, imaging the patient in real time as they move, and also being interactive with the patient, assessing their points of pain.

Magnetic resonance imaging (MRI) is a useful method for assessing the soft tissues for injury or mass, and the bones for occult injuries and bone marrow changes.

UPPER EXTREMITIES

FINGERS

For 2nd through 5th digits. Specifically to look at one finger for trauma, foreign body, or localized mass. A marker should be applied, particularly on the lateral projection at the finger of interest. Consider US for radiolucent foreign body. Consider MRI or US for mass or tendon lesion/injury.

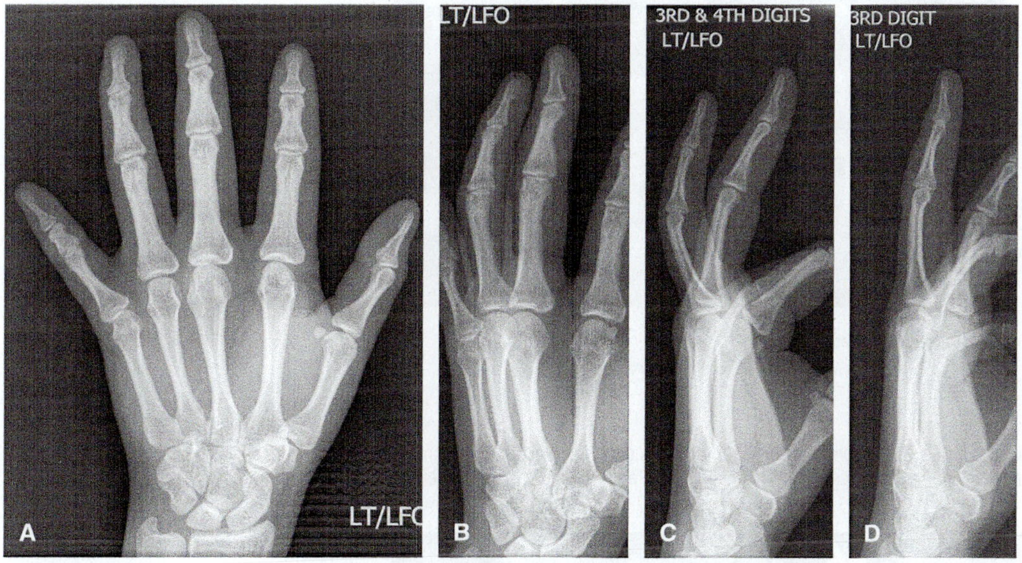

FIGURE 1. A: Posteroanterior (PA) view of hand. B: Oblique view of fingers. C, D: Lateral view of fingers.

THUMB

Specifically to look at the thumb for trauma, foreign body, or localized mass. Good for ulnar collateral ligament (UCL) avulsion. A marker should be applied. Consider US for radiolucent foreign body. Consider MRI or US for mass, UCL injury (without or with Stener lesion) or tendon lesion/injury. Stress views are no longer encouraged for acute UCL injury for fear of converting to a Stener lesion but maybe useful later to assess stability.

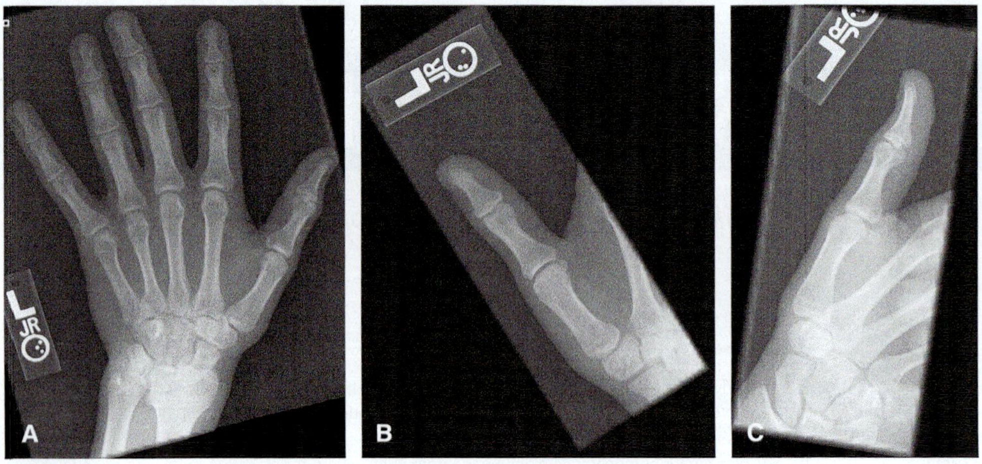

FIGURE 2. A: PA view of hand. B: PA view of thumb. C: Lateral view of thumb.

HAND
Routine

This includes an off-axis view of the wrist but should not be used to assess wrist alignment. Good overview for hand pain. May need additional wrist views if pain is proximal or difficult to localize. Important to have fingers spread on lateral view so that all volar plates are well visualized. MRI or US may be useful adjuncts to look at adjacent soft tissues.

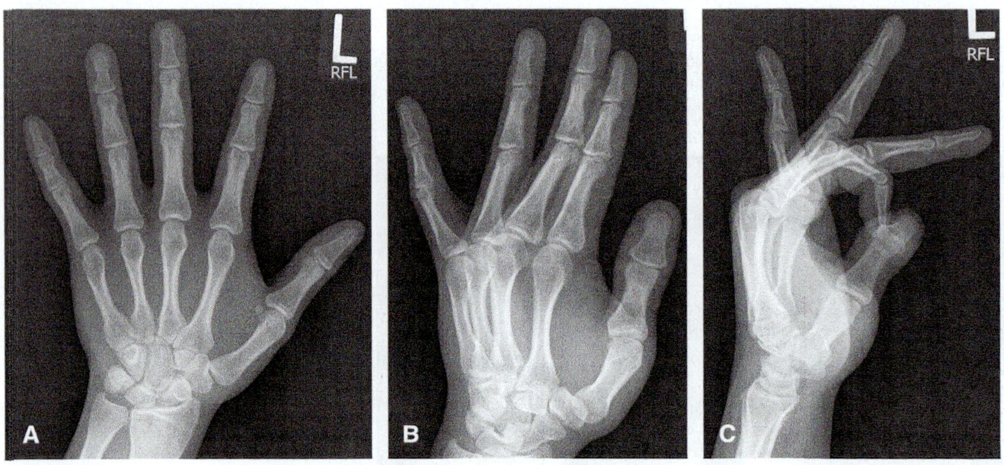

FIGURE 3. A: PA view of hand. B: Oblique view of hand. C: Lateral view of hand.

HAND
Arthritis Survey

Some centers prefer pronated obliques over supinated ball catcher (Norgaard) obliques. Both are good for overall assessment of arthritis, individual erosions, soft tissue swelling, and distribution. MRI or US are useful adjuncts to assess the soft tissues, for synovitis, joint fluid, and are said to be more sensitive for erosions.

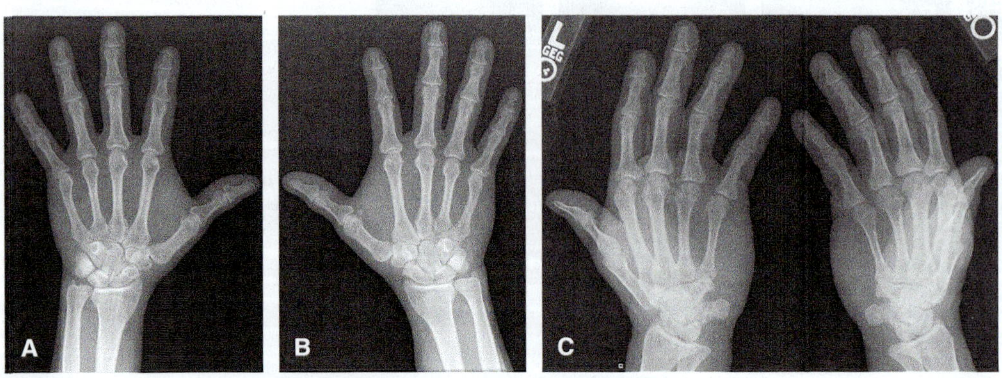

FIGURE 4. A, B: PA view of each hand. C: AP Norgaard projection (ball catcher's position).

HAND

Bone Age

Used to assess skeletal maturation in comparison to chronologic age. PA left hand and wrist radiograph is used to compare with the text of Greulich and Pyle.

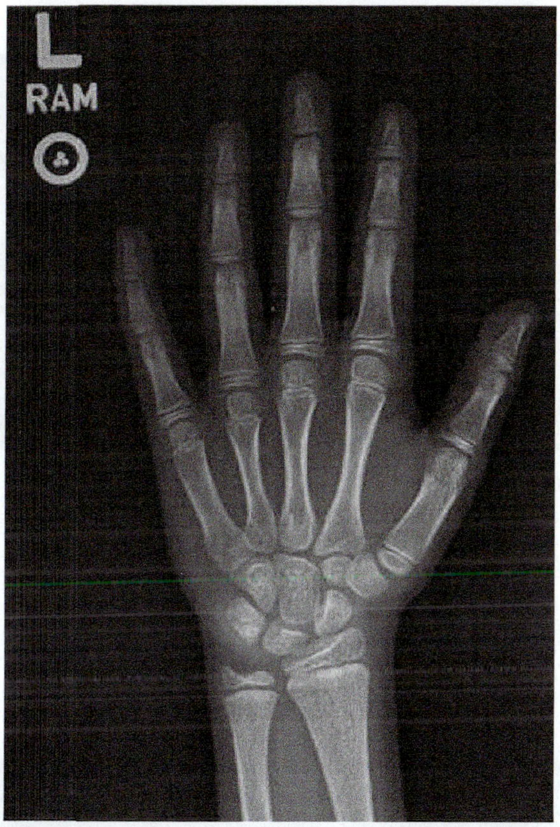

FIGURE 5. PA view of left hand and wrist.

WRIST

Nontrauma, Infection

For typical wrist pain evaluations including arthritis or mass. Good for carpal alignment. US: good for soft tissue masses, tendon pathology. CT scan may be a useful adjunct to assess for occult scaphoid fractures and for healing as well as other occult injuries such as hook of hamate fracture. CT scan is often used in the preoperative workup of intra-articular distal radial fractures. MRI is good for occult fractures, Kienböck disease, avascular necrosis (AVN) of lunate or scaphoid, triangular fibrocartilage tears, or intercarpal ligament injuries.

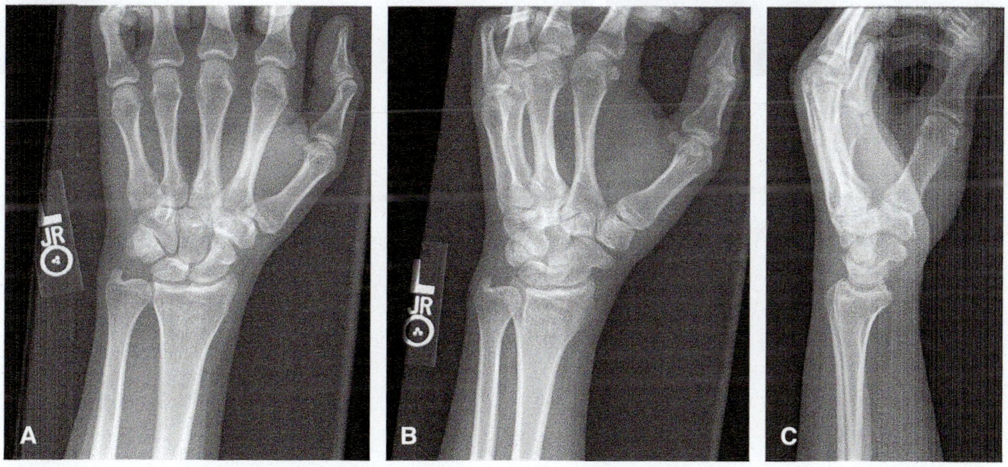

FIGURE 6. A: PA view of wrist. B: Ulnar oblique view of wrist. C: Lateral view of wrist.

WRIST

Trauma

Additional scaphoid views include oblique and ulnar/radial deviation with cranial angulation. These are good to assess for most aspects of trauma including fracture, subluxation, or dislocation. Of note the lateral view can only be used to assess alignment when the volar aspect of the pisiform projects between the volar aspects of the scaphoid and capitate. MRI is a useful adjunct to assess for occult injury, intercarpal ligament injury, triangular fibrocartilage complex injury, mass, or synovitis.

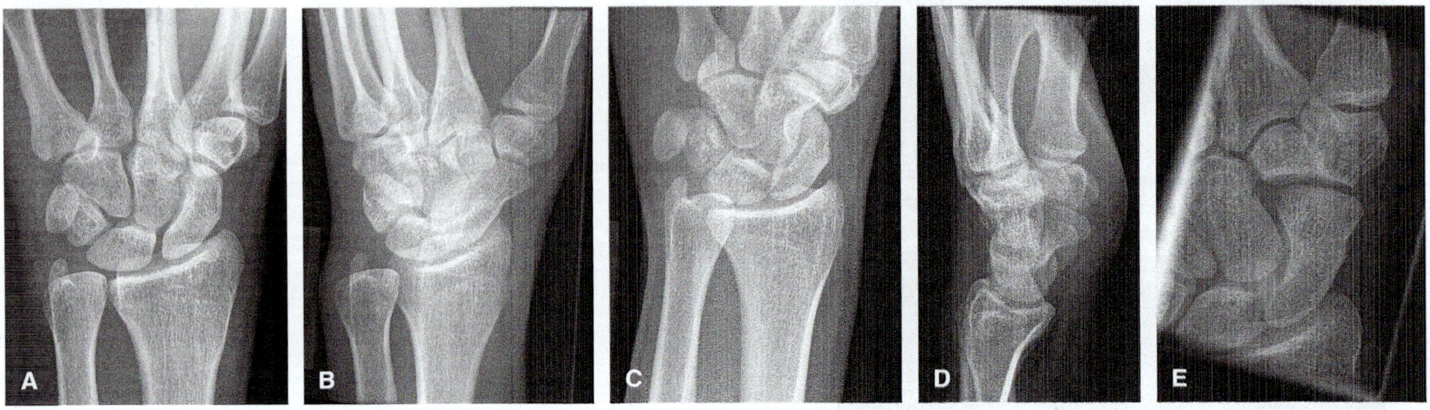

FIGURE 7. A: PA view of wrist. B: Ulnar oblique view of wrist. C: Radial oblique view of wrist. D: Lateral view of wrist. E: Navicular/scaphoid view.

WRIST

Additional Views

Clenched fist views; taken AP are useful for occult cases of scapholunate ligament disruption. Clenching the fist pushes the carpal bones apart. Carpal tunnel view; good for looking for hook of hamate, trapezial ridge fractures, or carpal tunnel syndrome posttrauma/wrist fracture. The carpal bridge view is a useful way to assess for dorsal carpal bone calcifications.

CT scan is another good way to assess for occult carpal fractures. MRI without or with intraarticular dilute Gadolinium is good to assess for internal derangement.

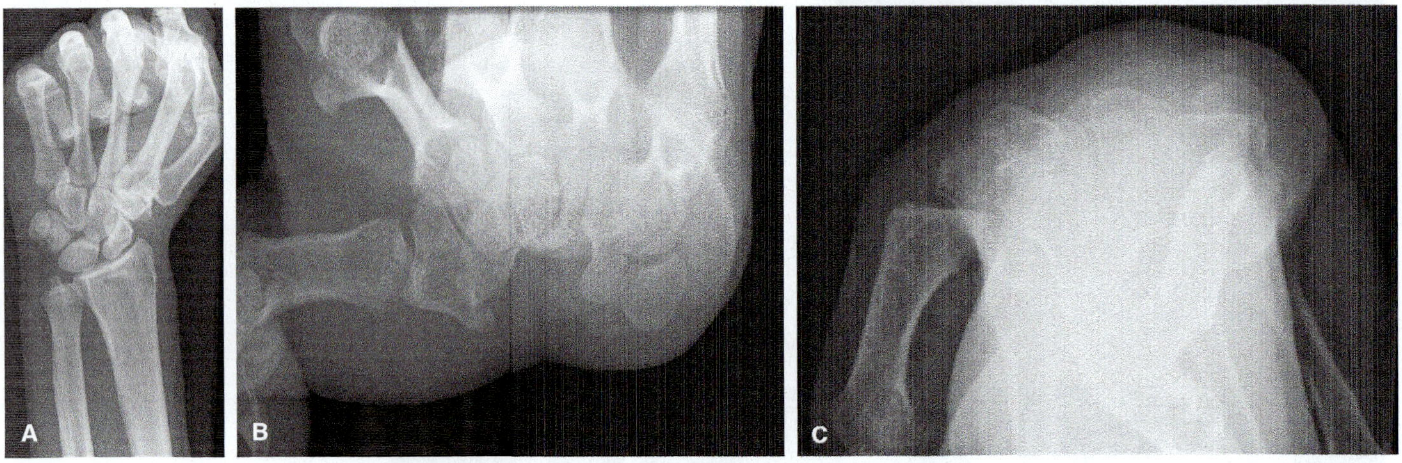

FIGURE 8. A: Clenched fist. B: Carpal tunnel. C: Carpal bridge.

FOREARM

Good for trauma, mass, foreign body, cellulitis/osteomyelitis, or abscess. It is important that the elbow rotates through 90 degrees between the AP and lateral so that two identical views of the ulna are not obtained. Consider US or MRI to assess for mass or soft tissue injury.

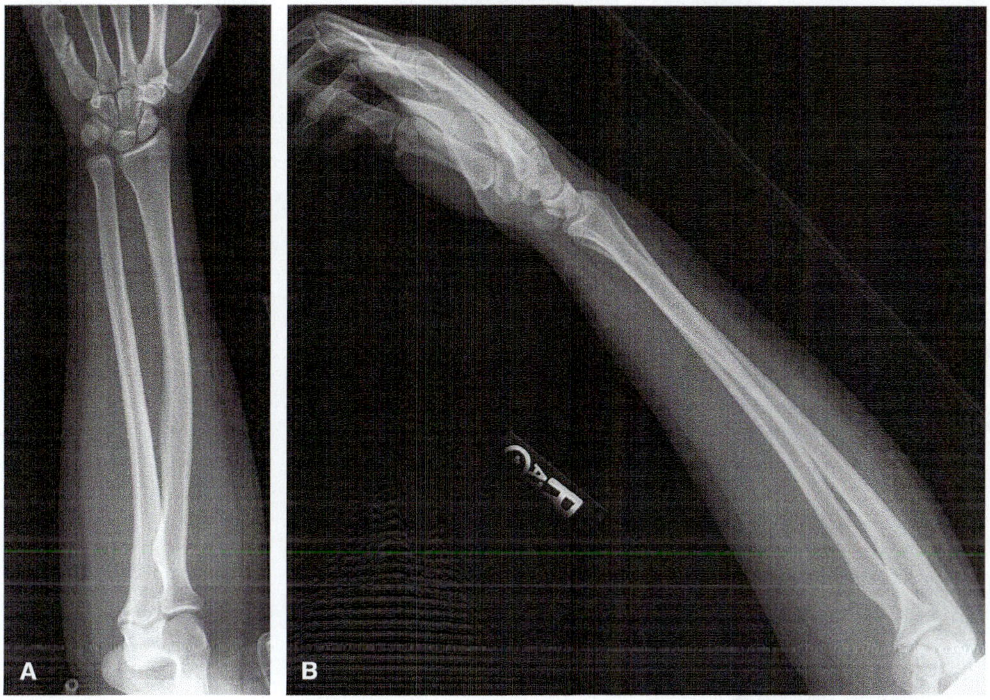

FIGURE 9. A: Anteroposterior (AP) view of forearm. B: Lateral view of forearm.

ELBOW

Nontrauma

Chronic injuries, arthritis, foreign bodies, and infection. Lateral is good for effusion and olecranon bursitis. AP is good for epicondylar enthesopathy and osteophytes. Consider US or MRI for soft tissue mass.

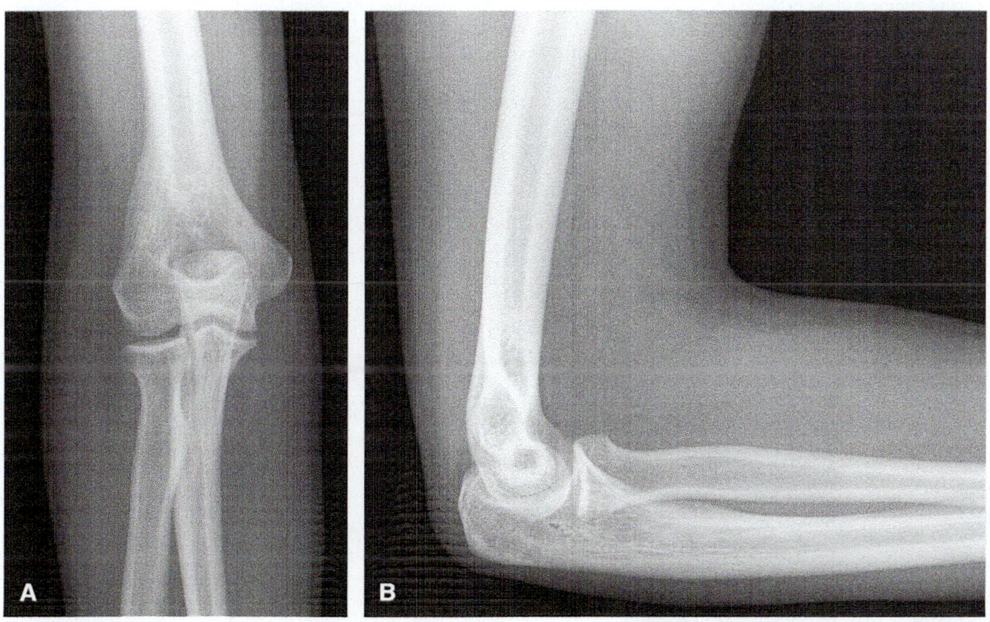

FIGURE 10. A: AP view of elbow. B: Lateral view of elbow.

ELBOW
Trauma

Good to assess for otherwise occult radial head fractures. Often, AP, lateral, and radial head are enough for trauma. US or MRI can assess for ligamentous or tendon injuries.

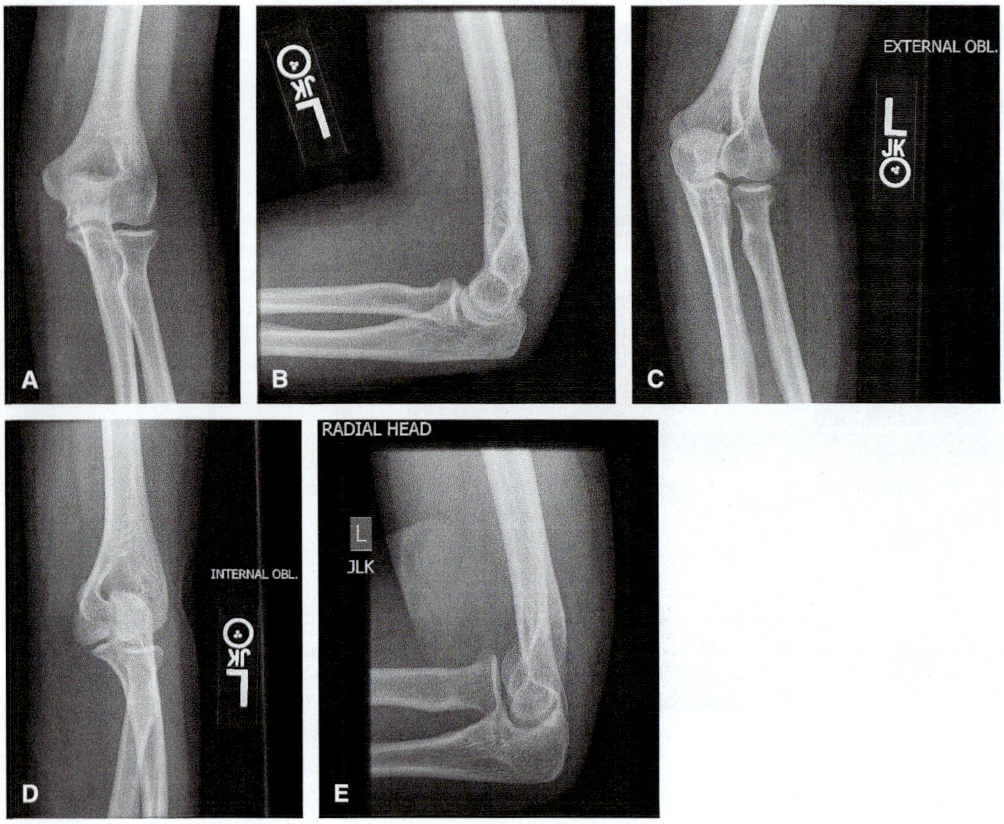

FIGURE 11. A: AP view. B: Lateral view. C: Lateral (external or radial) oblique view. D: Medial (internal or ulnar) oblique view. E: Radial head view.

ELBOW
Additional Views

Good to assess for radio opaque causes of cubital tunnel syndrome such as osteophytes. Consider US or MRI for further assessment of cubital tunnel.

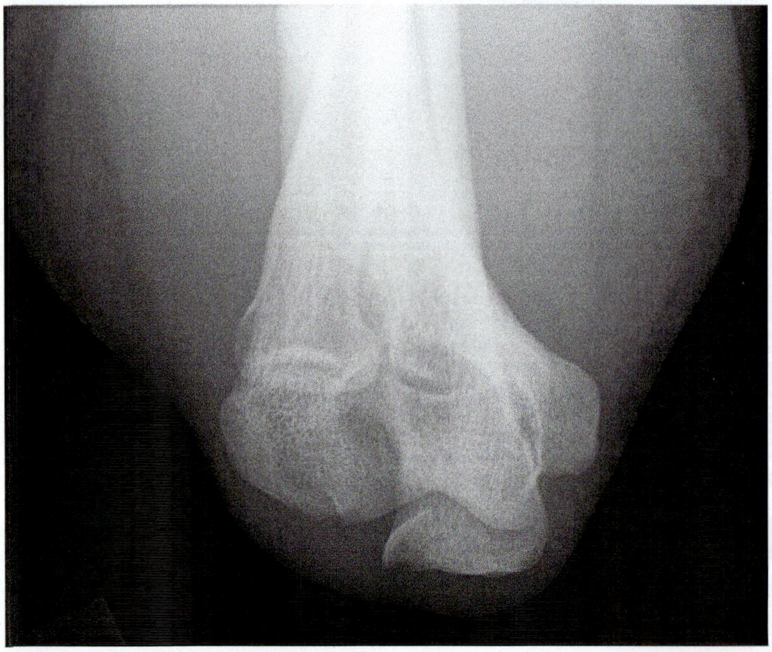

FIGURE 12. Cubital tunnel view.

HUMERUS

To assess for trauma, infection, mass, or foreign body. Both the shoulder and elbow should be included in the study in both projections, but they should not be over interpreted on such limited views.

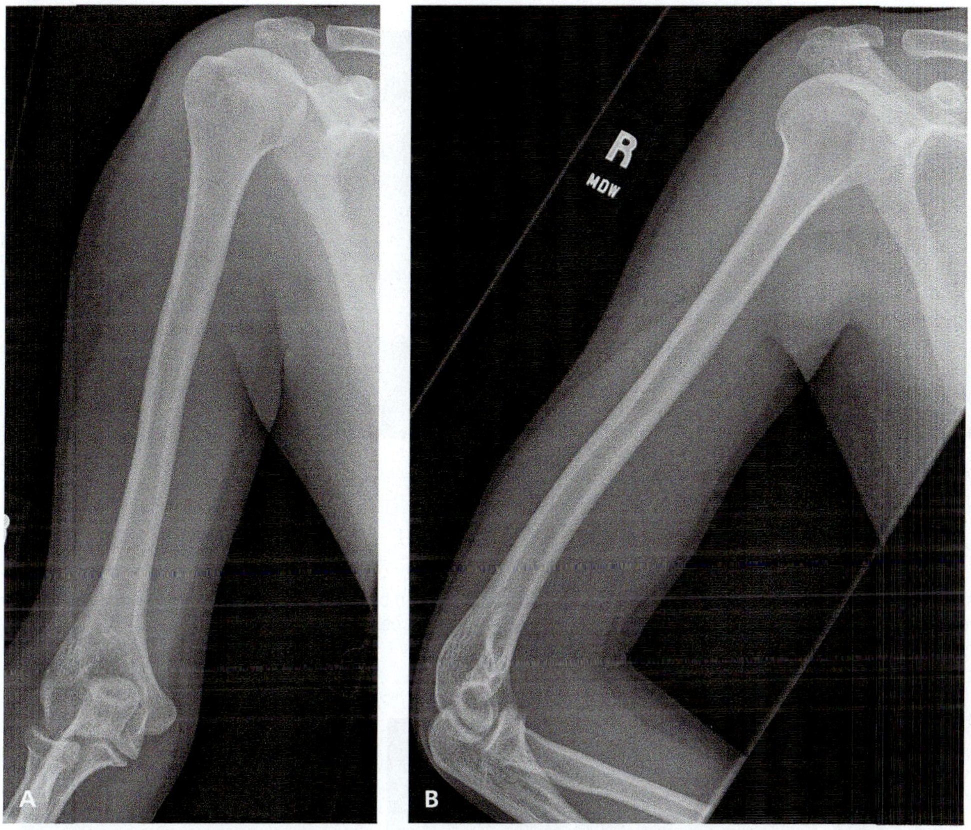

FIGURE 13. A: AP/external rotation view. B: Lateral/internal rotation view.

SHOULDER

Nontrauma, Chronic Pain

Shoulder series vary widely between institutions. Good to assess for location of hydroxyapatite, osteoarthrosis, and other degenerative changes. US or MRI is best to assess for rotator cuff tears. If a rotator cuff tear is seen on plain films by reduced acromiohumeral distance, then MRI is better than US to show the degree of retraction and atrophy, if the patient is a candidate for repair. MRI is best for glenoid labral pathology for which an MRI arthrogram will give additional information. CT scan is useful in the preoperative planning of shoulder arthroplasty to assess for bone stock, and any intra-articular glenoid fracture.

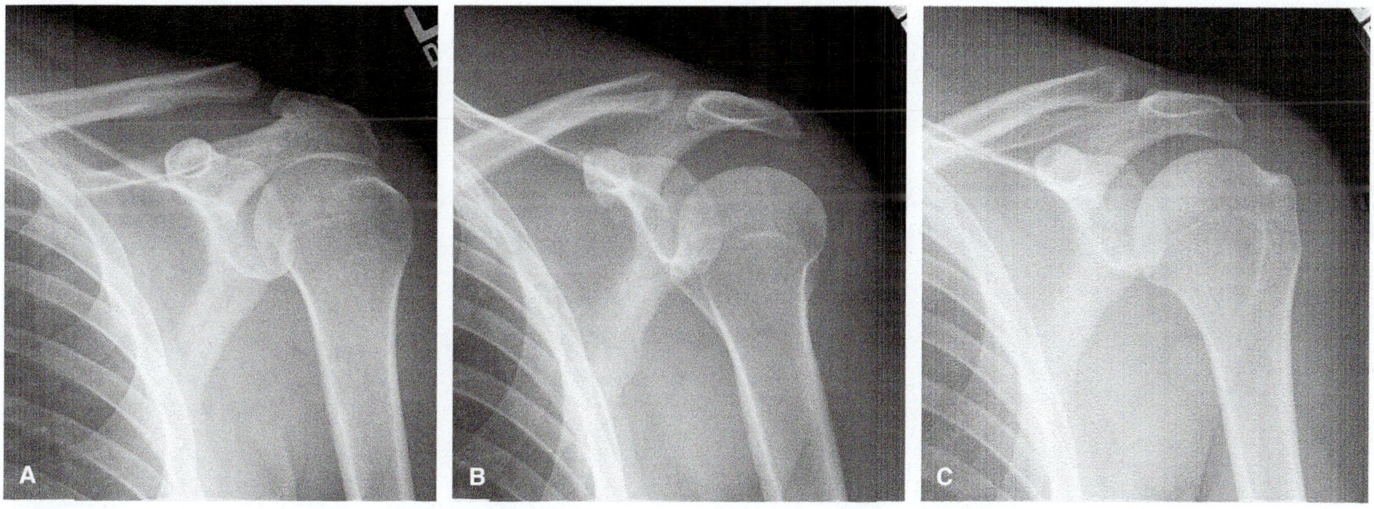

FIGURE 14. A: AP neutral rotation view. B: AP internal rotation view. C: AP external rotation view.

SHOULDER

Trauma, Acute Injuries

To evaluate for humeral neck/tuberosity fractures and shoulder dislocations. CT scan is useful to assess for Hill-Sachs lesions and bony Bankart. MRI can be difficult to interpret acutely due to blood tracking into the rotator cuff from tuberosity fractures. Subacutely, MRI may be useful to assess for accompanying internal derangement.

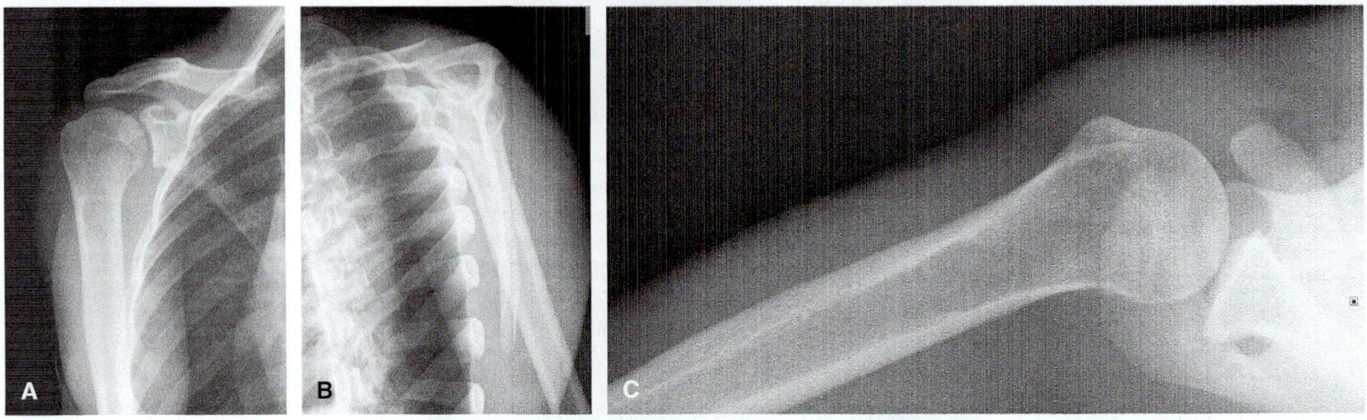

FIGURE 15. A: AP view of scapula, neutral rotation (Grashey). B: Lateral "Y" view. C: Axillary view, as tolerated by patient.

SHOULDER

Additional Views

Outlet view is good to look at subacromial space to assess for causes of external shoulder subacromial impingement. It can also be used to localize calcium in the rotator cuff. Stryker notch view is good for Hill-Sachs lesions, but most are seen on neutral rotation AP shoulder. Westpoint view is good for detecting bony Bankart lesions, but consider CT scan. Velpeau view; can be a useful adjunct to assess for dislocation in a patient who cannot raise their arm.

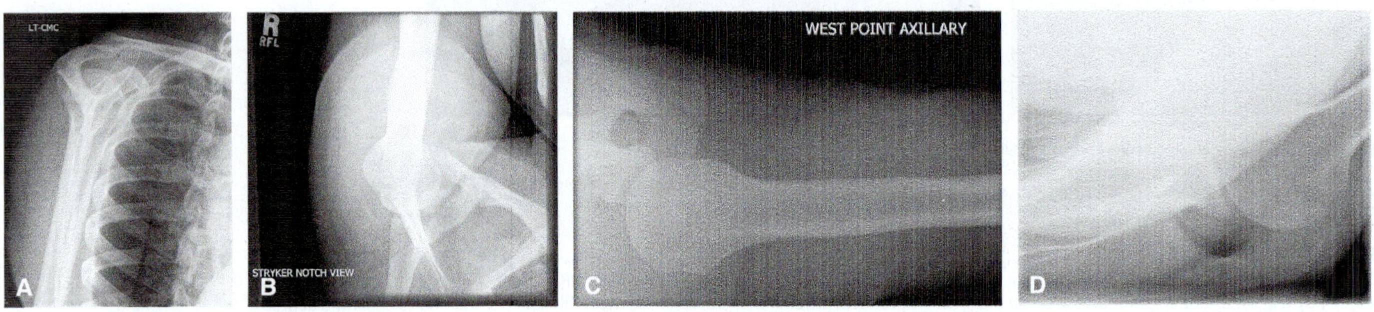

FIGURE 16. A: Supraspinatus view (outlet, Bigliani method). B: Stryker notch view. C: Westpoint view. D: Velpeau view.

SCAPULA

Good for trauma, scapulothoracic syndrome. Consider CT scan for trauma workup to assess for glenoid involvement. MRI can assess for scapulothoracic friction syndromes.

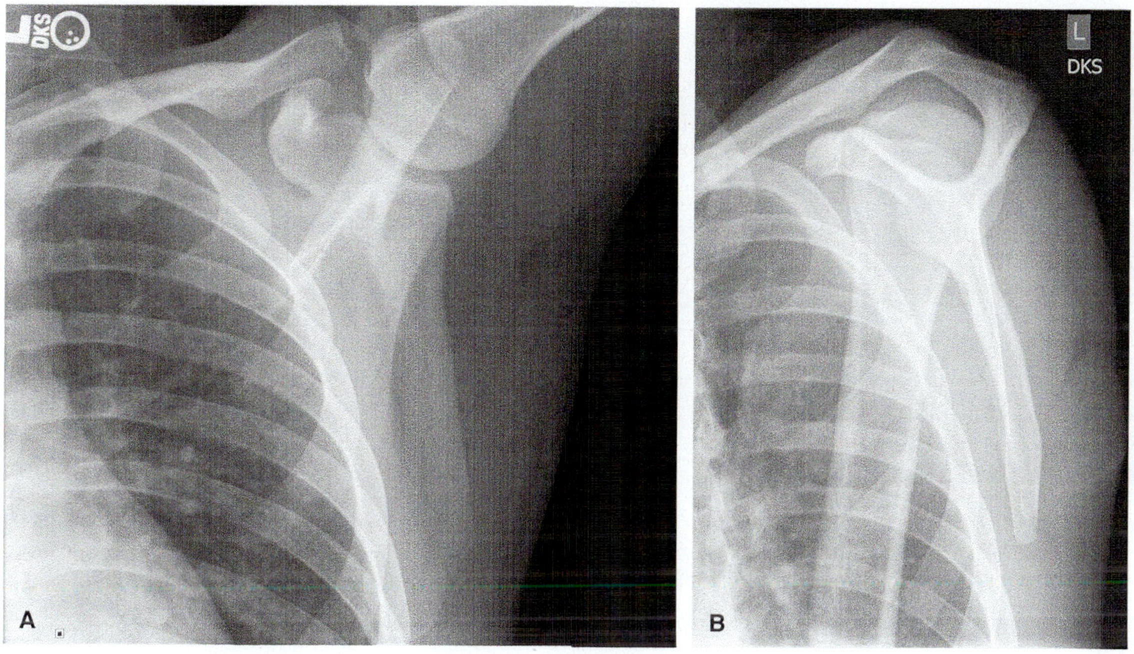

FIGURE 17. A: AP view of scapula. B: Lateral view of scapula.

ACROMIOCLAVICULAR JOINTS

These are routinely assessed on AP shoulder views. Views without and with weights to look for occult type 1 separations usually do not alter management but can make the diagnosis. May be useful in legal cases. Consider MRI to assess for deltotrapezial disruption in type 3 or higher injuries.

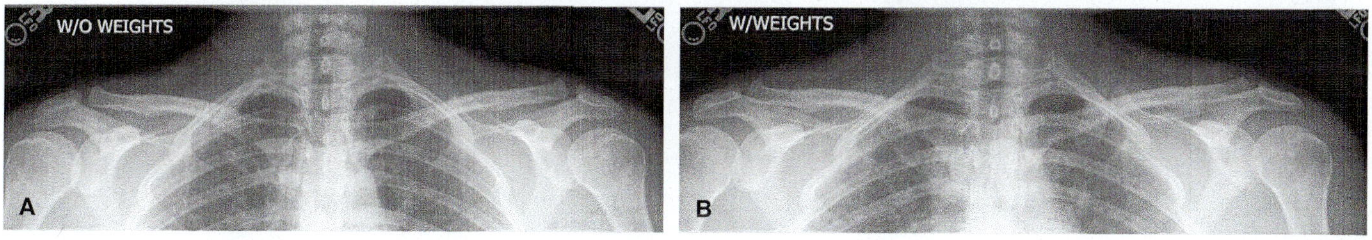

FIGURE 18. A: AP view without weights. B: AP view with weights.

ACROMIOCLAVICULAR JOINTS

Additional Views

The Zanca view centered at the acromioclavicular joint can give more precise information about alignment and degenerative change.

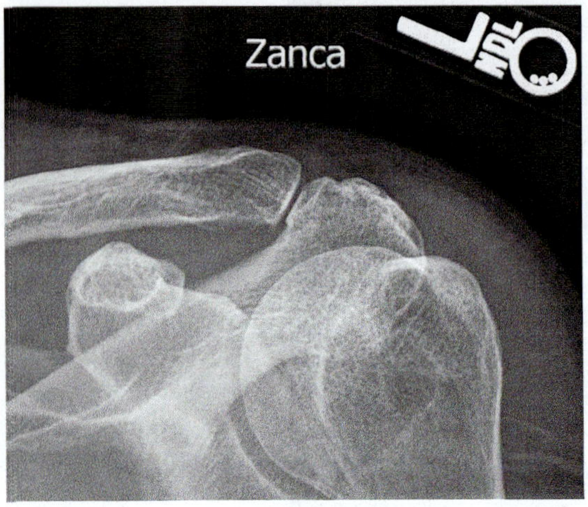

FIGURE 19. Zanca projection.

CLAVICLES

Good for clavicle fractures. Medial clavicle fractures can be difficult to see. Consider CT scan for possible medial clavicle fractures.

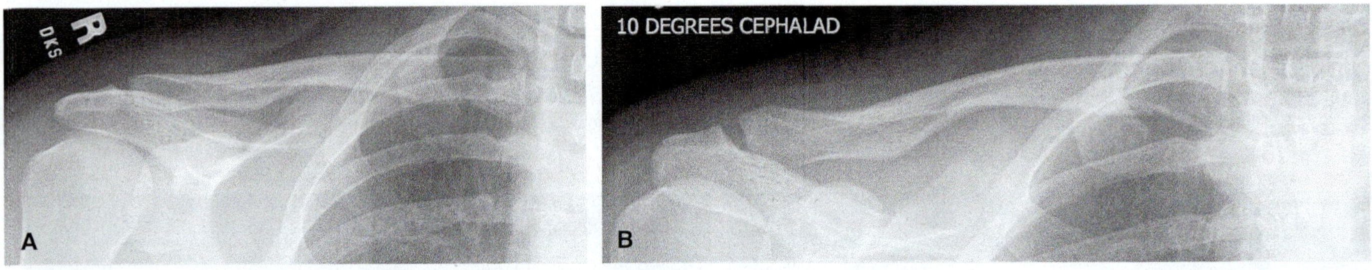

FIGURE 20. A: AP 0-degree tube angle view. B: AP 10-degree cephalad angle view.

LOWER EXTREMITIES

TOES

For 1st through 5th digits. Specifically, to look at one toe for trauma, foreign body, or localized mass. Socks off. A marker should be applied at the toe of interest. The lateral view should have the affected toe lifted or depressed clear of the others. Consider US for radiolucent foreign body. Consider MRI or US for mass or tendon lesion/injury.

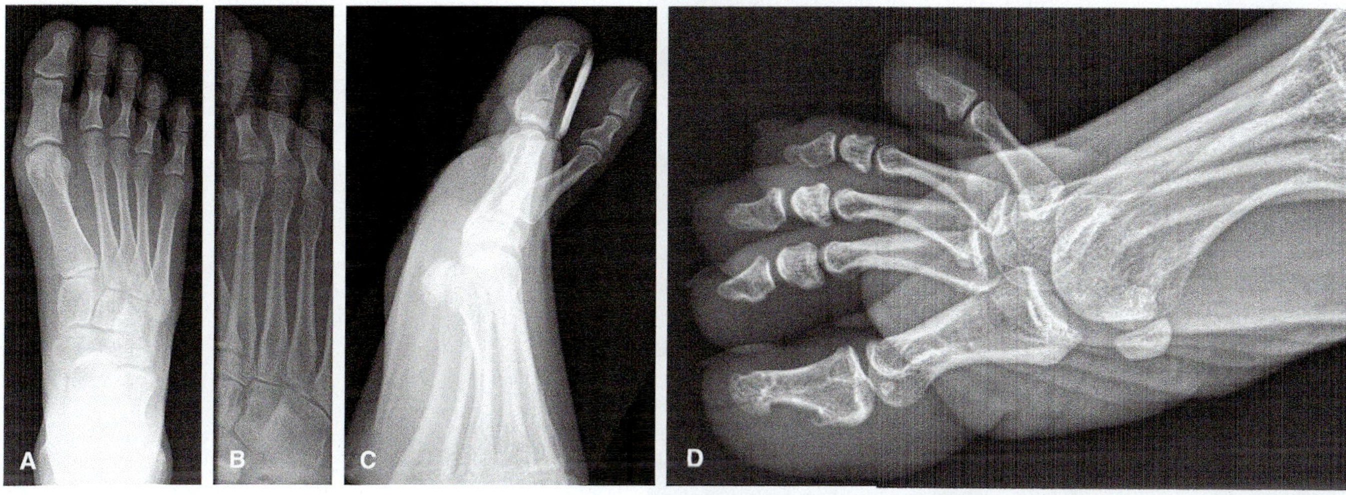

FIGURE 21. A: AP view of foot. B: Medial oblique view of affected toe(s). C. Lateral of toe(s). Wooden spatula between toe of interest and other toes. D: Alternate lateral method with toes splayed.

FOOT

Perform all three views for trauma and nontrauma cases. A limited two view foot is discouraged. Weight-bearing to assess foot alignment. Non–weight-bearing if painful to stand or looking for a foreign body or mass. Non–weight-bearing if ulcer and looking for osteomyelitis. Always remove socks. Consider US for Morton neuroma or plantar fasciitis, or superficial mass. CT scan is good for full assessment of Lisfranc injuries. MRI is good for occult fracture or mass.

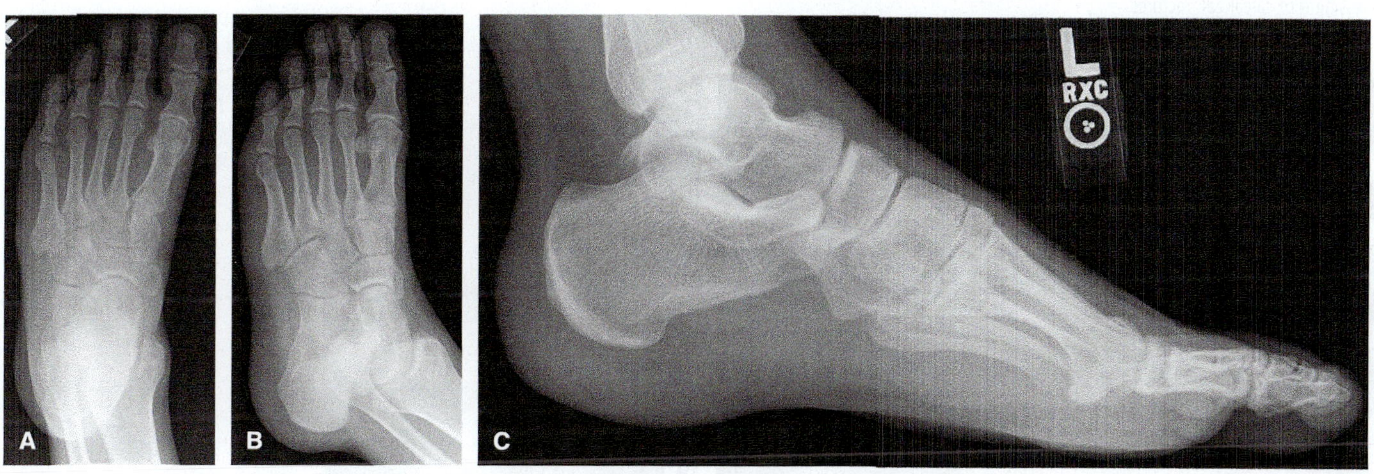

FIGURE 22. A: AP view (dorsoplantar). B: Medial oblique view. C: Lateral view (mediolateral projection).

Sesamoid View
Good to look at sesamoid alignment with metatarsal head in hallux valgus, to assess metatarsal sesamoid osteoarthrosis or to look for fracture of sesamoid.

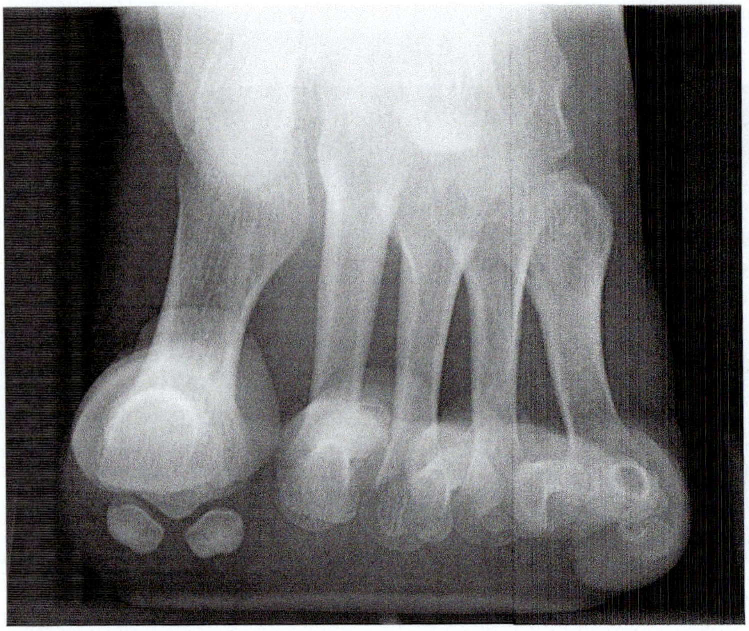

FIGURE 23. Sesamoid projection.

OS CALCIS
Weight-bearing for alignment or non–weight-bearing for mass or if too painful to stand. Good for trauma and heel alignment. This should be the preferred study for heal pain rather than a foot series. The posterior subtalar joint and middle subtalar facet are often well visualized on the axial or Harris-Beath view. Consider CT scan for full preoperative assessment of calcaneal fractures.

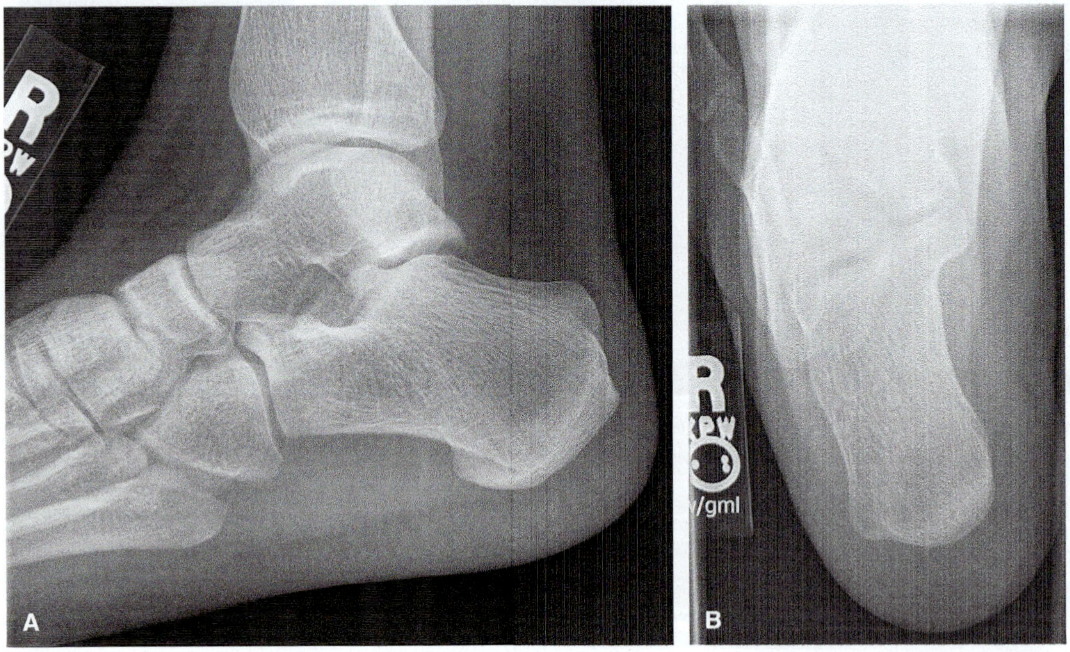

FIGURE 24. A: Lateral calcaneus mediolateral projection. B: PA axial plantodorsal view.

POSTERIOR SUBTALAR JOINT

The Broden view is a useful adjunct view to look at the posterior subtalar joint to assess for intraarticular fractures and arthritis.

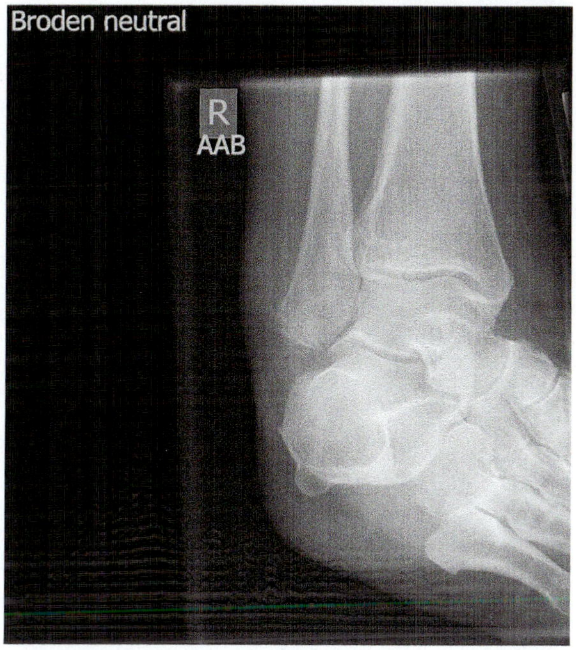

FIGURE 25. A: Broden view of posterior subtalar joint.

TALAR NECK

The Canale view or medial oblique axial talus view is a useful view when following up talar neck fractures to check alignment.

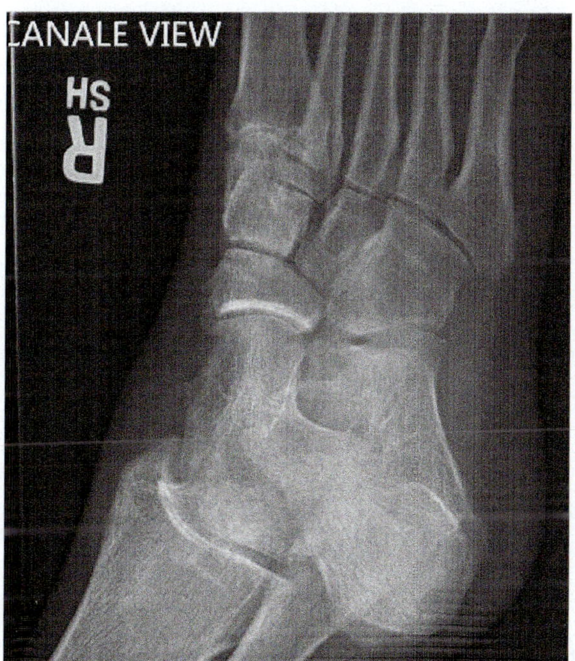

FIGURE 26. Canale view.

HINDFOOT ALIGNMENT

The Saltzman view, also known as the hindfoot alignment view, is a weight-bearing view to assess the angular relation of the talus and calcaneus.

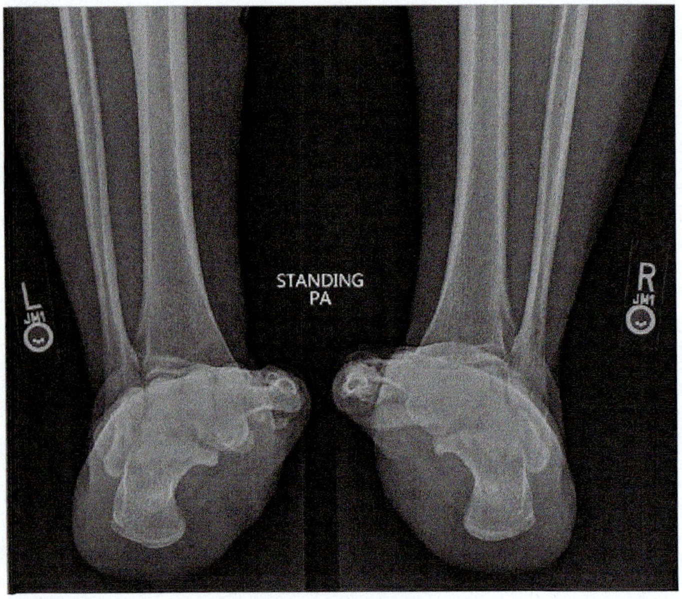

FIGURE 27. Saltzman view.

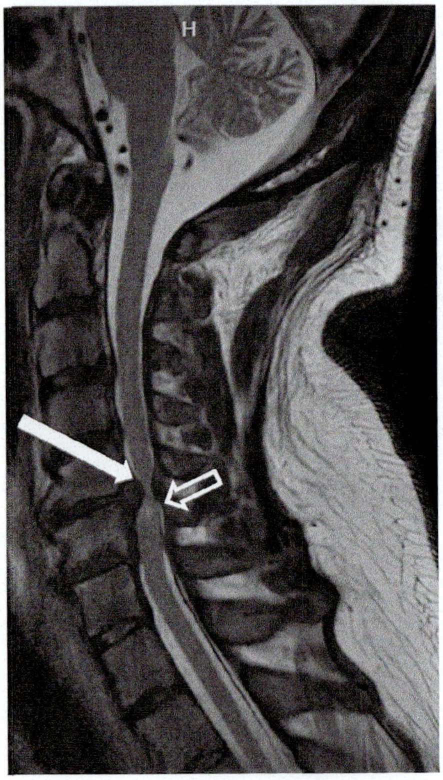

FIGURE 28. Cervical MRI T2-weighted sagittal view demonstrates cervical spinal stenosis at C5–C6 (*solid arrow*) with evidence of increased spinal cord signal consistent with myelopathic changes (*outlined arrow*).

ANKLE

Weight-bearing if alignment is being assessed, or non–weight-bearing if trauma, or if looking for mass. Ideal for all acute ankle injuries. The base of 5th metatarsal should be included in case the ankle pain originates from here. For heel pain, use heel or calcaneal projections. US is useful to assess tendon injuries. CT scan is good for complex hind foot fractures. MRI is good to assess the tendons and ligaments, for masses, and occult fractures.

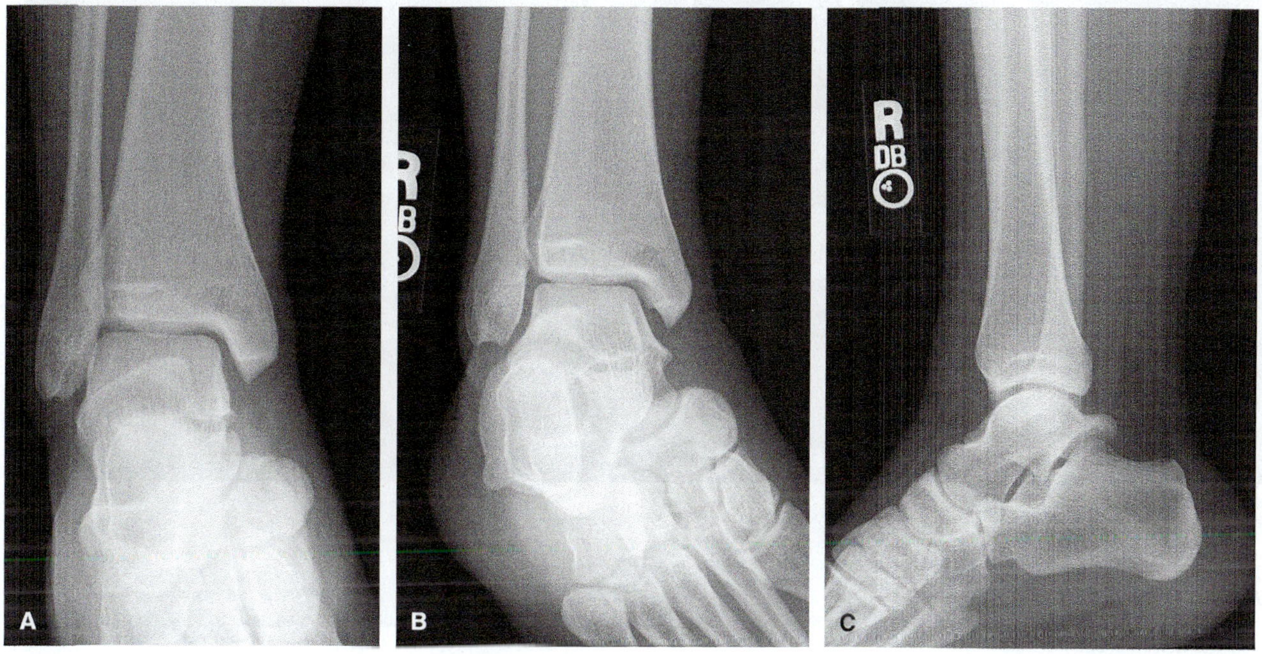

FIGURE 29. A: AP view of ankle. B: Mortise view of ankle. C: Mediolateral lateral view.

Weight-Bearing Views of the Ankle

Weight-bearing views are useful to eliminate the effects of a large joint effusion from widening or straightening the ankle mortise view and to assess hindfoot alignment.

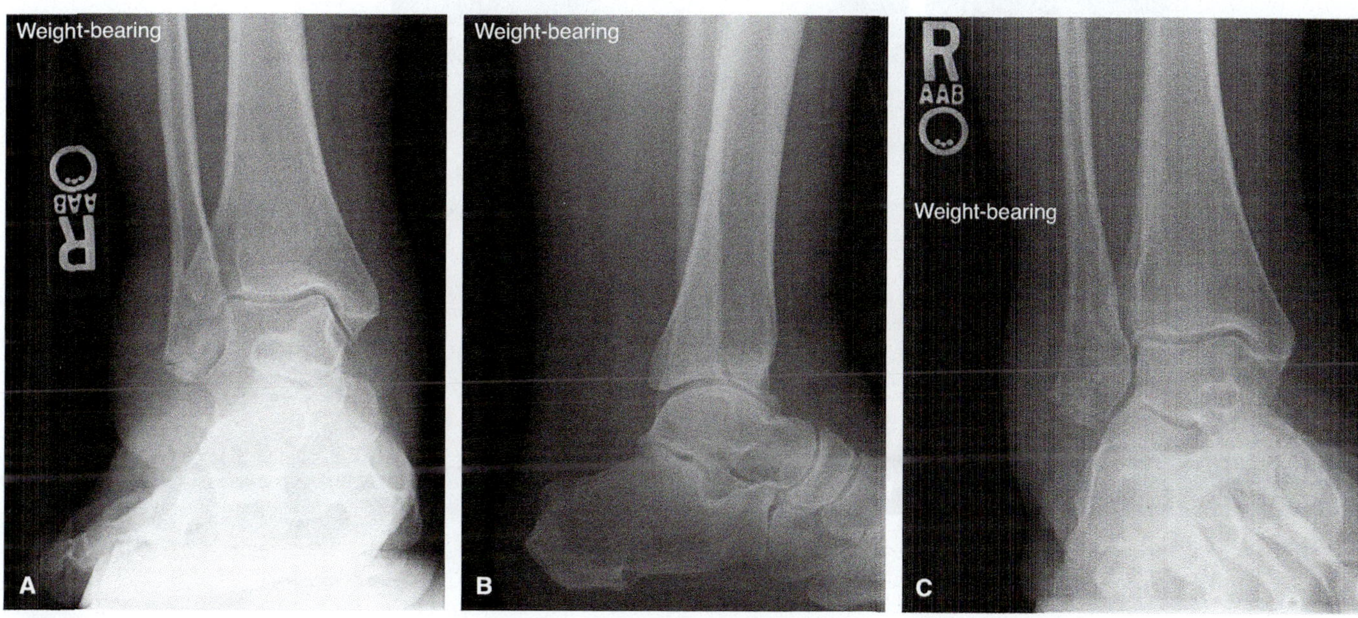

FIGURE 30. A: AP view of weight-bearing ankle. B: Mortise view of weight-bearing ankle. C: Mediolateral lateral view of weight-bearing ankle.

Stress Views of the Ankle

These give more functional information than MRI about ligamentous laxity and are useful in planning treatment for unstable ankles. In questionable cases, it can be useful to have the other side for comparison. These can be done by manual or gravity stress.

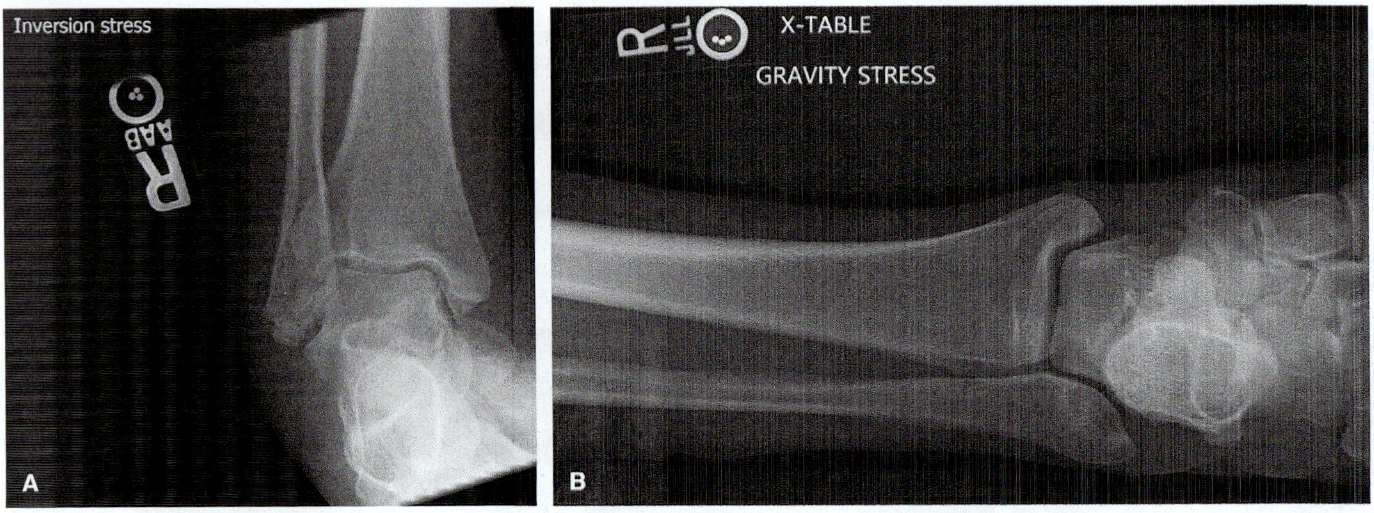

FIGURE 31. A: AP view of ankle with varus stress. B: AP decubitus view fracture side down to stress medial ligaments.

TIBIA/FIBULA

This should include both the ankle and knee joints. The ankle and knee should not be over interpreted on these off-axis views. Good for trauma, foreign body, mass, cellulitis. For occult stress fractures, consider MRI or bone scan.

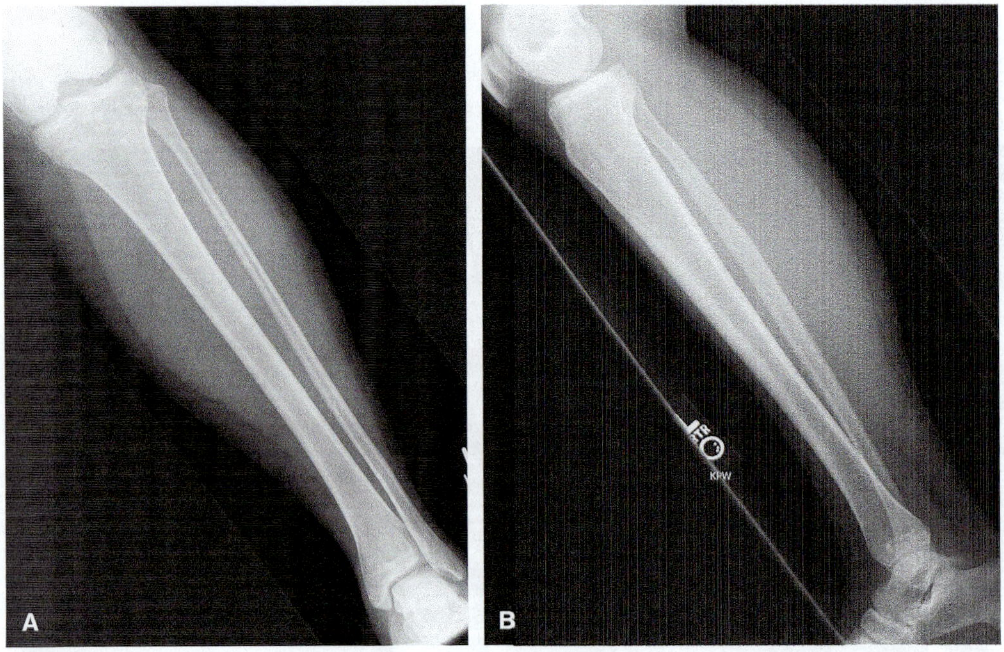

FIGURE 32. A: AP view. B: Mediolateral lateral view.

KNEE
Nontrauma, Chronic Injury
Good for initial arthritis assessment. MRI is useful to assess for internal derangement but is of less value when there is obvious osteoarthrosis on radiographs.

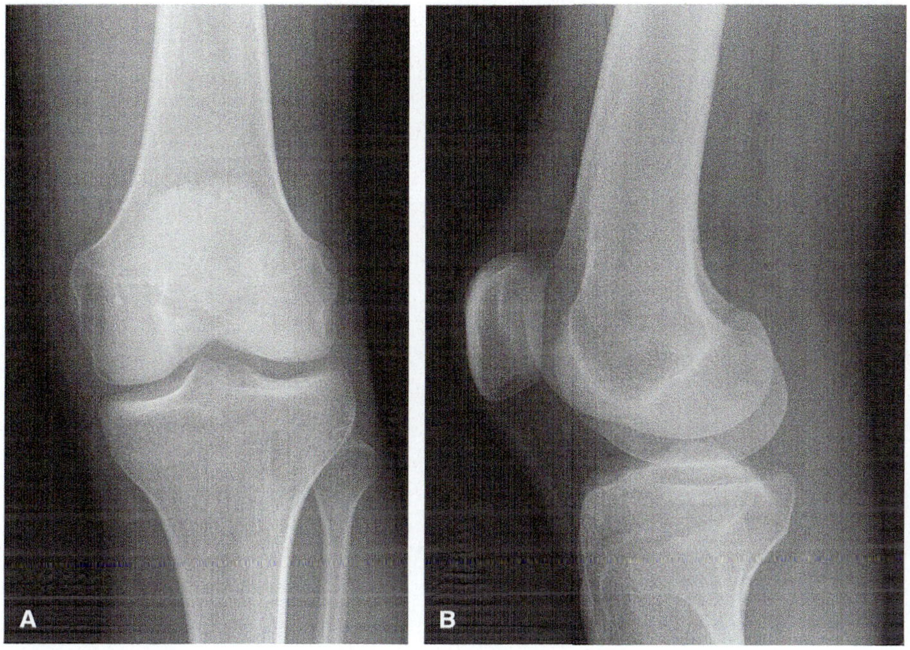

FIGURE 33. A: AP view. B: Mediolateral lateral view.

KNEE
Trauma, Acute Injury
Shoot through lateral added to assess for a lipohemarthrosis; if present, a fracture must be sought. CT scan is a useful adjunct to assess for occult tibial plateau fractures and to plan surgery with fractures seen on radiographs. MRI is being used increasingly to assess accompanying soft tissue injuries in cases of tibial plateau fractures.

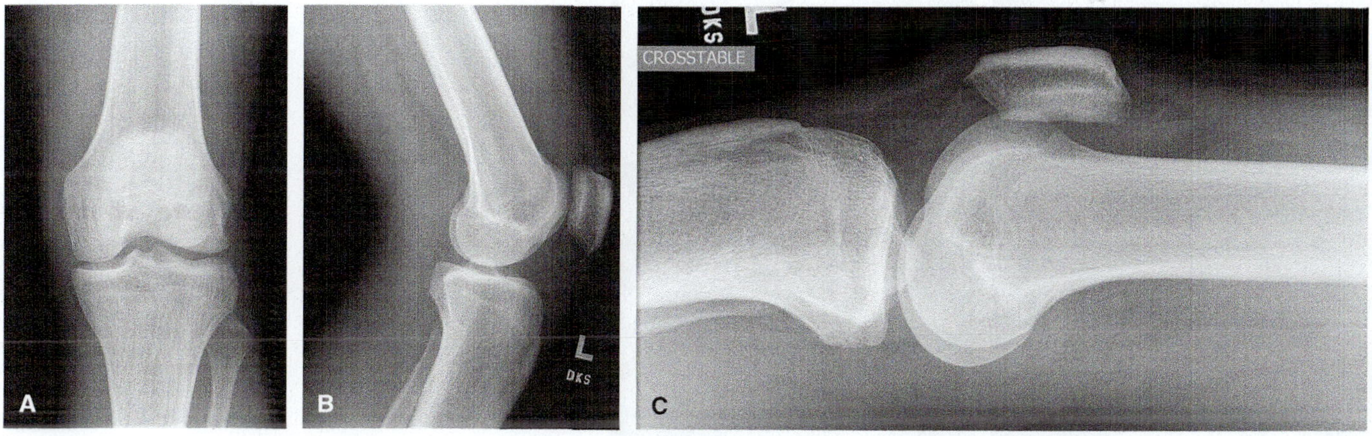

FIGURE 34. A: AP view. B: Mediolateral rolled lateral view. C: Lateromedial cross-table lateral view.

ADDITIONAL VIEWS

Knee Rosenberg View

This weight-bearing PA view with flexion is useful to show both the intercondylar notch and the joint space formed by the more posterior femoral condyle.

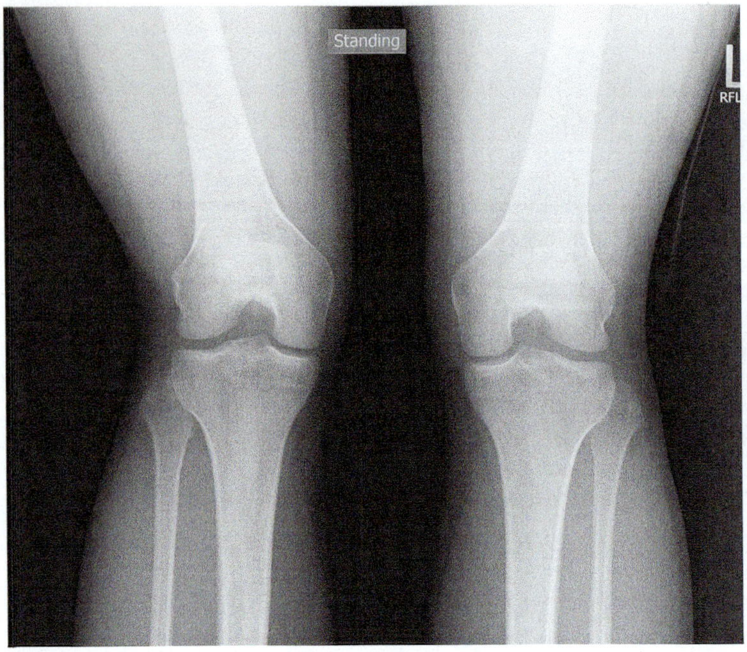

FIGURE 35. Rosenberg view.

KNEE

Oblique Views

Traditionally used to assess for occult tibial plateau fractures, still useful but now often replaced by CT scan or MRI.

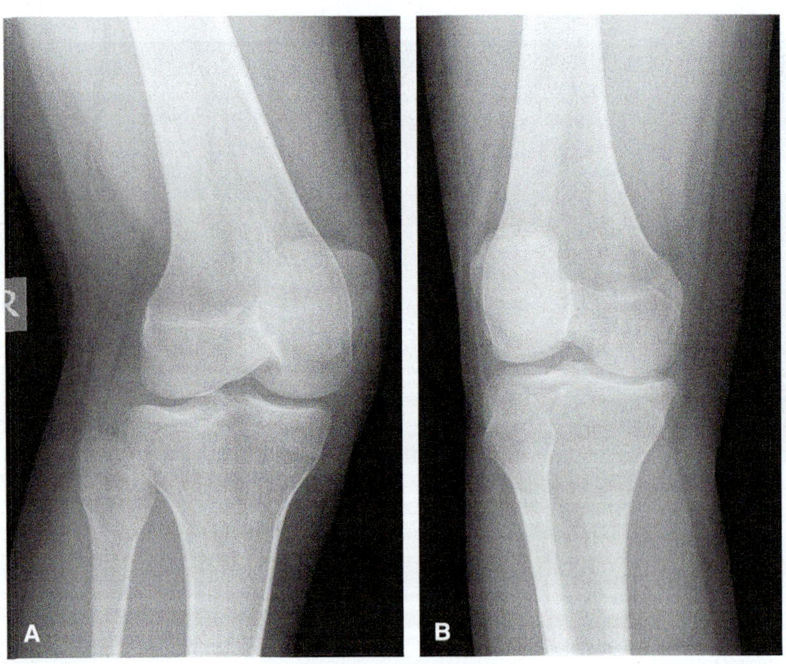

FIGURE 36. A: Medial oblique view. B: Lateral oblique view.

KNEE

Patella

Initially a routine knee is performed in cases of trauma.

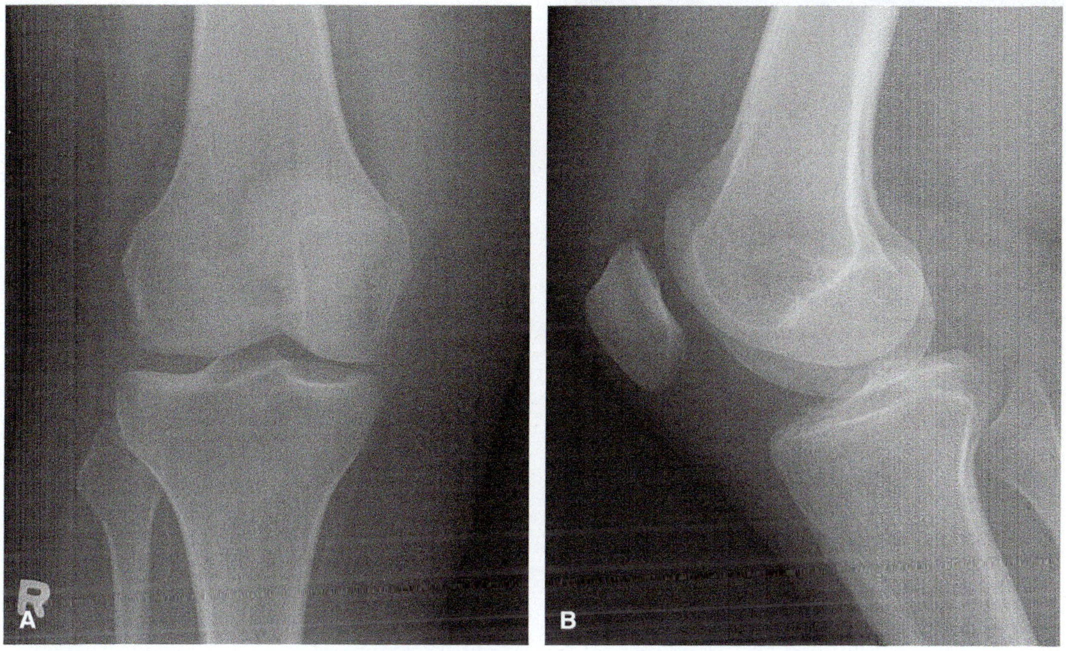

FIGURE 37. A: PA view of knee. B: Mediolateral lateral view.

PATELLA

Additional Views

Merchants view is good to assess patella alignment in cases of subluxation, dislocation, or tracking problems. These are taken at 30 degrees of flexion, the angle at which the patella is most unstable. It is taken caudal cranial and includes both knees. The sunrise axial projection is taken kneeling of just the affected the knee.

FIGURE 38. Merchants view (bilateral patellar view).

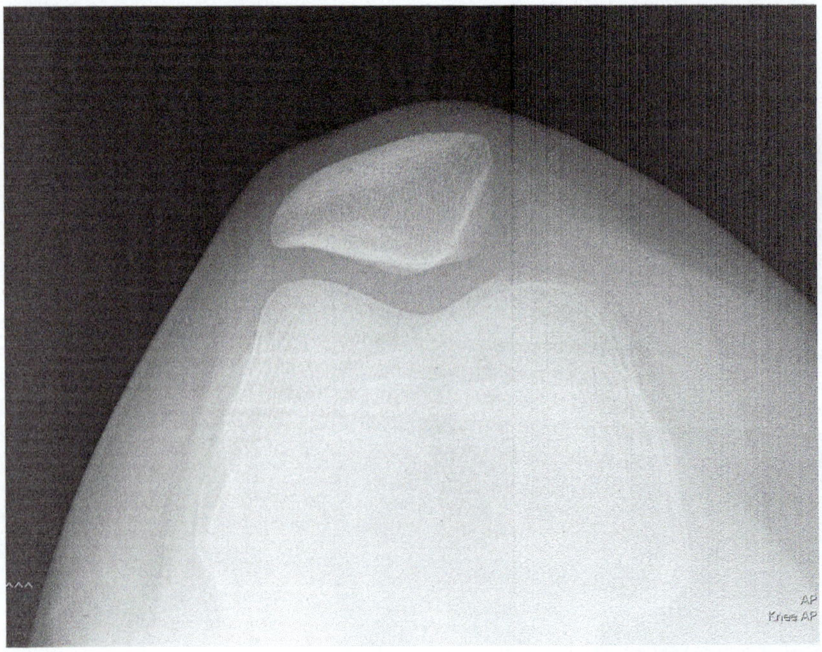

FIGURE 39. Axial projection (unilateral sunrise method).

FEMUR

Acute Injury, Trauma

Views of the femur should include both the hip and knee. The trauma series has a cross-table lateral of both the hip and knee so that the patient does not have to move.

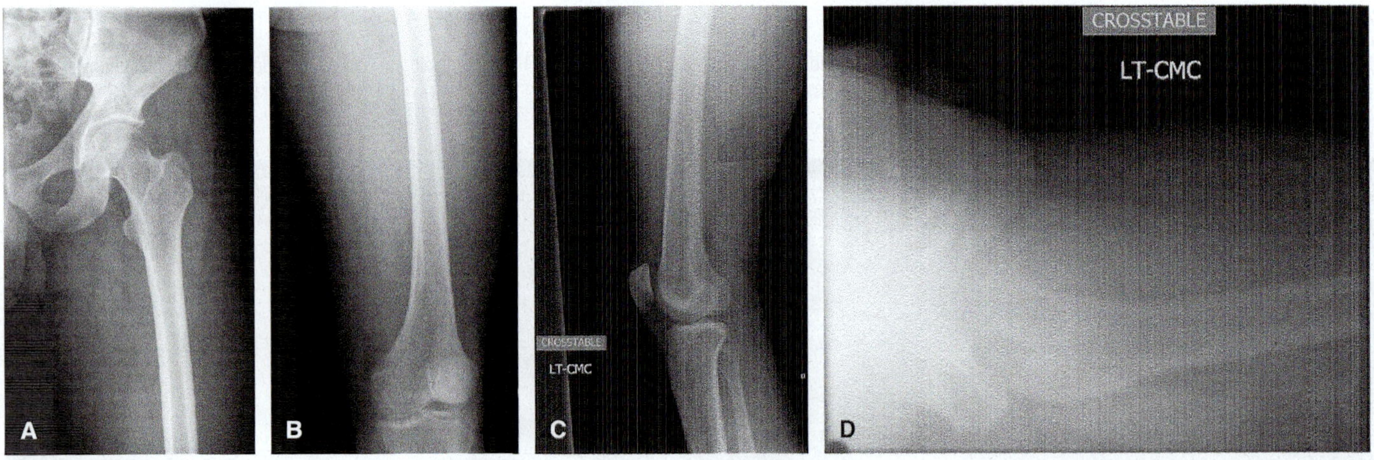

FIGURE 40. A: AP proximal view. B: AP distal view. C: Cross-table lateral view of femur to include knee joint. D: Inferosuperior lateral view to include proximal femur and hip joint for unilateral injury.

FEMUR

Nonacute Injury

The views include both the hip and the knee, but the hip is a frog lateral and the knee a rolled mediolateral. For soft tissue mass, consider MRI.

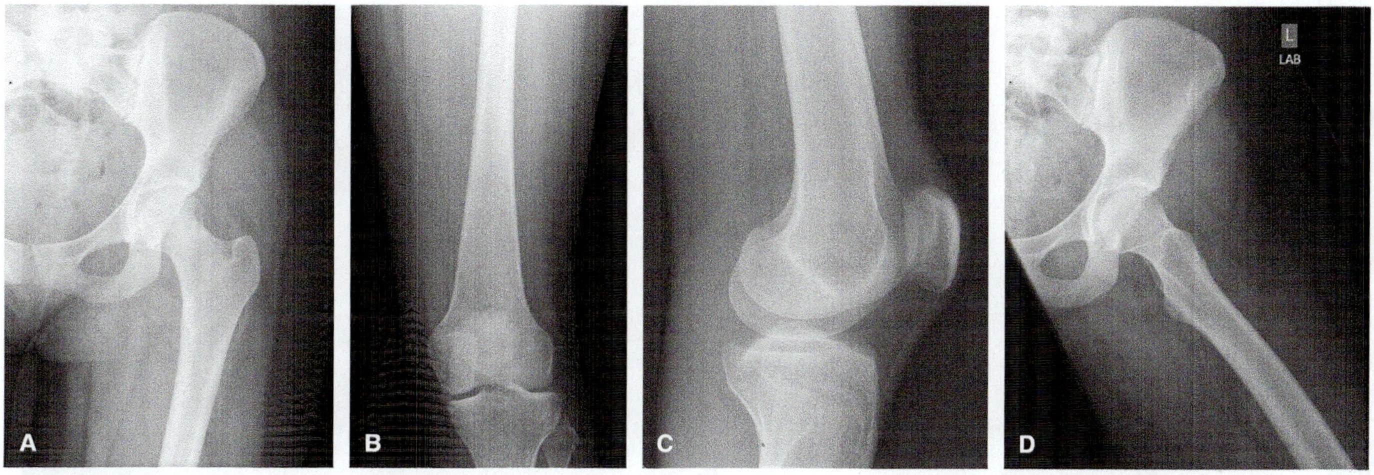

FIGURE 41. A: AP view to include hip and proximal femur. B: AP view to include knee and distal femur. C: Mediolateral lateral view to include knee. D: Lateral frog-leg hip view.

PELVIS

Include Both Hips on Image

Good initial screening test for acute trauma. Good for ill-defined pain or metastatic search. Consider CT scan for full assessment of pelvic trauma.

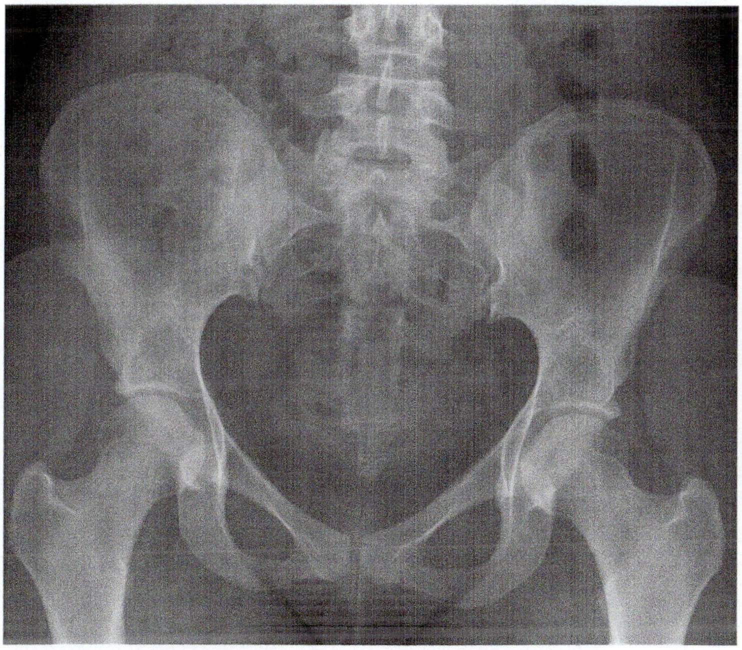

FIGURE 42. AP view of pelvis.

HIPS

Trauma, Acute Injury

AP pelvis and a cross-table lateral to assess for hip pain localized to the one side of the pelvis/hip.

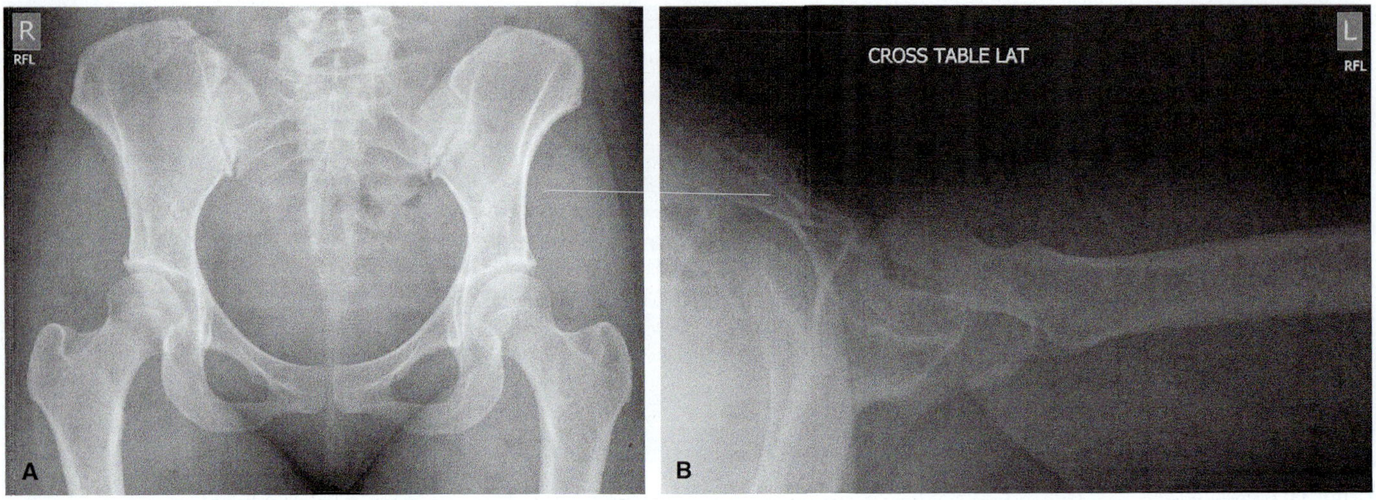

FIGURE 43. A: AP view of pelvis. B: Inferosuperior lateral oblique view to include proximal femur and hip joint for unilateral injury.

HIPS

Nontrauma, Chronic Injury

The cross-table lateral is replaced by a frog lateral. The frog leg can be bilateral or unilateral depending on the pain. MRI is an excellent way to assess hip pain if the radiographs show only minimal abnormality. MRI arthrogram can give useful additional information about the labrum.

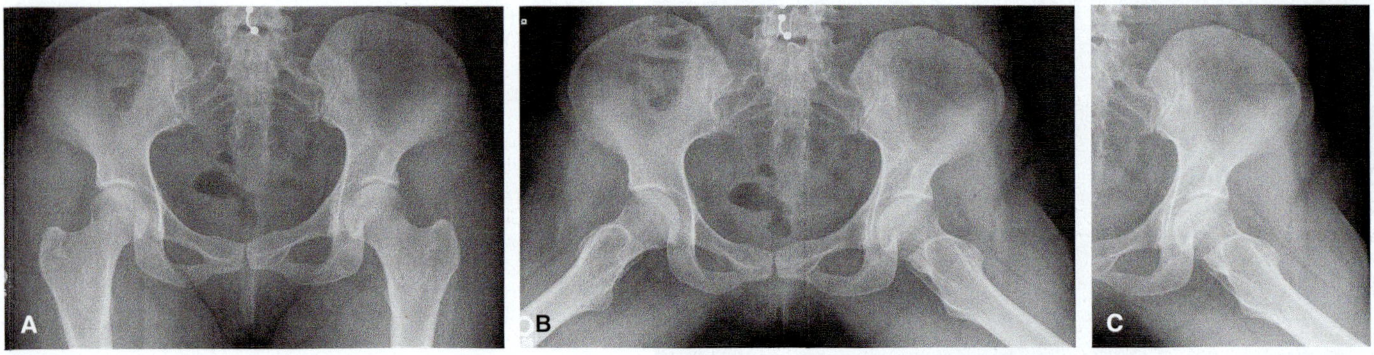

FIGURE 44. A: AP view of pelvis. B: Bilateral frog leg view. C: Frog-leg lateral view of affected hip.

HIPS

Additional Views

A Dunn view is useful in assessing for femoroacetabular impingement, particularly the presence of a cam lesion.

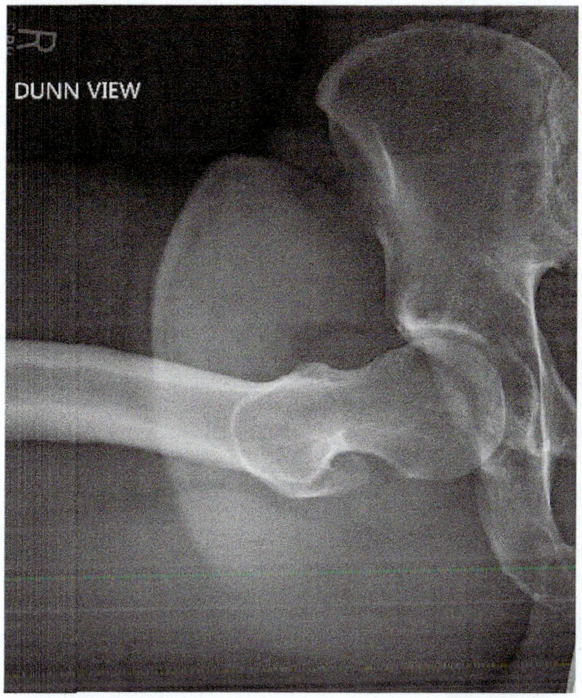

FIGURE 45. Dunn view.

SACROILIAC JOINTS

Good initial screening test for sacroiliitis. MRI is more sensitive and saves radiation to the gonads and intestines. An alternative is a PA view, which is more in the line of the sacroiliac joints and shows them magnified.

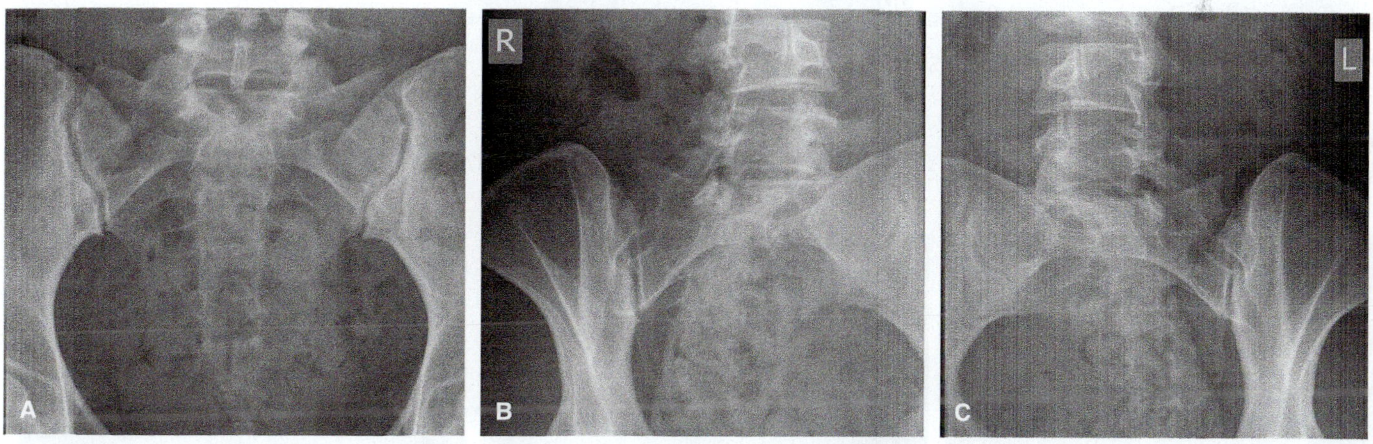

FIGURE 46. A: AP view of pelvis. B: AP oblique view of right sacroiliac joint. C: AP oblique view of left sacroiliac joint.

ACETABULUM (JUDET VIEWS)

Good for assessing acetabular fractures but now usually replaced by oblique images of whole pelvis; requires four images—two right posterior oblique (RPO) and two left posterior oblique (LPO) images, collimated to affected side only.

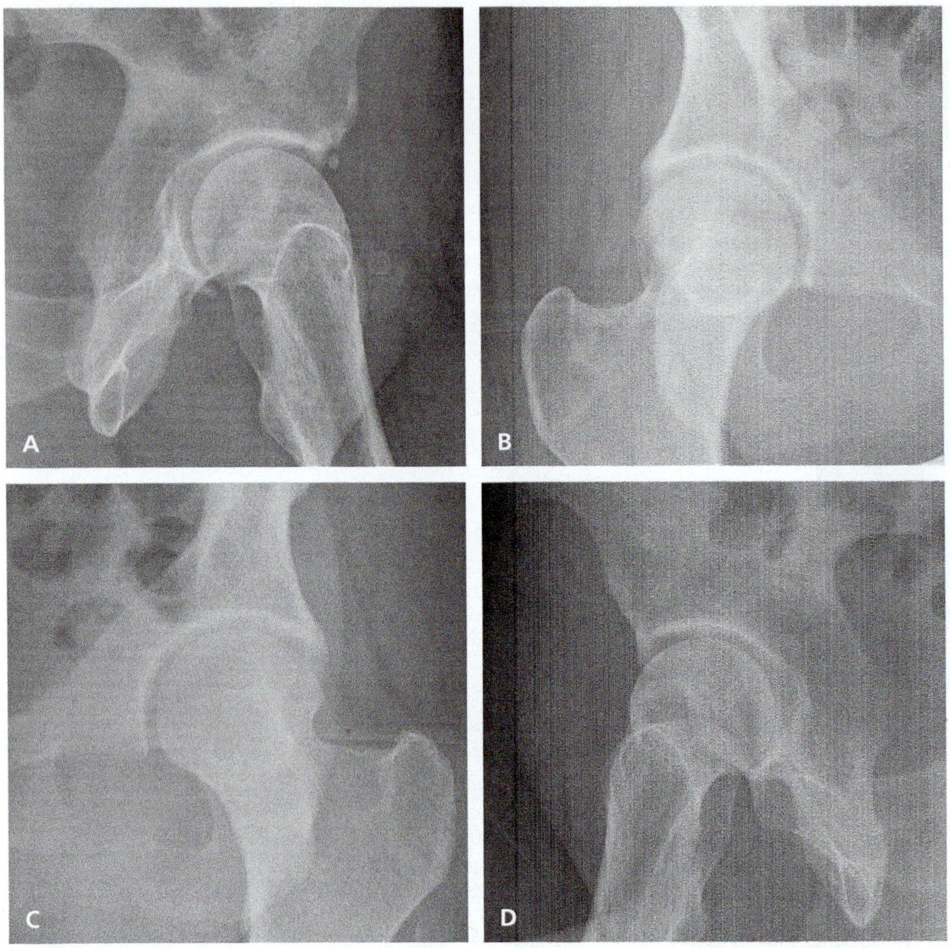

FIGURE 47. A: Left iliac LPO view. B: Left obturator RPO view. C: Right iliac RPO view. D: Right obturator LPO view.

OBLIQUE PELVIS

Also good for assessing fractures about the acetabular. CT scan is good for the initial assessment, but when there is a need to follow up fractures, oblique views are usually used.

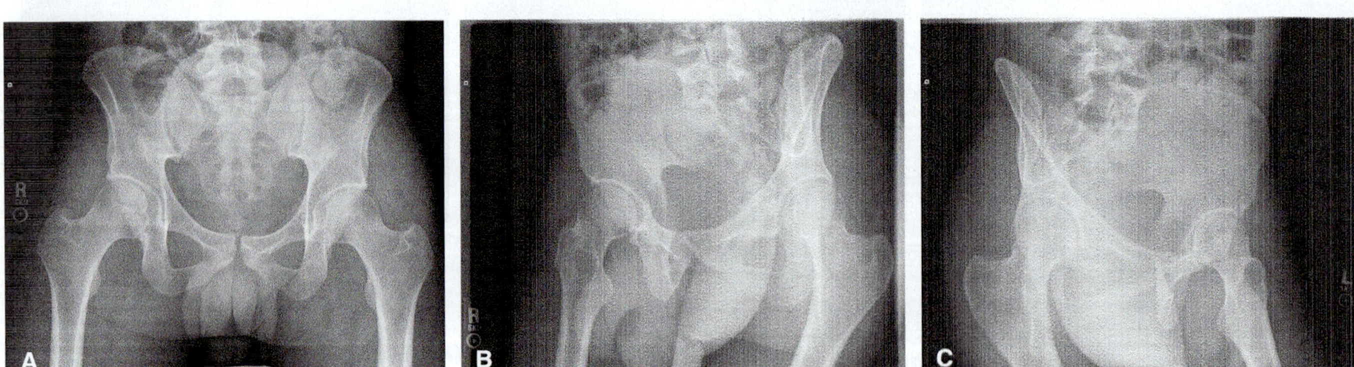

FIGURE 48. A: AP view of pelvis. B: RPO view. C: LPO view.

PELVIS

Inlet/Outlet

Good to assess for pelvic fractures involving the pubic rami and sacrum. CT scan is good for the initial assessment, but when there is a need to follow up fractures at these locations, inlet and outlet views are usually used.

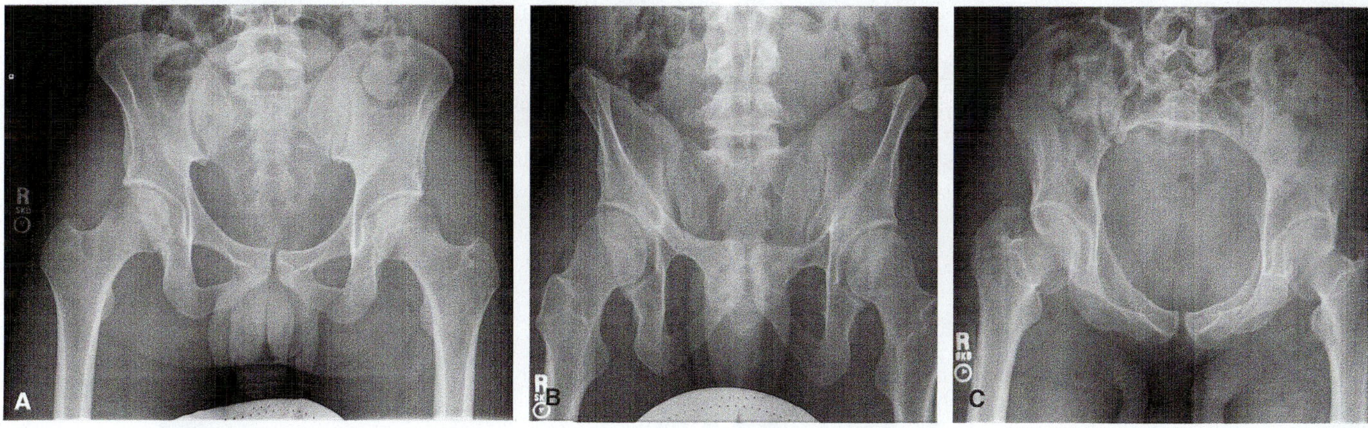

FIGURE 49. A: AP view of pelvis. B: AP axial outlet view. C: AP axial inlet view.

VERTEBRAL COLUMN

SKULL

Not used very often nowadays because most indications for a skull radiograph are better served by a CT scan; can still be used to assess shunt continuity.

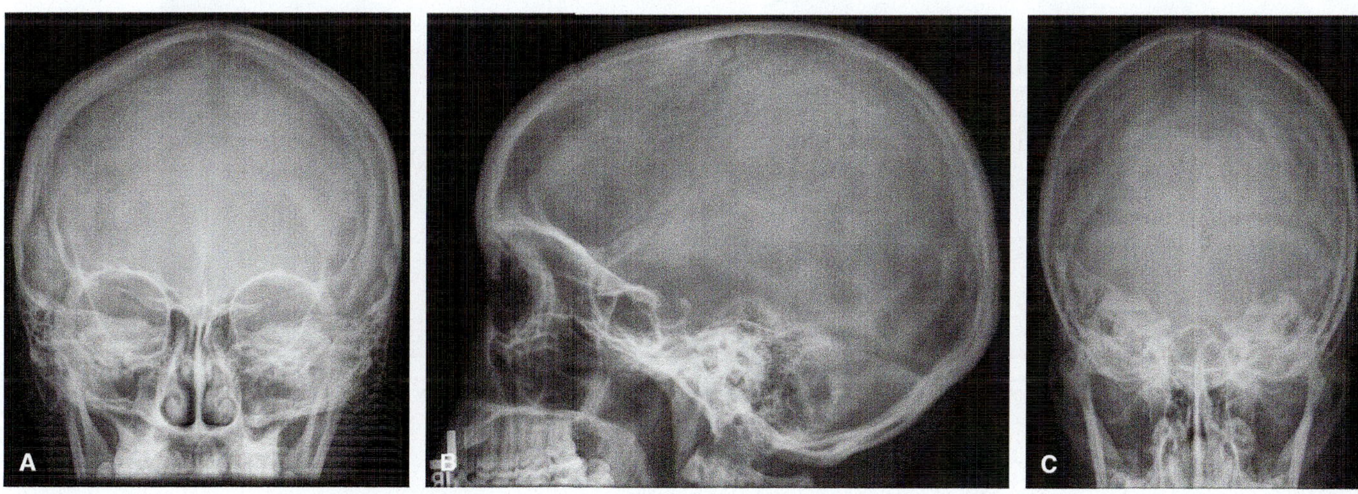

FIGURE 50. A: PA view of skull. B: Lateral view of skull. C: Townes view.

FACE

Good initial screening test for facial trauma. If found these will usually be followed up with CT scan to show the full extent.

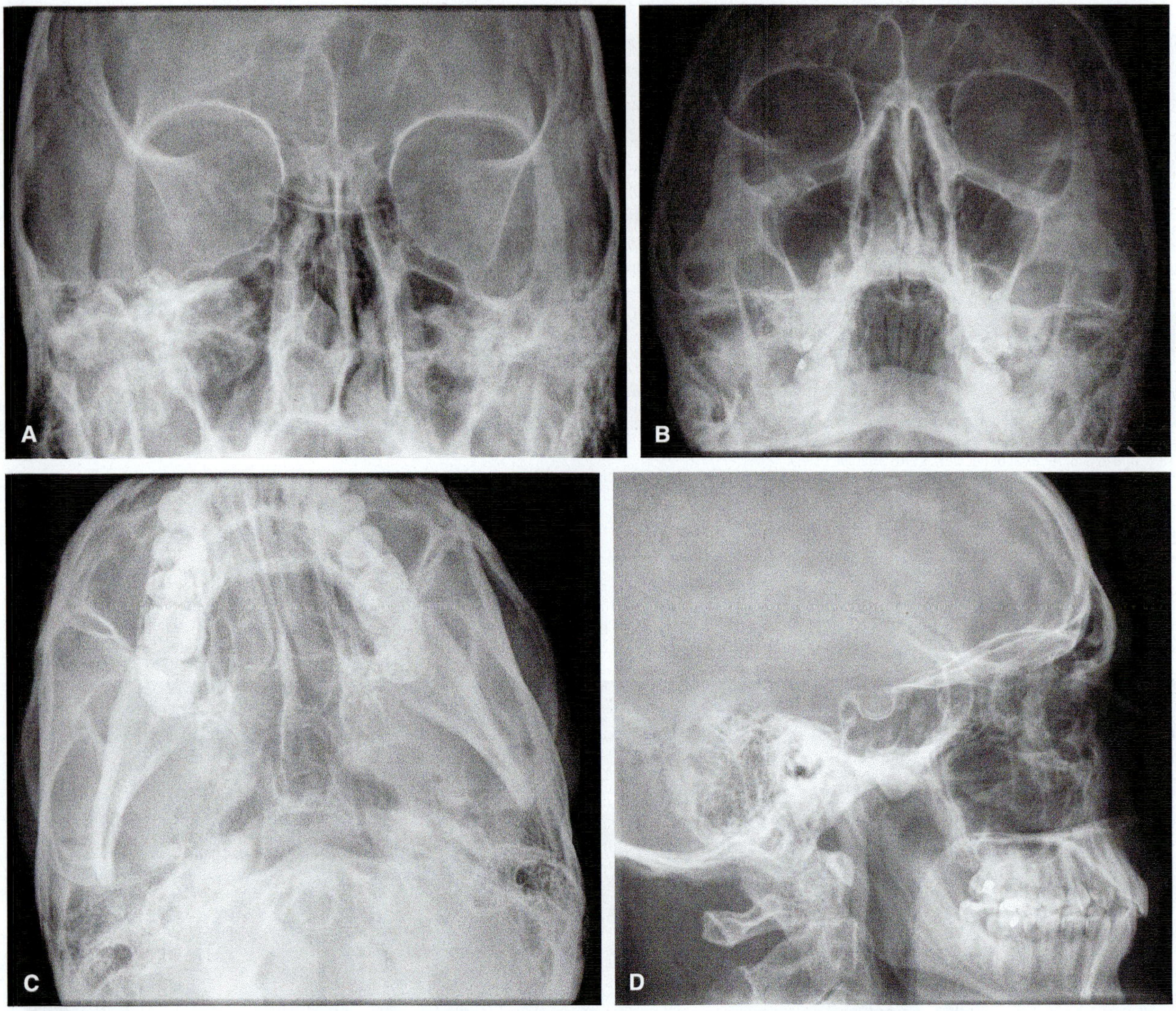

FIGURE 51. A: Occipitofrontal view. B: Occipitomental view. C: Occipitomental view with 30-degree cranial angulation. D: Lateral face view.

ORBITS

Useful to look for any destructive bony lesion about the orbit; replaced by CT scan when available.

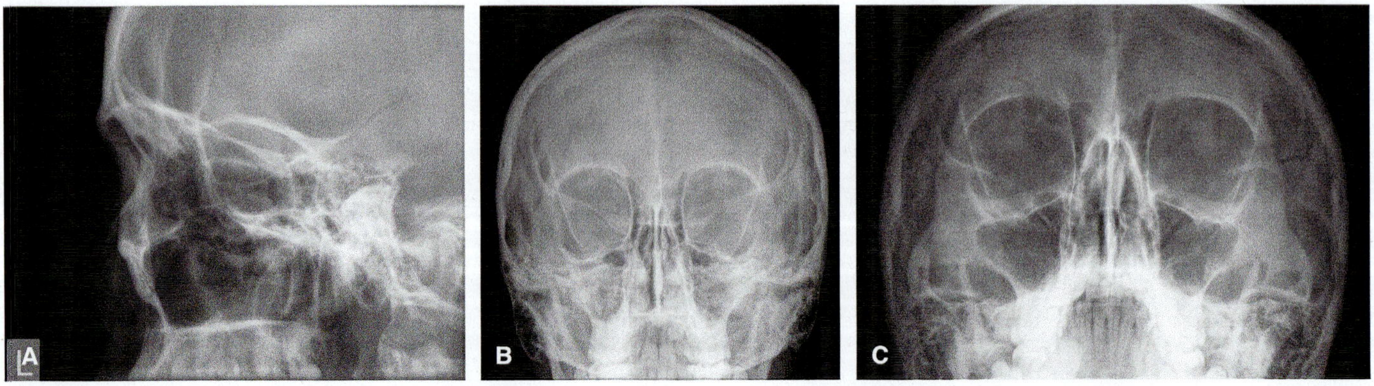

FIGURE 52. A: Lateral face view. B: Occipitofacial view. C: Occipitomental view.

EYES

Only indication would be to look for foreign body within the eye, usually prior to MRI. By just the eyes looking up and down, it is possible to see if the body moves with the globe or is elsewhere.

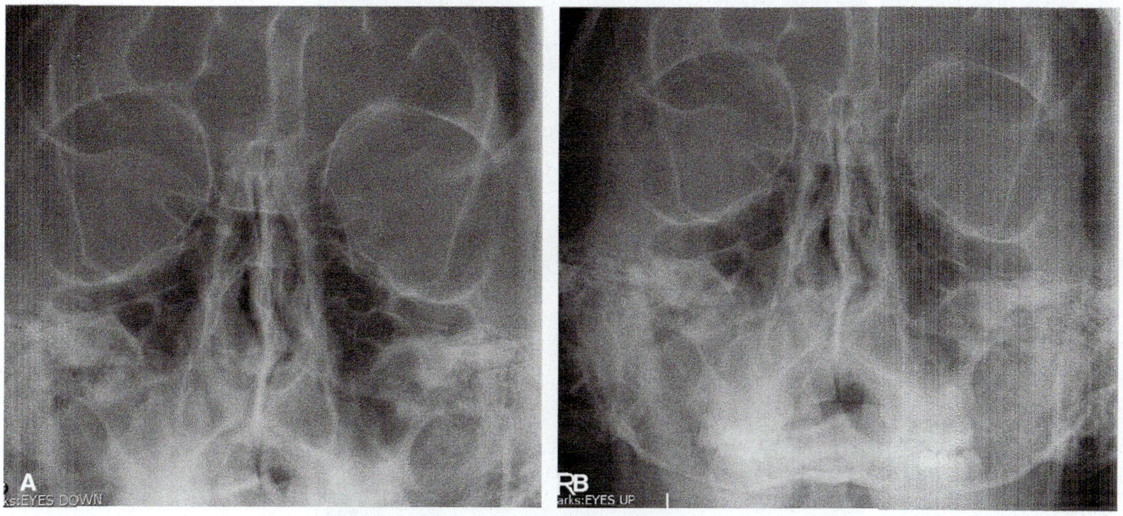

FIGURE 53. A: Occipitofacial view looking up. B: Occipitofacial view looking down.

TEMPOROMANDIBULAR JOINTS

These are taken with the mouth closed and open, coned down for each side with cranial angulation to prevent overlap.

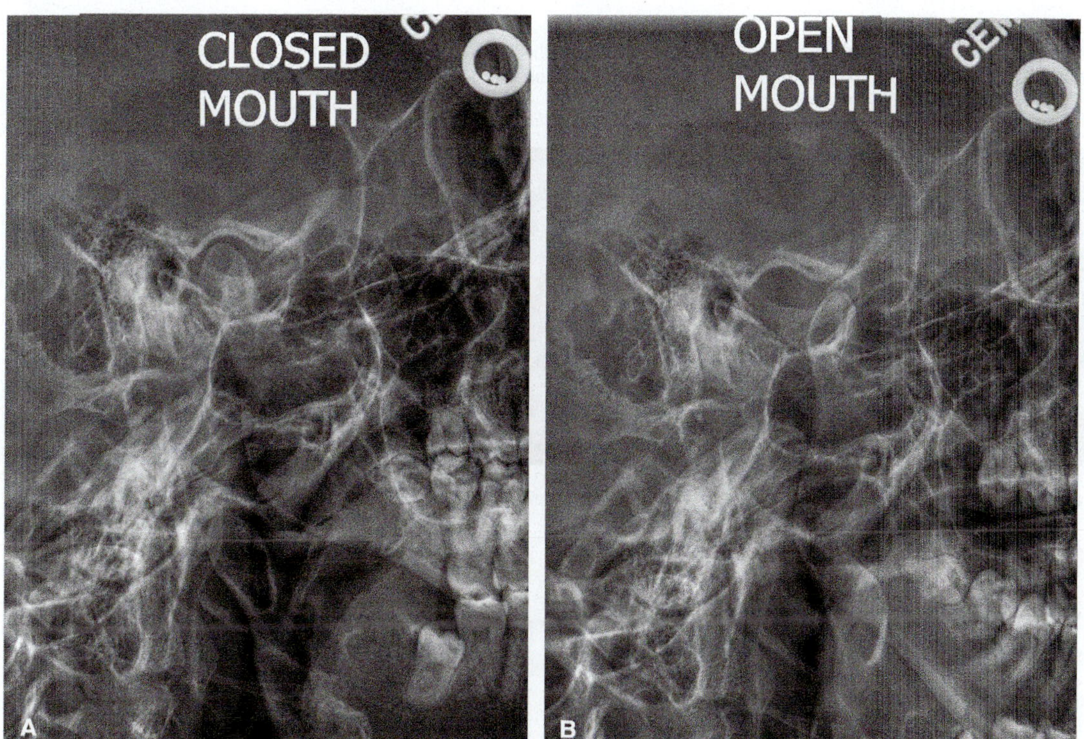

FIGURE 54. A: Left temporomandibular joint (TMJ) mouth closed. B: Left TMJ mouth open. *(continued)*

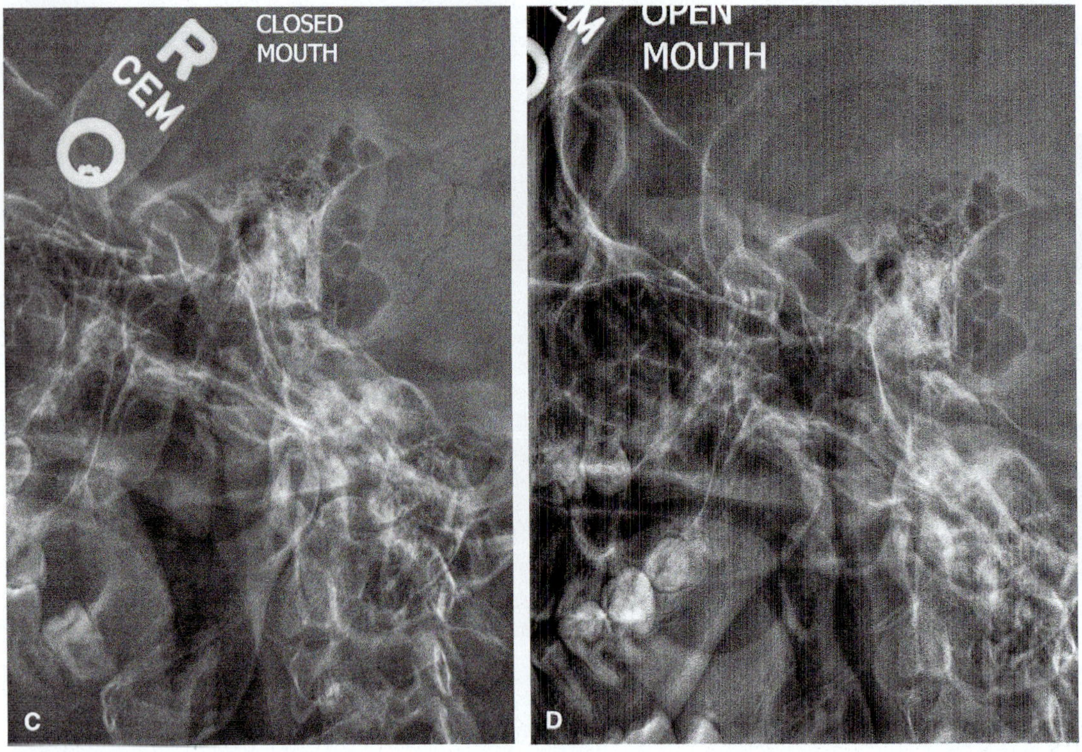

FIGURE 54. *(Continued)* C: Right TMJ mouth closed. D: Right TMJ mouth open.

MANDIBLE

The first investigation to look for mandible trauma but also used to look for disease related to the teeth and their sockets. CT scan is a useful adjunct for mandibular trauma. The oblique views are labeled, such that the side marker represents the inferiorly projecting side of the mandible.

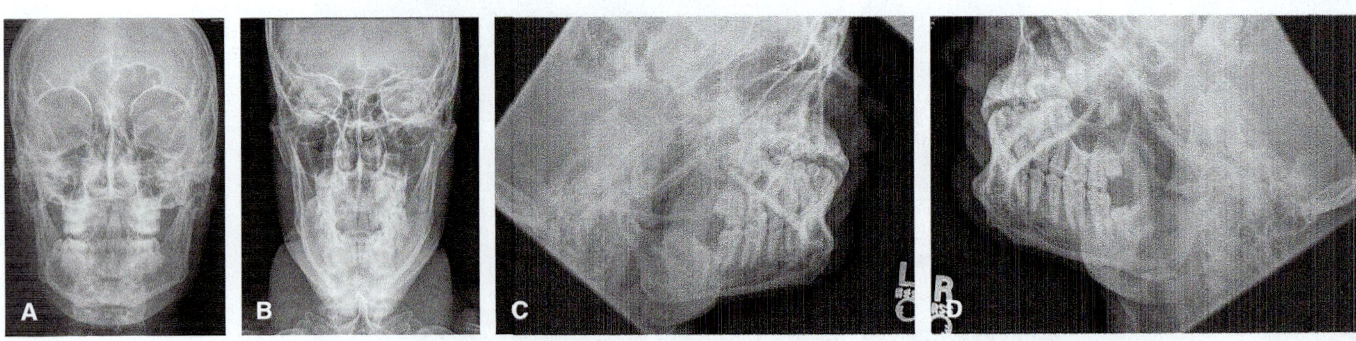

FIGURE 55. A: Occipitofacial view. B: AP axial view. C: Left inferosuperior oblique view. D: Right inferosuperior oblique view.

NASAL BONE

Used to assess for nasal trauma. Can also be used to show the septum in cases of nasal septal destruction but would usually be replaced by CT scan for the latter. Many advocate not radiographing the nose for 7 to 10 days until the swelling has subsided and then only if the patient is unhappy with the appearance. Bilateral lateral views are probably over-doing things.

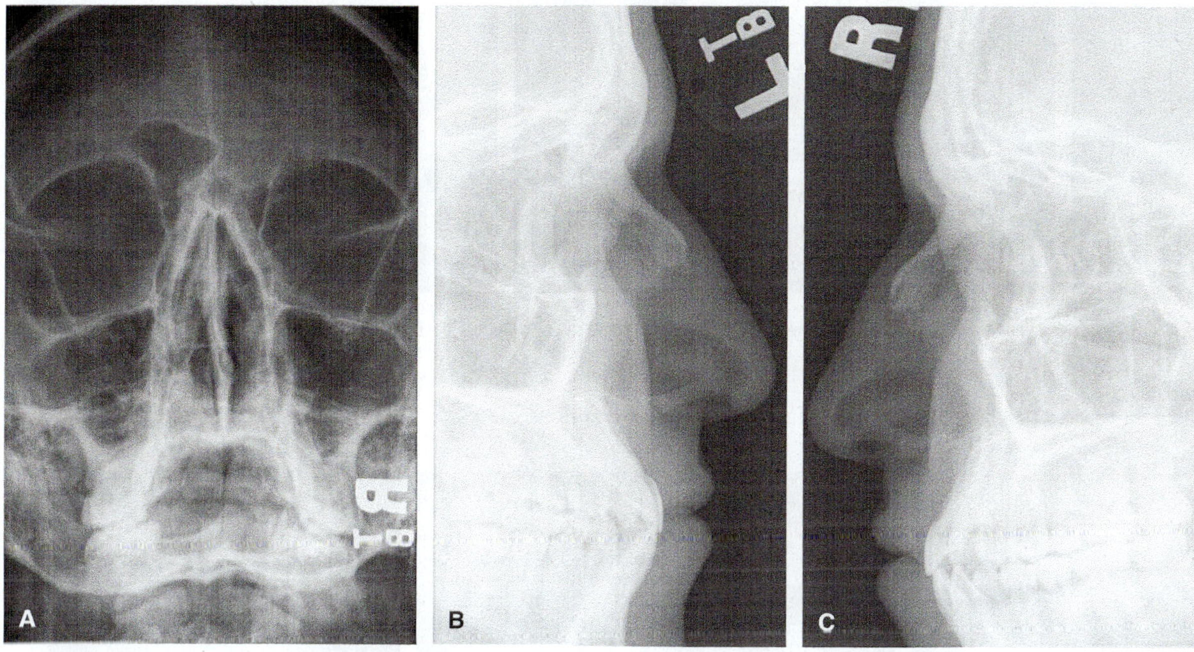

FIGURE 56. A: Coned-down occipitofacial view. B: Left lateral view of soft tissue exposure. C: Right lateral view of soft tissue exposure.

CERVICAL SPINE

Complete

Include a swimmer's view if C7–T1 junction is not well visualized on the lateral view, and a Fuchs view if the odontoid is suboptimal on the open mouth odontoid view. Such a full series is rarely used nowadays and would be replaced by CT scan for acute trauma and CT scan or MRI for chronic pain/radiculopathy. Oblique views such as these would be difficult in the trauma setting and would be done as trauma obliques with the patient supine and the beam angled obliquely. They can be useful to show the posterior elements, particularly at the cervicothoracic junction where it may otherwise be difficult.

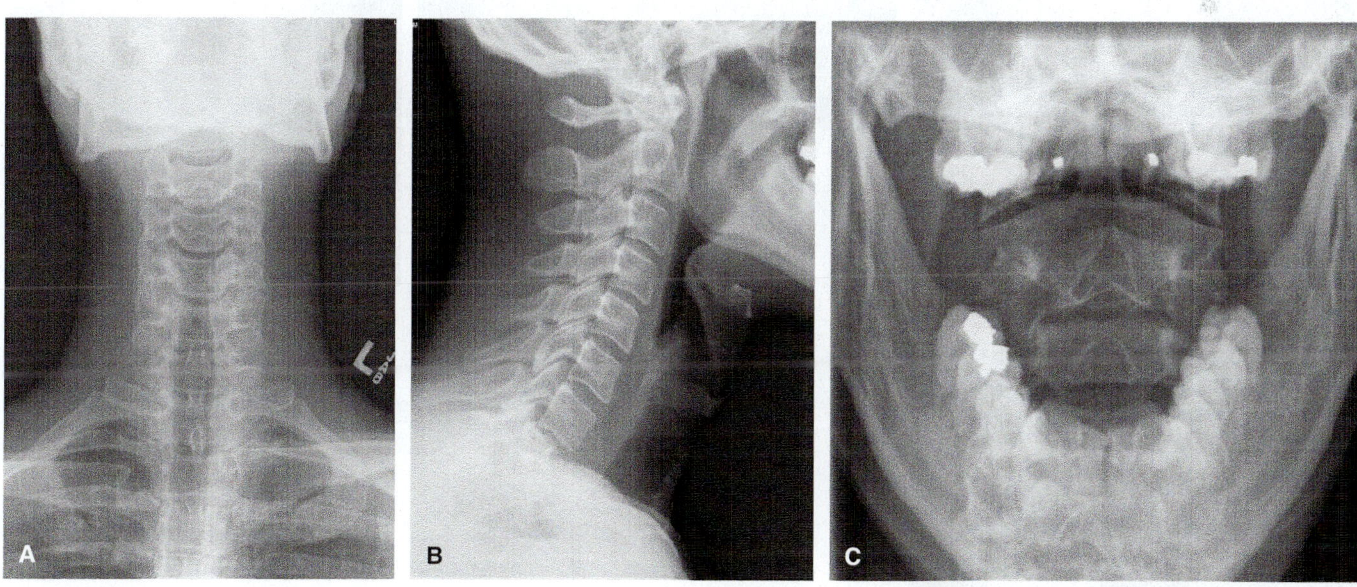

FIGURE 57. A: AP view. B: Lateral view. C: AP odontoid view (open mouth). *(continued)*

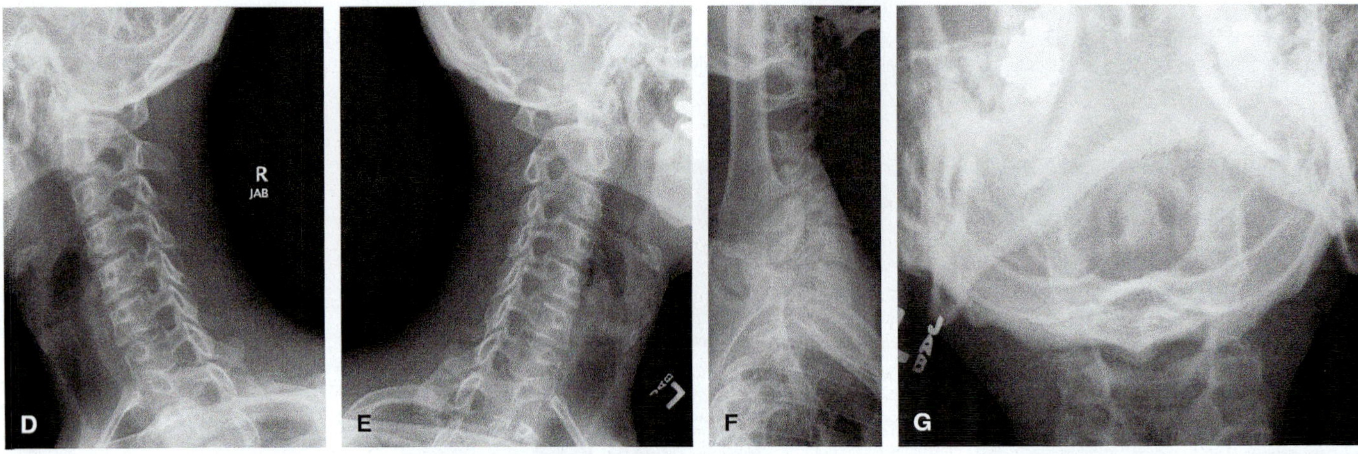

FIGURE 57. *(Continued)* D: Right anterior oblique view (wrongly labeled). E: Left anterior oblique view. F: Swimmer's view to visualize C7–T1. G: Fuchs view.

Cervical-Spine Limited

A more reasonable series for acute trauma. Follow-up or chronic pain would usually emphasize the area of interest.

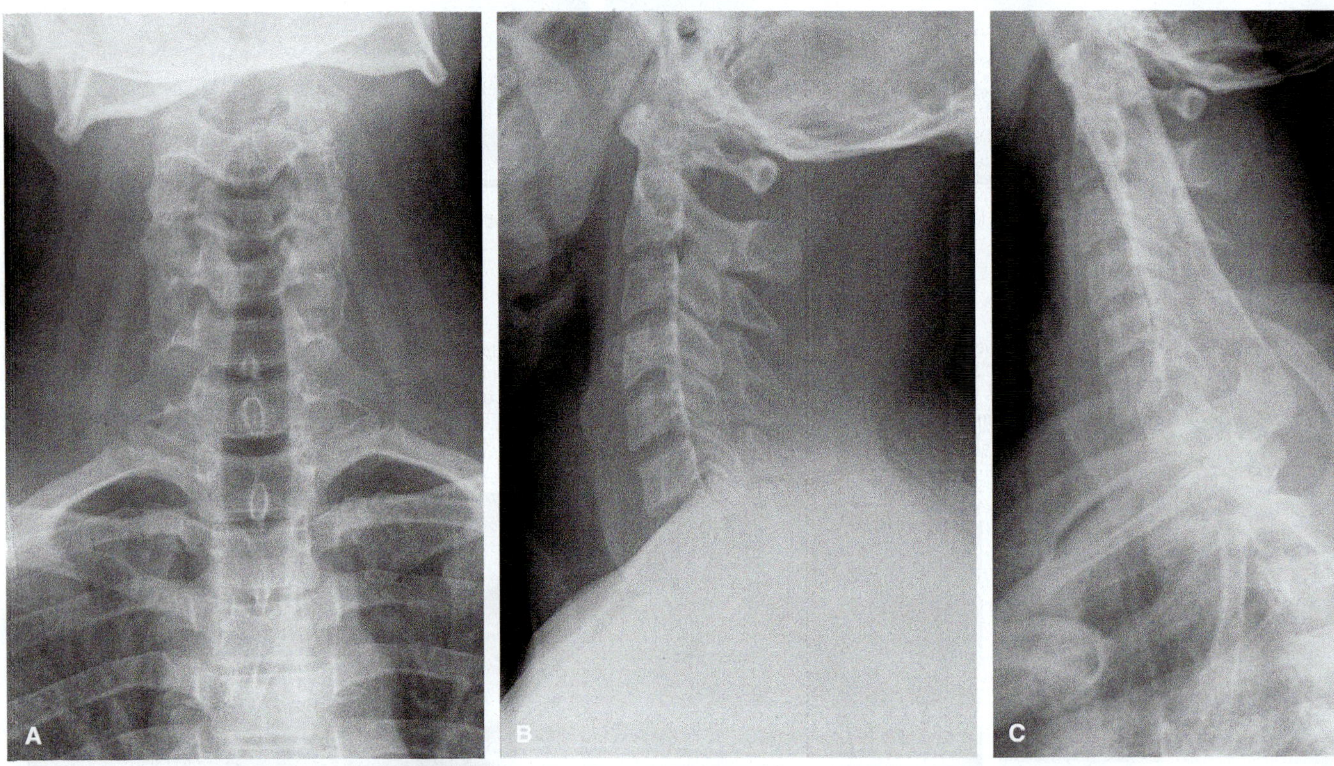

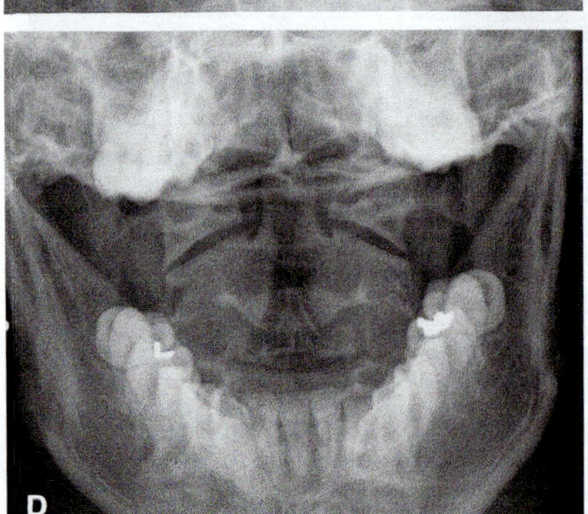

FIGURE 58. A: AP view. B: Lateral view. C: AP odontoid view (open mouth). D: Swimmer's view.

CERVICAL SPINE

Flexion–Extension Series

The best way to assess cervical stability. They cannot be obtained acutely after trauma when there will likely be spasm but should be delayed for 10 days.

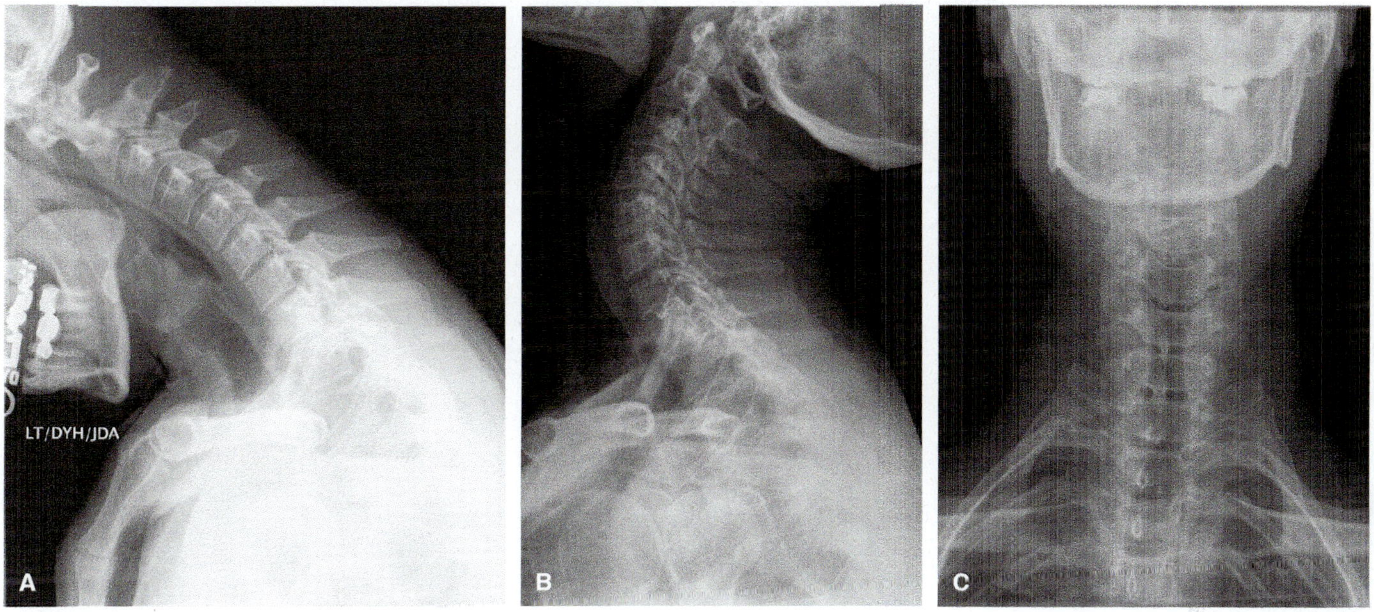

FIGURE 59. A: Flexion lateral view. B: Extension lateral view. C: AP view.

THORACIC SPINE

Guud Inltlal assessment of pain and trauma. The lateral view may need to be augmented by a swimmer's view to show the cervicothoracic junction.

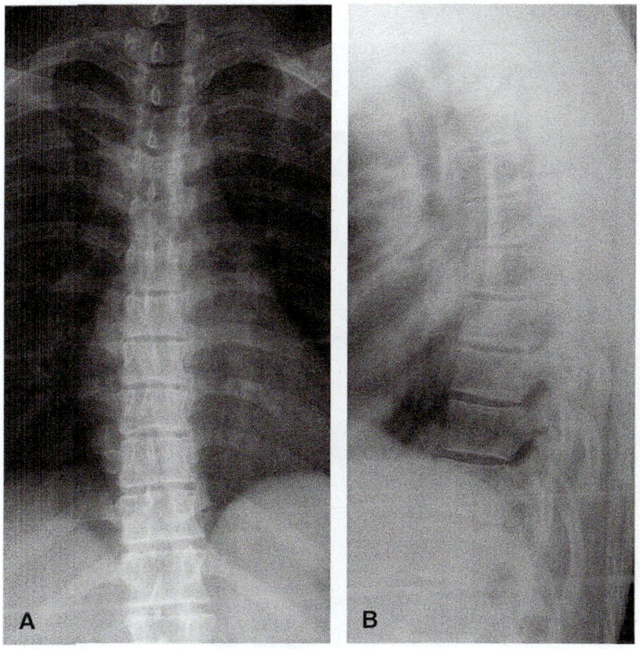

FIGURE 60. A: AP view of thoracic spine. B: Lateral view of thoracic spine.

THORACIC SPINE

Additional views

The lateral view may need to be augmented by a swimmer's view to show the cervicothoracic junction. CT scan is used to characterize any fractures seen and MRI in cases of long tract signs.

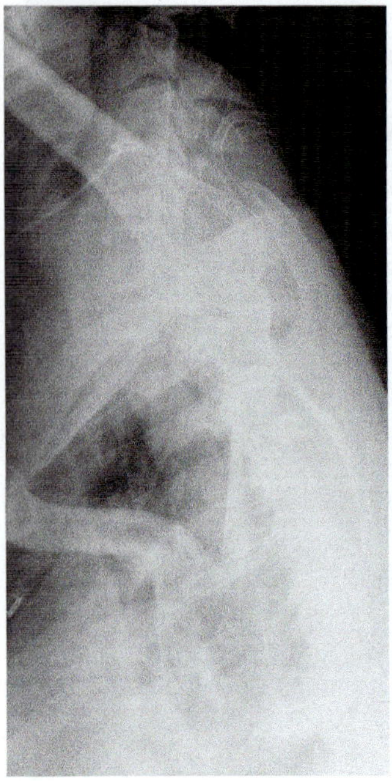

FIGURE 61. Swimmer's view of cervicothoracic junction.

LUMBAR SPINE

Routine Imaging

The images vary from center to center. Some will include an AP pelvis, others just AP, and lateral lumbar spine. Good to assess for acute trauma, alignment, spondylolysis, and spondylolisthesis. CT scan is usually performed if trauma is seen on the radiographs. MRI is useful in cases of radiculopathy.

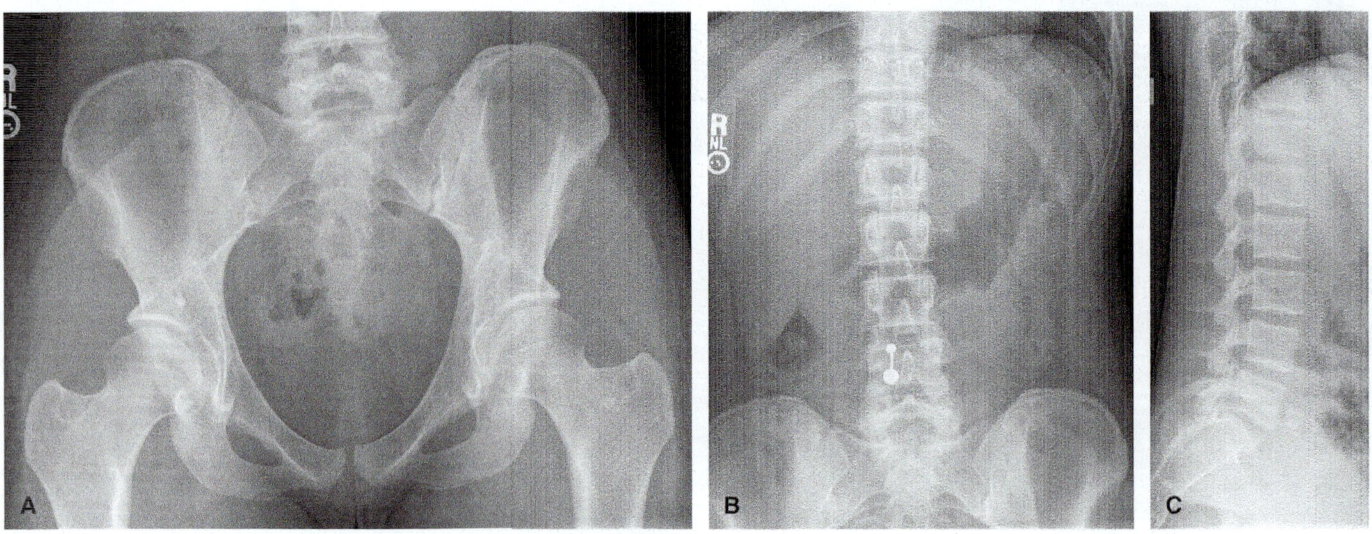

FIGURE 62. A: AP view of pelvis. B: AP view of lumbar spine. C: Lateral view of lumbar spine.

LUMBAR SPINE

Additional Views

For follow-up flexion–extension exams, a neutral lateral is not needed. These extra images start to incur a large radiation dose for little extra information and are not encouraged. Oblique views allow visualization of the facet joints and can show pars defects, although these are often better seen on the lateral view. The flexion–extension views are used to look for instability in the preoperative planning of possible spinal fusion or the postoperative assessment of fusion. The coned-down lateral view of the lumbosacral junction is useful because often this region is obliqued on the lateral lumber spine.

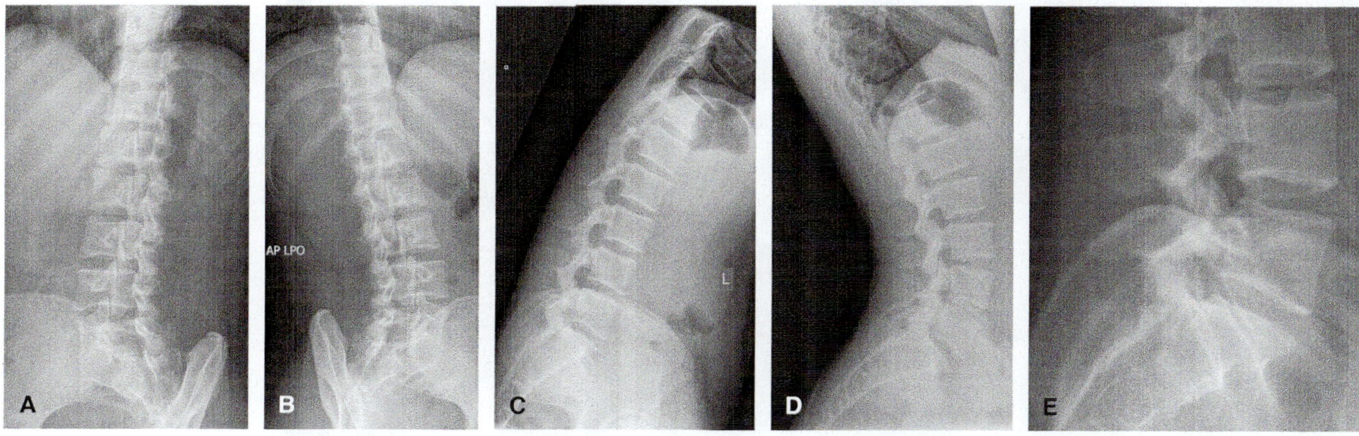

FIGURE 63. A: Right posterior oblique view of lumbar spine. B: Left posterior oblique view of lumbar spine. C: Flexion lateral view of lumbar spine. D: Extension lateral view of lumbar spine. E: L5–S1 lateral view.

SACRUM

Often difficult to see even with good radiographs due to bowel gas and feces. Not usually imaged separately from the pelvis in trauma. Can be used to look for lesions affecting the sacral plexus.

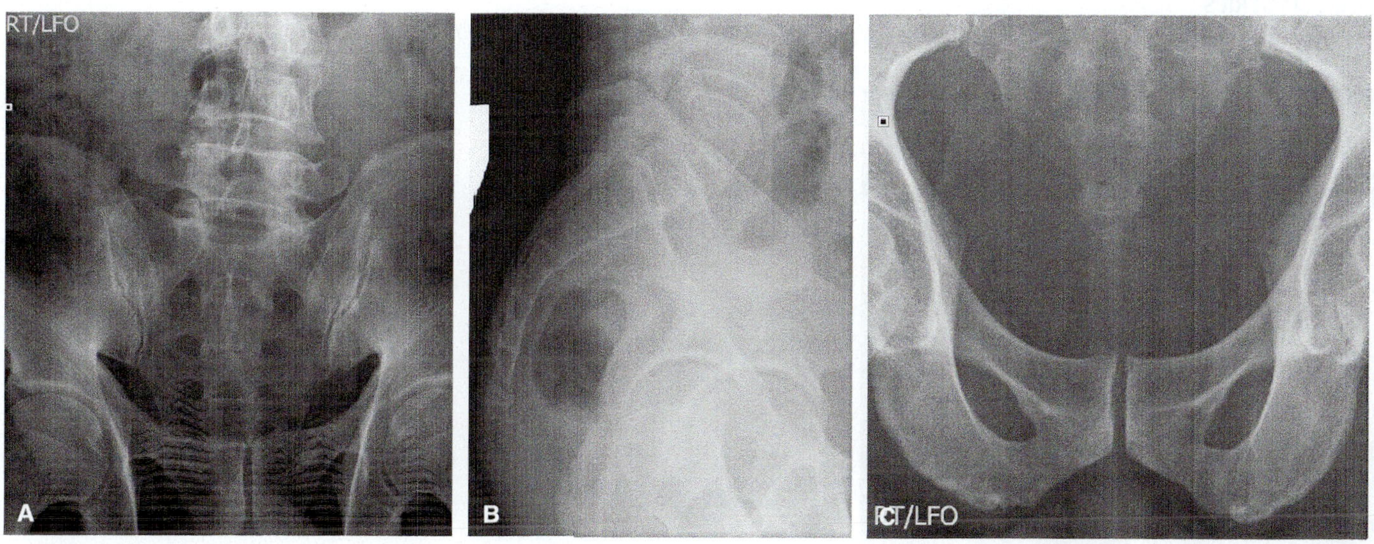

FIGURE 64. A: AP cranial view. B: Lateral view. C: AP caudal view.

COCCYX

Used in cases of coccydynia. The coccyx has a wide variety of shapes and angles and is often inconclusive for the radiation dose used.

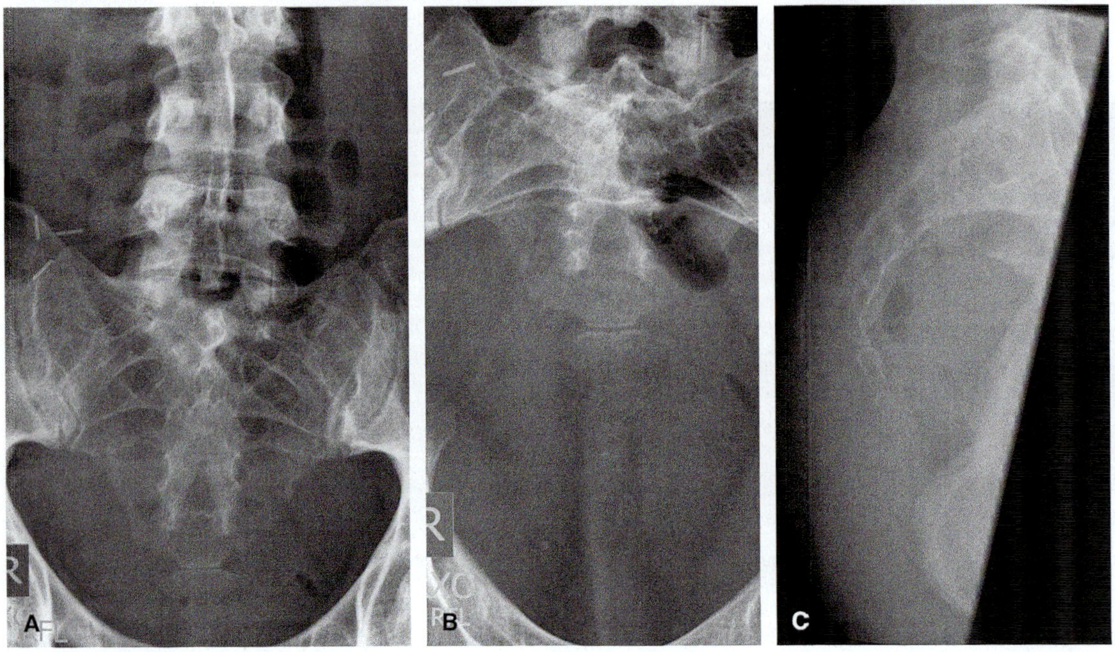

FIGURE 65. A: AP view. B: AP caudal view. C: Lateral view.

SCOLIOSIS SERIES

Used to measure the Cobb angle and look for progression. Also used to look for underlying congenital vertebral anomaly.

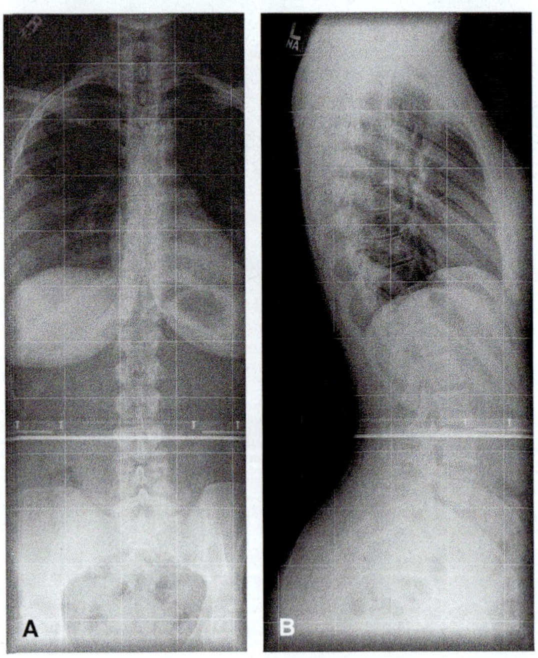

FIGURE 66. A: PA view of taken weight-bearing. B: Lateral view of taken weight-bearing.

SCOLIOSIS SERIES

Additional Views

Views taken erect, leaning to the left, and to the right are useful to look for mobile and fixed segments of scoliosis in planning surgery.

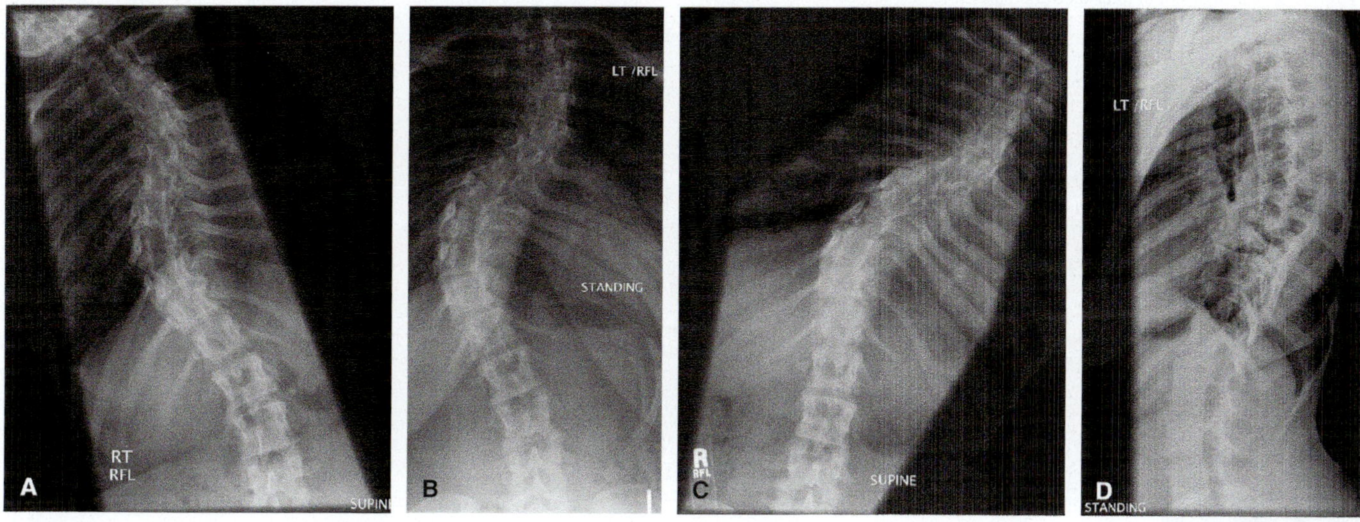

FIGURE 67. A: AP view of best bend right. B: AP view of erect. C: AP view of best bend left. D: Standing lateral view.

MISCELLANEOUS BONE STUDIES

SCANOGRAM

Used to measure leg length. Coned-down views are taken of the iliac crests, hips, knees, and ankles with a ruler behind the patient. The beam being centered on each area of interest will reduce artifact due to parallax.

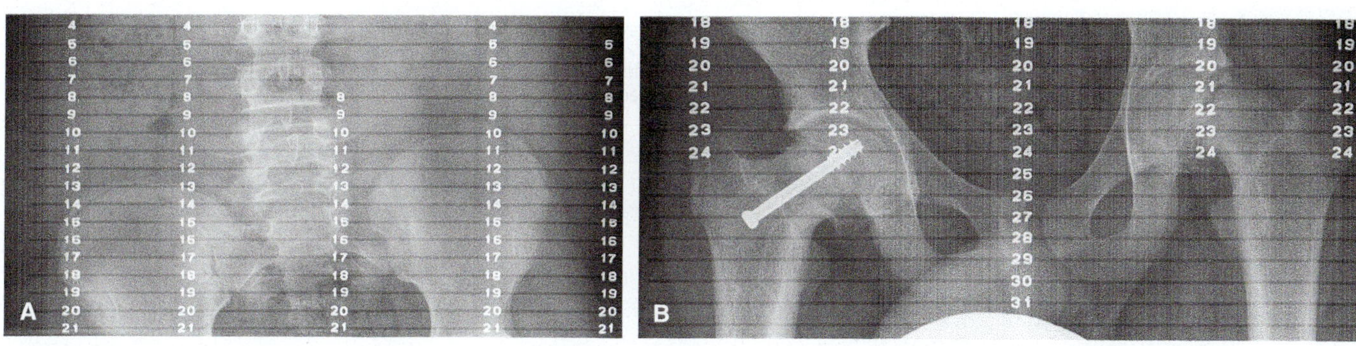

FIGURE 68. A: AP view of wing of pelvis. B: AP view of hip joint.

LEG ALIGNMENT

Include Joints from Hip to Ankle

Patient upright, equal weight in each foot. Both leg alignment and leg length can be assessed on this study if weight-bearing. The weight-bearing line passes from the middle of the femoral head to the middle to the tibial plafond and should pass between the tibial eminences. This determines varus or valgus deformity at the knees. Used for preoperative and postoperative assessment of total knee arthroplasty.

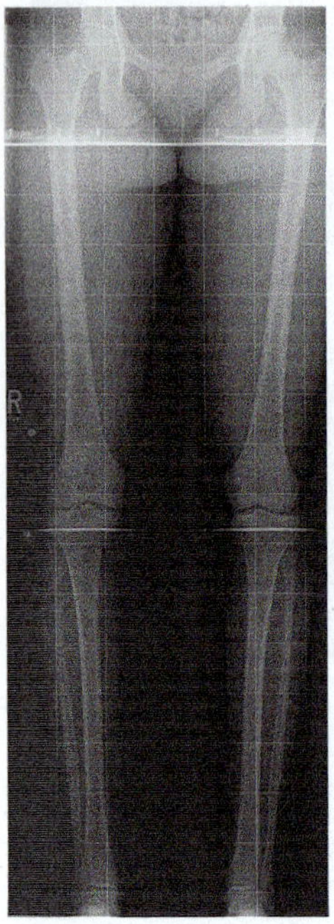

FIGURE 69. AP view of both legs.

ARTHRITIS JOINT SURVEY

This could include up to AP/lateral C-spine, AP/lateral T-spine, AP/lateral L-spine, AP bilateral shoulders, AP/lateral bilateral knees, AP pelvis, AP, oblique and lateral bilateral hands (to include wrists), AP/lateral bilateral ankles (include heel on lateral views), AP/oblique bilateral feet. Because this would be a large radiation dose it is often better to tailor this to the regions of pain.

METASTATIC BONE SURVEY

This varies from one center to another and could include from 5 to 30 images. The most important areas to image are the axial skeleton and the proximal appendicular skeleton. A full survey would include left lateral skull, AP/lateral C-spine, AP/lateral L-spine, AP/lateral bilateral humerus (to include shoulders), AP/lateral bilateral forearms, AP ribs, bilaterally, AP/lateral T-spine, AP pelvis, AP/lateral bilateral femurs, AP/lateral bilateral tibia/fibulas.

BONY THORAX

RIBS

For most acute rib injuries, the protocol is a PA erect chest exam to evaluate for pneumothorax. Only patients with pathologic fractures or patients who have undergone a bone scan should be imaged for rib fractures. Legal cases may also require documentation of fracture. It is important to have a "bb" at the site of pain and for the technologist to annotate if the bb is anterior or posterior.

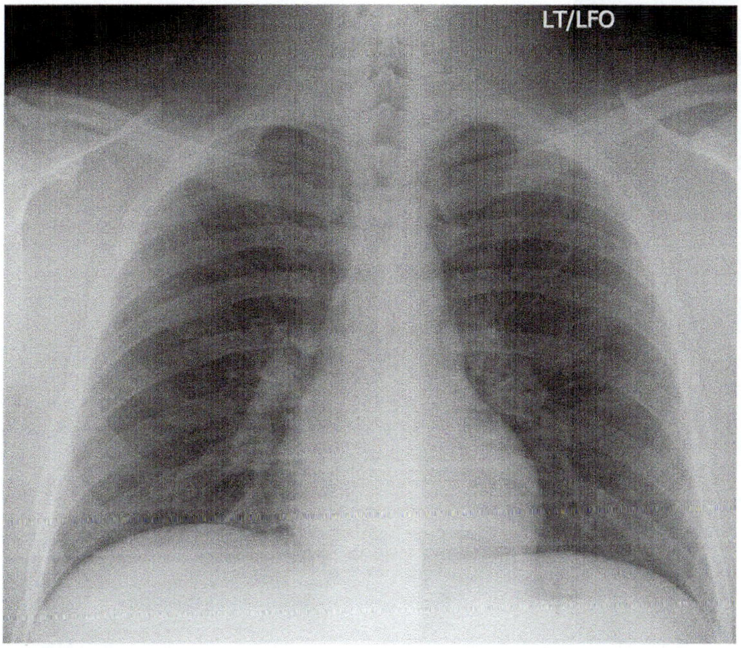

FIGURE 70. PA view of chest only, if history is acute rib injury.

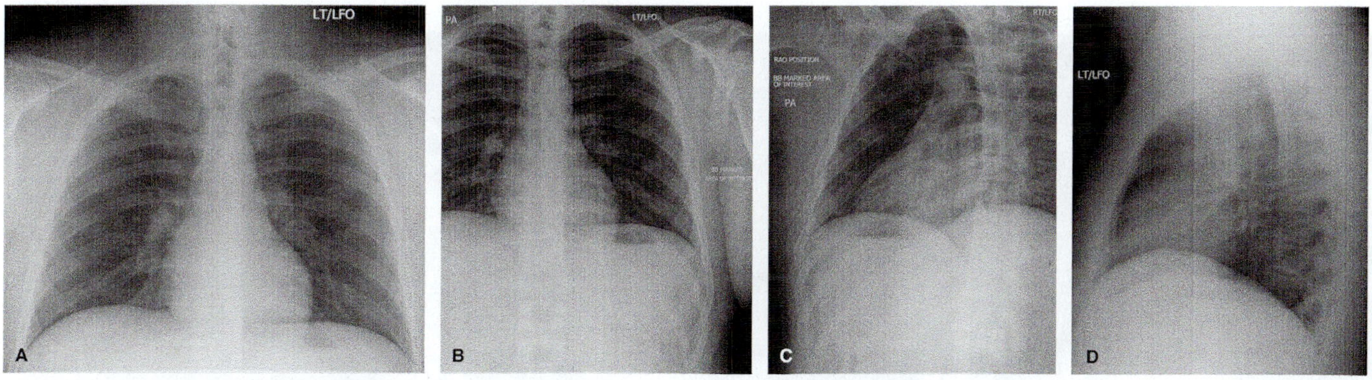

FIGURE 71. Post bone scan or pathologic fractures. A: AP or PA view of ribs—dependent on site of injury. B, C: Affected side closest to Bucky oblique ribs. D: Lateral ribs view.

STERNUM

Even on good radiographs, visualization of the sternum is limited. The study of choice is CT scan.

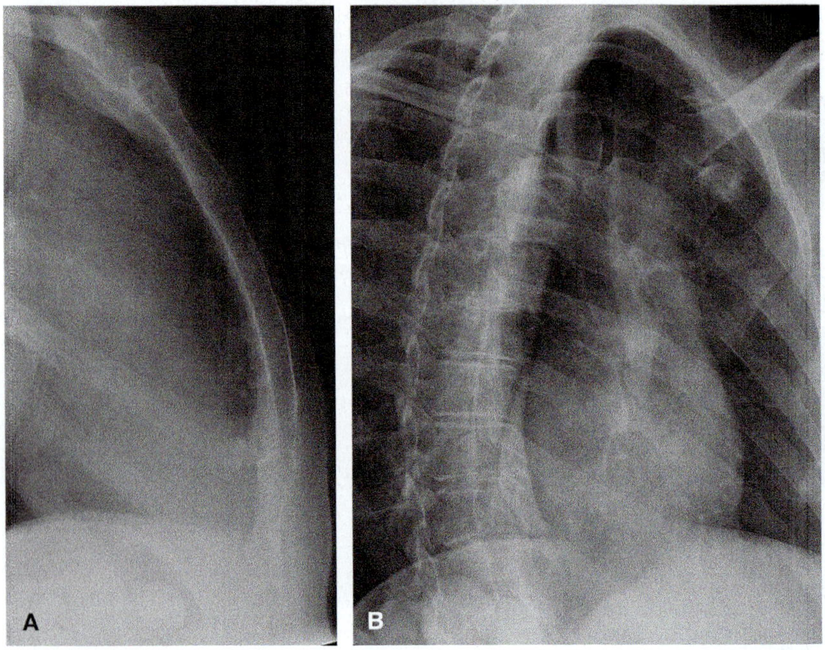

FIGURE 72. A: Lateral view. B: Right anterior oblique view.

STERNOCLAVICULAR JOINTS

Study of choice is CT scan. These are very poorly visualized radiographically. A useful sign is a difference in height of the anterior ends of the ribs.

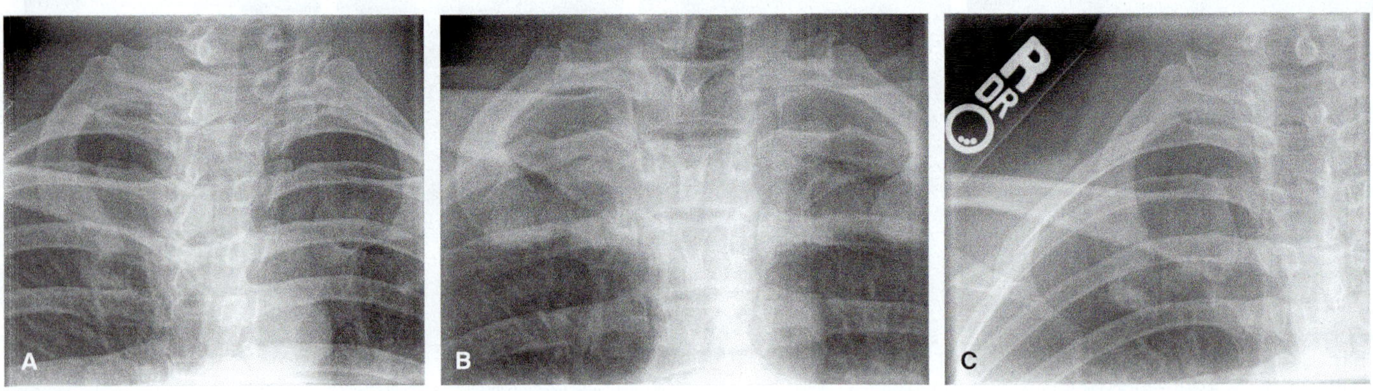

FIGURE 73. A: PA view. B: AP axial view. C: Coned-down PA view.

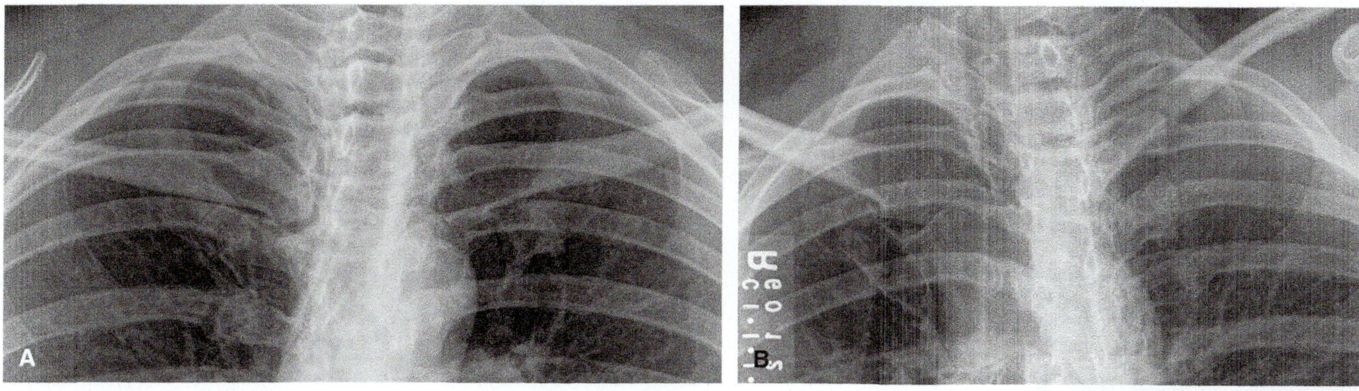

FIGURE 74. A, B: PA and oblique views.

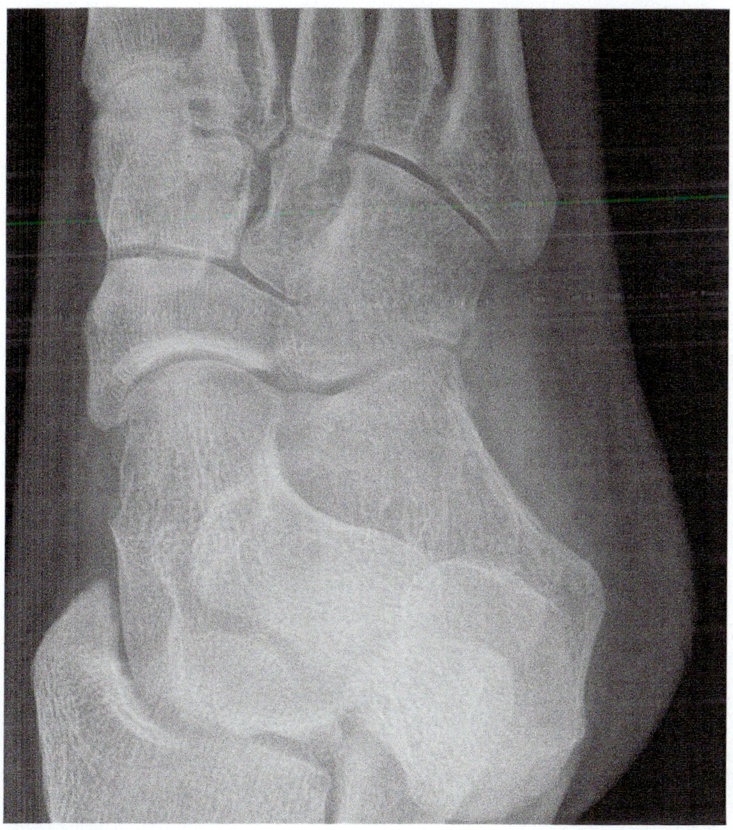

FIGURE 75. Cuboid avulsion.

DISTAL PHALANX FRACTURES

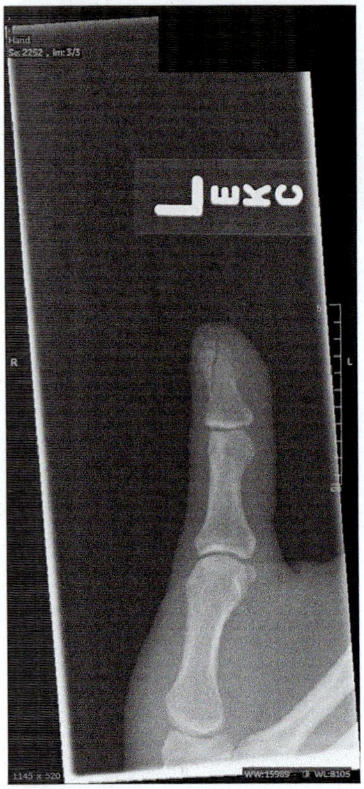

FIGURE 76. Longitudinal oblique view of distal phalanx fracture. (Photo courtesy of Drew Duerson, MD.)

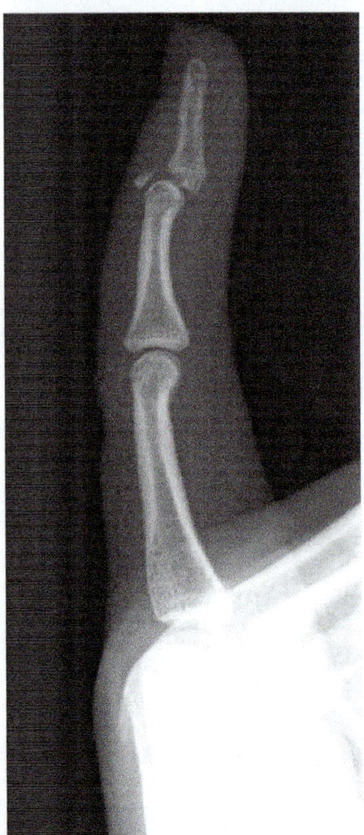

FIGURE 77. Mallet fracture. (Photo courtesy of Jonathan Napolitano, MD.)

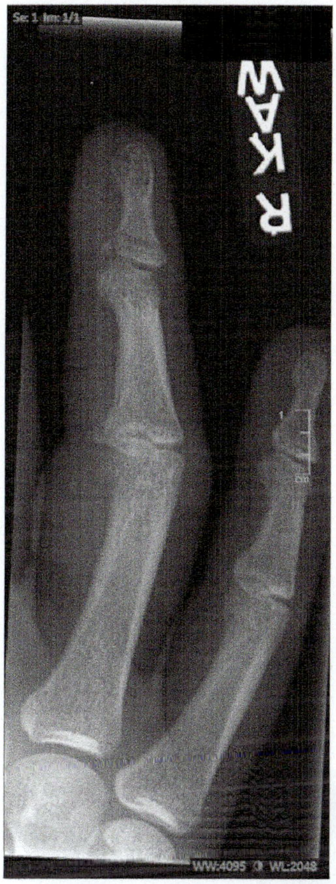

FIGURE 78. Jersey finger avulsion fracture. (Photo courtesy of Drew Duerson, MD.)

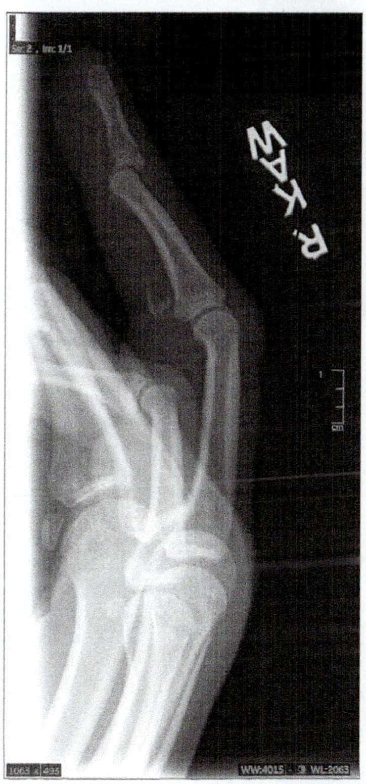

FIGURE 79. Proximally retracted or displaced jersey finger avulsion fracture. (Photo courtesy of Drew Duerson, MD.)

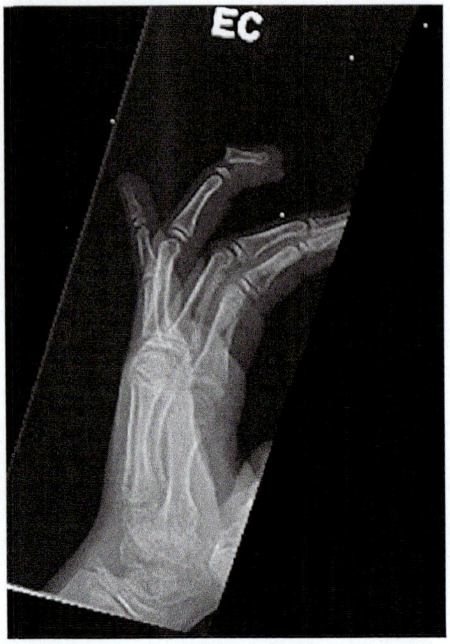

FIGURE 80. Seymour fracture. (Photo courtesy of Julie Samora, MD.)

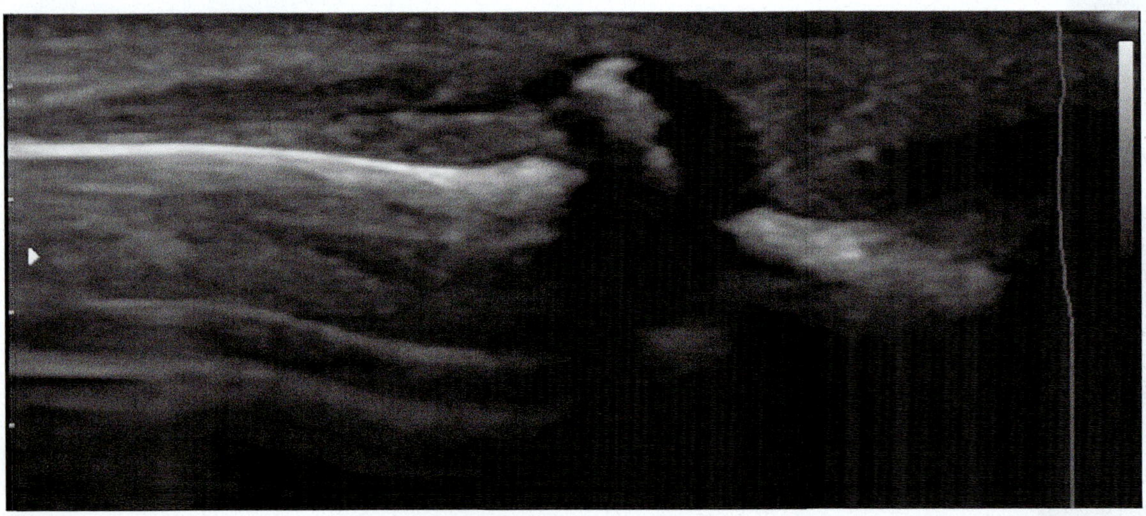

FIGURE 81. US of mallet fracture. (Photo courtesy of Jonathan Napolitano, MD.)

HOFFA FAT PAD

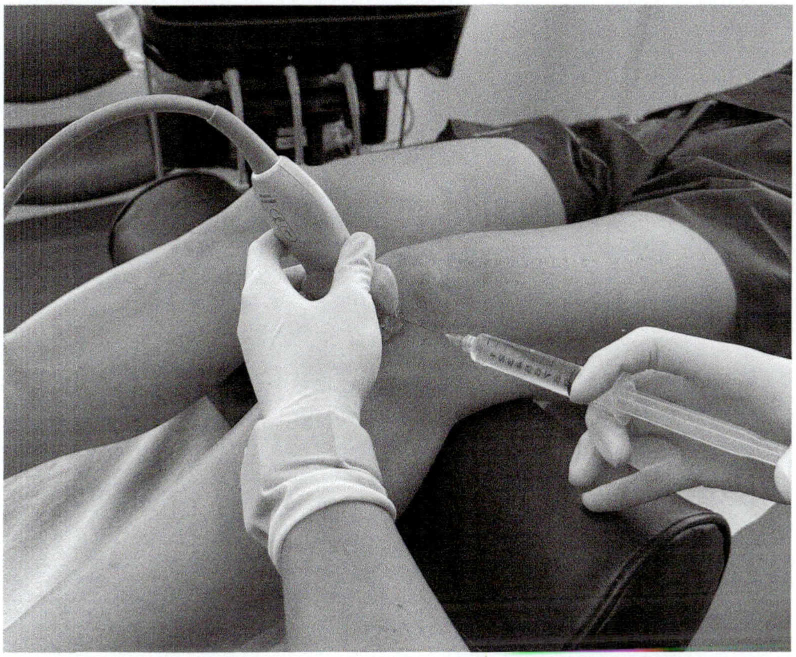

FIGURE 82. US probe positioned in short-axis relative to the patellar tendon and needle in plane to perform a US-guided Hoffa fat pad hydrodissection.

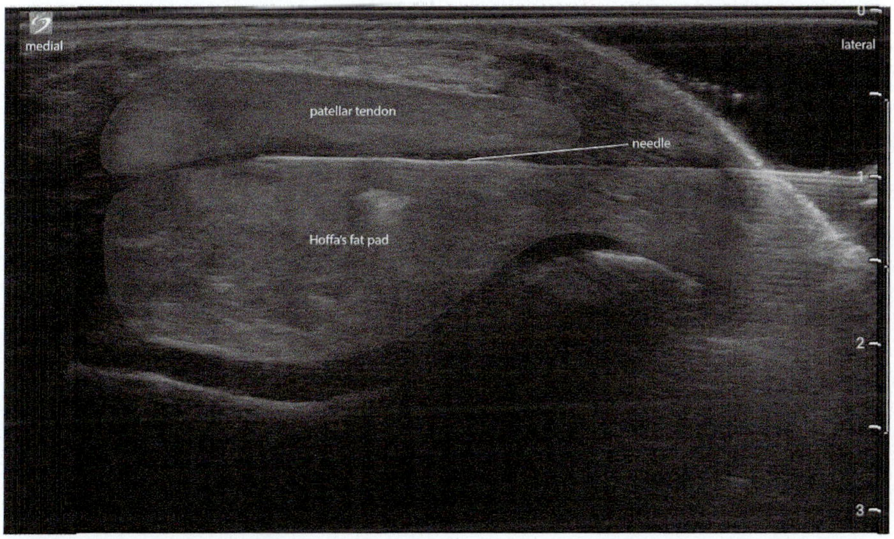

FIGURE 83. US image of guided Hoffa fat pad hydrodissection.

Appendix B

JOINT AND SOFT TISSUE INJECTION

Michal Kalli Hose, MD ▪ Anna P. Quan, MD

INTRODUCTION

Joint and soft tissue injections are valuable tools in the treatment of common musculoskeletal conditions. When musculoskeletal pain persists despite use of noninvasive modalities including oral and topical nonsteroidal anti-inflammatory drugs (NSAIDs), activity modification, splinting, ice, heat, and physical therapy, joint injections may provide temporary pain relief and improve function. Please note this chapter focuses on anatomic landmarks for joint injections which are most applicable to primary care clinics, rather than ultrasound guided procedures.

INDICATIONS FOR JOINT INJECTIONS

Diagnostic

- Injection of local anesthetic can provide temporary pain relief to allow more accurate musculoskeletal physical exam (e.g., evaluate for rotator cuff tear vs. weakness secondary to pain).
- Analysis of joint fluid aspirates can assist in the diagnosis of multiple conditions including:
  - Gout/pseudogout (crystal analysis)
  - Septic arthritis (elevated white blood cell [WBC] and/or positive Gram stain and culture)
  - Trauma (hemarthrosis)

Therapeutic

- Decrease pain
- Increase range of motion (ROM) and function
- Improve quality of life

Conditions

- Crystalline arthropathies
- Osteoarthritis
- Inflammatory arthritis
- Bursitis
- Tendinosis
- Ganglion cysts
- Nerve entrapments
- Fasciitis
- Trigger points

CONTRAINDICATIONS

Absolute

- Infection (overlying cellulitis)
- Lack of informed consent
- Allergy to injection medications
- Injection into and around weight-bearing tendons such as Achilles and patella due to high risk of rupture

Relative

- Brittle or uncontrolled diabetes
- Coagulopathy (safe in patients with international normalized ratio [INR] <3.5)
- Previous joint replacement/hardware
- History of avascular necrosis
- History of steroid or hyaluronic acid (HA) flare
- Injection around posterior tibialis tendon because of rupture risk

SUPPLIES

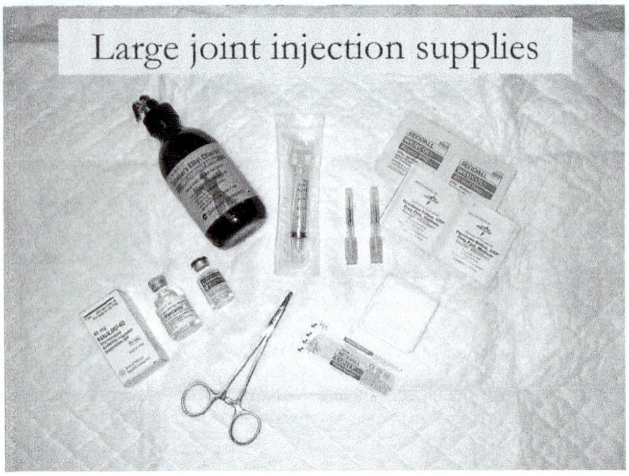

- Nonsterile gloves
- Syringes: 3 to 5 mL or larger volumes if aspiration is planned (10, 20, 60 mL)
- Needles:
  - 18 gauge for drawing up fluid or anti-stick needle/connector
  - 16 to 18 gauge for large aspirations or HA injections
  - 21 to 22 gauge 1.5 inches standard size for medium to large joints or HA injections
  - 25 gauge 1.5 inches or 25 gauge 5/8 inches standard size for small joints
  - 21- to 22-gauge 3.5-inch spinal needles often needed for ultrasound-guided hip injections and trochanteric bursa injections in large patients
- Povidone-iodine (Betadine) × 3 or chlorhexidine swabs × 45 seconds
- Alcohol swabs
- Gauze
- Adhesive bandages
- Topical vapocoolant spray, such as ethyl chloride
- Hemostat clamp

LOCAL ANESTHETIC

- Topical anesthetic can be useful for temporary pain relief or to aid in diagnosis.
- The choice of anesthetic depends on formulary availability and desired duration of action.
- In general, lidocaine has a quick onset of 3 to 5 minutes with 1- to 2-hour duration, and bupivacaine has a 5-minute onset with 3- to 4-hour duration.
- A growing number of studies demonstrate chondrotoxic effects of topical anesthetics; however, the clinical significance of these studies is still unclear. Anecdotally, we find patients tolerate arthrocentesis much better with the local anesthetic techniques described below. However, if patients or providers are concerned about the potential for chondrotoxicity, all procedures listed below can be performed without local anesthetic.
- Bupivacaine, ropivacaine, or lidocaine with epinephrine can be considered in large joints for possible prolonged benefit of the injection, but epinephrine should be avoided when injecting digits or smaller joints.

CORTICOSTEROID

- Corticosteroids can reduce inflammation which may decrease local pain and swelling.
- Lower solubility steroids have longer duration of action.
- To avoid suppression of hypothalamic-pituitary-adrenal axis, limit to 3 to 4 injections per year and be especially cautious for those with HIV on protease inhibitors.
- Based on in vitro, animal, and radiologic studies, intra-articular (IA) use of local anesthetics and cortisone may have detrimental effects on human articular cartilage and chondrocytes. Although the clinical significance of these studies is unclear, the clinical relationship between local anesthetic exposure and chondrolysis requires further study.

Table 1. Properties of Injectable Corticosteroids

Corticosteroid	Relative Anti-inflammatory Potency	Solubility	Biological Half-life
Hydrocortisone	1	High	8–12 h
Triamcinolone (Kenalog)	5	Intermediate	12–36 h
Methylprednisolone (Depo-Medrol)	5	Intermediate	12–36 h
Betamethasone (Celestone Soluspan)	25	Low/high	26–54 h
Dexamethasone (Decadron LA)	25	High	26–54 h

Reproduced with permission from McNabb JW, O'Connor FG. *A Practical Guide to Joint & Soft Tissue Injections.* 4th ed. Wolters Kluwer; 2022.

Table 2. Equivalent Dosages of Injectable Corticosteroids

Corticosteroid Preparation	Equivalent Dose/Volume
Kenalog	40 mg/mL
Depo-Medrol	40 mg/mL
Celestone Soluspan	6 mg/mL
Decadron LA	8 mg/mL

Reproduced with permission from McNabb JW. *A Practical Guide to Joint & Soft Tissue Injections*. 3rd ed. Wolters Kluwer; 2015.

VISCOSUPPLEMENTATION

- Sodium hyaluronate is a glycosaminoglycan found in normal joint fluid.
- In osteoarthritis, the concentration of sodium hyaluronate is lower.
- Synthetic formulations of sodium hyaluronate are derived from rooster combs.
- Available products:
  - Synvisc and Synvisc-One (Genzyme)
  - Gel-One (Zimmer)
  - Hyalgan (Fidia)
  - Supartz FX (Bioventus)
  - Orthovisc (Anika Therapeutics)
  - Euflexxa, previously named Nuflexxa (Savient)
  - Monovisc (Anika Therapeutics)
  - Gel-Syn (Institut Biochimique SA)
  - HYMOVIS (Fidia)
- Lack of high-powered evidence showing therapeutic efficacy
- Both the American College of Rheumatology (ACR) and the American Academy of Orthopaedic Surgeons (AAOS) have issued guidelines that do not recommend the routine use of HA injections for knee osteoarthritis, or, in some cases, actively recommend against it.
- Consider only for patients failing conservative therapy or when corticosteroids are contraindicated.
- Contraindicated in patients with allergies to avian proteins or eggs (those agents with avian proteins).

TECHNIQUE

- The specific techniques for each joint are discussed in each joint section.
- In general, the following techniques should be followed:
  - Identify the anatomic landmarks and mark the entry site with the cap of the needle.
  - Cleanse the area with alcohol followed by Betadine or chlorhexidine.
  - Spray topical ethyl chloride vapocoolant (if available) to decrease needle entry pain.
  - Insert the needle to the proper depth for the specific injection site.
  - Inject the steroid/analgesic mixture. There should be free flow (without resistance) of the medication.
  - Remove the needle and apply pressure with gauze.
  - Apply an adhesive bandage.

COMPLICATIONS

- Major risks of corticosteroid injections include bleeding, infection, tendon rupture, steroid flare, fat pad or soft tissue atrophy, and skin depigmentation.
- Steroid flare (crystal synovitis) is treated with rest, ice, and NSAIDs and usually resolves spontaneously after 24 to 36 hours.
- HA flare can also be treated with rest, ice, and NSAIDs and usually resolves spontaneously after several days. HA flare can be more drastic than steroid flare, and severe flares may require synovial aspiration and cultures to distinguish between pseudosepsis and true infection.
- The estimated risk of causing septic arthritis from arthrocentesis is low, on the order of 0.01%.

AFTERCARE

- While the local anesthetic is in effect, the patient will have less proprioceptive feedback from the joint, so patients are recommended to rest the injected joint for several hours.
- Educate the patient to monitor for signs or symptoms of infection including fever, erythema, warmth, or increasing pain.
- Ice is an effective modality for pain control following an injection.
- Activities can generally be resumed after 3 to 5 days as tolerated after a steroid injection. Patients may notice that HA has a longer lag time (1 to 2 weeks) before pain relief is noted.
- Encourage the patient to keep a pain and activity journal to record duration of pain relief and improved function. This information helps the patients make a personalized informed decision of whether to repeat injection therapy in the future.

INFORMED CONSENT

- Every invasive procedure (including joint aspirations or injections) should include a detailed informed consent.
- Lawsuits have occurred over complications to joint injections, and, in these situations, having an informed consent signed and kept with the patient's medical record is of utmost importance. Alternatives include careful informed consent discussed with the patient or guardians and documented in the record.
- The informed consent includes documentation that the patient is competent to make decisions and that a discussion of the risks and benefits of an injection have been reviewed.

BILLING/CODING

Current Procedural Terminology (CPT) and International Classification of Diseases (ICD) codes should be used to accurately assign the proper codes for the procedures performed.

BIBLIOGRAPHY

- Bhagra A, Syed H, Reed DA, et al. Efficacy of musculoskeletal injections by primary care providers in the office: a retrospective cohort study. *Int J Gen Med.* 2013;6:237–243.
- Bowman S, Awad ME, Hamrick MW, et al. Recent advances in hyaluronic acid based therapy for osteoarthritis. *Clin Transi Med.* 2018;7(1):6.
- Brophy RH, Fillingham YA. AAOS clinical practice guideline summary: management of osteoarthritis of the knee (nonarthroplasty), third edition. *J Am Acad Orthop Surg.* 2022;30(9):e721–e729.
- Brown GA. AAOS clinical practice guideline: treatment of osteoarthritis of the knee: evidence-based guideline, 2nd edition. *J Am Acad Orthop Surg.* 2013;21(9):577–579.
- Cardone DA, Tallia AF. Diagnostic and therapeutic injection of the elbow region. *Am Fam Physician.* 2002;66(11):2097–2100.
- Jackson DW, Evans NA, Thomas BM. Accuracy of needle placement into the intra-articular space of the knee. *J Bone Joint Surgery Am.* 2002;84(9):1522–1527.
- Kang MN, Rizio L, Prybicien M, et al. The accuracy of subacromial corticosteroid injections: a comparison of multiple methods. *J Shoulder Elbow Surg.* 2008;17(Suppl 1):61S–66S.
- Luc M, Pham T, Chagnaud C, et al. Placement of intra-articular injection verified by the backflow technique. *Osteoarthritis Cartilage.* 2006;14(7):714–716.
- Piper SL, Kramer JD, Kim HT, et al. Effects of local anesthetics on articular cartilage. *Am J Sports Med.* 2011;39(10):2245–2253.
- Tallia AF, Cardone DA. Diagnostic and therapeutic injection of the ankle and foot. *Am Fam Physician.* 2003;68(7):1356–1362.
- Tallia AF, Cardone DA. Diagnostic and therapeutic injection of the shoulder region. *Am Fam Physician.* 2003;67(6):1271–1278.
- Tallia AF, Cardone DA. Diagnostic and therapeutic injection of the wrist and hand region. *Am Fam Physician.* 2003;67(4):745–750.
- Webb CW, McLeod G, Nuti R. Injections of the hip and knee. *Am Fam Physician.* 2024;109(1):61–70.
- Zhang K, Li M, Yao W, et al. Cytotoxicity of local anesthetics on bone, joint, and muscle tissues: a narrative review of the current literature. *J Pain Res.* 2023;16:611–621.

TRIGGER POINT INJECTION

INDICATIONS

- Trigger points occur due to focal areas of muscular pain and spasm and often involve the back muscles.
- There is no clear evidence of benefit for trigger point injections, but anecdotally, some patients report reduced pain after trigger point injections.
- There are real risks of pneumothorax with legal actions taken against providers involved.

ANATOMY

- The anatomy depends on the location of the trigger point injection.
- The injection is performed over the tender nodule, which is usually in the muscles surrounding the scapula.

SUPPLIES

- Gloves
- Betadine or chlorhexidine and alcohol swabs
- 3-mL syringe with 25-gauge 5/8- to 1-inch needle
- 1 mL 1% lidocaine
- 0.5 mL (20 mg) triamcinolone suspension (Kenalog) or equivalent (optional)
- Ethyl chloride
- Gauze
- Adhesive bandage

TECHNIQUE

- Palpate the tender nodule and mark with needle cap.
- Cleanse the skin with alcohol swab and then Betadine × 3 or chlorhexidine × 45 seconds.
- Apply ethyl chloride until the skin turns white.
- Injection site is directly into the nodule.
- A fanning technique can be used to disperse the fluid in various directions, which can be helpful in large nodules.

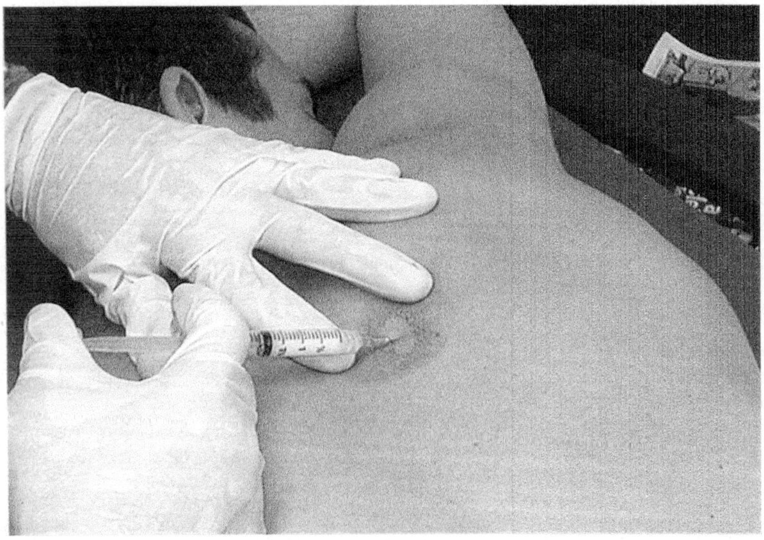

Reproduced with permission from McNabb JW. *A Practical Guide to Joint & Soft Tissue Injection & Aspiration: An Illustrated Text for Primary Care Providers.* 2nd ed. Lippincott Williams & Wilkins; 2010.

- Remove needle and apply pressure with gauze, gently massaging material.
- Apply adhesive bandage.

AFTERCARE

- Instruct patient that the area may be numb for several hours after the procedure and that pain may be present for several days.
- Instruct patient that the steroid usually takes effect within 72 hours.
- Instruct patient to return to your office if they develop redness, swelling, or increased pain at the injection site.

SUBACROMIAL INJECTION

INDICATIONS

- Subacromial injections are useful for diagnostic and therapeutic purposes.
- Any condition along the spectrum of rotator cuff diseases that cause subacromial pain syndrome may respond to corticosteroid injection.
- Injections are indicated once conservative therapy (activity modification, NSAIDS, physical therapy) has failed; however, in some cases, an injection given prior to physical therapy can allow patients to perform therapy better and with less pain.
- Subacromial corticosteroid injection provides short-term pain relief that is greater than placebo and at least equal to NSAID therapy—evidence rating B.

ANATOMY

- The subacromial space is bordered superiorly by the coracoacromial ligament stretching between the coracoid process and acromion.
- The contents of the subacromial space include the subacromial bursa, supraspinatus tendon, and tendon of the long head of the biceps.

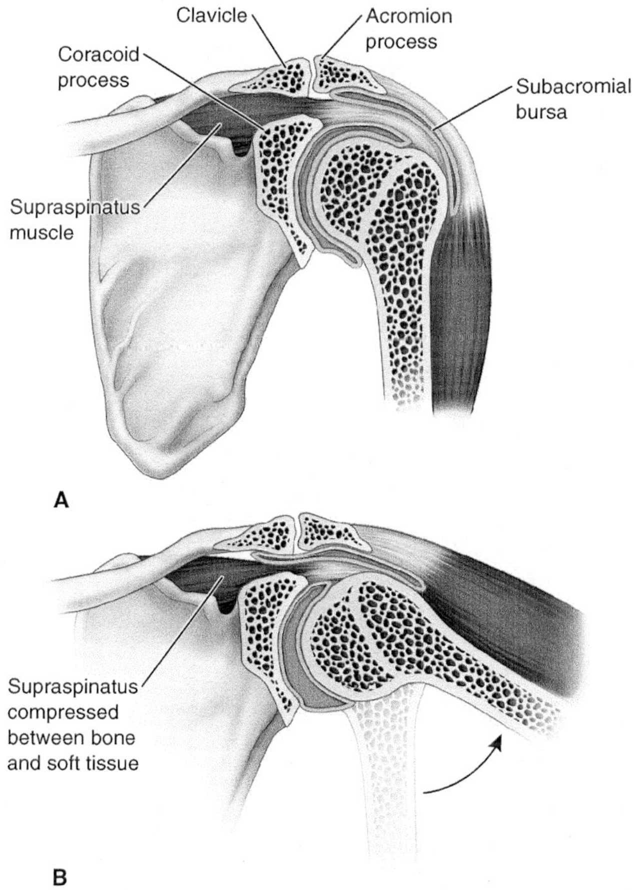

Reprinted with permission from Anderson MK. *Foundations of Athletic Training: Prevention, Assessment, and Management*. 7th ed. Wolters Kluwer; 2021.

SUPPLIES

- Gloves
- Betadine or chlorhexidine and alcohol swabs
- 5-mL syringe with 22-gauge or 25-gauge 1½-inch needle
- 4-mL anesthetic (can combine 2 mL 1% lidocaine and 2 mL 0.25% bupivacaine [Marcaine])
- 1 mL (40 mg) Kenalog or equivalent
- Ethyl chloride
- Gauze
- Adhesive bandage

TECHNIQUE

- There are three approaches to the subacromial injection: anterior, lateral, and posterolateral.
- Given the increased risk of pneumothorax with the anterior approach, we do not recommend this approach.
- Determine which approach you will use and mark the area with the needle cap.
- Lateral approach: The lateral edge of the acromion is palpated:
  - Cleanse the skin with alcohol swab and then Betadine × 3 or chlorhexidine × 45 seconds.
  - Apply ethyl chloride until the skin turns white.
  - The needle is inserted at the midpoint of the acromion and angled slightly upward under the acromion to full length (up to hub of needle).

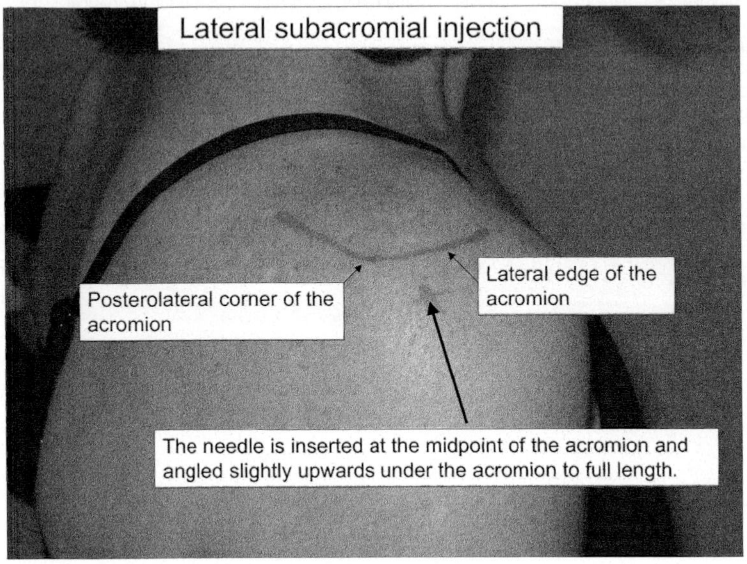

- Posterolateral approach: The distal, lateral, and posterior edges of the acromion are palpated, and the soft spot 1 cm below the posterolateral corner is marked:
  - Cleanse the skin with alcohol swab and then Betadine × 3 or chlorhexidine × 45 seconds.
  - Apply ethyl chloride until the skin turns white.
  - The needle is inserted 1 cm inferior to the posterolateral edge of the acromion. The needle is directed toward the opposite nipple (coracoid).

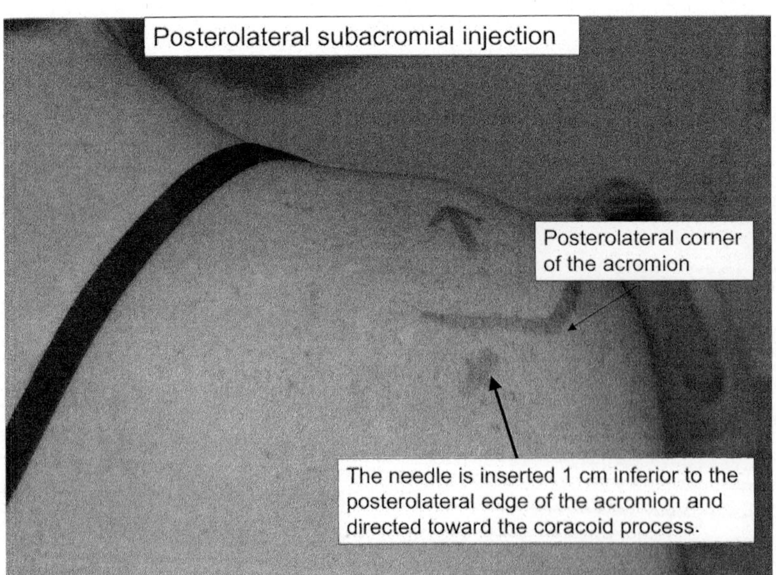

- Never inject under pressure—steroid injected directly into a tendon may cause tendon rupture.
- Remove needle and apply pressure with gauze.
- Apply adhesive bandage.
- Have patient perform Codman exercises or arm swings to disperse the fluid through the bursa.

AFTERCARE

- Instruct patient that the shoulder may be numb for several hours after the procedure and that pain may be present for several days.
- Instruct patient that the steroid usually takes effect within 72 hours.
- After 5 to 7 days, the patient can resume his or her regular activity, and you should recommend starting ROM and rotator cuff strengthening exercises.
- Instruct patient to return to your office if they develop redness, swelling, or increased pain at the injection site.

GLENOHUMERAL JOINT INJECTION

INDICATIONS

- Glenohumeral injections are useful for patients with shoulder pain secondary to osteoarthritis or rheumatoid arthritis.
- Glenohumeral injections can aid in improving ROM with physical therapy for patients with adhesive capsulitis or frozen shoulder.
- Injections are indicated once conservative therapy (activity modification, NSAIDs, physical therapy) has failed.

ANATOMY

- The glenohumeral joint is a ball and socket joint composed of the clavicle, scapula, and humerus.
- The glenoid cavity is very shallow but contains a lip of fibrous tissue called the glenoid labrum, which deepens the glenoid and increases shoulder joint stability.

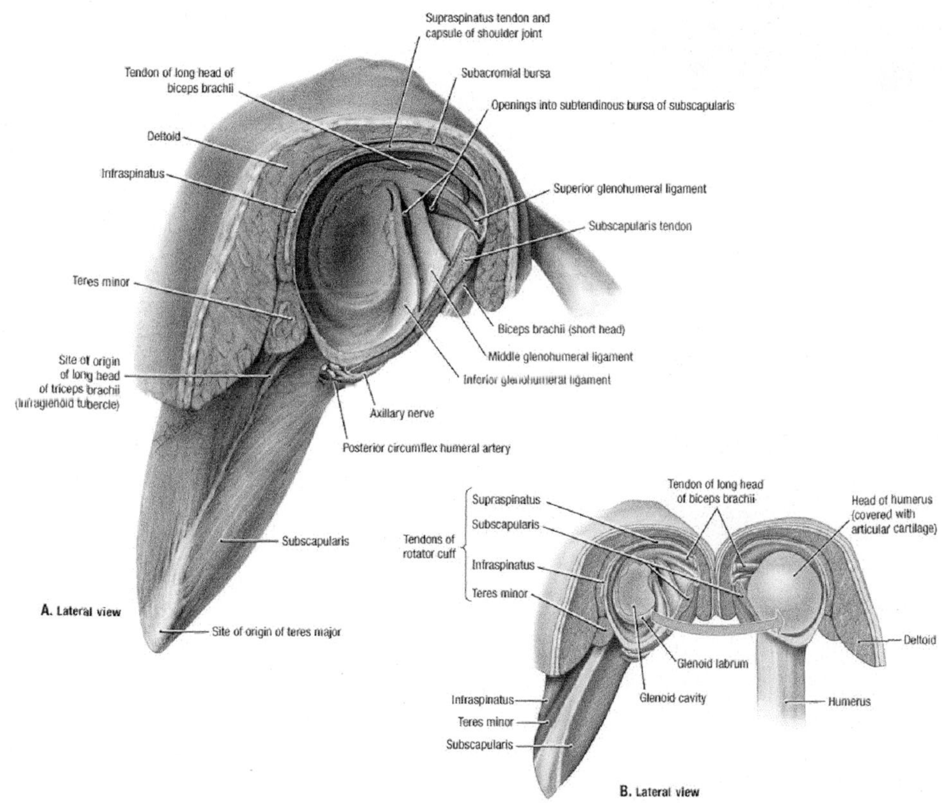

Reproduced with permission from Agur AMR, Dalley AF. *Grant's Atlas of Anatomy*. 15th ed. Wolters Kluwer; 2024.

SUPPLIES

- Gloves
- Betadine or chlorhexidine and alcohol swabs
- 3-mL syringe with 22-gauge or 25-gauge 1½-inch needle
- 1 to 2 mL anesthetic
- 1 mL (40 mg) Kenalog or equivalent
- Ethyl chloride
- Gauze
- Adhesive bandage

TECHNIQUE

- The glenohumeral joint can be approached from the anterior or posterior direction. Ultrasound-guided posterior approach improves the accuracy and safety of the procedure.
- The posterior approach is preferable because both subacromial and glenohumeral injections can be done through one needle stick.
- Posterior approach: The distal, lateral, and posterior edges of the acromion are palpated, and the soft spot 1 cm below the posterolateral corner is marked with the needle cap:
  - Cleanse the skin with alcohol swab and then Betadine × 3 or chlorhexidine × 45 seconds.
  - If available, have an assistant distract (pull down) and externally rotate the arm.
  - Apply ethyl chloride until the skin turns white.
  - The needle is inserted just inferior to the posterolateral edge of the acromion. The needle is directed anteriorly and may need to be walked into the joint.
  - Accuracy can be significantly improved with ultrasound guidance.

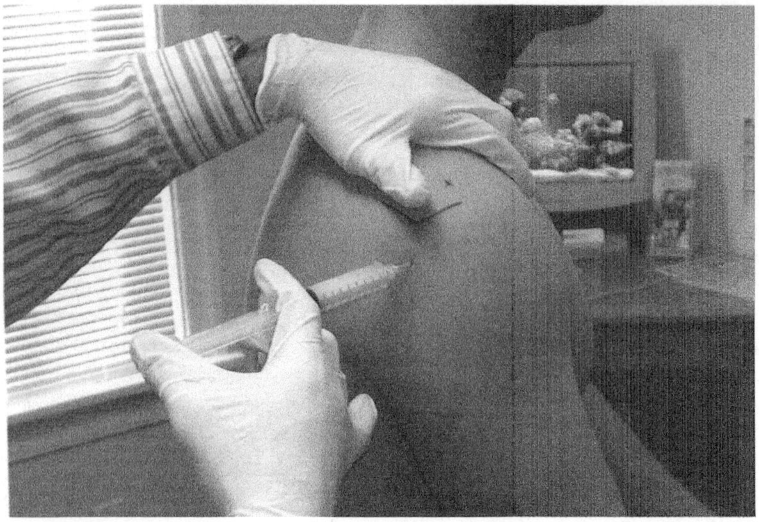

Reproduced with permission from McNabb JW. *A Practical Guide to Joint & Soft Tissue Injection & Aspiration*. Lippincott Williams & Wilkins; 2005.

- Anterior approach: The head of the humerus is palpated and the joint space determined and marked with the needle cap:
  - The needle should be placed just medial to the head of the humerus and 1 cm lateral to the coracoid process. The needle is directed posteriorly and slightly superiorly and laterally. If the needle hits against bone, it should be pulled back and redirected at a slightly different angle.

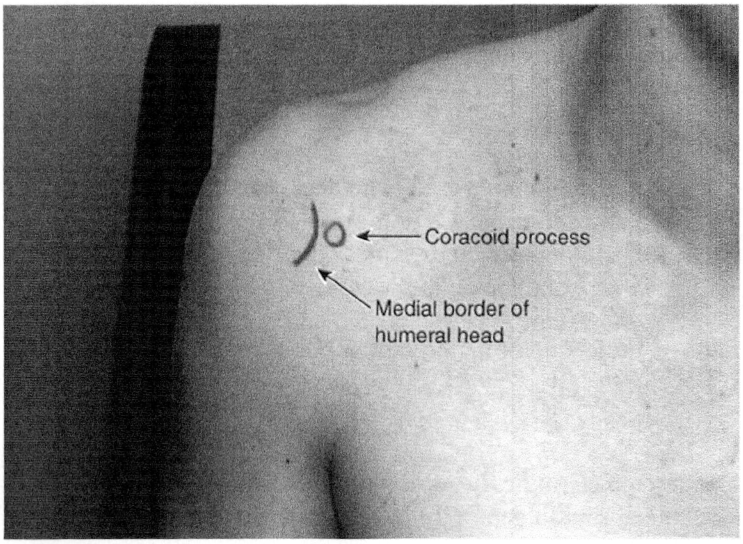

Reproduced with permission from McNabb JW. *A Practical Guide to Joint & Soft Tissue Injections*. 3rd ed. Wolters Kluwer; 2015.

- Never inject under pressure—steroid injected directly into a tendon may cause tendon rupture.
- Remove needle and apply pressure with gauze.
- Apply adhesive bandage.
- Have patient perform Codman exercises or arm swings to disperse the fluid through the glenohumeral joint.

AFTERCARE

- Instruct patient that the shoulder may be numb for several hours after the procedure and that pain may be present for several days.
- Instruct patient that the steroid usually takes effect within 72 hours.
- After 5 to 7 days, the patient can resume his or her regular activity.
- Instruct patient to return to your office if they develop redness, swelling, or increased pain at the injection site.

ACROMIOCLAVICULAR JOINT INJECTION

INDICATIONS

- Acromioclavicular (AC) joint injections are indicated for patients with shoulder pain due to pathology of the AC joint.
- Injections are indicated once conservative therapy (activity modification, NSAIDs) has failed.

ANATOMY

- The AC joint can be palpated as a narrow indentation at the distal end of the clavicle, about one thumb's width medial to the lateral edge of the acromion.
- The joint line runs obliquely medially at approximately a 20-degree angle.

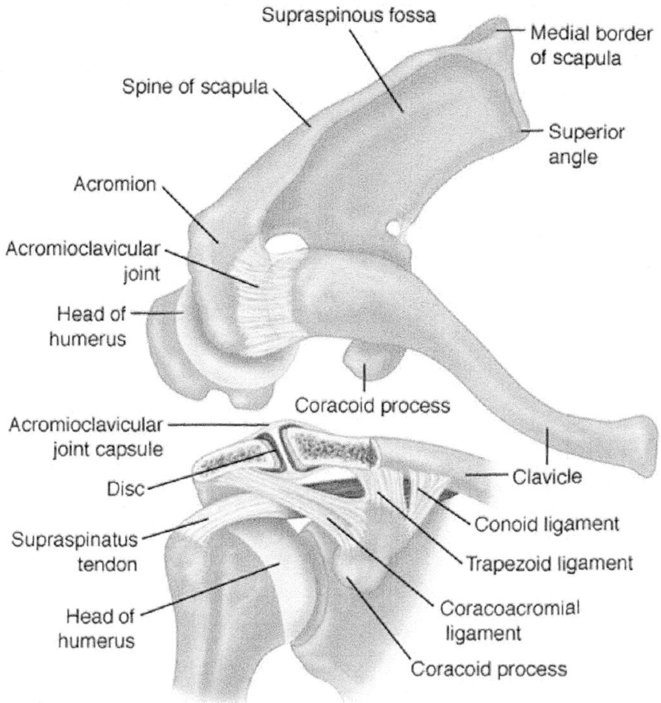

Reproduced with permission from Wiesel SW, Williams GR, Ramsey ML, et al. *Operative Techniques in Shoulder and Elbow Surgery*. 3rd ed. Wolters Kluwer; 2021.

SUPPLIES

- Gloves
- Betadine or chlorhexidine and alcohol swabs
- 3-mL syringe with 25-gauge 5/8- to 1-inch needle
- ½ mL 1% lidocaine
- ½ mL (20 mg) Kenalog or equivalent
- Ethyl chloride
- Gauze
- Adhesive bandage

TECHNIQUE

- Palpate the depression of the AC joint at the distal clavicle and mark it with the needle cap.
- Cleanse the skin with alcohol swab and then Betadine × 3 or chlorhexidine × 45 seconds.
- Apply ethyl chloride until the skin turns white.
- Insert the needle at a 15- to 20-degree angle (needle pointed more medially).

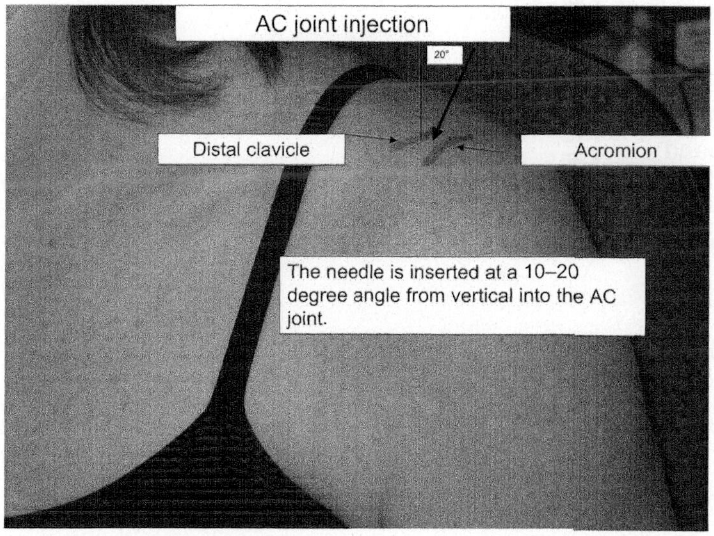

- Viewing the x-rays prior to injection can help determine the exact angle of the AC joint. Ultrasound guidance will dramatically help with accuracy and reduce pain of the injection.
- Inject the fluid into the joint.
- Remove needle and apply pressure with gauze.
- Apply adhesive bandage.

AFTERCARE

- Instruct patient that the shoulder may be numb for several hours after the procedure and that pain may be present for several days.
- Instruct patient that the steroid usually takes effect within 72 hours.
- Instruct patient to return to your office if he or she develops redness, swelling, or increased pain at the injection site.
- Avoid repetitive or heavy overhead lifting.

ELBOW JOINT INJECTION

INDICATIONS

- Elbow injections are useful for the treatment of elbow pain due to arthritis from either trauma, osteoarthritis, or rheumatoid arthritis.
- Injections are indicated once conservative therapy (activity modification, NSAIDs, physical therapy) has failed.

ANATOMY

- The elbow joint is composed of the ulnohumeral, radiocapitellar, and proximal radioulnar joints.
- The elbow joint can be approached via the triangle formed by the lateral olecranon, head of the radius, and lateral epicondyle.

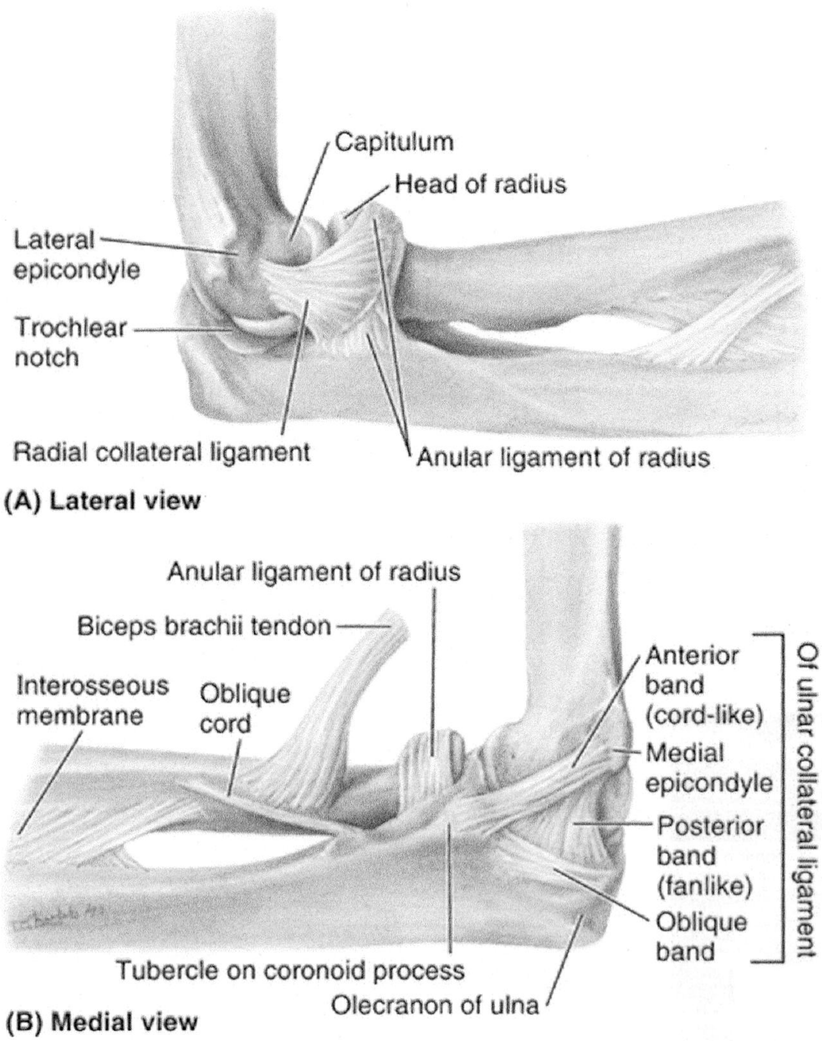

Reproduced with permission from Dalley AF, Agur AMR. *Moore's Clinically Oriented Anatomy*. 9th ed. Wolters Kluwer; 2023.

SUPPLIES
- Gloves
- Betadine or chlorhexidine and alcohol swabs
- 3-mL syringe with 25-gauge 1-inch needle
- 5- to 10-mL syringe with 20-gauge or 22-gauge needle if aspirating
- 1 mL 1% lidocaine without epinephrine
- ½ mL (20 mg) Kenalog or equivalent
- Ethyl chloride
- Gauze
- Adhesive bandage

TECHNIQUE
- Place the patient's arm on the table at a 45-degree angle.
- Mark the soft depression in the center of the triangle formed by the lateral olecranon, head of the radius, and lateral epicondyle with the needle cap.
- Cleanse the skin with alcohol swab and then Betadine × 3 or chlorhexidine × 45 seconds.
- Apply ethyl chloride until the skin turns white.
- The needle is inserted into the elbow joint between the lateral epicondyle and the radial head.

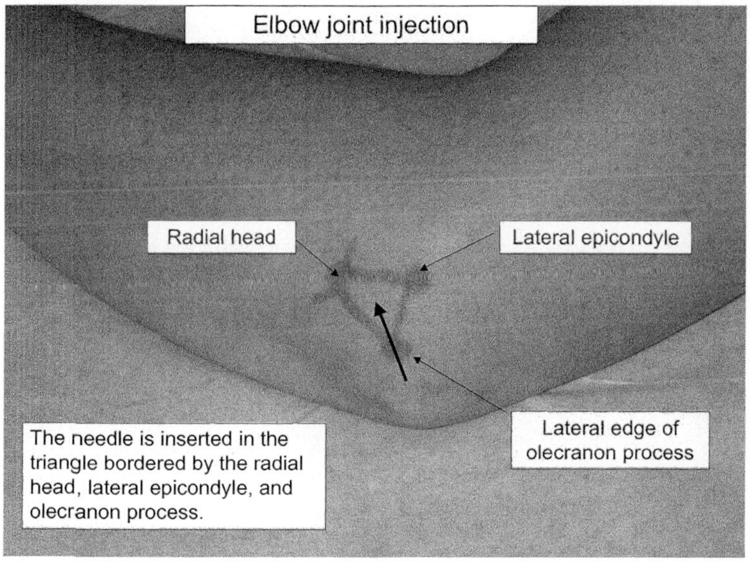

- If aspirating, remove as much fluid as possible and then stabilize the needle in the joint, twist off the syringe, and place the 3-mL syringe containing cortisone mixture on the needle.
- Inject the fluid into the joint.
- Remove needle and apply pressure with gauze.
- Apply adhesive bandage.
- Instruct the patient to perform flexion/extension ROM exercises to disperse the fluid within the joint.

AFTERCARE
- Instruct patient that the elbow may be numb for several hours after the procedure and that pain may be present for several days.
- Instruct patient that the steroid usually takes effect within 72 hours.
- After 3 to 5 days, the patient can resume his or her regular activity.
- Instruct patient to return to your office if they develop redness, swelling, or increased pain at the injection site.

EPICONDYLITIS INJECTION

INDICATIONS
- Epicondylitis corticosteroid injections are no longer routinely indicated for the treatment of lateral (tennis elbow) or medial (golfer's elbow) epicondylitis.
- Lateral epicondylitis injections used to be very common in primary care, but the frequency of these procedures has dramatically declined as evidence shows no long-term benefit.
- Injections are indicated only once conservative therapy (activity modification, NSAIDs, splinting, physical therapy) has failed and patient understands the temporary and limited benefit of lateral epicondyle corticosteroid injection.
- Corticosteroid injection reduces short-term (<6 weeks) symptoms from lateral epicondylitis, but physical therapy is superior to steroid injection after 6 weeks:
  - Evidence rating A

ANATOMY

- The origin of the common extensor tendon is at the lateral epicondyle.
- The origin of the common flexor tendon is at the medial epicondyle.
- The epicondyles are very superficial, which increases the risk of skin depigmentation and atrophy with cortisone injections.

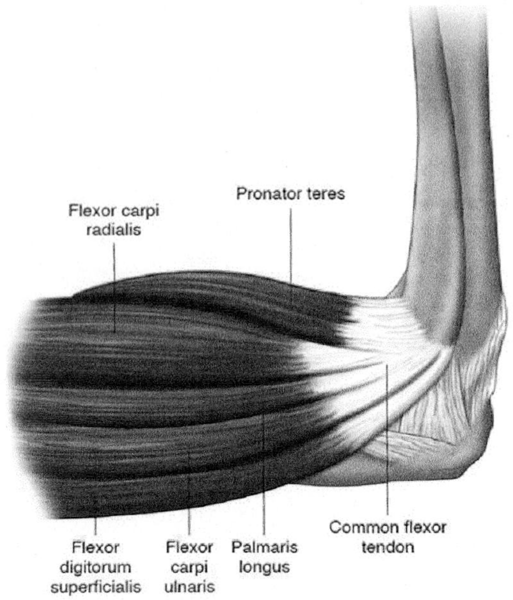

Reproduced with permission from Waldman S. *Waldman's Comprehensive Atlas of Diagnostic Ultrasound of Painful Conditions*. Wolters Kluwer; 2017.

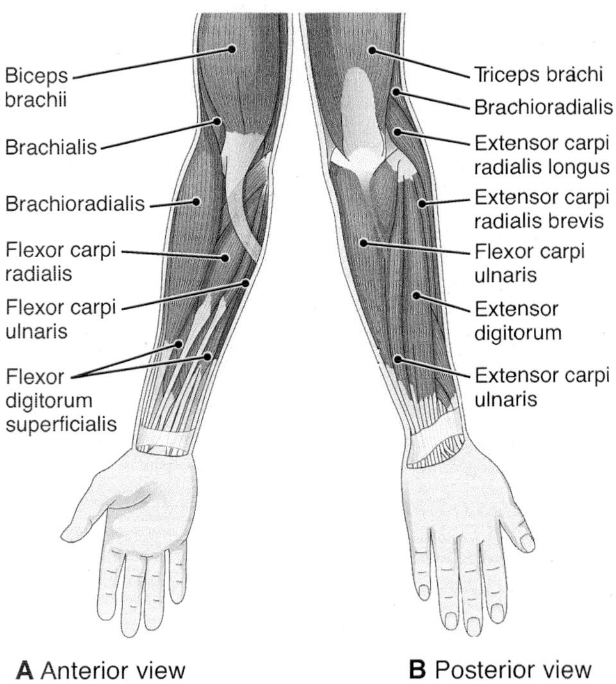

Reproduced with permission from Cohen BJ, Hull KL. *Memmler's The Human Body in Health and Disease*. 13th ed. Wolters Kluwer; 2014.

SUPPLIES

- Gloves
- Betadine or chlorhexidine and alcohol swabs
- 3-mL syringe with 25-gauge 5/8- or 1-inch needle
- ½ mL 1% lidocaine without epinephrine
- ½ mL (20 mg) Kenalog or equivalent

- Ethyl chloride
- Gauze
- Adhesive bandage

TECHNIQUE

- Lateral epicondyle: Place the patient's arm on the table at a 45-degree angle with the lateral elbow facing up:
  - Palpate the area of most tenderness over the epicondyle and mark this with the cap of the needle.
  - Cleanse the skin with alcohol swab and then Betadine × 3 or chlorhexidine × 45 seconds.

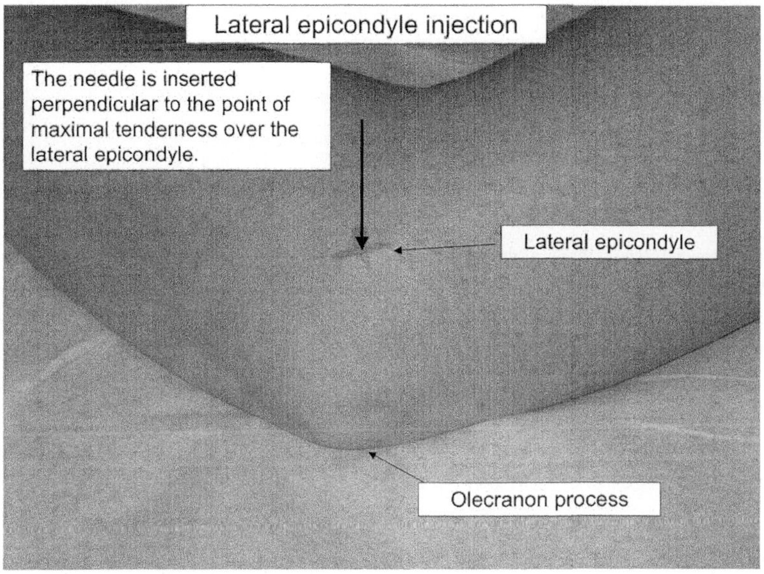

  - Apply ethyl chloride until the skin turns white.
  - The needle is inserted down to the bone of the lateral epicondyle.
  - Inject the fluid into the area. If there is resistance of flow, then back the needle slightly out so the hub of the needle is not against bone and then inject.
  - Take care not to inject cortisone while withdrawing the needle because this superficial tracking of cortisone can increase the risk of skin atrophy and depigmentation.
  - Remove needle and apply pressure with gauze.
  - Apply adhesive bandage.
- Medial epicondyle: Place the patient's arm on the table at a 45-degree angle with the medial elbow facing up:
  - Palpate the area of most tenderness over the epicondyle and mark this with the cap of the needle.
  - Cleanse the skin with alcohol swab and then Betadine × 3 or chlorhexidine × 45 seconds.
  - Apply ethyl chloride until the skin turns white.
  - The needle is inserted down to the bone of the medial epicondyle.

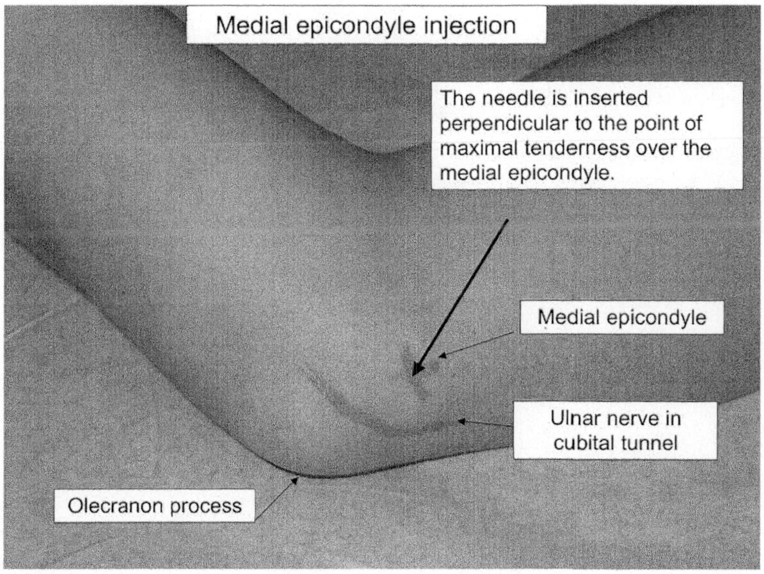

- Take care not to inject the ulnar nerve because it traverses posterior to the medial epicondyle in the cubital tunnel. If the patient experiences pain or numbness in the ulnar nerve distribution while the needle is inserted, then back out and reposition the needle more anteriorly before injecting cortisone. At this time, doing this injection without ultrasound guidance increases the risks of injury to the ulnar nerve.
- Of note medial epicondyle injections generally should be performed with ultrasound guidance to avoid ulnar nerve injury.
- Inject the fluid into the area. If there is resistance of flow, then back the needle slightly out so the hub of the needle is not against bone and then inject.
- Take care not to inject cortisone while withdrawing the needle because this superficial tracking of cortisone can increase the risk of skin atrophy and depigmentation.
- Remove needle and apply pressure with gauze.
- Apply adhesive bandage.

AFTERCARE

- Instruct patient that the elbow may be numb for several hours after the procedure and that pain may be present for several days.
- In addition, anesthetic spreading from the injection posteriorly may affect the ulnar nerve, and transient ring and pinky finger numbness may occur.
- Instruct patient that the steroid usually takes effect within 72 hours.
- NSAIDs and ice can be used to control post procedure pain.
- Consider an elbow extension splint to rest the elbow and/or wrist splint to avoid wrist flexion/extension for 1 to 2 weeks to allow the injection to take effect.
- The patient should avoid repetitive wrist extension or flexion.
- Instruct patient to return to your office if they develop redness, swelling, or increased pain at the injection site.

WRIST INJECTION

INDICATIONS

- Wrist injections are useful for the treatment of wrist pain due to arthritis from either trauma, osteoarthritis, or rheumatoid arthritis.
- Injections are indicated once conservative therapy (activity modification, NSAIDs, splinting, physical therapy) has failed.

ANATOMY

- The wrist joint capsule is not continuous but has septa, which makes the wrist injection sometimes difficult.
- The radiocarpal joint can be palpated just distal to the distal radius in a depression near the scapholunate articulation.

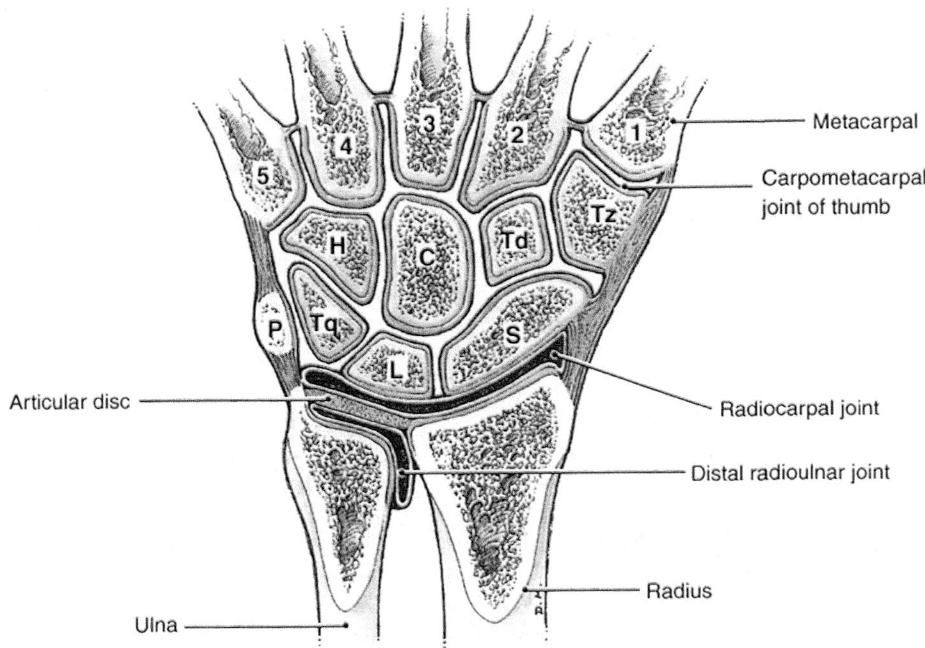

Reproduced with permission from Agur AMR, Dalley AF. *Grant's Atlas of Anatomy*. 16th ed. Wolters Kluwer; 2025;181. Figure 2.94E.

SUPPLIES

- Gloves
- Betadine or chlorhexidine and alcohol swabs
- 3-mL syringe with 25-gauge 5/8- or 1-inch needle
- 5- to 10-mL syringe with 20-gauge or 22-gauge 5/8- or 1-inch needle for aspiration
- ½ mL 1% lidocaine without epinephrine
- ½ mL (20 mg) Kenalog or equivalent
- Ethyl chloride
- Gauze
- Adhesive bandage

TECHNIQUE

- Palpate the depression distal to the distal radius near the scapholunate articulation.
- Mark this area with the cap of the needle.
- Cleanse the skin with alcohol swab and then Betadine × 3 or chlorhexidine × 45 seconds.
- Apply ethyl chloride until the skin turns white.
- The needle is inserted into the wrist joint.

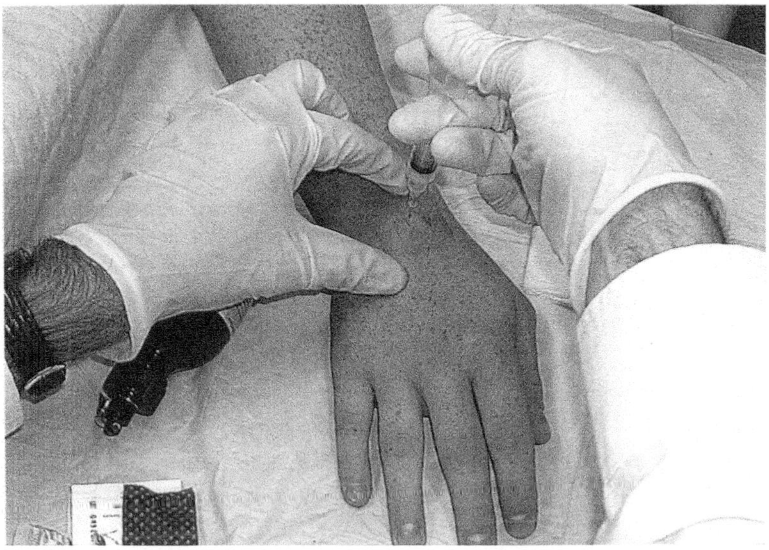

Reproduced with permission from McNabb JW. *A Practical Guide to Joint & Soft Tissue Injection & Aspiration*. Lippincott Williams & Wilkins; 2005

- If aspirating, withdraw fluid with 5- to 10-mL syringe, then stabilize needle, and exchange 3-mL syringe containing steroid mixture and inject.
- If injecting, use 3-mL syringe with 25-gauge 1-inch needle and inject fluid into joint.
- The fluid should flow easily without resistance. If there is resistance, reposition the needle by either advancing or withdrawing the needle until the flow of fluid is smooth.
- Remove needle and apply pressure with gauze.
- Apply adhesive bandage.
- Have patient perform wrist flexion and extension exercises to disperse the fluid through the wrist joint.

AFTERCARE

- Instruct patient that the wrist may be numb for several hours after the procedure and that pain may be present for several days.
- Instruct patient that the steroid usually takes effect within 72 hours.
- After 3 days, the patient can resume his or her regular activity.
- Consider use of wrist splint for 1 to 2 weeks after injection.
- Instruct patient to return to your office if they develop redness, swelling, or increased pain at the injection site.

DE QUERVAIN TENOSYNOVITIS INJECTION

INDICATIONS

- de Quervain tenosynovitis injections are indicated for the treatment of tenosynovitis over the radial aspect of the wrist.
- These injections are very common in primary care.
- Injections are indicated once conservative therapy (activity modification, NSAIDs, occupational therapy, splinting) has failed.

ANATOMY

- The dorsal wrist has six compartments containing tendons.
- The 1st dorsal compartment contains the abductor pollicis longus and the extensor pollicis brevis tendons.
- de Quervain tenosynovitis occurs when the tendon sheath becomes inflamed and thickened causing pain, swelling, and occasional triggering.

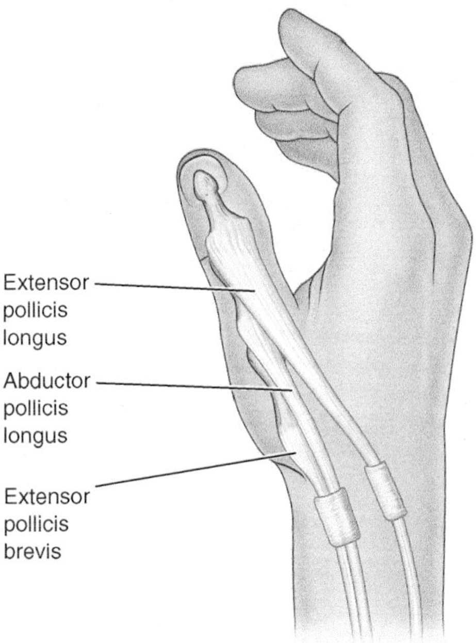

Reprinted with permission from Anderson MK. *Foundations of Athletic Training: Prevention, Assessment, and Management*. 7th ed. Wolters Kluwer; 2021.

SUPPLIES

- Gloves
- Betadine or chlorhexidine and alcohol swabs
- 3-mL syringe with 25-gauge 5/8- or 1-inch needle
- ½ mL 1% lidocaine without epinephrine
- ½ mL (20 mg) Kenalog or equivalent
- Ethyl chloride
- Gauze
- Adhesive bandage

TECHNIQUE

- Palpate the area of most tenderness over the 1st dorsal compartment and mark this with the needle cap.
- Cleanse the skin with alcohol swab and then Betadine × 3 or chlorhexidine × 45 seconds.
- Apply ethyl chloride until the skin turns white.
- The needle is inserted into the tendon sheath between the abductor pollicis longus and extensor pollicis brevis tendons at ~30-degree angle.
- Ultrasound dramatically increases accuracy of this injection and improves outcomes.

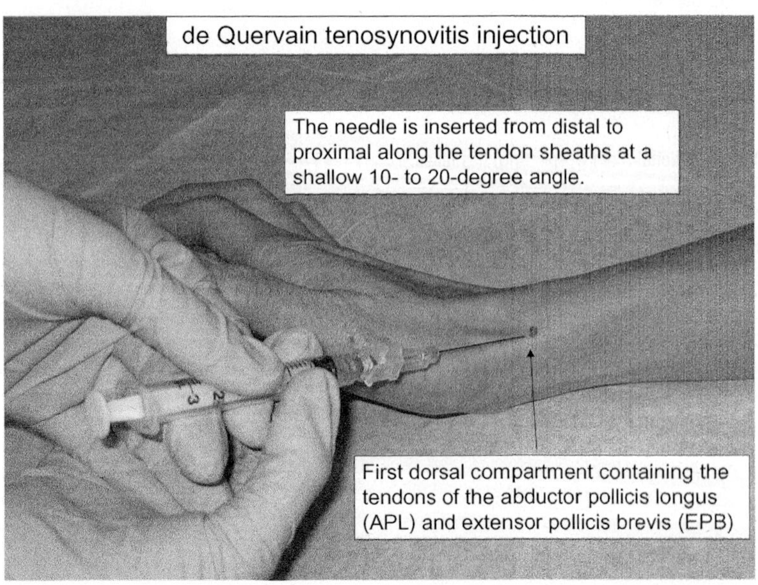

- Inject the fluid into the sheath. If there is resistance to flow, then the needle is likely in a tendon and should be backed slightly out until free flow is obtained.
- An elliptical shaped bulge occurs with the injection of the bolus of fluid into the sheath.
- Take care not to inject cortisone while withdrawing the needle because this superficial tracking of cortisone can increase the risk of skin atrophy and depigmentation.
- Remove needle and apply pressure with gauze.
- Gently massage the fluid up and down along the tendon sheath.
- Apply adhesive bandage.

AFTERCARE

- Instruct patient that the wrist may be numb for several hours after the procedure and that pain may be present for several days.
- Instruct patient that the steroid usually takes effect within 72 hours.
- NSAIDs and ice can be used to control postprocedure pain.
- Consider a thumb spica wrist splint to rest the tendons for 1 to 2 weeks to allow the injection to take effect.
- The patient should avoid repetitive thumb abduction and/or extension.
- Instruct patient to return to your office if they develop redness, swelling, or increased pain at the injection site.

1ST CARPOMETACARPAL JOINT INJECTION

INDICATIONS

- 1st carpometacarpal (CMC) (thumb) injections are useful for the treatment of thumb pain due to arthritis.
- Injections are indicated once conservative therapy (activity modification, NSAIDs, thumb spica splinting) has failed.

ANATOMY

- The thumb CMC joint is composed of the saddle-shaped base of the 1st metacarpal as it articulates with the trapezium.
- The thumb CMC joint can be approached on the extensor surface proximal to the 1st metacarpal, taking care to avoid the radial artery and extensor pollicis tendons.

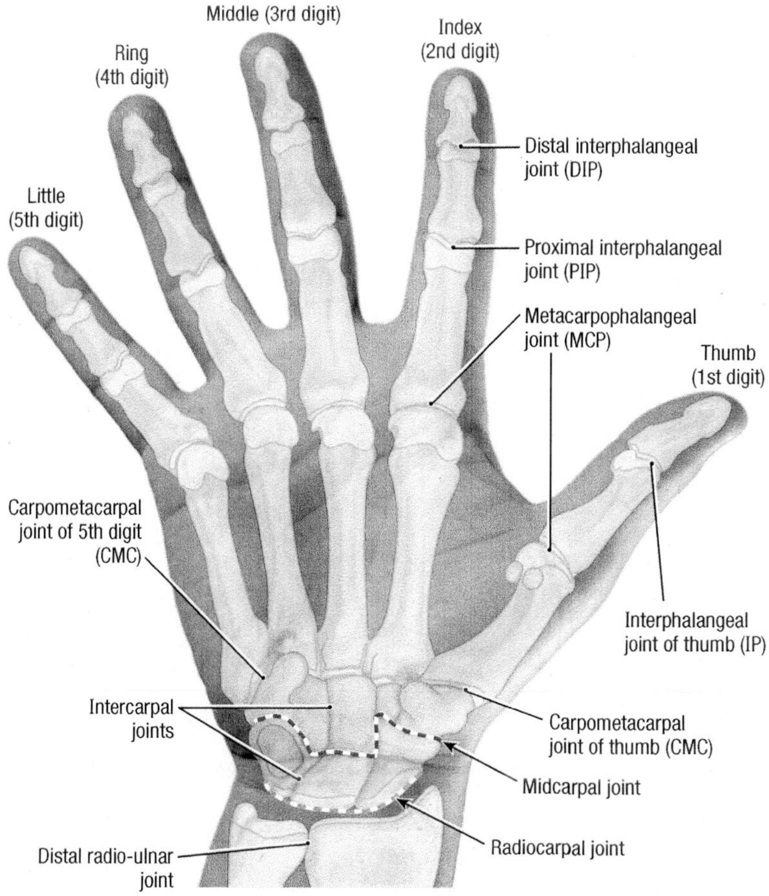

Reproduced with permission from Agur AMR, Dalley AF. *Grant's Atlas of Anatomy*. 15th ed. Wolters Kluwer; 2024.

SUPPLIES

- Gloves
- Alcohol swabs
- Betadine or chlorhexidine swabs
- 18-gauge needle for drawing up medications or Medic anti-stick needle
- 3-mL syringe with 25-gauge 1-inch needle for injection
- ½ mL 1% lidocaine without epinephrine (if using)

- ½ mL (20 mg) Kenalog or equivalent
- Ethyl chloride
- Gauze
- Adhesive bandage

TECHNIQUE

- Place the patient's hand and forearm on the table palm down.
- Palpate the CMC joint between the base of the 1st metacarpal and the wrist trapezium between the extensor pollicis longus and extensor pollicis brevis tendons.
- Mark the depression at the base of the 1st metacarpal with needle cap.
- Cleanse the skin with alcohol swab and then Betadine × 3 or chlorhexidine × 45 seconds.
- Apply ethyl chloride for topical cooling.
- To avoid the radial artery, the needle should enter on the ulnar side of the extensor pollicis brevis tendon. Distraction of the thumb can increase the space to get the needle into the joint.
- Corticosteroid alone can be injected without anesthetic, given the small size of the CMC joint. Usually, not more than ½ mL volume will fit into the joint space.

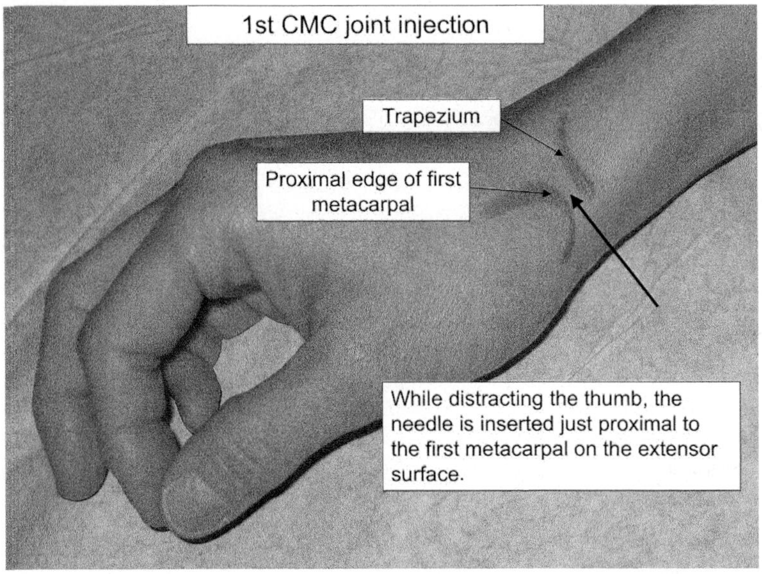

- Inject the corticosteroid into the CMC joint.
- Remove needle and apply pressure with gauze.
- Apply adhesive bandage.

AFTERCARE

- Instruct patient that the thumb may be numb for several hours after the procedure and that pain may be present for several days.
- Instruct patient that the steroid usually takes effect within 48 to 72 hours.
- Suggest the patient wear the thumb spica splint for the next 1 to 2 weeks with daily thumb extension stretches.
- After 3 to 5 days, the patient can resume his or her regular activity.
- Instruct patient to return to your office if they develop redness, swelling, or increased pain at the injection site.

CARPAL TUNNEL INJECTION

INDICATIONS

- Carpal tunnel injections are useful for the treatment of wrist pain due to median nerve compression at the carpal tunnel from either trauma, overuse, or rheumatoid arthritis.
- Injections are indicated once conservative therapy (activity modification, NSAIDs, splinting, physical therapy) has failed.
- Local corticosteroid injections for carpal tunnel syndrome provide greater symptom relief for 1 month after injection compared with placebo (number needed to treat [NNT] = 2) and oral corticosteroids. However, significant symptom relief after 1 month has not been demonstrated following injection.

ANATOMY

- The carpal tunnel is bounded by the carpal bones dorsally and the transverse carpal ligament (flexor retinaculum) ventrally.
- The contents of the tunnel include the median nerve and flexor tendons of the hand.

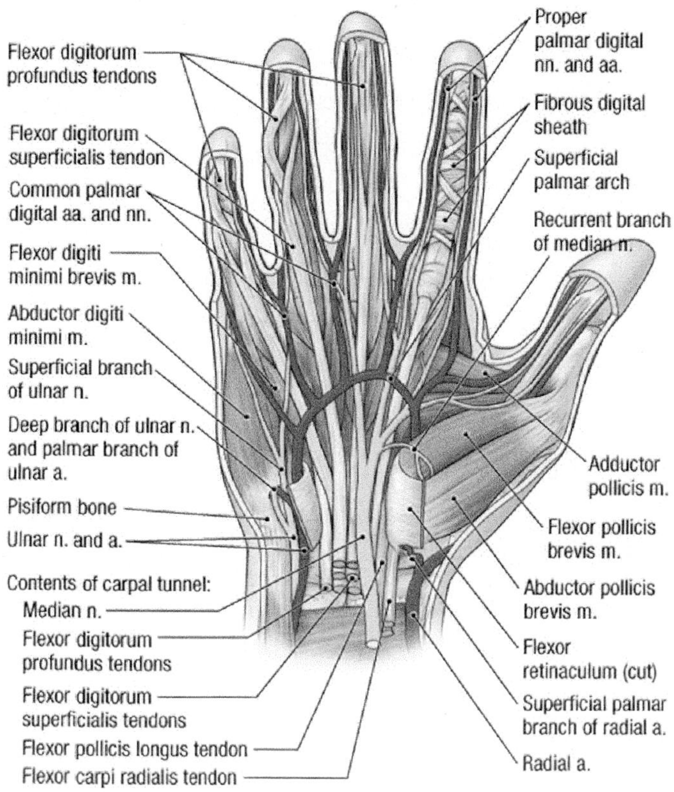

Reproduced with permission from Detton AJ. *Grant's Dissector*. 17th ed. Wolters Kluwer; 2023.

SUPPLIES
- Gloves
- Betadine or chlorhexidine and alcohol swabs
- 3-mL syringe with 25-gauge 1½-inch needle
- 1½ mL 1% lidocaine without epinephrine
- ½ mL (20 mg) Kenalog or equivalent
- Ethyl chloride
- Gauze
- Adhesive bandage

TECHNIQUE
- Have the patient lay the hand palm up on the table and make a fist with slight wrist flexion.
- Observe the tendons of the palmaris longus (10% of the population will not have one) and the flexor carpi radialis.
- Mark a spot with the needle cap 4 cm proximal to the distal palmar crease between the two tendons mentioned above.
- Cleanse the skin with alcohol swab and then Betadine × 3 or chlorhexidine × 45 seconds.
- With the fist clenched and the wrist slightly flexed, the needle is inserted at a shallow angle (~20 degrees) along the tendon sheath, aiming toward the ring finger. Have the patient slowly extend the wrist and fingers noticing the needle advance toward the carpal tunnel. This indicates proper needle placement.

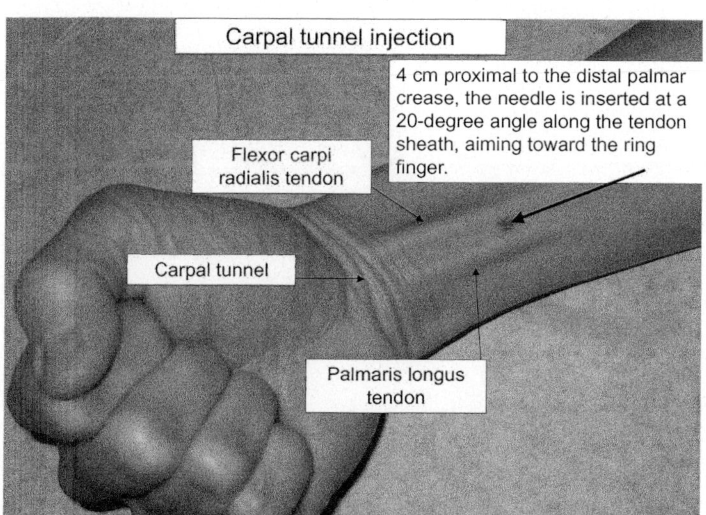

- Ask the patient if they feel any increased pain or numbness. If they do, remove the needle because it may be in the median nerve.
- *Do not inject into the median nerve.*
- The fluid should flow easily without resistance. If there is resistance, reposition the needle by repeating the technique from the beginning.
- Remove needle and apply pressure with gauze.
- Massage the fluid distally toward the carpal tunnel.
- Apply adhesive bandage.

AFTERCARE
- Instruct patient that the wrist may be numb for several hours after the procedure and that pain may be present for several days.
- Instruct patient that the steroid usually takes effect within 72 hours.
- After 3 days, the patient can resume his or her regular activity.
- Recommend continued use of wrist splint for 1 to 2 weeks after injection.
- Instruct patient to return to your office if they develop redness, swelling, or increased pain at the injection site.

TRIGGER FINGER INJECTION

INDICATIONS
- Trigger fingers occur when a flexor tendon nodule repetitively gets stuck under the annular pulley on the palmar aspect of the finger.
- Injections are indicated once conservative therapy (activity modification, splinting, NSAIDs) has failed.

ANATOMY
Nodule or thickening occurs in the flexor tendon, which catches on the A-1 proximal pulley making finger extension difficult.

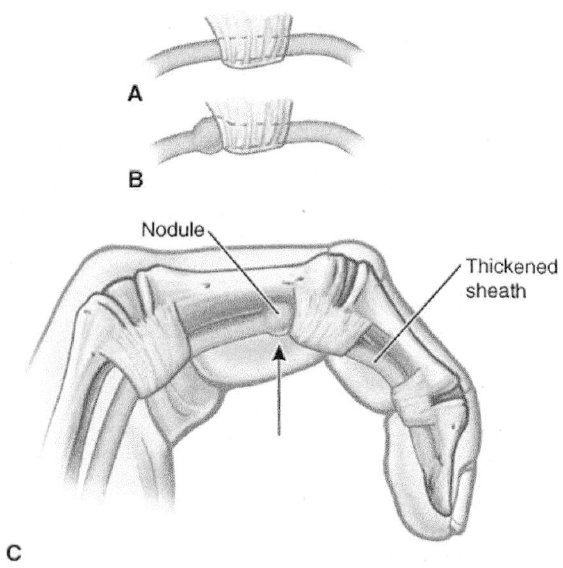

Reproduced with permission from Anderson MK. *Foundations of Athletic Training: Prevention, Assessment, and Management*. 7th ed. Wolters Kluwer; 2021.

SUPPLIES
- Gloves
- Betadine or chlorhexidine and alcohol swabs
- 3-mL syringe with 25-gauge 5/8- to 1-inch needle
- ½ mL 1% lidocaine
- ½ mL (20 mg) Kenalog or equivalent
- Ethyl chloride
- Gauze
- Adhesive bandage

TECHNIQUE
- Palpate the tender nodule on the palm of the hand and mark with needle cap.
- Cleanse the skin with alcohol swab and then Betadine × 3 or chlorhexidine × 45 seconds.
- Apply ethyl chloride until the skin turns white.
- Injection site is either directly into the nodule or at the proximal interphalangeal digital crease.

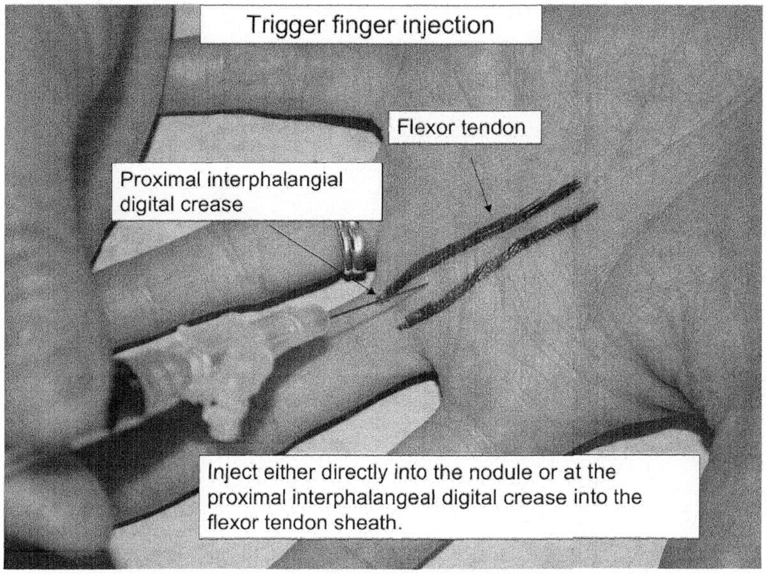

- Insert needle at a 45-degree angle—when you feel rubbery resistance, you are at the level of the tendon. Back needle out slowly until it is no longer in tendon and the fluid flows easily within the tendon sheath.
- Never inject under pressure—steroid injected directly into a tendon may cause tendon rupture.
- Remove needle and apply pressure with gauze, gently massaging material along tendon.
- Apply adhesive bandage.

AFTERCARE

- Instruct patient that the finger may be numb for several hours after the procedure and that pain may be present for several days.
- Instruct patient that the steroid usually takes effect within 72 hours.
- The use of a finger splint after an injection for 1 to 2 weeks can increase the efficacy of the injection.
- After 3 days, start extension exercises—hold finger in extension 10 seconds × 10 times for one set. Complete three sets per day.
- Instruct patient to return to your office if they develop redness, swelling, or increased pain at the injection site.
- Avoid repetitive gripping or use padded gloves for any vibrating tools (i.e., jackhammers).

GANGLION CYST INJECTION

INDICATIONS

- Most ganglion cysts resolve spontaneously, with conservative treatment including splinting. Home efforts to rupture the cyst by hitting it with a heavy book are not recommended.
- Aspiration and corticosteroid injection can be considered for ganglion cysts if patients complain of symptoms such as pain, limited ROM, paresthesias, or aesthetic considerations.
- Aspiration and steroid injection is effective without recurrence in 27–67% of cases.

ANATOMY

- Ganglion cysts are the most common soft tissue tumors of the hand and wrist, more commonly in women (3:1).
- These thick mucin-filled cysts may out pouch from synovial or tendon sheaths from trauma or repetitive irritation.
- Ganglion cysts are often connected to an underlying ligament or joint, most commonly at the scapholunate joint (60–70%), next most frequently at the volar wrist (20–25%), and thirdly at the palmar flexor tendon sheath (10–12%).

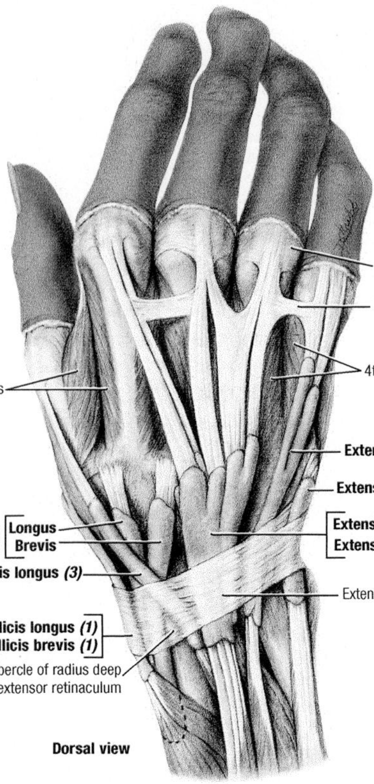

Reproduced with permission from Agur AMR, Dalley AF. *Grant's Atlas of Anatomy*. 15th ed. Wolters Kluwer; 2024.

SUPPLIES

- Gloves
- Alcohol swabs
- Betadine or chlorhexidine swabs
- 18-gauge needle for drawing up medications or Medic anti-stick needle
- 5- to 10-mL syringe with 18- to 22-gauge 1-inch needle if aspirating viscous cyst contents
- 3-mL syringe with 22-gauge 1-inch needle if injecting
- ½ to 1 mL 1% lidocaine without epinephrine (if using)
- ½ mL 40 mg/mL (20 mg) Kenalog or equivalent
- Ethyl chloride
- Gauze
- Adhesive bandage

TECHNIQUE

- Position the patient in sitting position with his or her arm on the table with the ganglion cyst facing upward.
- Cleanse the skin with alcohol swab and then Betadine × 3 or chlorhexidine × 45 seconds.
- Apply ethyl chloride for topical cooling.
- Aspirate using the 18-gauge needle—the thick mucoid cyst contents may be difficult to aspirate and may actually be more effectively milked out of the puncture site after the needle is removed.

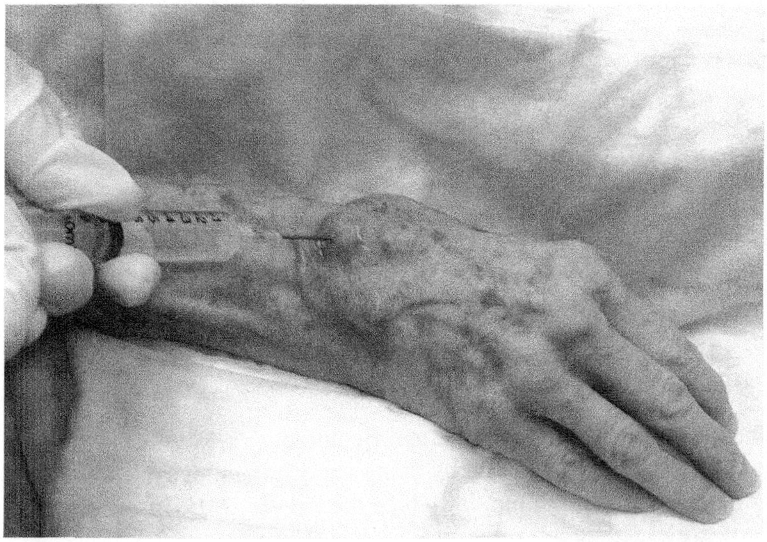

Reproduced with permission from McNabb JW. *A Practical Guide to Joint & Soft Tissue Injection & Aspiration: An Illustrated Text for Primary Care Providers*. 2nd ed. Lippincott Williams & Wilkins; 2010.

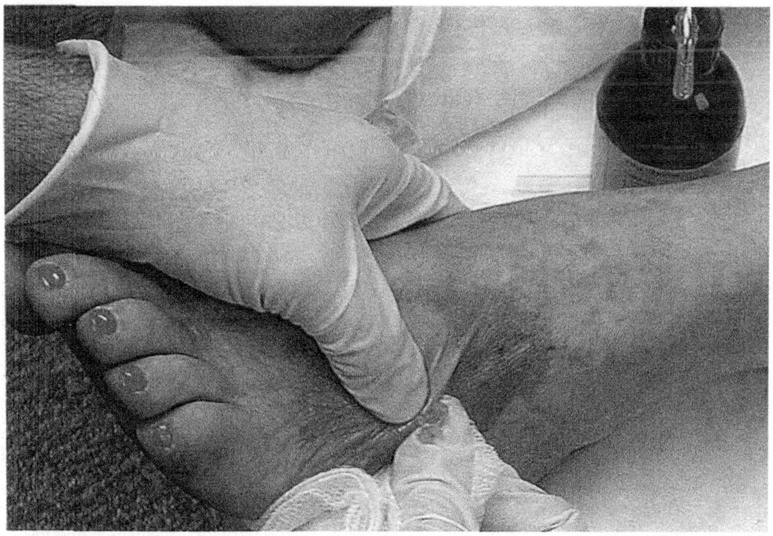

Reproduced with permission from McNabb JW. *A Practical Guide to Joint & Soft Tissue Injection & Aspiration*. Lippincott Williams & Wilkins; 2005.

- First, aspirate the cyst contents if possible and then stabilize the needle position with a hemostat, remove the aspiration syringe, secure the syringe with the steroid mixture, and inject.
- Remove needle and apply pressure with gauze.
- Apply adhesive bandage.

AFTERCARE

- Apply pressure dressing.
- Instruct patient to return to your office if they develop redness, swelling, or increased pain at the injection site.
- Ganglion cyst recurrence is common—consider referral to hand orthopedics for surgical ganglionectomy if patients continue to experience pain and discomfort from the ganglion cyst.

TROCHANTERIC BURSA INJECTION

INDICATIONS

- Corticosteroid injection is an accepted treatment for trochanteric bursitis or greater trochanteric pain syndrome caused by chronic hip pressure, limping, leg length discrepancies, acute trauma, hip surgery, or repetitive trauma, such as from iliotibial band friction.
- Trochanteric bursa injections are indicated if pain persists despite conservative therapy, including avoiding direct pressure and repetitive trauma, ice, NSAIDs, and stretching of the iliotibial band, tensor fascia lata, external hip rotators, hip flexors, and quadriceps.
- A randomized controlled trial showed prolonged benefit from early corticosteroid injection for trochanteric bursitis.
- Another randomized controlled study of patients who received trochanteric bursa corticosteroid injections demonstrated a 2.7 relative risk of recovery at 5 years, with the conclusion that early steroid injection may help prevent chronic bursitis pain.

ANATOMY

- The trochanteric bursa lies superficial to the greater trochanter of the femur, between the trochanteric process and the gluteus medius/iliotibial tract.
- Tenderness to palpation over the trochanteric process is the classic finding for trochanteric bursitis.

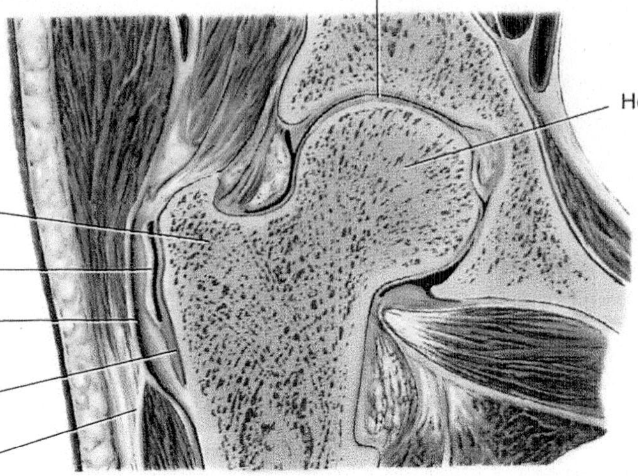

Reproduced with permission from McNabb JW, O'Connor FG. *A Practical Guide to Joint & Soft Tissue Injections*. 4th ed. Wolters Kluwer; 2022.

SUPPLIES

- Alcohol swabs
- Betadine or chlorhexidine swabs
- 18-gauge needle for drawing up medications or Medic anti-stick needle
- 6-mL syringe with 21- to 22-gauge 1½- to 2-inch needle for thin patients
- 21- to 22-gauge 3.5-inch spinal needle may be needed for heavier patients.
- 5 mL 1% lidocaine without epinephrine and/or 0.25% bupivacaine
- 1 mL 40 mg/mL (40 mg) Kenalog or equivalent
- Ethyl chloride
- Gauze
- Adhesive bandage

TECHNIQUE

- Lay the patient in lateral recumbent position, with the affected side up.
- Flex the patient's hip at 50 degrees, and flex the knees 60 to 90 degrees.
- Palpate the greater trochanteric process and identify the point of maximal tenderness, which usually corresponds well to the most superficial point of bony prominence. Mark this area with the needle cap.
- Cleanse the skin with alcohol swab and then Betadine × 3 or chlorhexidine × 45 seconds.
- Apply ethyl chloride for topical cooling.
- Position the needle perpendicular to the skin and advance toward the site of maximal trochanteric tenderness.
- Advance the needle until the tip reaches bone level to ensure delivery of the steroid below the tendon. Never inject under pressure, which may indicate placement within the tendon.
- Withdraw the needle 2 to 3 mm to remain within the trochanteric bursa.

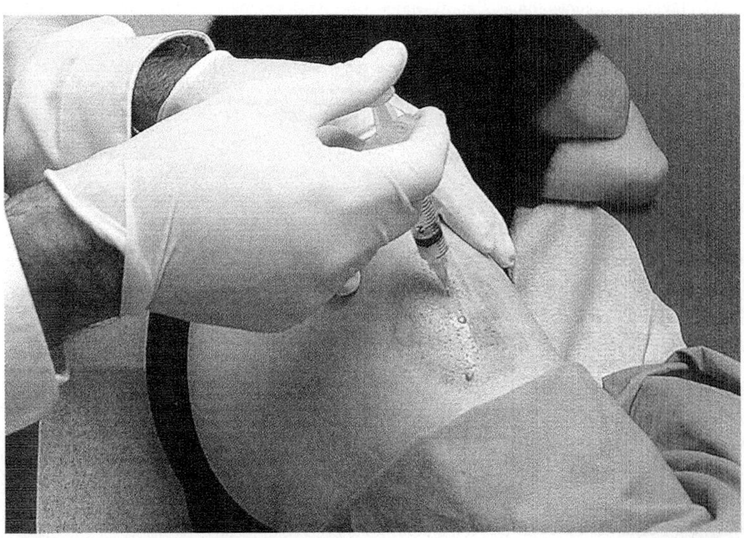

Reproduced with permission from McNabb JW, O'Connor FG. *A Practical Guide to Joint & Soft Tissue Injections*. 4th ed. Wolters Kluwer; 2022.

- For acute bursitis, the 5 to 6 mL of corticosteroid and lidocaine can be directly injected into the bursa.
- For chronic bursitis, a clockwise peppering motion may help break up scar tissue—each time, the needle should reach the level of bone and then inject.
- Crepitus can often be felt at the needle tip if chronic scarring/bursitis/tendonitis is present.
- Remove needle and apply pressure with gauze.
- Apply adhesive bandage.

AFTERCARE

- Warn patients that pain relief from the steroid anti-inflammatory effect may not start until 2 to 3 days postinjection.
- Avoid direct pressure or trauma to the trochanteric bursa.
- Rest 3 days and then restart stretches of the iliotibial band, hip flexors, and extensors.
- Instruct patient to return to your office if they develop redness, swelling, or increased pain at the injection site.
- Injection can be repeated in 6 to 12 weeks if pain relief was <50%.

OLECRANON BURSA INJECTION

INDICATIONS

- Olecranon bursa aspiration is useful to relieve swelling in acute bursitis or to diagnose gouty bursitis or infectious bursitis (most often *Staphylococcus aureus*). Olecranon bursa steroid injections are useful for the treatment of chronic bursitis.
- Most acute traumatic olecranon bursitis episodes are self-limited.
- Injections are indicated once conservative therapies (rest, ice, compression with elbow sleeve, elevation, avoidance of direct pressure, NSAIDs) have failed.

ANATOMY

- The olecranon bursa overlies the olecranon process at the proximal ulna.
- Olecranon bursitis is visible as posterior elbow swelling, often described as a golf ball or goose egg over the elbow tip.

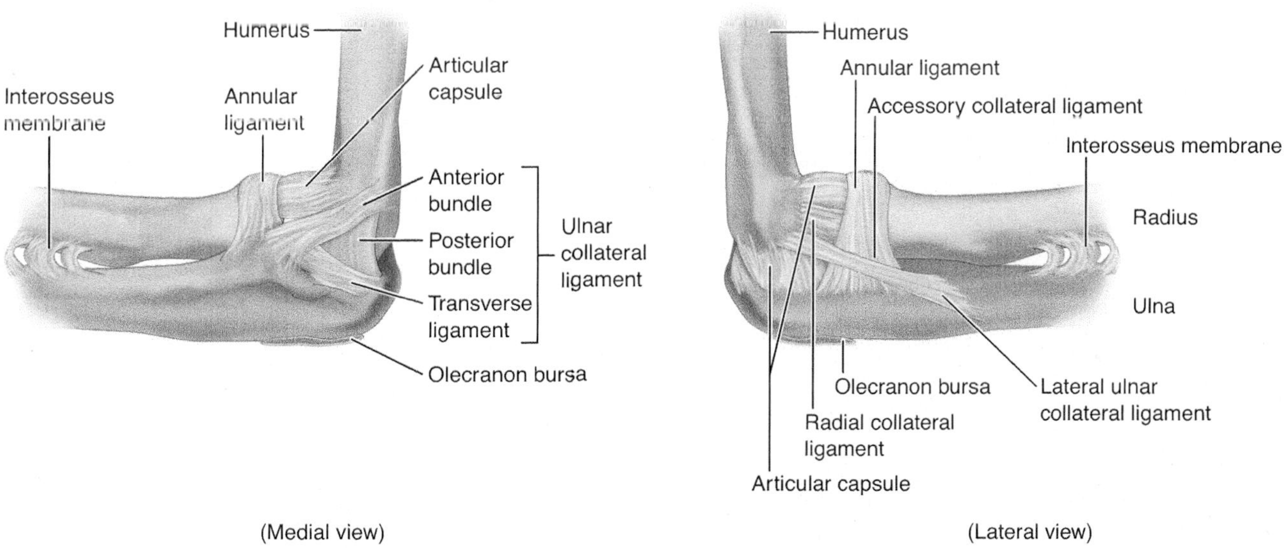

Reprinted with permission from Anderson MK. *Foundations of Athletic Training: Prevention, Assessment, and Management*. 7th ed. Wolters Kluwer; 2021.

SUPPLIES

- Gloves
- Alcohol swabs
- Betadine or chlorhexidine swabs
- 18-gauge needle for drawing up medications or Medic anti-stick needle
- 3-mL syringe with 25-gauge 1-inch needle if injecting
- 5- to 10-mL syringe with 18- to 22-gauge needle if aspirating
- 1 mL 1% lidocaine without epinephrine
- ½ mL 40 mg/mL (20 mg) Kenalog or equivalent
- Ethyl chloride
- Gauze
- Adhesive bandage

TECHNIQUE

- Place the patient's arm on the table at maximal elbow flexion to accentuate the swelling.
- Palpate over the olecranon bursa for fluctuance.
- Cleanse the skin with alcohol swab and then Betadine × 3 or chlorhexidine × 45 seconds.
- Apply ethyl chloride for topical cooling.
- Aim the needle perpendicular to the olecranon bursa.
- Aspirate bursa fluid until the bursa is flat.

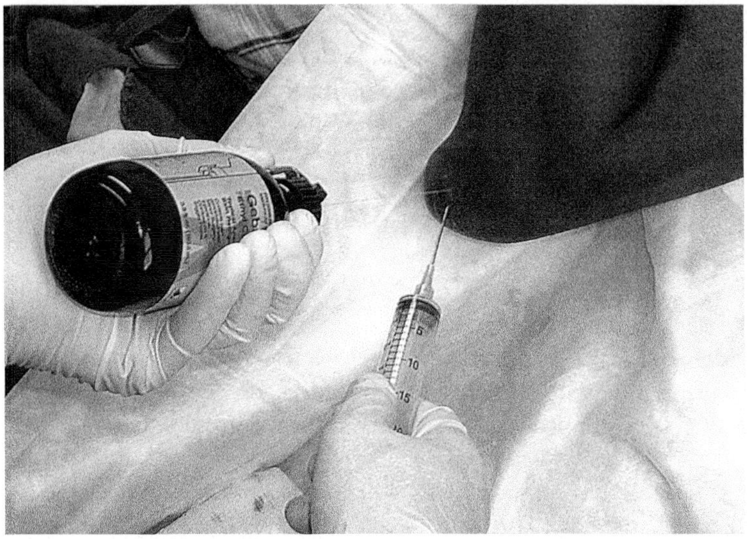

Reproduced with permission from McNabb JW. *A Practical Guide to Joint & Soft Tissue Injection & Aspiration: An Illustrated Text for Primary Care Providers*. 2nd ed. Lippincott Williams & Wilkins; 2010.

- If infection has been ruled out, inject steroid/lidocaine into bursa.
- Remove needle and apply pressure with gauze.
- Apply adhesive bandage.

AFTERCARE

- A compressive elbow sleeve may help prevent fluid reaccumulation.
- Avoid direct pressure or trauma to the elbow.
- For recalcitrant olecranon bursitis, consider a posterior splint or elbow pads for 1 to 2 weeks after the steroid injection.
- Instruct patient to return to your office if they develop redness, swelling, or increased pain at the injection site.

PREPATELLAR BURSA INJECTION

INDICATIONS

- Acute trauma, repetitive pressure, or rarely infection can cause inflammation and swelling in the prepatellar bursa.
- Prepatellar aspiration may be performed to relieve acute pressure and swelling.
- Corticosteroid injection is a second-line therapy for chronic prepatellar bursitis after the failure of conservative therapy, including avoidance of direct pressure, rest, ice, and NSAIDs.

ANATOMY

- The prepatellar bursa lies between the patella and the overlying skin.
- Prepatellar bursitis is visible as a well-circumscribed region of swelling over the patella.
- Prepatellar bursitis should be differentiated from patellar fracture or IA knee effusion.

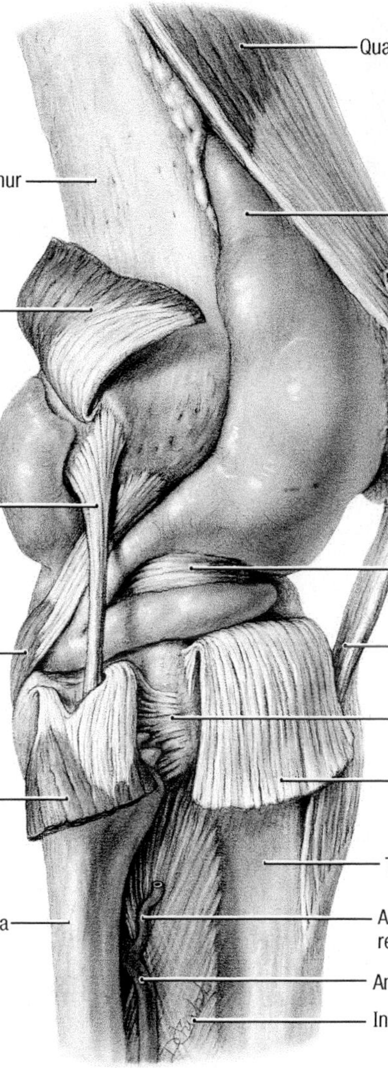

Lateral view

Reproduced with permission from Agur AMR, Dalley AF. *Grant's Atlas of Anatomy*. 15th ed. Wolters Kluwer; 2024.

SUPPLIES

- Gloves
- Alcohol swabs
- Betadine or chlorhexidine swabs
- 18-gauge needle for drawing up medications or Medic anti-stick needle
- 5- to 10-mL syringe with 18- to 22-gauge 1-inch needle if aspirating
- 1 mL 1% lidocaine without epinephrine (optional)
- ½ mL 40 mg/mL (20 mg) Kenalog or equivalent (optional)
- Ethyl chloride
- Gauze
- Adhesive bandage

TECHNIQUE

- Position the patient in supine position with the knee flexed at 30 degrees on a pillow.
- Position the affected leg with patella facing upward.
- Cleanse the skin with alcohol swab and then Betadine × 3 or chlorhexidine × 45 seconds.
- Apply ethyl chloride for topical cooling.
- The prepatellar bursa swelling should be clearly visible.
- Aspirate by approaching from the side of the visible prepatellar swelling.

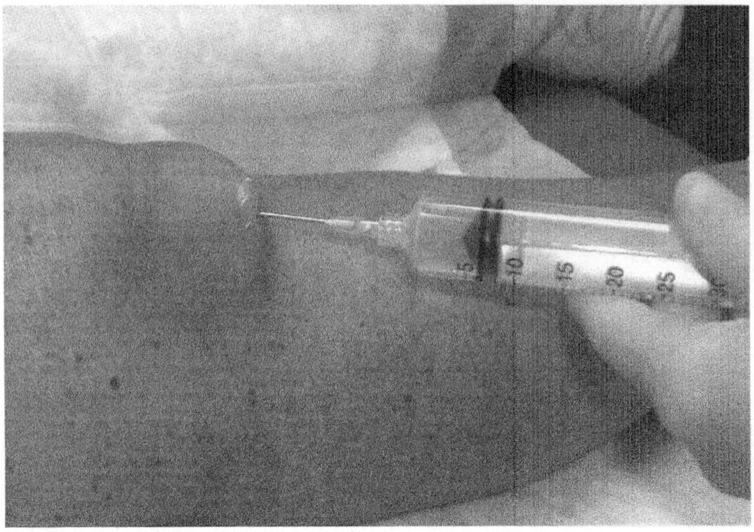

Reproduced with permission from McNabb JW. *A Practical Guide to Joint & Soft Tissue Injections*. 3rd ed. Wolters Kluwer; 2015.

- Aspirate first, then stabilize the needle position with a hemostat while changing to the syringe with the steroid/lidocaine mixture, and then inject.
- Remove needle and apply pressure with gauze.
- Apply adhesive bandage.

AFTERCARE

- Apply pressure dressing.
- Rest for 3 days.
- Continue the rest, ice, compression, and elevation (RICE) conservative therapy.
- Remind patients to avoid direct pressure on their patella's or to use knee pads if kneeling is required for work.
- Instruct patients to return to your office or urgent care if they develop redness, swelling, or increased pain at the injection site.

PES ANSERINE BURSA INJECTION

INDICATIONS

- Trauma or repetitive friction over the anserine bursa can cause inflammation that worsens with knee flexion or rotation.
- Corticosteroid injections may be considered early in the course of treatment for anserine bursitis, along with the conservative therapy of NSAIDs, rest, ice, and stretching.

ANATOMY

- The pes anserine bursa lies between the conjoined tendon of the sartorius, gracilis, and semitendinosus muscles and the tibial insertion of the medial collateral ligament.
- Diagnosis is made by tenderness to palpation over the anserine bursa, ~2 cm below the medial joint line at the proximal medial tibia.
- Swelling is not usually visible with anserine bursitis.

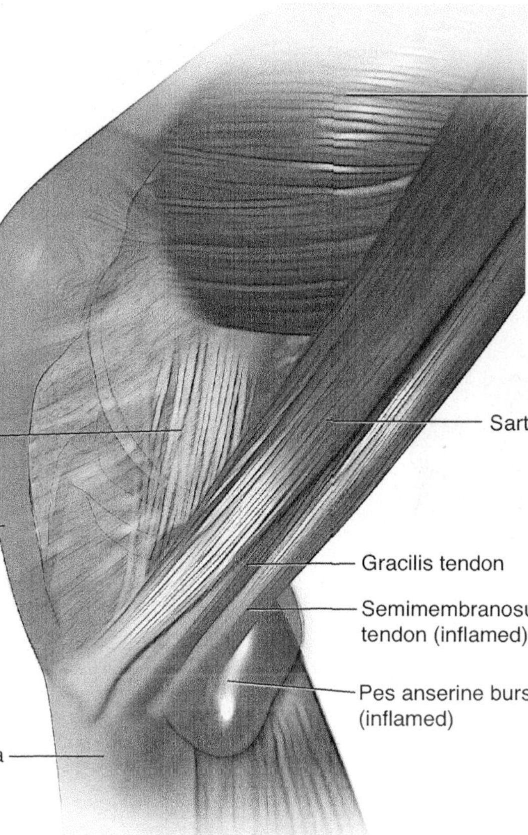

Reproduced with permission from Waldman S. *Waldman's Comprehensive Atlas of Diagnostic Ultrasound of Painful Conditions*. Wolters Kluwer; 2017.

SUPPLIES

- Gloves
- Alcohol swabs
- Betadine or chlorhexidine swabs
- 18-gauge needle for drawing up medications or Medic anti-stick needle
- 3-mL syringe with 25-gauge 1-inch needle
- 1 mL 1% lidocaine without epinephrine
- ½ mL 40 mg/mL (20 mg) Kenalog or equivalent
- Ethyl chloride
- Gauze
- Adhesive bandage

TECHNIQUE

- Lay the patient in supine position.
- Position the affected leg with the medial joint line accessible.
- Identify the anserine bursa 1 to 2 cm below the middle of the medial joint line.
- The point of maximal tenderness along the medial tibial plateau often serves to identify the ideal injection site—mark this site with the needle cap.
- Cleanse the skin with alcohol swab and then Betadine × 3 or chlorhexidine × 45 seconds.
- Apply ethyl chloride for topical cooling.
- Insert the needle perpendicular to the skin.
- Advance the needle to the level of bone to find the bursa space between the conjoined tendons and the tibia.
- Inject the steroid/lidocaine mixture into the bursa—resistance to flow should be minimal.

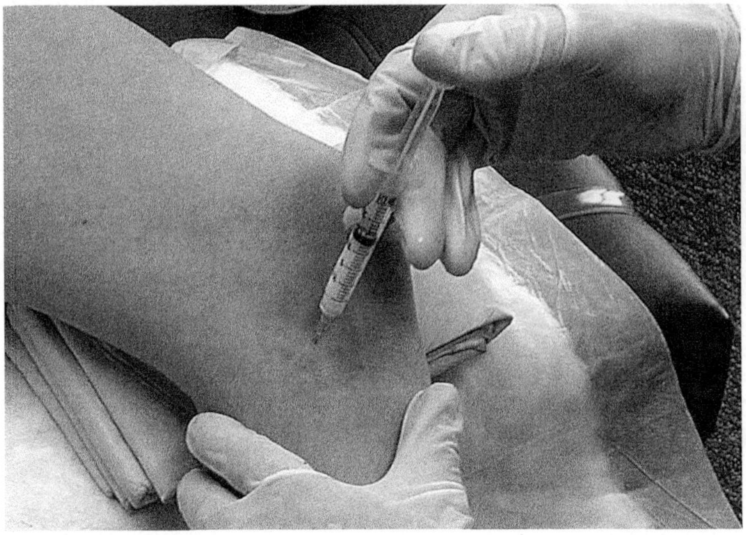

Reproduced with permission from McNabb JW. *A Practical Guide to Joint & Soft Tissue Injections*. 3rd ed. Wolters Kluwer; 2015.

- Remove needle and apply pressure with gauze.
- Apply adhesive bandage.

AFTERCARE

- Rest 3 days and then resume stretching exercises.
- A physical therapy referral to develop a stretching plan for the knee adductors and quadriceps, especially the vastus medialis, may help prevent recurrence.
- Sleeping with a cushion between the knees may help decrease direct pressure on the anserine bursa.
- Instruct patient to return to your office if they develop redness, swelling, or increased pain at the injection site.

KNEE JOINT INJECTION

INDICATIONS

- Knee joint aspiration is useful in the diagnosis of knee effusions (i.e., to diagnose crystalline disease, hemarthrosis, or rule out infection) and for the reduction of pain and pressure from effusions.
- Corticosteroid injection of the knee is indicated for the treatment of osteoarthritis, crystalline disease, or synovitis in rheumatoid arthritis.
- HA viscosupplementation injections are U.S. Food and Drug Administration (FDA)-approved for knee osteoarthritis but not recommended by many major medical organizations and some insurance companies.
- Knee injection therapy may be appropriate if knee pain continues despite evidence-based conservative therapy (activity modification, weight loss, acetaminophen, oral or topical NSAIDs, physical therapy, ice, heat).
- Strength of evidence for IA knee injection therapies is strongest for corticosteroid (Category 1A). In a recent large meta-analysis assessing pain relief at 3 months posttreatment, IA corticosteroid had a larger effect size than IA placebo, oral placebo, oral acetaminophen, and all other oral treatments.
- Strength of evidence for HA injections is more controversial because many of the HA studies were funded by pharmaceutical companies. 2012 guidelines by ACR list HA use as no recommendation, and current American Academy of Orthopedic Surgeons guidelines recommend against HA use, due to an effect size no better than NSAIDs, with higher risk of side effects. However, anecdotally, many patients report longer relief with HA injections than corticosteroid.
- No guidelines currently recommend use of newer injectable agents including platelet-rich plasma, immunologics, or botulinum toxin because evidence is still developing.
- Concerns regarding chondrotoxic effects from lidocaine, bupivacaine, or other IA anesthetics are mainly based on cell culture, animal studies, and high-dose exposure in operating room procedures. Evidence for harm in small doses in a single IA exposure is lacking. However, if patients are concerned, the knee injections can be done without IA anesthetic agents.

ANATOMY

The knee joint consists of the femoral–tibial and femoral–patellar joints, with stabilization from the anterior and posterior cruciate ligaments and the medial and lateral collateral ligaments.

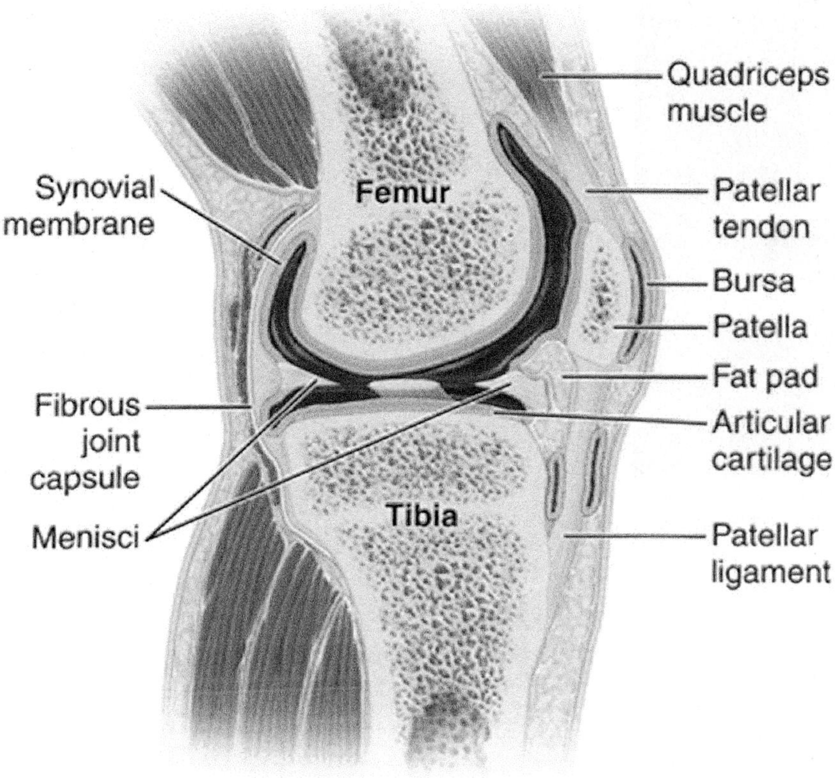

Sagittal section

Reprinted with permission from McConnell T, Hull KL. *Human Form, Human Function: Essentials of Anatomy & Physiology*. Lippincott Williams & Wilkins; 2011.

SUPPLIES

- Gloves
- Alcohol swabs
- Betadine or chlorhexidine swabs
- 18-gauge needle for drawing up medications or Medic anti-stick needle
- 3-mL syringe with 25-gauge 1-inch needle for injection
- 20- to 60-mL syringe with 18- to 22-gauge 1½-inch needle if aspirating
- 5- to 10-mL syringe with 21- to 22-gauge 1½-inch needle for injecting
- 5 to 7 mL 1% lidocaine without epinephrine and or 0.25% bupivacaine (if using)
- 1 mL 40 mg/mL (40 mg) Kenalog or equivalent
- Ethyl chloride
- Gauze
- Adhesive bandage

TECHNIQUE

- The knee joint can be aspirated or injected from multiple approaches, including the anterior medial or lateral approach with the knee flexed to 90 degrees, or a superior or midpatellar approach with the knee in extension.
- For the anterior approach, the patient is seated with the knee flexed at 90 degrees. The needle is inserted in the "soft spot" demarcated by the patella, patellar tendon, tibial plateau, and distal femoral condyle. The needle angle is parallel to the floor and aimed slightly posterior.

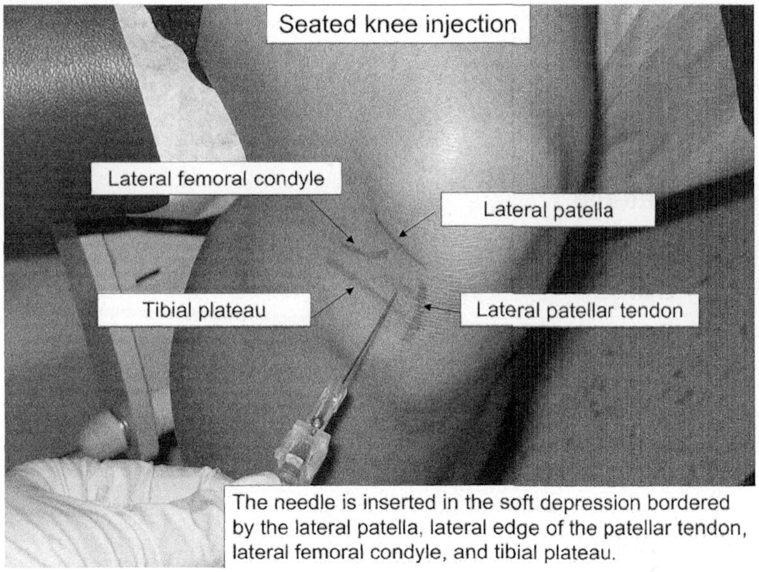

The needle is inserted in the soft depression bordered by the lateral patella, lateral edge of the patellar tendon, lateral femoral condyle, and tibial plateau.

- The anterior seated approach has the advantage of less bony discomfort but had a success rate of 70–75% in a trial comparing knee injection techniques. The supine lateral midpatellar approach had a higher success rate of 93% in the same study and may be a more reliable access to the knee joint in larger patients.
- For the supine medial or lateral midpatellar approach, position the patient's knee either in full extension, which gives the most patellar mobility, or slightly flexed at 5 degrees with a rolled towel supporting underneath. The needle is advanced parallel to the floor directed straight toward the patellar midpole.

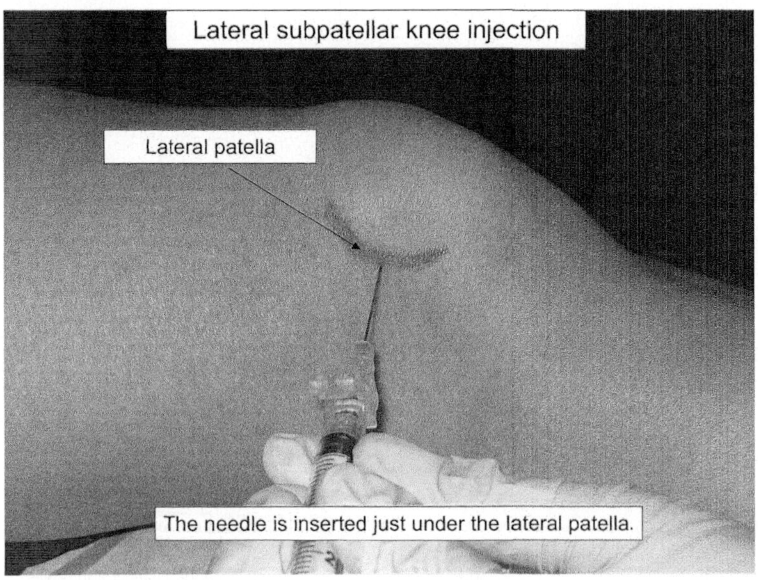

The needle is inserted just under the lateral patella.

- For the superior approach, draw lines from the superior and lateral borders of the patella—at the intersection of these lines, insert the needle at a 45-degree angle directed toward the middle of the patella.

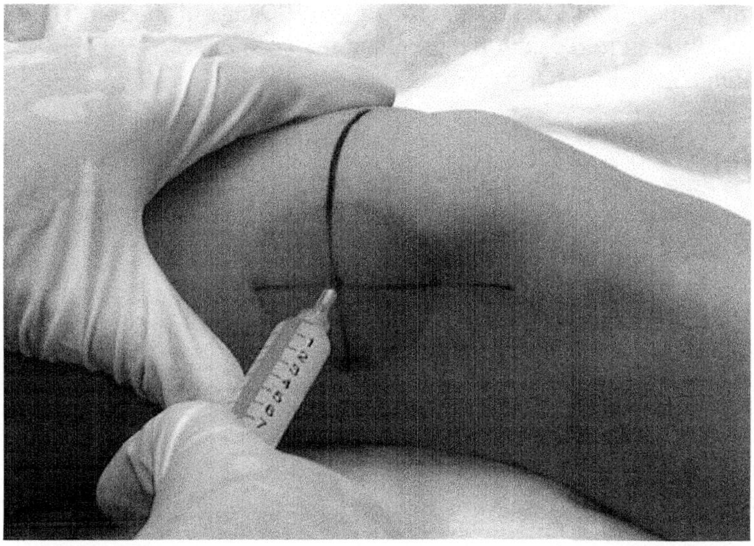

Reproduced with permission from McNabb JW. *A Practical Guide to Joint & Soft Tissue Injection & Aspiration*. Lippincott Williams & Wilkins; 2005.

- After selecting an injection approach, mark the entry point with a pen or needle cap.
- Cleanse the skin with alcohol swab and then Betadine × 3 or chlorhexidine × 45 seconds.
- Apply ethyl chloride for topical cooling.
- If draining an effusion, be careful not to move the needle during negative pressure aspiration.
- Keep the needle hub and syringe tip sterile during syringe transfers.
- Gentle pressure on the suprapatellar bursa may facilitate more complete drainage of the effusion.
- After aspiration, remove the aspiration syringe and connect the therapeutic syringe securely.
- Inject the therapeutic medication into the joint—there should be minimal resistance to flow.
- Remove needle and apply pressure with gauze.
- Apply adhesive bandage.

AFTERCARE

- Lidocaine lasts up to 4 to 6 hours; bupivacaine can last up to 12 hours—avoid heavy exercise while the IA anesthetics are in effect because the decreased proprioceptive feedback may increase risk of falls.
- Patients may have mild discomfort at the injection site and can use ice or NSAIDs to mitigate pain until the injection takes effect.
- Inform your patient that steroids may take 2 to 3 days, and HA may take up to several weeks to take effect.
- After 3 to 5 days, the patient can resume his or her regular activity and advance as tolerated.
- Instruct patient to return to your office if they develop redness, swelling, or increased pain at the injection site.
- Recommend continued isometric quadriceps strengthening, low-impact exercise, and weight loss.
- Repeat injection can be done after 3 months if the steroid injection afforded adequate pain relief—average duration of effect for joint steroid injections is 4 weeks.

ANKLE JOINT INJECTION

INDICATIONS

- Ankle aspiration is useful for the diagnosis of ankle effusions (i.e., to diagnose crystalline disease or rule out infection).
- Corticosteroid injection to the ankle is indicated for the treatment of ankle arthritis, crystalline disease, or synovitis in rheumatoid arthritis.
- Injections are indicated once conservative therapy (activity modification, NSAIDs, physical therapy) has failed.

ANATOMY

- The ankle joint consists of the articulation of the tibiotalar and talofibular joints.
- The ankle joint space can be approached either medially or laterally.

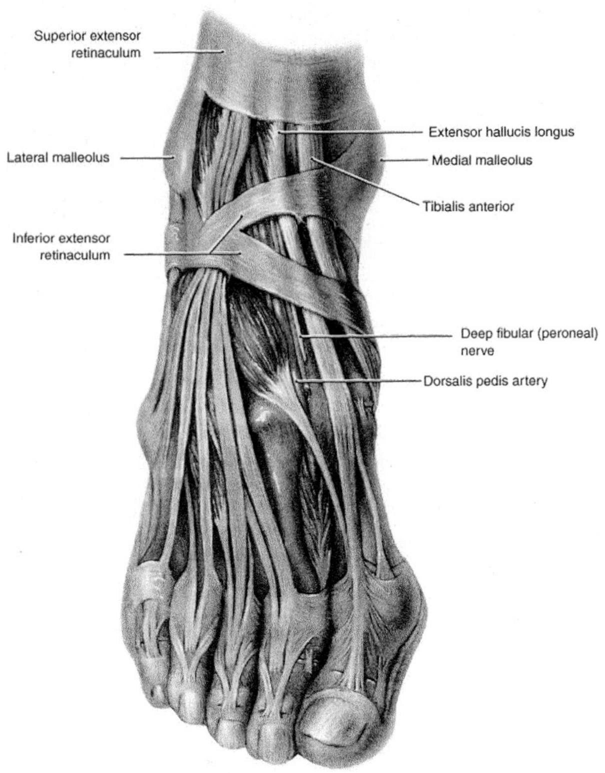

Reproduced with permission from Agur AMR, Dalley AF. *Grant's Atlas of Anatomy*. 16th ed. Wolters Kluwer; 2025:546. Figure 6.63B.

SUPPLIES

- Gloves
- Alcohol swabs
- Betadine or chlorhexidine swabs
- 18-gauge needle for drawing up medications or Medic anti-stick needle
- 3-mL syringe with 25-gauge 1-inch needle for injection
- Extra 3- to 5-mL syringes if needed for aspiration of effusion
- ½ to 1 mL 1% lidocaine without epinephrine (if using)
- ½ mL 40 mg/mL (20 mg) Kenalog or equivalent
- Ethyl chloride
- Gauze
- Adhesive bandage

TECHNIQUE

- The patient can be in a sitting or supine position.
- Medial approach: Identify the soft spot between the anterior tip of the medial malleolus and the medial edge of the tibialis anterior tendon:
  - Palpate down to feel the tibiotalar joint line—mark this site with the needle cap.
  - Cleanse the skin with alcohol swab and then Betadine × 3 or chlorhexidine × 45 seconds.
  - Apply ethyl chloride for topical cooling.

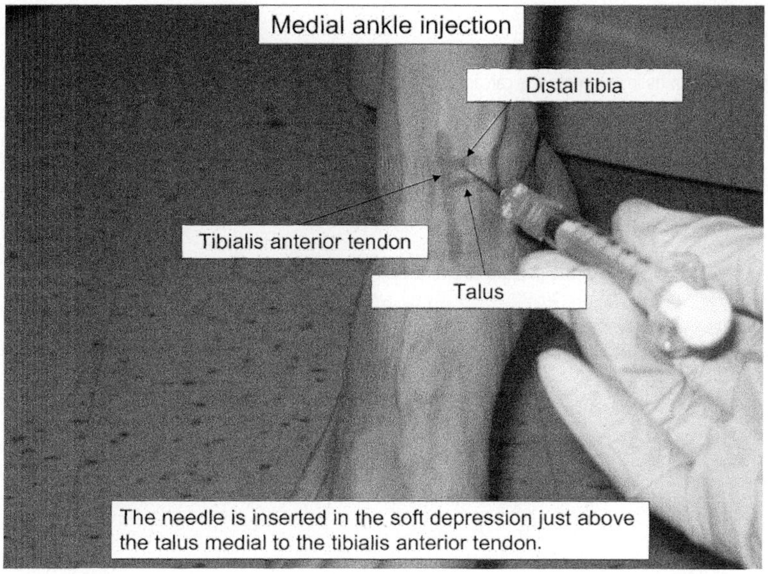

- Advance the needle in a posterolateral direction and inject.
- Having an assistant apply mild eversion/plantarflexion pressure may help to open the joint.
- Remove needle and apply pressure with gauze.
- Apply adhesive bandage.

- Lateral approach: Identify the triangular depression between the lateral tibia, fibula, and the talus:
  - Palpate down to feel the tibiotalar joint line—mark this site with the needle cap.
  - Cleanse the skin with alcohol swab and then Betadine × 3 or chlorhexidine × 15 seconds.
  - Apply ethyl chloride for topical cooling.
  - Advance the needle in a posteromedial direction.
  - If aspirating, remove as much fluid as possible, then stabilize the needle in the joint with a hemostat, and switch between the aspiration and therapeutic syringes. Keep the needle hub and syringe tips sterile.
  - After securing the therapeutic syringe, inject the steroid/lidocaine mixture.
  - Remove needle and apply pressure with gauze.
  - Apply adhesive bandage.

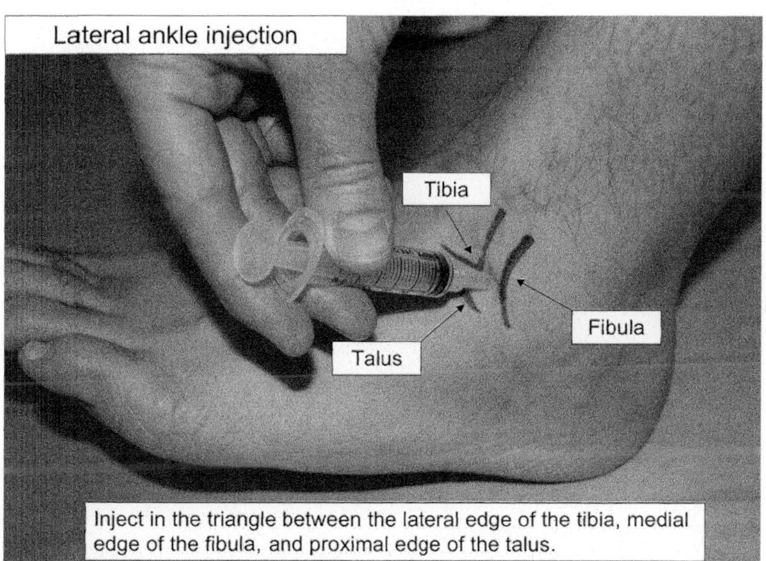

AFTERCARE

- Lidocaine lasts up to 4 to 6 hours; bupivacaine can last up to 12 hours—avoid heavy exercise while the IA anesthetics are in effect because the decreased proprioceptive feedback may increase risk of falls.
- Patients may have mild discomfort at the injection site and can use ice or NSAIDs to mitigate pain until the injection takes effect.
- Inform your patient that steroids may take 3 days to take effect.
- If pain is improved, start ankle rehabilitation with ROM exercises, strengthening band flexion/extension exercises.
- Instruct patient to return to your office if they develop redness, swelling, or increased pain at the injection site.
- Repeat injection can be done after 3 months if the steroid injection afforded adequate pain relief—average duration of effect for joint steroid injections is 4 weeks.

PLANTAR FASCIA INJECTION

INDICATIONS

- Excessive stretching and repetitive trauma can lead to microtears of the plantar fascia from its insertion on the calcaneus. These microtears can lead to chronic inflammation and pain at the calcaneal insertion or along the entire plantar fascia.
- Conservative treatment includes stretching, arch-supporting orthotics, heel pads, NSAIDs, and nighttime plantar fascia splints. Patients can roll pressure along their arch/heel with a tennis ball or frozen water bottle.
- Corticosteroid injection is a second-line therapy after the failure of conservative therapy, given the higher risk of complications, including fat pad atrophy and rupture of the plantar fascia.

ANATOMY

- The plantar fascia supports the medial longitudinal arch of the foot and stretches between the base of the phalanges and the medial tuberosity of the calcaneus.
- The plantar fascia lies deep to the fat layer of the heel.
- On physical exam, the plantar fascia insertion point on the calcaneus is usually markedly tender to palpation.

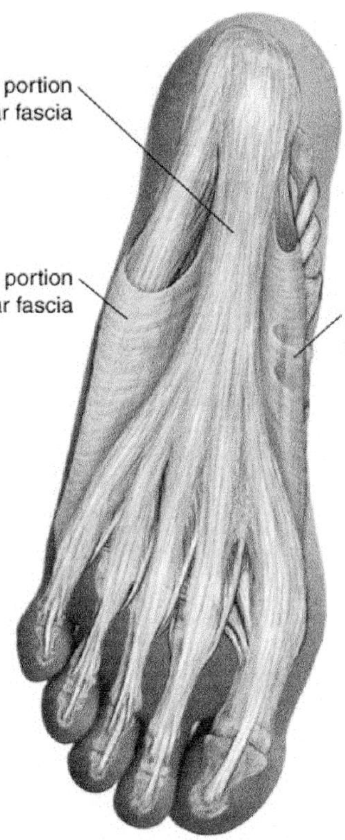

Reproduced with permission from Bucci C. *Condition-Specific Massage Therapy*. Lippincott Williams & Wilkins; 2012.

SUPPLIES

- Gloves
- Alcohol swabs
- Betadine or chlorhexidine swabs
- 18-gauge needle for drawing up medications or Medic anti-stick needle
- 3-mL syringe with 25-gauge 1½-inch needle for injection
- ½ mL 1% lidocaine without epinephrine (if using)
- ½ mL 40 mg/mL (20 mg) Kenalog or equivalent
- Ethyl chloride
- Gauze
- Adhesive bandage

TECHNIQUE

- Position the patient in the lateral recumbent position with the painful side down.
- Position the affected foot medial side up.
- Palpate the maximal point of tenderness at the plantar fascia insertion on the calcaneus, usually in the middle of the heel—this gives the injection target depth along the width of the heel.
- Find the medial edge of the calcaneus and mark with needle cap—this marks the injection point along the length of the foot.
- Cleanse the skin with alcohol swab and then Betadine × 3 or chlorhexidine × 45 seconds.
- Apply ethyl chloride for topical cooling.
- Inject perpendicular to the medial foot, aiming just distal to the calcaneal edge in order to avoid the heel fat pad.
- If the calcaneus is reached with the needle tip, walk the needle off the bony edge and then down to the depth of the point of maximal tenderness.
- Inject the steroid/lidocaine mixture.
- Remove needle and apply pressure with gauze.
- Apply adhesive bandage.

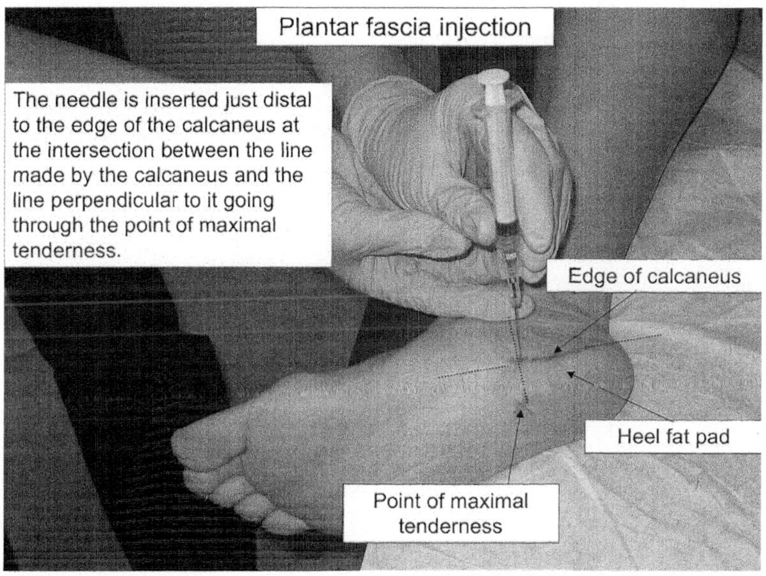

AFTERCARE

- Apply pressure dressing.
- Rest 3 days.
- Continue the RICE conservative therapy and consistent plantar fascia stretching.
- Instruct patient to return to your office if they develop redness, swelling, or increased pain at the injection site.

MORTON NEUROMA INJECTION

INDICATIONS

- Morton neuroma results from irritation of the interdigital nerve in the foot from repetitive compressive trauma, such as compression from tight or high-heeled shoes.
- Injections are indicated once conservative therapies (shoes with a wider metatarsal box, metatarsal pads, orthotic arch supports, NSAIDs) have failed.

ANATOMY

- Morton neuroma usually develops between the 2nd and 3rd or between the 3rd and 4th metatarsal heads.
- Tenderness to palpation between the metatarsal heads usually confirms the diagnosis.

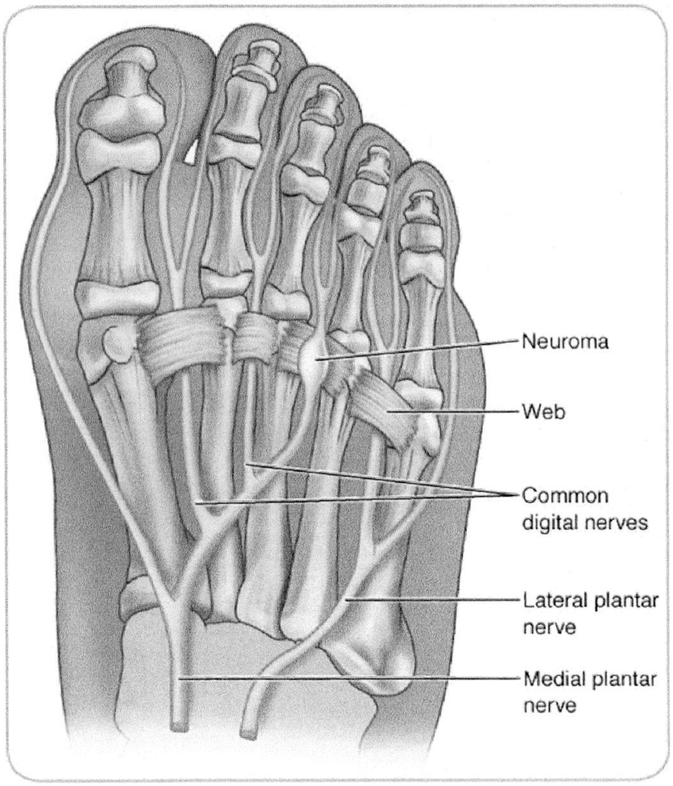

Reproduced with permission from Anderson MK. *Foundations of Athletic Training: Prevention, Assessment, and Management*. 7th ed. Wolters Kluwer; 2021.

SUPPLIES

- Gloves
- Alcohol swabs
- Betadine or chlorhexidine swabs
- 18-gauge needle for drawing up medications or Medic anti-stick needle
- 3-mL syringe with 25-gauge 1-inch needle for injection
- ½ mL 1% lidocaine without epinephrine (if using)
- ½ mL 40 mg/mL (20 mg) Kenalog or equivalent
- Ethyl chloride
- Gauze
- Adhesive bandage

TECHNIQUE

- Lay the patient in a supine position with a bent knee and the foot flat on the table.
- Identify the point of maximal tenderness between the metatarsal heads on the dorsal foot—mark entry site with needle cap.
- Cleanse the skin with alcohol swab and then Betadine × 3 or chlorhexidine × 45 seconds.
- Apply ethyl chloride for topical cooling.
- Advance the needle at a 45-degree angle proximally toward the point of maximal tenderness or nodule—aim toward the heel and stop at the level of the interdigital fullness.
- Do not inject at the level of the plantar fat pad to avoid fat pad atrophy.
- Remove needle and apply pressure with gauze.
- Apply adhesive bandage.

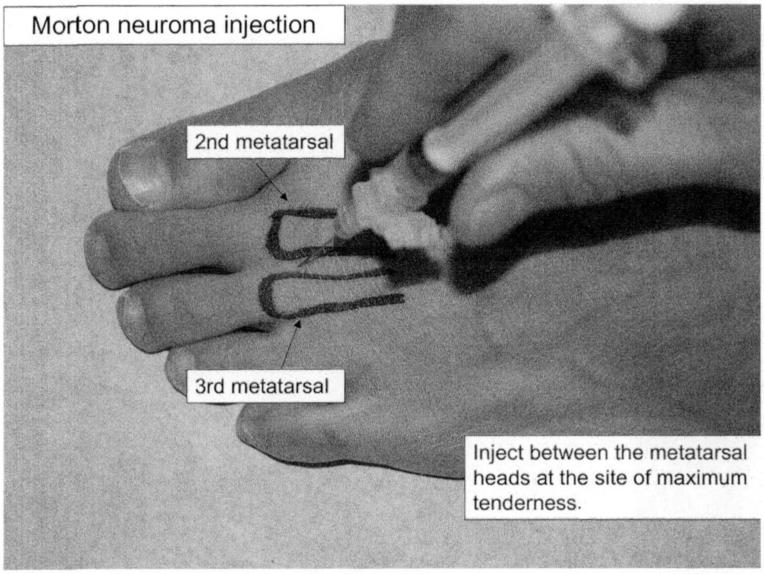

AFTERCARE

- Lidocaine lasts up to 4 to 6 hours; bupivacaine (Marcaine) can last up to 12 hours.
- However, steroid effect may take 2 to 3 days to decrease inflammation.
- Advise continued proper footwear, metatarsal pads, and orthotics. Gel toe spacers may relieve nerve pressure.
- Instruct patient to return to your office if they develop redness, swelling, or increased pain at the injection site.
- Repeat injection can be done after 3 months if the steroid injection afforded adequate pain relief—average duration of effect for joint steroid injections is 4 weeks.

1ST METATARSOPHALANGEAL INJECTION

INDICATIONS

- Aspiration of the 1st metatarsal phalangeal joint is useful in the diagnosis of gout and pseudogout.
- Therapeutic steroid injection can be a useful adjunct therapy for 1st metatarsophalangeal (MTP) osteoarthritis, rheumatoid arthritis, or crystal arthropathies.

ANATOMY

The MTP joint line is palpable on the dorsal surface of the foot.

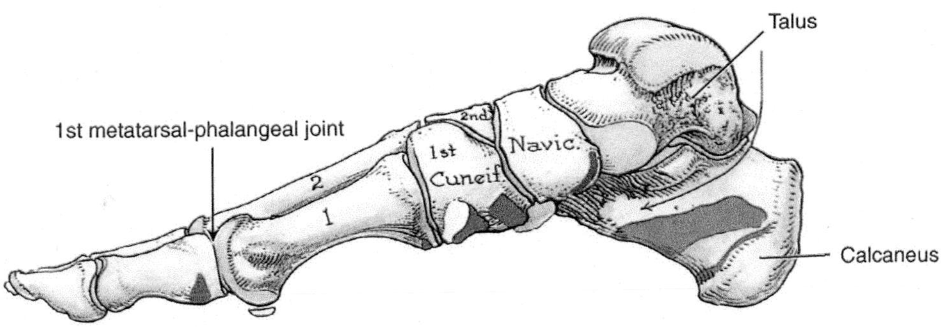

Reproduced with permission from Agur AMR, Dalley AF. *Grant's Atlas of Anatomy*. 16th ed. Wolters Kluwer; 2025:560. Figure 6.83B.

SUPPLIES

- Gloves
- Betadine or chlorhexidine and alcohol swabs
- 3-mL syringe with 25-gauge 5/8- to 1-inch needle
- 1 mL 1% lidocaine without epinephrine
- ½ mL (20 mg) Kenalog or equivalent
- Ethyl chloride
- Gauze
- Adhesive bandage

TECHNIQUE

- Lay the patient in a supine position with a bent knee and the foot flat on the table.
- Flex and extend the 1st MTP joint to identify the joint line and mark with needle cap.
- Cleanse the skin with alcohol swab and then Betadine × 3 or chlorhexidine × 45 seconds.
- Apply ethyl chloride for superficial numbing.
- Distal traction may help open the joint space.
- Aim the needle distally toward the toe and enter at a 60-degree angle to match the joint slope.
- The joint lies fairly superficially, and the injection solution should flow freely within the joint.
- Remove needle and apply pressure with gauze.
- Apply adhesive bandage.

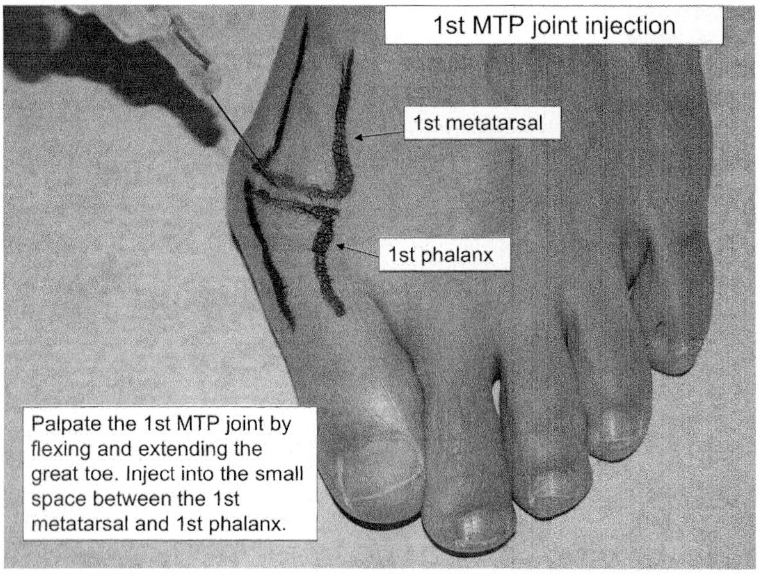

AFTERCARE

- Instruct patient that the toe may be numb for several hours after the procedure and that pain may be present for several days.
- Instruct patient that the steroid usually takes effect within 72 hours.
- Advise continued proper footwear and arch supports for proper walking mechanics.
- Instruct patient to return to your office if they develop redness, swelling, or increased pain at the injection site.
- If helpful, repeat injection can be done after 3 months—average duration of effect for steroid injections is 4 weeks.

INDEX

D

P

S

T

U

MPP1125